Patient-Centered Pharmacology:

Learning System for the Conscientious Prescriber

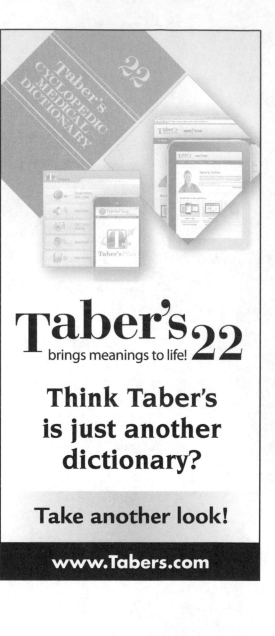
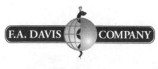

Patient-Centered Pharmacology:

Learning System for the Conscientious Prescriber

William N. Tindall, PhD, RPh

Professor Emeritus, Family Medicine
Wright State University
Boonshoft School of Medicine, Dept. of Family Medicine
Dayton, Ohio

Mona M. Sedrak, PhD, PA-C

Associate Dean, School of Health and Medical Sciences
Division of Health Sciences
Associate Professor, Physician Assistant Program
Seton Hall University
South Orange, New Jersey

John M. Boltri, MD, FAAFP

Professor and Chair
Department of Family Medicine and Public Health Sciences
Wayne State University School of Medicine
Detroit, Michigan

 F.A. Davis Company • Philadelphia

F. A. Davis Company
1915 Arch Street
Philadelphia, PA 19103
www.fadavis.com

Printed in the United States of America

Last digit indicates print number: 10 9 8 7 6 5 4 3 2 1

Acquisitions Editor: Andy McPhee
Manager of Content Development: George W. Lang
Developmental Editor: Patricia Gillivan
Art and Design Manager: Carolyn O'Brien

As new scientific information becomes available through basic and clinical research, recommended treatments and drug therapies undergo changes. The author(s) and publisher have done everything possible to make this book accurate, up to date, and in accord with accepted standards at the time of publication. The author(s), editors, and publisher are not responsible for errors or omissions or for consequences from application of the book, and make no warranty, expressed or implied, in regard to the contents of the book. Any practice described in this book should be applied by the reader in accordance with professional standards of care used in regard to the unique circumstances that may apply in each situation. The reader is advised always to check product information (package inserts) for changes and new information regarding dose and contraindications before administering any drug. Caution is especially urged when using new or infrequently ordered drugs.

Library of Congress Cataloging-in-Publication Data

Patient-Centered Pharmacology: learning system for the conscientious prescriber / [edited by] William N. Tindall, Mona M. Sedrak, John M. Boltri.
p. ; cm.
Includes bibliographical references and index.
ISBN 978-0-8036-2585-3
I. Tindall, William N., editor of compilation. II. Sedrak, Mona, editor of compilation. III. Boltri, John M., editor of compilation.
[DNLM: 1. Pharmaceutical Preparations. 2. Drug Therapy. QV 55]
RM300
615.1—dc23
2013007350

Dedication

I dedicate this book to my three grandchildren, Aidan, Cameron, and Kendall Taylor, who light my days with their love, wonder, and joy; my daughters, Christine and Laura, who continue to teach me the meaning of unconditional love; and my best friend and loving wife, Sylvia, for all she has sacrificed in support of me, my career, and my many pursuits.

William N. Tindall

I dedicate this book first and foremost to my parents Edward and Marcelle Naim. Mom and Dad, you gave me the courage and the confidence to dream big, reach for the stars and beyond, and to never give up. Also, I dedicate this book to the one I lost and that I hope to find fully again one day. Working on this project helped keep me sane when I found solace in little else. My precious child, you were with me in each word I wrote and each page I turned, as you are now and will forever be.

Mona M. Sedrak

I dedicate this book to my wife and best friend, Shelley; to my children, Mark, Joe, and Mary; and to my parents, Lillian and Mario. You have all taught me the meaning of love and what is really important in life—to love and be loved.

John M. Boltri

This textbook is designed to be used as a learning system about medications for students who will one day possess prescribing rights. We believe every clinician should be a *conscientious prescriber*. To us, *conscientious prescribing* refers to a thoughtful process that always places the patient's well-being first, ahead of every prescribing decision, *before* any prescription is written, and includes appropriate follow-up after the patient has completed the course of medication.

Being a conscientious prescriber is based on the following tenets:

1. That each time a medication is chosen, the choice should be based on a substantial body of literature supporting the decision.
2. That for most patients, monotherapy is a better choice than polytherapy.
3. That low doses are preferred over high doses.
4. That short term therapy is preferred over long-term therapy.
5. That although newer medications may have promotional advantages, there is not always the best evidence available to support these advantages until clinical trials are conducted to prove the existence of significant "risk-benefit" advantages.
6. That *before any prescription is written*, the clinician must consider the patient's lifestyle behaviors, adherence issues, economic issues, mind-body-spiritual issues, health-risk issues, age, weight, and other physical issues that might affect pharmacodynamic and pharmacokinetic parameters and hence final outcomes.
7. That after a prescription is written, treatment failure can be the result of inappropriate prescribing, dosing or dosage errors, misdiagnoses of its need, interference by other illnesses, administration of concurrent foods or drugs, environmental factors, or genetic issues.
8. That a conscious effort should be made to confirm a patient's response to a medication, manage adverse reactions, change the dosage, or discontinue the medication.
9. That patient education is vital for compliance.
10. That all patients should know *at least* the following drug information before they leave the clinician's office: name of the medication, indication, expected side effects, and contraindications.
11. That sophisticated clinical, financial, and administrative systems in health care can change quickly, requiring clinicians to remain vigilant about therapeutic decisions and be focused on which treatments benefit the patient's health most effectively.

Our approach is based on the belief that clinicians must always put the patient first in any decision regarding drug choices. Putting the patient first allows you to assess the patient as a unique individual in need of your skills as a conscientious clinician.

Organization

The text is designed as a teaching tool and not as a reference, with our goal of making you think twice before prescribing once. In other words we hope to make you a more conscientious prescriber. Whereas a typical college course in pharmacology focuses on the pharmacokinetics and pharmacodynamics of drugs by grouping similar chemical classes of medications together, this textbook presents similar information, but groups medications by the patient's clinical problem(s) or issues, thereby emphasizing the clinical application of the information presented.

The book is divided into three units. The first unit presents basic pharmacological principles that, once mastered, make it easier to assimilate the rest of the text. The second unit contains chapters that focus on the treatment of patients with common diseases and disorders seen in primary care, such as hypertension, diabetes, infections, and so forth. The third unit focuses on the treatment of patients that fall under specific patient populations with special considerations. These include pediatric patients, women, men, and the elderly.

Each chapter progresses from general information that clinicians need to know about the drugs discussed in the chapter, including conscientious prescribing and patient education points applicable to all drugs in a particular class. It covers specific information about individual drugs, including mechanism of action, pharmacokinetics, dosage and administration, clinical uses, adverse reactions, interactions, contraindications, conscientious considerations, and patient and family education.

Here are other elements to the chapters:

■ Generic and trade names are given for each drug in this format: generic name (Trade Name).
■ Adverse reactions are listed by system. Life-threatening adverse reactions are printed in capital letters, whereas common side effects are printed in regular text. These lists are not exhaustive; readers are advised to consult a drug guide for a complete list of adverse reactions.
■ Conscientious Considerations are clinical tips for clinicians.
■ Patient/Family Education content conveys information that clinicians should communicate to patients about the drugs they are prescribed.

- Spotlight features focus on treating specific conditions with the drugs discussed in the chapter.
- Special Case boxes discuss treatment of uncommon conditions such as digitalis and cyanide toxicity.
- Other boxes and tables highlight and summarize important information for easy access.
- Implications for pregnant, pediatric, and geriatric patients are given for each class of drugs discussed.
- Learning Exercises present case studies related to the chapter content and are followed by critical thinking questions designed to apply the content to real-world prescribing situations. Answers to the critical thinking questions are found at the end of the book.

Each chapter coordinates with the companion online website, providing a comprehensive learning system that reinforces key concepts.

Web Resources for Instructors

The Instructor's area on DavisPlus (http://davisplus.fadavis.com Keyword Tindall) provides online support through chapter outlines and learning objectives, PowerPoint presentations for each chapter, additional case studies for class discussion or homework assignments, and a test bank for each of the 26 chapters.

Web Resources for Students

Because the patient should be your first consideration in the clinical application of any medication, you as a learner are the first consideration in our learning program. Thus, the authors have prepared a unique group of ancillary learning products to support you as a learner and help you improve your understanding of the clinical application of pharmacological principles.

The Web resources include chapter outlines and learning objectives, pre- and post-study chapter quizzes, additional case studies for independent study, links to helpful websites, and a "Create Your Own Formulary and Drug Card" system. We firmly believe that our approach will help further develop your basic problem-solving and decision-making skills related to prescribing medications, thereby improving your critical thinking skills.

Real-World Constraints

No teaching text can cover every drug used in a modern society, especially when new drugs are continuously being introduced. However, this textbook and its companion pieces are designed to focus your attention on common medicinal agents likely to be encountered in primary care settings and also likely to be found on a typical prescription benefit list. Any attempt to build a working knowledge of drug therapy will be tempered by real-world constraints such as the following:

- Alternative therapies
- Guidelines and algorithms suggested by government agencies
- Use of some medicines based on local habits and customs
- Therapeutic choices that vary by health plan benefits

- Accepted knowledge that any patient at any time may change his or her medication regimen due to individual economics, compliance behavior, health risks, multiple therapeutic needs, and other demands.

Importance of Study

We study medications to prepare for that ultimate clinical act of prescribing a medication in such a way that the patient will adhere to its regimen and ultimately obtain the best benefit. The mental gymnastics that go into this process are *conscientious*, and when done so illuminate a path to better patient care. We need to fuse pharmacology, therapeutics, practical realities, market realities, and the human side of medicine together in the learning process. You can then see at the onset of your career how your choice of drugs to prescribe can affect health outcomes.

Studying pharmacology is much different from studying other scientific and medical topics. Many students are tempted to use rote memorization to learn drug actions, names, side effects, contraindications, and so forth. Approaching the study of pharmacology in this manner is, frankly, a waste of time. We believe the best way to truly learn pharmacology is to focus on distinguishing information about each class of drugs. You then can better understand similar drugs used to treat similar conditions. For example, if agents used to treat cancer seek out and destroy fast-growing cells, is it not logical to assume they would do the same to the host taking them? Of course. So cells in the blood, gastrointestinal tract, hair, and certain other organs bear the brunt of those agents and tend to manifest as side effects—such a bone marrow suppression, enteritis, and hair loss—all related to damage done to fast turnover cells.

As you undertake the important task of becoming a conscientious prescriber, instead of trying to memorize facts, ask yourself a series of questions.

- If this is what a drug is doing to combat a disease, what is the body doing to combat the presence of the drug?
- How much of this drug should I give to achieve the desired outcome and not harm the patient?
- What information do I need to know about the patient and the patient's health status to prescribe safely?
- What information do I need to tell the patient about his or her health and prescribed regimen so that the patient feels like a partner in health-care decisions and is encouraged to take responsibility for his or her health?

We hope that this approach and the approaches we offer throughout the book afford you the ability to separate the forest from the trees and understand that, at the end of the day, every day, it is truly all about the patient. Providing patient-centered medicine, putting the patient first, and prescribing conscientiously are at the root of providing quality patient care. We thank you for allowing us to play a small, yet important, part in your education.

WILLIAM N. TINDALL, PhD, RPH
MONA M. SEDRAK, PhD, PA-C
AND JOHN M. BOLTRI, MD

Contributors

Richard Ackermann, Sr., MD, Geriatrician, Family Practitioner

Family Health Center
Director, Geriatric Fellowship
Macon, Georgia

Justin B. Beverly, MD, Pediatrician

Family Health Center
Primary Pediatrics of Macon
McDonough, Georgia

Florence T. Baralatei, MD, Geriatrician, Family Practitioner

Family Health Center
Macon, Georgia

David E. Burtner, MD, Family Practitioner

Family Health Center
Macon, Georgia

Edward K. Clark, MD, Pediatrician

Children's Health Center
Macon, Georgia

Y. Monique Davis-Smith, MD, Family Practitioner

Health Services of Central Georgia
Director, Residency Program
Macon, Georgia

Sabry A. Gabriel, MD, Family Practitioner

Mercer Health Systems
Professor, Family Medicine, Mercer University
Macon, Georgia

Fred S. Girton, MD, Family Practitioner

Health Services of Central Georgia
Professor and Chairman, Dept. Family Medicine,
    Mercer University
Macon, Georgia

Alice A. House, MD, Family Practitioner

Byron Family Health Care
Byron, Georgia

Steven A. House, MD, Family Practitioner

Family Practice Physicians
Associate Professor, Assistant Director, Family Residency
University of Kentucky
Glasgow, Kentucky

Kathy A. Kemle, MS, PA-C, Family Practitioner

Health Services of Central Georgia
Assistant Professor, Assistant Director, Division of
    Geriatrics, Mercer University
Macon, Georgia

Hugh L. McLaurin, MD, Family Practitioner

Family Health Center
Assistant Professor of Family Medicine
Macon, Georgia

Dipesh R. Patel, MD, Geriatrician and Family Practitioner

Family Health Center
Assistant Professor, Family Medicine
Macon, Georgia

W. Patrick Roche, III, MD, Family Practitioner & Internal Medicine

Family Health Center
Macon, Georgia

Roberta J. Weintraut, MD, Family Practitioner

Family Health Center
Assistant Professor
Macon, Georgia

Ancillaries

Mary Banahan, MS, PA-C, LCCE

Chair, Physician Assistant Admissions Committee,
    Assistant Professor
Touro College Physician Assistant Program
Manhattan, New York

Georgina Ferriero, MSPA PA-C

Hospitalist Physician Assistant
Evangelical Community Hospital
Lewisburg, Pennsylvania

Pamela Gregory-Fernandez, MS, PA-C, GEA, DFAAPA

Assistant Professor–Industry Professional
College of Pharmacy and Health Sciences
Physician Assistant Education
St. John's University
Queens, New York

Sandra Kaminski, MS, PA-C

Assistant Professor, PA Program
School of Health and Medical Sciences
Seton Hall University
South Orange, New Jersey

Krisie Kupryk, MS, PA-C

Emergency Department, Physician Assistant
Overlook Hospital
Summitt, New Jersey

Michelle McWeeney, MS, PA-C

Assistant Professor, PA Program
School of Health and Medical Sciences
Seton Hall University
South Orange, New Jersey

Raffi Manjikian, MS

Adjunct Instructor
Department of Physics
Seton Hall University
South Orange, New Jersey

Jurga Marshall, MS, PA-C

Clara Maass Medical Center Emergency Department
St. Mary's Hospital Emergency Department
Belleville, New Jersey

Jennifer Hofmann Ribowsky, MS, RPA-C

Academic Faculty/Pre-clinical Coordinator
Pace University–Lenox Hill Hospital Physician
    Assistant Program
New York, New York

Denise Rizzolo, PhD, PA-C

Associate Professor, PA Program
School of Health and Medical Sciences
Seton Hall University
South Orange, New Jersey

Abby Saunders, MS, PA-C

Assistant Professor, PA Program
School of Health and Medical Sciences
Seton Hall University
South Orange, New Jersey

Lauren Seavy, MPA, PA-C

Instructor, PA Program
School of Health and Medical Sciences
Seton Hall University
South Orange, New Jersey

Sue Wulff, MS, PA-C

Chair, Physician Assistant Department
School of Education and Health Sciences
University of Dayton
Dayton, Ohio

Marcie L. Baird, MS, RN, FNP-C

Assistant Professor
School of Nursing
Indiana Wesleyan University
Marion, Indiana

Julie P. Balk, DNP, FNP-BC

Associate Professor
School of Nursing and Health Sciences
Westminster College
Salt Lake City, Utah

Jeffrey A. Bates, PharmD, CGP

Assistant Professor
Pharmaceutical Sciences
College of Pharmacy
Ferris State University
Big Rapids, Michigan

Clint C. Blankenship, PharmD, PA-C

Assistant Professor
Medical University of South Carolina
Charleston, South Carolina

Gilbert A. Boissonneault, PhD, PA-C

Professor
Division of Physician Assistant Studies
University of Kentucky
Lexington, Kentucky

Anthony Brenneman, MPAS, PA-C

Director of Clinical Education
Assistant Professor
Physician Assistant Program
University of Iowa
Iowa City, Iowa

James B. Caputo, PharmD

Assistant Professor
Physician Assistant Program
Morosky College of Health Professions and Sciences
Gannon University
Erie, Pennsylvania

DeShana Collett, MSPAS, PA-C

Professor
Physician Assistant Studies
University of Kentucky
Lexington, Kentucky

Theresa E. Coyner, RN, MSN, NP

Nurse Practitioner
Randall Dermatology
West Lafayette, Indiana

Deborah A. Crowe, DNP, FNP-BC

APRN, Adjunct Faculty
Nursing Department
Indiana Wesleyan University
Glennallen, Arkansas

Randy D. Danielsen, PhD, PA-C

Dean and Professor
AT Still University
Mesa, Arizona

Amy M. Drab, MPAS, PA-C

Associate Professor
Physician Assistant Department
Kettering College
Kettering, Ohio

Katherine Erdman, MPAS, PA-C

Assistant Director and Assistant Professor
School of Allied Health Sciences
Baylor College of Medicine
Houston, Texas

Alison C. Essary, MHPE, PA-C

Program Director, Associate Professor
Physician Assistant Program
Midwestern University
Glendale, Arizona

Cynthia L. Fritz, FNP, BC, NP-C

Nurse Practitioner
IU Goshen Physicians
Elkhart, Indiana

Jennifer Gentry, RN, MSN, ANP BC, GNP, ACH PN, FPCN

Nurse Practitioner
Advanced Clinical Practice and Palliative Medicine
Duke University Hospital
Durham, North Carolina

Larry E. Gerson, PhD, MS, MPAS, PA-C

Director of Clinical Education
Physician Assistant Studies
Trevecca Nazarene University
Nashville, Tennessee

Darla Gowan, RN-BC, MN, FNP-BC

Assistant Professor for Graduate Nursing
Primary Care Coordinator
Graduate Nursing Studies, Division of School of Nursing
Indiana Wesleyan University
Marion, Indiana

Joellen W. Hawkins, RN, WHNP-BC, PhD FAAN, FAANP

Professor Emeritus
Maternal Child Health Department
William F. Connell School of Nursing
Boston College
Auburndale, Massachusetts

Jill Isaacs, APRN, NP-C

Instructor
School of Nursing
Creighton University
Omaha, Nebraska

Monica M. Jones, DNP, FNP-BC

Assistant Professor of Nursing
School of Nursing
Delta State University
Cleveland, Mississippi

Jamiley Maynard, PhD, FNP, BC

Adjunct Professor
Nursing Department
Indiana Wesleyan University
Terre Haute, Indiana

Melissa M. Menacho, ACNP, MSN

Critical Care Nurse Practitioner
Medicine-Neurology Department
Duke University Medical Center
Durham, North Carolina

Charlene M. Morris, MPAS, DFAAPA

Physician Assistant
Family Medicine Department
Pamlico Medical Center
Bayboro, North Carolina

Jacqueline A. Morse, PharmD, BCPS

Assistant Professor
Pharmacy Practice Department
Ferris State University
Grand Rapids, Michigan

John T. Musser, MD

Physician
Emory University
Atlanta, Georgia

Shannon R. Myatt, RN, MSN, CPNP

Nurse Practitioner
Adolescent Medicine Department
Cincinnati Children's Hospital Medical Center
Cincinnati, Ohio

Terry Neal, EdD, MSN, FNP-BC

Associate Professor
Division of Graduate Studies in Nursing
Indiana Wesleyan University
Marion, Indiana

Joan M. Nelson, ANP, BC, DNP

Associate Professor
College of Nursing
University of Colorado
Aurora, Colorado

Diane Nunez, RN, MS, ANP-C

Clinical Associate Professor
College of Nursing and Healthcare Innovation
Arizona State University
Phoenix, Arizona

Debra Perlsweig, PharmD

Independent Consultant
Aston, Pennsylvania

Megan Rourke, PA-C

Certified Physician Assistant
Avon, Connecticut

Jeb Sheidler, PA-C, MPAS, DFAAPA, ATC

Associate Professor
Physician Assistant Department
Kettering College
Kettering, Ohio

Sharon Schulling, PhD, MSN, FNP-BC

Associate Professor, Research Coordinator
Graduate School of Nursing
Indiana Wesleyan University
Marion, Indiana

Richard Seides, EdD, NP-C

Assistant Professor
Nursing Department
Seton Hall University
S. Orange, New Jersey

Emily K. Sheff, CMSRN, FNP, BC

Instructor
School of Nursing
Massachusetts General Hospital Institute of Health
    Professions
Braintree, Massachusetts

Laurel R. Spence, MS, PA-C

Assistant Professor
School of Allied Health Sciences
Physician Assistant Studies
Baylor College of Medicine
Houston, Texas

Betty J. Sylvest, DNS, RN, CNE

Robert E. Smith School of Nursing
Delta State University
Cleveland, Mississippi

Donald H. Yager, DHSc, PA-C, MT(ASCP)

Director of Clinical Studies
School of Physician Assistant Studies
South College
Knoxville, Tennessee

Acknowledgments

To complete a project of this size is impossible without the help of a dedicated team of individuals. Many people work behind the scenes and rarely get proper acknowledgment. Thus, the authors wish to thank first and foremost Patricia Gillivan, developmental editor, for all her efforts in seeing to the development and publication of this manuscript. The road has been a long and bumpy one, and your guidance and input has been invaluable. We thank God that you were assigned to this project and that you were brave enough to take us on!

We would like to thank the students and faculty at Kettering College PA Program, Kettering, Ohio, because they were the first to be subjected to the content of this textbook. Your continual feedback informed us of the merits of this project and taught us how to be better educators.

Additionally, we would like to give special thanks to all our contributing authors at Mercer University Department of Family Medicine and elsewhere. Without your dedication and willingness to share your clinical expertise, this project would not have been possible. Your trust, insights, and belief in teaching pharmacology using a patient-first approach have truly made this book possible. Thanks to each and every one of you.

Finally, the authors wish to acknowledge the support given by their spouses, Sylvia Tindall, Samy Sedrak, and Shelley Boltri, who sacrificed much by allowing us to use family time to complete this immense project.

Contents

Unit 3

Conscientious Prescribing for Special Populations

Conscientious Prescribing in the 21st Century

Conscientious and Rational Prescribing in the 21st Century

chapter 1

H. Patrick Roche III, William N. Tindall, John M. Boltri, Mona M. Sedrak

CHAPTER FOCUS

This chapter introduces the concept of conscientious prescribing and a patient-centered approach to delivery of health care. It discusses why a patient-centered approach builds sound prescribing habits and lowers the incidence of medication errors. Because clinicians who prescribe or administer drugs must adhere to certain regulations and covenants, this chapter introduces the statutory and professional requirements involved in prescription writing, as well as some of the disciplined and conscientious thinking a clinician must employ before writing any prescription.

OBJECTIVES

After reading and studying this chapter, the student should be able to:

1. List six steps clinicians can take to adopt a rational approach to drug therapy.
2. Understand why medication errors result from faulty systems not faulty people.
3. List the reasons why medication errors occur as described by the Institute for Safe Medication Practices (ISMP).
4. Recall the components of a legal prescription and how each component communicates different information to both patients and dispensing personnel.
5. Describe practical ways to improve adherence to a prescribed regimen.
6. Discuss the impact of the Controlled Substances Act on prescribing habits.
7. List and describe the FDA's pregnancy categories for drugs.
8. State Latin abbreviations for prescriptions in common use today and recall those abbreviations to be avoided.
9. Explain what differentiates a prescription medication from an over-the-counter medication.

Key Terms

Adherence and Compliance

Algorithms

Conscientious prescribing

Controlled Substances Act (CSA)

C-I, C-II, C-III, C-IV, C-V

Durham-Humphrey Amendment (1951)

Food and Drug Administration (FDA)

Generic

High-Alert Medication List

Legend drug

Managed care

OTC (over-the-counter) drug

Pharmacy and Therapeutics (P&T) Committee

Rational prescribing

Treatment guidelines

Several millennia after natural substances were first used to treat illnesses and cure diseases, we continue to search for better and better remedies. Like their ancestors who wrote the first prescriptions on clay tablets in Sumeria some 5,000 years ago, clinicians today need the best information available about the pharmacological agents in use, and they must be able to rationally apply that information in a manner that meets one covenant of their profession: First do no harm.

What has changed over the millennia is the amount of information available about medications used today, especially regarding their ability to do harm or to do good. The ancient Egyptians wrote their prescriptions on papyrus and applied to patients what little medical knowledge they had of natural healing substances. They used their religious beliefs as a way of explaining much of what they did not know and prayed that their patients would come to no harm. The ancient Greeks also used natural healing substances along with incantations to specific gods such as *Hygeia,* the goddess of health, and *Panacea,* the goddess of treatment, both daughters of *Asclepius,* the god of healing, to help protect patients from harm. Today, healers have access to a phenomenal body of scientific literature on which to rely and have access to tools such as the Internet to help them search texts, latest journal articles, and other scientific (and sometimes nonscientific) resources. There is no reason a clinician of today should not be able to make a decision using the most up-to-date information about exactly how prescribed agents work and how they should be used.

Around the year 500 BC, Hippocrates taught that the body had a wealth of recuperative powers and that disease resulted when the natural processes that keep one healthy went astray. Hippocrates became revered as the Father of Medicine, and many of his beliefs are still in favor today. For example, his belief that the role of a clinician is to assist in the healing or recuperative process is still being taught some 2,500 years after he introduced it.

Paracelsus (1493–1541), a physician, alchemist, astrologer, and general occultist, believed that diseases are actual entities that can be combated with the right remedies. He introduced new remedies and improved therapeutics. His influence is also still felt today, especially his scientific approaches to medication use, which led to a decrease in the prevalence of overdosing, a common problem in his day.

Another, somewhat primitive approach to clinical pharmacology was taken in 1829 when Johannes Evangelista Purkinje advocated that the most desirable results of pharmacotherapy could be obtained only if clinicians took the drugs themselves. As a result, he studied the effects of digitalis, camphor, and belladonna on himself. Later, in the 1960s, Sir Malcolm Lader, a psychiatrist, stressed that a clinician should always taste a drug before prescribing it so that those who prescribe it may have some of the same experiences a patient has. Perhaps because his audience was medical students, his advice was not taken seriously.

Overview of Federal Drug Regulation

In the United States, the first Federal Food, Drug, and Cosmetic Act (FDCA) was passed in 1906. This act established the U.S. **Food and Drug Administration (FDA)** and its responsibilities to protect the public from drugs that cause harm because they are *adulterated* and/or *mislabeled.* This law made it a federal offense to introduce into interstate commerce any contaminants in drugs (adulterations) or drugs that had false and misleading advertising (mislabeling). The FDA reports to Congress and has authority over the process of drug research and the process by which drugs flow into the marketplace through Investigational Drug Applications (IDA) and New Drug Application (NDA) approvals.

By definition, a contaminant was defined as anything in a drug that was not stated on its label. In 1906 the vehicles used to dilute the active ingredients of many drugs were very suspect. For example, a medication that stated it was 5% methyl salicylate might also be found to contain dirt, insect parts, or other contaminants. Because it was adulterated, it could be legally removed from the market. Misleading labeling referred to a list of things for which manufacturers could not advertise a cure, such as cancer. It was also common to advertise medications as being good for curing things such as miasma, vapors, female complaints, and a host of symptoms that were difficult to define.

In 1906 the FDCA gave the power to enforce official standards for drug potency and identification to The United States Pharmacopeia, Inc. (USP), a Washington DC agency that is still run as a private sector–government collaboration. The USP sets standards for the assay of drugs and for making available consumer and professional information about them. It does this by drawing upon the knowledge of the best scientists and practitioners in the country.

In 1938 the FDCA was amended to protect people from drugs being marketed before they had been proved to be safe. The amendment was enacted to protect the public from ingesting harmful agents as a result of a product that brought harm, in one case a liquid product that resulted in the death of about 150 pregnant women. This harmful agent was marketed as Elixir of Sulfanilamide. It did contain one of the first sulfa drugs ever marketed, but its label stated that it was an elixir, which by definition is an alcohol-based solution. Actually, sulfanilamide, the active ingredient, was dissolved in a solution of propylene glycol, the ingredient used to make antifreeze. The FDA quickly removed this product from the market because it was mislabeled, but in the process discovered it would be better for the public to have a drug's safety proven before it entered the market. Thus began a new era of requiring all manufacturers of medicines to file safety data before releasing any product to the public.

In 1951, the **Durham-Humphrey Amendment** passed, which had been sponsored by Minnesota Senator Hubert H. Humphrey and North Carolina Congressman Carl Durham, both pharmacists. Also known as the Prescription Drug Amendment, the Durham-Humphrey Amendment established, under the authority of the Food, Drug, and Cosmetic Act, two classes of drugs—legend and over-the-counter (OTC) drugs. **Legend drugs** could only be sold in pharmacies under a valid prescription order. Legend drugs had to be labeled with either the symbol "Rx only" in a special font and size or the statement "Caution: Federal law prohibits dispensing without a prescription." **OTC drugs** do not require a prescription and are labeled in such a manner that, if users follow the label instructions, they should come to no harm by self-medicating.

Prior to the passage of the Durham-Humphrey Amendment, drug manufacturers were generally free to determine to which category each drug belonged, but the Durham-Humphrey Amendment gave the FDA the authority to categorize drugs as those that:

■ Need a prescription because they are habit-forming.
■ Are generally considered unsafe except when used under the supervision of a clinician.
■ Are new drugs and thus subject to a New Drug Application (NDA) approval process set down by the FDA, the rules of which require the manufacturer to conduct trials to demonstrate safety in humans.

Since 1951, all 50 states have enacted legislation that parallels the federal FDAC legislation. This was done because the FDA does not have jurisdiction over all state licensing bodies due to the powers vested in the U.S. Constitution pertaining to health, education, and welfare of citizens. Therefore, violations of laws regarding prescription medications are handled at the state level.

Part of the labeling required of a legend drug includes adequate directions for the clinician to use to prescribe it. Because of the space limitations on small prescription bottles, the FDA allows manufacturers to attach a lengthy package insert (PI) to, or place in the box with, the bottle of medication for the clinician to read. The PI includes highly detailed information about the effects of the drug as well as its pharmacodynamics. It also contains the information that must be approved by the FDA before the drug is marketed, including the drug's side effects, dosage and administration, and cautions for its use.

Information in a package insert is different from the information given in the patient information leaflet (PIL) placed on the package when a drug is dispensed. The patient information leaflet contains drug and dosage information in language that can be easily understood by the consumer. The source of patient information is usually the USP or a private drug information company that sells its leaflets to pharmacies and takes responsibility for its content. By contrast the professionals' package insert is information approved by the FDA.

An OTC drug is one that can be purchased by patients without a prescription. Manufacturers must place general directions for its use directly on its label and packaging. Additionally, as a general rule, OTC drugs are used by purchasers to self-treat conditions, and these drugs have been proven to meet higher safety standards required for those who are self-medicating. Many new OTC drugs had at one time been prescription-only drugs, but the FDA has approved the marketing of lower strengths of their active ingredient(s) than are available in their prescription counterparts. OTC medications such as antibiotic ointments, steroid creams, and cough and cold preparations are usually one-tenth to one-half the strength of their prescription counterparts. A good example is the pain-alleviating medication ibuprofen. It has been widely available as an OTC painkiller in 200-mg strength since the mid-1980s, yet it is still available by prescription in doses up to four times the strength of the OTC

dose. Much of this has been a marketing ploy as health insurance formularies took hold in the marketplace. Thus, it is not uncommon for a clinician to tell patients to take double the dose of the OTC form of the medication so that they take a "prescription strength" dose at OTC prices.

Additional Federal Regulation and Safety Measures

In the early 1960s, the thalidomide tragedy was a catalyst for additional safety regulation of medications. Thalidomide, a tranquilizer marketed in Europe during the late 1950s, was responsible for serious birth defects among thousands of infants after pregnant women took the drug to treat nausea and morning sickness associated with pregnancy. Because the FDA had not approved the use of this drug, it was not distributed in the United States; nevertheless, some incidents of birth defects caused by this drug did occur in the United States because patients obtained the medication from abroad. In response, in 1962 Congress enacted the Kefauver-Harris Amendment, also called the Drug Efficacy Amendment, as yet another modification to the FDCA. This amendment required that during the lengthy approval process to market a drug in the United States, its manufacturer not only had to prove it was safe, but also had to prove the drug was effective for the purpose(s) stated.

The FDA applied the Kefauver-Harris Amendment retroactively and required all drugs sold in the United States to demonstrate the efficacy requirement. This was done on a case-by-case basis for all prescription drugs that had been approved for use between 1938 and 1962. The FDA signed a contract with the National Academy of Science and the National Research Council to have them study all claims for drugs introduced into the U.S. market since 1932. The result was that hundreds of drugs were withdrawn from the market owing to lack of evidence to support their claimed or advertised use.

Today, all manufacturers must demonstrate to the FDA that the drugs they produce are:

■ Free from adulteration.
■ Free from misbranding.
■ Safe for use.
■ Efficacious for the indicated disorder.

Regulation of Herbals, Vitamins, Minerals, and Food Supplements

Herbals, vitamins, minerals, and food supplements are not regulated by the FDCA. Additionally, they are not subject to the stringent labeling necessary for prescription or OTC products because federal regulations for dietary supplements are very different from those for prescription and OTC drugs. For example, a dietary supplement manufacturer does not have to prove that its product is safe and effective before it is marketed. Dietary supplements are defined in a law passed by Congress in 1994 called the Dietary Supplement Health and Education Act (DSHEA) as an amendment to the FDCA. This gave the term *dietary supplement* its own definition and a regulatory framework for their marketing.

By creating the DSHEA, Congress emphasized the importance of diet and nutrition to the American people including their use of dietary supplements for promoting health and reducing the risk of disease. The significance of the DSHEA is that it provided broad access to dietary supplement information to patients and recognized a rational regulatory framework under which the FDA has authority to remove these products from the marketplace if they pose a "significant or unreasonable risk to consumers," if they are adulterated, or if they are marketed with inaccurate labeling.

Congress defined *dietary supplement* to mean products that are intended to supplement the diet because they contain one or more dietary ingredients such as the following:

- A vitamin or a mineral.
- An herb or other botanical.
- An amino acid.
- A dietary substance for use by humans to supplement the diet by increasing the total dietary intake.
- A concentrate, metabolite, constituent, or extract.
- A combination of the preceding ingredients.

Unlike in 1962 when the efficacy requirement was applied retroactively for all prescription drugs, Congress considered dietary ingredients marketed prior to passage of the DSHEA to be generally safe and permitted dietary supplements to be freely marketed, just as if they were regular foods.

Herbal supplements are considered as one type of dietary supplement. A herb is a plant or plant part (such as leaves, flowers, or seeds) that is used for its flavor, scent, and/or therapeutic properties. The term *botanical* is often used as a synonym for *herb*. A herbal supplement may contain a single herb or a mixture of herbs. When taking a drug history of any patient, clinicians should ask if that patient is taking any herbal substances because many patients do not think of them as "drugs."

Nearly 18% of the U.S. public takes supplements each year. Although they seem innocuous, substances such as iron, vitamin B_{12}, vitamin K, and many others are the source of many drug interactions and adverse effects with prescription medications. For example, many laxatives may bind to a recently ingested active ingredient in a prescription pill to the point that the medication becomes ineffective.

The Concept of Off-Label Prescribing

Clinicians may legally prescribe drugs for uses other than those officially listed in package inserts approved by the FDA. This is known as *off-label* or *unapproved* usage. However widespread this practice may be, manufacturers may not promote or market drugs for any type of off-label use. It is estimated that anywhere between 18% and 60% of all prescriptions written today are for these unapproved uses, with the majority being written to help with either chemotherapy or pediatric prescribing. These off-label uses have not been approved because chemotherapy and pediatric groups are the hardest to assemble for clinical trials. The fact that this practice is widespread raises legal and ethical questions centered on the question of whether off-label use is a form of human experimentation and a practice that removes safeguards established to protect human life. There are those who maintain, however, that it is the clinician's prerogative to use his or her professional judgment and should not be interfered with because clinicians are acting in the best interests of their patients.

Federal Control of Opioids, Narcotics, and Other Dangerous Drugs

In 1914 the Harrison Narcotic Act was passed. It was the first federal law aimed at curbing drug addiction or drug dependence, a growing national concern and one that had been increasing since the Civil War. It was this law that gave us the term *narcotic* and regulated the importation, manufacture, and sale of such substances using a tax stamp system. The Harrison Narcotic Act was superseded in 1971 by the Comprehensive Drug Abuse and Control Act, also called the **Controlled Substances Act (CSA)**. Besides providing for research into the issues of drug dependence and rehabilitation, its goal was to improve the manufacturing, distribution, prescribing, and dispensing of controlled substances by legitimate clinicians in health care. It was also aimed at stopping the widespread diversion of these agents into illicit or "street" channels.

The CSA states that any drug with a potential for drug abuse, drug dependence, or both falls under its purview. Such drugs include all opiates and their synthetic analogues, sedatives, stimulants, and hallucinogens; these drugs are collectively referred to as *controlled substances*. As a consequence, controlled substances are placed into one of five categories or schedules according to their relative potential for abuse or addiction. Thus, controlled substances are referred to as *scheduled drugs* (Table 1-1). Manufacturers of controlled substances must place on their prescription bottle a label with large bold letters that indicate what category or schedule the drug fits into using the abbreviations **C-1, C-II, C-III, C-IV, and C-V.** Sometimes additional state regulations exist regarding the format of prescriptions for scheduled drugs, how refills are to be managed, and record-keeping of the prescribing and dispensing of the medication, as well as how the medications are stored (in a locked place).

Today, the Drug Enforcement Agency (DEA) and the Department of Justice have jurisdiction over controlled substances. The CSA states that it is unlawful for any person to possess a controlled substance unless it has been obtained by a valid prescription or its possession is pursuant to actions in the regular course of professional conduct (a pharmacy inventory). Finally, the CSA brings drug wholesalers, manufacturers, hospitals, physicians, pharmacists, pharmacies, nurses, and others to task for a host of accountability regulations that affect the flow and distribution of these agents right down to the administration of one individual dose. This is why most health institutions have very rigid protocols for safeguarding narcotics once they possess them. Furthermore, the DEA has a registration requirement specifically for physicians, physician assistants, nurse practitioners, and pharmacies authorized by state or federal law or regulation to prescribe, dispense, or administer controlled substances. Clinicians must also comply with state regulations regarding the format of prescriptions for scheduled drugs, how refills are managed, record-keeping of the prescribing and

TABLE 1-1	DEA Categories of Scheduled Drugs		
SCHEDULE	DEFINITION	RESTRICTIONS	EXAMPLES
SCHEDULE I (C-I)	High potential for abuse.	No accepted medical use in the United States.	Heroin, LSD, marijuana, and mescaline.
SCHEDULE II (C-II)	High potential for abuse, psychic or physical, with severe dependence or liability.	Prescriptions must be written in ink or typed and signed by clinician. Verbal orders must be confirmed in writing within 72 hours and given only in true emergencies. No refills.	Certain narcotics, stimulants and depressants: hydromorphone (Dilaudid), meperidine (Demerol), methadone, fentanyl, oxycodone, morphine. Non-narcotic amphetamines (amphetamine, methamphetamine, and Ritalin [methylphenidate], pentobarbital and secobarbital).
SCHEDULE III (C-III)	Some potential for abuse: Substances in this schedule have an abuse potential less than those in Schedules I and II and include compounds containing limited quantities of certain narcotic and non-narcotic drugs. Their abuse may lead to moderate or low physical dependence or high psychological dependence.	Prescriptions may be oral or written. Up to five renewals are permitted within 6 months.	Codeine (Tylenol with Codeine), hydrocodone combination products, butalbital, ketamine, pentobarbital combination products, anabolic steroids (dihydrotestosterone).
SCHEDULE IV (C-IV)	Low potential for abuse: Substances in this schedule have an abuse potential less than those listed in Schedule III, which may lead only to limited physical dependence or psychological dependence.	Prescriptions may be oral or written. Up to five renewals are permitted w/in 6 months.	Butorphanol (Stadol), chloral hydrate, diazepam, flurazepam, midazolam (Versed), pemoline (Cylert), phenobarbital, sibutramine (Meridia), triazolam (Halcion), zaleplon (Sonata), zolpidem (Ambien), dextropropoxyphene dosage forms and pentazocine (Talwin-NX), Darvocet.
SCHEDULE V (C-V)	Subject to state and local regulation: These substances have an abuse potential less than those listed in Schedule IV and consist primarily of preparations containing limited quantities of certain narcotic and stimulant drugs generally for antitussive, antidiarrheal, and analgesic purposes.	Prescriptions may not be required.	Lomotil and Robitussin AC or other cough syrups with codeine.

Note: The drugs listed in this table are a brief compilation of the agents over which the DEA exerts control. For a complete list of all controlled substances, please consult the DEA website, www.deadiversion.usdoj.gov/schedules/orangebook, or for a fuller look at the Controlled Substances Act itself, go to www.justice.gov/dea/pubs/csa.html.

dispensing of medications, and how the medications are stored (in a locked place).

The Emergence of Rational Prescribing

In the late 20th century, the European office of the World Health Organization (WHO) reported its concern regarding drugs not being used as efficiently and as safely as they should. Several European countries looked into the matter and concluded that it takes the same kind of expertise to prescribe a drug for a diagnosis as it takes to make a diagnosis. Since then the Europeans have collectively reported on the ethical, effective, safe, and economic use of drugs and have worked to establish an academic discipline known as *clinical pharmacology* in their medical schools. These efforts have resulted in a gradual decline in morbidity and mortality of many drugs; this information, gained as a result of clinical trials, is reported in the highly respected *European Journal of Clinical Pharmacology*, now free and available online to any subscriber.

In 1994 the World Health Organization (WHO) published its *Guide to Good Prescribing*, which advocated a global approach to prescribing. (We present a similar approach to that of WHO but prefer to use the word *conscientious*.) At the time the WHO released its recommendations for **rational prescribing**, it asked that clinicians first create a personal formulary containing a few effective medications that they frequently use and then use those medications in a manner that ensures they have done the following:

■ Defined the problem.
■ Addressed a specific therapeutic objective.
■ Ensured that any medication in the personal formulary is safe and effective for the patient under consideration.
■ Informed the patient about the risks and benefits of the medication.
■ Monitored the results of the treatment.
■ Stopped the drug when the treatment period is over.

In 1999 a landmark report titled *To Err is Human: Building a Safer Health System* was issued by the Institute of Medicine (IOM) of the National Academies of Health. This report pointed to the statistic that nearly 98,000 Americans die each year from preventable medical errors, many of them drug related. At that time a goal was set to achieve a target of a 50% reduction in medical errors by 2010. Unfortunately, the Centers for Disease Control and Prevention (CDC) report that the number of preventable medical errors is still approximately 100,000 annually and is growing, largely because of methicillin-resistant *Staphylococcus aureus* (MRSA) and preventable hospital errors.

The Extent of Medication Errors

Few reliable estimates of the true costs of medication errors in the United States exist. However, in 2006 the IOM found that about one adverse drug event (ADE) per day occurs in every hospital throughout the United States and that it costs about $8,750 per event. The IOM also found there are about 530,000 preventable ADEs per year among outpatient Medicare patients and about 800,000 preventable ADEs occurring per year in long-term care facilities. Finally, 1 in 3 Americans have suffered from a medical mistake, of which 28% were due to medication errors (Institute of Medicine, 2007).

Because most medication errors result from multiple events that compound themselves, rather than from a single act committed by a single careless person, medication errors tend to be a function more of faulty systems, not faulty people. For this reason, the IOM advocates moving to a system of computerized prescribing, or "e-prescribing," to avoid the mistakes that accompany handwritten prescriptions. In fact, it is becoming more common for patients visiting a medical office today to leave not with a prescription, but with a postcard-size document advising that a prescription has been electronically sent to the pharmacy of their choice (Fig. 1-1).

According to the Institute for Safe Medication Practices (ISMP), a nonprofit organization of clinicians dedicated to educating the health-care community and consumers about safe medication practices, most medication errors are latent, which

> **To Our Patients**
> *We are committed to the safety, security, and accuracy of your prescription. This is why we send your prescriptions electronically to your pharmacy using a secure network. Please show your pharmacist this card to ensure he/she is aware that your prescription has been sent electronically.*

FIGURE 1-1 Postcard advising a patient that a prescription has been sent to his or her pharmacy.

means they have delayed effects or results. Medication errors are often caused by the following:

■ Failed communications. Handwriting and oral communications are a common source of errors. For instance, when communicating a drug order by telephone, errors can occur when drugs have similar names. Poor handwriting and hastily written prescriptions can have missing or misplaced zeros and decimal points. Errors can also occur due to the use of nonstandard abbreviations or the writing of ambiguous or incomplete orders.
■ Poor drug distribution practices—mail. Many patients receive medications by mail. Patients must be counseled to review their medications carefully upon receiving them and to call the pharmacy or clinician if the medication looks different from what they have previously taken or if they receive another patient's order in error.
■ Complex or poorly designed technology. At times even the best systems may fail. Human errors can occur even when using the most up-to-date technology; clinicians still must be careful to select the correct drug and dosage before printing a prescription or electronically sending it to the pharmacy.
■ Access to drugs by nonpharmacy personnel—samples. Errors may occur if the clinician relies on other personnel in the office to choose and distribute drug samples to the patient. The wrong medication or dosage may inadvertently be given to the patient.
■ Lack of information about the patient (no medication history). Errors can easily occur if the clinician is in a hurry and does not take an adequate patient history. For instance, the clinician may forget to ask if the patient has a medication allergy. Furthermore, clinicians may fail to tailor drug dosages for patients with abnormal renal or hepatic function or fail to look for interactions with other medications a patient may be taking.
■ Allowing the patient to leave without checking the patient's understanding of therapy. Patients do not always understand the directions written on their medicine bottle. Do not leave patient education to the pharmacy. It is the clinician's duty to make sure patients fully understand why they are taking medications and how they are to take them (ISMP, 2012).

IOM Recommendations: Safe Medication Practices

The IOM has laid out a comprehensive strategy by which government, clinicians, industry, and patients can reduce preventable medical errors. The IOM made the following three recommendations:

1. Implementation of safe medication practices, such as having the FDA provide oversight over safety issues associated with similarly named drugs. Today, the FDA reviews drug names for confusion and rejects approximately one-third of proposed names for medications because of their potential for confusion. As an example, Kapidex was to be the brand name of a proton pump inhibitor used to treat heartburn and other conditions. After review by the FDA, the manufacturer had to change this brand name to Dexilant to help prevent medication errors (U.S. FDA, 2010).

2. Creation of two national reporting systems for medication errors. One of these systems was to be voluntary, which would provide confidential feedback to health professionals so they could learn from the mistakes of others. The second national reporting system was to be mandatory and would make medication errors known to the public. A decade after these recommendations were made, 24 states have implemented medical error reporting systems, but most of them do not report facility-specific information in a public venue.

3. Creation of a center for patient safety. This center was to be set up as another federal oversight agency within the federal Agency for Healthcare Research and Quality (AHRQ). However, its work was hindered by the lack of reliable reporting that would give it the data needed to monitor the problem reliably and accurately (IOM, 1999).

High-Alert Medications

The ISMP publishes The High-Alert Medication List, a list of drugs likely to cause harm if used in error. The ISMP publishes another list of drugs entitled ISMP's List of Confused Drug Names (available at http://ismp.org). The drugs on this list have been involved in medication errors reported to ISMP and/or appear on The Joint Commission's (TJC) list of look-alike/sound alike (LASA) drug names. Furthermore, the USP's National Coordinating Council for Medication Error and Reporting Program (NCC MERP) publishes the following list of recommendations to improve the accuracy of prescription writing to prevent medication errors (NCC MERP, 2005):

1. All prescription documents must be legible. Verbal orders should be minimized.

2. Prescription orders should include a brief notation of purpose (e.g., for cough), unless considered inappropriate by the clinician. Notation of purpose can help further ensure that the proper medication is dispensed and creates an extra safety check in the process of prescribing and dispensing a medication. The council does recognize, however, that certain medications and disease states may warrant maintaining confidentiality.

3. All prescription orders should be written in the metric system except for therapies that use standard units such as insulin, vitamins, etc. Units should be spelled out rather than writing *U*. The change to the use of the metric system from the archaic apothecary and avoirdupois systems will help avoid misinterpretations of these abbreviations and symbols and miscalculations when converting to metric measurements, which are used in product labeling and package inserts.

4. Clinicians should include age and, when appropriate, weight of the patient on the prescription or medication order. The most common errors in dosage occur in pediatric and geriatric populations. The age (and weight) of a patient can help dispensing clinicians in their double-check of the appropriate drug and dose.

5. Medication orders should include drug name, exact metric weight or concentration, and dosage form. Strength should be expressed in metric amounts, and concentration should be specified. Each order for a medication should be complete. The pharmacist should check with the prescribing clinician if any information is missing or questionable.

6. Whenever a dosage strength is indicated, a leading zero should always be used for the decimal expression of a quantity less than 1. For example, write "0.5 gm" for a half-gram dose rather than ".5 gm." Using the leading zero is likely to result in fewer errors. Likewise, a terminal or trailing zero should never be used after a decimal because 10-fold errors in drug strength and dosage have occurred with its use. For example, it is better to write 5 gm rather than 5.0 gm.

7. Clinicians should avoid the use of abbreviations, including those for drug names (e.g., MOM for milk of magnesia or HCTZ for hydrochlorothiazide) and Latin directions for use.

8. Clinicians should not use vague language, such as "take as directed" or "take/use as needed" as instruction for use.

Presently, the ISMP, USP, and FDA collect and track medication errors and make information available to clinicians and the public. Information and alerts about confusing drug names may be obtained from these organizations' websites: www.ismp.org, www.usp.org, and www.fda.gov. However, it remains vital for all health professionals to work together to establish practices that reduce the potential for harm resulting from ordering, dispensing, or administering the incorrect drug.

Writing Prescriptions to Avoid Errors

Although prescriptions are not difficult to write, great care and diligence should be taken when writing any prescription to avoid the potential for errors. Prescription formats have changed little over the centuries and have as their basis roots in Latin. Thus, even today, when prescriptions are printed on paper or are used in electronic formatting, there is little variation in their appearance across the United States because of their generally accepted traditional composition and because, in most states, there is a state law that defines who can prescribe and what is expected of a prescription. State law usually parallels federal law, but in some states, to help prevent forgeries, stolen prescriptions, and other crimes, the size of a prescription pad is mandated, and in some states only certain approved printers are allowed to print prescription pads for the professional. Even *who* may write prescriptions is a matter of state law. For instance, medical practitioners, veterinarians, dentists, and podiatrists have prescribing rights, and in all states certified physician assistants (PA-C) have prescribing rights, although there are some limitations depending on the state. In many states nurse practitioners also have full prescribing rights, whereas clinical pharmacists may have limited prescribing rights. In several states clinical psychologists (PhDs) who have special training are also given limited rights to prescribe. Health economists in the United States frequently assert that although health-care spending per capita might be higher in the United States than in other high-income countries, the long-term rates of spending growth have been similar, and it is institutional factors that contribute most to increases in spending. These institutional factors include policies that offer "free" or low-cost prescription benefits with both public and private health insurance plans. Thus on a global basis, all countries that offer health-care benefits are experiencing increases in health-care spending, especially for prescription drugs (White, 2007). The result of all this new spending activity in the United States was that, in the decade between 1997 and 2007, the number of prescriptions rose 72% whereas the population rose only 11% (Aitken, Berndt, & Cutler, 2009).

Figure 1-2 shows the conventional format for a written prescription that helps clinicians and dispensers avoid errors when it is written legibly. The clinician identification (Fig. 1-2A), which includes the clinician's name, professional degree, office address, and telephone number, is required on all prescriptions. Also, patient identifiers (Fig. 1-2B) are required and include the patient's name and address. Some providers also include the patient's age, sex, and drug allergies on their prescriptions.

This is a good idea, especially when prescribing medications for children and infants, because it alerts the dispensing pharmacist to be sure the dosage is correct.

All the drug information and directions (Fig. 1-2C) for its use are placed in the center of the prescription form. The name of the drug and its strength are known as the *inscription* (Fig. 1-2C-1). The Rx symbol is also here. This symbol has been used since early recorded Egyptian times and is seen on the walls of ancient hieroglyphics. Its literal interpretation is simply "take thou," as instructions to the pharmacists. Here the word *strength* refers to the strength of each dosage unit, not the total dose to be taken. Abbreviations may be used only if the clinician is certain the pharmacist will understand them. There is much encouragement today to use the **generic** name of the drug (the name that is not trademarked), but use of the trademarked (trade), or brand, name is still in prevailing use. It is only outside the United States that generic names on prescriptions are used more than brand names because of health insurance plans.

Each state also has a drug substitution law that either permits or mandates that a pharmacist substitute a generic bioequivalent drug for a brand name one stated on a prescription. Clinicians can also exercise their prerogative that a substitution *not* be made by writing "dispense as written," or DAW, on the prescription or by signing in the correct box on the prescription. Most preprinted prescriptions contain two spaces for the clinician's signature to indicate his or her wishes in this matter. In the preceding example, note the space on the bottom left indicating "substitution permitted" (Fig. 1-2G) and the other space (Fig. 1-2H), bottom right, indicating the clinician wants the pharmacist to dispense as written (Fig. 1-2H). Today, the practice of brand and generic substitution is widely accepted. However, there are drugs for which bioequivalence studies indicate that once a patient has started on a particular manufacturer's brand of a drug, biologically significant fluctuations can be observed when brands or manufacturers are switched or substituted (Box 1-1). When this is known, providers must indicate that no substitution should be made for the brand they have selected.

Since the early 1970s, generic substitution has grown considerably despite concerns about the bioavailability and safety of

A	**John Smith, MD** **123 Main Street** **Uptown, VA** **(123) 456-7890**	Allergies: _____ Age: _____ Sex: _____	
B	Patient Name Patient Address		
C	(1) Inscription: Brand/ generic name and strength (2) Subscription: Quantity to be dispensed (3) Signa: Instruction to the pharmacist as to what directions they should give the patient for taking the medication. Latin abbreviations are used (BID, TID)		
D Refill: 0 1 2 3 PRN		E Date:	F DEA#:
G Sign name here (substitution permitted)		H Sign name here (dispense as written)	

FIGURE 1-2 Components of a written prescription.

BOX 1-1 Examples of Medications that Should not be Substituted

Quinidine

Theophylline

Warfarin

Conjugated estrogens

Chlorpromazine

Dicumarol

Digitalis (Lanoxin)

Phenytoin

Levothyroxine

generic drugs. For most drugs, bioequivalence testing should have confirmed that it was generally safe for a clinician to request a generic product in place of the innovator's product, and in most cases this has been the case. However, for narrow therapeutic drugs or highly variable drugs with strict dosing parameters, this is not true, and many generic drugs have proved to be problematic when it comes to bioequivalence. Since 1989 the FDA stepped up its generic testing and instituted a large postmarketing surveillance system to keep watch over generic usage. The FDA publishes its findings on generic bioequivalence in its *Orange Book: Approved Drug Products with Therapeutic Equivalence Evaluations*, commonly known as the *Orange Book* (available at www.accessdata.fda.gov/scripts/cder/ob/default.cfm). In the *Orange Book*, drug products are rated as A (substitutable) or B (noninterchangeable). Secondary letters indicate the type of study by which a product was determined to be bioequivalent, for example, in vitro or in vivo studies, or the type of formulation that is not considered bioequivalent.

Instructions to the pharmacist regarding dosage form and number of dosage units to dispense is known as the *subscription* (Figure 1-2C-2). This should be specific to the dosage form (tablet, capsule, suspension) and to the quantity (e.g., 4-oz syrup or 30-gm tube). For controlled substances, quantities should be written in words as well as numbers to guard against alteration (i.e., dispense thirty [30] tablets). There are countless cases in which drug-seeking individuals have obtained a prescription for 10 tablets of a controlled substance, and by the time it reaches the pharmacy for dispensing, the number 10 has been changed to 100 by adding another zero. For a precompounded drug in the form of tablets, the subscription is generally a number, commonly preceded by the symbol #. To avoid confusion, Arabic numbers (50) are preferred to Roman numerals.

In the case of a suspension or liquid medication, the dispensing can be in milliliters (mL) or cubic centimeters (cc), but the milliliter measurement is preferred today. When the pharmacist is mixing components for a specific cause, the mixture may be specified. In the case of prescription orders for extemporaneously compounded products, this portion of the prescription may include phrases such as "make sugar free" or "mix and divide into 30 capsules." Extemporaneous compounding is the pharmacist's art of preparing a drug product for a specific patient using a physician's prescription, a drug formula, or a recipe. In these cases calculated amounts of ingredients are measured and made into a homogenous (uniform) mixture. Extemporaneous compounding is typical when certain medical needs of an individual cannot be met by the use of a commercial drug product. Some examples of extemporaneous compounding include making a pediatric dosage form of a medication when only an adult dosage form is available or fulfilling a dermatologist's prescription for the clinician's own special formula for an acne patient.

Signa on a prescription form indicates the instructions the clinician has given to the patient (Fig. 1-2C-3). Signa is the abbreviation for the Latin word *signatura* and tells the pharmacist what words to "sign" on the prescription label as directions for use. These patient instructions should be simple, complete, and specific as possible and include how much to take, when to take it, and why it is being taken. The pharmacist will write whatever the clinician has directed him or her to write in this area on the medication container. Directions such as "use as directed" and "usual directions" should be avoided because they are confusing, dangerous, and illegal in some states. Every clinician must commit to memory common Latin abbreviations that have been used for centuries (Table 1-2). However, keep in mind there are often local habits and conventions that are used. Nevertheless, there are also several Latin abbreviations used in prescription writing that can cause errors and confusion when hastily or sloppily used.

Refill information (Fig. 1-2D) indicates the number of times (or time period) that the patient may renew the prescription without authorization. Prescriptions for schedule II controlled substances may not be refilled. Schedule III to V controlled substances have a five-refill or 6-month limit. The date the prescription is written (Fig. 1-2E) should be included on all prescriptions, and the clinician's DEA number (Fig. 1-2F) should be included when necessary. Unless otherwise specified by the clinician, medications will be dispensed in childproof containers, which may be difficult for elderly or arthritic patients. Patients may request that the pharmacist put the medication in an easy-to-open container.

To reduce medication errors, many clinicians add the diagnosis to the instructions, for example, "Take one tablet daily for blood pressure" or "Apply to affected area twice a day for poison ivy." Clinicians must also be very careful when writing dosages and must ensure that the units are written clearly. Standardization of approved abbreviations is now required in most hospitals, and prescriptions are returned when unacceptable abbreviations are written. Finally, clinicians must make the effort to write legibly if they are still handwriting prescriptions.

Federal Regulations Protecting Pregnant Women

Because drug testing and clinical trials have produced better information than in decades past, the FDA has assigned "Pregnancy Safety Categories" for all drugs that have been studied in humans and animals (Table 1-4). Should any untoward reactions occur in pregnant animals, the data is extrapolated to include humans. This is done because it would be impossible to ask a pregnant woman if she would like to be part of a drug study that could be harmful to an unborn child, especially because teratogenicity caused by drugs is a well-known phenomenon. Congenital malformations, which are often thought to be the result of genetic factors or environmental factors (such as smoking or taking drugs), occur in 3% to 4% of live births. Clinicians must be aware of the risks when prescribing for the pregnant patient because they are prescribing for two patients, the fetus and the mother (CDC-NBDPN, 2008). The FDA's drug-pregnancy rating system takes all available information and weighs the risks and benefits to the pregnant patient. The rating system was introduced in 1979 and was based on a model put into practice in Sweden in 1978.

TABLE 1-2 Common Abbreviations Used in Prescription Writing as Taken From the Original Latin

ABBREVIATION	MEANING	ORIGINAL LATIN	ABBREVIATION	MEANING	ORIGINAL LATIN
DOSING			qd	every day	*quoque die*
tsp	teaspoon	(English)	qh	every hour	*quoque hora*
tbsp	tablespoon	(English)	qid	four times a day	*quart in die*
g, gm, Gm	gram	*grammae*	q.o.d or q.a.d	every other day	*quoque alternis die*
gr	grain	*granum*	stat	at once, immediately	*statim*
Gtts	drops	*guttae*			
mcg	micrograms	(English)	tid	three times a day	*ter in die*
mg	milligram	(English)	tiw	three times a week	*ter in septimane* or 3 in 7 (**Note:** There is no Latin word for "week.")
ROUTE OF ADMINISTRATION					
ad	right ear	*auris laeva*			
as	left ear	*auris sinistra*	ut dict	as directed	*ut dictum*
au	both ears	*auris utraque*	*MISCELLANEOUS ABBREVIATIONS*		
od	right eye	*oculus dexter*	aa	of each	*ana*
os	left eye	*oculus sinistra*	aq	water	*aqua*
ou	each/both eye	*oculus uterque*	cap	capsule	*capsulae*
po	by mouth	*per os*	et	and	*et*
p.r.	per rectum	(English))	fl	fluid	*fluidus*
PV	vaginally	*per vaginum*	c	with	(English)
FREQUENCY OF ADMINISTRATION			mitte	mix	*mitte*
ac	before meals	*ante cibos*	n.r.	no refill	*non repetatur*
ad lib	take freely, at your pleasure	*ad libitum*	qs	add a sufficient amount	*quantum sufficit*
am	in the morning	*ante meridian*	Rx	take	*recipe*
bid	twice a day	*bis in die*	rep	repeat, refill	*repateur*
BM	bowel movement	(English)	ss	one-half	*semis*
Cc	with food	*cum cibos*	s	without	*sine*
d/c	discontinue	(English)	s.a.	use your own discretion	*secundum artem*
h	hour	*hor*			
hs	at bedtime	*hora somni*	sig	mark on label	*signatura*
pc	after meals	*post cibos*	tab	tablet	*tabletae*
prn	as needed	*pro re nata*	w/o	without	(English)
q	every	*quoque*			

Sources: Osborn, O. T. (1906). *Introduction to Materia Medica and Pharmacology*. Philadelphia: Lea Brothers; Davis, N. M. (2007). *Medical Abbreviations: 28,000 Conveniences at the Expense of Communication and Safety*. Warminster, PA: Neil M. Davis Associates.

Not all drugs have been rated, and the FDA list is not all inclusive. In addition, not all drugs reported as being teratogenic (agents that can interfere with normal embryonic development) are; animal studies used may not transfer to humans, and the dosages used in the studies may not be the same as those used in humans. Thus, every clinician has to be extremely conscientious when prescribing for pregnant patients and must remember to consider the following:

■ Not all teratogenic agents cause malformations with every exposure.
■ There are large variations in teratogenicity between species.
■ There are wide variations in susceptibility among humans.

■ Damage brought about by teratogenic agents is usually a function of dosage, length of exposure, and a window of opportunity, that is, the first weeks or trimester of pregnancy.
■ Teratogenicity itself is not fully understood.

Conscientious Prescribing and a Patient-Centered Approach: A Perfect Partnership

In *De Medicina*, Aulus Cornelius Celsus (ca 25 BC–50 BC), a Roman encyclopedist, wrote that "the art of medicine should be rational, drawing on evident causes." Although this statement seems self-explanatory, not everyone interprets it the

TABLE 1-3 Six Timeless Questions to Improve Prescription Safety and Efficacy Every Prescriber Should Answer Before Any Prescription Leaves with a Patient

1. Have you thought through the reason why you are prescribing any particular medication?

   If you are thinking in a "patient first" manner, you will more conscientious about whether or not your prescription is treating a symptom or an underlying pathology. Have you thought about nonprescription alternatives as treatment options before any prescription is written?

2. Have you enough experience with any one drug to know its expected outcomes in a population of patients?

   Most clinicians stick with prescribing drugs they have experience with rather than use a wide range of drugs that may not be common in their scope of practice. They tend to avoid prescribing drugs newly on the market, but rather they wait for evidence-based clinical studies to point the way. Conscientious clinicians do not play roulette with certain drugs because they see them as a clinical trial of one; instead, they are always aware of the drug's risk-benefit ratio, thus are you aware of the risks versus benefits of your prescription drug?

3. Are you prescribing this drug as a result of a telephone consultation or e-mail, or have you really examined the patient?

   All too often patients ask for drugs over the telephone. This is especially true of drugs used for pain and for antibiotics. Often long-term drugs, such as those used for hypertension, are refilled without recent evidence of their dosing schedule, dosages, and adherence patterns. Additionally, some patients may have a disease state relapse because they have stopped a drug, and they are now are asking for higher doses. Do you have a good read on the patient's history and on the patient's adherence behaviors?

4. Have you talked enough with this patient so that you are comfortable that the dosing schedule has been shared and agreed upon?

   Many drugs should be taken four times a day, but this may not mean every 6 hours in a 24-hour period. Thus, don't leave it to the patient to interpret any of the directions you may put on a prescription. This can become a real issue if more than one drug is added to a patient's already busy drug regimen or if it is interfered with due to patients' lifestyle issues. Thus are you considering the patients need for a "conservative" approach to drug-taking and that they do not want you to add more drugs with complex regimens?

5. Have you considered the long-term effect of your prescribing a particular drug and when you want the patient to stop taking it?

   On occasion a patient may need therapy for a considerable length of time. Any new drug may offer only marginal benefit at first, but until it has clinical evidence produced over several years, it is best to stick with the tried-and-true therapy despite advertising that induces patients to ask for it. The conscientious clinician will also conduct a review of any drugs used for any considerable length of time to assess whether they can be discontinued.

6. Before doing anything, do you have an accurate medication history on this patient?

   Before starting any drug, patients should be asked if they are seeing any other clinicians, and if so, for what, and what other medications (Rx and OTC) might they be taking. An accurate medication history is also a great tool to discover drugs that produce unsuccessful outcomes as well as a means to discover potential drug-drug and drug-food interactions.

TABLE 1-4 United States FDA Pharmaceutical Pregnancy Safety Categories

CATEGORY	DEFINITION
A	Adequate and well-controlled studies indicate no risk to the fetus in the first trimester of pregnancy, and there is no evidence of risk in later trimesters.
B	Animal reproduction studies indicate there is no risk to the fetus, yet there are no well-controlled studies in pregnant women.
C	Animal reproduction studies have reported adverse effects on a fetus; there are no well-controlled studies in humans, but potential benefits may indicate the use of the drug in pregnant women despite potential risks.
D	Positive human fetal risk has been reported in investigational or marketing experience or human studies. Considering potential benefit versus risk may, in selected cases, warrant the use of these drugs in pregnant women.
X	Fetal abnormalities reported and positive evidence of fetal risk in humans is available from animal or human studies. The risks clearly outweigh the potential benefits. These drugs should not be used in pregnant women.

same way. Thus, learning the tenets of conscientious prescribing is important. To the authors of this text, **conscientious prescribing** means "a thoughtful process that always places the patient's well-being first, ahead of every prescribing decision made *before* any prescription is written and includes appropriate follow-up *after* that patient has taken any course of medication." (See Table 1-3.)

Individualizing health care so that it is more conscientious and patient-centered is a movement gaining strong support in the United States. Great strides are being made to focus health systems on being more responsive to patient's needs, preferences, and values rather than on systems of payment set by insurance models. Some of that impetus comes from studies and reports issued by organizations such as The Institute of Medicine (IOM), The Commonwealth Fund, the American Association of Family Practice (AAFP), the American Academy of Pediatrics (AAP), the Agency for Healthcare Research and Quality (AHRQ), the American College of Physicians (ACP), and the American Osteopathic Association (AOA). Some of this impetus also comes from what has been learned from abroad. For example, in Denmark, every clinician is given responsibility to care for about 1,500 patients. Patients are assigned to a medical home where they are assured patient-centered services, such as same-day appointments, walk-in appointments, electronic prescribing systems connected to local pharmacies, off-hour telephone services, electronic access to patient health records, patient reminder systems, and patient surveys to assess quality of care.

Although U.S. health care is making great strides to be more responsive to patients' needs, values, and preferences, the process is slow. Patients want access to the same information their clinician has so that they are better able to be an active partner in shared treatment decisions. Clinicians need to supply information in an unbiased way that meets the patient's right to make an informed decision. When clinicians and patients share in the decision-making process, patients are more likely to adhere to the prescribed medication regimen (Campaign for Effective Patient Care, n.d.).

This textbook provides students with a sound foundation for learning the fundamentals and foundations of practical pharmacology, but its ultimate goal is to help future clinicians begin to apply a conscientious process to their eventual prescribing habits by adopting a patient-centered philosophy. Conscientious prescribing involves applying pharmacological knowledge to benefit patients while considering the many factors related to the individual and the drug choices that may impact the choice of prescription, such as the following:

- Patient factors. These factors include age, gender, weight, culture, health beliefs, mental status, ability to adhere to a regimen, and ability to understand the benefits and risks of the medication.
- Disease factors. Also considered are drug-disease compatibility, liver or renal disease that affects drug action, goal of therapy (long term or short term), the presence of comorbidities and multiple medical problems that may lead to polypharmacy and its resultant drug interactions and adverse reactions.
- Drug factors. Clinicians should consider such drug factors as similar mechanisms of action, adverse risks, drug interactions, ability to monitor, alternatives available, contraindications, precautions, dosage regimen and duration, hypersensitivities and allergies, therapeutic window, blood levels, drug half-life, speed of onset, and bioavailability.
- Social factors. Clinicians should also consider cost of medications (generic versus brand name), insurance limitations, patient lifestyle and accountability, and drug formularies that limit alternatives.
- Knowledge factors. Sources of information that can be trusted such as evidence from randomized controlled clinical trials, evidence from clinical practice guidelines, evidence from systematic reviews, published drug references, drug product monographs, and electronic drug information databases should be used when choosing the best drug to prescribe.
- Third-party factors. In the 21st century, **managed care** insurance programs are partners in many of the decisions regarding drug usage. Formularies (lists of approved drugs that insurance companies will pay for) often dictate what may or may not be a drug benefit. The patient's share (copay) in that benefit also requires the clinician to adhere to commonly accepted **algorithms**, or pathways, for selecting or limiting drug choices. This oversight has some benefits. The **Pharmacy and Therapeutics (P&T) Committee** of many managed care organizations (MCOs) acts as a watchdog over prescribing habits. For example, proton pump inhibitors (PPIs) are best used for treatment of peptic ulcer disease (PUD) and should not to be used for routine relief of dyspepsia. Thus, many health plans dictate that after 6 weeks of therapy they will no longer pay for the routine use of PPI because any PUD should have healed by then. This has resulted in PPIs becoming OTC drugs rather than prescription drugs.
- Government and learned society factors. Government agencies such as the Agency for Health Care Research and Quality (AHRQ), the National Institutes of Health (NIH), and the National Heart Lung Blood Institute (NHLBI) influence prescribing habits by spelling out treatment algorithms offering the best evidence available for treating certain diseases. Other learned societies and organizations such as the American Cancer Society (ACS), the American Heart Association (AHA), and the American College of Obstetrics and Gynecology (ACOG) also provide **treatment guidelines** and algorithms that their most respected and credentialed experts agree on as guidelines for choosing appropriate treatment or best practices.
- Collaborating colleagues. Conscientious clinicians realize that the body of health-care information available today is too much for one person to digest and apply alone. They collaborate with other members of the health-care team to provide high-quality care. It has been a longstanding habit

of primary clinicians to consult with specialists and colleagues. Today's health-care delivery system is an even more expanded model of collaboration because nurses, physicians, pharmacists, physician assistants, dentists, nurse practitioners, midwives, and others all realize they need each other to provide high-quality patient care.

This team collaboration model has become even more important in the era of managed care in which knowledge and experience shared from several perspectives helps everyone achieve best practices and best patient-focused outcomes.

Steps That Lead to Being a More Thoughtful and Conscientious Prescriber

Former Surgeon General C. Everett Koop has often been quoted as saying "Drugs don't work in people who don't take them." Drugs also don't work unless someone prescribes them—and prescribes the right ones. Writing the correct prescription, however, is much easier said than done because clinicians today have to wade through a sea of drug options and thoughtfully choose an appropriate medication for each patient. Most clinicians who have prescription rights receive a basic education in pharmacology in the classroom and then learn how, what, and when to prescribe as they undergo clinical training. During clinical training, many learn prescribing routines of medication selection by observing, copying, or discarding the behavior of experienced clinicians or by applying and monitoring clinical guidelines advocated by professional societies.

Prescribing is an art as well as a science. Most clinicians are familiar with at least one drug as their first choice for conditions they see regularly. Confidence in this choice is based on a real understanding of the drug's therapeutic uses, common side effects, pharmacokinetics, pharmacodynamics, common dosages, efficacy under common circumstances, likely adverse events, safety profile, and cost. There are about 8,000 marketed drugs in the United States, and a clinician can't know all there is about all of them. Thus, it makes sense that a clinician should pick 30 or 40 drugs and know them very well. For example, a clinician may use a certain medication consistently to treat new-onset hypertension but has another medication in mind if the patient also has a history of diabetes or is African American. Clinicians become familiar with drugs through clinical experience and being open to using the best evidence written about drugs, as well as by collaborating with trusted colleagues and relying on their experienced clinical judgment.

Conscientious prescribing is a thoughtful process. Clinicians should ask themselves the following 10 questions before writing any prescription, especially if they want to be more conscientious about exercising their prescription privileges and honoring their covenant between professional and patient (Boxes 1-2 and 1-3).

BOX 1-2 Ten Questions for Clinicians to Ask Themselves Before Prescribing

1. Have I selected the most appropriate drug and drug dosage?
2. Have I weighed all the risks and benefits?
3. Have I addressed the need to monitor the effects of this medication?
4. Am I fully informed about this patient's condition, other medications, comorbidities, allergies, and adverse events with other medications?
5. Have I made the prescription as legible to the pharmacist as it is to me?
6. Have I done all I can to assure the patient will be compliant?
7. Have I considered what the medication will cost the patient?
8. Have I considered the health literacy of the patient?
9. Have I involved my patient in a shared decision-making process?
10. Have I done all I can to minimize errors and increase patient safety?

BOX 1-3 Six Suggestions for Better Prescription Writing

1. Think Beyond Drugs.

   Seek nondrug alternatives as the first rather than the last resort.

   Treat underlying causes rather than solely treating symptoms.

   Look for prevention opportunities rather than exclusively focusing on established disease or symptom amelioration.

2. Practice More Strategic Prescribing.

   Defer nonurgent drug treatment whenever possible and desirable.

   Use only a few drugs; learn to use them well.

   Avoid drug switching without compelling evidence-based reasons.

Continued

BOX 1-3 Six Suggestions for Better Prescription Writing—cont'd

---

Be circumspect and skeptical about "individualizing" therapy when trials suggest little evidence of benefit in the studied cohort.

Be cautious about telephone or e-mail prescribing.

Whenever possible, start drug treatment with only one new drug at a time.

3. Maintain Heightened Vigilance About Adverse Effects.

Maintain a high index of suspicion for adverse drug effects.

Educate patients about potential adverse effects to ensure more timely recognition.

Be alert to clues of drug withdrawal symptoms masquerading as disease "relapses."

4. Exercise Caution and Skepticism Regarding New Drugs.

Learn about new drugs and new indications from unbiased sources such as randomized trials and from colleagues with reputations for conservative prescribing.

Do not rush to use new drugs because new adverse effects often emerge later.

Be certain drugs improve clinical outcomes rather than solely modify a surrogate marker.

Do not stretch indications away from trial-based evidence.

Avoid seduction by elegant pharmacology or physiological mechanisms in the absence of demonstrated clinical outcomes benefit.

Beware of selective reporting or presentation of studies.

5. Work with Patients Using a Shared Agenda

Do not reflexively succumb to patients' requests for new drugs they have heard advertised or recommended.

Avoid prescribing additional drugs for "refractory" problems, failing to appreciate possible nonadherence.

Obtain accurate medication histories to avoid repeat prescriptions for drugs previously tried unsuccessfully.

Discontinue drugs not working or no longer needed.

Work with and promote patients' desires for conservative therapy.

6. Consider Long-Term, Broader Impacts.

Think beyond short-term effects; consider longer-term benefits and risks.

Seek better prescribing systems (computerized physician order entry, reliable laboratory monitoring) rather than just new drugs as ways to improve pharmacotherapy. The implication here is that an improved drug or drug delivery system may offer only marginal benefits over an established system or drug.

Adapted from: Schiff D, Galanter WL, Duhig J, Lodolce AE, Koronkowski MJ, Lambert BL, Principles of conservative prescribing. *Archiv. Intern. Med.2011Sep.12; 171*(16):1433-1440 also available at www.ncbi.nlm.nih.gov/pubmed/21670331

Ten Questions to More Conscientious Prescribing

1. Have I selected the most appropriate drug and drug dosage for this patient in this setting? Once the decision to prescribe has been made, the clinician has to determine the most appropriate drug and dose for a given individual. In most clinical settings, the decision about the choice of drug is influenced substantially by the confidence the clinician has in the accuracy of the diagnosis. There will generally be several medications that could be used in a given situation, but conscientious clinicians learn to master a short list of useful drugs and make an effort to use them. When possible, the clinician should use the agent that is least toxic, most efficacious, and least expensive in a given situation.

The initial dosage regimen is based on published standards and is determined by estimation of the pharmacokinetic properties of the drug in the individual receiving the prescription. Occasionally, the level of certain drugs is measurable in the laboratory, but more often, it is not. Even when the plasma level of a drug is in the target range, there can be considerable variation among patients in the response they have to the drug being used. Every therapeutic plan is an experiment, and the clinician should recognize this, establish clinical goals when possible, and then monitor the patient for the desired outcome or any adverse event. Rational therapy is based on observing a patient through time and adjusting the medication accordingly.

2. Have I weighed all the risks and benefits to my patient? Although many patient problems can be treated by prescription drugs, many common complaints can be treated by OTC agents and nondrug alternatives that are safe and effective. It is important to ask if the patient has tried OTC medications or nondrug alternatives to alleviate symptoms before prescribing. For instance, take the time to explain to your patients that not every cold or flu-like illness requires an antibiotic or prescription cough medication. Also, when prescribing, keep in mind the age and comorbidities of your patient. Generally, the very old or very young will be more sensitive and have more side effects to medications and will be at increased risk for adverse outcomes.

Any patient with comorbidities, including psychiatric or mental illness, may be at high risk for untoward consequences of medications. Patients who use many medications on a long-term or chronic basis seem to be more prone to the adverse drug events (ADE) that occur most frequently when starting a prescription. When any patient is at a higher risk for an ADE, the starting dose should be the lowest possible to see how the patient will react, or as it is said in the popular idiom, "When in doubt, start low and go slow." (Silva, n.d.)

Often, clinicians are faulted for treating an individual's symptoms without addressing the disease. Many complaints come from patients with diseases that are not being effectively addressed. When symptoms are treated in isolation and the disease (the big picture) is not being confronted, the risks often exceed the benefits of treatment. Clinicians will lessen risk by using fewer drug treatments to control symptoms and focusing instead on treating underlying causes. An example is treating the joint pain of rheumatoid arthritis rather than addressing the disease state and offering medications that could effectively yield remission.

There are obviously many occasions in which a prescription is clearly in the patient's best interest—situations in which the benefit of taking a prescribed medication dwarfs the risk of an adverse event. Common wisdom is to use penicillin in the diagnosis of strep throat to shorten the duration of symptoms and to eradicate the small risk of late sequelae, such as rheumatic fever. In these situations, it is foolish to delay prescribing. But much of the time, prudence favors waiting to prescribe until the patient is more fully known to the clinician and the illness is better defined, perhaps by seeking more history or perhaps through repeated examinations or diagnostic testing. A dictum for conscientious prescribing may be to be patient with the patient, recognizing fully there is a downside to any prescription. Always remember the possibility of bringing harm with the prescription and act cautiously.

3. Have I addressed the need to monitor the effects of this medication? Because any therapeutic plan is, in essence, a clinical trial in which one individual is the subject (and there is no control), objectives should be established and the patient should be monitored for the expected end result of therapy. These therapeutic objectives should be clearly stated to the patient, with an expected time frame in which they might be realized. Obviously, the purest experiment will involve introducing or withdrawing one medication at a time, and clinicians should avoid attempting to treat several illnesses simultaneously. The clinician (or the staff) should routinely monitor the patient for good and bad effects, and this monitoring implies knowledge of common side effects and awareness of adverse events. Practitioners should be quick to discontinue medications that are not working or that are no longer needed.

The conscientious clinician should also monitor his or her own patterns of prescribing in an effort to stay apprised of therapeutic strengths and weaknesses and to discover what influences those prescribing patterns. In many health insurance plans, individuals now have a pharmaceutical benefit that will notify prescribing doctors of their patients' medication profiles, with suggestions of how they may be improved. Some computer databases can tabulate a clinician's most common therapeutic choices. Other prescription services may notify clinicians if they have failed to prescribe enough medication in certain disease states, as measured against evidence supporting certain drugs for certain diagnoses. One example of this is the clinician who, while caring for a newly diagnosed type 2 diabetic, receives notice from the patient's insurance company that the patient might benefit from adding a cholesterol-lowering medication, as recommended by the National Cholesterol Educational Program (NCEP), to the other medications being prescribed (see *Third Report of the National Cholesterol Educational Program Expert Panel on Detection, Evaluation and Treatment of High Blood Cholesterol in Adults (ATPIII)*, published by the National Institutes of Health [NIH], available at www.nhlbi.nih.gov/guidelines/cholesterol/atp3xsum.pdf). Health-care insurers frequently send their suggestions to clinicians, as they too are looking to see that best practices are being used in the care of their insured individuals.

Although it is considered a wise practice to be skeptical and cautious in the use of new drugs brought into the market, it may also be foolish to neglect using a new medication until large numbers of scientific studies with large populations have proven its safety. In short, clinicians may find it prudent not to be the first to use the new therapeutic agent, but they may also find it unwise to be the last to adopt its use. When using new drugs, prescribing should be more limited, and it should target patients with indications and situations for which benefit has been established. In a recent *Journal of the American Medical Association* article, Dr. Gordon Schiff, associate professor of medicine at Harvard Medical School, stated, "More training in pharmacokinetics and drug dosing is all to the good. But trainees also need to acquire a set of guiding principles to help them become more careful, cautious, evidence-based, and frankly skeptical prescribers throughout their careers." (Schiff & Galanter, 2009.)

4. Am I fully informed about this patient's condition, other medications, comorbidities, allergies, and adverse events with other medications? Because several of the most popular reference texts (*Physicians' Desk Reference, Epocrates*) are compendiums of package inserts published by the pharmaceutical manufacturing industry, unbiased and evaluated literature can be difficult to obtain. *Facts and Comparisons*, a lengthy and annually updated information resource for clinicians, is a reliable resource of unbiased information. It offers comparisons of drugs within classes and is available in many forms, ranging from print to electronic media (see www.factsandcomparisons.com). *The Sanford Guide to Antimicrobial Therapy*, 41st edition, is another resource that is available in print and electronic formats (see www.sanfordguide.com/Sanford_Guide/Home.html).

In periodicals, *The Medical Letter* (http://secure.medicalletter.org), which has been published since 1959, and *The Prescriber's Letter* are two publications edited by learned boards whose members have been vetted for lack of manufacturer bias, and each newsletter has loyal followings. *The Prescriber's Letter* (www.prescribersletter.com) is a concise monthly newsletter that provides large amounts of information about drug therapy categorized by medical specialty and disease states. Perhaps most importantly, this newsletter presents the information in an interesting and helpful manner that is well matched to the needs of practitioners. Finally, the federal government provides a source of unbiased online drug information at *Medline Plus–Drug Information* at www.nlm.nih.gov/medlineplus/druginformation.html.

A great deal of excessive prescribing can be attributed to patient demands for specific medications, which are often driven by direct-to-consumer (DTC) advertising. This type of marketing encourages patients to believe that there is a pill for every ill and has led to the unnecessary use of antibiotics, analgesics, oral contraceptives, weight loss medicines, and medications for sleep and mood disturbances. We now recognize that highly resistant bacterial strains, high rates of addiction to prescription drugs and narcotics, and unsupervised use of psychotropics have been deleterious to society. Clinicians today find themselves in a conundrum, balancing patient demand for advertised drugs against societal problems spawned by medical permissiveness.

5. Have I made the prescription as legible to the pharmacist as it is to me? In writing a prescription, legibility is of utmost importance. As mentioned earlier in this chapter, countless errors have been caused by poor handwriting that was incorrectly translated into the wrong prescription. Because these have been publicized, there has been an increased drive to have all prescriptions typed into the electronic record and transmitted to the pharmacist electronically in an effort to lessen errors. Given that the current system allows for handwritten prescriptions, the first rule is to practice legibility or to use a typed version. Furthermore, prescriptions should be written in indelible ink.

6. Have I done all I can to assure the patient will be compliant? Medication **adherence** can be improved by educating a patient about the following:

■ The name of the medication.
■ What the medication is used for.
■ When the medication should be taken and the expected duration of therapy.
■ Any special instructions on using the medication.
■ Some of the common adverse effects and how they can be handled.
■ Any interactions with other medications or OTC products.

Remember that the clinician's job as a patient educator is not done until the clinician has asked for feedback. Ask patients to repeat the preceding information to make sure that they understand what you have told them. Many patients know that the clinician is busy and will answer "yes" when asked if they understand, even though they really do not, so try to ask feedback questions in an open-ended way.

7. Have I considered what the medication will cost the patient? Even though many patients have prescription plans that assist them in the payment of hefty pharmacy bills, it is still a smart practice to first use older, less expensive medications when they are available and are considered to be reasonable approaches. In these circumstances, generic drugs will be much cheaper. Learn to prescribe generics when there are no clear indications not to do so, and prescribe them until they have failed to work. Some drug store chains now offer generic medications for a few dollars per month or for a 3-month supply.

It is appropriate to query patients about their ability to pay and to discuss the cost of medication with them before they leave your office. Many Web-based programs allow the conscientious clinician to learn the costs of the prescribed medication and to compare them with costs of similar agents. This guidance prevents sticker shock in the pharmacy and helps the patient respond regarding his or her ability to comply with treatment recommendations.

A word of caution about the use of samples: Many clinicians attempt to save the patient money by offering sample medications that have been donated by the pharmaceutical sales force. Most of these medications are under patent protection, so after samples are exhausted, the patient will pay a premium for the same product in the drug store. If the clinician intends to prescribe the medication long term or for a chronic illness, he or she should be aware of the costs of the medications dispensed as samples and understand the ability of the patient to purchase or procure the medication with insurance. A wonderful new medication that is unaffordable is a poor choice for the indigent or uninsured patient.

8. Have I considered the health literacy of my patient? Many clinicians assume their patient can read and write and is somewhat literate about their disease and thus don't ask questions to determine the patient's health literacy. The prevalence of illiteracy in medical settings is an issue and one that is important to uncover. This may be as simple as asking patients if they have difficulty reading or writing. Or, you may ask the patient to read the written or printed prescription back to you. Unfortunately, in a fast-paced ambulatory practice, this component of ensuring therapeutic understanding is often discounted and discarded; consequently, many patients will not adhere to the prescribed regimen of their clinician.

9. Have I involved my patient in a shared decision-making process? Sharing the decision-making process with the patient gains the patient's confidence in the treatment regimen and assures **compliance** to the regimen. There have been over 50 randomized clinical trials on the topic of shared decision-making showing that it offers significant benefits for the clinician, patient, and health system. Patients report less decisional conflict and better satisfaction with the health-care system when they are made to feel part of it (International Alliance of Patients' Organizations, 2005). Even more important, though, is that greater patient compliance with medication occurs, especially for chronic conditions (Campaign for Effective Patient Care, n.d.). Involving the patient begins with telling the patient what you think is causing the problem, why you think that, and what you hope to do with treatment (or what you want to treat in order to avert a future problem). It is important to define what your patient already knows, where he or she gained the information, and what the patient's concerns might be about treatment. When further education is warranted, brochures may be helpful; in cases of illiteracy, clinicians can suggest audio or videotapes; occasionally, there are appropriate computer programs to effectively educate the patient. However, before providing DVDs, websites, or any educational material requiring technical means to view or use it, the prescriber should ask if the patient has the required equipment and skills.

There are also numerous nonprofit organizations that will assist with patient education, but the clinician should always offer the patient a chance to ask questions and listen to the concerns the patient may have about the medication being offered as therapy. There is a corollary here: Avoid reflexively prescribing to patients who self-diagnose and request a particular (advertised) medication. There is always a risk to any medication, which may not be realized by a patient who has learned of a medication through an advertisement or from another patient. Each patient has factors that make him or her unique, factors that the conscientious clinician needs to learn before succumbing to the demands of a (partially) educated patient. The discussion about risks and benefits, side effects, and cost will often lead to nonpharmacological alternatives for problems identified by consumers of health care. A conscientious clinician should be confident enough to refuse a treatment that is unnecessary.

10. Have I done all I can to minimize errors and increase patient safety? As discussed throughout this chapter, a number of pitfalls can occur when a prescription is written, received, translated in a pharmacy, labeled, dispensed, and then used by the patient receiving it. Some of the errors previously discussed have to do with prescribing the wrong medication after incomplete evaluation of the patient, performing inadequate patient education, writing illegibly, using inappropriate abbreviations, and failing to share the decision of how to treat an identified problem. There are many errors every year that lead to serious injury, hospitalization, and some deaths. Much effort is now taken to reduce errors in medical therapeutics, inside and outside of hospitals.

The use of an electronic medical record (EMR) designed to allow the clinician to write electronic prescriptions from a computer can eliminate illegible handwriting; avoid transcription errors; improve response time, accuracy, and completeness; and improve coordination and continuity of care. With decision support systems in place, software can alert a clinician to improper doses or schedules, allergies, drug duplications, interactions, and other contraindications. However, empirical evidence about the potential of computerized systems to reduce medication errors has been limited, despite implied benefits. Two studies found that although computer prescription order entry may prevent errors from reaching and harming patients, there is no evidence that facilities with computer prescription order entry have fewer medication errors than those without it (Devine, Wilson, Lawless, et al., 2010; Ford, McAlearney, Phillips, et al. 2008).

There are, however, national imperatives to mandate prescribing electronically and to implement electronic medical records so that these techniques will improve communication across the health-care team and limit outpatient prescription forgery.

Short of the EMR, which has an imbedded program for writing and sending e-prescriptions, many clinicians use handheld computers or personal digital assistants (PDAs) to navigate the voluminous formularies they are confronted with in the course of their practices. Much of the software is free, readily downloaded from an Internet connection, and often are available for use with a handheld device. For example, applications such as Epocrates assist the clinician with doses, schedules, adverse effects, contraindications, costs, and pill color and shape. These devices have largely replaced textbooks in the rapid office practice, though they lack the depth of the textbooks described previously.

Lastly, there is no substitute for the pharmacy consultant. Most hospitals and many retail pharmacies have a consulting pharmacist available 24 hours a day, and it is prudent for a conscientious clinician to consider a pharmacist as a resource. Often, the time spent in conversation with a resourceful pharmacist will prevent an error in prescribing and save the clinician embarrassment and liability. Pharmacists are trained today to be more than excellent dispensers; they are well equipped to help with medication therapy management, and some insurance companies and even Medicare are paying for their interventions. It behooves clinicians to form a collegial relationship with a pharmacist.

It is important to develop a routine to remain current and vigilant over shifting and evolving drug therapy as well as the many clinical guidelines put forth by learned societies and organizations. Most clinicians are voracious readers, especially on the subjects of new techniques, updates, therapies, and protocols. The pharmacology learned today will be out of date fairly soon if the FDA continues its approval of 20 to 30 new drugs per year. Quality clinicians engage in self-learning and continuing professional/medical education (CPE/CME) as a well-disciplined activity. Clinical guidelines are offered by many societies and often appear as algorithms to guide the clinician in drug selection. However, they are just that—guidelines—and are not absolutes. They may point to appropriate drugs, but they do not select the dose and duration, leaving that to the judgment of the clinician. Five sources of clinical guidelines that clinicians often find helpful are shown in Box 1-4.

BOX 1-4 Examples of Clinical Guideline Resources Available for Clinicians

- **National Guideline Clearinghouse.** The federal government has listed guidelines for the treatment of obesity, asthma, cholesterol, and hypertension. They are part of an activity called the National Guideline Clearinghouse (NGC), a public resource for evidence-based clinical practice guidelines useful in health-care decision-making. www.guideline.gov
- **The American College of Clinical Endocrinologists.** This organization publishes guidelines on treatment of menopause, osteoporosis, hyperthyroidism, diabetes, male sexual dysfunction, and other health issues. www.acce.com/clin/guidelines
- **The Agency for Health Care Research and Quality.** A series of 19 clinical practice guidelines are available from this agency. Each guideline is electronically retrievable and in sections. www.ahcrq.gov/clinic

Continued

BOX 1-4 Examples of Clinical Guideline Resources Available for Clinicians—cont'd

■ **The National Library of Medicine.** The National Library of Medicine has a free searchable collection of large, full-text clinical practice guidelines. Its guidelines come from a number of credible government and private sector providers, and because its access is free and open, it is a public site. http://hstat.nlm.nih.gov

■ **The American College of Cardiology.** Evidence-based clinical statements and guidelines developed by leaders in cardiovascular medicine are available. Access to and downloads of clinical documents are free, but reprints are $10.00 each. www.acc.org

■ **The National Heart, Lung, and Blood Institute (NHLBI).** The NHLBI has published clinical guidelines for asthma, cholesterol and cholesterol screening, hypertension, and obesity. www.nhlbi.nih.gov/guidelines/index.htm

---

LEARNING EXERCISES

1. Mrs. Jones asks you if the ibuprofen in her prescription arthritis medication is the same as the ibuprofen sold over-the-counter in a pharmacy, and if so, why can't she just buy the ibuprofen without a prescription? How do you answer her?

2. A patient says, "I just overheard two nurses saying that there is a new legend drug on the market." What exactly is a legend drug?

References

Aitken, M., Berndt, E., & Cutler, D. M. (2009). Prescription drug spending trends in the United States: Looking beyond the turning point. *Health Affairs, 28*(1), w151-w160.

Campaign for Effective Patient Care. (n.d.). *Shared decision making FAQs.* Retrieved January 31, 2011, from www.safecarecampaign. org/For-Patients.html, info can be found at www.patients-association.com/Default.aspx?tabid=237

Centers for Disease Control and Prevention and National Birth Defects Prevention Network (CDC-NBDPN). (2008). *Preventing birth defects.* Retrieved January 30, 2012, from www.nbdpn.org/current/2008pdf/PrevBDBroch.pdf

Devine, E. B., Wilson, J. L., Lawless, N. M., Hollingsworth, W., Hansen, R. N., Fisk, A. W., Sullivan, S. D. The Impact of Computerized Provider Order Entry on Medication Errors in a Multispecialty Group Practice, J.Am.Inform.Assoc (January 2010) 17(1) 78-84.

European Association for Clinical Pharmacology and Therapeutics. (1993). Aims of European Association for Clinical Pharmacology and Therapeutics [Electronic version]. *British Journal of Clinical Pharmacology, 36*, 183-184. Retrieved January 31, 2011, from http://eacpt.org/?q=node/2

Ford, E. W., McAleearney, A. S., Phillips, M. T., Menachemi, N., Rudolph, B. Predicting Computerized Physician Order Entry System Adoption in US Hospitals: can the federal mandate be met. Int.J.Med Info. (August 2008). 77(8) 539-45.

Institute for Safe Medication Practices (ISMP). (2012). *Root-cause analysis of medication-related sentinel events.* Retrieved January 30, 2012, from www.ismp.org/Consult/rootcause.asp

Institute of Medicine. (1999). *To err is human: Building a safer health system.* Washington, DC: The National Academies Press.

Institute of Medicine. (2007). *Preventing medication errors: Quality chasm series.* Washington, DC: The National Academies Press.

International Alliance of Patients' Organizations (IAPO). (2005). *What is patient-centred healthcare?: A review of definitions and principles.* Retrieved January 30, 2012, from www.patientsorganizations.org/pchreview

National Coordinating Council for Medication Error Reporting and Prevention (NCC MERP). (2005). *Recommendations to enhance accuracy of prescription writing.* Retrieved January 30, 2012, from www.nccmerp.org/council/council1996-09-04.html

Schiff, G. D., & Galanter, W. L. (2009). Promoting more conservative prescribing, *Journal of the American Medical Association, 301*(8), 865-867.

Silva, S. (n.d.). *How to avoid medication side effects.* Retrieved January 31, 2011, from www.wellsphere.com/mental-health-article/how-to-avoid-medication-side-effects-start-low-go-slow/782450

U. S. Food and Drug Administration (FDA). (2010). *FDA approves name change for heartburn drug Kapidex* [Press release]. Retrieved January 30, 2011, from www.fda.gov/NewsEvents/Newsroom/PressAnnouncements/2010/ucm203096.htm

White, C. (2007). Health care spending growth: How different is the United States from the rest of the OECD? *Health Affairs, 26*(1), 154-161.

Resources

The High-Alert Medication List. Published by the Institute for Safe Medication Practices (ISMP), this is a list of drugs likely to cause harm if used in error. Available at www.ismp.org/Tools/highalertmedications.pdf

At one time The Joint Commission (TJC) published a list of drugs with look-alike or sound-alike names, along with specific safety strategies to avoid the confusion that may result from these similarities in names. In 2012 they no longer maintain that list and they now direct people to the Institute for Safe Medication Practices (ISMP) website for its List of Confused Drug Names, at www.ismp.org/Tools/confuseddrugnames.pdf

The National Coordinating Council for Medication Error and Reporting has published a list of confusing drug name sets available from the USP by contacting USP's Practitioner and Product Experience department at (800) 487-7776.

The Institute for Safe Medication Practices, USP, and the FDA collect and track medication errors and make information available to clinicians and the public at www.ismp.org, www.usp.org, and www.fda.gov

An Introduction to Pharmacodynamics and Pharmacokinetics

chapter 2

William N. Tindall, John M. Boltri, Mona M. Sedrak

CHAPTER FOCUS

Every successful prescriber requires a working knowledge of pharmacodynamics and pharmacokinetics as well as an understanding of how genetics, age, risk factors, and diseases affect drug activity. All of this information and knowledge enhances the rational decision-making that maximizes benefits and minimizes risks associated with selecting a medication on behalf of a particular patient. This chapter reviews the general properties of drug action (pharmacodynamics) and how a body treats the presence of a drug (pharmacokinetics) to help the learning clinician think more critically when it comes to drug selection, prescribing, and administration.

OBJECTIVES

After reading and studying this chapter, the student should be able to:

1. Describe how drug receptors work and explain their roles.
2. Differentiate between an agonist and an antagonist.
3. Differentiate between a drug's efficacy, affinity, and potency.
4. Differentiate between a receptor-mediated drug activity and a second-messenger drug activity.
5. Explain how ion channels, enzymes, and transporter systems behave as sites of drug activity.
6. Define what is meant by a drug's median effective dose (ED50), median lethal dose (LD50), median toxic dose (TD50), and its therapeutic index (TI).
7. Describe how the body absorbs, distributes, metabolizes, and eliminates drugs.
8. Describe the blood-brain barrier and explain its significance in drug action.
9. Explain why a drug's potency is a factor in its dosing.
10. Describe how drug clearance, volume of distribution, and half-life can be used to monitor patient therapy.

Key Terms

Absorption
Adrenergic
Adverse effects
Affinity
Agonist
Antagonist
Blood-brain barrier
Brand name
Chemical name
Competitive antagonist
Cytochrome P450 system
Dose response curve
Distribution
Drug
Drug receptors
Effective dose (ED50)
Efficacy
Excretion
False substrate
Generic name
Half-life (t$_{1/2}$)
Lethal dose 50 (LD50)
Metabolism
Meta-analysis
Noncompetitive antagonist
Pharmacodynamics
Pharmacokinetics
Potency
Sympathomimetic
Therapeutic index
Toxic dose 50 (TD50)
Trade name
Volume of distribution

19

For centuries, people learned what drugs did to the body by direct observation—that is, by administering a substance, usually a plant or chemical, and making observations of what they perceived that plant or chemical was doing to the body as they attempted to treat or cure diseases (or, in some cases, to poison their enemies!). Hippocrates, who lived five centuries before Christ, stated, "Diseases result from natural causes and can best be understood by observing natural laws." For centuries afterward, medicines were often described in observational terms such as, in 1902 when "Opium, when given as two teaspoons of tincture, will dull the pain of a broken leg," (Potter, 1902) or as William Withering, a physician, pharmacologist, and botanist wrote in 1775, "When given as four ounces of tea made from ground digitalis sativa leaves, we notice a strengthening of heart beat." (Withering, 1775)

This method sufficed when students had only the therapeutic benefits of a medicinal derived from plant, animal, or mineral resources to study. Clinicians today, however, have access to manufactured drugs and are aware of the physiological effects of a drug on the body, including side effects, drug interactions, and other adverse events. They are better equipped to do the following:

■ Compare one drug with another as a means of making drug choices, based on a clear knowledge of the risks and benefits, indications, and contraindications.

■ Predict potential problems with the use of a particular drug based on a patient's age, sex, current or new disease states, other comorbidities, drug interactions, concurrent use of other medications, and risk factors.

■ Develop a uniform means of communicating with other clinicians involved in the care of the patient using a commonly accepted nomenclature in pharmacology. For example, because there is a widely accepted agreement regarding the definition of terms such as *agonist*, clinicians are better able to talk with each other about classes of drugs that *are* agonists. Likewise, how a drug is named often tells us a great deal about its characteristics and in turn helps us to compare and contrast it with other pharmacological agents with similar properties. For example, drugs that are in the class of drugs known as penicillins primarily have names that end with "cillin," and drugs that are angiotensin-converting enzyme (ACE) inhibitors have names that end in "pril," such as "lisinopril." Clinicians who recognize and understand this consistent nomenclature are able to talk with other clinicians about the dozens of drugs in these drug classes.

■ Rationally select a drug and its appropriate dose and dosing interval. Clinicians understand that there is a time period between when target sites are affected (e.g., by a few molecules of the drug) and the body's ability to distribute, circulate, metabolize, and eliminate remaining drug molecules.

Drug Nomenclature

For the purposes of this textbook, a **drug** is any substance that is used for the diagnosis, cure, treatment, or prevention of a disease or condition. Whether it is prescribed or not, before it is approved by a governmental agency for sale in the marketplace it acquires three names: its chemical name, its generic name, and its trade, or brand, name. The **chemical name** is, as implied, the precise description of a drug's chemical structure. It is a name that is meaningful for a research chemist but has little meaning for a clinician, patient, or pharmacist. Two examples of chemical names are *N*-4 hydroxyphenol acetamide and *N*-methyl-3-phenyl-3-[4-(trifluoromethyl) phenoxyl] propan-1-amine. Imagine trying to remember these names and writing them on a prescription. Thus, a shorter name, the **generic name**, derived from the chemical name, is commonly used. The generic names for the two examples given previously are *acetaminophen* and *fluoxetine*.

To bring a drug into the market in the United States, the manufacturer must apply to a quasi-government agency called the United States Adopted Name Council (USAN) and register the generic name. By convention, manufacturers typically choose a name that is easy for people to remember or that makes it easy to remember which class of medication the drug fits into. Because the USAN name is considered an official name, it is the one used in official references such as in the United States Pharmacopeia (USP). The USP is the accepted reference or compendium for all drugs marketed in the United States. However, because even a generic name is often hard to use, manufacturers use names that will make the product they are marketing stand out in a crowd of similar products. Thus, they will register with the U.S. Trademark office a **brand**, or **trade, name** to go along with the generic name and have it protected for advertising purposes.

In the two previous examples, the drugs acetaminophen and fluoxetine were given the brand names of Tylenol and Prozac (Table 2-1). After heavy marketing, the brand names are the names usually used by clinicians to write a prescription because these names have been heavily promoted and popularized. However, so many brand names have look-alike and sound-alike names that prescription errors have occurred when one brand name is mistaken for that of another drug. Also, numerous brand names exist for the same generic product, adding more confusion.

In this textbook, both generic and trade names are listed for all drugs. The generic name is listed first in lower case followed by the brand name or trade name in parentheses, for example, fluoxetine (Prozac).

TABLE 2-1 Chemical, Generic, and Trade Names for Two Drugs		
CHEMICAL NAME	GENERIC NAME	TRADE NAME
N-4 hydroxyphenol acetamide	acetaminophen	Tylenol
N-methyl-3-phenyl-3-[4-(trifluoromethyl) phenoxy]propan-1-amine	fluoxetine	Prozac

Introduction to Basic Pharmacology Principles

Pharmacology is a word derived from two Greek words, *pharmakos*, meaning "medicine" or "drug," and *logos*, meaning "study." Pharmacology is a not an exact science; it is a constantly evolving body of knowledge involving much research to understand how medications work. Some of this work is quite accurate, but most is based on logic and theoretical underpinnings, some more so than others. The accuracy of some pharmacological information is somewhat tenuous. This is why current standards of practice and published literature are often at variance and why a learning resource of this nature *cannot* be a definitive reference book. It is the responsibility of every clinician to evaluate the current scientific findings and theories behind a drug's action using the context of the clinical situation and tempering it with information from primary literature or meta-analysis of a large number of reputable studies. **Meta-analysis** is the mathematical combination of the results of several studies.

Understanding Pharmacodynamics

Pharmacodynamics is the study or science of the effects of medications on the human body, including the actions and effects of drugs in relation to their chemical structure. In other words, pharmacodynamics attempts to answer "What does a particular drug do to the body, biochemically and physiologically, and how does it do it?" Throughout this text you will see the phrase *mechanism of action (MOA)*, followed by an explanation of how a drug achieves its effect at the site of action. It is because of the drug's mechanism of action that a reaction occurs between a functionally important living system and a medicinal agent. For a response to occur, the receptor must recognize the drug, respond in an efficient manner, have enough receptors responding to make a difference, and have the drug be potent enough to make the response happen. By studying drug action at its biochemical and physiological levels, the clinician can better determine the magnitude of a drug's effect on the human body.

The Peculiar Nature of Drug Receptors

All bodily functions are mediated by control systems that involve a host of chemotransmitters, neurotransmitters, hormones, enzymes, receptors, and specialized molecules such as DNA. Medications alter the body's control systems by binding to a constituent of a cell or organ to alter its function and affect the physiological system to which it is attached. A **drug receptor** is any portion of a tissue or cell (i.e., a cell macromolecule) to which a drug can bind and initiate its macromolecular effect(s). It is important to remember that receptors can cause an effect when activated or blocked because, in essence, they are sensing elements that help to coordinate the functions of all the different cells in the body.

Drugs alter the body's control systems by the doing following:

- Attaching to a cell membrane and acting on a specific receptor.
- Interfering with ion passage through or across a membrane.
- Inhibiting a membrane-bound enzyme and ion pumps.
- Acting on metabolic processes within a cell, such as inhibiting carrier molecules (transport processes), incorporating into larger molecules, or altering metabolic processes.
- Acting outside the cell to change its environment.
- Acting inside a cell on cellular proteins or cellular constituents such as amino acids.

The exact nature of drug receptors remains unknown, but scientists know they exist and that drug receptors, once bound, show amazing selective or nonselective effects. When a drug is able to bind with a specific cell site, either on its cell membrane or within the cell, this is known as *specificity*. Some cell receptors are able to bind to more than one drug. Thus, the role of drug receptors is as follows:

- Set the quantitative relationship between the dose of a drug and its pharmacological effect.
- Mediate between blocking a drug's effect (**antagonist**) and stimulating a drug's effect (**agonist**).

Drug Receptor Responses: Affinity, Efficacy, Potency, Quantity

Four factors determine the way a receptor will respond to a drug: (1) the receptor's affinity for the drug, (2) the quantity of receptors available and the amount of the drug presented to the receptors, (3) the efficacy of the drug, and (4) the potency of the drug. **Affinity** refers to the strength of the binding between a drug and its receptor. Most drugs have high-affinity binding to receptors, which means the fit between the drug and binding site is so good that only low concentrations of the drug are needed to cause agonist or antagonist actions. The more receptors that are bound, the greater the effect of the drug. The amount of any drug bound to a receptor is determined by the quantity of receptor binding sites available, the receptor and tissue type, and the amount of drug available. For example, drugs that are highly lipophilic are highly bound to blood serum proteins. It is assumed that only a small fraction of the circulating drug (the "free drug concentration") is able to cross cell membranes, especially the blood brain barrier and endothelial cells of the heart, and find its way onto active receptor sites.

Efficacy refers to the ability of a drug to initiate a biological effect or stimulate its receptor in a way that produces a pharmacological response after it has bound itself to a receptor. Some drugs may have a high degree of affinity or selectivity to bind to a receptor, but once they are bound, they are not very efficient or efficacious in producing the desired response.

Potency is a measure of the ability of a set dose of an agonist or antagonist to produce its maximum pharmacological effect. For example, if drug A and drug B are both agonists, and drug A produces a maximum pharmacological response at half the dose of drug B, then drug A is deemed twice as potent as drug B.

Receptor Agonists and Antagonists

When drugs act on receptors, they do so as either agonist or antagonist endogenous mediators. Agonists have an affinity for activating cell receptors because they resemble a naturally occurring hormone, transmitter, or enzyme. They mimic or induce the same response produced by the endogenous substance. Agonists have value in clinical situations because they can resist degradation and act for longer periods of time than can the natural substances they are designed to mimic. Following are some examples of agonists:

- Albuterol acts as a bronchodilator having longer activity than naturally occurring epinephrine.
- Terbutaline (Brethine), salmeterol (Serevent), and albuterol (Proventil) are **sympathomimetic** drugs (drugs that are capable of stimulating the sympathomimetic nervous system to produce the same physiological effects as its natural stimulants such as epinephrine [adrenalin]). Drugs such as terbutaline, salmeterol, and albuterol are useful in the treatment of asthma and chronic obstructive pulmonary disease (COPD) because they act on specific beta-2 (pulmonary) **adrenergic** receptors to induce bronchodilation by blocking the effects of natural epinephrine.
- Norepinephrine stimulates beta-1 receptors on the SA node of the heart; it is used to increase heart rate just as naturally occurring adrenalin does.

Agonists possess both affinity for a particular receptor and efficacy, which is a measure of how efficient they are as agonists. There are two types of agonists:

- Full agonist: an agonist with maximal efficacy.
- Partial agonist: an agonist with less than maximum efficacy or one that shows a low degree of activation.

Antagonists are also called blockers because they are similar enough to the naturally occurring agonists to be recognized by the receptor and to occupy the receptor site, but they don't turn on the receptor's natural effect. These drugs can bind to the receptor in a relatively specific manner and with high affinity, but they do not activate the receptor because they lack some critical component in their molecular design. Simplistically, we would assume that antagonists produce no effect because they do not activate the receptor. However, antagonists do cause biological effects by blocking the normal stimulation of the receptor as would be seen by agonists. Thus, the antagonist produces an effect indirectly by blocking or nullifying endogenous agonist activation of the receptor.

Antagonists *do not* change the receptor; they only bind to it and block the action of an endogenous agonist. For example, a drug such as propranolol (Inderal) is a beta adrenoreceptor antagonist, or as it is most often called, a beta blocker. It blocks beta-1 receptors on the SA node, effectively decreasing heart rate and causing vasodilatation and subsequently lowering blood pressure. A second example would be diphenhydramine (Benadryl), which blocks histamine receptors on cells to block the release of histamine and thus prevent allergic reactions from occurring. A dramatic example of an antagonist is naloxone (Narcan), which blocks opiate receptors in the respiratory center and quickly reverses the respiratory depression caused by a drug abuser's overdose by narcotics.

Antagonists are further classified as being either being competitive or noncompetitive. A **competitive antagonist** (reversible antagonist) is a drug that competes with an agonist for binding to a receptor. The agonist response is abolished or diminished as long as the antagonist can successfully compete with the agonist for the receptor site. This competition can be overcome by flooding the receptor site with increasing concentrations of an agonist. A **noncompetitive antagonist** (irreversible antagonist) is a drug that binds to a receptor and stays bound; it cannot be displaced by increasing the concentration of agonists. Thus, the effect is irreversible because the drug does not let go of its receptor. This effect is similar to that of a competitive antagonist, but as more and more receptors are bound (and essentially destroyed), the agonist drug becomes incapable of eliciting its maximal effects.

What Determines the Ability of a Drug to Bind to a Receptor?

Drugs bind to a receptor, whether agonist or antagonist, much like a key fits a lock (see Fig. 2-1). This analogy has some merit because, as with a lock, many keys can enter the lock's keyhole, but only certain keys will actually unlock the device. Similarly, among those many keys (agonists and antagonists) that enter the lock, only agonists can activate/unlock the lock whereas many other keys will fit the lock but do nothing (antagonists). Whereas, the antagonist keys fit the lock but do not activate it, they block other keys from fitting in the lock because they are occupying the space another key could have used. Scientists worked hard to explain just how a drug "sticks" to its receptor. That answer is complex and involves more than just the right "key" to "open or fit" to a receptor site. In essence, however, drugs fit to their receptor sites by many different types of bonding, three of which are quite common: ionic bonding, van der Waals bonding, and hydrogen bonding.

IONIC BONDING Although not as powerful as the covalent bond, the ionic bond is reversible. The ionic bond is the attraction between two truly charged atoms—one positively charged and one negatively charged. In the case of drug-receptor interactions, the powerful ionic bonds are probably the causative agent of bringing the drug to the receptor and the initial "fitting" of the drug into the binding site of the receptor.

VAN DER WAALS BONDING These very weak, electrostatic bonds are also known as *forces*. These forces are formed by the partial charges of an atom's nucleus (weak positive charge) and its electron (weak negative charge) as the electron spirals around its nucleus. These van der Waals interactions tend to be quite common in drug-receptor interactions, and although very weak, they are theorized to be forces that precisely position a drug to its binding site on the receptor. To prove these forces are not just

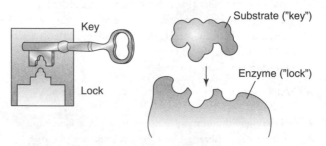

FIGURE 2-1 Drug binding to a receptor site.

theory, recently scientists were able to measure the adhesion forces between a calcium channel blocker drug and its receptor in living cells by using an atomic force microscope.

HYDROGEN BONDING A hydrogen bond is the attraction of a hydrogen atom with an electronegative atom like oxygen. Scientists speculate that what determines an agonist from antagonist is probably a combination of all three bonding systems. For example, an agonist has the necessary combination of ionic, hydrogen, and van der Waals bonds to fit into the receptor (key) and activate it (unlock it), and the antagonist has a different combination of bonds that allow it to fit into the receptor (key) but not to activate it (remains locked). Further evidence suggests that a drug's effect is reversible when the drug leaves the receptor because the receptor has changed while the drug is bound to it and it returns to how it was once the drug has left. Obviously the fact that a drug's effect is reversible is very important—especially to the patient.

Selectivity and Dosage

Two more principles of pharmacology are *selectivity* and *dosage*. Drug action can be either selective or nonselective. Selective drugs have a preference for acting at certain binding sites or receptors. Selectivity is highly desirable for any drug, because it usually means the drug is likely to have fewer side effects. For example, drugs such as beta-adrenergic receptor blockers, or beta blockers, affect only beta-adrenoreceptors. Nonselective drugs, on the other hand, affect all adrenoreceptors, regardless of whether they are alpha or beta receptors. Not surprisingly, receptors are divided again into subgroups, and their locations are being mapped as drug target sites. This allows more specific targeting for drug activity if, for example, a drug can be created that distinguishes between alpha-1, alpha-2, beta-1, beta-2, and beta-3 receptors. It also allows for the creation of drugs that have fewer adverse side effects.

The right dosage of a drug is just as important as a drug's mechanism of action, for as Paracelsus (1493–1541) said, "It is the dosage of a drug alone that determines if something is a poison." Receptor activation determines the nature of a drug's effect and the number of receptors activated determines the magnitude of that effect, whether good or bad. Thus, a drug that is highly selective for certain receptors is an easier drug to manage than one that is highly nonselective. For example, sildenafil (Viagra) is highly selective for only one of the 10 types of phosphodiesterase inhibitor sites in the body. Its side effects occur because it has some selectivity for other phosphodiesterase receptors. In practice, the clinician then wants to give a patient a drug that is highly selective, and at the right dose, so that any additional unwanted or **adverse effects** will be minimal.

General Rules of Drug Behavior

It is because of drug-receptor research that most of today's new drugs have been developed. This research has demonstrated some rules that define how drugs behave. For example, see the following:

- All of a given type of receptor is identical and equally accessible to drugs.
- Intensity of response is proportional to the number of receptors occupied.
- The amount of drug that combines with a receptor is negligible.
- A drug's intensity and duration of effect is *reversible* because the forces holding the drug to its receptor are weak.
- A drug can produce *numerous effects*, if more than one set of receptors will respond to it.
- Receptors may exist on a cell membrane or inside a cell on any of its structures. In many cases drug effects result from a combination of both extracellular and intracellular receptors being activated. For example, some drugs react with extracellular receptors because they cannot cross, or cross very slowly, into cell cytoplasm (lipid soluble). Reacting with cell surface receptors invokes a response that allows the drug to enter the cell where there may be numerous subtypes of receptors that, when activated, produce the desired or an undesired response (e.g., the opiates).

Other Methods of Drug Action

There are numerous types of receptors in the human body, and scientists engaged in molecular pharmacology have been investigating them to better understand how diseases occur and how medications can be used to reverse them. For example, some receptors are triggered by endogenous stimulants, and their effects can last milliseconds (synaptic transmissions) or hours or days (thyroid and steroid hormones). We know that catecholamines act in seconds and peptides take longer to exert their effects, thus scientists look for drugs that will either turn off or turn on a biological effect for more than a few milliseconds. Not all biological responses, however, result from a simple yet direct drug-receptor activity. Some other systems of drug action follow.

THE TRANSMEMBRANE G-PROTEIN COUPLED RECEPTOR These are the most common receptor types found in humans and include receptors for many hormones, acetylcholine, adrenoreceptors, and chemokines. Because they are so common, they are constantly being studied by scientists working to make clinically useful drugs. The G-protein receptor complex is external to a cell, and it has a protein crossing back and forth across the cell membrane. A G-protein complex consists of three subunits—an alpha and a tightly integrated beta and gamma subunit. The alpha subunit in the resting state is associated with quanosine (the G-protein). When a drug binds to the G-protein receptor on the extracellular side of the membrane, it alters the three-dimensional conformation of the receptor protein, which in turn produces an intracellular signal that alters the functioning of the cell. Scientists have identified several types of G-proteins; for example, G-stimulatory proteins activate calcium channels and adenylyl cyclase, and G-inhibitor proteins activate potassium channels and inhibit adenylyl cyclase.

G-O protein inhibits calcium channels, and G-Q activates phospholipase C. In essence, G-protein receptors are somewhat like second messenger stimulants and are responsible for how certain drugs, such as those associated with insulin, various cytokines, growth factors, and natriuretic factors, work.

SECOND MESSENGER SYSTEMS Some drugs pass all the way through a cell membrane where they are able to influence a physiological system inside the cell. They initiate what is referred to as a second messenger system by triggering a cascade of events, typically through protein systems inside a cell. For example, a number of drugs once inside a cell are able to produce either an increase in cyclic adenosine monophosphate (cAMP), change calcium concentrations, or affect phosphoinositide.

ION CHANNELS Scientists have discovered that when drugs act on ion channels, they do so as either as blockers or modulators of an ion channel. On a molecular level, they increase or decrease the opening of the ion channel to let ions pass in and out of the cell. One example of a drug that influences ion channels as its mechanism of action is the diuretic hydrochlorothiazide. This drug is a blocker of renal tubule sodium channels. A second example is aldosterone, which also is a modulator of renal tubule sodium channels.

Intracellular concentrations of the cations Na^+, K^+, Ca^{2+}, and Cl^- are controlled by *ion pumps* that move specific ions from one side of the cell membrane to the other and *ion channels* that allow selective transfer of ions down their concentration gradients. As they diffuse into a cell, they cause depolarization of excitable tissue. As Cl^- and K^+ diffuse out of a cell, depolarization is inhibited; this is an important factor for drugs such as digoxin, phenytoin, and omeprazole that move cations, especially potassium (K^+) in and out of cardiac cells. It is important for people who take drugs such as digitalis to replace potassium that is being lost; if it is not replaced, the person could suffer cardiac arrest when the cationic pump stops working.

Finally, there is a family of *nuclear receptors* that regulates genes. They are receptors for steroid hormones, thyroid hormones, and various substances such as retinoic acid and vitamin D.

ENZYMES Drugs may act on enzymes as inhibitors, suppressing the normal effect of the enzyme; false substrates, producing an abnormal metabolite; or prodrugs, resulting in the production of an active drug. Sarin, a nerve gas, and Malathion, an insecticide, are irreversible inhibitors of the enzyme acetylcholinesterase because they stop the regulatory/physiological responses of the nervous system. The cholesterol-lowering drugs 3-hydroxy-3-methylglutaryl-coenzyme A (HMG CoA) reductase inhibitors, which inhibit a key enzyme in the biosynthesis of cholesterol, and protease inhibitors, which prevent the maturation of the HIV virus, are examples of reversible inhibitors. Penicillin is another enzyme inhibitor; its bacteriocidal activity is due to inhibition of an enzyme necessary for bacterial cell wall synthesis.

The combination of carbidopa and levodopa used in Parkinson's disease (PD) inhibits the enzyme dopa decarboxylase and methyldopa by acting as a false substrate for dopa decarboxylase. A **false substrate** undergoes chemical transformation in the body to form an abnormal product that subverts the normal metabolic pathway being targeted.

A prodrug presents the clinician with a unique strategy, which is to administer a drug in an inactive, or a significantly less active, form. Once absorbed, the drug is transformed in vivo to its more active form (a process called biotransformation). Examples of prodrugs include valacyclovir, which is activated by an esterase enzyme to its active form acyclovir; heroin, which is deactivated by an esterase to the more potent morphine; prednisone, which is activated by a liver enzyme to its active form prednisolone; and enalapril, the ACE inhibitor (ACEI) that is biotransformed by an esterase to its active form enalaprilat.

ANTIMETABOLITES Many anticancer drugs are known as antimetabolites. They act by blocking the conversion of a metabolic pathway (purine, pyrimidine) or by preventing DNA from being synthesized and cell division from occurring. The popular drugs aspirin, ibuprofen, and others known as NSAIDs are other examples of drugs that are enzyme inhibitors because they inhibit two enzymes known as cyclooxygenase 1 (COX-1) and cyclooxygenase 2 (COX-2). In the 1990s, researchers discovered these two different COX enzymes. COX-1 is present in most tissues. It is present in the gastrointestinal tract where it maintains the normal lining of the stomach, and it also is involved in kidney and platelet function. COX-2 is primarily present at sites of inflammation. Both COX-1 and COX-2 convert arachidonic acid to prostaglandin. NSAIDs inhibit COX-2, which makes NSAIDs and aspirin desirable for the relief of pain and inflammation. However, the ability of NSAIDs to also inhibit COX-1 makes them have undesirable side effects (stomach and intestinal adverse effects) as well as raises the risk for problems with kidneys, heart, and blood vessels.

TRANSPORTERS These types of drugs have a mechanism of action that is either to aid normal transport or to block normal transport of ions and small organic molecules across a cell. Examples include digitalis (Digoxin), a cardiac glycoside that inhibits the Na^+/K^+ pump, or the diuretic furosemide (Lasix), which inhibits the transport of $Na^+/K^+/Cl^-$ in Henle's loop. The transport of ions and small organic molecules across a cell membrane generally requires a carrier protein because the permeating molecule is often too lipidic to penetrate the membrane on its own. These drugs are generally responsible for transport of glucose and amino acids into cells, the transport of ions into and out of the renal tubules, and the uptake of neurotransmitters, such as noradrenaline and serotonin.

It is through much effort and devotion to the science of molecular biology that the knowledge of specific sites of drug action has come such a long way over the past few decades. As knowledge of drug receptors grows, it has become well established that these cellular macromolecules may be either in or on the cell membrane to react with an extracellular agent, either as a stimulant (agonist) or as a depressant (antagonist). In addition, these receptors may trigger intracellular changes directly, by inhibiting an intracellular process; indirectly, by interacting with DNA to alter synthesis of cellular products such as proteins or DNA; or by changing a normal intracellular signaling agent (second messenger) that in turn controls another physiological process.

Quantifying the Relationship Between a Given Dose and Its Biological Response

The more receptors activated by a drug, the greater the response is to that drug, up to a point; drug receptors can become overstimulated or saturated. However, if drug receptor activation rises with the amount of drug given, then the relationship between the dose of a drug and its biological response should be easily quantified. If a drug's response can be quantified relative to the amount of drug given, then a graph, the **dose response curve,** can be drawn to illustrate it.

In practice, a dose response curve is drawn using a logarithmic drug dose scale on the x-axis. This log scale is used because any pharmacological responses mediated by receptors occur over a wide range of doses and also because any response to a drug increases with its dose. By using a log scale, the central portion of the dose response curve will appear as a straight line, making it easier to understand and to apply to clinical situations. Thus, the typical dose response curve illustrates how a drug response develops slowly, enters its linear phase over a wide range of dosages, and then plateaus at the highest dosages of the drug. The shape of this S-curve provides a fairly accurate illustration of how drugs and receptors respond to each other. For instance, the slow or delayed start represents the buildup to a threshold effect, and below that threshold there are drug-receptor reactions so low that they are rare, ineffective, or more likely, below the ability to be measured. As the dosage of a drug increases, more receptors become bound to the drug, and activation occurs as a measurable response. At some later point, all of the receptors are occupied or the response is maximal and the dose response curve plateaus. Note that the plateau may be related to either all the receptors being occupied or the effect being maximized or even lethal.

Figure 2-2 shows four dose response curves for agonists. The leftmost curve is considered to be representative of the most potent agonist as its effects occur with the lowest drug doses. The shorter third curve is still that of an agonist, but it is an agonist that does not produce as great an effect as do the other three. Compared to the other drugs in this illustration, this drug is not as effective in producing the response. It is important to remember that no matter how much of this drug is administered, the maximal effect will never exceed that shown on the curve. Thus the slopes of these curves are important because curves with similar slopes suggest that the drugs they represent work through similar mechanisms, and the height of the curves on a dose response graph tell us a lot about the drug efficacy. There are many types of dose response curves available; they vary *only* in the response.

It is important for any clinician to be able to read a dose response curve. Note in Figure 2-2 the point at which there is the maximal effect of the drug. This flattening of the curve reveals the magnitude of response that a particular drug is capable of producing. In many cases it is specific to the drug being tested, but when drugs within a class of drugs are being compared, it will reveal the maximal effect they produce. This is a measure of the effectiveness of one drug over another. In Figure 2-2 a dose of the example agonist at about 5 mg produces the same effects as a dose of 100 mg. Thus, clinicians would use the 5-mg dose and realize any larger dose is likely to produce untoward or unwanted side effects and very little, or no, beneficial effects compared with the lower dose.

Another important aspect revealed to a clinician by observing the dose response curves in Figure 2-2 is their midpoints. At these midpoints, they are not half the scale of the graph but rather half of the maximal response for the drug. Just as drugs will vary in maximal response produced, the 50% response point will vary accordingly. This point—or rather the dose that produces half the maximal response for that particular drug—is known as its **effective dose,** or ED50. The ED50 is specific for a drug; when it is used, it is important to compare it with similar drugs in its class as a comparative measure of its potency among similar drugs (see following section in this chapter on ED50).

A third characteristic of the dose response curve is the slope of the curve. Although the slope of a dose response curve of a single drug may be of interest, it is the comparison of the slopes of the curves of different drugs that is of interest to the clinician. Whereas dose response curves are used to illustrate the relationships between dosing and responses, their usefulness is to help define the terms that quantify a drug's action relative to that drug's potency, efficacy, and toxicity:

- Effective dose 50 (ED50).
- Lethal dose 50 (LD50).
- Toxic dose 50 (TD50).
- Therapeutic index (TI).

Effective Dose 50

ED50 refers to the median effective dose, or the dose at which 50% of the test subjects in a population or sample will respond with a predefined or expected effect. Put another way, ED50 is the dose that produces half of the maximal beneficial response for a given drug. ED50 is used clinically to set recommended doses because it is an indicator of a drug's potency when given to a diverse group of individuals.

In pharmacology, efficacy is far more important than potency. *Potency* deals with the size of the dose needed, whereas *efficacy* deals with the response possible from each specific agent. In clinical use the ED50 is the one parameter normally cited to characterize therapeutic effects, but even this is somewhat nebulous because therapeutic effects are brought about by a wide range of doses and what is effective in one patient may not be effective in another. This is evident when, for example, a clinician is dosing both a 100-lb, 90-year-old woman with very little body fat and a 400-lb obese individual with a significant

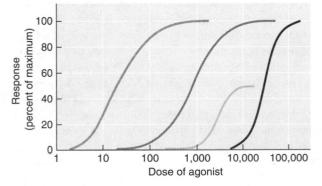

FIGURE 2-2 Typical dose response curve for an example agonist.

percentage of body fat in which to store a lipid-soluble drug. Clinicians think of ED50 as a recommended guideline, not an absolute policy.

Lethal Dose 50

Other measures of quantifying a drug's effect are the **lethal dose 50** (LD50) and the toxic dose 50 (TD50). These measurements are *estimates*, typically made using animal studies. Obviously, no one wants to (nor could) truly measure the dose at which 50% of a population of human test subjects would die from taking a drug or how long one should continue taking a drug in order to reach its toxic endpoint. The problem is not the endpoint per se, but rather defining the endpoint. As an example, consider the effects of tobacco smoking. Death from smoking can be the result of induced lung cancer, throat cancer, or other soft tissue cancer, but these occurrences each have other variables, such as risk factors and genetics, that can result in different likelihoods of cancer. It therefore becomes difficult to predict how much nicotine one would have to ingest to produce a measurable LD50. For this reason, some drugs have a different LD50 value, depending on the parameters being measured and the animals being tested, and in many cases they are best guesses using scientific models.

Toxic Dose 50

The designation **toxic dose 50 (TD50)** is used to indicate the dose (exposure) that will produce signs of toxicity in 50% of animals being tested, typically at least three species whose metabolism closely resembles humans. The larger the TD50, the more of the drug it takes to produce signs of toxicity (nausea, vomiting, diarrhea, skin rash). The toxicity of a drug is an inherent property of the drug itself, and each drug causes different toxic effects at different dosages. For this reason, when using the TD50 as a reference, clinicians must also know the precise definitions for the type of toxicity that was measured and the dose and route of administration that was used to determine it. For example, drugs given intravenously can be more toxic than those given orally (PO); thus, the TD50 is lower for IV drugs.

Therapeutic Index

With the therapeutic index (TI) of a drug—or as it is now more often called, its therapeutic window—data derived from dose response curves are used to put the LD50 and the ED50 into a more useful and meaningful perspective for the proper and safe prescribing and administration of a drug. The **therapeutic index** is a ratio of the LD50 to the ED50.

$$TI = LD50/ED50$$

By definition, if a drug has a very low value for its therapeutic index, it is said to have a *narrow therapeutic window* (Fig. 2-3). This means that there is a small difference between the dose of the drug that produces desired effects and the dose of the drug that produces toxic effects. It is usually better for everyone if a drug has a high therapeutic index or a *wide therapeutic window* because it means there is a high margin of safety between the dose needed to produce benefits and the dose that will produce harm (Fig. 2-4).

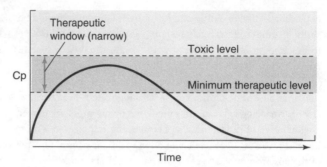

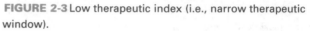

FIGURE 2-3 Low therapeutic index (i.e., narrow therapeutic window).

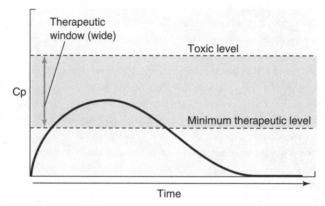

FIGURE 2-4 High therapeutic index (i.e., wide therapeutic window).

The dose response values of ED50, TD50, and LD50 are terms that require very careful exploration and thorough understanding so that they will have meaning and clinical applicability for a clinician. Additionally, the comparisons of a drug's potency should never be done without also including comparisons of its efficacy. Remember, there is the ongoing problem of determining lethality and toxicity. Also, keep in mind that for the TI, the larger the value, the safer a drug is considered to be. As a general rule, and for most drugs, the number 100 is considered the base value of a TI acceptable for clinically used drugs. However, for some drugs, using the therapeutic index as a measure for determining safety is ignored because of the risk involved. For example, some drugs that are used to treat cancers are very risky and the dosing of these drugs deals with a very fine line between the dose to harm and the dose to benefit. Both are quantifiably close, but because of the dangers and risks of cancers, these drugs are used with the hope that the cancer can be controlled or cured. In several cases of cancer-fighting drugs, their effective dose occurs at the same dose that toxicity occurs, necessitating special monitoring and administration. Another example in which applying the TI would be important is in the case of medications used to induce sleep: If a drug's lethal dose and its effective dose were very close, a person could wake up after the effect of the drug had started to wear off, still feel the need for sleep, and easily retake the tablets, thus harming himself or herself.

Some drugs have overlapping dose response curves, where the ED50 curve overlaps the LD50 curve. This overlap could be either large or small. For instance, it is possible that the dose of a certain drug at which half the people find the drug effective (ED50) is the same dose at which 15% find it to be lethal (LD50). This suggests that although the TI of a drug is commonly used, it may not always be a reliable descriptor of a drug's safety. Finally, an entire field of toxicology is devoted to expanding knowledge of dose response studies by using animals to accurately predict health risks associated with drug exposure in humans.

Understanding Pharmacokinetics

Pharmacodynamics is essentially the study of how drugs affect the body; **pharmacokinetics** is the study of how the body affects a drug over time. Pharmacokinetics describes the movement of a drug throughout the body and includes the process by which it enters the body (absorption), is distributed throughout the body, and is removed from the body. This knowledge helps clinicians decide on patient instructions for using a drug. For example, a drug with a long half-life of 12 hours should be dosed about twice a day if its pharmacokinetic characteristics have reduced the circulating active drug to 50% of its effective dose. By convention, clinicians, pharmacists, scientists, and the health community at large use a specific selection of terms when talking about the pharmacokinetic characteristics of a drug. These terms are: absorption, distribution, metabolism, excretion, (ADME) and half-life (Table 2-2).

It is important for clinicians to realize that pharmacodynamics and pharmacokinetics are intertwined and that drug molecules are coursing throughout the body in a constant stream of motion and activity (Fig. 2-5). For example, while a drug is being metabolized, it is also being eliminated—and at the same time it is trying to stick to its receptor sites. If it cannot stick to a re-

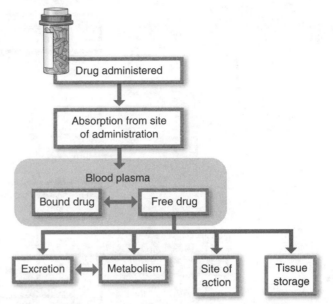

FIGURE 2-5 The relationship between drug administration, absorption, distribution, metabolism, and elimination.

ceptor site, it is either stored until a later time or it remains in the blood circulation until the receptor site becomes available. In many cases the drug has to compete with other drugs for the same site. Finally, it should be pretty obvious now that whatever drug receptors are involved following a drug's administration, very few of its molecules are actually attached to a receptor at any one time and that over time, because of pharmacokinetics (what the body does to the drug), very few drug molecules actually reach their intended receptor site (Fig. 2-6).

Factors Influencing Drug Absorption

Absorption is the process by which a drug moves from its site of administration, such as the muscle (given as an intramuscular drug), digestive tract (given as a swallowed pill), rectum (given as a suppository), lungs (as an inhaled aerosol), or skin (applied as an ointment), and into the circulatory system. How a drug is administered affects its absorption. For example, about 75% of any given oral drug is absorbed in 1 to 3 hours unless physiology or formulation factors alter this. Such factors include gastrointestinal (GI) motility, hepatic blood flow, drug particle size, and drug formulation (sustained release). A drug administered intravenously (IV) is ready to go to work immediately versus a drug given in tablet form, which requires time to disintegrate and for the active ingredient to be absorbed.

Since the IV route is best, why isn't it used more often? Eighty percent of all medications are taken orally (PO, or by mouth) because it is convenient and economical and because drugs remain stable in tablet forms over a long period of time. A drug can be given *sublingually* where it is dissolved under the tongue and absorbed through the mucous membranes and into bloodstream very quickly. An example of this is nitroglycerin tablets given when a person is experiencing angina.

TABLE 2-2	The Five Basic Parameters of Pharmacokinetics
TERM	DEFINITION
Absorption	The uptake of substances into or across tissues or the manner of how drugs enter the body
Distribution	The pattern by which drugs are distributed throughout various tissues after the drug has entered the circulatory system and is on its way to its site of action
Metabolism	The process by which the body breaks down (metabolizes) and converts (biotransformation) drugs into inactive substances
Excretion	The rate and method by which drugs or their metabolites are eliminated from the body
Half-life	The time it takes for the plasma concentration of a drug to reach half of its original concentration

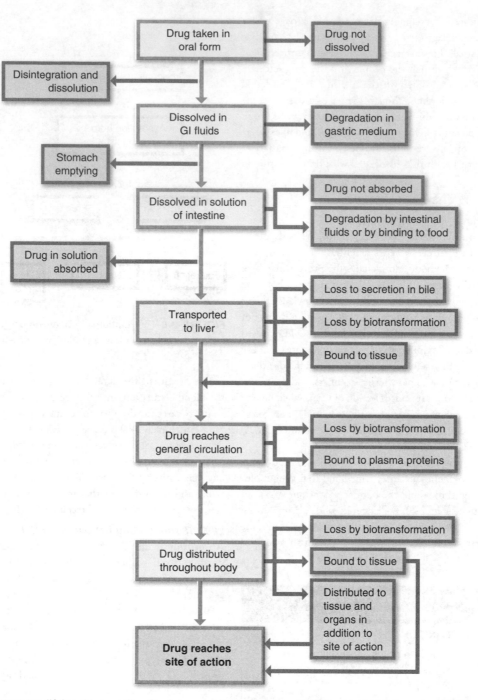

FIGURE 2-6 Factors modifying the quantity of a drug reaching a receptor site following a single oral tablet.

Drugs are also given using the *transdermal* route. A patch containing the drug is applied to the skin, which absorbs the drug. The transdermal route provides continuous, long-acting therapy, but some drugs can be expensive when supplied in patches, and the adhesive used to adhere the patch to the skin can cause local irritation.

Drugs are also administered in a suppository form via the rectal and vaginal route. They are absorbed efficiently through the mucous membrane of the rectum into a rich supply of blood vessels. This route is indicated for patients who are experiencing nausea and vomiting and cannot take medications by mouth.

Compazine, which is prescribed for nausea, is an example of a popular drug administered using the rectal route.

Inhalation is another means of drug administration. Today, inhaled drugs are administered as a gas or an aerosol and are an effective and popular route for drugs that act on lung tissue, such as bronchodilators and steroids. Although these drugs provide fast action, some, such as Primatene Mist (epinephrine for inhalation), can irritate lung tissue.

Intranasal administration means the drug is absorbed through the mucous membranes in the nasal passage and then into the bloodstream. Calcitonin-salmon (Miacalcin) and oxymetazoline (Afrin) are two examples of drugs administered intranasally. Some routes of administration combine topical as well as systemic effects. For example, inhalation of asthma drugs (topical) may be for targets on bronchial and airway sites, yet inhalation of anesthetics is done so they reach targets in the brain (systemic effect).

Parenteral administration includes intravenous, intramuscular, subcutaneous, and sometimes rectal administration. Parenteral administration routes provide more rapid responses than oral or rectal routes, and they are especially helpful ways to administer drugs to unconscious or uncooperative patients. However, giving drugs parenterally often causes pain at an injection site, and once a drug has been administered to a patient, the drug cannot be retrieved. Parenteral administration is not synonymous with intravenous administration. It can be intra-arterial (into an artery), intramuscular (into a muscle), intracerebral (into the brain), intracardiac (into the heart), intradermal (into the skin), intrathecal (into the spinal canal), intravesical (into the bladder), or intracavernosal (into the base of the penis). Rectal administration of drugs, by strict definition, is also considered parenteral because the effects are systemic. For example, antinauseant suppositories can be given to a person in a rectally administered form for their antiemetic effect, which happens systemically once it is absorbed from the rich blood supply of the anal region. This is also a common way to administer medications to an unconscious patient.

Factors other than the form of the drug and how it is administered affect drug absorption:

■ Blood flow. Highly vascularized organs such as small intestines have the greatest absorbing ability.
■ Surface area available. Absorption is directly proportional to surface area available.
■ Solubility of the drug. Ratio of hydrophilic-to-lipophilic properties determines the drug's ability to permeate cell membranes.
■ Drug drug interactions. Drugs can inhibit or enhance absorption of other drugs.
■ pH. A drug's acidity or alkalinity affects its charge, which affects absorption. Many drugs are either weak acids or have a weak base, which means the pH of the GI tract can affect absorption.

How Drugs Are Absorbed from the GI Tract and Into Cells

To be absorbed from inside the lipid membrane of the GI tract and into the bloodstream, a drug must be in a lipid-soluble state. Drugs exist in a lipid-soluble form or a non-lipid-soluble form, depending on their chemistry. Because the pH environment of the GI tract differs in the various areas of the GI tract, so does drug absorption as a drug is taken from a particular dissolved pill. Some pills are designed to dissolve in an acidic pH and some are designed to dissolve in more of a basic pH. Thus, some drugs absorb better from the stomach and some better from the intestine. If a drug is particularly susceptible to destruction by the acid environment of the stomach, it will typically be formulated to dissolve in the more basic pH of the intestine. Therefore, one would see a therapeutic effect at a later time than if the drug was absorbed from the stomach or lungs.

There are several means by which small molecules can cross through the lipid cell membranes. First, they can diffuse directly through the cell membrane itself. Second, they can diffuse through the aqueous pores formed by special proteins on a cell membrane that "open up" in the presence of a drug molecule. Thirdly, they can combine with a transmembrane carrier protein that binds to the drug molecule and transfers it on one side of the membrane, then releases it back to its active form once it has transferred to the other side of the membrane.

The stomach is highly acidic and favors absorption of weak acidic drugs. Aspirin is a weak acid and is converted to a non-charged molecule in the stomach. Thus, it can be absorbed through the lipid membrane of the stomach. The intestine is slightly alkaline and favors absorption of weak basic drugs. The intestine is a huge site of drug absorption due to its large surface area.

How Drugs Are Distributed Throughout the Body

Because of differences in pH, lipid content, cell membrane functions, and other individual tissue factors, most drugs are not distributed equally in all parts of the body. For example, the acidity of aspirin influences its distribution pattern so that it is different from that of an alkaline drug such as an amphetamine. Drugs transfer between regions of the body not only relative to characteristics of the drug itself, but also because of the nature of various tissues and blood flow. For instance, once absorbed, a drug may stay in the vascular system, or it may be distributed throughout all body water, or it may concentrate in a specific tissue. If the drug stays in the vascular system, it is likely a high-molecular-weight entity or it is being tightly bound to plasma protein. If the drug is distributed in body water, it is typically a low-molecular-weight substance, such as alcohol. Some drugs concentrate themselves in specific tissues. Two classic examples of this are the drugs tetracycline, which concentrates in bones and teeth, giving teeth a mottled appearance, and iodine, which concentrates in the thyroid gland. In addition, some drugs, such as fat-soluble vitamins, are highly lipid soluble and concentrate in fat tissues.

Once absorbed into the bloodstream, drugs will circulate in plasma and bind reversibly with plasma proteins (albumin, lipoproteins). This plasma protein-binding profile determines the extent of a drug's distribution throughout the body and also its elimination rate. Only unbound, or free, drugs may diffuse through capillary walls, produce a pharmacological affect, and be metabolized and excreted. Because only a free drug is capable of being excreted, some bound drugs disassociate from plasma proteins to reestablish the equilibrium between free and bound drugs. This circulating drug reservoir is what gives a drug its long duration of action. It is interesting to note that drugs that compete for the same plasma protein-binding sites may displace each other, causing drug-drug interactions (e.g., warfarin and aspirin).

The process by which a drug leaves the bloodstream and enters the interstitium of tissue cells is called *drug distribution*. The time that it takes for a drug to be distributed into all of the body tissues that it is physically able to is called the *distribution phase* and is typically quite rapid. The drug is said to distribute into an imaginary volume, called its *volume of distribution* (VD). The VD is based upon sampling and modeling a drug's concentration in standard reference fluids (serum or plasma) shortly after dosing on the assumption that a drug is uniformly distributed throughout the human body. However, nature does not always follow models and assumptions. For example, if a drug easily transfers into fat tissues, its plasma concentration after dosing will be quite low and its **volume of distribution** will appear quite high; in fact, it could be larger than the plasma volume in the human body. However, the term *volume of distribution* is useful for understanding just where a drug goes once it is ingested.

From a clinician's viewpoint, drug distribution depends on physical and chemical characteristics of the drug such as the following:

- Its ability to permeate capillaries.
- Its ability to bind to plasma proteins, such as albumin, which in turn determines the extent of drug distribution and its rate of elimination.
- Its fat-soluble or water-soluble characteristics: Small lipophilic molecules distribute to more sites than do large polar molecules. Only unbound, or free, drug may diffuse through capillary walls, produce a pharmacological effect, be metabolized, and be excreted.
- Drug dissolution: Inert ingredients and tablet formulations determine how rapidly and completely a tablet will dissolve and be ready to be absorbed in the GI tract.

Drug distribution also depends on the environment of the GI tract. Food, calcium, iron, and other elements can bind a drug and cause it to be excreted in feces. For instance, absence of too much hydrochloric acid in the stomach prevents dissolution of drugs having a basic pH.

Drug distribution is a complex process and the rate by which a drug is distributed is proportional to the drug's ability to pass through a membrane and the blood perfusion occurring at target tissues. It seems logical that because blood perfusion is the greatest in the brain, kidney, heart, and liver, these are tissues likely to be affected by many drugs.

In summary, when considering the extent to which drug distribution occurs, the most important factors are lipid solubility, the drug's pH-pK$_a$ or solubility ratio, its ability to bind to plasma protein, and its ability to undergo intracellular binding. Finally, it is part of nature's grand design to protect the human body by having a **blood-brain barrier**, a unique barrier that restricts transfer of lipid-soluble drugs into the brain, whereas elsewhere in the body capillary walls are easily permeated by lipid-soluble drugs.

Understanding the Blood-Brain Barrier

Some parts of the body do *not* follow the rules of other parts of the body. For example, drugs tend to be poor at penetrating into the central nervous system because they are actively pumped out, are highly charged molecules, or have a high molecular weight and cannot pass through lipid membranes. This is especially true for drugs entering the cerebral spinal fluid (CSF) and drugs that transfer across the placenta, or into breast milk, or into genital secretions. For example, some *lipophilic* drugs, such as morphine, can concentrate in breast milk because of its high fat content.

Drug penetration into the brain is another example of specialized drug penetration. The capillary endothelial cells in the brain have no pores to allow diffusion of drugs; consequently, the brain is inaccessible to many drugs, such as anticancer drugs and antibiotics such as aminoglycosides. In addition, there is glial connective tissue attached to the basement membrane of the capillary endothelial cells. Taken together, these structural modifications are called the blood-brain barrier. Thus ionized molecules cannot enter the brain, but nonionized molecules not bound to plasma proteins can enter the brain easily because they are lipid soluble. However, inflammation of the brain can disrupt the blood-brain barrier, allowing substances that are normally impervious to enter the brain. An example of this occurs when penicillin, if given intravenously, penetrates into the brain and is useful as an antibiotic to treat bacterial meningitis, which causes intense inflammation.

Drug Bioavailability

Bioavailability refers to the ability of a drug to reach the systemic circulation after an oral dosage. It is generally a good indication of the amount of medication that is absorbed into the bloodstream of the patient. Drugs having low oral bioavailability are either poorly absorbed in the GI tract, or they are partially metabolized by the liver.

Bioavailability values are typically used to determine drug dosages for adults, but they can be useful in estimating the likelihood that a fetus or breastfed infant may absorb enough of a drug taken by the mother to provide clinically significant plasma concentrations and to produce adverse consequences. For example, if a drug is destroyed in the GI tract, it is not usually available in a mother's breast milk. In addition, if a drug is substantially metabolized in the liver on its first pass through it, this will diminish the likelihood of the drug passing on to harm an infant or fetus.

Since bioavailability is an expression of how much drug reaches the circulation after administration, it makes sense that a drug administered by injection is 100% bioavailable. The same drug given by oral tablets may only be 10% bioavailable because much of it is destroyed by stomach acid; thus a clinician is required to prescribe higher maintenance doses of the oral drug to maintain the drug's bioavailability to the systemic circulation.

Drug Metabolism

The primary sites for drug metabolism are the liver and enterohepatic recirculation, the kidney, and biliary excretion. The liver and its enterohepatic recirculation is the route that detoxifies and eliminates most substances from the body. Enzymes in the liver, especially the cytochrome P450 set of enzymes, are responsible for biochemically changing drugs and other foreign substances. Most enzymes detoxify the foreign agent or produce substances that can be active. These end products of metabolism are then bound to other substances for excretion through the lungs or bodily fluids such as saliva, sweat, breast milk, and urine, or through reabsorption by the intestine to be acted on again.

Metabolism of drugs is primarily through one or more biochemical modifications, using specialized enzyme systems, resulting in a more lipophilic compound better able to be a more readily excreted polar product. It stands to reason then that the rate with which this happens determines the duration and intensity of a drug's activity, especially if the drug is converted to an active compound and subject to hepatic recirculation.

A person's genetics is responsible for the type, potency, and quantity of enzymes in the liver and which enzymes are used to metabolize many drugs. The group of liver enzymes responsible for most oxidative reactions of drugs is called the **cytochrome P450 (CYP450) system**. In essence, this superfamily of proteins contains a heme factor and uses a number of small or large molecules as substrates in causing enzymatic reactions. They appear in all tissues of the body, but most are membrane-associated proteins appearing in mitochondria or endoplasmic reticulum of cells. Humans have 57 genes and more than 59 pseudogenes divided among 18 families of CYP450 genes and 43 subfamilies. For humans, CYP450 enzymes play important roles in hormone synthesis and breakdown (CYP21A2), synthesis of cholesterol (CYP51A1), and vitamin D synthesis (CYP24A1). One or more of these isomers will metabolize a specific medication or many medications.

About 75% are metabolized by one of six common CYP450 isomers even though there are 11,000 or more of them that are known to exist in all forms of life. In humans, for example, the CYP2D6 isomer, a subset of CYP450 enzymes, is responsible for the metabolism of tricyclic antidepressants and other common drugs such as metoprolol (Lopressor), verapamil (Calan), and codeine. The CYP450 subset CYP1A2 is responsible for metabolizing substances such as caffeine and SSRIs such as venlafaxine (Effexor). CYP2C9 metabolizes ibuprofen (Motrin). Probably the most common CYP450 substrate involved in drug interactions is the substrate CYP3A4, which metabolizes about 36% of all drugs placed into the human body. CYP3A4 can either deactivate a drug or enhance its excretion. It is found primarily in the liver, but it is also found in the intestine where it can activate a prodrug and assist in its absorption (e.g., terfenadine). Interestingly, a neonate does not express CYP3A4 and does not have it in abundance until after 1 year of life, making the administration of drugs to these special patients a job for the well informed and skilled. Classes of drugs that are affected by the CYP3A4 enzymatic system include most chemotherapeutic agents, SSRIs, antipsychotics, opiates, statins, macrolides, antifungals, and anticonvulsants.

Some people are poor metabolizers of certain drugs, meaning they lack a gene to produce the CYP450 enzyme or they produce a poor-quality enzyme. Similarly, some people are extensive metabolizers and are able to metabolize a drug normally. Fortunately, poor metabolizers are a distinct minority among the world's population, and the only common factor among these poor metabolizers is their genetic makeup relative to race.

For example, knowledge of these metabolic differences has become quite common and recently the FDA (2010) has required the maker of clopidogrel (Plavix) to issue a warning on its label that patients who are poor metabolizers of clopidogrel do not efficiently convert it to its active form and thus may not receive its benefits. In addition, the FDA points out that tests are available to determine whether or not an individual's CYP2C19 isomers enzyme (the enzyme that converts clopidogrel [Plavix] to its active form) is working or not.

These enzymes lower the concentration of a drug circulating in the bloodstream by two effects: the first pass effect and induction/inhibition of drug metabolism. *First pass effect* occurs when drugs enter the bloodstream from the GI tract, then enter the liver via the hepatic portal vein before entering the general circulation. The first pass effect allows the liver to metabolize the drugs into less active or inactive metabolites/drugs before they are distributed throughout the body (e.g., heroin, which is potent, is converted to morphine, which is less potent).

Another way enzymes lower the concentration of a drug is through induction or inhibition. Enzymes in the liver that metabolize drugs may be induced or inhibited by the presence of other drugs, leading to drug-drug interactions. Whether or not an enzyme is induced (stimulated by the presence of a drug molecule) or inhibited (by the presence of another drug molecule) is not only important for explaining drug interactions, but it also explains why some drugs with a narrow therapeutic window produce side effects with small increases or decreases in circulating drug amounts. For example, a drug molecule may inhibit the work of a CYP450 enzyme by being competitive, noncompetitive, uncompetitive, or partially competitive. Thus, its half-life, elimination, and metabolism can be affected. However, in the presence of two or more drugs acting on the same enzyme substrate, serum levels can be increased to the point of adverse effects or toxicity. The classic example is the anti-epilepsy drug phenytoin (Hydantoin) because it inhibits the work of four of the CYP450 isomers (CYP1A2, CYP2C9, CYP2C19, and CYP3A4). Patients who take this drug chronically to ward off seizures may find themselves in trouble if they take medications such as amiodarone (Cordarone) because the blood plasma concentration of amiodarone will be decreased as a result of an enzyme induction reaction.

Knowing which cytochrome P450 enzyme is responsible for metabolizing a drug is useful when predicting or understanding how drug interactions occur. For example, if a person is taking a drug such as Quinidine, which is a potent inhibitor of the isoenzyme CYP2D6, then is started on a tricyclic antidepressant, that person will be unable to metabolize the tricyclic drug, and toxic amounts could, and likely will, build up as both drugs compete for metabolism by the same enzyme. Such potential interactions are not confined only to the concurrent use of other drugs. For example, because nicotine stimulates the production of CYP3A4 isoenzyme, a smoker who takes a drug such as verapamil (Calan), which is an inhibitor of CYP3A4, will experience a drug interaction. In fact, verapamil has been found to have drug interactions with about 490 drugs. Nicotine also induces (inhibits) CYP1A2 enzymes. This is problematic in an asthmatic patient who needs the same enzymes to metabolize theophylline. Patients who smoke have decreased serum levels of theophylline and have poorly controlled asthma.

Drug interactions can also result from CYP450 substrates acting on the protein that carries a drug into the liver. For example, the major protein in the body that helps transport drugs across cell membranes is P-glycoprotein (P-gp). P-gp is found in many organs, including the GI tract, liver, brain, gonads, and kidney. It is responsible for the transport of hydrophobic substances into the GI tract, out of the brain, into urine, into bile, out of the gonads, and out of other organs. Thus, P-gp plays a large role in the distribution, as well as elimination, of drugs. It is also implicated as the causative agent in the multidrug resistance seen with anticancer drugs. It is well-known that prescription drugs, over-the-counter (OTC) drugs, and food may inhibit or affect these protein transporters. Researchers in Canada found that P-gp proteins played a significant role in making a blood pressure drug almost toxic when taken with a glass of grapefruit juice because bioactive compounds in the grapefruit juice interact with the P-gp to either increase or decrease the bioavailability of numerous drugs (Romiti, Tramonti, Donati, & Chieli, 2004). Although the interaction of grapefruit juice and many drugs lasts up to 24 hours, it is greatest when given 4 hours before taking a medication. The bottom line is that if a patient is given two different drugs that rely on P-gp transport to enter the liver, GI tract, or kidney, or to exit the brain, they will compete for transport and result in decreased absorption of the drug, decreased biliary secretion of the drug, or decreased renal elimination of the drug.

Finally, because certain medications and foods, such as grapefruit juice, can inactivate or lessen the metabolic activity of CYP450 isoenzymes, the clinician must change the dosage of these drugs to compensate for their higher levels in the circulation. The rate that people metabolize a drug can, and will, vary significantly. Factors such as genetics, body weight, environment, nutrition, and age also influence drug metabolism. For example, infants and the elderly often display a reduced capacity to metabolize certain drugs and because of this may require lower dosages.

How Drugs Are Eliminated and Excreted

Excretion is the removal of waste substances from body fluids. Removal predominantly occurs by way of urine formed in the kidneys. Other routes of excretion to eliminate drugs from the body can include using bile, saliva, sweat, tears, feces, breast milk, and exhaled air. Most drugs are first metabolized prior to being excreted, yet some drugs (aminoglycoside antibiotics, for example) are polar compounds and thus can be excreted by the kidneys without first being metabolized. When drugs are excreted by the kidney, they are done so by one of three processes: glomerular filtration, tubular secretion, and tubular reabsorption. Unfortunately, high-molecular-weight drugs, such as heparin, or drugs that are tightly bound to plasma protein are poor candidates for excretion by glomerular filtration. Most drugs are filtered out through the kidney by tubular secretion. In tubular secretion two carrier systems come into play, one for carrying drugs with a base pH, such as amiloride HCL (Midamor), and one for carrying drugs with an acidic pH, such as propranolol HCL (Inderal).

Not all drugs and their metabolites are eliminated from the body; some are reabsorbed back into the bloodstream via tubular reabsorption. It is part of the normal physiological process (stasis) that most water that enters the kidney is reabsorbed back into the bloodstream as a means of conserving body fluids and ions. In so doing some drugs are carried back into the bloodstream attached to a molecule of water. *Clearance* is the rate of elimination of substances from the blood, whereas renal clearance (Cl_r) is the total amount of drug excreted over a specific time. Renal clearance depends on how well glomerular filtration, tubular secretion, and tubular reabsorption are working. All drugs have published renal clearance rates, and this is an important factor in determining drug dosage. For example, if a drug has a high clearance rate, meaning that it is eliminated from the blood rapidly by the kidneys, higher doses are needed to keep the active compounds working. Other drugs have a low clearance rate, possibly due to inefficient excretion rates, and lower dosage levels can be used to maintain therapeutic levels in the blood.

Finally, the pH of urine has a great influence on whether a drug is excreted quickly or slowly. In some clinical situations, urinary pH is adjusted to control the excretion of certain drugs from the body. Urinary pH is important because most drugs are either weak acids or weak bases. In alkaline urine, acidic drugs are more readily ionized. In acidic urine, alkaline drugs are more readily ionized. Because ionized substances are more soluble in water, they readily dissolve in body fluids, thus they are easily excreted into the urine. One practical example of this is the use of cranberry juice to shift the pH of a women's urine so that the sulfa drug she is taking to treat a urinary tract infection becomes more concentrated in urine where it can do the most good.

The lipophilic properties that allow drugs to pass through the cell membranes of the GI tract will hinder elimination of a drug if it is not "modified" to pass through the lipophilic membranes of the kidney into water-soluble urine or into bile where it can mix with feces. Drug metabolism takes place primarily in the liver through catabolic reactions (oxidation, reduction, hydroxylation, acetylation, glucuronidation) and other enzymatic processes. Drugs are then excreted as active, inactive, or partial metabolites. If these liver enzymes, as they do their work, also make the drug metabolite into a more water-soluble compound, it can be eliminated by glomerular filtration or tubular excretion in the urine. If, on the other hand, it is metabolized to a less water-soluble compound, it will be excreted into bile and can then be eliminated in feces. In some cases, especially when an active metabolite is made, the metabolite enters the small intestine to be reabsorbed into the general circulation, returned to the liver, and excreted once again into bile (enterohepatic recirculation).

Understanding the Role of Half-Life

The **half-life** ($t_{1/2}$) of a drug is the measure of how long it takes for half of a drug to be eliminated from the bloodstream. One practical example of applying half-life information is found with the class of antidepressants known as selective serotonin reuptake inhibitors (SSRIs). Patients taking SSRIs that have short half-lives, such as fluvoxamine (Luvox; $t_{1/2}$ 13–15 hours), are much more likely to experience SSRI discontinuation syndrome. This is a type of *withdrawal syndrome* that occurs following the interruption of dosing, the lowering of dosages, or the discontinuation of regular SSRI use. This condition often begins between 24 hours to 1 week from the last dose taken and can be predicted upon knowing the half-life of the drug. The prescribing literature of SSRIs acknowledges the existence of "intolerable discontinuation reactions," and some patients have extreme difficulty discontinuing their use of SSRIs, especially those drugs with short half-lives (Warner, Bobo, Warner, Reid, & Rachal, 2006).

Clinicians and patients can use the general rule, commonly known as the six half-life rule: It takes six half-lives for the concentration of a medication to reach a point at which it stops causing effects. However, because the rule is only a rough estimate, there is no literature to validate it or attest to its scientific merit, nor is there an author to lay claim to inventing it. According to the six half-life rule, if the half-life of a drug is 24 hours, the plasma concentration over time as it is eliminated will be as follows:

- Day 1: 50% of its dose or fraction remaining 1/2.
- Day 2: 25% of its dose or fraction remaining 1/4.
- Day 3: 12.5% of its dose or fraction remaining 1/8.
- Day 4: 6.25% of its dose, or fraction remaining 1/16.
- Day 5: 3.12% of its dose still circulating or fraction remaining 1/32
- Day 6: 1.56% of its dose is circulating but likely to cause no clinically discernible effect, or fraction remaining 1/64.

This six half-life ($t_{1/2}$) rule has clinical significance in that it tells a clinician that if a patient experiences adverse effects from a drug and the clinician stops the drug, then the patient could expect these effects to disappear in about 5 or 6 days (assuming that the 3.12% or 1.56% of the drug left in the body does not produce noticeable effects). In some cases the half-life elimination is a linear process, as just illustrated, and in other cases it is curved, with more drug being eliminated at the beginning of the dosing period.

Thus half-life is important because knowing the manner in which a drug's plasma concentration rises or falls once dosing has begun (or is readministered or discontinued) provides the clinician with a rational means of controlling a drug's effect by first determining a starting dose and then setting a maintenance dose and the intervals between them. If untoward effects arise, the clinician also has a rule of thumb to help the patient understand when the adverse effects can be expected to cease after the drug is discontinued. In medical practice, many clinicians use this half-life rule as a means of "washing out" one drug before starting another.

Half-life is important not only because it helps determine dosing intervals but also because of the time it takes to reach steady state, the time at which serum concentrations are at their peak efficiency during continuous dosing. Under normal circumstances, it takes three half-lives for serum concentrations to reach 90% of peak steady state values. Thus clinicians say, "Experience has taught me that three to five half-lives is when you are likely to feel the effects of this drug because then it is working at it best efficiency." However, this model only roughly corresponds with real life.

Monitoring Drugs in Patients

Clinicians often monitor the plasma concentrations of certain drugs that have the following characteristics (Table 2-3):

- Drugs that have a low therapeutic window.
- Drugs with active metabolites.
- Drugs whose concentrations are not predictable from dosing parameters.
- Drugs that are often taken in overdose.
- Drugs whose effects are dangerous when the patient compliance/adherence is poor.

Knowing more precisely the pharmacokinetic measurements of a certain drug in an individual patient will help the clinician decide if it is the best drug to use, what its first (loading) and subsequent doses will be, and the interval between those subsequent doses. Clinical pharmacists are often employed as part of the clinical team to do the testing when these drugs are used.

Putting Pharmacodynamics and Pharmacokinetics To Use

With a good understanding of both pharmacodynamics and pharmacokinetics, clinicians can better understand, determine, and monitor the magnitude of a drug's effect on the body. Conscientious prescribing is a complex process. Misuse of medications by either a patient or clinician can be disastrous. Think about the allegations of medication abuse and misuse that surround the deaths of stars such as Michael Jackson.

The pharmacokinetic properties (ADME) of a drug determine how quickly and to what extent a drug will appear at its

TABLE 2-3	Common Drugs for Which Blood Testing Is Recommended
CLASS	**DRUG**
ANTI-CONVULSANT	carbamazepine (Tegretol) phenytoin (Dilantin) phenobarbital valproic Acid (Depakote)
ANTIARRHYTHMICS	amiodarone digitalis (Digoxin)
ANTIBIOTICS	gentamicin vancomycin
ANTICOAGULANTS	warfarin (Coumadin)

target site of action, stay there, be neutralized, and leave the body. Pharmacodynamics will determine the pharmacological effect the drug will have once it reaches its target site. By knowing a few facts about the pharmacokinetics and pharmacodynamics that apply to the majority of drugs in a particular drug class, the task of learning a huge body of information becomes manageable and allows the student or clinician the opportunity to focus on the exceptions. For example, when learning about antipsychotic drugs, it is common knowledge that they all exhibit similar pharmacokinetic characteristics:

■ They are all are readily absorbed.
■ They are all metabolized by the hepatic cytochrome P450 system, thus they are all prone to drug interactions.
■ Their $t_{1/2}$ is generally 20 hours, except for ziprasidone (Geodon) and quetiapine (Seroquel).
■ Dosing adjustments must be made in the elderly and for any others with renal and/or hepatic impairment.

Clinicians refer to standard reference texts, such as the *Physician's Desk Reference* (PDR), to guide their medication recommendations. The PDR, which is fundamentally a compilation of medication package inserts), provides information about the properties of a particular pharmaceutical (e.g., molecular weight, pH, protein-binding, etc.). Such information has been approved by the FDA, but it is written without reference to the drugs' use in practice and may be outdated. There is a host of primary literature available today for the clinician that presents the best evidence that clinical research can supply. However, what every patient ultimately relies on is the good judgment of his or her clinician.

LEARNING EXERCISES

1. Assume a patient takes a 100-mg tablet, goes to bed, falls asleep, and wakes up 3 hours later. How much drug is left in his body if the 100-mg tablet has a $t_{1/2}$ of 1 hour?

2. What is the primary site of drug absorption for a drug given in tablet form?

3. A new drug hits the market, and you read that its half-life is 20 hours. This drug is to be dosed once a day. You find that a patient taking this drug is experiencing nausea and vomiting. How long should the patient be told it will take until these adverse effects disappear?

References

Potter, S.O. L. *Opium: A Compendium of Materia Medica, Therapeutic, and Prescription Writing* (1902). Self-published in 1902.

Romiti, N., Tramonti, G., Donati, A., & Chieli, E. (2004). Effects of grapefruit juice on the multidrug transporter P-glycoprotein in the human proximal tubular cell line HK-2. *Life Science, 76*(3), 293-302.

U. S. Food and Drug Administration (FDA). (2010, March 12). *FDA drug safety communication: Reduced effectiveness of Plavix (clopidogrel) in patients who are poor metabolizers of the drug.* Retrieved February 3, 2011, from www.fda.gov/Drugs/DrugSafety/Postmarket DrugSafetyInformationforpatientsandProviders/ucm203888.htm

Warner, C. H., Bobo, W., Warner, C., Reid, S., Rachal, J. (2006). Antidepressant discontinuation syndrome. *American Family Physician, 74*(3), 449-456. Retrieved February 3, 2011, from www.aafp.org/afp/2006/0801/p449.html

Withering, W. (1785). An account of the foxglove and some of its medical uses: with practical remarks on dropsy and other diseases. London: J and J Robinson.

Communicating with Patients About Medications: A Patient-Centered Approach

chapter 3

William N. Tindall, Mona M. Sedrak

CHAPTER FOCUS

The purpose of this chapter is to present the importance of efficiency and effectiveness in communication between patients and clinicians regarding medication selection and use. The chapter discusses how openness and trust are essential components of **patient-centered care** and how these qualities can be developed by setting the correct environment, using active listening skills, responding empathetically to patients, using open-ended questioning techniques, and setting professional boundaries. The chapter further gives attention to effective dialogue with children and their caregivers, adolescents, the elderly, and those who may display characteristics of polypharmacy, drug-seeking behaviors, or nonadherence to medication regimens.

OBJECTIVES

After carefully reading and studying this chapter, the student should be able to:

1. Describe how a shifting health-care environment has created the opportunity for patient-centered communications to flourish.
2. Describe the reasons for the development of patient-centered care and how it contributes to better health-care delivery.
3. Describe the personal barriers that hinder a clinician's ability to have an effective dialogue with patients.
4. Analyze the effectiveness of patient-centered communication in preventing noncompliance with medications.
5. Define empathy and recall how it can be employed to improve the clinician-patient relationship.
6. Describe the differences between open-ended and closed-ended questions and how best to use open-ended questions to help prevent medication errors.
7. State how I-messages are constructed and used to help set boundaries with patients.

Key Terms

Active listening

Closed-ended questions

Covenants

Empathic responding

I-messages

Nonadherence

Open-ended questions

Patient-centered care

Patient-centered communication

Polypharmacy

In health care today, clinicians are experiencing profound changes in the ways they deliver patient care. The ongoing evolution of the health-care environment has challenged centuries-old covenants and relationships between clinicians and patients owing to limitations of care and services enforced by managed care and the growth and application of technology in the delivery of health care. Furthermore, patients have become more active in dealing with their own health needs, asking for more autonomy, improved services, and partnerships with clinicians to achieve desired outcomes.

Most states regulate certain prescribing behaviors, but they do not regulate communication patterns between clinicians and patients. Traditional covenants such as the Oath and Prayer of Maimonides, the Hippocratic Oath, the Oath of the Physician Assistant, and the Nightingale Pledge for Advanced Practice Nurses (APNs) regulate communication patterns. However, **covenants** are pledges to use learned professional judgment to guide interpersonal communication between themselves and patients; they are not contracts. Every clinician develops a personal communication style that deeply impacts his or her patient-clinician relationships. Patient satisfaction, trust in the clinician, and compliance with treatment regimens often stem directly from the clinician's ability to communicate effectively.

To ensure successful patient-centered care, all clinicians must understand the principles of effective communication and become skilled communicators. Communication between patients and clinicians is complex and is affected by a patient's life experience, culture, age, sex, language, religious preferences, and previous experiences with clinicians. Nevertheless, effective communication is a *skill* that can be learned and practiced. Many practitioners believe that achieving effective patient-clinician communication requires spending more time with patients, but this is not true. By developing smarter communication methods, it is possible to see patients in *less* time and still be an effective communicator. Poor communication leads to the development of poor patient-clinician relationships. Patients who do not believe that their clinician is making time available to speak with them and is truly demonstrating an interest in their health care tend to hold back critical pieces of information necessary for their care, especially when they have not been encouraged to speak openly.

Patient-Centered Communication

Patient-centered care means that patients are treated as partners in health-care decision-making and encouraged to take responsibility for their health (Box 3-1). Today, health insurance companies, group practices, institutions, universities, and health agencies are measuring patient-centered care practices because they are considered an important component of quality health care. For example, patients are more likely to be compliant when there is the following:

- A realistic assessment of their knowledge, and they are allowed to help shape their dosing regimens.
- Clear and effective communication with their clinician.
- Nurturance of trust in the therapeutic relationship (Martin, Williams, Haskard, & DiMatteo, 2005; Commander & Stambaugh, 2008).

BOX 3-1 The Developing and Still Evolving Philosophy of Patient-Centered Care

Early to Mid-20th Century: Biomedical Model of Care
Integration of medical science and technology caused a gradual shift away from patients' existential concerns about illness and a shift in the power structure between patient and physician so that physicians became the "experts."

Mid-20th Century: Biopsychosocial Model of Care
Concerns over equity in civil and human rights led to changes in care and promotion of a more collaborative and collegial care model, which shifted the balance of power in professional relationships.

Late 20th Century, Early 21st Century: Patient-Centered Model of Care
The biopsychosocial model of care expanded to include the contextual concerns of patients and their daily lives, such as cultural concerns, philosophical approaches and beliefs, attitudes toward the organization of the health system, community concerns, and the impact of limited resources and payment systems. It also includes understanding an array of other factors, such as practitioner and patient approaches to preventive health. Today much of patient-centered delivery of health care is based on three maxims:

"The needs of the patient come first."

"Nothing about me without me."

"Every patient is the only patient."

Patient-centered communication is only one component of delivering patient-centered care. Similar to patient-centered care, **patient-centered communication** focuses on the patient's needs, values, and wishes. Patients often have unaddressed concerns and worries that they do not share with their clinician. Between 30% and 80% of patients' expectations are not met in the primary care visit (Kravitz, 1996). Clinicians often begin communication by asking open-ended questions but redirect their patients within less than 30 seconds of the patient's expressing a concern (Marvel, Epstein, Flowers, & Beckman, 1999). Many clinicians do not involve their patients in the decision-making process about their health. As many as 40% of clinical recommendations made by clinicians are forgotten or ignored by patients because the patients have differences of opinions and expectations that are not reconciled during the visit (Martin, Williams, Haskard, & DiMatteo, 2005). Thus, it is not surprising that adherence to treatment protocols is poor and problems persist even with the best of intentions of both parties.

Barriers to Effective Communication

Improving communication begins with understanding the barriers to effective and efficient communication. There are many types of barriers, and they differ from person to person and practice to practice.

Physical Barriers

In every medical setting where care is delivered, there are many distractions that can impede the free flow of dialogue between a clinician and a patient. Telephones, pagers, or cell phones may ring, or staff may be conversing in the hallways. Strong or inadequate lighting may affect a person's perceptions. Sometimes the biggest physical barrier is the personal space or distance between the patient and the clinician. If the space is too close, the patient may feel hemmed in; if it is too far, the patient may feel depersonalized. In many cases a large desk between patient and caregiver is seen as a barrier, hence it impedes open dialogue. The best-case scenario is for each person to be sitting or standing in a private and quiet area where eye-to-eye contact can be made.

One of the least considered barriers is the white coat. Many patients experience "white coat syndrome," in which they see a white coat and become very anxious, unable to fully express their concerns to the clinician. Others see the white coat as an authority symbol and feel that they should not bother the busy clinician or should not speak until they are asked a question. In both scenarios the patient leaves the office without concerns and questions having been addressed. Thus, patients should be encouraged to bring in a list of questions that they created before their visit so that all their questions are addressed.

Language Barriers

Language barriers can impede effective dialogue. Technical phrases, concepts, and medical jargon can be confusing to patients. The clinician should determine each patient's understanding of medical terms as well as the patient's level of education. Clinicians can use language that is appropriate for that particular patient, avoiding either talking down or talking above the patient's level of understanding. Language barriers due to English as a second language and cultural differences are also important to understand and are discussed later in this chapter.

To determine whether a patient fully understands his or her medical problem and management, clinicians should ask if the patient understands or has further questions. For example, one useful patient-centered technique is to state, "I want to be sure I have not forgotten to tell you something important. Can you tell me the name of your medicine and what you are taking it for? What can you expect while taking this medication?" If the patient is refilling a medication, state, "I would like to know how the medicine is working for you." By asking these types of questions, the clinician will be able to determine the patient's level of understanding and commitment to taking the medications appropriately.

Personal and Emotional Barriers

Preconceived attitudes are another barrier to effective dialogue. Like all people, clinicians have personal and professional situations that can affect their ability to provide quality care. Most patients do not think of their clinician as being subject to the frailties and ambiguities of life. When they interact with a clinician, they do so with the belief that at the time of their visit they have the clinician's full attention. It is important that clinicians become aware of their own attitudes and emotional health and their ability to provide care daily. If patient-centered care is to flourish, it requires clinicians to have insight into their own behaviors and make a cognizant effort to focus on the patient's needs, purposefully leaving their own problems and attitudes outside the room.

Techniques for Effective Communication

Active listening/**empathic responding**, use of open-ended questions, and use of I-messages are communication techniques that enhance patient care, establish trust, and help patients with medication management. These techniques can be learned and mastered and are effective at improving listening and interviewing skills.

Active Listening

Active listening is a structured form of listening and responding that focuses the clinician's attention on the speaker. It is a simple concept that starts with listening attentively, repeating what the patient has said in the patient's own words, then asking the patient if this is what he or she said. This style of responding demonstrates the clinician's understanding of the patient's message and allows the patient to clarify any misunderstandings. Instead of just repeating the words, the clinician is encouraged to interpret the patient's words in terms of feelings to show that he or she understands the patient's emotional response to the event. The five key elements of active listening are as follows:

1. Pay attention: Give patients your undivided attention and acknowledge what they are saying by looking at them directly, putting aside distracting thoughts, and observing their body language. Reading body language is a skill in itself, but over time people can become good at distinguishing whether or not someone with crossed arms is closed to further communication or is just someone with crossed arms. Nonverbal communication, such as facial expressions, posture, dress, and appearance, sends messages that are just as strong as verbal messages. In fact, many clinicians trust the nonverbal messages more than some verbal messages. A good example is the patient who states that he has quit smoking while a pack of cigarettes protrudes from a jacket pocket. Additionally, many nonverbal behaviors are cultural. For example, although making eye contact with a clinician is considered acceptable and expected behavior in certain cultures, it may be considered disrespectful in others.

2. Show that you are listening: Use your body language and gestures to show that you are giving the patient your full attention. Occasionally nod, smile, and use other facial expressions to indicate that you are listening empathetically. Encourage the patient to continue talking by making brief comments like "yes" or "I see." Also, be aware of your posture and appearance and make sure that it sends the message that you are approachable and not that you are frustrated or in a rush.

3. Provide feedback: Our personal assumptions, judgments, training, and beliefs can change what we hear. As a clinician your role is to understand what is being said and to

reflect upon it. You can do this by paraphrasing what the patient has said: "What I hear you say is. . ." You also can ask questions to clarify certain points, and you can summarize the patient's comments periodically.

4. Respond appropriately and empathically: To develop a trusting relationship with the patient, be respectful and nonjudgmental. Deliver your response in a candid, open, and honest manner, and give the patient time to ask questions or comment on your response. Responding empathically means communicating your understanding of the patient's situation, feelings, and motives, for example: "I understand your problem and how you feel about it."

Using Open-Ended Questioning

Closed-ended questions are those that typically elicit a "yes" or "no" or other brief response. For example, a clinician may ask, "Did you understand what I just said?," and the patient may respond with a simple "yes." Closed-ended questioning is of little value in patient-centered care because it does not probe deeply enough to acquire essential information that may help improve patient outcomes. Although closed-ended questions may save time, they may also inhibit the patient's desire to share more information or emotions.

Open-ended questions are worded to encourage patients to share information and emotions. They begin with words such as *who*, *what*, *when*, *where*, *why*, and *how*. Open-ended questions contribute to positive health-care outcomes, patient satisfaction, and an increased interest in adherence to health and medication regimens (Beardsley, Kimberlin, & Tindall, 2011). Open-ended questioning invites patients to provide details, clarify a notion or belief, and elaborate on their behaviors and attitudes. Table 3-1 provides examples of closed- and open-ended questions.

An important part of patient-centered communication is trying to pinpoint the patient's concerns and then identifying which concern should be addressed first. Often clinicians believe that the first concern a patient mentions is the most important one. Even more deceiving is that they feel that patients will spontaneously report all of their fears and concerns. Neither assumption is true. Patients should be given license to speak freely at the beginning of the visit by the clinician asking, "What brings you in today?" Ask patients with multiple complaints, "Which of these issues would you like to start with today?" Then negotiate the agenda for the rest of the visit. At the end of the visit, ask, "Have I addressed all your concerns today?" or "Do you have any other concerns that we should address today?" If patients have their health concerns addressed during the visit and understand their medical problems and management, they may have fewer negative outcomes and may make fewer calls and follow-up visits to the office.

Establishing Boundaries Using I-messages

I-messages express the clinician's thoughts and feelings; what behaviors, words, or actions gave rise to certain feelings; and what effect the conversation is having on the clinician. I-messages are constructed as follows:

"**I feel** _____ (insert feeling word)____, **when you do** ____ (insert action verb)___, **because it makes me feel** _____(insert effect word) **about** _____ (insert situation)."

I-messages are used to establish boundaries and maintain the control and direction of patient-centered conversations. The following case exemplifies the use of I-messages.

CASE A patient with chronic obstructive pulmonary disease (COPD) comes into the clinic for a refill of a bronchodilator and an inhaled corticosteroid. He has a pack of cigarettes in his shirt pocket. This patient has not stopped smoking, started a smoking cessation program, or accepted counseling and medication, even though these topics have been discussed during prior visits. Today he asks if it is really necessary for him to quit smoking. He also asks, "Are the warnings about cigarettes written on the package really true, or are they just scare tactics?" In response the clinician states the following I-message:

"I feel really upset and concerned when I see that you continue to smoke. I care about what happens to you. When I see cigarettes in your pocket, it makes me feel like my advice is not worth anything."

Some people would respond to the preceding case with a you-message. A you-message would focus on the behavior seen right now by placing blame, making a judgment, or making a belittling remark. An example of a you-message might be:

"I'm not sure what you're looking for here! We have talked about this so many times, and you have deliberately ignored my advice about smoking. I know you are going to do whatever you want anyway, regardless of what I say. To tell you the truth, you are acting incredibly foolishly and irresponsibly and I will not be held accountable if you die from smoking."

The use of an I-message will do much more to encourage a conversation than the finger-pointing and anger expressed in the you-message, which will likely end any further helpful conversation. Once an I-message has been stated, it can be followed up with a message that establishes boundaries for the relationship. For example, for the preceding case, the clinician could establish his or her boundaries by adding on to the end of the I-message:

"I feel really upset and concerned when I see that you continue to smoke. I care about what happens to you. When I see cigarettes in your pocket, it makes me feel like my advice is not worth anything. I know that

TABLE 3-1	Open-Ended Questions vs. Closed-Ended Questions	
OPEN-ENDED QUESTIONS	**CLOSED-ENDED QUESTIONS**
How may I be of help to you?	Can I help you?
What kind of medication information can I provide?	Do you know what this med is for?
What are you expecting to happen when you take this?	You know the side effects, right?
What is it you want to know about ___?	Can you be more specific?
Why are you taking this medication?	You know the reason for this, don't you?

stopping smoking is a difficult process, and I want you to attend a smoking cessation program where all your questions can be answered."

Medication Safety and Communication

Patients often accept prescriptions that they will never fill and fill prescriptions that they will never take. Many times this is due to misunderstandings about the prescription and its benefits or fear of side effects and adverse reactions. An important part of patient education and counseling is teaching patients how to correctly manage their medications.

Maintaining an accurate, up-to-date, and accessible medication list in the patient's chart is the essence of effective patient management. In many offices, medical assistants and nurses help take the medication history. However, it is still the responsibility of the treating clinician to verify the medical history and to review medication lists with patients at every visit.

Clinicians can start taking a drug history by asking open-ended questions of their patients, such as, "Can you tell me what medications you are taking at this time?" Patients who cannot name their medications can be prompted by discussing their chronic medical problems and medications that they may be taking for those problems. Ask patients if they have been seeing other clinicians who prescribed medications for them and what those medications may be. Also ask about any over the counter medications such as analgesics, ibuprofen (Advil, Motrin), and acetaminophen (Tylenol), which are commonly used by individuals for pain. If the patient is using any over-the-counter medications, take the time to get a thorough history of quantity and frequency. It is also imperative to ask about vitamins, herbals, and other supplements. Finally, when taking a drug history, consider cultural and religious implications and ask about home remedies that patients may be using for management of medical problems. Patients are often reluctant to talk to their clinician about these issues, and it is up to the clinician to develop a nonjudgmental relationship with the patient in keeping with the patient-centered medicine philosophy.

It is important that medication lists and records be maintained as patient medications change. Medication lists that are maintained well and clearly written become a vital part of the chart and make the clinician's job much easier. Commonly overlooked medications in the medication list include birth control pills, inhalers, eyedrops, patches, herbal medicine, and medications prescribed by other clinicians. There are a variety of forms available to record this information (Fig. 3-1). Regardless of the format chosen, it is advisable to write the drug's brand name, generic name, strength, and frequency in the appropriate fields on the form and to include the date reviewed. Any clinician or staff person reviewing a patient's medications should initial next to the current date. There should also be an area on the form where notes can be made indicating when the medication was discontinued and why.

Benefits to using a medication list include the following:

1. Efficient charting and electronic medical records: Medication lists can be updated with a few checkmarks, and documentation is made easier and quicker. This saves time from visit to visit.
2. Safer refills: By keeping the medications list up-to-date, prescription refills can be handled more efficiently by clinicians and nurses.
3. Communication with other clinicians: The medication list can be copied and sent to other clinicians who see the patient, which improves information sharing and prevents medication errors.
4. Information recall: The medication list is a snapshot of a patient's medical history, which helps the clinician easily recall past treatment and recurring medical problems.
5. Allergy documentation: Allergies should be documented in one place in the chart and in every SOAP note. (SOAP is an acronym for subjective, objective, assessment, and plan.) They should also be listed in the medication list. The allergic reaction should be described, and the date it first occurred should be noted.

Patient Name: _____	Allergies: ___ Reaction ___ Date ___
Date Of Birth: _____	1. _____
MRN#: _____	2. _____
	3. _____

Date started	Date D/C	Medication brand/generic	Dosage strength/frequency	Date reviewed/initialed						

FIGURE 3-1 Medication management review.

Culturally Competent Communication

Racial, ethnic, and cultural disparities are clearly demonstrated and documented in health care in the United States. Certain racial and ethnic groups have higher rates of particular diseases (e.g., cardiovascular disease in African American population, diabetes in American Indian and Hispanic American population) (Smedley, Stith, & Nelson, 2002). It is important that clinicians and organizations be responsible for providing culturally competent health care. Understanding how to communicate with diverse populations is an important part of eliminating health-care disparities and providing quality health care to all patients. Culturally competent communication refers to the clinician's ability to communicate with awareness and knowledge of health-care disparities and to understand the sociocultural factors that have important effects on health beliefs and behaviors. These issues are so important that the Institute of Medicine (2002) identified cross-cultural training as a key recommendation for reducing health-care disparities in its report, *Unequal Treatment: Confronting Racial and Ethnic Disparities in Health Care.*

Whereas clinicians bring to the health-care encounter their medical expertise and empathy, patients bring their cultural backgrounds, beliefs, practices, and languages, all of which affect communication in the delivery of health care. For instance, patients and clinicians have different understandings of illness and disease. A disease is something that the health-care clinician understands and diagnoses, while an illness is something that the patient experiences. For some patients this difference in defining a medical problem affects their view and understanding of their illness, symptoms, etiology, expectations about appropriate treatment, and what is expected of them in the healing process.

When patients and clinicians speak the same language, patients are more likely to have positive health outcomes. However, when patients cannot communicate in the clinician's language, or vice versa, delays in positive outcomes can occur because of missed appointments, nonadherence to therapy, and medical errors. Clinicians may not be able to fully understand the scope of a medical problem and the symptoms that accompany the problems. Trained translators are not always available, and clinicians must rely on relatives for translation. However, numerous studies have documented problems with this approach, ranging from poor translation to patient unwillingness to disclose sensitive but important information in the presence of a family member or stranger (Karliner, Jacobs, Chen, & Mutha, 2007).

When communicating with individuals and families who have limited English proficiency, keep in mind that this limited proficiency is not indicative of a patient's intellectual level and has no bearing on the patient's ability to communicate effectively in his or her language of origin. In fact, patients may or may not be literate in their own language or in English. Clinicians must determine how well their patients can understand and participate in health-care decisions. Using bilingual/bicultural staff, personnel, or volunteers may help with medical interpretation during treatment, interventions, and other events. When the patient cannot understand the clinician, other forms of communication may be necessary, such as use of simplified written diagrams, patient education leaflets in the patient's native language, or computer translators that instantly convert English comments into many other languages.

Communicating with Children and Adolescents

Children and adolescents are important consumers of medication, but communication with them is much different from that with adults. First, communication with children and adolescents is typically a three-way process: the child, the child's parent(s) or caregivers, and the health professional. Secondly, children and adolescents, especially younger children, need to be communicated with on a level that is appropriate to their age and cognitive development. However, it is important to use a patient-centered style with children and adolescents because they too would like to ask more about their medicines, but they will not ask questions if they are not given the opportunity to do so (Erickson, Gerstle, & Feldstein, 2005). If given the opportunity to talk about their medications, they are more likely to adhere to their medication regimens, especially if they are taught something about their disease and its treatment (Bush, 1999).

Children want to know how medicines are made, how they work, and especially how they go to various parts of the body. In addition, they want general questions answered, such as why some medicines can be used for more than one purpose and why some medicines are only for children while some are only for adults. Clinicians should also negotiate the transfer of responsibility for medication use, when appropriate, to the child in a way that respects both the parents' and the child's capabilities.

Some helpful techniques for communicating with and empowering children and adolescents are to do the following:

1. Always introduce yourself and give your name to the child first, then tell the parent that you are going to talk directly to the child. This is important for approaching children of any age.
2. Start with asking a few general questions to gain some appreciation for the cognitive level of the child or adolescent. Once a child is 5 or 6 years old he or she can be more actively involved in the medication regimen. Often a good way to get started is to ask about a child's hobby or favorite TV show so as to assess his or her ability to understand cause-and-effect relationships.
3. Use open-ended questions and simple declarative sentences. When using a declarative sentence, ask for feedback. For example, you might say, "It's important that you work with your mom and dad in taking this medication. Do you know what I mean by that?"
4. Ask the child or adolescent if he or she has questions for you. If none are forthcoming, give examples of questions other patients have asked you and tell the child whether such questions might apply to him or her.
5. Pay special attention to any nonverbal behavior. If you are not getting through to a child or adolescent, wait a minute

and try again. Children are especially tuned in to nonverbal behavior and will interpret it before interpreting verbal behavior. If you appear bored, rushed, or not fully committed to helping a child or adolescent, the child will interpret this to mean, "This person does not care about me, so why should I trust what he says?"

Communicating with Older Patients

The U.S. population is aging at a rapid pace. By the year 2030, 71 million Americans will be age 65 or older. Those 65 or older now account for 12.9% of the total population (U.S. Census Bureau, 2010). Older Americans consume more health resources on a daily basis. In the United States it is estimated that individuals over the age of 65 visit their clinician an average of eight times more per year than does the general population (Thompson, Robinson, & Beisecker, 2004). Thus, clinicians need to learn how to communicate effectively with this aging population.

Communicating with older patients can be challenging because they actually are a more heterogeneous population than a younger population (Tindall & Clasen, 2007). Older patients come with a wide variety of life experiences and cultural backgrounds that affect their perception of health and illness and their willingness to adhere to medication regimens. Communication may be more difficult owing to the normal aging process, which includes sensory loss, slower processing of information and decline in memory, and other chronic medical conditions that may impact the patient's ability to communicate and understand his or her health concerns. It is unfortunate that at the time these patients require the most care from their clinicians, they may be hindered from sharing their concerns because of factors out of their control. Clinicians must be aware of the obstacles that exist and work to improve communication with older patients, thus avoiding medical errors and improving the quality of health care for the elderly.

Older patients may feel that they are a burden on their families as well as the health-care system. They may be less willing to share their complicated medical history and medication regimens with new clinicians. Furthermore, older patients may be reluctant to ask questions regarding their health and medication regimens, feeling that to do so would be to insult the clinician. This may lead to misunderstandings and nonadherence to medication regimens. Therefore, clinicians must give their patients the opportunity to ask questions and must verify that patients understand their medical problems and their management before leaving the office.

The following tips are useful when communicating necessary information and instructions to older patients:

1. Allow extra time and schedule older patients early in the day.
2. Minimize visual and auditory distractions.
3. Sit face to face with patients.
4. Listen without interrupting.
5. Speak slowly, clearly, and loudly enough to ensure being heard.
6. Use short, simple words and sentences.
7. Stick to one topic at a time.
8. Simplify and write instructions.
9. Use charts, models, and pictures to illustrate the message.
10. Give patients a chance to ask questions.

Communicating with Older Patients About Polypharmacy and Adverse Drug Reactions (ADR)

Polypharmacy is defined as the concurrent use of several drugs at the same time. This is not uncommon in the elderly, but it does increase their risk of adverse drug reactions and drug-drug interactions. Other clinical consequences of polypharmacy include **nonadherence**, increased risk of hospitalizations, and medication errors. A number of researchers have studied the problem of polypharmacy. According to Gurwitz et al. (2003), taking two drugs increases the risk of an adverse event by only 6%, but taking eight medications raises the risk of an adverse drug reaction to 100%. At any given time, an elderly patient takes, on average, four or five prescription drugs and two over-the-counter medications; thus, the risk of having an adverse drug reaction (ADR) or adverse drug event (ADE) is virtually a given (Gurwitz et al., 2003). According to Beers (2009), polypharmacy is a real problem among the elderly, and it is believed that adverse reactions to medicines as a result of polypharmacy are at the root of 5% to 17% of hospital admissions. ADRs cause 100,000 deaths yearly and are the fourth leading cause of death, ahead of pulmonary disease, diabetes, AIDS, and automobile accidents. As people age, their use of medications increases to the point that the ambulatory elderly use 9 to 13 prescriptions a year concurrently, and individuals over age 65 use 2 to 6 prescription drugs and 1 to more than 3 OTC drugs.

When caring for older patients, clinicians should keep in mind the possibility of drug-induced disease and adverse drug reactions. The most common adverse drug reactions are confusion (especially with beta blockers, H_2 blockers, anticholinergics, and sedatives/hypnotics); urinary frequency (often erroneously attributed to incontinence or aging); dry mouth; indigestion; dizziness; rash; diarrhea; depression; and fatigue.

Patients should bring all of their prescribed and OTC medications to each visit to check for outdated medications or those with potential for drug-drug interactions and ADR. Conduct a comprehensive medication history and be vigilant for duplicate medications, such as generic and trade drugs, or two medications from the same drug family taken at the same time. A drug review session is also a good time to look for stockpiled medications, especially if an expensive medication has been discontinued and the patient chooses not to dispose of it. Failure to dispose of medications often leads to patients taking outdated medication. A drug review is also a good time to check on drugs with a long half-life because they are cleared very slowly from the body and the risk of drug interaction will persist for a considerable time after they are stopped. For example, an interaction with fluoxetine (Prozac) can occur up to 6 weeks after it has been discontinued. This is also the time to discuss such things as the use of antacids, vitamins, and herbal remedies, because many patients do not consider them drugs.

Whenever possible, patients should be encouraged to use only one pharmacy. With modern computerized drug databases, pharmacists can stop drug interactions before they occur. Every pharmacy in the United States is connected to one of a few reliable and referenced databases that automatically check interactions. In addition, the pharmacist can keep for each patient a computerized record of all medications prescribed by several different clinicians as well as OTC drugs and herbal remedies. Patients with impaired vision can request large-letter labels to reduce the likelihood of a medication error at home. Some pharmacies even print labels in non-English formats.

Elderly patients can suffer adverse drug reactions with doses that may be normal. Advise all patients to report any new symptoms to their clinician, because many patients often attribute the signs and symptoms of polypharmacy or adverse drug reactions to their disease or getting older. Instruct all patients that the medication prescribed is a course of therapy and that they should not stop taking it without medical advice. Finally, besides looking for polypharmacy, keep in mind that street drugs and alcohol are drugs as well, especially because alcohol interacts with up to one-half of all medications.

Communicating About Noncompliance

Noncompliance to a prescribed medication regimen is a complicated and complex issue. It is an observed behavior in patients of all ages, positions, education levels, economic statuses, and health beliefs. Many studies have attempted to predict which patients will enter a state of noncompliance, but they have failed because of the difficulty of addressing in any one study all of the following factors that affect noncompliance, as follows:

■ The patient's perception of the medication and its regimen
■ The relationship between the patient and the prescribing or dispensing clinician
■ Any faults and weaknesses in the health-care delivery system

Responsibility for complying with a medication regimen is shared by the patient and clinician. For the patient, impaired vision, hearing, or mobility may affect compliance, as will medical illiteracy and the patient's health beliefs. The clinician influences compliance by educating the patient regarding the benefits of medications, establishing a trusting relationship with the patient, and considering the impact of the cost of medications on the patient.

Whatever the cause of medication noncompliance, the problem is all too prevalent, and it is all too problematic in that it reduces the effectiveness of prescribed drugs. Following are five simple strategies that any clinician can use to improve medication adherence:

1. Use the least number of medications possible and use a simple dosing schedule, preferably one that has been agreed to by the patient.
2. Help correct compliance by seeing it as a problem requiring a team effort. Be an example to everyone (physician, physician assistant, nurse, receptionist, and so forth) in the clinic by taking the time to talk to a patient and ask, "What questions do you have about your medications that I can answer for you?"

3. Develop an inquiring approach to individualizing medication regimens, keeping a focus on the patient's needs, desires, beliefs, motivations, challenges, experiences, issues with costs, memory, and disabilities, and help the patient develop strategies to deal with any issues.
4. Develop a plan for follow-up, monitoring and modifying a medication plan once one has been mutually arranged.
5. Always be mindful that if a patient is noncompliant, it will take more than a one-time encounter to address and correct this because patients do not change their behavior simply because they are told to do so.

Communicating About Medication Costs

A study of 660 older adults with chronic diseases found that as many as 32% of the participants admitted underusing prescribed medications during the previous year because they could not afford them (Piette, Heisler, & Wagner, 2004). More than half of these patients never told their clinicians that they could not afford their medications. Many were not asked by their clinician if they could afford them. In the same study, almost 60% of patients did not tell their physician because they thought that there was nothing their clinician could do to help them obtain the medications they needed. Of the patients who chose to discuss the topic with their clinician, three-fourths stated that the discussion was helpful, but one-third stated that their clinician would not make any changes to generic or less expensive medications or help them in other ways.

The elderly are not the only ones who cannot afford their medications. Many people, especially in today's economic climate, have no health insurance for themselves or their family members. This problem hits all age brackets and across all cultural lines. Even patients who have health insurance that covers some of their health-care needs may still have to shoulder much of the burden for buying their own outpatient medications. Those patients with limited incomes may have to choose between buying groceries and filling their prescriptions. Thus, their prescriptions often go unfilled. It is important that clinicians take necessary steps to make sure that their patients, regardless of their age, sex, or employment status, have access to the medications they need.

Often clinicians are in a rush or uncomfortable with asking patients if they can afford their medications. A good way to determine if patients are purchasing and taking their medications is to get into the habit of reviewing their medication list each and every time you see patients and asking, "Are you taking this medication?" Also, when prescribing a medication, instead of asking "Can you afford this medication?," clinicians can phrase the question differently, such as, "Do you have any concerns about filling this prescription today?" Phrasing the question in this manner provides the opportunity for the patient to discuss whether the medication's affordability, as well as other issues, may affect the patient's compliance. If a patient cannot afford to fill a prescription, the clinician must ask a series of follow-up questions to determine the situation. This may lead to a greater understanding of factors affecting the patient's overall well-being. Finally, patients may need to be assured that their financial information will be kept private by you and your staff members.

There are other things that clinicians can do to assist their patients with the affordability of medications, including the following:

1. Consider nonmedical treatments such as lifestyle changes: weight loss, smoking cessation, exercise, and relaxation. By practicing sound preventative medicine, you can keep your patients healthier without prescribing as many medications.
2. Prescribe generics whenever possible, because the cost savings may be as much as 90% compared with the cost of the brand-name version of the same drug, and many are just as effective (Sagall, 2006). However, know the differences and the effectiveness of brand-name versus generic medications, because not all medications can be substituted with the same effectiveness.
3. Learn drug prices, and be honest with your patient.
4. Try older drugs first, and do not be seduced by every new drug on the market. Although sometimes they are beneficial, frequently the newer drugs are not much better and are definitely more expensive than older medications.
5. Prescribe half a pill. The price of some medications does not increase very much for a higher dose pill, which can be cut in half for the appropriate dose. Be sure your patient understands how to take the medication appropriately.
6. Keep up-to-date with pharmaceutical patient assistance programs (PAPs). Many pharmaceutical companies have programs that are designed to help those individuals who have no insurance coverage for certain medications. All of these programs require some clinician involvement, and all you have to do is provide a prescription or sign a form. Many prescribed medications are available through pharmaceutical companies' PAPs (Table 3-2).

Understanding Drug-Seeking and Overprescribing Behaviors

Misuse of prescription medication is a common problem in today's health-care environment, especially because so many medications are available, such as analgesics, hypnotics, sedatives, and appetite and mood stimulants. It has become increasingly important to correctly identify patients who display drug-seeking behavior as opposed to those who truly need treatment.

The term *drug seeking* is rarely defined. However, it is used to refer to the behavior of those who seek medications for their own use or to give to friends and family. Approximately 30% of prescription narcotics are diverted to illegal use by someone other than the person for whom they are prescribed (Longo, Parran, Johnson, & Kinsey, 2000; Pretorius & Zurick, 2008). Many are sold to dealers or strangers. This method of obtaining and selling drugs is becoming increasingly popular. The American Medical Association describes someone who becomes involved in these types of behavior as one who is "dated (i.e., out of touch), duped, dishonest, or disabled" (Parran, 1997).

Clinicians can use the following steps to identify patients exhibiting drug-seeking behaviors and to limit their access to drugs (Longo, Parran, Johnson, & Kinsey, 2000; Pretorius & Zurick, 2008):

1. If controlled substances must be prescribed, write prescriptions in such a way that they cannot be tampered with, and stick to a systematic treatment plan. For example, write the prescription for only enough drug to last until the next appointment, and write out the quantity to be dispensed, for example, "ten," not "10," to which another zero could be added. If available, review state-provided controlled substance databases, which can easily be accessed by conducting an Internet search.
2. Keep current on the pharmacodynamics, pharmacokinetics, drug interactions, signs of toxicity, and signs of withdrawal of medicines that can be abused as well as the epidemiology of abuse behavior.
3. Institute a "one clinician–one pharmacy" treatment plan in which the patient can only see one clinician in the practice and the clinic will send the patient to only one pharmacy.
4. Consult with all peers, staff, and others to raise the awareness level and to restate the position that the clinic will take in case of administrative or legal action.
5. Because any medication has a potential for abuse, the clinician can require the patient to sign a consent form to document the decision-making process, so that any deviation from the advised treatment plan is done voluntarily and at the patient's risk.

TABLE 3-2 Medications Available Through PAPs		
BRAND NAME	**GENERIC NAME**	**COMPANY PROGRAM**
ACCOLATE	Zafirlukast	Astra Zeneca
Advair	Fluticasone propionate	GlaxoSmithKline
Amaryl	Glimepiride	Sanofi-Aventis
Glucotrol	Glipizide	Pfizer
Accupril	Quinapril	Pfizer
Calan	Verapamil	RX Outreach
Lipitor	Atorvastatin calcium	Pfizer
Zoloft	Sertraline	Pfizer
Valium	Diazepam	Roche
Prozac	Fluoxetine	Eli Lilly

LEARNING EXERCISES

Case 1

MS is a 68-year-old man who comes to the clinic complaining of urinary frequency and urgency. He thinks he has a urinary tract infection (UTI). You check his records before seeing him and notice that he is also being treated for hypertension. You also see a notation in his chart, "Patient told to quit smoking, start diabetic diet, and exercise 30 minutes per day." As you begin your interview with MS, you notice a tobacco odor on his clothes and breath.

1. How should you address this issue?

2. Should you address the issue of his smoking even though he came to see you for a UTI?

3. What would be a good approach for you to use to gain his trust?

Case 2

TG presents at the clinic with a recurring ear infection. He is from Turkey and speaks little English. As you begin to give him instructions on taking the oral antibiotic you are prescribing, you find that he is becoming agitated and frustrated. In broken English, he asks why he would need to swallow tablets when it's his ear that hurts.

1. How should you proceed?

2. What measures can you take in a busy practice to meet the needs of patients whose culture is different from yours?

Case 3

LD is a 76-year-old female. She is seeing you today for a sleep problem. On reviewing her chart, you note that she has hypertension, type 2 diabetes mellitus, and osteoporosis. Her chart also reveals she had a "small stroke" 2 years ago and that she is taking five different classes of medication. She also takes several OTC medications: a multivitamin, fish oil capsules, glucosamine, and chondroitin. She states, "For the past 6 months I have had trouble sleeping, so every night I take a Benadryl and drink chamomile tea because they make me feel good." She also took something that her neighbor gave her, but it did not work.

1. What should you do to establish trust and rapport with LD?

2. How would you deal with some of the challenges that LD may have, such as her ability to learn, her diminished senses, and the psychosocial factors in aging?

References

Beardsley, R. S., Kimberlin, C. L., & Tindall, W. N. (2011). *Communication skills in pharmacy practice* (6th ed.). Philadelphia: Lippincott, Williams, & Wilkins.

Beers, M. H. (1998, December). Aging as a risk factor for medication-related problems. *The Consultant Pharmacist.* Presented at the Gerontological Society of America Annual Meeting Post-Conference Symposium, Philadelphia.

Bush, P. J. (1999). *Guide to developing and evaluating medicine education for children and adolescents.* Washington, DC: United States Pharmacopeia.

Commander, C., & Stambaugh, T. (2008). *Patient-centered models in medication adherence: Reducing costs and non-compliance through health behavior change* (p. 39). Wall Township, NJ: Healthcare Intelligence Network.

Erickson, S. J., Gerstle, M., & Feldstein, S. W. (2005). Brief interventions and motivational interviewing with children, adolescents, and their parents in pediatric health care settings: A review. *Archives of Pediatrics & Adolescent Medicine, 159*(12), 1173-1180.

Gurwitz, J. H., Field, T. S. Harrold, L. R., Rothschild, J., Debellis, K., Seger, A. C., et al. (2003). Incidence and preventability of adverse drug events among older persons in the ambulatory setting. *Journal of the American Medical Association, 289*(9), 1107-1116.

Institute of Medicine. (2002, March 20). *Unequal treatment: Confronting racial and ethnic disparities in health care.* Retrieved February 9, 2011, from www.iom.edu

Karliner, L. S., Jacobs, E. A., Chen, A. Hm., & Mutha, S. (2007). Do professional interpreters improve clinical care for patients with limited English proficiency? A systematic review of the literature. *Health Services Research, 42*(2), 727-754.

Kravitz, R. L. (1996). Patients' expectations for medical care: An expanded formulation based on a review of the literature. *Medical Care Research and Review, 53,* 3-27.

Longo, L. P., Parran, T., Johnson, B., & Kinsey, W. (2000). Identification and management of the drug-seeking patient, part II. *American Family Physician, 61,* 2121-2128.

Martin, L. R., Williams, S.L., Haskard, K.B., & DiMatteo, M.R. (2005). The challenge of patient adherence. *Journal of Therapeutics and Clinical Risk Management, 1*(3), 189-199.

Marvel, M. K., Epstein, R. M., Flowers, K., & Beckman, H. B. (1999). Soliciting the patient's agenda: Have we improved? *Journal of the American Medical Association, 281,* 283-287.

Parran, T. (1997). Prescription drug abuse: A question of balance. *Medical Clinics of North America, 8,* 967-978.

Piette, J. D., Heisler, M., & Wagner, T. H. (2004). Cost-related medication underuse: Do patients with chronic illnesses tell their doctors? *Archives of Internal Medicine, 164,* 1749-1755.

Pretorius R.W., & Zurick GM. (2009) A systematic approach to identifying drug-seeking patients. *Family Practice Management, 15*(4), A3-A5.

Sagall, R. J. (2006). Can your patients afford the medications you prescribe? *Family Practice Management, 13*(4), 67-69. Retrieved February 9, 2011, from www.aafp.org/fpm/2006/0400/p67.html

Smedley, B. D., Stith, A. Y., & Nelson, A. R. (Eds.) (2002). *Unequal treatment: Confronting racial and ethnic disparities in health care.* Committee on Understanding and Eliminating Racial and Ethnic Disparities in Health Care, Board on Health Sciences Policy, Institute of Medicine. Washington, DC: National Academies Press.

Thompson, T. L., Robinson, J. D., & Beisecker, A. E. (2004). The older patient-physician interaction. In J. F. Nussbaum, & J. Coupland (Eds.), *Handbook of communication and aging research* (2nd ed.). Mahwah, NJ: Lawrence Erlbaum Associates.

Tindall, W. N., & Clasen, M. E. (2007). *Medication needs of the ambulatory elderly in geriatric pharmacotherapy: A guide for the helping professional.* Washington, DC: American Pharmacists Association.

U. S. Census Bureau. (2010). American Fact Finder. Retrieved October 2, 2011, from http://factfinder2.census.gov/faces/nav/jsf/pages/searchresults.xhtml

A Body Systems Approach to Conscientious Prescribing

Drugs Used in the Treatment of Bone and Joint Disorders

chapter 4

Sabry Gabriel, Mona M. Sedrak, James R. Davis

CHAPTER FOCUS

Rheumatoid arthritis (RA), osteoarthritis (OA), and gout, all of which may produce pain in one or more joints, are discussed in this chapter. There is no cure for these conditions; thus, medical treatment focuses on alleviating joint pain and improving joint mobility and function. NSAIDs and cyclooxygenase (COX-1, COX-2) compounds are prescribed for pain. Disease-modifying anti-rheumatic drugs (DMARDs), gold salts, and tumor necrosis factor (TNF) agents are used to improve joint mobility and function, and colchicine, allopurinol (Zyloprim), probenecid (Benemid), and sulfinpyrazone (Anturane) are used to treat gout.

OBJECTIVES

After reading and studying this chapter, the student should be able to:

1. State the pharmacological interventions involved in treatment algorithms for osteoarthritis and rheumatoid arthritis.
2. Recall the uses of NSAIDs, their appropriate doses, and their common adverse effects and contraindications.
3. Describe salicylism, its symptoms, and its treatment.
4. Explain COX-1 and COX-2 enzyme activity.
5. Describe DMARDs, give examples of them, and state how they are used to treat rheumatoid arthritis.
6. Explain how gold salts are used as anti-rheumatic drugs.
7. Describe two TNF treatments that are made by DNA synthesis and used in rheumatoid arthritis.
8. Describe the pharmacology of the drugs used to treat gout.

Key Terms

Agranulocytosis
Antipyretic
Cyclooxygenase
Disease-modifying anti-rheumatic drugs (DMARDs)
Gout
Interleukin-1
Lipoxygenase
Monoclonal antibodies
NSAID
Osteoarthritis (OA)
Rheumatoid arthritis (RA)
Salicylism
Tumor necrosis factor (TNF)

DRUGS USED FOR THE TREATMENT OF COMMON BONE AND JOINT DISORDERS

Drugs Used in the Treatment of Osteoarthritis
NSAIDs
  acetaminophen
  aspirin
  meclofenamate (generic)
  diclofenac (Voltaren)
  indomethacin (Indocin)
  sulindac (Clinoril)
  ibuprofen (Motrin)
  ketoprofen (Orudis)
  naproxen (Anaprox)
  oxaprozin (Daypro)
  meloxicam (Mobic)

  piroxicam (Feldene)
  nabumetone (Relafen)
  ketorolac (Toradol)
  etodolac (Lodine)
Cyclooxygenase-2 (COX-2) Inhibitors
  celecoxib (Celebrex)
Drugs Used in the Treatment of Rheumatoid Arthritis
Disease-Modifying Anti-rheumatic Drugs (DMARDs)
  methotrexate (Folex, Rheumatrex)
  leflunomide (Arava)
  hydroxychloroquine (Plaquenil)
  penicillamine (Cuprimine)

Gold Salts
  auranofin (Ridaura)
  aurothiomalate (Myochrysine)
  aurothioglucose (Solganal)
Tumor Necrosis Factor (TNF) Modifiers
  etanercept (Enbrel)
  infliximab (Remicade)
  anakinra (Kineret)
Drugs Used in the Treatment of Gout
  allopurinol (Zyloprim)
  colchicine
  probenecid (Benemid)
  sulfinpyrazone (Anturane)

DRUGS USED IN THE TREATMENT OF OSTEOARTHRITIS

NSAIDs

Of the drugs sold in the United States, **NSAIDs**, including aspirin and acetaminophen, are sold the most because of their effect on pain, inflammation, and fever, three clinical signs of many diseases. The fact that NSAIDs do not rely on opiate analgesics to reduce pain is another advantage. Aspirin differs from other NSAIDs in that it has antiplatelet properties in addition to **antipyretic** (fever reducing), analgesic, and anti-inflammatory properties.

Conscientious Prescribing of NSAIDs

- Acetaminophen, in doses up to 1 gm, four times a day, may be prescribed for mild to moderate pain. If the pain progresses to moderate or severe, however, then NSAIDs are more effective because they provide both analgesic and anti-inflammatory actions.
- Chronic high-dose (greater than 2 gm a day) acetaminophen consumption may increase the risk of bleeding in patients on warfarin or hepatotoxicity in patients who abuse alcohol.
- The choice of NSAIDs is typically determined through trial and error and is affected by factors such as adverse effects, cost, duration of action, and patient preferences.
- For patients who have significant gastrointestinal (GI) upset or GI adverse events, an H$_2$ blocker is often prescribed concurrently with an NSAID.
- Ibuprofen and aspirin are the drugs of choice for reduction of fever, but they should not be used for more than 3 days without further evaluation.
- Acetaminophen is the preferred drug for mild to moderate pain if there is no accompanying inflammation, but its use should be limited to no more than 5 days in children and no more than 10 days in adults because it is associated with increased risk of hepatic reactions.
- Age-related decreases in renal and hepatic dysfunction raise the risk of adverse reactions.

Patient/Family Education for NSAIDs

- Compliance is essential. It may take up to 2 weeks to see improvement in arthritic conditions.

- Taking higher-than-recommended doses does not increase the effectiveness of the NSAID, but it does increase the probability of side effects.
- Take with food or milk or antacids if GI side effects occur.
- Take with a full glass of water and remain upright for 15 to 30 minutes afterward.
- Tablets can be crushed and mixed with fluids or water.
- For a more rapid effect, take NSAIDs 30 minutes before food or 2 hours after meals.
- If a dose is missed, take it as soon as possible; however, if it is close to the time of the next dose, skip the missed dose and return to the regular schedule.
- Contact the clinician if signs of hepatic failure (fatigue, lethargy, pruritus, jaundice, upper right-quadrant tenderness, persistent headache, visual disturbances, weight gain, and flu-like symptoms) or GI ulceration (usually manifested as black tarry stool, skin rash, edema, or weight gain) occur.
- Caution patients that consumption of alcohol while using NSAIDs may increase the risk of GI bleeding.
- Coadministration with opioid analgesics may have additive analgesic effects.
- Caution patients to wear sunscreen and protective clothing to avoid photosensitivity reactions.

Mechanism of Action

Wherever inflammation occurs in the body, its destruction of cell membranes results in the release of chemical mediators (cytokines, histamine, leukotrienes, prostaglandins) that can be produced only in the presence of special enzymes (**cyclooxygenase**-1, or COX-1; cyclooxygenase-2, or COX-2; and lipoxygenase). COX-1 is expressed systematically and continuously and is present in all tissues and cells, where it has a role in regulation of platelets, endothelium, and cells of the GI tract and kidney. Because it regulates gastric acid secretion and mucous protection by the lining of the stomach, it is understandable that use of NSAIDs, which inhibit COX-1, can result in adverse effects on the GI tract and kidney. COX-2 is an inducible enzyme that is synthesized in response to pain and inflammation. Most NSAIDs are specific for COX-1 enzymes (aspirin, indomethacin, piroxicam), whereas some are selective for the COX-2 enzyme (celecoxib) and inhibit the synthesis of prostaglandins required for inflammation to occur.

Pharmacokinetics

■ Absorption: Rapidly and completely from the GI tract.
■ Distribution: Crosses the placenta; naproxen enters breast milk; ibuprofen does not enter breast milk; protein binding for all is 90% to greater than 99%.
■ Metabolism: Mostly metabolized by the liver.
■ Excretion: In urine.
■ Half-life: Children (under 8 years), 8 to 17 hours; adolescents (8 to 14 years), 8 to 10 hours; adults (over 14 years), 10 to 20 hours.

Clinical Uses

■ Reduction of body temperature in febrile patient (antipyretic).
■ Relief of mild to moderate pain (analgesic).
■ Suppression of inflammation (anti-inflammatory) due to sprains, strains, or chronic pain.

Dosage and Administration of Common NSAIDs

Chemical Class	Generic Name	Trade Name	Route	Typical Dosage
PROPIONIC ACIDS				
	ibuprofen	Advil, Motrin	PO	200–800 mg 3–4 times/day
	ketoprofen	Orudis	PO	25–75 mg 3–4 times/day
	oxaprozin	Daypro	PO	600–1,800 mg/day
	naproxen	Naprosyn Aleve	PO	250 mg 4 times/day
ACETIC ACIDS				
	diclofenac	Voltaren, Cataflam	PO	50–75 mg 2–3 times/day
	indomethacin	Indocin	PO	25 mg 2–3 times/day
	sulindac	Clinoril	PO	150–200 mg 2 times/day
FENAMIC ACID				
	meclofenamate		PO	50–100 mg every 6 hr
	mefenamic acid	Ponstel	PO	500 mg STAT, then 250 mg 4 times/day
OXICAMS				
	meloxicam	Mobic	PO	7.5–15 mg/day
	piroxicam	Feldene	PO	20 mg/day
PYRROLIZINE CARBOLIC ACID				
	ketorolac	Toradol	PO	10 mg every 4–6 hr, max 40 mg/day
NAPTHYL- ALKANONES				
	nabumetone	Relafen	PO	500–1,000 mg 2 times/day
PYRANO- CARBOXYLIC ACID				
	etodolac	Lodine	PO	300–500 mg 2 times/day
COX-2 INHIBITORS				
	celecoxib	Celebrex	PO	100–200 mg 1–2 times/day

Adverse Reactions

DERM (dermatological): Rashes.
EENT (ear, eye, nose, and throat): Amblyopia, blurred vision, tinnitus.
GI (gastrointestinal): GI bleed, nausea, vomiting, peptic ulcerations, abdominal pain, diarrhea, flatulence, dyspepsia.
GU (genitourinary): Cystitis, hematuria, renal failure.
HEM (hematological): Coagulation disorders, prolonged bleeding times.
META (metabolic): NSAIDs uncouple oxidative phosphorylation, which results in energy being wasted as heat or fever. Severe metabolic (ketolactic) acidosis with compensatory respiratory alkalosis, which may be acute or chronic, may develop with severe salicylate intoxication (salicylism, Box 4-1).
MISC (miscellaneous): Allergic reactions, including anaphylaxis.
NEURO (neurological): Headache, dizziness, drowsiness, psychic disturbances.
SALICYLISM: Poisoning by NSAIDs and salicylates.

Interactions

■ May limit cardioprotective effect of low-dose aspirin.
■ May increase hypoglycemic effects of insulin and oral hypoglycemics.

BOX 4-1 Salicylism

Salicylism is mild, chronic salicylate intoxication that may occur after repeated administration of high doses of NSAIDs. It is common among those who self-medicate with any drug in this class. Symptoms consist of headache, dizziness, tinnitus, hearing loss, mental disturbances, sweating, thirst, hyperventilation, nausea, vomiting, and sometimes diarrhea. More marked CNS effects, including excess stimulation, incoherent speech, vertigo, tremor, delirium, hallucinations, convulsions, and coma; skin eruptions of various types; and changes in acid-base balance develop with more severe intoxication. Hyperthermia is usually present, and dehydration often occurs. Nausea, vomiting, and abdominal pain are commonly present.

The onset of chronic salicylism may be insidious; elderly individuals may consume an increasing amount over several days to alleviate arthralgias, subsequently becoming confused because salicylate pharmacokinetics change at higher concentrations. This may lead to a perpetual spiral of increased salicylate consumption and increased confusion. Similar scenarios occur in persons with underlying psychiatric disorders. A mortality rate of 1% can be expected, and a morbidity rate of 16% is usually associated with patients having acute overdose of NSAIDs.

Treatment must begin immediately and is currently aimed at augmenting elimination of salicylate via the urine or, in more severe cases, directly from the blood by hemodialysis or exchange transfusion. Gastric lavage or induction of emesis will prevent further absorption if performed within 1 to 2 hours after ingestion. Activated charcoal may be given to absorb medication left in the stomach.

■ May see additive adverse effects with concurrent administration of aspirin (ASA), other NSAIDs, corticosteroids, or alcohol.

■ May see increased risk of bleeding with Cefotan, valproic acid, thrombolytics, warfarin, and drugs affecting platelet function.

■ Increased risk of bleeding with natural products such as arnica, chamomile, garlic, ginger, ginseng, ginkgo, and others.

Contraindications

■ Comorbid factors that increase the risk of NSAID-induced GI bleeding are a history of ulcer disease, advanced age, poor health, smoking, and alcohol use.

■ Patients with renal impairment, heart failure, or hypertension (HTN) should not take NSAIDs.

■ Cross-sensitivities exist with other NSAIDs, including aspirin, especially for persons with asthma, ulcer disease, or chronic alcohol use.

■ Women who are pregnant may find persistent pulmonary hypertension in their newborn infants. NSAIDS are contraindicated during the third trimester as they may cause the premature closure of the ductus arteriosus, which connects the pulmonary artery to the heart, soon after the baby's birth.

■ Use cautiously in patients who are elderly, chronic alcohol users, or have ulcer disease.

Acetylsalicylic acid (Aspirin)

Discovered in the late 1800s, aspirin's exact mechanism of action was not known until the discovery of prostaglandins almost 100 years later. Acetylsalicylic acid (aspirin) serves as the prototype drug for the nonnarcotic analgesics. It possesses analgesic, antipyretic, anti-inflammatory, and antiplatelet properties. It is also considered an NSAID.

Mechanism of Action

Aspirin (acetylsalicylic acid) is a weak organic acid with a pKa of 3.5. The breakdown of acetylsalicylic acid into acetic acid and salicylate often leads to the vinegar-like odor of old aspirin tablets. Aspirin has five dose-related actions:

1. Analgesic action: Aspirin relieves low- to moderate-intensity pain, such as headache, myalgia, arthralgia, and other pains arising from integument structures. Aspirin may also be effective against chronic postoperative pain or pain associated with inflammation.

2. Antipyretic action: Aspirin lowers elevated body temperature. Body temperature is maintained at a set point that is regulated by the hypothalamus; during fever, the set point is at a higher level. The salicylates reset the "thermostat" for normal temperature, and heat loss is enhanced as a result of cutaneous vasodilation and sweating. Salicylates do not reduce exercise-induced hyperthermia.

3. Anti-inflammatory effects: Salicylates are used in the treatment of rheumatic diseases. Again, inhibition of prostaglandin and thromboxane synthesis is the mechanism of anti-inflammatory action. Generally, higher doses are required for effective anti-inflammatory action, as compared to analgesic and antipyretic doses. This may be related to the concept that COX-2 plays a more prominent role than does COX-1 in the inflammatory process and that aspirin is a much more effective inhibitor of COX-1 than is COX-2. COX-2 is induced by cytokines and other mediators of nflammation. Aspirin does not inhibit the formation of leukotrienes via the **lipoxygenase** pathway.

4. Antiplatelet effect: Aspirin significantly reduces the incidence of stroke and myocardial infarction in patients at risk. In even the lowest therapeutic doses, aspirin produces a measurable prolongation of bleeding time. This effect is due to alteration of platelet aggregation.

5. Acetylation effect: Aspirin covalently acetylates a serine at the active site of platelet cyclooxygenase, thereby reducing the formation of thromboxane A2, which promotes platelet aggregation. Because the acetylation of the enzyme is irreversible, the inhibitory effect of aspirin on platelet aggregation lasts for up to 8 days, until new platelets are formed.

Pharmacokinetics

■ Absorption: Orally ingested salicylates are rapidly absorbed, partly from the stomach and mostly from the upper small intestine. Significant plasma concentrations are found at 30 minutes after ingestion; peak concentrations may be seen at 1 to 2 hours after ingestion. Absorption occurs by passive diffusion of the nonionized form. Absorption from enteric-coated preparations may be erratic and slow.

■ Distribution: Salicylates rapidly distribute throughout the body, primarily by pH-dependent passive diffusion. Salicylate is highly bound to plasma proteins (primarily albumin but also beta-globulins), and it cross the placenta and enters breast milk.

■ Metabolism: Metabolism of salicylates takes place primarily in the liver microsomal system and mitochondria. The primary metabolites are conjugated with glycine (salicyluric acid) and glucuronic acid (an ether glucuronide and an ester glucuronide). Salicylate metabolism demonstrates biphasic kinetics; at high and toxic doses metabolism is limited and occurs according to zero-order kinetics, whereas at lower doses metabolism proceeds according to first-order kinetics. This difference in rate of metabolism is very important from the standpoint of drug accumulation with repeated administration of high doses.

■ Excretion: Salicylate is excreted in the urine as the free compound and as conjugate metabolites. The amount of unchanged salicylate excreted may vary between 10% (acid urine) and 85% (alkaline urine). As the pH of the urine increases (alkalization), procedures can markedly enhance salicylate clearance from a low of 2% to 3% up to 80%.

■ Half-life: The half-life for salicylate is 3 to 6 hours in low doses and 15 to 30 hours at high doses.

Clinical Uses

■ Anti-inflammatory
■ Antipyretic

■ Analgesic
■ Cardiovascular disease

Dosage and Administration

Generic Name	Trade Name	Route	Dose	Indication
acetylsalicylic acid (aspirin)	Aspirin (generic)	PO	325 mg–650 mg 4–6 times/day, 40–80 mg/day	Relief of mild pain and fever
				Antiplatelet
			1 gm 4–6 times a day	Moderate arthritic pain

Adverse Reactions

CV (cardiovascular): Hypotension, tachycardia, dysrhythmias, edema.

DERM: Rash, angioedema, urticaria.

EENT: Hearing loss, tinnitus.

GI: Nausea, vomiting, dyspepsia, heartburn, GI ulceration, gastric erosions, duodenal ulcers, hepatotoxicity, increased transaminases, hepatitis.

GU: Interstitial nephritis, proteinuria, blood urea nitrogen (BUN) and serum creatinine increases, papillary necrosis.

HEM (hematological): Prolonged prothrombin times, iron-deficiency anemias, thrombocytopenia.

MISC: ANAPHYLAXIS, Reye's syndrome, low birth weight, STILLBIRTH, prolonged labor.

MS (musculoskeletal): Rhabdomyolysis, weakness.

NEURO: Fatigue, insomnia, nervousness, agitation, confusion, dizziness, headache, lethargy, hyperthermia, coma.

PUL (pulmonary): Asthma, bronchospasm, dyspnea, hyperpnea, tachypnea, respiratory alkalosis

Interactions

■ At low doses, aspirin can block the actions of probenecid (a gout medication).
■ Aspirin displaces plasma proteins and may affect concentrations of other NSAIDs.
■ Aspirin blocks active transport of penicillin from cerebrospinal fluid (CSF) to blood.

Contraindications

■ Treatment of acute cases of gout.

Acetaminophen (Tylenol)

Acetaminophen (Tylenol) is an alternative to aspirin because of its analgesic and antipyretic properties. This agent is ineffective as an anti-inflammatory agent and is not considered useful as the sole long-term therapy in rheumatic disease. Acetaminophen lacks several of the undesirable effects of aspirin; however, in situations of acute overdose it can cause fatal hepatotoxicity.

Mechanism of Action

Acetaminophen does not produce the gastric irritation, erosion, and bleeding characteristic of aspirin, nor does it show cross-hypersensitivity, yet its mechanism of action remains elusive. Because it has no action on COX-1 and COX-2, acetaminophen has no anti-inflammatory action and, more important, does not cause GI adverse events. Acetaminophen inhibits a previously unknown COX-3 substance in the brain and spinal cord, which explains its ability to reduce fever and pain without causing the unwanted GI side effects (Botting & Ayoub, 2005). Acetaminophen inhibits the synthesis of prostaglandins that serve as mediators of pain and fever, primarily in the central nervous system (CNS).

Pharmacokinetics

■ Absorption: Absorption is incomplete and varies by dosage form.
■ Distribution: 8% to 40% is bound to protein.
■ Metabolism: At normal doses acetaminophen is converted by microsomal enzymes in the liver to sulfate and glucuronide metabolites.
■ Excretion: Metabolites are excreted in the urine.
■ Half-life: 1 to 4 hours; may be prolonged in elderly.

Clinical Uses

■ Relief of mild to moderate pain.
■ Reduce fever.

Dosage and Administration

Generic Name	Trade Name	Route	Dose	Indication
acetamino-phen	Tylenol, generic	PO	Adults and children > 14 years: 325–650 mg every 4–6 hr	Mild to moderate pain and fever
			Not to exceed 4 gm/day in patients with renal impairment	
			Children <12 years should receive not more than (NMT) 5 doses/24 hr without guidance from a health professional	
			Adults: up to 1 gm 4 times/day, not to exceed 4 gm/day	Osteoarthritis

Adverse Reactions

DERM: rash, urticaria.

GI: hepatic failure, hepatotoxicity (overdose).

GU: renal failure in high doses or chronic use.

Interactions

■ Chronic high doses increase the risk of bleeding.
■ Hepatotoxicity is additive with other drugs, especially alcohol.
■ Barbiturates increase the risk of liver damage.

Contraindications

■ Products containing alcohol, aspartame, sugar, saccharin, or tartrazine should be avoided in those with sensitivities or intolerance to them.
■ Use cautiously in those with hepatic or renal disease.

Conscientious Considerations

■ Overall health and alcohol use should be assessed before recommending/prescribing.
■ Overall prescription use should be reviewed before recommending.

Patient/Family Education

■ Advise patients to take exactly as recommended and *not* to exceed recommended dosages.
■ Remind patients that excessive use is more than 4 gm a day, and it can lead to hepatotoxicity. (Box 4-2).
■ Adults should not take for more than 10 days and children for more than 5 days.

BOX 4-2 Acetaminophen Poisoning (Tylenol Toxicity)

In acute overdose, acetaminophen produces a dose-dependent, potentially fatal hepatic necrosis that runs a course of 7 to 8 days:

Day 1: nausea, vomiting, diaphoresis, vomiting

Day 1–2: liver enzymes, alanine aminotransferase (ALT), bilirubin, and prothrombin rise

Day 3–4: peak hepatotoxicity

Day 7–8: death or recovery

Acute acetaminophen toxicity should be referred to a Poison Control Center hospital. If that is not possible, obtain a serum concentration of acetaminophen as soon as possible and perform gastric lavage if it has been less than 4 hours since ingestion of the drug. Renal tubular necrosis may occur as well as anemia, neutropenia, pancytopenia, and thrombocytopenia. Normally, acetaminophen is metabolized through conjugation either as a sulfate or as a glucuronide. With toxic doses, this system is saturated, and microsomal enzymes produce other metabolites, which can bind sulfhydryl groups on cell constituents. These metabolites are normally inactivated by glutathione. If glutathione stores are depleted by large amounts of metabolites resulting from toxic doses, then hepatic damage ensues.

Treatment of acute overdose of acetaminophen must begin immediately and includes removal of the remaining drug from the stomach, supportive therapy, and initiation of therapy to protect against hepatic damage.

The hepatotoxicity caused by acetaminophen is delayed, and the patient may appear to improve after initial GI symptoms subside (24 to 48 hours after ingestion). However, after 36 to 72 hours, hepatic enzymes, bilirubin, and prothrombin time become abnormal as hepatic injury occurs.

Protection against hepatic damage may be obtained by early administration of sulfhydryl compounds to inactivate the toxic metabolites. *N*-acetylcysteine (Mucomyst, Mucosal; 10% or 20% Acetadote solution) is effective if given less than 24 hours after ingestion of acetaminophen, and it is even more effective when administered within 10 hours.

■ Remind patients to avoid alcohol (more than three glasses a day increases risk of hepatotoxicity).
■ If parents are giving liquid preparations to children, be sure they know understand the dosage. Incorrectly measured amounts and misunderstanding of "cc," "mL," and "tsp" measurements have led to many hospitalizations.
■ If patient is diabetic, acetaminophen may alter blood glucose.
■ If routine fever or pain is not relieved in 3 days, the clinician should be contacted.

Misoprostol (Arthrotec, Cytotec)

The gastric mucosal injury produced by NSAIDs, including aspirin, especially in those patients at high risk (aged patients, those with a history of ulcers, debilitated patients), can be prevented by an agent that increases the production of mucus lining the stomach (a cytoprotective effect) and by decreasing gastric acid secretion (antisecretory effect).

Mechanism of Action

Misoprostol is a synthetic prostaglandin (E_1) analogue with antisecretory and mucosal protective properties. Misoprostol affects basal and nocturnal acid secretion to protect against antiprostaglandin synthesis of NSAIDs and prevent the gastric ulceration that NSAIDs are known to create.

Pharmacokinetics

■ Absorption: Rapid after oral administration.
■ Distribution: Good oral bioavailability because of its methyl group.
■ Metabolism: Misoprostol acid, the chief active metabolite, occurs in parietal cells.
■ Excretion: Urine.
■ Half-life: 20 to 40 minutes.

Clinical Uses

■ Patients with OA at high risk of developing gastric and duodenal ulcers.

Dosage and Administration

Generic Name	Trade Name	Route	Dose	Indication
misoprostol	Arthrotec, Cytotec	PO	200 mcg 4 times/day orally, with or after meals and at night	Antiulcer

Adverse Reactions

GI: Abdominal pain, diarrhea, dyspepsia, nausea, flatulence, vomiting.
NEURO: Headache.
OB/GYN: Miscarriage, menstrual disorders.

Interactions

■ May see increased toxicity of methotrexate, digoxin, cyclosporine, lithium.
■ May increase K+ when used with K+-sparing diuretics.

Contraindications

- Pregnancy: Increases uterine contractility.
- Do not use in patients sensitive to prostaglandins.

Conscientious Considerations

- Avoid use of antacids with magnesium salts because diarrhea usually occurs.

Patient/Family Education

- Patient should be instructed to take medication as a full course of therapy. If a dose is missed, the patient should take it as soon as remembered but not double the dose.
- Emphasize that patients should not share this medication.
- Inform patients that this medication may induce spontaneous abortion. They must use more than one form of contraception throughout therapy; if pregnancy is suspected, they should stop taking misoprostol and notify their clinician.
- Patients should be informed that they may experience diarrhea or black tarry stools that may persist for up to a week.
- Advise patients to avoid alcohol and any other foods that can cause an increase in GI irritation.

Ibuprofen (Advil, Motrin, Nuprin)

Ibuprofen is primarily used for its anti-inflammatory properties but also because of its effectiveness at relieving mild to moderate pain. Ibuprofen also has antipyretic properties. Its antiplatelet activity exists only while the NSAID is in the blood; thus, NSAIDs are not used for antiplatelet therapy, as is aspirin.

Mechanism of Action

Ibuprofen belongs to the group of propionic acid derivatives that inhibits the enzyme cyclooxygenase (prostaglandin synthesis), which catalyzes the transformation of unsaturated fatty acids to prostaglandins. The inhibition of prostaglandin synthesis is the reason for the analgesic, antipyretic, and anti-inflammatory actions of the drug.

Pharmacokinetics

- Absorption: Absorbed and rapidly bound to protein (usually albumin).
- Distribution: Hepatic (hydroxylate and carboxylate derivatives).
- Metabolism: Hepatic metabolism via oxidation.
- Excretion: Renal.
- Half-life: 2 to 4 hours.

Clinical Uses

- Mild to moderate pain.
- Musculoskeletal aches and pains (joint pain, back pain) because of its anti-inflammatory properties.
- Antipyretic.
- Rheumatoid arthritis.
- Osteoarthritis.
- Dysmenorrhea.

Dosage and Administration

Generic Name	Trade Name	Route	Dose	Indication
ibuprofen	Advil, Motrin, Nuprin	PO	400, 600, or 800 mg 3–4 times/day, not to exceed 3.2 gm/day	Osteoarthritis Rheumatoid arthritis
			400 mg every 4–6 hr	Mild to moderate pain
			Children 6 mo–12 years 5 mg/kg for temp <39.1°C (102.5°F)	Fever reduction

Adverse Reactions

CV: Arrhythmias, edema.
DERM: Rashes.
EENT: Amblyopia, blurry vision, tinnitus.
HEM: Prolonged bleeding time, thrombocytopenia.
GI: GI bleeding, hepatitis, constipation, dyspepsia, nausea, vomiting.
MISC: Anaphylaxis.
NEURO: Headache, dizziness, drowsiness, psychic disturbances.

Interactions

- May limit the cardioprotective effect of low-dose aspirin.
- May increase the hypoglycemic effects of insulin and oral hypoglycemics.
- May see additive adverse effects with concurrent administration of ASA, other NSAIDs, corticosteroids, or alcohol.
- May see increased risk of bleeding with Cefotan, valproic acid, thrombolytics, warfarin, or drugs affecting platelet function.
- Increased risk of bleeding with natural products such as arnica, chamomile, feverfew, garlic, ginger, ginseng, gingko, and others.
- **Note:** All NSAIDs have drug interactions with anticoagulants, beta adrenergic blockers, hydantoins, lithium, loop diuretics, probenecid, and salicylates.

Contraindications

- Cross-sensitivity in those sensitive to ASA and other NSAIDs.
- Use cautiously in patients with CV, renal, or hepatic disease, especially the elderly.
- Chewable tablets of ibuprofen contain aspartame, which is contraindicated in those sensitive to it and those with phenylketonuria.

Conscientious Considerations

- Use caution when prescribing NSAIDs for those on multiple drug therapy because drug interactions are many.
- Use with caution in pregnancy.
- Even though isolated cases of severe gastric complications in association with ibuprofen use are observed, this is the anti-rheumatic agent with the best tolerance. Its handicap is its short duration, which can be circumvented with slow-release preparations. The anti-inflammatory effect usually only

commences after a few days of treatment with high doses. Slow-release preparations have low GI side effects (compared with aspirin and indomethacin) and mid-level potency.

Meloxicam (Mobic)

Meloxicam is another popular NSAID used as a nonopioid analgesic.

Mechanism of Action

By increased inhibition of the enzyme cyclooxygenase, meloxicam (Mobic) decreases biosynthesis of prostaglandin.

Pharmacokinetics

- Absorption: Plasma levels peak at 4 to 5 hours.
- Distribution: Unknown.
- Metabolism: Cytochrome P450 enzymes in liver metabolize to inactive metabolites.
- Excretion: Metabolites are excreted in urine and feces.
- Half-life: 15 to 20 hours.

Clinical Uses

- Rheumatoid arthritis, including juvenile rheumatoid arthritis.
- Osteoarthritis.
- Anti-inflammatory.
- Analgesic.
- Antipyretic activity.

Dosage and Administration

Generic Name	Trade Name	Route	Dose
meloxicam	Mobic	PO	7.5 mg daily, but some patients benefit at 15 mg once daily (do not exceed 15 mg)

Adverse Reactions

CV: Edema.
DERM: Stevens-Johnson syndrome, toxic epidermal necrosis.
GI: GI bleeding, abnormal liver function tests, diarrhea, dyspepsia, nausea.
HEM: Anemia, leukopenia, thrombocytopenia.

Interactions

- May reduce antihypertensive effects of ACE inhibitors.
- May reduce diuretic effects of furosemide and thiazide diuretics.

Contraindications

- Cross-sensitivity with other NSAIDs.

Conscientious Considerations

- Significantly less GI toxicity when compared with other NSAIDs such as piroxicam.
- Use cautiously in those with cardiovascular disease or impaired renal function, especially the elderly.

Patient/Family Education

- Same as for acetaminophen and NSAIDs listed previously.

Cyclooxygenase-2 (COX-2) Inhibitors

Although the COX-1 and COX-2 isomers each play a role in the production of prostaglandins from arachidonic acid, COX-2 is released on initiation of inflammation, whereas COX-1 is present in all cells. COX-1 and COX-2 inhibitors both blunt the effects of inflammation and provide analgesia, but the COX-2 agents are relatively free of GI side effects. However, COX-2 inhibitors may produce NSAID-associated nephrotoxicity because the human kidney expresses COX-2, which means it plays a role in maintaining normal physiological function.

Celecoxib (Celebrex)

Celecoxib (Celebrex) is the only remaining COX-2 inhibitor on the market; rofecoxib (Vioxx) and valdecoxib (Bextra) were removed from the market by the Food and Drug Administration (FDA) in 2005 and 2009 following lengthy court proceedings.

Mechanism of Action

Celebrex inhibits prostaglandin synthesis by decreasing the activity of the enzyme COX-2. At therapeutic levels there is little to no effect on COX-1 because this is a highly selective COX-2 inhibitor. Celebrex does not exhibit any antiplatelet activity, which is an advantage over other NSAIDs.

Pharmacokinetics

- Absorption: Orally with good absorption; peak plasma levels at 2 to 4 hours.
- Distribution: Bound extensively to plasma proteins.
- Metabolism: Metabolized by the CYP2C9 enzyme in the liver.
- Excretion: Carboxylic acid and glucuronide metabolites are excreted in urine and feces.
- Half-life: 11 hours.

Clinical Uses

- Rheumatoid arthritis.
- Osteoarthritis.
- Dysmenorrhea.

Dosage and Administration

Generic Name	Trade Name	Route	Dose
celecoxib	Celebrex	PO	100–200 mg 1–2 times/day for arthritis

Adverse Reactions

CV: Lower extremity edema and HTN, increased risk of myocardial infarction (MI) and stroke.
DERM: Rash; swelling of the hands, feet, ankles, or lower legs; itching.
GI: Stomach pain, diarrhea, heartburn, black and tarry stools, red blood in stools, bloody vomit, unexplained weight gain, GI bleeding.
GU: Renal toxicity is worse than with other NSAIDs because of high expression of COX-2 in the kidney.

MISC: Extreme tiredness, flu-like symptoms.

NEURO: Headache.

Interactions

■ Can enhance the effects of warfarin when used in conjugation with it.

■ Interacts with diazepam, glyburide, norethindrone, ethinyl estradiol, omeprazole, dextromethorphan, and aspirin.

Conscientious Considerations

■ Use cautiously in those with renal failure and cardiovascular disease.

Patient/Family Education

■ Patients should be instructed to take this medication exactly as prescribed and be advised that increasing its dosage does not increase its effectiveness.

■ Ask patients to notify their clinician if signs of hepatotoxicity occur, such as nausea, fatigue, flu-like symptoms, jaundice, lethargy, pruritus, and upper right-quadrant tenderness.

■ Ask patients to report if pregnancy is planned or suspected.

PRACTICAL PHARMACOLOGY OF DRUGS USED IN THE TREATMENT OF RHEUMATOID ARTHRITIS

Treatment options for RA have expanded widely with the introduction of biological DMARDs, which are designed to prevent further joint damage and loss of joint function and decrease the amount of pain at the joint. In mild cases of RA, NSAIDs, glucocorticoid joint injections, or low doses of prednisone may be indicated. However, as the disease progresses, patients with RA who stay on NSAIDs are twice as likely as patients with OA on NSAID therapy to have serious NSAID complications. Since NSAIDs are not a cure, do not alter the course of the disease, and do not prevent joint destruction, other options should be sought.

DMARDs are a diverse group of chemicals that alter the course and progression of RA. The American College of Rheumatology classifies DMARDs as biological response modifiers (BRMs), such as **tumor necrosis factor (TNF)** agents that restore or repair the immune system so that it can fight arthritis and rheumatic disease, or as nonbiological DMARDs. Examples of TNF agents are etanercept (Enbrel), adalimumab (Humira), anakinra (Kineret), abatacept (Orencia), efalizumab (Raptiva), infliximab (Remicade), leflunomide (Arava), rituximab (Rituxan), golimumab (Simponi),

▌SPOTLIGHT ON OSTEOARTHRITIS

Osteoarthritis (OA), the most common joint disorder in the United States, affects 70 million people. Complicating their osteoarthritis is the fact that patients with arthritis tend to be sedentary, which leads to other debilitating conditions such as obesity, heart disease, diabetes mellitus, and hypertension (HTN). Although there is no known cure for OA, there are many pharmacological and nonpharmacological treatment options, leading to a great deal of self-medication. Nonpharmacological treatments include weight loss, range of motion exercises, strength training exercises, and prosthetics that maintain joint function and minimize pain. The use of pain-relieving drugs is guided by the degree of joint dysfunction and pain. For example, if joint pain is mild, then acetaminophen (Tylenol) up to 1 gm, four times a day, will likely control the discomfort, but when the pain moves from mild to moderate, then NSAIDs are usually administered. NSAID use in OA is primarily based on patient preference, trial and error, cost, observable duration of action, and lack of adverse reactions, especially GI upset. The use of NSAIDs has increased progressively, owing in part to their availability without a prescription. Despite their common ability to cause gastrointestinal side effects, they are assumed to be well tolerated and are used by millions of people throughout the United States as therapy for mild pain and mild inflammation; however, NSAIDs have been implicated in approximately 7,600 deaths and 76,000 hospitalizations annually in the United States (Frech & Go, 2009). Such statistics have led scientists to pursue new agents to treat pain syndromes, leaving clinicians to treat patients with agents that protect the gastric mucosa. For example, misoprostol, a synthetic prostaglandin analogue, was once commonly used, but serious side effects were seen

with therapeutically effective dosages; thus, its clinical application has become limited.

Medications provide only temporary symptom relief; they do not cure osteoarthritis. Clinicians must educate patients who take certain agents intended for short-term use about the serious adverse reactions that may occur if the drug is taken for a prolonged period of time. Patients also need to know that externally applied medications, such as the warming agent methyl salicylate or the cooling agent camphor or menthol, do very little to warm or cool deeper layers of skin where arthritis is a problem. These agents also may have a strong odor and leave the skin feeling greasy, especially if they have an ointment base.

Osteoarthritis causes more people to seek alternative therapy than any other condition. For example, the use of glucosamine, which is found in oyster and crab shells, and chondroitin, which comes from shark and cow cartilage, became popular in the 1990s. It is believed that the effect of both drugs on chondrocytes is to increase production of proteoglycans and in so doing possibly yield an anti-inflammatory effect and regenerate articular cartilage. The mechanism of action of chondroitin remains theoretical, but it may produce compounds that improve viscoelasticity and hydration properties within the joint. Chondroitin does exert anti-inflammatory effects and inhibits extracellular proteases that metabolize connective tissues. The net effect of both drugs is to control cartilage matrix integrity and bone mineralization, but a paucity of evidence exists to prove this. However, both drugs are free of serious side effects so there is little risk in their use. All clinicians have a role in helping patients with osteoarthritis understand the appropriate roles of rest, exercise, and diet and that they should be careful using unproven therapies. A treatment algorithm for osteoarthritis is shown in Figure 4-1.

Continued

SPOTLIGHT ON OSTEOARTHRITIS—cont'd

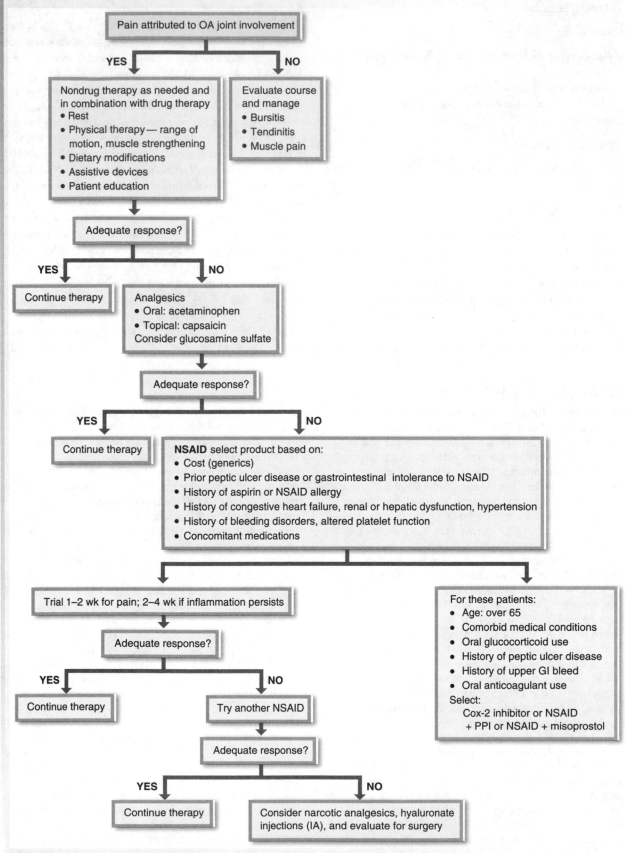

FIGURE 4-1 Osteoarthritis treatment algorithm. *Courtesy of American College of Rheumatology.*

and natalizumab (Tysabri). Examples of nonbiological DMARDs are NSAID/hydroxychloroquine, methotrexate (Azithroprine), gold salts, prednisone, and cyclophosphamide.

It is hoped that within 1 year of taking a DMARD, the patient will experience a 50% improvement in symptoms; thus DMARD therapy is long-term. The American College of Rheumatology (ACR) has updated its guidelines on using DMARDs and suggests that most patients start on a treatment regimen using either methotrexate or leflunomide (Arava) and that patients with a high level of disease or poor prognosis may be given DMARDs as first-line treatment (American College of Rheumatology Press Release, 2010).

Disease-Modifying Anti-rheumatic Drugs

DMARDs influence the disease process of rheumatoid arthritis by preventing bone loss and cartilage erosion. Depending on patient responses, it is not uncommon to administer one or more of these drugs at the same time. DMARDs can be lifesaving and effective, but drugs such as methotrexate may produce only an 18% to 20% reduction in symptoms after 1 year (Katz et al., 1997). As the practice of rheumatology has developed, it has been shown that the earlier DMARDs are introduced into the treatment regimen, the better the patient outcomes; thus, early diagnosis of the disease is critical. Physicians who specialize in treating RA were very cautious about DMARD use until research showed that the DMARD side effect profile is no worse than that of NSAIDs (O'Dell, 1997).

Conscientious Prescribing of DMARDs

- When DMARDs are used as monotherapy, they are ineffective. Thus, they are prescribed in combination with biological modifiers (etanercept, infliximab) or in multiple drug regimens, including NSAIDs, other DMARDs, and sometimes corticosteroids, in all but the mildest forms of RA.
- NSAIDs as monotherapy should be given a trial of no longer than 3 months before adding a DMARD is considered in patients who do not achieve adequate response to NSAIDs alone. If adequate response is achieved with a DMARD, an NSAID can be used as needed in many patients.
- Corticosteroids can be used in these three situations: early in treatment to provide symptomatic relief while waiting for a DMARD to work, in low doses chronically for patients who fail to get an adequate response from a DMARD, and in bursts to treat acute flare-ups of disease.

Patient/Family Education for DMARDs

- Pharmacotherapy is only a part of the therapeutic regimen, which should include physical therapy, exercise, and rest. Assistive devices and orthopedic surgery also may be necessary in some patients.
- Patients require careful monitoring for toxicity and therapeutic benefit for the duration of treatment.

Methotrexate (Rheumatrex)

Methotrexate is an antimetabolite; thus, it is used as an antineoplastic and an immunosuppressive as well as a DMARD. It can be used alone or in combination with other treatment modalities.

Mechanism of Action

Methotrexate is a folate antimetabolite that inhibits DNA synthesis. Its mechanism of action is unknown when used in the treatment of arthritis, but it appears to act as a cell antiproliferative with multiple effects.

Pharmacokinetics

- Absorption: Readily absorbed from the GI tract in small doses; large doses are somewhat incompletely absorbed.
- Distribution: Slow delivery to body spaces, and certain sites may act as a storage and slow-release area for the drug.
- Metabolism: Minimally metabolized because hepatic enzymes convert methotrexate to an inactive metabolite.
- Excretion: Up to 90% of any unchanged dose and metabolites are excreted in the urine.
- Half-life: 3 to 10 hours (low doses); 8 to 15 hours (high doses).

Clinical Uses

- Psoriasis.
- Systemic lupus erythematosus.
- Sarcoidosis.
- Antifolate chemotherapeutic drug in treatment of lung, head and neck, and breast cancers and leukemia.
- Rheumatoid arthritis.

Dosage and Administration

Generic Name	Trade Name	Route	Dose
methotrexate	Rheumatrex	PO or IM	7.5 mg–25 mg weekly

Adverse Reactions

EENT: Blurred vision, transient blindness.
DERM: Alopecia, photosensitivities, pruritus, urticaria.
GI: Nausea, mucosal ulceration, hepatotoxicity, anorexia, stomatitis, vomiting.
GU: Infertility.
HEM: Anemia, leukopenia, thrombocytopenia.
MISC: Nephropathy, chills, fever, soft tissue necrosis.
MS: Hyperuricemia, osteonecrosis, stress fractures.
NEURO: Dizziness, headache, malaise, drowsiness.
PUL: Pulmonary fibrosis.

Interactions

- Hematological toxicity increases when given with high doses of salicylates, NSAIDs, oral hypoglycemics, tetracyclines, or sulfonamides.
- Liver or kidney disease may be induced when methotrexate competes with any drug for excretion.
- Concomitant use with herbals such as echinacea and melatonin interfere with immunosuppression.
- Caffeine will lower the effect of methotrexate.

Contraindications

- Methotrexate is teratogenic; women must wait one menses before trying pregnancy, and men should wait 3 months.

Conscientious Considerations

- Methotrexate has a low incidence of side effects when prescribed on a low-dose, weekly schedule.
- Although it may decrease the efficacy of treatment, leucovorin can be used to reduce the toxicity of methotrexate (does not reverse neurotoxicity).
- Elderly people are at risk because of decreased renal and hepatic function.

Patient/Family Education

- Instruct patients to take dosages exactly as prescribed.
- Instruct patients to report *any* side effects.
- Instruct patients to avoid crowds and persons with any infections.
- Instruct patients to use a soft toothbrush and an electric shaving razor and to avoid falls.
- Instruct patients to ask their clinician before using any over-the-counter medications.
- Instruct patients to use sunscreen to avoid photosensitivity reactions.
- Instruct patients to refrain from receiving any vaccinations unless they first talk with their clinician.

Leflunomide (Arava)

Leflunomide is an immunomodulator drug that was introduced in 1998 to reduce the signs and symptoms of rheumatoid arthritis and to slow the progression of its associated joint damage.

Mechanism of Action

This DMARD inhibits de novo ribonucleotide synthesis and triggers p53 translocation to the nucleus of the cell (arrests the cell in the G_1 phase). In effect, this agent inhibits an enzyme required for pyrimidine synthesis, which in turn allays pain and inflammation, slows structural progression of the disease, and improves joint function.

Pharmacokinetics

- Absorption: 80% rapidly absorbed.
- Distribution: 99% bound to protein.
- Metabolism: Rapidly converted to an active metabolite.
- Excretion: About one-half in feces; about one-half in urine.
- Half-life: 14 to 18 days.

Clinical Uses

- To slow progression of rheumatoid arthritis and joint destruction.

Dosage and Administration

Generic Name	Trade Name	Route	Dose
leflunomide	Arava	PO	Loading dose is 100 mg daily for 3 days, then 20 mg/day. If intolerance develops, decrease dose to 10 mg/day

Adverse Reactions

DERM: Alopecia, pruritic rash, dry skin.
EENT: Rhinitis, sinusitis.

HEM: T and B cells undergoing rapid DNA synthesis; cell turnover is affected the most severely by the drug's actions.
GI: Diarrhea, nausea, abdominal pain, abnormal liver enzymes, hepatotoxicity.
META: Hypokalemia, weight loss.
MISC: Paresthesia, flu-like symptoms, infections.
MS: Back pain, arthralgia, leg cramps, synovitis.
NEURO: Headache, dizziness, weakness.
PUL: Bronchitis, cough.

Interactions

- Concurrent use with any hepatotoxic drug will increase the likelihood of hepatotoxicity.

Contraindications

- Pregnancy or the possibility of pregnancy.
- Liver disease.

Conscientious Considerations

A patient's range of motion and degree of swelling and pain in affected joints must be assessed before and during therapy. Watch for elevated bilirubin and elevated alkaline phosphatase.

Patient/Family Education

- Instruct patients to take exactly as directed.
- Caution patients of childbearing age that leflunomide has teratogenic effects.
- Explain that the patient may experience dizziness and should avoid tasks requiring alertness or driving until the medication's effect is known.
- ASA, NSAIDs, or low-dose corticosteroids may be continued during therapy, but clinicians need to know *all* other drugs the patient is taking.
- Discuss the potential for hair loss and how to cope with it.
- Instruct patients to avoid vaccinations.

Hydroxychloroquine (Plaquenil)

This drug has been used for decades to suppress malaria and is now used in the treatment of severe rheumatoid arthritis and systemic lupus erythematosus.

Mechanism of Action

It is unclear how hydroxychloroquine works in rheumatoid arthritis, but it is suspected that it decreases the T-cell response to mitogens.

Pharmacokinetics

- Absorption: The drug is absorbed rapidly in the GI tract. It is safer given orally than intramuscularly or subcutaneously.
- Distribution: Relatively slow rate.
- Metabolism: Liver CYPs (cytochrome P450s) create two active metabolites through biotransformation.
- Excretion: Renal clearance of the active metabolites in the urine.
- Half-life: 30 to 60 days.

Clinical Uses

- Antirheumatic.
- Systemic lupus erythematosus.

Dosage and Administration

Generic Name	Trade Name	Route	Dose
hydroxychloroquine	Plaquenil	PO	Usually dosed at 5 mg/kg/day to initiate therapy in RA: 400–600 mg 1 time/day, then maintain at 200–400 mg/day divided 2 times/day

Adverse Reactions

DERM: Skin rashes, pruritus, exacerbation of psoriasis, bleaching of hair, alopecia.
EENT: Ototoxicity, tinnitus, visual disturbances, retinopathy.
GI: Cramps are common; anorexia, diarrhea, vomiting, hepatic failure.
HEM: Agranulocytosis, aplastic anemia.
MS: Myopathy.
NEURO: Seizures, aggressiveness, anxiety, apathy, fatigue, headache, irritability, personality changes, psychoses.

Interactions

■ May increase risk of hepatotoxicity when administered with drugs with biliary excretion .
■ May increase risk of dermatological reactions when administered with any drug having a known risk of such a reaction.

Contraindications

■ History of liver or renal disease or use of alcohol.

Conscientious Considerations

■ Eye examinations should be performed frequently because hydroxychloroquine can cause irreversible retinopathy with resultant blindness.
■ Not often used as a first-line treatment choice, but rather as a drug to try when others have failed.

Penicillamine (Cuprimine)

Penicillamine is a heavy-metal DMARD that chelates copper, iron, mercury, and lead to form complexes, resulting in the promotion of copper excretion. It also combines with cystine-forming complex to reduce formation of cystine stones and prevent renal calculi.

Mechanism of Action

Its mechanism of action as a DMARD is unknown, but it is thought to decrease cell-mediated immune responses and inhibit new collagen formation, thus acting as an anti-inflammatory.

Pharmacokinetics

■ Absorption: When given orally, about one-half of the dose is absorbed.
■ Distribution: Protein binds to albumin.
■ Metabolism: Hepatic biotransformation in small amounts.
■ Excretion: Metabolites found in both feces and urine, but mostly it is excreted unchanged.
■ Half-life: 1.7 to 3.2 hours.

Clinical Use

■ Rheumatoid arthritis.

Dosage and Administration

Generic Name	Trade Name	Route	Dose
penicillamine	Cuprimine	PO	500–700 mg/day as a maintenance dose; start with 125–250 mg/day and increase over 1–3 months

Adverse Reactions

DERM: Rash.
GI: Anorexia, nausea, vomiting, altered taste, oral ulcers, glossitis.
GU: Proteinuria, nephrotoxicity, hematuria.
HEM: Leukopenia, aplastic anemia, agranulocytosis, and thrombocytopenia; may see white papules at venipuncture
MISC: Hot flashes, drug fever.
NEURO: Headache.

Interactions

■ Cross-reactivity with penicillin may cause urticaria or produce macular reactions.
■ Magnesium and aluminum hydroxide antacids block absorption.

Contraindications

■ Pregnancy.
■ Aplastic anemia.
■ Renal failure.

Conscientious Considerations

Although it is rarely used, approximately 75% of patients respond to this metal chelator, but the effect takes months to establish.

Gold Compounds

Gold salts such as auranofin (Ridaura), aurothioglucose suspension (Solganal), and sodium aurothiomalate (Myochrysine) have been used for over 65 years to treat inflammation in patients who do not respond to other drug therapies. However, because these agents are very slow acting and toxic, they are agents of last resort. Myochrysine is used in treating juvenile arthritis. Gold salts are rarely used today because TNF agents are available.

Mechanism of Action

The mechanism of action (MOA) by which gold compounds alter cellular mechanisms such as collagen biosynthesis, enzyme synthesis, and immune responses remains unclear. Some believe the compounds interfere with **interleukin-1** (IL-1), a protein that is a major mediator of joint disease, and TNF-alpha. One popular theory is that gold is taken up by mononuclear cells and inhibits their phagocyte function, which in turn reduces the release of anti-inflammatory mediators. Gold salts administered orally have a slower onset of action than gold salts given intramuscularly (IM), and whereas oral gold is less efficacious, it is better tolerated. IM gold salts are used for suppression of synovitis during the active stages of rheumatoid arthritis, but they are not a cure.

Pharmacokinetics

■ Absorption: Auranofin is 29% gold and is moderately absorbed from the GI tract; aurothioglucose is 50% gold with slow, erratic absorption after IM administration.

■ Distribution: Gold readily binds to albumin (95% to 99%) and accumulates in many tissues, especially liver, kidney, bone marrow, spleen, and lymph nodes, as well as the synovium of inflamed joints.
■ Metabolism: Gold sodium thiomalate is metabolized in the liver; others are not.
■ Excretion: It is excreted largely by the kidney, and sometimes by the liver.
■ Half-life: Aurothioglucose, 3 to 27 days; auranofin, 21 to 31 days due to extensive tissue binding; gold sodium aurothiomalate, 5 days.

Clinical Uses
■ Rheumatoid arthritis.
■ Juvenile arthritis.

Dosage and Administration

Generic Name	Trade Name	Route	Dose
aurothioglu-cose	Solganal	IM injection for rheumatoid arthritis	10 mg to start, then 25 mg for 2 doses, then 50 mg weekly thereafter. If there are no signs of toxicity or patient improves, give 50 mg at 3- or 4-month intervals for many years
Gold sodium	Myochrysine	IM injection	Initially 10 mg IM, then 25 mg IM for 2 doses, then auroth-iomalate 50 mg weekly until a total dose of 0.8–1 gm is given. Maintain at 25–50 mg every 2 weeks for next 2–20 weeks
Auranofin	Ridaura	PO	6 mg/day as a single dose or 2 times/day

Adverse Reactions

DERM: Allergic skin rash.
EENT: Oral ulceration.
GI: Nausea, vomiting, GI discomfort, altered taste (very common), constipation.
GU: Proteinuria, nephritic syndrome.
HEM: Blood dyscrasia, agranulocytosis, aplastic anemia.
NEURO: Encephalopathy, peripheral neuropathy.
SERIOUS REACTIONS: Gold toxicity is a possibility, and signs such as decreased hemoglobin (Hb), leukopenia, reduced granulocytes, proteinuria, throat ulcers, and other reactions must be monitored.

Interactions

■ None.

Contraindications

■ Any history of blood dyscrasias.
■ Congestive heart failure (CHF).
■ Dermatitis.
■ Colitis.
■ Concurrent use of antimalarials.

Conscientious Considerations

■ Currently, the use of gold compounds is on the decline, and they are mostly used as second-line drugs. Besides their many toxic effects, they are also expensive. However, benefits have been noted in treating juvenile arthritis with gold compounds.
■ *Any* appearance of side effects, no matter how minor, should be cause for discontinuance.
■ Regular monitoring of urine protein and blood counts should be carried out during treatment.
■ Pruritus is a warning sign for cutaneous reactions.
■ Metallic taste is a warning sign for stomatitis.

Patient/Family Education

■ Unwanted effects will occur in about one-third of patients. They should be taught to watch for mouth ulcerations and skin rashes and to report any such signs to their clinician.
■ If therapy is stopped when the early symptoms appear, the risk of other toxicities appearing is low.

Tumor Necrosis Factor (TNF) Inhibitors

With new drugs such as etanercept (Enbrel), infliximab (Remicade), and anakinra (Kineret), clinicians have access to anticytokine therapy, which is able to target the rheumatoid process. These agents have gained in popularity, but they all have different moieties. Etanercept (Enbrel) is a TNF receptor joined to a human IgG molecule. Infliximab (Remicade) is a mouse/human monoclonal antibody, and anakinra (Kineret) is an agent that blocks interleukin-1. Although there are many other agents on the market, three of the most common are discussed here.

Mechanism of Action

The three DMARDs are similar yet different. Etanercept (Enbrel) is a protein that acts as a TNF inhibitor. It was developed by recombinant DNA synthesis and is designed to interfere with the inflammatory cascade initiated by TNF-alpha and thereby lower circulating cytokines, making them inactive and unable to mediate the inflammatory response of cell surface receptors found in the synovial fluid of patients with rheumatoid arthritis.

Infliximab (Remicade) is a chimeric **monoclonal antibody** (variable murine region linked to common human region) target to TNF-alpha and is specific to the human form only. It neutralizes and prevents the activity of TNF-alpha, resulting in anti-inflammatory and antiproliferative activity.

Anakinra (Kineret) is an antirheumatic agent that acts by blocking the action of interleukin-1, which is found in excessive amounts in the joints of patients with RA. Anakinra is used in moderate to severe RA where, as an antagonist of IL-1 receptors, it reduces pain and inflammation because it is an immunomodulator.

Pharmacokinetics

■ Absorption: Anakinra, no accumulation in tissues or organs is observed after daily subcutaneous doses; etanercept, well absorbed after subcutaneous (SC) administration, Infliximab: IV administration gives complete bioavailability.
■ Distribution: Remains unknown.
■ Metabolism and excretion: Remains unknown.
■ Excretion: Anakinra, in urine; others are unknown.
■ Half-life: Anakinra, 4 to 6 hours; etanercept, 115 hours; infliximab, 7.7 to 9.5 days.

Clinical Uses

■ Etanercept and infliximab are used in moderate to severe RA or for those with an inadequate response to other DMARDs. They may be used concurrently with methotrexate.
■ Crohn's disease that is moderate to severely active.

Dosage and Administration

Generic Name	Trade Name	Route	Dose
etanercept	Enbrel	SC	25 mg twice a week
infliximab	Remicade	IV using sterile technique	3 mg/kg followed by 3 mg/kg 2 and 6 weeks after initial dose, then every 8 weeks thereafter. May be adjusted every 4 weeks depending on patient response.
anakinra	Kineret	SC	100 mg once a day

Adverse Reactions

DERM: Erythema.
GI: Abdominal pain, nausea, vomiting, constipation, flatulence, oral and tooth pain.
GU: Dysuria.
HEM: Neutropenia.

MISC: Life-threatening infections, pain and pruritus at injection site, infusion reactions.
MS: Low back pain, involuntary muscle spasm, myalgia.
NEURO: Headache, fatigue, anxiety, paresthesia.
PUL: Bronchitis, cough, dyspnea, increased upper respiratory infections (URIs), rhinitis.

Interactions

■ None.

Contraindications

■ Patients with serious infections.
■ Use in children.
■ Hypersensitivity to proteins in the formulations.
■ Pregnancy.
■ People with infections or tuberculosis.

Conscientious Considerations

■ Use cautiously in patients who have been treated for more than 2 years.
■ TNF has a key role in host defense mechanisms. It is believed its long-term suppression might increase infections or malignancies, but few instances are reported in the literature as yet.
■ Patients must be screened for latent or active tuberculosis as a precautionary measure.
■ Assess patients for pain and range of motion prior to and periodically after beginning use of these agents.

Patient/Family Education

■ Advise patients of potential adverse reactions (myalgia, rash, fever, pruritus), which can occur 3 to 12 days after administration.
■ Patients on either etanercept or infliximab should be cautioned against getting infections.
■ Advise patients to contact their clinician if any symptoms of toxicity occur.
■ Because these drugs may cause dizziness, caution is required until response is known.

SPOTLIGHT ON RHEUMATOID ARTHRITIS

Rheumatoid arthritis (RA) affects 1.3 million Americans (Helmick et al., 2008), and one in three people who are diagnosed with RA become severely disabled. It affects 2.5 times as many women as it does men, and the average age of onset is 66.8 years (Helmick et al., 2008). The joint changes associated with rheumatoid arthritis represent an autoimmune reaction characterized by the following three signs:
a) Increased presence of inflammatory cytokines (interleukin 1 (IL-1), and tumor necrosis factor (TNF-alpha) both of which play a central role in regulation of immune and inflammatory responses).
b) Proliferation of the synovium.
c) Erosion of cartilage and bone.
　Although NSAIDs relieve pain and inflammation of rheumatoid arthritis, they do nothing to halt the loss of bone. DMARDs are a chemically diverse group of drugs that slow the progression of joint erosion; all DMARDs have different capabilities, mechanisms of action, and applications for use.
　The benefits of DMARDs were discovered by serendipity and clinical intuition. Their effects have resulted in more bewilderment than understanding, even after decades of experimentation. DMARDs take weeks to months to exert their effects and are often used in combination with other DMARDs and NSAIDs. In the past, DMARDs were used only when NSAIDs had failed. Current thinking is to employ them early for aggressive treatment of the disease. The cost of treating a patient suffering from RA is about $10,000 per year, and use of drugs such as etanercept or infliximab can add another $12,000. This is one reason why sales of alternative therapies are flourishing. A treatment algorithm for rheumatoid arthritis is shown in Figure 4-2.

Continued

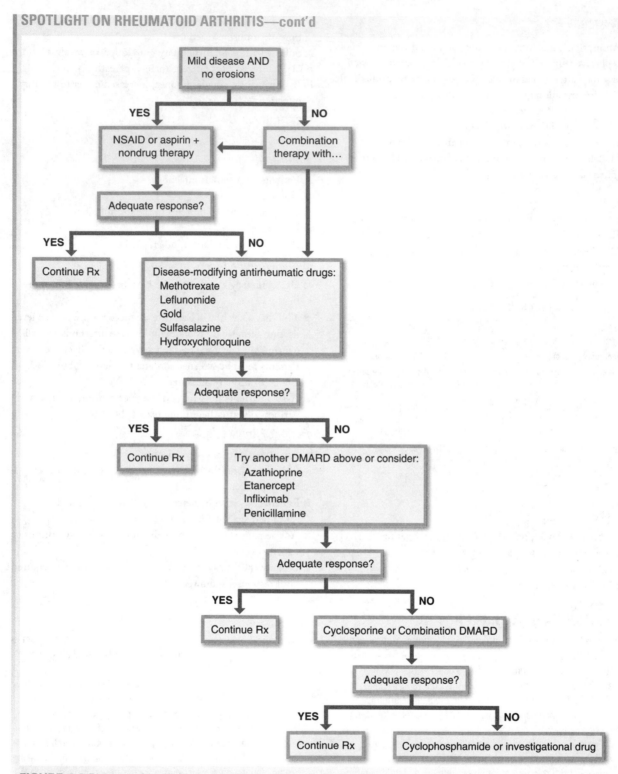

FIGURE 4-2 Rheumatoid arthritis treatment algorithm. *From Rindfleish, A. J. (2005). Diagnosis and Management of Rheumatoid Arthritis. American Family Physician, 72(6), 1037. Copyright 2005 by American Academy of Family Physicians. Reprinted with permission.*

DRUGS USED TO TREAT GOUT

Gout is a disorder associated with an inborn error of uric acid metabolism, which results in high levels of circulating levels of uric acid in the blood. As the amount of uric acid circulating in the blood rises, it tends to deposit as uric acid crystals in the cartilage of the body, especially the big toe, ankle, instep of the foot, knee, and elbow. The crystals deposited into these joints tend to grow larger to the point that they can become quite painful. They may be seen as deposits along the margin of the ear (tophi), but they can also deposit in the kidney (nephritis) and cause scarring of blood vessels (sclerosis). They are also a cause of arthritis.

Drugs used to treat gout are designed to end a painful attack, prevent the formation of uric stones in the kidney, and prevent complications from uric stone (calculus) formation in the joints. The drugs used to treat an acute attack include colchicine, probenecid (Probalan), allopurinol (Zyloprim), sulfinpyrazone (Anturane), the corticosteroids, and the NSAIDs. The NSAIDs have no effect on the underlying uric acid metabolism, but they do relieve the pain of an acute gout attack.

Conscientious Prescribing of Drugs Used to Treat Gout

- All health professionals need to be aware that any patient taking low doses of aspirin is at risk for an attack of gout because aspirin interferes with uric acid excretion.
- A clinician should first determine the cause of the hyperuricemia and then decide how to treat it. For example, certain foods, such as bananas and peaches, are high in urates and can raise blood levels. Dietary changes, along with medication, may be necessary.

Patient/Family Education

- Patients must be educated to avoid alcohol because it increases serum levels of urates.

Allopurinol (Zyloprim)

Allopurinol is a structural analogue of the natural purine base hypoxanthine. It is used to prevent gout and renal calculi caused by either uric acid or calcium oxalate and to treat uric acid nephropathy, hyperuricemia, and some solid tumors. It has been on the market for decades, and there are at least 65 branded products and countless generic manufacturers.

Mechanism of Action

Allopurinol inhibits the enzyme xanthine oxidase, blocking the conversion of the oxypurines hypoxanthine and xanthine into uric acid. Allopurinol also facilitates the incorporation of hypoxanthine and xanthine into DNA and RNA, resulting in further reductions of serum uric acid concentrations.

Pharmacokinetics

- Absorption: Orally ingested and absorbed rapidly from the GI tract (better than 90%).
- Distribution: Peak plasma concentrations occur within 60 to 90 minutes, but protein binding is negligible. Allopurinol does enter breast milk.
- Metabolism: Metabolized in the liver to oxypurinol, a metabolite with a long half-life.
- Excretion: Excreted either unabsorbed in the feces or unchanged in the urine. Oxypurinol is excreted in the urine.
- Half-life: 1 to 2 hours for allopurinol; 18 to 30 hours for oxypurinol.

Clinical Uses

- Chronic gouty arthritis.
- Prevention of uric acid calculi.

Dosage and Administration

Generic Name	Trade Name	Route	Dose
allopurinol	Zyloprim	PO	Management of gout: 100 mg/day to start, maintain at 100–200 mg 2–3 times/day
		IV	Management of hyperuricemia: 600–800 mg/day in divided doses

Adverse Reactions

DERM: Rash following injection; if the rash is severe, consider it toxic; urticaria.
GI: Diarrhea, hepatitis, nausea, vomiting.
GU: Renal failure.
HEM: Bone marrow depression.
MISC: Sensitivity reactions possible after prolonged use.
NEURO: Drowsiness.

Interactions

- Increases the half-life of probenecid and enhances its uricosuric effect. Probenecid increases the clearance of the active oxypurinol; therefore, dosages must be increased when a patient is taking probenecid.
- Allopurinol inhibits metabolism of azathioprine and 6-mercaptopurine, which require normal purine synthesis for action.
- With angiotensin-converting enzyme (ACE) inhibitors, allopurinol has produced Stevens-Johnson syndrome (fever, arthralgias, skin eruptions).
- Aluminum hydroxide antacids inhibit the response to allopurinol.

Contraindications

- Nursing mothers and children.
- Patients with a history of hypersensitivity reactions.

Conscientious Considerations

- May see increased attacks of gout during initial treatments.
- Serum uric acid needs to be monitored, and normal levels may take 1 to 3 weeks to achieve.

Patient/Family Education

- Take with food and a full glass of water.
- Avoid alcohol.
- Check to see if patient is taking dicumarol because allopurinol increases the anticoagulant effect.

Colchicine (generic)

Even after several hundred years of use, this is a drug whose mechanism of action remains unknown. Because its anti-inflammatory properties have been observed over a long period of time, its use continues while research on its mechanism continues. Colchicine does not affect levels of uric acid in the circulatory system.

Mechanism of Action

Colchicine is a plant alkaloid believed to interfere with the ability of white blood cells (leukocytes) to perpetuate an inflammatory response resulting from monosodium urate crystal deposits in the synovial fluid of joints.

Pharmacokinetics

- Absorption: Occurs rapidly but varies with peak plasma concentrations and ranges from 0.5 to 2 hours.
- Distribution: Highest concentrations are in liver, spleen, and kidney with protein binding 30% to 50%, but it concentrates in white blood cells (WBCs).
- Metabolism: Colchicine reenters the biliary tract by biliary secretion and is reabsorbed by the intestines.
- Excretion: Excreted primarily in feces with some in urine.
- Half-life: 20 minutes in plasma, 60 hours in WBCs.

Clinical Use

Use is mostly restricted to the treatment of acute gout attacks. Relief is usually seen in affected joints in 12 hours, with all symptoms disappearing by 48 hours.

Dosage and Administration

Generic Name	Route	Dose
colchicine	IV	2 mg initially, then 0.5 mg every 6 hr
	PO	0.6–1.2 mg at onset of attack; repeat each hr until relief of acute attack, up to 2–3 days

Adverse Reactions

DERM: Alopecia.
GI: Nausea, vomiting, diarrhea, abdominal pain.
GU: Anuria, hematuria, renal damage.
HEM: Agranulocytosis, aplastic anemia, leukopenia, thrombocytopenia.
MISC: Phlebitis at injection site.
NEURO: Peripheral neuritis.

Interactions

- May see additive GI effects when combined with any NSAID.

Contraindications

- Patients with cardiac, renal, hepatic, or GI diseases because toxicities may be cumulative.
- Avoid use in those with renal impairment; if must be used, reduce dosage.
- Safety has never been established in lactating women.

Conscientious Considerations

- Colchicine overdose can be fatal.
- Once dosing limit has been reached, do not take any colchicine for 21 days.

Patient/Family Education

- Patient must review administration schedule and understand that if a dose is missed, it should be taken ASAP but not doubled.
- Patients taking prophylactic colchicine should not increase doses if a gouty attack occurs. It is preferable to get a steroid injection (intrasynovial) or use an NSAID.
- Patient must follow the clinician's advice regarding diet, weight loss, and alcohol consumption.
- Patient should stop medication if *any* type of GI symptoms appears.
- Surgery or dental work can precipitate gouty attacks; thus, confer with a clinician at least 3 days before any procedure.

Probenecid (Probalan)

Probenecid is an agent used to treat hyperuricemia and chronic gouty arthritis. It lowers serum levels of urates by competitive inhibition in the renal tubules. This ability gives it a role to play in increasing circulating levels of antibiotics as an adjunct to antibiotics such as penicillin and some of the cephalosporins. This competitive inhibition of probenecid at both renal and proximal tubules results in increased serum concentrations and effectiveness of these antibiotics, which is important when treating sexually transmitted diseases (STDs) such as gonorrhea, pelvic inflammatory disease (PID), and syphilis.

Mechanism of Action

- Inhibits renal tubular reabsorption of uric acid, thus promoting its renal secretion and preventing high serum levels of uric acid.

Pharmacokinetics

- Absorption: Occurs completely after oral administration. Peak plasma concentrations present at 2 to 4 hours.
- Distribution: Will cross the placenta.
- Metabolism: Hydroxylated to metabolites that retain their carboxyl function and uricosuric activity.
- Excretion: Only a small amount is released in the urine.
- Half-life: Ranges from less than 5 hours to more than 17 hours.

Clinical Uses

- Chronic gout.
- Patients with gonorrhea or neurosyphilis (by delaying the excretion of penicillin).

Dosage and Administration

Generic Name	Trade Name	Route	Dose
probenecid	Probalan	PO	500 mg 2 times a day for 7 days

Adverse Reactions

DERM: Flushing, rashes.
GI: Nausea, vomiting, abdominal pain, diarrhea, sore gums, drug-induced hepatitis.
GU: Uric acid stones, urinary frequency.

HEM: Aplastic anemia.
NEURO: Headache, dizziness.

Interactions

■ Blood levels of many drugs are increased in the presence of probenecid.
■ Probenecid increases the clearance of the active form of allopurinol.

Contraindications

■ Patients with renal failure.

Conscientious Considerations

Monitor patients' intake and output of fluids for urate stone formation.

Patient/Family Education

■ Patients should be instructed not to take aspirin or other salicylates because they decrease the effects of probenecid.
■ Patients should be told that erratic dosing schedules may cause raised levels of uric acid and precipitate an attack of gout.
■ Any side effects, particularly bruising, should be reported immediately to the clinician.
■ Patients may be given sodium bicarbonate or potassium citrate to alkalize the urine.
■ Patients need to drink 2,000 to 3,000 mL of fluid per day.

Sulfinpyrazone (Anturane)

This agent is similar in action to probenecid, but it inhibits reabsorption of urates only at the proximal tubule, thus increasing urinary uric acid excretion.

Mechanism of Action

Inhibits the renal tubular reabsorption of uric acid, thus increasing its secretion and thereby decreasing serum blood levels of uric acid.

Pharmacokinetics

■ Absorption: Occurs completely after oral administration. Peak plasma concentrations present at 2 to 4 hours.
■ Distribution: Widely in serum.
■ Metabolism: Metabolized in liver to four active metabolites that contribute to its effect.
■ Excretion: About 50% is released unchanged in the urine. The rest is excreted as the active metabolites.
■ Half-life: Between 2.7 and 6 hours.

Clinical Use

Uricosuric agent used in the treatment of chronic gout.

Dosage and Administration

Generic Name	Trade Name	Route	Dose
sulfinpyrazone	Anturane	PO	100–200 mg PO initially, then increase to 1 dose of 400–800 mg every other day

Adverse Reactions

DERM: Rash, flushed face.
GI: Nausea, vomiting, stomach pain.
GU: Frequent urge to urinate.
HEM: Agranulocytosis and aplastic anemia. **Note:** Sulfinpyrazone is a sulfonamide; thus, like any sulfonamide, it can cause agranulocytosis, aplastic anemia, and other hemolytic disorders in patients who are deficient in glucose-6-phosphate dehydrogenase.
NEURO: Headache, dizziness.

Interactions

■ Will interact with acetaminophen, causing increased risk of toxicity.
■ Reduces hypotensive effect of beta blockers.
■ Inhibits warfarin metabolism.

Contraindications

■ Patients with underlying blood dyscrasias.
■ Patients with renal failure.

Conscientious Considerations

Clinicians need to monitor complete blood count (CBC) and WBC.

SPOTLIGHT ON GOUT

Gout results from the precipitation of urate crystals within the tissues. It can arise from the overingestion, underexcretion, or overproduction of urate. Hyperuricemia sets up an environment that limits solubility and encourages the high concentration of urate to begin to crystallize. Gout attacks can be quite painful without proper medication, and these attacks usually occur at the base of the first toe. The treatment depends on whether the patient is dealing with an acute attack or a chronic case. In the acute phase, treatment should focus on managing inflammation. Although it may seem counterintuitive, patients must avoid drugs that could dissolve the urate crystals and alter serum uric acid levels. Acute treatment eases the inflammatory response without spreading the urate crystals throughout the body. Also, it is important to remember to avoid aspirin and other salicylates that may enhance uric acid reabsorption by the kidney at low doses. Chronic treatment includes inhibiting the production of and enhancing elimination of uric acid. Generally, clinicians should counsel patients to avoid foods that are high in purines, such as sweetbreads, anchovies, sardines, liver, kidneys, meat, poultry, fish of all kinds, spinach, oatmeal, and bran, and to limit alcohol intake.

Patient/Family Education

■ Patients can take with milk or food to decrease GI upset.
■ Patients need to be counseled to drink plenty of fluids.
■ Patients should avoid ASA and other salicylates.

Implications for Special Populations

Pregnancy Implications

When prescribing for pregnant females, clinicians should carefully consider their choice of drugs.

Following is a selected list of antiarthritic and antigout drugs, along with their assigned FDA safety category.

FDA PREGNANCY SAFETY CATEGORY	DRUGS
B	Etanercept, infliximab, anakinra, penicillamine, ibuprofen, diclofenac, and other NSAIDs
C	Allopurinol, aurothiomalate, aurothioglucose, hydroxychloroquine, celecoxib, etodolac
D	Colchicines, methotrexate
X	Leflunomide
Unclassified	Probenecid, sulfinpyrazone

Pediatric Implications

NSAIDs are a low-risk alternative for children. The FDA has approved aspirin, ibuprofen, naproxen, and tolmetin for use in children. These agents are used in the treatment of juvenile rheumatoid arthritis and many musculoskeletal syndromes, such as tendinitis. All clinicians should advise patients and their families to minimize GI distress with these agents by giving them with food. Also, because kidney, neurological, and GI adverse events such as pediatric inflammatory bowel disease are associated with these drugs, their use needs to be monitored by the clinician and parents.

Geriatric Implications

Anti-inflammatory drugs such as the NSAIDs have been associated with increased blood pressure among the geriatric population, especially when they have been used in high doses or for long periods of time. They have also been implicated as a contributor in Alzheimer's disease. For the safe use of NSAIDs in the elderly, conduct a BUN and creatine level every 3 months, substitute acetaminophen if possible, and educate the patient to use the lowest dose possible on an as-needed basis. If patients experience an acute flare of arthritis, they should take an NSAID for no longer than 7 to 10 days, then discontinue it. Indomethacin is poorly tolerated by geriatric patients.

DMARDs require 1 to 3 months of use before the patient begins to show signs of improvement. In the elderly, however, normal declines in physiology due to the aging process require their use to be individualized to meet the severity of the disease and any attendant comorbidity. This makes RA treatment in the elderly challenging because of the changes in renal and hepatic function that must be taken into account.

LEARNING EXERCISES

Case 1

J.D. is a 64-year-old African American female taking captopril for the treatment of hypertension. She has recently started taking a nonprescription form of ibuprofen for the aches and pains of osteoarthritis. During her last office visit, her blood pressure was found to be higher than usual at 155/110 mm Hg. Explain the drug interaction and suggest ways to overcome the problem.

Case 2

A.B. is a 65-year-old male who comes to your office for a medical checkup before a big trip. A.B. presents with one complaint. He states, "My left knee and hip hurt more often, but I guess that's a part of getting older." He states that he takes Tylenol, 500 mg about four times a day, when it gets bad, and he tries to walk it off. You check his medical record and find that he also has a mild case of CHF and some mild renal failure (CLcr [creatinine clearance] 50 mL/min). He has also complained of dyspepsia, which he controls by taking an antacid (Mylanta). You discover in the medical record that he has been prescribed lisinopril, 10 mg two times a day, for his mild CHF.

1. **What are the risks and/or advantages of prescribing a conventional NSAID or a COX-2 selective NSAID for A.B.?**

2. **What over-the-counter products should A.B. avoid or use only with caution?**

References

American College of Rheumatology. (2005). *Guidelines for the medical management of osteoarthritis of the joint and hip.* Retrieved December 10, 2012, from www.rheumatology.org/practice/clinical/guidelines/oa-mgmt.asp

American College of Rheumatology. (2010). Press release. *DMARDs, glucocorticoids, and biologics, equally effective for rheumatoid arthritis. Study shows biologics can be reserved for treatment resistant patients.* Retrieved December 10, 2012, from www.rheumatology.org/about/newsroom/2010/2010_01_28.asp

Botting, R., & Ayoub, S. S. (2005). COX-3 and the mechanism of action of paraceptamol/acetaminophen. *Prostoglandins, Leukotrienes, and Essential Fatty Acids, 72*(2), 85-87.

Frech, E. J., & Go, M. F. (2009). Treatment and chemoprevention of NSAID-associated gastrointestinal complications. *Therapeutics and Clinical Risk Management, 4*(1), 65-73.

Helmick, C., Felson, D., Lawrence, R., Gabriel, S., Hirsch, R., Kwoh, C. K., et al. (2008). Estimates of the prevalence of arthritis and other rheumatic conditions in the United States. *Arthritis & Rheumatism, 58*(1), 15-25.

Donahue, K. E., Gartlehner, G., Jonas, D. E., Lux, L. J., Thieda, P., Jonas, B. L., et al. Systematic Review: Comparative Effectiveness and Harms of Disease-Modifying Medications for Rheumatoid Arthritis. *Ann Intern Med.* (2007 Nov. 19).

O'Dell, J. (1997). Combination DMARD therapy for rheumatoid arthritis: apparent universal acceptance. *Arthritis & Rheumatism, 40*(Suppl. 9), 50.

Drugs Used in the Treatment of Eye and Ear Disorders

chapter 5

David E. Burtner, William N. Tindall, Mona M. Sedrak

CHAPTER FOCUS

This chapter focuses on common outpatient disorders of the ears and eyes. These conditions are confronted by clinicians almost daily in primary care settings as inflammatory conditions, acute infections, or allergies. This chapter discusses the anti-infective, anti-inflammatory, and analgesic medications that are commonly prescribed in the clinical setting, as well as ophthalmic agents that are more typically prescribed by ophthalmologists than by primary care clinicians.

OBJECTIVES

After reading and studying this chapter, the student should be able to:

1. Describe the common disorders of the ear and suggested therapy for infections, pain, inflammation, and cerumen impaction.
2. Describe the common diseases of the eye such as conjunctivitis, blepharitis, and glaucoma and suggest a course of therapy for each.
3. Recall the pharmacology and pharmacokinetics of the drugs involved in treating glaucoma.
4. Explain the differences between a mydriatic and a miotic and include examples of each and when each is used.
5. Recall the drugs used to treat dry eyes.
6. Describe the pharmacology of prostaglandin analogues, carbonic anhydrase inhibitors, alpha adrenergic blockers, sympathomimetics, and beta blockers.
7. Describe the pharmacology of the osmotic agent mannitol, including how and when it should be used.

Key Terms

Cellulitis
Cerumen
Conjunctivitis
Corneal abrasion
Cycloplegia
Empirically
Exudative
Miotics
Muscarinic
Mydriatics
Narrow-angle
  glaucoma
Open-angle
  glaucoma
Osmotic
Ototoxicity
Periosteum
Primary and
  secondary
  glaucoma
Rebound congestion

DRUGS USED TO TREAT COMMON EAR DISORDERS

Agents Used in the Treatment of Otitis Externa

Topical Anti-Infectives
ofloxacin (Floxin)
ciprofloxacin with hydrocortisone (Cipro HC Otic)
ciprofloxacin with dexamethasone (Ciprodex)
neomycin/polymyxin B (Cortisporin)
chloroxylenol/pramoxine/hydrocortisone (Cortane)

Acid and Alcohol Solutions
acetic acid/aluminum acetate (Domeboro Solution, Burrow's Solution)
acetic acid/propylene glycol (VoSoL Otic)
isopropyl alcohol/glycerin (Swim-Ear)
isopropyl alcohol/propylene glycol (Ear Sol)

Otic Analgesics
benzocaine/antipyrine/glycerine (Auralgan Otic)
benzocaine/antipyrine/propylene glycol (Tympagesic)

Agents Used in the Treatment of Otitis Media
amoxicillin (Amoxil)

Agents Used in the Treatment of Cerumen Impaction
carbamide peroxide (Debrox, Murine Ear, Auro Ear Drops)
triethanolamine (Cerumenex drops)

DRUGS USED TO TREAT COMMON EYE DISORDERS

Ophthalmic Anesthetics
tetracaine (Pontocaine)
proparacaine (Ophthaine, Ophthetic)

Agents Used in the Treatment of Conjunctivitis

Ophthalmic Anti-Infectives
tobramycin (Tobrex)

sulfacetamide (Bleph-10)
erythromycin
ciprofloxacin (Ciloxan)
gentamicin (Garamycin)

continued

DRUGS USED TO TREAT COMMON EYE DISORDERS—cont'd

moxifloxacin (Vigamox)
polymyxin B/bacitracin (Polysporin)
Ophthalmic Mast Cell Stabilizers
nedocromil (Alocril)
cromolyn sodium (Opticrom, Corlon)
lodoxamide (Alomide)
Ophthalmic Antihistamines
antazoline (Vasocon)
azelastine (Optivar)
epinastine (Elestat)
emedastine (Emadine)
ketotifen (Zaditor)
levocabastine (Livostin)
olopatadine (Patanol)
ketotifen (Refresh Eye Itch Relief, Zaditor)
Ophthalmic Vasoconstrictors
naphazoline
oxymetazoline
tetrahydrozoline
Agents Used to Maintain Ocular Hydration
mineral oil/ white petrolatum (Refresh, Lacri-Lube)

polyvinyl alcohol/povidone (Nature's Tears, Murine Tears)
methylcellulose (Lacrisert)
Agents Used in the Treatment of Glaucoma
Direct and Indirect Acting Miotics
carbachol (Isopto Carbachol)
pilocarpine (Isopto Carpine)
echothiophate (Phospholine)
Prostaglandin Analogues
bimatoprost (Lumigan)
latanoprost (Xalatan)
travoprost (Travatan)
unoprostone (Rescula)
Carbonic Anhydrase Inhibitors
acetazolamide (Diamox Sequels)
brinzolamide (Azopt)
dorzolamide (Trusopt)
methazolamide (Neptazane)
Sympathomimetics
dipivefrin (Propine)
epinephrine (Epifrin, Glaucon)

Alpha-Adrenergic Agonists
brimonidine tartrate (Alphagan)
apraclonidine (Iopidine)
Beta antagonists (blockers)
betaxolol (Betoptic)
carteolol (Ocupress)
levobunolol (Betagan)
metipranolol (OptiPranolol)
timolol (Timoptic)
Osmotics
mannitol
Agents Used for Pupillary Dilation
Alpha-Agonists
phenylephrine
muscarinic antagonists
atropine sulfate
cyclopentolate hydrochloride
homatropine hydrobromide
tropicamide
Ophthalmic Diagnostic Agent
fluorescein

Medications used to treat common eye and ear disorders are often the same as medications used systemically, except that they are packaged in sterile delivery systems for application to the eye and ear. This is especially true of the anti-infectives, analgesics, and anti-inflammatory drugs used to treat ocular infections, inflammation, or other common disorders of the eye and ear. Many internal medicine, geriatric, and family medicine clinicians treat glaucoma; thus, these medications are highlighted in this chapter. Many of these medications can be absorbed systemically and can cause adverse reactions or interact with other medications that the patient may be taking. This chapter also discusses drugs used as eye lubricants, antihistamines, and vasoconstrictors. It is important for every clinician to be aware of drugs that can cause ototoxicities, and these medications are presented as well.

DRUGS USED TO TREAT COMMON EAR DISORDERS

Typical disorders of the ear canal include otitis media, otitis externa, inflammatory conditions, and cerumen impaction. Antibiotics are used to treat bacterial infections, corticosteroids are used to reduce inflammation, local anesthetics are used to reduce pain, and miscellaneous agents such as emulsifiers are used to treat cerumen impaction. Agents such as glycerin, mineral oil, and olive oil emollients are used to relieve pruritus.

Conscientious Prescribing of Otic Preparations

■ Ototopical preparations are both more effective and safer than systemic preparations when used appropriately. Not all ototopical preparations are the same. Two ototopical formulations containing the same antibiotic may differ in pH, viscosity, and the presence of steroids. Consequently, substitution of one preparation for the other is not recommended. For example, substituting a solution of ciprofloxacin for a solution of ofloxacin is more reasonable than choosing a suspension of ciprofloxacin with low pH and high viscosity as a substitute. This type of substitution is reasonable because you are choosing between two compounds of the same chemical classification (i.e., fluroquinolones), thus side effects, mode of action, clinical utility, kinetic activity, etc., will be similar. Ciprofloxacin has better activity against gram-negative bacilli, an advantage which may be negated by ofloxacin's longer half-life and higher serum levels. Therefore, while both drugs are effective as treatments for infections due to gram-negative organisms, ofloxacin is also appropriate in the treatment of infections where both aerobic gram-negative rods and *staphylococci* or *Streptococcus pneumoniae* are documented or suspected, or in urethritis, particularly when *Chlamydia trachomatis* is documented or suspected. In this case, infection of eye and ears respond well to either of these two fluroquinlones. Furthermore, substituting a combination of tobramycin and dexamethasone for a drop containing ciprofloxacin and hydrocortisone may be more appropriate, even though the active agents are different. These drops share the features of low pH and high viscosity, and they are combination products.

■ Before using topical agents, the clinician should ensure that the tympanic membrane is not ruptured.

Patient/Family Education for Otic Preparations

■ A clean cotton plug can be used to keep topical medications in the ear.

■ To prevent contamination, the patient should not touch the applicator to any surface, including the ear.

Agents Used to Treat Otitis Externa

Otitis externa is inflammation of the outer ear canal. One of the key diagnostic signs of otitis externa is pain on movement of the pinna. The ear epithelium is highly innervated, has a close association with the **periosteum**, and has minimal subcutaneous tissue. There is often a history of swimming or other exposure to contaminated water. In these cases, otitis externa is usually caused by a mixed infection of gram-negative rods and fungi.

Therapy should consist of an analgesic as well as an antibiotic. The inflammation and edema of otitis externa can be so severe that they interfere with topical applications of medication, and a cotton wick must be used to deliver it. If the infection seems deep-seated and is classified as **cellulitis** involving the areas around the ear proper, then systemic antibiotics should be used. In these cases fluoroquinolones are often chosen because of their effectiveness against the *Pseudomonas* species. Severe otitis externa with underlying osteomyelitis is called *malignant external otitis* and will generally require hospitalization and parenteral antibiotics. This disease has a high morbidity and mortality, but fortunately it is rare.

Topical Otic Anti-Infectives

The anti-infectives include agents such as mild acids and alcohol that simply make the environment inhospitable for pathogens to reproduce. Fluoroquinolones have broad coverage and affect *Pseudomonas* species. The corticosteroids aid in reducing inflammation and relieving patient symptoms as well as giving better access for topical medicines. Although many over-the-counter (OTC) topical antibiotics contain formulations with Neomycin, this antibiotic has been implicated as the source of serious ototoxicity (Box 5-1), especially when the tympanic membrane has been perforated. Neomycin can also cause contact dermatitis.

Mechanism of Action

Topical anti-infectives work as bacteriostatic agents or bactericidal agents, as do their systemic counterparts. The inclusion of a corticosteroid in these products accounts for their anti-inflammatory, antipruritic, and antiallergenic effects.

Pharmacokinetics

The topically applied antibiotics used to treat bacterial infections are not absorbed through the skin. The amount of any antibiotic that finds its way into the systemic circulation is minimal, and it occurs only if the skin is denuded or abraded or the antibiotic is applied to a large area (such as a burn). Because these antibiotics are not absorbed, the method of metabolism and excretion of these drugs when applied topically remains unknown.

Dosage and Administration

	Generic Name	Trade Name	Route	Usual Adult Daily Dose
ANTI-INFECTIVES WITHOUT STEROIDS	ofloxacin	Floxin	Top.	10 drops in ear daily for 7 days
	neomycin	Myciguent	Top.	Apply up to 3 times/day
	bacitracin	Baciguent		Apply up to 3 times/day
	mupirocin	Bactroban		Apply up to 3 times/day
	polymyxin B/neomycin/ bacitracin (OTC)	Neosporin		Apply up to 3 times/day
ANTI-INFECTIVES WITH STEROIDS	ciprofloxacin/ hydrocortisone	Cipro HC Otic	Top.	3 drops in ear 2 times/day for 7 days
	ciprofloxacin/ dexamethasone	Ciprodex	Top.	4 drops in ear 2 times/day for 7 days
	hydrocortisone/ neomycin/ polymyxin B	Cortisporin Otic	Top.	4 drops in ear 3–4 times/day
	hydrocortisone/ neomycin/ colistin	Cortisporin-TC Otic	Top.	5 drops in ear 3–4 times/day
	chloroxylenol/ pramoxine/ hydrocortisone	Cortane-Aqueous	Top.	4 drops in ear 3–4 times/day

Clinical Uses

■ Inflammatory skin diseases and pruritic dermatoses.

Adverse Reactions

EENT: Ear pain, ear discomfort or irritability, ear residue; OTOTOXICITY with neomycin, which is reversible.

Interactions

■ None

Contraindications

■ Hypersensitivity to the active ingredients or the vehicle

Conscientious Considerations

■ If the product contains the antibacterial Neomycin, it has the potential for ototoxicity, especially if the tympanic membrane has perforated. It also commonly causes contact dermatitis.

■ As with other antibacterial preparations, use of these products may result in overgrowth of nonsusceptible organisms, including yeast and fungi. If the infection is not improved

---

BOX 5-1 Selected Drugs that Cause Ototoxicity

Many systemic drugs affect the ear and hearing. Following is a brief list of common agents that can induce **ototoxicity** (damage to hearing or balance) ranging from reversible tinnitus to irreversible hearing loss.

Analgesics	Aspirin and NSAIDs
Antibiotics	Aminoglycosides
	Clarithromycin
	Erythromycin
	Vancomycin
	Neomycin
Antineoplastic	Cisplatin
	Mechlorethamine
Loop Diuretics	Bumetanide
	Ethacrynic acid
	Furosemide

after 1 week of treatment, cultures should be obtained to guide further treatment.

■ If two or more episodes of ear infections occur within 6 months, further evaluation is recommended to exclude an underlying condition such as cholesteatoma, presence of a foreign body, or a tumor.

Patient/Family Education

■ Instruct patients on the proper way to instill eardrops. The patient should be instructed to lie down or tilt the head so that the affected ear faces up. For adults, gently pull the earlobe up and back to straighten the ear canal. For children, gently pull the earlobe down and back to straighten the ear canal. Drop the medicine into the ear canal. Keep the ear facing up for several minutes so that the medicine can run to the bottom of the ear canal.

■ Instruct patients not to miss any doses. If they miss a dose of this medicine, they should use it as soon as possible. If it is almost time for the next dose, they should skip the missed dose and go back to the regular dosing schedule.

Acid-Alcohol Solutions

One of the defense mechanisms of the ear is keeping an acidic environment that is inhospitable to common pathogens. The ear normally maintains a slightly acidic pH, and these agents supplement this effect. The alcohol also induces a drying out of cellular infective agents.

Mechanism of Action

The inclusion of acetic acid, isopropyl alcohol, propylene glycol, and aluminum acetate (a topical astringent) provides a topical, antibacterial, and antifungal effect. Acetic acid, a weak acid that can inhibit carbohydrate metabolism, causes the subsequent death of the organism.

Pharmacokinetics

■ With these topical agents, systemic pharmacokinetics is not an issue because plasma concentrations are not great enough to be a concern.

Dosage and Administration

Generic Name	Trade Name	Route	Usual Adult Daily Dose
acetic acid/ aluminum acetate	Domeboro Otic Burrow's Otic	Top.	4–6 drops every 3–4 hr until burning sensation stops
acetic acid/ propylene glycol	VoSoL Otic	Top.	5 drops 4 times/day
acetic acid/ propylene glycol/ hydrocortisone	Emadine	Topical	5 drops 4 times/day or 3 times/day for 7–10 days
isopropyl alcohol/glycerine	Swim Ear	Topical	4–6 drops in each ear after swimming or bathing
isopropyl alcohol/propylene glycol	Ear Sol	Topical	6–8 drops in each ear 2 times/day

Clinical Uses

■ Treatment of superficial infections of the external auditory canal caused by organisms susceptible to the action of the antimicrobials and complicated by inflammation (e.g., otitis externa, commonly known as "swimmer's ear").

Adverse Reactions

EENT: stinging or burning due to the acidic pH, local irritation (rare)

Interactions

■ None

Contraindications

■ None

Conscientious Considerations

■ Clinicians must be aware of the important considerations that apply to all otic preparations (see p. 66, Conscientious Prescribing of Otic Preparations).

Patient/Family Education

■ The advisories for patients who are taking these medications (acid alcohol solutions) are the same as for patients taking any other otic preparations (see p. 66, Patient/Family Education Regarding the Use of Otic Preparations).

Otic Analgesics

Topical antipyrine and benzocaine are the most common otic analgesics used. Topical agents must reach the affected area to be effective. Two products commonly used today are combinations of acetic acid and benzocaine/antipyrine/glycerine, sold in a dropper bottle as Auralgan Otic, and benzocaine/antipyrine/propylene glycol drops, sold as Tympagesic.

Mechanism of Action

Antipyrine is an older agent that affects the prostaglandin system and thus has anti-inflammatory effects. It is not used systemically. Benzocaine is one of the anesthetics that works by blocking the nerve sodium channel and terminating signal propagation. It is for topical use only. Glycerin is in these products because it is hygroscopic (attracts or absorbs moisture from the air).

Pharmacokinetics

■ These topical agents develop no serum/plasma concentrations; thus, they are not a pharmacokinetic concern.

Dosage and Administration

Generic Name	Trade Name	Route	Usual Adult Daily Dose
acetic acid/ benzocaine/ antipyrine/ glycerine	Auralgan	Top.	Fill ear canal and insert cotton plug. Repeat every 1–2 hr as needed.
benzocaine/ antipyrine/ propylene glycol	Tympagesic	Top.	Fill ear canal and insert cotton plug. Repeat every 2–4 hr as needed.

Clinical Uses

■ For the treatment of mild pain along external auditory canal

Adverse Reactions

■ None

Interactions

■ None

Contraindications

■ Hypersensitivity
■ Perforation of the tympanic membrane

Conscientious Considerations

■ Ear pain can be quite severe and should not be under-treated. Systemic analgesics are often indicated for symptom relief. Acetaminophen, NSAIDs, and narcotics should be made available as appropriate.
■ Repeated use of topical benzocaine risks sensitizing the patient to subsequent use of an important class of drugs.
■ Clinicians must be aware of the important considerations that apply to all otic preparations (see p. 66, Conscientious Prescribing of Otic Preparations).

Patient/Family Education

■ Advise patients to hold the bottle of medication in their hands for a few minutes to warm it up. Some patients let the bottle sit in a glass of warm water if they want an even warmer sensation.
■ The advisories for patients who are taking these medications (acid alcohol solutions) are the same as for patients taking any other otic preparations (see p. 66, Patient/Family Education Regarding the Use of Otic Preparations).

SPOTLIGHT ON ACUTE OTITIS MEDIA (AOM)

The middle ear is an air-filled cavity directly connected to the nasopharynx by the eustachian tube. It is often involved in acute, self-limiting infections known as acute otitis media (AOM). Although AOM is most common in children, it also affects many adults. AOM is defined as an inflammatory process in the middle ear that produces pain, fever, malaise, feelings of pressure in the ear, and acute hearing loss. Obstruction of the eustachian tube is the most prevalent event associated with AOM. Many times this is triggered by an upper respiratory tract infection (URI) involving the nasopharynx. Although the triggering inflammation is usually viral in origin, approximately half of AOM cases in children are triggered by pathogenic bacteria found in the effusion, with four types predominating: *S. pneumonia, Haemophilus influenzae, Moraxella catarrhalis, and Streptococcus pyrogenes.* Differentiation between bacterial and viral causes of AOM is difficult; thus, clinicians tend to overtreat it with antibiotics, especially when parents and/or patients believe that an antibiotic is necessary for relief of AOM symptoms.

   A number of clinical studies have shown that in uncomplicated cases of AOM using systemic antibiotics produces no better outcome than letting the infection run its course and not treating it with antibiotics. Thus, the American Academy of Pediatrics (AAP) and the American Academy of Family Physicians (AAFP) issued the following guidelines for treatment of AOM:

1. Accurately diagnose AOM and differentiate it from otitis media with effusion (OME), which requires different management.
2. Relieve pain, especially in the first 24 hours, with ibuprofen or acetaminophen.
3. Minimize antibiotic side effects by giving parents of select children the choice to have their children fight the infection on their own for 48 to 72 hours, then starting antibiotics if they do not improve.
4. Prescribe initial antibiotics for children who are likely to benefit the most from treatment.
5. Encourage families to prevent AOM by reducing risk factors. For babies and infants, these factors include breastfeeding for at least 6 months, avoiding bottle propping, and eliminating exposure to passive tobacco smoke.
6. If parents and clinicians agree that antibiotic treatment is best, prescribe amoxicillin for most children (AAP & AAFP, 2004).

Agents Used to Treat Cerumen Impaction

Although the ear is usually self-cleaning, some patients are genetically prone to developing thicker cerumen, which is a combination of cellular debris and material from the glands in the ear canal. Accumulation of cerumen can lead to conductive hearing loss, impaction, and an environment conducive to infections.

   When removing cerumen, clinicians must be conscious of the tender nature of the ear canal and avoid trauma to the tympanic membrane. If irrigation is performed, the water temperature may affect the inner ear canal and trigger a vertigo reaction.

   Ceruminolytics can be used to soften and remove cerumen from the external auditory canal. Ceruminolytics are classified as water-based, oil-based, or non–water-based/non–oil-based. Ceruminolytic products contain carbamide peroxide (Debrox, Murine Ear, Auro Ear Drops), which softens and emulsifies the wax. Some also contain triethanolamine 10% (Cerumenex drops), which is a mineral oil–type compound that softens the wax. Another ceruminolytic contains isopropyl alcohol and glycerin (Swim Ear).

Mechanism of Action

The water-based agents are thought to soften wax by swelling dried ear canal epithelium, which is the major component of cerumen. Oil-based solutions soften cerumen by placing oily glandular material in solution. The cerumen is then removed by either natural cleaning mechanisms or syringe irrigation.

Pharmacokinetics

■ With these topical agents, systemic pharmacokinetics is not an issue because plasma concentrations are not great enough to be a concern.

Dosage and Administration

Generic Name	Trade Name	Route	Usual Daily Administration For Use In Children
carbamide peroxide 6.5%	Debrox Murine Ear	Top.	For children, 1–5 drops per ear 2 times/day; adults, 510 drops per ear 2 times/day.
triethanolamine polypeptide oleate	Cerumenex Drops	Top.	Fill the ear canal with drops and hold the agent in place with a cotton plug to soften the earwax, then flush with warm water.

Clinical Uses

■ Removal of excess or impacted cerumen

Adverse Reactions

EENT: Mild itching, burning, ear pain, erythema of the ear canal

MISC: ALLERGIC REACTIONS—HIVES; DIFFI-CULTY BREATHING; SWELLING OF FACE, LIPS, TONGUE, OR THROAT (REQUIRES EMERGENCY MEDICAL ASSISTANCE)

Interactions

■ None because agent is inert and applied topically.

Contraindications

■ Perforated eardrum
■ Ear discharge, pain, rash, or irritation around the ear

Conscientious Considerations

■ Continue using triethanolamine polypeptide if mild itching, burning, ear pain, or mild erythema of the ear canal occurs. This typically happens if the drops are left in the ear canal for prolonged periods or if the ear is not syringed properly. When the drops remain in the ear for longer than 30 minutes, inflammation occurs.
■ Once softened or emulsified, the cerumen can be removed by irrigation with warm water or saline.
■ Patients who are genetically prone to cerumen occlusion might benefit from preventive scheduled irrigations.

Patient/Family Education

■ Patients who use cotton swabs or other probes often push cerumen farther back into the ear.
■ Patients should be reassured that it is acceptable to get clean, soapy water in their ears.
■ If the ear canal is excoriated, application of steroid or antibiotic drops for 7 to 10 days will prevent otitis externa from developing.
■ If Debrox is used, the patient may hear a bubbling sound inside the ear caused by the foaming action of carbamide peroxide releasing oxygen from the cerumen.
■ Do not use carbamide peroxide for longer than 4 days. Use beyond 4 days can damage the tympanic membrane.
■ Patients should be instructed to wash their hands before and after use of the medications.

DRUGS USED TO TREAT COMMON EYE DISORDERS

The eye, like other areas of the body, is subject to infection, inflammation, allergies, hypersensitivities, pain, and other disorders, such as glaucoma, that affect its ability to function. Many common eye infections such as conjunctivitis, blepharitis, and hordeolum can be treated in the primary care setting. Systemic antibiotics are commonly used to treat these disorders.

Conscientious Prescribing of Common Ocular Preparations

■ Monitor the effectiveness of any therapy, especially if there is a possibility that intraocular pressure (IOP) could become elevated. If IOP does become elevated, referral to a specialist may be necessary.
■ Choice of antibiotics depends on the organism suspected of causing the infection. For example, when *H. influenza* is suspected, sulfacetamide is a good choice. If bacterial conjunctivitis is suspected, bacitracin/polymyxin B (Polysporin) and trimethoprim/polymyxin B (Polytrim) provide antibiotic combinations that are effective against most organisms that cause this infection.
■ In infants and children, erythromycin is effective, and its ointment form is easier to administer than drops.
■ Patients who develop an allergy or other reaction to the preservative in eyedrops may need to use a formulation without a preservative. Many eyedrops are also available in single-use disposable containers.

Patient/Family Education for Common Ocular Preparations

■ Instruct patients on how to use eyedrops before giving them a prescription so that they avoid overuse or underuse of the medication, two common reasons for therapy failure (Box 5-2).
■ Advise patients to avoid touching the dropper to the eye or any other surface to avoid contamination.

Ophthalmic Anesthetics

The word *anesthetic* comes from the Greek word *anaisthesia*, which means loss of sensation. The use of topical anesthetics has been common practice for well over 100 years. Cocaine was first used in the 1860s, procaine in 1904, and tetracaine in 1920, and lidocaine was introduced in 1943 as a means of overcoming the side effects of the others, especially hypersensitivity/allergic reactions (bronchospasm and angioedema). These medications are used to ensure that patients undergoing cataract surgery and other eye procedures are free from pain. There are two classes of drugs used as topical anesthetics, the amino esters (tetracaine, proparacaine) and the amino-amides (lidocaine). At one time, the use of topical cocaine was common, but its use has waned once cocaine became a popular drug of abuse and became tightly regulated. When not used properly, ophthalmic anesthetics can cause deep corneal infiltrates, ulceration, and perforation. These agents are reserved for hospital and clinic use only.

BOX 5-2 Patient Education: Proper Instillation of Eyedrops and Eye Ointment

- Wash your hands with soap and water.
- Look toward the ceiling with both eyes open.
- Pull lower lid down and steady your hand on your forehead.
- Put a drop of medicine or small strip of ointment (¼ inch) in the sac behind the lashes of the lower lid.
- Avoid touching the eyeball with the tip of the dropper or ointment tube.
- Do not give more than one eye medicine at a time. Wait 5 minutes between medicines.
- When using both ointments and drops, use the ointment *after* the drops.
- Try to keep your eyes closed for 1 minute after instilling the drops to obtain maximum benefit from medications.
- Store eyedrops in a cool, dry place.
- Do not keep eyedrops beyond the printed expiration date.
- Always check the label before instilling eyedrops to be sure you are using the right medication.

Mechanism of Action

When ophthalmic anesthetics such as tetracaine (Pontocaine) and proparacaine (Ophthaine, Ophthetic) are applied, these agents penetrate to sensory nerve endings in corneal tissue. Tetracaine and proparacaine are derivatives of para-aminobenzoic acid (PABA) and lidocaine is an amide derivative; all three are able to locally stabilize and block initiation and conduction of nerve impulses by decreasing the neuronal membrane's sensitivity to sodium ions. Thus, once bound to receptor sites within the sodium channels, ion movement is blocked through the membrane's pores, inhibiting depolarization, which results in a failure of the nerve to transmit the impulses that render the sensation of pain. Once applied topically, these anesthetics work within 20 to 30 seconds and for a period of up to 15 minutes. For example, the more popular tetracaine, when used as a 0.5% solution, requires only one or two drops to produce anesthesia within 30 seconds.

Pharmacokinetics

- Absorption: Rapidly absorbed via conjunctival capillaries to act locally. Any systemic absorption is directly related to the surface area to which the anesthetic is applied and the duration of the application.
- Distribution: Protein binding is high should any systemic absorption occur.
- Metabolism: It is not known if these agents are metabolized while on the surface of the skin or eye. If systemically absorbed, proparacaine is hydrolyzed by plasma esterases, and tetracaine is hydrolyzed by cholinesterase in the plasma, and to a much lesser extent in the liver, to a PABA metabolite.

These metabolites are active. The metabolism of lidocaine remains unknown.

- Excretion: Lidocaine remains unknown; tetracaine and proparacaine are excreted in the bile.
- Half-Life: Procaine is short acting, lidocaine is intermediate in action, and tetracaine is longer acting.

Dosage and Administration

Generic Name	Trade Name	Route	Usual Adult Daily Dose
proparacaine 0.5% solution	AK-Taine Ophthaine Alcaine	Top.	For removal of foreign bodies: 1–2 drops in eye produces anesthesia for up to 25 min.
tetracaine 0.5% solution	Amethocaine Pontocaine	Top.	For removal of foreign bodies: 1–2 drops in eye produces anesthesia for up to 25 min.
lidocaine	Akten	Top.	2 drops applied just before procedure; may be reapplied

Clinical Uses

- To produce local anesthesia of short duration for ophthalmic procedures, including measurement of intraocular pressure (tonometry), removal of foreign bodies and sutures, and conjunctival and corneal scraping in diagnosis and gonioscopy.
- To produce local anesthesia prior to surgical procedures such as cataract extraction, usually as an adjunct to locally injected anesthetics.

Adverse Reactions

EENT: Tetracaine may cause burning or stinging sensation when first applied. Proparacaine may cause severe keratitis, opacification, and scarring of the cornea resulting in loss of vision (with repeated use of these agents over several days).

Interactions

- None

Contraindications

- None

Conscientious Considerations

- Proparacaine is highly toxic if it enters systemic circulation.
- These agents interfere with healing processes when use is prolonged in acute injuries.

Patient/Family Education

- Patients should be told to expect a brief burning or stinging sensation when tetracaine is first applied. Proparacaine is relatively free of these effects.
- Patients should be instructed on how to use eyedrops (see Box 5-2) before they are given a prescription so that they avoid overuse and underuse of the medication, two common reasons for therapy failure.

Agents Used to Treat Conjunctivitis

Conjunctivitis, inflammation of the conjunctiva, is caused by sources ranging from allergens to infections. Allergic conjunctivitis is common and can be seasonal. It is often pruritic and symmetrical, with discharge that is watery or crusty in the morning. If an **exudative** discharge is present, other causes should be considered. It is often associated with allergic rhinitis.

Infectious forms are viral, bacterial, or, rarely, fungal. Bacterial infections should be suspected when discharge is purulent. Acute conjunctivitis (pinkeye) is usually caused by a virus. Viral conjunctivitis is caused by many viruses. Adenovirus is the most common, but herpes zoster and herpes simplex are the most threatening. The course of the disease usually runs 10 to 15 days. Patients with herpes infections of the eyes should be referred to an ophthalmologist because of the serious consequences of these infections. They can be recognized by their severity, vesicular nature, corneal involvement or nerve distribution, and patient population. Contact lens use suggests a greater possibility of fungal infection requiring referral to an ophthalmologist. If deeper infection of the globe or eye socket is suspected, referral to an ophthalmologist and aggressive systemic therapy are indicated.

To treat allergic conjunctivitis, immune modulators such as antihistamines, NSAIDs, leukotriene inhibitors, and corticosteroids are applied topically or systemically. If associated with allergic rhinitis, a nasal and ophthalmic topical agent or systemic treatment should be given.

Simple viral conjunctivitis is often treated with sulfacetamide 10% solution or ointment applied four times a day. This treatment is a relatively benign intervention. The most appropriate treatment is supportive. Viral infections are best treated by simple saline drops, warm compresses, and time. They are often highly contagious, so common hygienic practices, such as thorough hand washing, using hand sanitizers, and keeping hands away from face and eyes, should be followed.

Staphylococcus aureus, Streptococcus pneumoniae, and *Haemophilus influenzae* are the organisms that most commonly cause bacterial conjunctivitis. Suspected organisms usually guide the choice of antibiotic, but even these bacterial infections can resolve on their own. They are usually treated **empirically** (before a definitive diagnosis is made) with topical antibiotics such as sulfacetamide, but *not* if *H. influenzae* is the suspected organism. Trimethoprim/polymyxin B or a fluoroquinolone provides good coverage against most organisms causing bacterial conjunctivitis. Because most cases of infective conjunctivitis are not bacterial, they are therefore unresponsive to the usual antimicrobials.

Ophthalmic Anti-infectives

Like their systemic counterparts, ophthalmic anti-infectives are either bacteriostatic or bacteriocidal. Ophthalmic anti-infectives such as tobramycin (Tobrex), sulfacetamide (Sulamyd, Bleph-10), and sulfacetamide/prednisolone (Blephamide) remain the mainstay for fighting ophthalmic gram-positive and gram-negative organisms. Fluoroquinolones (ciprofloxacin, gatifloxacin, levofloxacin, moxifloxacin, norfloxacin, ofloxacin) are also used as ophthalmic bactericides. Polymyxin B is also used in ophthalmic preparations.

Mechanism of Action

- Sulfacetamide is a synthetic sulfonamide that inhibits bacterial dihydrofolate synthesis. It is effective against *Escherichia coli, Klebsiella,* and *Neisseria gonorrhoeae.*

- Ophthalmic sulfa drugs, like their systemic counterparts, are bacteriostatic, blocking the synthesis of folic acid in susceptible bacteria.
- Tobramycin is a water-soluble, broad-spectrum aminoglycoside and thus lends itself to topical ophthalmic use. However, its exact mechanism as a bacteriocidal agent is unknown.
- Bacitracin is bacteriostatic and works by inhibiting the incorporation of amino acids and nucleotides into the bacterial cell. Its wide spectrum of activity makes it useful against many gram-positive and gram-negative bacteria.
- Erythromycin is used in many topical otic preparations because it is a bacteriostatic agent (it binds to the 50S ribosomal subunit), preventing protein synthesis in the bacteria. As with its systemic counterpart, the ophthalmic use is mainly against gram-positive organisms (*Streptococcus pyogenes, S. pneumoniae, S. viridans,* and *Corynebacterium diphtheriae*).
- Fluoroquinolones inhibit DNA synthesis in the invading bacteria, and this somehow leads to cell death. Their spectrum is mostly gram positive, and they are active against staphylococci, *S. pneumoniae, H. influenzae,* and some species of *Enterobacter* and *Pseudomonas.*
- Polymyxin B is used in ophthalmic preparations because of its high affinity for phospholipids in the cell wall. By binding to these lipids, cell wall permeability is increased, leading to cell death.

Pharmacokinetics

- These anti-infective agents are not absorbed to any appreciable extent through denuded skin, broken skin, wounds, or mucous membranes. Pharmacokinetic issues are not applicable for these topical formulations of systemic drugs.

Dosage and Administration

Generic Name	Trade Name	Route	Usual Adult Daily Dose
sulfacetamide solution and ointment	Sulamyd Bleph-10	Top.	Solution: 1–2 drops every 2–3 hr during the day, less often at night Ointment: Use a small amount 3–4 times a day
erythromycin ointment	E-Mycin Ilotycin	Top.	½–¼-inch ribbon of ointment applied 2–3 times/day
tobramycin ointment and drops	Tobrex	Top.	½ inch ribbon of ointment applied 2–3 times/day; 1–2 drops every 4 hr for mild to moderate infections
ciprofloxacin ophthalmic drops	Ciloxan	Top.	1–2 drops every 2 hr while awake, for 2 days, then 1–2 drops every 4 hr while awake for the next 5 days
polymyxin B/trimethoprim ophthalmic	Polytrim	Top.	1 drop every 3 hr for 7–10 days. Up to 6 doses/ day
polymyxin B/bacitracin ophthalmic ointment	Polysporin Ophthalmic	Top.	Apply a ½-inch ribbon every 3–4 hr
gentamicin ophthalmic	Garamycin	Top.	Apply a ½ inch ribbon 2–3 times/day; 12 drops every 4 hr
moxifloxacin	Vigamox	Top.	1 drop 3 times/day for 7 days

Clinical Uses

■ Bacterial infections of the eye

Adverse Reactions

EENT: local irritation, super infections with long-term use
MISC: Hypersensitivity reactions to sulfacetamide possible

Interactions

■ None for topical formulations

Contraindications

■ Ophthalmic tobramycin should not be used if systemic aminoglycosides are also being prescribed because serum concentrations may be affected, leading to toxicities.

Conscientious Considerations

■ Ophthalmic sulfacetamide may lose its effectiveness in the presence of exudates or other topical agents; thus, the surface to which it is applied should be clean of any debris before application.
■ With the use of ophthalmic tobramycin, the clinician should monitor the patient for hypersensitivity reactions, which include lid itching, erythema, and congestion of the conjunctiva.
■ *All* of the ophthalmic anti-infective preparations may cause some local irritation on application, but this usually dissipates quickly.
■ Bacitracin may induce transient blurry vision upon application.
■ The fluoroquinolones have been found to create a white crystalline deposit/precipitate along the edges of the cornea.
■ Clinicians must be aware of the important considerations that apply to all ocular preparations (see p. 70, Conscientious Prescribing of Ocular Preparations).

Patient/Family Education

■ Patients should be cautioned that instillation of the drops may cause some discomfort.
■ Patients should be cautioned that if sulfacetamide solution has turned a dark color, then it has lost its potency and should be discarded.
■ Patients should be informed that sulfacetamide is incompatible with any other drops that include thiomersal or silver preparation (see Special Case: Thiomersal and Silver Nitrate).

SPECIAL CASE: Thiomersal and Silver Nitrate

Thiomersal products are increasingly being removed from products as preservatives because they are irritating to the eye and do not completely sterilize the preparations in which they are used.

Two drops of a 1% silver nitrate solution is used only as a routine prophylactic against *gonorrhea ophthalmia neonatorum*. In the past it has been required by law that this agent be administered to all neonates right after birth because gonococcus organisms are particularly susceptible to it. Silver nitrate solution can cause a severe chemical conjunctivitis. Topical 1% silver nitrate, 0.5% erythromycin, and 1% tetracycline are considered equally effective for prophylaxis of ocular gonorrhea infection in newborn infants.

Ophthalmic Mast Cell Stabilizers

Ophthalmic mast cell stabilizers are used for allergic eye disorders such as allergic conjunctivitis and keratitis. Patients may present with symptoms of excessive tearing, itching, redness, or a purulent discharge. Examples of ophthalmic mast cell stabilizers include nedocromil (Alocril), cromolyn sodium (Opticrom), and lodoxamide (Alomide). These agents can also be found in combinations with a corticosteroid such as prednisolone or dexamethasone to further help with reduction of inflammation.

Mechanism of Action

Mast cell stabilizers inhibit the degranulation of mast cells after exposure to a specific antigen. Mast cell inhibition prevents inflammation because histamine and the slow-releasing substance of anaphylaxis are unable to produce their profound characteristics.

Pharmacokinetics

■ Ophthalmic mast cell stabilizers are not absorbed and therefore have no pharmacokinetic properties. With these topical agents, systemic pharmacokinetics is not an issue because plasma concentrations are not great enough to be a concern.

Dosage and Administration

Generic Name	Trade Name	Route	Usual Adult Daily Dose
nedocromil 2% solution	Alocril	Top.	1 drop in each eye, 2 times/day
cromolyn sodium 4% solution	Opticrom	Top.	1 drop in each eye, 2 times/day
lodoxamide 0.1% solution	Alomide	Top	1 drop up to 4 times/day

Clinical Use

■ Allergic conjunctivitis

Adverse Reactions

EENT: Transient stinging or burning on application, blurry vision, photophobia mydriasis, rhinitis, and sinusitis
NEURO: Headache

Interactions

■ None

Contraindications

■ None

Conscientious Considerations

■ Referral to an ophthalmologist for evaluation is warranted in refractive or serious cases to rule out herpes keratitis.

Ophthalmic Antihistamines

A host of products are available as antiallergenic ophthalmics, and the list of products is growing. Some popular products are antazoline (Vasocon), azelastine (Optivar), epinastine (Elestat), emedastine (Emadine), ketotifen (Zaditor), levocabastine (Livostin), and olopatadine (Patanol).

Mechanism of Action

Topical antihistamine agents work in the same way that systemic antihistamines do: They are either mast cell stabilizers or histamine (H_2) blockers. Rather than acting systemically, they act at the cellular level when applied directly as ointments, creams, gels, and lotions, where they block the effects of histamine released during allergic reactions and blunt its symptoms.

Pharmacokinetics

■ Ophthalmic antihistamines are not absorbed and therefore have no pharmacokinetic properties. With these topical agents, systemic pharmacokinetics is not an issue because plasma concentrations are not great enough to be a concern.

Dosage and Administration

Generic Name	Trade Name	Route	Usual Adult Daily Dose
azelastine	Optivar	Top.	1 drop in each eye 2 times/day
epinastine	Elestat	Top.	1 drop in each eye 2 times/day
emedastine	Emadine	Top.	1 drop every 6 hr
ketotifen	Zaditor	Top.	1 or 2 drops every 8–12 hr
levocabastine	Livostin	Top.	1 drop 4 times/day for up to 2 weeks
olopatadine	Patanol	Top.	1–2 drops 2 times/day at 6- to 8-hr intervals

Clinical Uses

■ For temporary relief of the itching associated with seasonal and typical allergic conjunctivitis

Adverse Reactions

EENT: Transient stinging or burning on application, blurry vision, photophobia, mydriasis, rhinitis
NEURO: Headache

Interactions

■ None

Contraindications

■ None

Conscientious Considerations

■ Clinicians must be aware of the important considerations that apply to all ocular preparations (see p. 70, Conscientious Prescribing of Ocular Preparations).

Patient/Family Education

■ Instruct patients to use the medication only as prescribed.
■ Advise patients not to wear contact lenses while using ophthalmic antihistamines and to replace the contact lenses if the eyes are red. They should wait at least 15 minutes after administration before reinserting the contact lenses.

Ophthalmic Vasoconstrictors

Ophthalmic vasoconstrictors, such as naphazoline 0.03%, oxymetazoline 0.02%, and tetrahydrozoline 0.012%, are available as OTC preparations, but naphazoline 0.1% is available only by prescription.

Mechanism of Action

These agents are weak sympathomimetic agents; thus, they act by constricting the blood vessels in the conjunctiva.

Pharmacokinetics

■ Because they are topical, there is no information on their pharmacokinetics other than observable half-lives, which are as follows: naphazoline: 3 to 4 hours; oxymetazoline: 4 to 6 hours; tetrahydrozoline: 1 to 4 hours. With these topical agents, systemic pharmacokinetics is not an issue because plasma concentrations are not great enough to be a concern.

Dosage and Administration

Generic Name	Trade Name	Route	Usual Adult Daily Dose
naphazoline	Privine	Top.	1–2 drops 4 times/day, as needed. Do not use beyond 3–4 days without consultation
oxymetazoline	Afrin Dristan	Top.	1–2 drops in eye 2–4 times/day, but not to exceed every 6 hr
tetrahydrozoline	Visine	Top.	1 or 2 drops in eye not to exceed 4 times/day

Clinical Uses

■ Used to provide temporary relief of redness in the eye caused by minor irritants or allergic conjunctivitis.

Adverse Reactions

EENT: Transient burning or stinging (on application), transient blurry vision, **rebound congestion** or redness (with frequent administration)

Interactions

■ Increase in pressor effects if used with monoamine oxide inhibitors (MAOIs) and tricyclics.

Contraindications

■ In patients with **narrow-angle glaucoma**, ophthalmic vasoconstrictors may induce, as a side effect, an increase in intraocular pressure or hypersensitivity in people who may be sensitive to any of their ingredients.

Conscientious Considerations

■ Ophthalmic vasoconstrictors are used for relief of eye redness; they must not be confused with ophthalmic lubricants.
■ Clinicians must be aware of the important considerations that apply to all ocular preparations (see p. 70, Conscientious Prescribing of Ocular Preparations).

Patient/Family Education

■ Warn patients that heavy continual use of these agents can lead to rebound congestion.
■ Instruct patients on how to use eyedrops (see Box 5-2) before they are given a prescription so that they avoid overuse and underuse of the medication, two common reasons for therapy failure.

Cyclosporine (Restasis-Ophthalmic)

Cyclosporine is a polycyclic peptide that inhibits both cellular and humeral immune responses by inhibiting interleukin-2, a proliferative factor needed for T-cell activity. The main use of this drug is to prevent organ rejection following transplant surgery and as an ophthalmic preparation (0.05%) to prevent rejection of corneal transplants.

Agents Used to Maintain Ocular Hydration

Ophthalmic lubricants contain agents that provide hydration, maintain moisture, and protect the eye. These agents may be viscous (e.g., ointment formulations) or nonviscous. Nonviscous agents do not cause blurring of vision. Examples of ophthalmic lubricants are demulcents (e.g., polyethylene glycol and propylene glycol); hygroscopic agents (e.g., glycerin); hypertonicity agents (e.g., sodium chloride) like those found in ocular lubricants used for the relief of corneal edema; polymers (e.g., HP-guar, polyvinyl alcohol, povidone), which are viscosity-increasing agents; and surfactants (e.g., polysorbate 80). Ocular lubricants are buffered to adjust pH, and they contain a balanced solution of salts to maintain tonicity of the eye, viscosity enhancers to prolong contact with the eye, and a preservative to keep the solution sterile.

Mechanism of Action

Ophthalmic lubricants are formulations that contain combinations of the following five types of inert agents:

1. Demulcents, which form a protective film on the ocular surface to allow epithelial repair.
2. Hygroscopic agents, which draw water into the corneal cells to protect against hyperosmotic stress.
3. Hypertonicity agents, which are placed in ocular lubricants for the relief of corneal edema.
4. Polymers (e.g., HP-guar, polyvinyl alcohol, povidone), which act as viscosity-increasing agents that bind to natural tears and to the mucosal surface of the eye to form a protective, lubricant film. Polymers also prolong the contact time of the ophthalmic agent on the ocular surface. Polymers act similarly to endogenous ocular mucin and adhere to the mucosal surface of the eye to stabilize and thicken the tear film and maintain moisture. One such polymer is carboxymethylcellulose (CMC), which has been shown to bind to epithelial cells beneath the ocular surface to lessen dehydration and osmotically protect against hypertonic stress.
5. Surfactants are surface active agents that act as wetting agents to lower fluid surface tension and lubricate the eye.

Pharmacokinetics

■ Ophthalmic lubricants are not absorbed and therefore have no pharmacokinetic properties. With these topical agents, systemic pharmacokinetics is not an issue because plasma concentrations are not great enough to be a concern.

Dosage and Administration

Ophthalmic lubricants are used by the patient as needed. Most come with instructions to instill one to two drops into the eye up to three or four times a day. There are 45 to 50 products being sold on the market today as artificial tears and that are advertised to relieve dry eyes and discomfort caused by wind and sun. Table 5-1 presents a representative list of those products.

TABLE 5-1 Administration of Ophthalmic Lubricants (Artificial Tears)

INGREDIENTS	PRODUCT BRAND NAME	APPLICATION AND COMMENTS
42.5% mineral oil, 58.5% white petrolatum, chlorobutanol as preservative	Refresh Lacri-Lube eye ointment	Designed for nighttime use to provide relief of intense dry, irritated eye. Apply thin film at bedtime.
Methylcellulose with no preservatives	Lacrisert (60 inserts per package)	A sterile, translucent, rod-shaped, water-soluble insert to be placed in the inferior cul-de-sac of the eye once a day; pull down eyelid and insert 1/4 inch of lubricant.
Carboxymethylcellulose, calcium chloride, potassium chloride, water, sodium chloride, sodium lactate	Allergen's Refresh Celluvisc	For relief of moderate to severe dry eye(s). No preservatives and a thicker formulation that can be applied as many times a day as the user wants.
Polyvinyl alcohol 1%, polyethylene glycol 1%, edetate disodium, dextrose, water, benzalkonium chloride	HypoTears	Instill 1–2 drops of this hypertonic solution in affected eye as needed for relief of burning of the eye due to irritation, sun exposure, or wind exposure.
Glycerin 0.2%, hypromellose 0.2%, polyethylene glycol 400 1% Inactive ingredients: ascorbic acid, benzalkonium chloride, boric acid, dextrose, disodium phosphate, glycine, magnesium chloride, potassium chloride, purified water,; sodium borate, sodium chloride, sodium citrate, sodium lactate	Visine Tears	Apply 1–2 drops as needed (remember to remove contact lenses before using).
Polyvinyl alcohol/povidone, also benzalkonium chloride, disodium edetate, potassium chloride, water, sodium bicarbonate, sodium chloride, sodium phosphate chloride	Nature's Tears All Natural Eye Mist, Murine Tears	Hold dispenser 10–15 inches from face. While keeping eyes open, press actuator and mist across both eyes in a single sweep. This application may take 1–2 seconds.

Clinical Uses

■ Supplement natural tears when relief of dry eyes is needed or to wash away eye irritations.

■ Act as viscosity enhancers to promote increased contact time of the ophthalmic agent with the ocular surface.

■ Sooth corneal edema secondary to certain ocular diseases, overwear of contact lenses, or ocular surgery, trauma, infection, or inflammation.

Adverse Reactions

EENT: Mild stinging on application, transient blurry vision; vision changes, prolonged redness, and discharge with long-term use

Interactions

■ None

Contraindications

■ Hypersensitivity to the agent or a preservative

Conscientious Considerations

■ Clinicians must be aware of the important considerations that apply to all ocular preparations (see p. 70, Conscientious Prescribing of Ocular Preparations).

Patient/Family Education

■ Advise patients to call their clinician if there are prolonged vision changes, headache, prolonged redness, or a discharge.

■ Instruct patients on how to use eyedrops (see Box 5-2) before they are given a prescription so that they avoid overuse or underuse of the medication, two common reasons for therapy failure.

■ Patients who use artificial tears more frequently than once every 3 hours should choose a brand without preservatives or one with special nonirritating preservatives.

Agents Used to Treat Glaucoma

Glaucoma is the third most frequent cause of blindness in the world and the second most frequent cause of blindness in the United States. Glaucoma is at once quite simple yet very complicated. The simple definition of glaucoma is abnormally elevated intraocular pressure. The resulting negative impact that elevated IOP has on retinal function and the optic nerve is complicated and not clearly correlated with increased IOP, but if IOP is sufficiently high and persistent, it may lead to irreversible blindness. Glaucoma is primarily a disease of middle age, affecting about 2% of people over the age of 40.

There are two types of glaucoma: primary and secondary. **Primary glaucoma**, also called *closed-angle glaucoma, acute congestive glaucoma,* and *chronic simple glaucoma,* accounts for about 10% of cases. It results from a physiological or anatomical predisposition by which the angle of the anterior chamber of the eye is reduced, limiting the outflow of aqueous humor. This limited outflow leads to a painful acute attack. Closed-angle glaucoma is of more rapid onset and can cascade until the IOP reaches levels that rapidly damage the optic nerve and retina. It is an emergency and requires rapid intervention to salvage sight in the involved eye. An acute unilateral painful eye without any other clear explanation for the symptoms necessitates IOP measurement.

Secondary glaucoma, also called **open-angle glaucoma**, occurs in about 90% of cases, but it does not have a clear cause. It is considered secondary glaucoma because the IOP occurs secondary to an increased production of aqueous humor or a degenerative change in the outflow system. It is insidious in its development because production and outflow are normally so well balanced that IOP varies by less than 2 mm Hg. Secondary glaucoma is often the result of eye disease, or it may follow cornea extraction.

To treat primary glaucoma, rapid intervention with acetazolamide and pilocarpine, as well as **osmotic** agents, is appropriate. "Osmotic" refers to the ability of a solution having high solute concentration (osmolality) to draw through a semi-permeable membrane a solution having a low solute concentration. In this case the FDA has classified mannitol (Osmitrol) as a drug able to reduce intercranial pressure, reduce blood pressure, and reduce intraocular pressure by how it draws water and sodium out of the body through the kidney's nephrons. Mannitol is given IV. Definitive therapy is surgical intervention with acute laser iridotomy, opening an avenue for the fluid to flow into the anterior chamber. There are two primary methods for treating secondary glaucoma: decreasing the amount of aqueous humor that comes into the eye and increasing the amount of aqueous humor that leaves the eye. Aqueous humor flows out of the eye using two pathways: one that is sensitive to pressure (the trabecular pathway) and one that is independent of eye pressure (the uveoscleral pathway). In all cases, the choice of any agent to treat glaucoma is based on the patient's characteristics and comorbidities, the ability to avoid adverse effects, the ability to use once-a-day dosing to improve adherence, and the ability to monitor IOP and progression of the glaucoma.

Aqueous humor production may be decreased by using a carbonic anhydrase inhibitor such as acetazolamide. Aqueous humor production is also mediated by autonomics, so both alpha-2 adrenergic stimulation and beta-adrenergic blockade are effective in reducing IOP. Outflow is stimulated by nonselective alpha agonists such as epinephrine. Prostaglandins such as latanoprost also stimulate outflow. Because the ciliary body and the iris can occlude the outflow tract when the iris is dilated, agents that stimulate the cholinergic parasympathetic receptors of the eye, such as pilocarpine and carbachol, are useful in chronic or open-angle glaucoma.

Direct-Acting and Indirect-Acting Miotics

Several cholinergic medications are useful as **miotics**, agents that cause the pupils to constrict. They are applied topically to treat open-angle glaucoma. There are two types of miotic drugs: direct-acting (carbachol [Isopto Carbachol]) and pilocarpine (Isopto Carpine). The indirect-acting, irreversible cholinesterase inhibitor is echothiophate (Phospholine).

Mechanism of Action

Miotics are chemicals related to acetylcholine, the neurotransmitter that mediates nerve transmission at all cholinergic (parasympathetic) nerve endings. When applied to the eye, miotics cause the sphincter muscle of the iris to contract, resulting in constriction of the pupil (miosis). As the pupil is constricted, it also contracts the ciliary muscles attached to the trabecular meshwork, which in turn opens up Schlemm's canal, increasing the outflow of aqueous humor and dropping IOP. As expected, when the ciliary muscle is contracted, it will affect the accommodation reflex of the eye, leaving it in a state of near vision.

The direct-acting miotic drugs carbachol and pilocarpine inhibit the enzymatic destruction of acetylcholine by deactivating cholinesterase and permitting acetylcholine to continue working on the iris sphincter and ciliary muscle so that a state of miosis is induced. The indirect-acting miotic, echothiophate (Phospholine), is considered an irreversible agent because it binds to cholinesterase in a covalent bond that does not hydrolyze. For ophthalmic activity to return to normal, new cholinesterase must be synthesized, or it must be drawn from other parts of the body. As a result, its effects last for days or weeks once administered.

Pharmacokinetics

With these topical agents, systemic pharmacokinetics is not an issue because plasma concentrations are too low to be a concern. Their duration of effect, however, is known: carbachol, 6 to 8 hours; echothiophate, several days to weeks; and pilocarpine, 4 to 6 hours.

Dosage and Administration

Generic Name/Strength	Route	Usual Adult Daily Dose
echothiophate powder for solution when reconstituted is 0.03%, 0.06%, 0.12%, or 0.25% solution	Top. drops	Start with 0.03% 2 drops in eye in the morning and 2 drops at night
carbachol, 0.75%–3% solutions	Top. drops	Titrate strength and dose to that which works best, usually 1 drop 4 times/day
pilocarpine solutions, 0.4%–8%	Top. drops	Use any strength that works, from 0.4% up to 8%; administer 4 times/day

Clinical Uses

■ Treatment of glaucoma
■ Pilocarpine used to treat dryness of the eyes caused by Sjögren's syndrome

Adverse Reactions

EENT: Transient discomfort on application, blurry vision, or photophobia
GI: Abdominal cramps, diarrhea, watering mouth, excessive sweating
GU: Urinary incontinence
MS: Muscle weakness.
MISC: ALLERGIC REACTIONS MANIFESTING AS SHORTNESS OF BREATH; SWELLING OF LIPS, FACE, AND TONGUE; HIVES; IRREGULAR HEARTBEAT

Interactions

■ None

Contraindications

■ Active inflammation of the eye

Conscientious Considerations

■ Miosis makes it difficult for patients to adjust to shifts in light. Thus, elderly patients who may have light adaptation and visual acuity reductions may find nighttime particularly hazardous, especially if trying to drive a car.

Patient/Family Education

■ Advise patients to contact their clinician immediately if any decrease in vision or an increase in floaters in the visual field is noticed.
■ Patients should watch for signs of hypersensitivities and allergic reactions and quickly report any that occur to their clinician.

Topical Prostaglandin Agonists

Topical prostaglandin agonists (latanoprost, bimatoprost, unoprostone, and travoprost) are stabilized synthetic analogues of prostaglandin. They are the newest agents (since 1996) approved by the U.S. Food and Drug Administration to increase the outflow of intraocular aqueous humor and thus lower IOP. The four analogues currently available are considered safe and effective, although their most common side effect is hyperemia. (The incidence varies among them and among patients.) Their prescribing should be left to the skill and experience of an ophthalmologist.

Mechanism of Action

These agents are selective agonists of a prostaglandin receptor known as the RF receptor. By acting on this receptor, they increase the outflow of aqueous humor and cause a subsequent drop in IOP. However, their exact mechanism of action on the RF receptors is unknown. They drop IOP about 6 to 8 mm HG, or 23% to 35%.

Pharmacokinetics

■ Absorption: Latanoprost and bimatoprost are absorbed through the cornea where they are hydrolyzed to become an active compound. Travoprost and unoprostone are not absorbed but are active on the cornea; once hydrolyzed by corneal esterases they are absorbed.
■ Distribution: Bimatoprost, approximately 80% protein bound; latanoprost, about 4 hours in aqueous humor, then about 1 hour in plasma; travoprost, about 1 hour in plasma then rapidly eliminated; unoprostone, not reported.
■ Metabolism: Latanoprost is hydrolyzed in the liver; bimatoprost is oxidated in the liver; travoprost and unoprostone are hydrolyzed by esterases in the cornea to active free acid and are then inactivated when absorbed.
■ Excretion: Latanoprost and bimatoprost are excreted in the urine; travoprost and unoprostone are rapidly eliminated in the urine and have unmeasurable levels within an hour; unoprostone is excreted in the urine.
■ Half-life: Latanoprost: 45 minutes; bimatoprost: about 45 minutes; travoprost: 45 minutes; unoprostone: unreported.

Dosage and Administration

Generic Name	Trade Name	Route	Usual Adult Daily Dose
latanoprost 0.005% solution	Xalatan	Top. drops	Once a day
bimatoprost 0.3% solution	Lumigan	Top. drops	Once a day
travoprost 0.004% solution	Travatan	Top. drops	Once a day
unoprostone 0.15% solution	Rescula	Top. drops	Once a day

Clinical Uses

■ Treatment of open-angle glaucoma

Adverse Reactions

EENT: Sensation of a foreign body in the eye; permanent discoloration of the iris with a brown pigment (when used over a period of months), eyelash changes, conjunctival hyperemia

PUL: Systemic absorption, which could lead to bronchospasm

Interactions

■ Latanoprost, when applied at the same time as thiomersal, will precipitate out of the solution.

Contraindications

■ Topical prostaglandin agonists are labeled as pregnancy category C and should not be used during lactation.
■ These drugs are not to be used in children.
■ They are contraindicated in patients with Raynaud's disease, asthma, chronic obstructive pulmonary disease (COPD), or any other pulmonary disease because patients may experience bronchospasm, which could be fatal.

Conscientious Considerations

■ Latanoprost should not be administered while the patient is wearing contact lenses, and the patient should wait at least 15 minutes before replacing them.
■ These drugs can permanently discolor the iris with a brown pigment when used over a period of months, especially in hazel or dark green eyes. The discoloration of the pigment is due to an increased amount of melanosomes in melanocytes.
■ One effect is an increase in the length and number of eyelashes, which has resulted in a product called bimatoprost ophthalmic solution 0.03% (Latisse), widely advertised for use in hypotrichosis or as an eyelash growth product for women who have thin or short eyelashes.

Carbonic Anhydrase Inhibitors

Carbonic anhydrase inhibitors (CAIs) were developed during the middle of the 20th century and are used as diuretics. In the latter half of the century, acetazolamide and methazolamide were developed as orally administered glaucoma drugs when numerous attempts to formulate them into eyedrops proved unsuccessful. Today, the CAIs are a drug class of alternative medications for patients who do not achieve control with topical antiglaucoma agents or who fall under one of the contraindications to first-line therapy with beta-adrenergic antagonists.

Currently, there are two carbonic anhydrase inhibitors that can be applied topically to the eye: brinzolamide 1% suspension (Azopt) and dorzolamide 2% solution (Trusopt). Acetazolamide, 125 mg and 250 mg (Diamox), and methazolamide, 25 mg and 50 mg (Neptazane), are CAIs that are given orally. Acetazolamide, taken orally for short-term use, has some application as an adjunct in open-angle glaucoma; however, it is considered an agent of last resort if long-term management of closed-angle glaucoma is needed.

Mechanism of Action

The carbonic anhydrase inhibitors act to decrease the volume of sequestered fluid, especially aqueous humor, by slowing the action of the enzyme carbonic anhydrase. Carbonic anhydrase reduces formation of hydrogen and bicarbonate ions from carbon dioxide and water. This has the effect of preventing the reabsorption of bicarbonate, sodium, potassium, and water in the proximal tubules and in turn increases tubular osmotic pressure (through a reduction in available sodium ions), leading to osmotic diuresis of an alkaline pH urine. Through a feedback mechanism, this leads to decreased production of aqueous humor (by as much as 50%) and a subsequent decrease in IOP. The orally administered tablets are just as effective as the topically administered eyedrops for lowering IOP.

Pharmacokinetics

■ Absorption: Oral acetazolamide and methazolamide are rapidly absorbed; brinzolamide and dorzolamide ophthalmic drops are applied topically and reach the systemic circulation.
■ Distribution: Acetazolamide and methazolamide are distributed throughout body bound to serum protein, erythrocytes, and kidney tissue. Once dorzolamide and brinzolamide are applied topically and reach the systemic circulation, nearly 60% is distributed because they are attached to red blood cells (RBCs).
■ Metabolism: Acetazolamide is not metabolized; methazolamide is metabolized in the liver. The metabolism of methazolamide and brinzolamide remains uncertain.
■ Excretion: Acetazolamide, dorzolamide, and brinzolamide are excreted unchanged in urine and are removed by hemodialysis; methazolamide is excreted in urine.
■ Half-life: Acetazolamide: 2.5 to 5.8 hours; methazolamide: 14 hours, dorzolamide: 120 days (4 months); brinzolamide: 111 days (nearly 4 months).

Dosage and Administration

Generic Name	Trade Name	Route	Usual Adult Daily Dose
brinzolamide 1% solution	Azopt	Top.	1 drop 3 times/day
dorzolamide 2% solution	Trusopt	Top.	1 drop 4 times/day
methazolamide, 25- to 50-mg tab	Neptazane	PO	50–100 mg taken 2–3 times/day
acetazolamide, 250- to 500-mg tab	Diamox	PO	250–500 mg 1–4 times/day

Clinical Uses

■ Treatment of open-angle glaucoma

Adverse Reactions

DERM: Rash, alopecia, STEVENS-JOHNSON
 SYNDROME
GI: Anorexia, a bitter or altered sense of taste with dorzolamide
 and brinzolamide
GU: Kidney stones (crystalluria).
HEM: Blood dyscrasias, bone marrow depression
META: Metabolic acidosis
MISC: Overall weakness and myalgia (especially in overdosing
 situations and in the elderly), groin or leg pain, malaise,
 fatigue
NEURO: Depression, headache, increased nervousness,
 numbness or tingling

Interactions

■ None known for brinzolamide and dorzolamide.
■ Acetazolamide and methimazole are sulfa derivatives and
 thus have drug interactions with salicylates, phenytoin,
 quinidine, and cyclosporine.

Contraindications

■ Allergy or sensitivity to sulfonamides

Conscientious Considerations

■ Use cautiously in patients with diabetes mellitus, gout, or
 pulmonary disease.
■ Watch for patients with sulfonamide sensitivity or allergy,
 Addison's disease, hypokalemia, kidney disease, or a history
 of renal calculi.

Patient/Family Education

■ Patients should be educated about adverse events associated
 with carbonic anhydrase inhibitors.
■ Patients should be taught that if they miss a dose, they should
 take the next dose as soon as they can and that they should
 not apply extra medicine to make up for a missed dose.
■ Patients using eyedrops should be taught to store the
 bottle upright, and, if using other eyedrops, to wait at
 least 10 minutes before administering them.

Sympathomimetic Agents

Two sympathomimetic agents are now available to treat open-
angle glaucoma. These sympathomimetic agents are dipivefrin
0.1% (Propine) and epinephrine 0.5% to 1% and 2% (Epifrin,
Glaucon). Dipivefrin is a *prodrug*, a drug that has to undergo
metabolic conversion to become an active pharmacological agent;
it is converted to epinephrine by enzyme hydrolysis in the eye.
Side effects of these agents are rare and not troublesome, but systemic side effects can occur (tachycardia, palpitations, hypertension, increased sweating, tremors, or lightheadedness). The
liberated epinephrine resulting from the prodrug dipivefrin is a
more efficient way of delivering epinephrine, and it produces
fewer side effects than does conventional epinephrine therapy.

Mechanism of Action

Dipivefrin (Propine) is readily absorbed through the cornea and
into the anterior chamber of the eye because it is a more

lipophilic compound than is epinephrine. It is converted by
enzyme hydrolysis to epinephrine in the eye's ocular fluid, where
it serves as a direct-acting sympathomimetic to lower intraocular
pressure by decreasing aqueous humor production, dilating
pupils, and constricting conjunctiva blood vessels (**mydriatic**
effect), thus increasing intraocular fluid outflow.

Pharmacokinetics

■ Absorption: When placed onto the eye, the local mydriatic
 effect and systemic absorption increase the outflow of
 aqueous humor.
■ Distribution: Both dipivefrin and epinephrine are well
 distributed and bound to plasma.
■ Metabolism: Dipivefrin is metabolized by hydrolysis into
 epinephrine. Both are rapidly metabolized, and their action is
 terminated by enzymatic action while they are on the cornea
 or, if they are absorbed, by rapid hydrolysis in the liver.
■ Excretion: Both drugs are excreted in the kidneys as inactive
 metabolites.
■ Half-life: Unknown, but for epinephrine onset of mydriatic
 action is 1 hour, and it lasts up to 24 hours. Dipivefrin's
 mydriatic effect occurs within 30 minutes, with a peak effect
 in 1 hour.

Dosage and Administration

Generic Name	Trade Name	Route	Usual Adult Daily Dose
dipivefrin 0.1%	Propine	Top.	1 drop in eye every 12 hr
epinephrine 1%–2%	Epifrin Glaucon	Top.	1 drop, 1–2 times/day

Clinical Uses

■ Treatment of open-angle glaucoma by reducing elevated IOP
■ Can also be used to treat ocular hypertension

Adverse Reactions

CV: Tachycardia, palpitations, hypertension.
EENT: Stinging, eye irritation, increase in tears, and brow
 pain. Colored spots on the inner lining of the eye or the
 surface of the eye may develop following chronic use, but
 are harmless.
NEURO: Sweating, tremors, lightheadedness, nervousness.

Interactions

■ If significant systemic absorption of ophthalmic epinephrine
 occurs, then concurrent use of cyclopropane, halothane, or
 possibly chloroform may increase the risk of severe ventricular
 arrhythmias. This may occur because these anesthetics greatly
 sensitize the myocardium to the effects of sympathomimetics.
■ Concurrent use of tricyclic antidepressants may potentiate
 the cardiovascular effects of the epinephrine, possibly resulting in arrhythmias, hypertension, or tachycardia.
■ Concurrent use of ophthalmic betaxolol, levobunolol, or
 timolol with ophthalmic dipivefrin may provide a beneficial
 additive effect in lowering intraocular pressure.
■ Concurrent use of digitalis glycosides may increase the risk
 of cardiac arrhythmias.

■ Concurrent use of systemic antihistamines (diphenhydramine, chlorpheniramine) may result in potentiated effects of the epinephrine.

Contraindications

■ Hypersensitivities
■ Cerebrovascular insufficiencies
■ Cardiovascular disease (angina, arrhythmia)
■ Diabetes
■ Hyperthyroidism
■ Parkinson's disease
■ Hypertension

Conscientious Considerations

■ Because of the risk of severe ventricular arrhythmias with the anesthetics cyclopropane, halothane, and chloroform, therapy with dipivefrin should be interrupted prior to a patient's receiving general anesthesia.
■ Epinephrine is available in many forms, concentrations, and percentages. Packaging labels can be easily confused, leading to patient harm and fatalities.

Patient/Family Education

■ Patients need to be instructed in proper application of these drops.
■ Patients should be told that after a period of use, or at times immediately after instilling the drop, the eye may become red and that this occurs because epinephrine dilates the blood vessels in the eye. Patients should be assured that the redness is harmless.
■ Advise patients that if their eyes begin to itch and/or hurt, they may be having an allergic reaction to the medication, which should be reported to the clinician.

Alpha-2 Adrenergic Agonists

Two alpha-2 adrenergic agonists are available today to lower intraocular pressure in patients with open-angle glaucoma. These two agents are brimonidine tartrate 0.2% solution (Alphagan) and apraclonidine 0.5% and 1% solution (Iopidine). The term *brimonidine* has often been confused by clinicians with *bromocriptine* because they have look-alike and sound-alike names. Clinicians must ensure use of the correct term when prescribing these agents.

Mechanism of Action

■ Alpha-2 adrenergic agonists mimic, by their direct action, the activity of epinephrine on the dilator muscle of the iris, causing it to dilate (mydriasis), and by doing so, it decreases congestion in the blood vessels of the conjunctiva. The net effect is reduction of IOP by reducing the production of aqueous humor and by increasing its outflow.

Pharmacokinetics

■ With these topical agents, systemic pharmacokinetics is not an issue because plasma concentrations are not great enough to be a concern.
■ Their duration of effect, however, is known: apraclonidine, 7 to 12 hours; brimonidine, 12 hours.

Dosage and Administration

Generic Name	Trade Name	Route	Usual Adult Daily Dose
apraclonidine 0.5%, 1%	Iopidine	Top.	1 or 2 drops in eye 3 times/day
brimonidine 0.2%	Alphagan	Top.	1 drop in eye 3 times/day

Clinical Uses

■ Treatment of glaucoma; also used as a prophylactic measure to prevent IOP spiking following laser surgery.

Adverse Reactions

EENT: Lid retraction, mydriasis, local irritation, conjunctival blanching, oral dryness
CV: Orthostatic hypotension, vasovagal attacks
NEURO: Headache, fatigue

Interactions

■ CONCURRENT USE OF ALPHA-2 ADRENERGIC AGONISTS WITH MAOIs MAY PRECIPITATE A HYPERTENSIVE CRISIS.
■ Because tricyclic antidepressants can interfere with circulating amines, taking them concurrently with alpha-2 adrenergic agonists can lead to depression of pulse and blood pressure.
■ Alpha-2 adrenergic agonists also interact with CNS depressants, alcohol, cardiac glycosides, beta blockers, and antihypertensives.

Contraindications

■ Contraindicated if there is concurrent use of MAOIs
■ Contraindicated in children and infants

Conscientious Considerations

■ Although not proven with topically applied alpha-adrenergic blockers, systemically used alpha-adrenergic blockers affect vascular smooth muscle, causing a reduction in blood pressure. This blood pressure drop is greater in people who have renal disease; thus, caution should be used when prescribing these topical medications for people with any kind of kidney impairment.

Patient/Family Education

■ These agents are typically prescribed with other antiglaucoma drops. Instruct patients to wait at least 10 minutes between administering two different agents to prevent washout of the first drug applied.

Beta-Adrenergic Antagonists (Beta Blockers)

Beta blockers remain the most commonly used agents to treat open-angle glaucoma. Although beta blockers are very effective and safe when used in eyedrops, the clinician should watch for a number of side effects when beta blockers are used for long periods of time. Side effects are more commonly seen with nonselective beta blockers, such as Timoptic, than with selective beta blockers, such as Betoptic. However, Timoptic is better at lowering IOP by as much as 20% to 25%, whereas the selective beta blocker, Betoptic, lowers IOP only 15% to 20%. One side effect from long-term use is bronchospasm. Thus, it would be best to avoid the use of these drugs in the glaucoma patient who smokes.

Mechanism of Action

Beta blockers reduce IOP by interfering with cyclic adenosine monophosphate (cAMP), which is used to help produce aqueous humor in the ciliary process of the eye. (See the following Dosage and Administration table for a list of agents.) The exact mechanism of this action is not known, but when administered, these agents reduce IOP in patients in whom it is elevated or normal by reducing aqueous humor formed in the ciliary body. It is interesting that visual acuity, pupillary size, and the accommodation reflex are not affected by these ophthalmic beta blockers.

Pharmacokinetics

■ The pharmacokinetics of beta blockers is also unknown except for their duration of activity, which in the case of the selective beta blockers betaxolol (Betoptic) and carteolol (Ocupress) is 12 hours and in the case of the nonselective beta blockers levobunolol and timolol is about 12 to 24 hours.

Dosage and Administration

Generic Name	Trade Name	Route	Usual Adult Daily Dose
betaxolol	Betoptic	Top. drops	1–2 drops 2 times/day
carteolol solution	Ocupress	Top. drops	1–2 drops, 2 times/day
levobunolol	Betagan	Top. drops	1 drop in affected eye 1–2 times/day
timolol 0.25% and 0.5% in Ocudose dispenser	Timoptic		Start with 0.25% and administer 2 drops twice a day; increase to 0.5% if response in not adequate

Clinical Uses

■ Treatment of glaucoma

Adverse Reactions

EENT: Burning and stinging upon application
CV: Bradycardia, hypotension
PUL: Bronchospasm after long-term use

Interactions

■ Systemic and ophthalmic beta blockers should not be used concurrently because additive effects, such as bradycardia and asystole, have occurred.

Contraindications

■ Because beta blockers can suppress conduction through the AV node, the topical beta blockers are contraindicated in patients with glaucoma who also have bradycardia, AV block, or heart failure (HF).
■ Beta blockers are contraindicated in patients with diabetes because these agents interfere with glycogenolysis.
■ They are contraindicated in patients with hyperthyroidism because these agents can mask its symptoms.

■ If the patient has Raynaud's disease or any other peripheral vascular disorder, these conditions may become exacerbated in the presence of these agents.

Conscientious Considerations

■ Because of the potential for systemic drug absorption, the patient should be monitored for bradycardia and hypotension as well as bronchospasm if he or she is asthmatic or a smoker.

Patient/Family Education

■ Because multidose vials have been associated with bacterial contamination, patients should be taught how to care for their medications.
■ Patients should be told not to wear soft contact lenses while using these medications because they may absorb benzalkonium chloride, which is used as a preservative.

Ophthalmic Osmotics

Osmotic agents such as mannitol are used for acute interventions until more definitive, usually surgical, treatment is available. Mannitol (Osmitrol, Resectisol) is a parenteral agent. When there are situations of extremely high IOP, such as acute attacks of angle-closure glaucoma or cerebral edema, mannitol is useful because it mobilizes excessive interstitial fluid and does not allow excessive fluid and electrolytes to be reabsorbed by the kidney.

Mechanism of Action

Mannitol makes osmotic pressure of the glomerular filtrate hypertonic, allowing water and electrolytes to be pulled passively out of cellular and interstitial spaces. Those electrolytes are sodium, potassium, chloride, calcium, phosphorus, magnesium, urea, and uric acid. Mannitol prevents the kidney from reabsorbing these electrolytes and excessive interstitial fluid. To equalize the solute gradient, excess fluid is excreted in the urine. Because its effect occurs fairly quickly, mannitol is used parenterally to interrupt an acute attack of glaucoma or in emergencies of hypertensive crisis.

Pharmacokinetics

■ Absorption: IV administration produces complete bioavailability
■ Distribution: Confined to the extracellular space; does not cross the blood-brain barrier or the eye
■ Metabolism: Excreted by the kidneys; minimal liver metabolism
■ Excretion: Excreted by the kidneys into the urine
■ Half-life: 100 minutes

Dosage and Administration

Generic Name	Trade Name	Route	Dosage
mannitol	Osmitrol Resectisol	IV	0.25–2 gm/kg as a 15%–25% solution given IV over 30–60 min

Clinical Uses

■ Treatment of edema; reduction of oliguric renal failure; reduction of intracranial and intraocular pressure

Adverse Reactions

EENT: Blurred vision, rhinitis
CV: Transient volume expansion, chest pain, edema, tachycardia
GI: Nausea, vomiting, thirst
GU: Renal failure
META: Dehydration, hyperkalemia, hypernatremia, hypokalemia, hyponatremia
MISC: Phlebitis at injection site
NEURO: Confusion, headache

Interactions

■ Hypokalemia may result, which increases the risk of digitalis/digoxin toxicity.

Contraindications

■ Drug hypersensitivity
■ Cardiac impairment
■ Severe liver function impairment
■ Dehydration
■ Any intracranial bleeding
■ Kidney impairment

Conscientious Considerations

■ Administration requires constant monitoring of vital signs and neurological status.
■ Administer a test dose to see if urine flow is increased.
■ Infuse over 30 minutes if trying to reduce IOP.
■ Explain the purpose of the therapy to the patient, if the patient has cognitive ability, to reduce unneeded anxiety.
■ Effectiveness of therapy will be assessed by monitoring urine output of the patient (being 30 to 50 mL/hr), reduction in intracranial pressure, and reduction of IOP.

Agents Used for Pupillary Dilation

Cyclopentolate, homatropine, and tropicamide are agents used to dilate the pupil (mydriasis) for an examination of the retina. These agents allow the pupil to respond to a fixed light and relax the ciliary muscle, and they paralyze the accommodation reflex (**cycloplegia**).

Mechanism of Action

These **muscarinic** antagonists produce mydriasis by blocking parasympathetic receptors that if stimulated, would normally cause pupils to constrict (miosis). The result is an overbalance toward sympathetic input; thus, there is a dilation of the pupil.

Pharmacokinetics

■ Because these drugs are used topically, there are no pharmacokinetic parameters of concern except their duration of action, which affects dosing.
■ Cyclopentolate: one drop of a 0.5% to 2% solution will produce a peak effect of mydriasis in 25 to 75 minutes that lasts 6 to 24 hours.

■ Homatropine will produce mydriasis and cycloplegia that persists for 24 to 72 hours.
■ Tropicamide's peak effect occurs in 20 to 30 minutes, with its cycloplegia lasting 2 to 6 hours and its mydriasis effect lasting up to 7 hours.

Dosage and Administration

Generic Name	Trade Name	Route	Usual Adult Daily Dose
cyclopentolate 0.5%, 1%, 2% solution	Cyclogyl AK-Pentolate Cylate	Top.	1 drop of selected solution, repeated every 5–10 min for 3 doses for approximately 45 min before the eye examination. Use the 2% for heavily pigmented iris.
homatropine, 1%, 5% solution	Isopto Homatropine	Top.	1–2 drops of a 2% solution before procedure, or 1 drop of the 5% solution. Repeat at 5- to 10-min intervals during the eye examination, as needed.
tropicamide	Mydral Mydriacyl	Top.	1–2 drops; may repeat in 5 min. Examination must be completed within 30 min of second dose; if not, instill an additional drop.

Clinical Use

■ Used as a cycloplegic before eye examinations

Adverse Reactions

CV: tachycardia
DERM: flushing
EENT: blurry vision, photophobia
GI: dry mouth
NEURO: slurred speech, drowsiness, hallucinations
PUL: congestion

Interactions

■ None

Contraindications

■ Closed-angle glaucoma

Conscientious Considerations

■ These agents must be used with caution in patients with a history of glaucoma.
■ Homatropine is used for cycloplegic refraction in children because the mydriasis is too long acting to be used in adults. (Effects on accommodation may last up to 6 days.)
■ Tropicamide is effective but may require repeated dosing in patients with dark-colored irises.
■ Clinicians must always be aware of the risk of precipitating closed-angle glaucoma with any mydriatic because dilation of the iris can occlude the outflow of aqueous humor at the periphery of the anterior chamber of the eye. This acute blockage of aqueous humor increases intraocular pressure. As IOP and pain increase, the iris is pushed forward and can further impede outflow by contracting the lens and blocking flow to the anterior chamber.

Patient/Family Education

■ Inform the patient that the examination should last no more than 30 minutes. Patients should report any pain or discomfort to the clinician.

Fluorescein (Fluorescite) is an ophthalmic diagnostic agent used by clinicians to detect corneal defects and abrasions on the corneal surface. It is a yellow, water-soluble dibasic-acid xanthine dye supplied in a single-use 5-mL vial. It does not stain the corneal surface but is used to detect corneal abrasions and defects. When placed on a **corneal abrasion** (a scratched or torn area of the cornea) or a defect, it will appear bright yellow-green, especially when a Wood's lamp, which makes the defect fluoresce under the ultraviolet spectrum of the lamp, is used. Fluorescein is not absorbed, but it can stain soft contact lenses if left on the cornea. Before reinserting contact lenses, the patient must wait an hour after insertion of the fluorescein, and the eyes must be flushed with saline.

IMPLICATIONS FOR SPECIAL POPULATIONS

Pregnancy Implications

When prescribing drugs affecting the eyes and ears for the pregnant female, clinicians should carefully consider their choice of drugs. Below is a selected list of drugs along with the assigned FDA safety category. Please note that most of these topically applied agents have not had adequate animal studies done on which to base use during human pregnancy.

FDA PREGNANCY SAFETY CATEGORY	DRUGS
B	emedastine (Emadine), nedocromil (Alocril), cromolyn sodium (Opticrom, Crolom), lodoxamide (Alomide), tobramycin ophthalmic, sulfacetamide (Bleph-10), acetazolamide (Diamox Sequels), brinzolamide (Azopt), dorzolamide (Trusopt), methazolamide (Neptazane), dipivefrin (Propine), epinephrine (Epifrin, Glaucon)
C	antazoline (Vasocon), azelastine (Optivar), epinastine (Elestat), ketotifen (Zaditor), levocabastine (Livostin), olopatadine (Patanol), ketotifen (Refresh Eye Itch Relief, Zaditor), flurbiprofen (Ocufen), suprofen (Profenal), diclofenac ophthalmic (Voltaren), ketorolac (Acular), naphazoline ophthalmic (Albalon, Clear Eyes), oxymetazoline ophthalmic (Visine L.R., Visine Long Lasting, Ocuclear), tetrahydrozoline ophthalmic (Visine, Murine Plus), tetracaine (Pontocaine), proparacaine (Ophthaine, Ophthetic), benzocaine/antipyrine/glycerine (Auralgan Otic), benzocaine/antipyrine/propylene glycol (Tympagesic), carbamide peroxide (Debrox, Murine Ear, Auro Ear Drops), cyclosporine (Restasis Ophthalmic), phenylephrine atropine sulfate, cyclopentolate hydrochloride, homatropine hydrobromide betaxolol (Betoptic), carteolol (Ocupress), levobunolol (Betagan), metipranolol (OptiPranolol), timolol (Timoptic), tropicamide, carbachol (Isopto Carbachol), pilocarpine (Isopto Carpine), echothiophate (Phospholine), bimatoprost (Lumigan), latanoprost (Xalatan), travoprost (Travatan), unoprostone (Rescula), dipivefrin (Propine), epinephrine (Epifrin, Glaucon), mannitol, fluorescein
D	
X	
Unclassified	

Pediatric Implications

Ear, nose, and throat problems are more common in children and adolescents than in the elderly, and this is true especially for ear infections. Children need help in applying both eye and ear medications. It may be difficult to keep younger children still while eye medications are being administered. One technique is to have the child and the person administering the medication sit on the floor, with the child between the adult's legs, and the child's legs pointing in the same direction as the adult's legs. This way the adult can use his or her legs to steady the child, with the child's arms below the adult's thighs. This leaves both of the adult's hands free to administer the medication to a somewhat immobile child and to do so in a few seconds.

Geriatric Implications

Most changes in the eye and ear as a function of aging are not associated with any disease process. However, the elderly do suffer more from failing near vision (presbyopia), macular degeneration, cataracts, and glaucoma than do younger populations, as well as having more hearing loss. It is common for clinicians to ask elderly patients to demonstrate how eye and ear medications will be used and to repeat how often they will be used to ensure that patients understand how to administer the medication. This is especially important if the elderly patient has trouble reading the small print on labels. Geriatric patients should be encouraged to have an annual eye examination as well as an otoscopic examination for impacted cerumen.

LEARNING EXERCISES

Case 1

Mrs. M.J. has been a patient at your ophthalmology clinic for some time. She has been diagnosed with open-angle glaucoma, and for 2 years she has been coming every 90 days to have her IOP checked. During these 2 years, her IOP has been consistent, and her headaches and vision issues seem controlled. However, the last few times she was in the clinic, wide fluctuations were noticed in her IOP. Her record indicates that she is using pilocarpine 0.04%, and you begin to wonder if she may need a stronger dose because at this visit her IOP is near symptom-producing levels. As you interview her, she states that she has been using her medication as prescribed and rarely forgets a dose. Is it possible that the drug's effect is wearing off, or might it be possible that Mrs. M.J. has become noncompliant?

Case 2

Mr. J.T. comes to see you and presents with red, inflamed eyes and excessive tearing for the past month. He states, "Every spring when there is pollen in the air this itching, burning, redness, and soreness in my eyes just drives me nuts. What can you prescribe for me that will relieve my suffering?"

1. What is Mr. J.T.'s likely diagnosis?

2. What treatment could be suggested?

3. Of what medication side effects should the patient and clinician be aware?

References

American Academy of Pediatrics (AAP) & American Academy of Family Physicians (AAFP). (2004). Clinical practice guidelines: Diagnosis and management of acute otitis media. Retrieved January 21, 2011, from http://aappolicy.aappublications.org/cgi/content/full/pediatrics;113/5/1451

Drugs Used in the Treatment of Cardiovascular Disorders

chapter 6

Alice A. House, Mona M. Sedrak

CHAPTER FOCUS

This chapter focuses on medications used to treat common cardiovascular disorders including cardiac glycosides, digitalis, antiarrhythmics, nitrates, and peripheral vasodilators. Although diuretics, angiotensin-converting enzyme inhibitors (ACEIs), angiotensin II-receptor blockers (ARBs), and calcium channel blockers (CCBs) are discussed in detail in Chapter 7, they are also discussed here because they are important in treating cardiovascular disorders. The drugs discussed in this chapter improve oxygenation of heart muscle, decrease remodeling of heart muscle following a myocardial infarction (MI) or heart failure (HF), are easily dosed as oral agents, and are agents with relatively few adverse effects.

OBJECTIVES

After reading and studying this chapter, the student should be able to:

1. Describe the role of digitalis in the treatment of atrial and ventricular arrhythmias and heart failure (HF).
2. Describe the modified Vaughan Williams classification of antiarrhythmic drugs.
3. Compare and contrast the effects of available antiarrhythmic drugs on ventricular conduction velocity, refractory period, automaticity, and inhibition of specific myocardial ion channels.
4. Apply knowledge of the mechanism of action, clinical use, and dosing of nitroglycerin and nitrates for the routine treatment of angina.
5. List the advice a clinician should give to patients or patients' caregivers concerning the use of digoxin, nitrates, nitroglycerin, and antiarrhythmics.
6. Describe the pharmacology of ranolazine, a unique cytoprotective agent used for chronic angina.
7. Describe the use of beta-adrenergic blockers in treating cardiac arrhythmias.
8. Describe the treatment of digitalis toxicity with Digibind.
9. Describe the essential first steps in initiating drug therapy for drugs used in life-threatening cardiovascular situations.

Key Terms

Angina pectoris
Arrhythmia
Automaticity
AV (atrioventricular) node
Bradycardia
Chronotropic effect
Heart failure (HF)
Inotropic effect
NA^+/K^+ ATPase Pump
Narrow therapeutic range
Paroxysmal supraventricular tachycardia (PSVT)
SA (sinoatrial) node
Tachycardia

DRUGS USED IN THE TREATMENT OF CARDIOVASCULAR SYSTEM

Cardiac Glycosides	Class Ia: Na+ Channel Blockers	Class Ic
digoxin IM	quinidine (Quinidex, Cardioquin)	propafenone (Rythmol)
digoxin IV	procainamide (Pronestyl, Procan SR)	flecainide (Tambocor)
digoxin PO	disopyramide (Norpace)	**Class II: Beta-Adrenoreceptor Blocker**
Digoxin Antidote	**Class Ib**	propranolol (Inderal)
digoxin immune FAB (Digibind)	lidocaine (Xylocaine)	metoprolol (Lopressor, Toprol)
Antiarrhythmics	mexiletine (Mexitil)	nadolol (Corgard)
	tocainide (Tonocard)	atenolol (Tenormin)

continued

DRUGS USED IN THE TREATMENT OF CARDIOVASCULAR SYSTEM—cont'd

acebutolol (Sectral)	**Class IV: Ca++ Channel Blocker**	*Antianginal Drug for Chronic Angina (Cytoprotective)*
pindolol	nondihydropyridines	ranolazine (Ranexa)
sotalol (Betapace)	diltiazem (Cardizem)	*Peripheral Vasodilators*
timolol	verapamil (Isoptin, Calan)	hydralazine (Apresoline)
esmolol (Brevibloc)	*Nitrates*	minoxidil (Loniten)
Class III: K+ Channel Blocker	nitroglycerin (NTG)	
sotalol (Betapace)	isosorbide dinitrate (Isordil)	
amiodarone (Cordarone)	isosorbide mononitrate (Monoket,	
bretylium	IMDUR)	

Using medications to treat cardiovascular disorders requires specialized knowledge, skills and insights about management of heart failure (HF), antiarrhythmic drugs, antianginal drugs that affect the renin-angiotensin-aldosterone system, and other vasoactive substances. Understanding the use and action of calcium channel blockers (CCBs), angiotensin-converting enzyme inhibitors (ACEIs), beta blockers, diuretic drugs, anticoagulants, antiplatelets, and fibrinolytic drugs, as well as drugs to fight hypercholesterolemia and coronary heart disease (CAD), is also critical. The pharmacokinetics of these drugs can be challenging, especially to clinicians as they try to improve patients' quality of life while lowering morbidity and mortality.

RATIONAL DRUG TREATMENT OF HEART FAILURE

Some literature still refers to heart failure as congestive heart failure (CHF), but because heart failure can occur without congestion, the more correct term is *heart failure*. **Heart failure** is the inability of the heart to maintain adequate coronary output (CO) to meet the metabolic demands of the body (NLM, 2011). Each year, about a half million new cases of HF occur in the United States, leading to an average population of 5.5 million cases of heart failure, coronary heart disease, stroke, and high blood pressure prevalent at any one time in the United States (American Heart Association, 2012).

Although there are modest gains in HF survival rates, optimal strategies for its treatment still need work, especially because the older adult population in America is growing (Curtis et al., 2008). HF is a syndrome, not a disease, and it is brought on by abnormalities in myocardial contraction (systolic dysfunction), ventricular relaxation and filling (diastolic dysfunction), or both. These abnormalities are usually secondary to hypertension (HTN) and CAD. Other causes of heart failure include diseases of the heart valves, metabolic diseases, infectious diseases, and toxic drugs. Classification of the various stages of heart failure helps a clinician determine the severity of the condition and the effectiveness of his/her treatment as patients move into and out of the various stages. Typically a clinician uses two measures or scales of heart failure because one focuses on the symptoms (NYHA) and one focuses on the hearts physical functionality. The NYHA is more widely used as it classifies heart failure patients into one of four categories according to symptoms which

then becomes a tool to assess whether or not the heart failure is worsening, getting better, or staying the same following treatment. The second system (a joint effort of the American College of Cardiology and American Heart Association) used the letter A-d to define the heart's condition including a category for people who may be at risk. The point of this classification is that if a patient's risk factors are known intervention can be prescribed to lessen or prevent a deadly episode of heart failure.

The New York Heart Association (NYHA) classifies symptoms according to how they affect a person's ability to function. Unlike the AHA/ACC staging system, the NYHA classification system allows for movement between classifications based upon symptoms responding to therapy so that as symptoms improve or worsen, the patient's classification can be adjusted (NYHA, 1994).

Pharmacological treatment of heart failure is aimed at antagonizing the neurohormones that are increased in HF patients using drugs such as vasodilators and beta-adrenergic blockades. Bisoproprolol, carvedilol, and metoprolol are three beta blockers commonly used today. Diuretics are used to relieve volume overload. Vasodilators such as hydralazine act directly on arterial smooth muscle to produce vasodilation and reduce afterload, which is the tension or stress developed in the wall of the left ventricle during ejection. When used in combination with nitrates (e.g., isosorbide dinitrate), vasodilators have proven to produce life-saving outcomes in HF. No matter the cause of HF, it is likely that the patient will be on a multidrug regimen to prolong life expectancy and control symptoms. For example, a combination of hydralazine and isosorbide dinitrate with a beta blocker and ACEI has been shown to reduce mortality in African Americans (Taylor et al., 2004).

The drug most commonly used to treat HF is the digitalis glycoside digoxin (Lanoxin). It is still used after three centuries because it increases cardiac contractility and may also attenuate the neurohormonal activity that occurs with HF. Digitalis has proven to be the one drug that decreases the number of HF patients requiring hospitalization without any increase in mortality. If it is discontinued when patients become stabilized, those people tend to enter a state of clinical deterioration. However, digitalis is not used ubiquitously to treat heart failure. There are other, more effective drugs that have been shown to reduce mortality, such as carvedilol (Coreg), which is indicated for treatment of heart failure of ischemic or cardiomyopathic origin in a narrow group of patients (mild to moderate heart failure or NYHA class II or III). To halt the progression of HF, carvedilol is given in conjunction with diuretics and angiotensin-converting enzyme (ACE) inhibitors. Again, there is no simple drug treatment when it comes to advanced HF. At that time it is important for the clinician to determine if therapy is optimal to prevent systolic dysfunction because many patients may not have had trials of ACEIs and beta blockers. With careful and slow titration of these drugs, it is often possible to reach stabilization; however, when a beta blocker is started in a decompensated state or contraindications to its use have been found, it often must be stopped. If the patient remains in a NYHA class III state, clinicians should consider using an aldosterone antagonist or the addition of an angiotensin-receptor blocker (ARB) such as candesartan or valsartan in addition to the ACEI, all of which have been shown to reduce morbidity and mortality when used. However, a quadruple combination of an ACEI, ARB, aldosterone antagonist, and beta blocker is not recommended for use in patients with heart failure because there is insufficient safety data from clinical trials. The addition of digoxin also has a place in the management of advanced HF, but in patients who have HF and abnormal sinus rhythm there is an overall neutral effect on mortality. However, there is evidence that digoxin reduces hospitalizations for HF in patients with sinus rhythm, especially in those with large ventricles who were being hospitalized frequently. It, of course, maintains a role in those with advanced HF and atrial fibrillation, where rate control may improve symptoms.

Often patients with advanced HF cannot tolerate blockade of the renin-angiotensin-aldosterone system due to worsening renal failure. Very often, the patient must stop using ACEI/ARB/aldosterone antagonists to allow renal dysfunction, hypotension, and diuresis to reoccur and then restart the drugs. However, should this prove to be impossible, offloading can be aided by adding hydralazine and isosorbide dinitrate. African American patients (who are known to be less responsive to ACE/ARB therapy than are Caucasians) with NHYA III/IV HF and systolic dysfunction may respond to treatment with an ACEI or ARB plus beta blocker and the addition of hydralazine and isosorbide dinitrate. Whether this approach is useful in non–African American populations remains unknown.

There are also different treatments for those who have either systolic or diastolic heart failure. Most people think of HF as a condition in which the heart does not pump out enough blood: This is systolic heart failure. However, many people have heart failure that is caused by the heart not fully relaxing so that it does not fill properly with blood. This is called diastolic heart failure (DHF). In mild DHF, shortness of breath and fatigue usually occur during stress or activity, but more severe DHF causes many of the same symptoms of systolic heart failure (SHF). A person with DHF has high pressure in the arteries of their lungs, their heart's pumping chambers may not be enlarged, and their "ejection fraction" may be normal, but they still have the same symptoms as a person with SHF. In people with DHF, metoprolol (Toprol-XL) may be a better beta blocker than carvedilol (Coreg) because it does not lower blood pressure as much as metoprolol does. Interestingly, drug treatments for SHF are based on large, properly executed and scientifically sound clinical trials, but unfortunately, no such trials exist for DHF. Thus, guidelines for treatment of DHF are the result of smaller trials and the clinician's experience and understanding of the disease using the following goals:

■ Treatment should reduce CHF symptoms, mainly by reducing heart size (diuretics, sodium restriction, dialysis), reducing pulmonary blood pressure through maintaining good pumping in the heart's upper chambers (atriums), and slowing the heart rate (use of a pacemaker).

■ Treatment should target the underlying cause, if possible. For example, high blood pressure should be controlled, remodeling should be reversed, the aortic valve should be replaced if necessary, and any ischemia should be treated by increasing blood flow to the heart and reducing its need for oxygen.

■ Treatment should target the bodily systems changed by the disease, mainly the neurohormonal systems. With few exceptions, many of the drugs used to treat systolic heart failure are also used to treat diastolic heart failure. However, the reasons for choosing one drug over another and choosing the doses used will vary because the doses are often different for DHF. For example, in DHF, beta blockers are used to make filling the heart with blood take longer and to change the heart's response to exercise. In SHF, beta blockers are used to increase pumping power and reverse heart remodeling. Diuretic doses for DHF patients are usually much smaller than for SHF. Calcium channel blockers have no place in SHF treatment but may help DHF. Thus, most clinicians use beta blockers and calcium channel blockers (CCB) to slow heart rate in DHF patients, but they are wary of slowing a person's heart rate too much because it can reduce cardiac output (CO) despite the better filling of heart chambers. This is why patients with SHF need very individualized treatment, especially when an initial goal might be a resting heart rate of about 60 beats per minute. Because beta blockers and CCBs increase the time it takes for the heart to fill with blood, these drugs decrease pulmonary hypertension. However, these drugs also reduce the heart's ability to relax, leaving the clinician with the task of finding the right dosage to balance and minimize symptoms in the patient with DHF. Finally, the long-term effect of CCBs on patients with DHF remains unknown; it is known, however, that all calcium channel blockers except amlodipine (Norvasc) increase mortality in patients with SHF.

The cardiac glycosides remain a favorite subject of pharmacology classes, and a beginning student will discover that they are popular subjects on examinations. In practice, however, the use of glycosides, and other agents, to treat heart failure is a balancing act requiring clinical experience and consultation with colleagues to truly help a patient have both a better quality of life and a longer life.

Pharmacology of the Cardiac Glycosides

Cardiac glycosides are among the oldest known drugs used in the treatment of heart failure. Records from the 1700s indicate that a tea made from the plant *Digitalis purpurea*, or foxglove, has a history of use as a tonic for the heart. This purple flowering plant remains popular today in many home gardens. There are three main glycosides in *D. purpurea*, but the purified extract, known as digoxin, is its most abundant glycoside. Digoxin (Lanoxin) is an oral tablet used most frequently in medical applications owing to its convenient routes of administration, monitoring, and pharmacokinetics. The four goals of digoxin treatment are as follows:

1. To strengthen the heart beat
2. To slow the heart rate
3. To convert any irregular sinus rhythm
4. To arrest the ventricular rate to between 70 to 80 beats per minute (BPM)

After nearly 300 years, digoxin therapy remains controversial owing to debate over its risk verses benefits profile, especially when it is used in patients with systolic heart failure. However, it has proven to be beneficial when heart failure results from uncontrolled hypertension or severe aortic stenosis.

Conscientious Prescribing of Cardiac Glycosides

■ Ten percent of individuals have intestinal bacteria that can inactivate digoxin in the gut, greatly reducing bioavailability and requiring higher than average doses to produce a therapeutic response.

■ Generic tablet preparations have a bioavailability of 70% to 80%; bioavailability is 90% to 100% for digoxin elixir and encapsulated gel.

■ Because of the narrow safety margin between therapeutic effects, loss of effect, and toxicity, small variations in bioavailability can have serious consequences. It is best to prescribe one brand and ensure that the pharmacy does not substitute.

■ Digoxin should be used cautiously in patients with kidney impairment.

■ Hypothyroidism and chronic renal failure decrease the volume of distribution of digoxin, necessitating a decrease in both loading and maintenance doses.

■ Digoxin should be used cautiously in patients with electrolyte abnormalities because the concentration of potassium, calcium, and magnesium affects sensitivity to cardiac glycosides and may result in toxicity.

■ ST-T wave changes on an ECG do not correlate directly with serum drug levels of digoxin; therefore, these readings should not be used as an indication of toxicity.

■ When switching from parenteral to oral dosing forms, a dosing adjustment will always be needed because of the pharmacokinetic variations in the percentage of digoxin absorbed.

■ Digoxin has a very narrow therapeutic index, or dosing range. Many errors have occurred with this medication, including miscalculations of pediatric and geriatric dosage adjustments.

Patient/Family Education for Cardiac Glycosides

■ Instruct patients on how to take their own pulse and to see a clinician if the pulse rate is less than 60 or greater than 120.

■ Review signs and symptoms of digitalis toxicity with patients and family.

■ Advise patients to keep digoxin tablets in their original prescription container and not to mix them with pills of other kinds.

■ Caution patients that sharing their medication with someone could be fatal.

■ Advise patients to wear a medical identification bracelet or necklace that states the name of the drug they are taking and/or the disorder for which it is being taken.

■ Advise patients that taking digoxin with a high-fiber meal or after a meal results in reduced total absorption of the drug.

■ Instruct patients that digoxin should be taken exactly as prescribed and at the same time each day. Missed doses need to be taken within 12 hours of the scheduled dose or not at all. If doses are missed for 2 days or more, a clinician should be consulted.

■ Advise patients to eat a diet high in potassium unless they are also taking a potassium-sparing diuretic. Patients should also consume moderate amounts of calcium.

■ Advise patients to store the drug in its original tightly covered, light-resistant container.

■ Inform patients that antacids and antidiarrheal drugs should not be taken within 1 hour of taking the cardiac glycosides.

Mechanism of Action

Digoxin increases the force of myocardial contractions by prolonging the refractory period of the AV node and decreasing conduction through the **SA** (sinoatrial) and **AV** (atrioventricular) **nodes**. The net effect of digoxin is to increase cardiac output (a positive **inotropic effect**) and slow the heart rate (a negative **chronotropic effect**). Digoxin is able to decrease **automaticity** (the pathological phenomenon of spontaneous and repetitive firing of heart muscle cells that give the heart its rhythm as well as arrhythmias) and conduction velocity through the AV node by central vagal stimulation and facilitation of muscarinic transmission at the cardiac muscle cell.

Digoxin is a potent inhibitor of the Na/K-adenosine triphosphatase (ATPase) pump (Fig. 6-1). By inhibiting **NA⁺/K⁺-ATPase Pump**, cardiac glycosides such as digitalis and digoxin cause intracellular sodium concentration to increase. This then leads to an accumulation of intracellular calcium via the Na^+-Ca^{++} exchange system. In the heart, increased intracellular calcium causes more calcium to be released, causing more calcium to be available to bind to troponin-C, which increases the force of contractility. Inhibition of the Na^+/K^+-ATPase in vascular smooth muscle causes depolarization, which causes smooth muscle contraction and vasoconstriction. By mechanisms that are not fully understood, digitalis compounds also increase vagal efferent activity to the heart. This parasympathomimetic action of digitalis reduces sinoatrial firing rate (decreases heart rate; negative chronotropy) and reduces conduction velocity of electrical impulses through the atrioventricular node. Thus, digoxin also allows conduction of electrical impulses between the atria and ventricles to be slowed, and because of its slowing of ventricular contractions, it is used to treat ventricular arrhythmias.

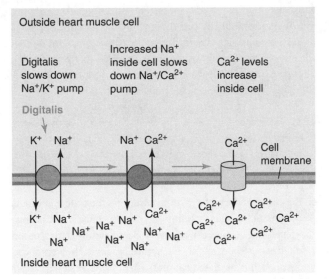

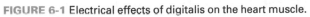

FIGURE 6-1 Electrical effects of digitalis on the heart muscle.

Pharmacokinetics

- Absorption: Absorbed well from the gastrointestinal (GI) tract when taken orally. Note that although 80% of digoxin is absorbed from intramuscular (IM) sites, the IM route of administration is not recommended owing to extreme pain and irritation.
- Distribution: Widely distributed to the tissues including the CNS. Highest tissue concentrations are found in the heart, kidney, and liver. It will cross the placenta and enter breast milk.
- Metabolism: Not extensively metabolized, and digoxin is excreted virtually unchanged.
- Excretion: Almost entirely unchanged by the kidneys into the urine.
- Half-life: 36 to 48 hours, but increased if there is renal impairment.

Dosage and Administration

Generic Name	Route	Onset	Peak	Duration	Dose
digoxin	PO	30–120 min	2–8 hr	2–4 days	Loading dose: Adults: 0.75–1.5 mg given as ½ of first loading dose and then ¼ in each of 2 doses at 6- to 12-hr intervals. Maintenance dose: 0.125 mg–0.5 mg/ day
digoxin	IV	5–30 min	1–4 hr	2–4 days	Adults: A larger loading or digitizing dose of 0.5–1.0 mg as ½, then ¼ each, as 2 doses at 6- to 12-hr intervals.
digoxin	IM	30 min	4–6 hr	2–4 days	Dosing: Not recommended

Clinical Uses

- Treatment of HF. Although no longer the first-line drug for treatment of HF, digoxin is still central to the treatment for patients with severe systolic dysfunction.
- Digoxin is also used in treating paroxysmal atrial **tachycardia** (rapid heart rate that starts and stops abruptly), tachyarrhythmias, such as atrial flutter and atrial fibrillation, because it slows the ventricular rate.

Adverse Reactions

CV: ARRHYTHMIAS, **bradycardia** (slow heart rate), ECG changes
EENT: Blurry vision, yellow or green blurry vision, halos around lights
ENDO: gynecomastia
GI: anorexia, nausea, vomiting, diarrhea
HEM: thrombocytopenia
META: electrolyte imbalances, especially potassium, with acute digoxin toxicity
NEURO: headache, weakness, disorientation, hallucinations

Interactions

- Quinidine, amiodarone, benzodiazepines, and verapamil reduce renal clearance and can double the serum concentration, resulting in digoxin toxicity.
- Potassium and cardiac glycosides interact by inhibiting each other's binding to the Na$^+$/K$^+$ ATPase.
- Excessive use of laxatives may cause hypokalemia and increase the risk of digoxin toxicity.
- Blood levels of digoxin may be reduced by aminoglycosides, antimetabolites, fibrates, antacids, and bismuth subsalicylate (Kaopectate).
- Thyroid hormones will decrease the therapeutic effect of digoxin.
- Macrolide antibiotics kill bacteria in the GI tract, which in turn raises serum levels of digoxin to toxic levels. It may be necessary to lower the dosage of digoxin for patients taking macrolide antibiotics for up to 9 weeks.
- Licorice and aloe increase the risk of potassium depletion.
- St. John's wort decreases digoxin levels and its effect.
- Ingestion of a high-fiber meal reduces digoxin absorption.

Contraindications

- Cardiac glycosides are contraindicated in AV block and uncontrolled ventricular arrhythmias because their action on the AV node may worsen the arrhythmia.
- Cardiac glycosides are contraindicated in those with hypersensitivities.
- Patients who are hypokalemic, hypercalcemic, or hypomagnesic may find themselves at greater risk of digoxin toxicity.
- Geriatric patients are at increased risk of toxicity because they are highly sensitive to digoxin (see Special Case: Digitalis Toxicity and Digibind).

SPECIAL CASE: Digitalis Toxicity and Digibind

Digitalis toxicity is commonly caused by excessive administration of cardiac glycosides; too much diuresis, resulting in hypokalemia; concurrent development of renal insufficiency; or drugs that interfere with the excretion of digoxin. Digitalis toxicity is especially common in older adults because they are the most sensitive to it.

Clinical and laboratory data are used to diagnose digitalis toxicity. Serum levels alone are insufficient to diagnose toxicity because there is considerable overlap in serum concentrations between those with and without evidence of toxicity. Toxicity is diagnosed for serum levels greater than 2 ng/mL. Toxicity commonly presents with arrhythmias, neurological and GI symptoms (nausea, vomiting, diarrhea, loss of appetite), and visual disturbances (blurred vision, blind spots, yellow and green halos seen around lights). Other symptoms include atrial arrhythmias and atrial tachycardia with AV block, decreased consciousness, decreased urine output, difficult breathing when supine, irregular pulse, and overall swelling

Treatment of digitalis toxicity may include potassium administration, lidocaine, atropine, or digoxin immune fab (Digibind). Digibind is an antibody that is produced in sheep. It has the property of binding to unbound digoxin in serum, allowing for its ultimate removal and prevention of toxic effects. It is administered only by IV, thus it is 100% bioavailable and is widely distributed throughout extracellular spaces. It is excreted by the kidneys as the bound complex (i.e., digoxin immune fab plus digoxin). Digibind has a half-life of 2 to 6 hours. During that time, its adverse effects may be the reemergence of atrial fibrillation or HF. It starts reversing symptoms of digoxin toxicity within 30 minutes. Digibind is expensive; it may cost $2,000 to $3,000 per patient. Digibind is made from sheep protein; it is wise to do a skin test on patients at high risk of being allergic.

Pharmacology of Antiarrhythmics

Abnormalities in heart rhythm are called **arrhythmias**. These may result in abnormally fast (tachyarrhythmia) or slow (bradyarrythmia) heart rates. Therapeutic options for clinical management of arrhythmias have been expanding at a rapid rate and include drugs; devices, such as pacemakers and defibrillators; and transcatheter therapies. Currently available antiarrhythmic drugs work by one of two mechanisms: They either directly alter the function of ion channels that participate in a normal heartbeat or they interfere with neuronal control. The function of antiarrhythmic drugs is to restore normal sinus rhythm and/or suppress initiation of abnormal rhythms. These drugs are used for all forms of tachycardia, although they are not effective for long-term therapy of symptomatic bradycardia. They may be administered intravenously (IV) acutely or orally for long-term prophylaxis.

Although much is known about the current ion channels that regulate cardiac function, the precise action of many of the antiarrhythmic drugs is not completely understood. Antiarrhythmic drugs affect normal cardiac function and have the potential for many serious side effects. Because of the potential for serious adverse effects, clinician vigilance is required to ensure proper dosing. A thorough knowledge of drug-drug interactions and close follow-up by clinicians is important.

The choice of antiarrhythmic drugs is usually based not only on its the benefit, but also on its risks. Benefits may also be assessed by electrophysiological tests because the more potentially lethal an arrhythmia shows itself to be, the more acceptable the risks of drugs to prevent it. The presence of other diseases and other organ systems may also dictate the choice of drugs based on the effects of the antiarrhythmic drugs on the system affected. Also, costs and frequent monitoring may affect decision-making.

There is no universally accepted classification algorithm or guidelines for choosing antiarrhythmic agents; however, the Vaughan Williams classification, which was first described in 1970 and then expanded into its present form (Table 6-1), is still used in spite of the limitations caused by its complexity. This classification assigns the appropriate drug for any given arrhythmia based on its electophysiological effects on myocardial targets, that is, myocardial sodium, myocardial potassium, myocardial calcium channels, and myocardial beta-adrenergic receptors. Thus, the Vaughn Williams classification of antiarrhythmics is a grouping of pharmaceuticals used to suppress arrhythmias. It consists of four classes:

- Class I: Sodium channel blockers, which block voltage-gated sodium channels.
- Class II: Beta blockers, which have sympathetic blocking action.
- Class III: Potassium channel blockers, which prolong action potential duration and refractoriness.
- Class IV: Calcium channel blockers, which have calcium channel–blocking properties.

This classification system is complicated by the fact that many drugs have multiple actions and multiple effects on many targets. Thus, the classification uses an oversimplification of the effects of these drugs, but because it is easy to use, the classification remains useful for the clinician who is experienced, understands that these drugs have overlapping effects, and understands that the classification has inaccuracies. For example, Quinidine is classified as Vaughn Williams 1a sodium channel blocker, but it also has a Class III effect, blocking of potassium, and thus could lead to torsade de pointes, a serious consequence.

Conscientious Prescribing of Antiarrhythmics

- Take a thorough medication history to determine whether the patient is receiving any prescription or nonprescription drugs that can cause or contribute to the development of an arrhythmia.
- Monitor the patient's serum electrolyte concentration to determine the presence or absence of hypokalemia, hyperkalemia, hypomagnesemia, or hypermagnesemia.
- Because the margin between therapeutic efficacy and toxicity is narrow and the knowledge needed to prescribe these

TABLE 6-1 Vaughn Williams Classification of Antiarrhythmic Agents			
CLASS	GENERIC NAME	TRADE NAME	ROUTE
Class I: sodium channel blockers (3 groups)			
Class Ia	quinidine	Quinidex, Quinora	PO, IV
	procainamide	Pronestyl, Procan SR	PO, IV
	disopyramide	Norpace	PO
Class Ib	lidocaine	Xylocaine	IV
	tocainide	Tonocard	
	mexiletine	Mexitil	PO
Class Ic	propafenone	Rythmol	PO
	flecainide	Tambocor	PO
Class II: beta-adrenergic blockers	propranolol	Inderal	IV, PO
	metoprolol	Lopressor	PO
	nadolol	Corgard	PO
	atenolol	Tenormin	PO
	acebutolol	Sectral	PO
	pindolol		PO
	timolol		PO
	esmolol	Brevibloc	IV
Class III: potassium channel blockers	bretylium	Bretylol	
	amiodarone	Cordarone	PO, IV
	sotalol	Betapace	PO
	dofetilide	Tikosyn	
	ibutilide	Corvert	IV
Class IV: calcium channel blockers	verapamil	Calan	PO
	diltiazem	Cardizem	PO, IV

drugs is extensive, it is best to refer patients to cardiologists for initiation of therapy.

■ Potassium concentration and extracellular spaces are the major determinant of resting membrane potential and membrane stability; thus, potassium levels should always be checked for patients with rhythm disturbances.

■ Renal and hepatic function should be watched because they are the principal routes of excretion for antiarrhythmic drugs. Intervals for testing depend on the drug class.

■ Antiarrhythmic agents tend to have a **narrow therapeutic range** (difference between the therapeutic and lethal dose) and are often given to patients who are taking other drugs. This may lead to drug interactions and increased risk of toxicity or lack of efficacy.

■ Monitor serum drug levels at regular intervals after steady state is achieved.

■ Monitor 12-lead electrocardiogram for indications of efficacy and toxicity.

Patient/Family Education for Antiarrhythmics

■ Advise patients of possible adverse reactions such as dizziness, which is a common reaction. Advise patients to change positions slowly when arising from a lying position.

■ Caution patients to be careful driving or engaging in other activities that require alertness until the response to the medication is known.

■ Instruct patients on how to take their own pulse and blood pressure.

■ Advise patients to immediately contact the clinician to report hypotension and slow, rapid, or irregular heart rate.

■ Instruct patients to report fever, chills, sore throat, or unusual bruising.

■ Advise patients that it is critical to keep follow-up appointments to monitor efficacy and adverse reactions.

■ Advise patients to wear a medical identification bracelet or necklace that states the name of the drug they are taking and/or the disorder for which it is being taken.

Class I Antiarrhythmic Drugs

Class I drugs are the sodium channel blocking agents. Quinidines inhibit ventricular automaticity and slow conduction velocity. Due to differences in the potency of the drugs to slow conduction velocity, this class of drugs is subdivided into class IA, IB, and IC.

Class IA drugs—quinidine (Quinidex, Quinora); procainamide (Pronestyl, Procan SR); and disopyramide (Norpace)—lengthen the duration of action potential and prolong the ventricular refractory period. They also reduce the speed of conduction and block parasympathetic nervous discharge, resulting in increased conduction rates at the AV node.

Class IB drugs—lidocaine (Xylocaine IV); tocainide (Tonocard); and mexiletine (Mexitil)—slow conduction and shorten the action potential and non-disease tissue. These drugs act on the polarized myocardium binding to sodium channels in the inactivated state.

Class IC drugs—propafenone (Rythmol) and flecainide (Tambocor)—act in the refractory period in the Purkinje fibers without altering the refractory period in the adjacent myocardium. They have a propensity for severe exacerbation of arrhythmias, even in normal doses, in patients after MI.

The class I antiarrhythmics have different adverse effects and precautions because their mechanisms of action differ. Given the nature of arrhythmias and their treatment risks and benefits, a cardiologist should be consulted for anyone with a rhythm disturbance because the choice and use of drugs is based on assessment by electrophysiological studies and not by empiric means. These agents are expensive, and the margin between their therapeutic toxicity and efficacy is very narrow, which again necessitates use by cardiologists.

Procainamide (Procan SR, Pronestyl)

A wide range of arrhythmias, including both ventricular and atrial arrhythmias, may be suppressed by procainamide, making it a popular agent.

Mechanism of Action

Procainamide increases the effective refractory period and decreases conduction velocity in the atria and ventricles. It also increases the threshold for cardiac excitability in the atria and ventricle as well as the slowing phase for depolarization.

Pharmacokinetics

- Absorption: Well absorbed following IM administration. A sustained-release (SR) oral preparation is more slowly absorbed.
- Distribution: Rapidly and widely distributed.
- Metabolism: Converted by the liver to an active compound.
- Excretion: That which is not converted to an active metabolite (40% to 70%) is excreted unchanged in the kidneys.
- Half-life: 2.5 to 5 hours.

Dosage and Administration

Generic Name	Trade Name	Route	Dose
procainamide	Pronestyl	PO	Non-life-threatening symptoms: 1.25 gm initially, then 750 mg 2 hr later, then 0.5–1 gm every 2–3 hr, followed by maintenance dose of 0.5–1 gm every 4–6 hr.
		IV	Life-threatening symptoms: 100 mg every 5 min until arrhythmia is abolished.
		IM: Only when IV and oral routes are unavailable	50 mg/kg/day in divided doses every 3–6 hr.

Clinical Uses

- Treatment of atrial arrhythmias such as premature atrial contractions, paroxysmal atrial tachycardia, and atrial fibrillation of recent onset

- Effective for maintaining normal sinus rhythm after conversion from atrial flutter or fibrillation

Adverse Reactions

CV: Hypotension, AV BLOCK, VENTRICULAR ARRHYTHMIAS, COMPLETE HEART BLOCK
DERM: Rashes
GI: Anorexia, diarrhea, bitter taste, nausea, vomiting
HEM: AGRANULOCYTOSIS, leukopenia, thrombocytopenia
MISC: Chills, fever
NEURO: SEIZURES, confusion, dizziness

Interactions

- Other antiarrhythmics will produce an additive effect.
- Antihypertensives and nitrates will potentiate hypotension effect.
- Drugs with anticholinergic properties will produce an additive anticholinergic effect, such as dry mouth, wheezing, urinary retention, and orthostatic hypotension.
- Ranitidine, cimetidine, quinidine, or trimethoprim will increase the effects of procainamide.

Contraindications

- Hypersensitivity
- AV block and myasthenia gravis
- Hypersensitivity to tartrazine dye (FD&C Yellow no. 5)

Conscientious Considerations

- Due to its proarrhythmia risks, treatment should be limited to hemodynamically significant data with ECG, pulse, and blood pressure (BP) monitored. If patient is given IV procainamide, he or she should remain supine throughout the procedure.
- Oral procainamide should not be used longer than 3 months without a complete blood count (CBC) check every 2 weeks.

Patient/Family Education

- A drug-induced lupus reaction (fever, chills, joint pain, rash); leukopenia (sore throat, gums, mouth); or thrombocytopenia (unusual bleeding or bruising) may occur, requiring that medication be discontinued.
- Routine follow-up examinations are necessary to monitor progress.

Lidocaine (Xylocaine)

This agent, commonly known as the topical anesthetic lidocaine or Solarcaine, is used in many popular over-the-counter (OTC) preparations. It can also be given IM and IV as an antiarrhythmic drug.

Mechanism of Action

Given IM or IV, lidocaine suppresses automaticity and spontaneous depolarization of the ventricles during diastole by altering the flux of sodium ions across cell membranes with little or no effect on heart rate. Given topically, it produces local anesthesia by inhibiting transport of ions across neuronal membranes, thereby preventing initiation and conduction of normal nerve impulses.

Pharmacokinetics

- Absorption: Well absorbed after administration into the deltoid muscle (IM).
- Distribution: Widely distributed concentrating in adipose tissue. Crosses blood-brain barrier and enters breast milk.
- Metabolism: Metabolized in the liver.
- Excretion: Metabolites excreted in urine.
- Half-life: Has biphasic half-life; first is 7 to 30 minutes, followed by terminal phase of 90 to 120 minutes.

Dosage and Administration

Generic Name	Trade Name	Route	Dose
lidocaine	Xylocaine	IV in hospital	1–1.5 mg/kg as a bolus; repeat every 5–10 min up to total dose of 3 mg/kg, then start continuous infusion of 1–4 mg/kg/min as antiarrhythmic in adults
lidocaine	LIDOJECT	IM self-injected when no IV is available	300 mg/3 mL self-injection; may repeat in 60–90 min

Clinical Uses

- Used exclusively for ventricular arrhythmias, especially those associated with acute myocardial infarction.
- Not effective in treatment of supraventricular arrhythmias such as atrial flutter or fibrillation.
- Treatment of digitalis-induced arrhythmias.

Adverse Reactions

Note: These reactions apply to systemic, not topical, use.

CV: CARDIAC ARREST, arrhythmia, bradycardia, hypotension
GI: Nausea, vomiting
MISC: Allergic reactions, ANAPHYLAXIS
NEURO: CONVULSIONS, confusion, drowsiness, dizziness, nervousness, slurred speech, tremor
PUL: Respiratory depression

Interactions

- May have additive or antagonistic effects anti-arrhythmics.

Contraindications

- Hypersensitivity
- Heart block

Conscientious Considerations

- DURING ADMINISTRATION ECG, BP, AND RESPIRATORY RATES MUST BE MONITORED.
- Serum lidocaine levels should be monitored periodically to watch for signs of toxicity if lidocaine therapy is to be prolonged.

Patient/Family Education

- Because lidocaine may cause dizziness, patients should call for assistance if walking or being transferred in a facility.

- Lidocaine is available as LidoPen, an autoinjector for use outside a hospital. If symptoms occur, patients should know how to self-administer it: (1) remove safety cap, (2) place back end of autoinjector on back of thigh or deltoid muscle, (3) press hard until needle prick is felt, (4) hold in place for 10 seconds, (5) massage area for another 10 seconds. Patients should call for help and not drive after an injection.

Flecainide (Tambocor)

Flecainide is a class IC medication that stabilizes membranes and depresses the action potential phase. This drug comes with a black box warning because there is an increased risk of mortality and nonfatal cardiac arrest rate when used in non-life-threatening ventricular arrhythmias in patients who have had MIs 6 days to 2 years previously.

Mechanism of Action

Flecainide slows conduction in cardiac tissues by altering transport of ions across cell membranes; thus, it can suppress arrhythmias because it affects automaticity of the SA node and slows AV node of conduction.

Pharmacokinetics

- Absorption: Well absorbed from GI tract following oral administration
- Distribution: Widely distributed
- Metabolism: Mostly metabolized in the liver, but liver disease may increase free drug levels
- Excretion: Metabolites and unchanged drug (30%) in the urine
- Half-life: 13 hours

Dosage and Administration

Generic Name	Trade Name	Route	Dose
flecainide	Tambocor	PO	For ventricular tachycardia (sustained or life threatening): 100 mg every 12 hr initially; increase by 50 mg 2 times/day until response is obtained. Maximum dose is 400 mg. Some patients require dosing every 8 hr for paroxysmal supraventricular tachycardia (PSVT): 50 mg every 12 hr; increase by 50 mg 2 times/day every 4 days until effective. Maximum dose 300 mg/day.

Clinical Uses

- Sustained ventricular tachycardia
- **Paroxysmal supraventricular tachycardia (PSVT)** (occasional rapid heart rate)

Adverse Reactions

CV: May slow conduction in a reentrant circuit without terminating it. This may lead to accelerating the ventricular rate during atrial flutter because fewer atrial beats are blocked owing to the slower cyclic link. It may also lead to converting a rapid, but self-limited, AV reentrant tachycardia into a slower but persistent arrhythmia.

EENT: Diplopia, tinnitus, blurred vision.
GI: Nausea, constipation.
MS: Asthenia (loss of strength).
NEURO: Dizziness, headache, tremor.

Interactions

- Calcium channel blockers, beta blockers: Increase arrhythmia risk, additive myocardial depression
- Digoxin: Increases digoxin levels
- Amiodarone: Doubles serum flecainide levels
- Acidifying agents, foods that decrease urine pH less than 5, acidic juices: Increase renal elimination, decrease effectiveness

Contraindications

- Hypersensitivities
- Preexisting AV block, cardiogenic shock (sustained decrease in cardiac output despite adequate blood volume as occurs with myocardial infarction causing the heart to not deliver adequate blood to the organs), CAD

Conscientious Considerations

- Use with extreme caution in patients with structural heart disease and anyone with potential for myocardial ischemia.
- This is not considered first-line therapy and should be kept in reserve for resistant arrhythmias.
- Must monitor plasma levels in patients with renal disease and HF.

Patient/Family Education

- Watch for dizziness and blurred vision.

Class II Antiarrhythmic Drugs

Class II antiarrhythmic drugs are beta blockers, which reduce adrenergic activity in the heart. This class of drugs includes beta-1 selective drugs that act mainly on cardiac muscle and nonselective beta-1 and beta-2 drugs that also act on lung, arterial, pancreatic, kidney, adipose, and liver tissues, resulting in a wide range of adverse responses. The antiarrhythmic properties of beta-adrenergic receptor agonists results from two major actions. These drugs increase the threshold potential and prolong the effective refractory period (ERP), and thus they decrease heart rate and conduction velocity. They also exert a significant negative inotropic effect that reduces the force of contraction. A more complete discussion of these drugs is provided in Chapter 7 (Drugs Used to Control Blood Pressure) .

Class III Antiarrhythmic Drugs

The class III drugs bretylium (Bretylol) and amiodarone (Cordarone) are used for arrhythmia emergencies, whereas sotalol (Betapace) is used primarily in family medicine. Dofetilide (Tikosyn) and ibutilide (Corvert) prolong the action potential and refractory period of myocardial cells and act directly on all cardiac tissue. These drugs often block potassium channels, which results in a decreased AV and sinus node function as evidenced by a lowering of ventricular ectopic beats and suppression of arrhythmia. Dofetilide and ibitilfide are used in hospitals and nursing homes to maintain normal sinus rhythm in patients following conversion from atrial fibrillation or flutter. Dosing requires an individualized regimen using a seven-step dosing algorithm dependent on calculated creatine clearance and QT interval measurements.

Amiodarone (Cordarone)

A class III antiarrhythmic drug, amiodarone (Cordarone), prolongs the rapid repolarization phase of myocardial tissue (phase 3); however, it has an FDA black box warning stating that patients should be hospitalized while it is being administered and its use should be restricted to life-threatening arrhythmias (recurrent ventricular fibrillation or ventricular tachycardia)owing to the possibility of drug-associated toxicity and the need for constant monitoring. Alternative agents should be tried first. Even though an oral form of amiodarone is available for use with outpatients, patients should be hospitalized when amiodarone is initiated because of its complicated pharmacokinetics and unpredictable onset of arrhythmia.

Mechanism of Action

Amiodarone acts directly on all cardiac cells to inhibit adrenergic stimulation (both alpha- and beta-blocking properties) affecting sodium, potassium, and calcium channels, thereby prolonging the action potential and the refractory period. The resulting effect is suppression of arrhythmias as the AV and sinus node functioning are depressed.

Pharmacokinetics

- Absorption: IV administration means complete bioavailability. PO administration results in slow and variable absorption (35% to 65%).
- Distribution: Accumulates slowly in all body tissues but reaches higher levels in fat tissues, muscle, liver, lungs, and spleen.
- Metabolism: In the liver to several metabolites, one of which is active.
- Excretion: In the bile.
- Half-life: 13 to 100 or more days; metabolite 611 days.

Dosage and Administration

Generic Name	Trade Name	Availability	Adult Dose Ventricular Arrhythmia	Adult Dose IV For Ventricular Arrythmia
amiodarone	Cordarone, Pacerone	200-mg and 400-mg tabs 50 mg/mL in 3-mL ampoules	600–800 mg/day in 1–2 doses, then 600–800 mg/day in 1–2 doses for a month, then 400 mg/day maintenance	10 mg/kg/day for 10 days until response or adverse effects occurs, then 5 mg/kg/day for several weeks, then decrease to 2.5 mg/kg/day as maintenance dose

Clinical Uses

- It suppresses life-threatening ventricular and supraventricular arrhythmias that are refractory to other drugs.
- Given PO, it is indicated in management of supraventricular tachyarrhythmias. Given IV, it is part of the Advanced

Cardiac Life Support (ACLS) and Pediatric Advanced Life Support (PALS) treatment guidelines for ventricular fibrillation and pulseless ventricular tachycardia after cardiopulmonary resuscitation and/or defibrillation have failed.

Adverse Reactions

CV: WORSENING OF HF OR ARRHYTHMIAS, hypotension, heart block, bradycardia

DERM: Photosensitivity, rash, slate-blue skin, TOXIC EPIDERMAL NECROSIS

ENDO: Hypothyroidism, hyperthyroidism (because iodine is an element in this drug, about 5% of patients with underlying predisposition to thyroid disease may develop thyrotoxicosis or hypothyroidism, thus a thyroid function test is ordered before therapy begins)

GI: Anorexia, nausea, vomiting, constipation, abnormal sense of taste, LIVER FUNCTION ABNORMALITIES

GU: Decreased libido, epididymitis

NEURO: Dizziness, fatigue, malaise, headache, insomnia, ataxia, parathesia, neuropathy, poor coordination, tremors

PUL: Pulmonary fibrosis

Interactions

- Digoxin: Increases blood levels and toxicity risk.
- Class I antiarrhythmics: Increase blood levels and toxicity risk.
- Beta blockers, calcium channel blockers: Increase the risk for bradyarrhythmias, sinus arrest, and AV block.
- Cholestyramine: May decrease amiodarone blood levels.
- Quinolones, macrolides, and azoles: Increased risk of QT prolongation.
- St. John's wort: Induces enzymes that metabolize amiodarone and thus decrease serum levels and effectiveness.
- GRAPEFRUIT JUICE TAKEN CONCURRENTLY INCREASES SERUM LEVELS AND CHANCE OF TOXICITY because it has an enzyme that inhibits GI tract metabolism of the amiodarone.

Contraindications

- Use cautiously in patients with a history of HF.
- Do not use in patients with cardiogenic shock, severe sinus node dysfunction, or severe AV block and bradycardia.

Conscientious Considerations

- SHOULD ONLY BE ADMINISTERED BY CLINICIANS WITH EXPERIENCE IN TREATING LIFE-THREATENING CONDITIONS because an ECG will have to be monitored continuously during IV therapy.
- Monitoring parameters need to be introduced to check on pulmonary toxicity (chest X-ray), electrolytes, liver function tests, ECG, QT intervals, central nervous system (CNS) symptoms.

Patient/Family Education

- Inform patient that side effects may not occur until weeks or years after starting therapy and may persist for several months after withdrawal.

- Teach patients how to monitor their pulse rate on a daily basis.
- Advise patients of potential photosensitivity reactions and how to prevent them.
- Inform patients that a bluish tinge to face, neck, and arms is possible after prolonged use and that it is reversible and will fade over time.
- Inform male patients of possible epididymitis (pain and swelling in scrotum), which may require a reduction in dose.
- Emphasize the importance of follow-up exams.

Sotalol (Betapace)

Sotalol is both a class II and a class III antiarrhythmic. It is a beta-adrenergic blocking agent that prolongs action potential, effective refractory period, and QT interval.

Mechanism of Action

- It decreases heart rate and AV node conduction and increases AV node refractoriness.

Pharmacokinetics

- Absorption: Well absorbed following oral administration
- Distribution: Crosses the placenta and enters breast milk
- Metabolism: None
- Excretion: Unchanged in the urine
- Half-life: 12 hours

Dosage and Administration

Generic Name	Trade Name	Route	Dose
sotalol	Betapace	PO	MANAGEMENT OF LIFE-THREATENING ARRHYTHMIA: usually 80 mg 2 times/day to start; may increase up to 240 mg/day

Clinical Uses

- Management of life-threatening ventricular arrhythmias

Adverse Reactions

CV: BRADYCARDIA, HF, PULMONARY EDEMA, ARRHYTHMIAS

DERM: Itching, rashes

EENT: Blurred vision, dry eyes, nasal stuffiness

ENDO: Hyperglycemia, hypoglycemia

GI: Constipation, diarrhea, nausea

GU: Erectile dysfunction, decreased libido

MS: Arthralgia, back pain, muscle cramps

NEURO: Paresthesia, fatigue, weakness, drowsiness, memory loss, mental status changes, nervousness, nightmares

PUL: Bronchospasm, wheezing

Interactions

- Not recommended with other drugs in its class or may be increased risk of CV events.
- May alter the effects of insulin or oral hypoglycemics.
- Ingestion of nitrates or other antihypertensives with alcohol may cause additive hypotension.
- User of amphetamines or cocaine may result in excessive hypertension.

Contraindications

- Bronchial asthma
- Cardiogenic shock
- Prolonged QT syndrome

Conscientious Considerations

- Monitor BP and pulse frequently.
- Monitor intake and output ratios and weight to assess patient for fluid overload.

Patient/Family Education

- Refer to Patient/Family Education for Antiarrhythmics on page 91.
- Tell patients to look for signs of overdose, especially bradycardia, dizziness, severe drowsiness, and bluish fingernails, and report these to the clinician.
- Inform patients that initial therapy may cause drowsiness and that they should avoid driving until effects are known.
- Advise patients to check pulse daily and BP biweekly. If heart rate is under 50 BPM, they should contact a clinician.
- Instruct patients with diabetes to closely monitor blood sugar, especially if weakness, malaise, irritability, or fatigue should occur.

Bretylium tosylate (Bretylium)

This class III antiarrhythmic directly affects myocardial cell membranes, contributing to suppression of ventricular tachycardia.

Mechanism of Action

Bretylium tosylate works by way of an electrophysiological effect that results in prolongation of the action potential and lengthening of the ERP, which ends in an increase in myocardial contractility. This drug is also taken up by the adrenergic nerve terminals where, after an initial release of epinephrine, it prevents further release, thereby increasing the threshold for antifibrillation.

Pharmacokinetics

- Absorption: Given IV or IM
- Distribution: Only 1% to 6% protein bound
- Metabolism: Not metabolized at all
- Excretion: Unchanged in the urine
- Half-life: 6 to 13 hours

Dosage and Administration

Generic Name	Trade Name	Route	Dose
sotalol	Betapace	PO tablets	Ventricular arrhythmia: 80 mg 2 times/day to start, then moves up to a maintenance dose of 160–320 mg/day in 2–3 divided doses. Atrial fibrillation: 80 mg 2 times/day; increase using careful monitoring up to 120 mg 2 times/day if necessary.

Clinical Uses

- For the prophylaxis and treatment of ventricular arrhythmias.

Adverse Reactions

CV: ARRHYTHMIAS, BRADYCARDIA, HF, PULMONARY EDEMA, orthostatic hypotension, peripheral vasoconstriction
DERM: Itching, rashes
EENT: Blurry vision, dry eyes, nasal stuffiness
ENDO: Hyperglycemia
GI: Constipation or diarrhea, nausea, vomiting, bitter taste
GU: Impotence, decreased libido
MISC: Paresthesia of fingers and toes, hand tremors, weakness, drug-induced lupus syndrome
NEURO: Fatigue, weakness, anxiety, dizziness, drowsiness, insomnia, memory loss, depression, nervousness, nightmares
PUL: Cough, breathing difficulties (due to neuromuscular blockade)

Interactions

- Catecholamines and digoxin may have enhanced effects resulting from some norepinephrine release.

Contraindications

- Use with caution in patients with aortic stenosis, severe pulmonary hypertension, and kidney function impairment.

Conscientious Considerations

- Patients need constant monitoring, especially ECGs, electrolytes, and BP.

Patient/Family Education

- Advise patients of the risks and benefits.
- Refer patients to education sources to learn about taking antiarrhythmics and sotalol.
- This medication may mask tachycardia and increased blood pressure as signs of hypoglycemia, but dizziness and sweating may still occur.

Class IV Antiarrhythmics

These drugs are calcium channel blockers (CCBs). Examples are verapamil (Calan) and diltiazem. They are used as antianginal, antiarrhythmic, and antihypertensive agents. As antiarrhythmics they inhibit the movement of calcium ions across cardiac and smooth muscle membranes. The result is a dilation of coronary arteries, peripheral arteries, and arterioles, ending in decreased heart rate as myocardial contractility and AV and SA conduction. Also, decreased peripheral vascular resistance results through vasodilation. They also have been used for treating idiopathic left ventricular tachycardia. These drugs are fully discussed in Chapter 7. They are included here because they are used to temporarily control rapid ventricular rates in atrial fibrillation or flutter or to achieve conversion of paroxysmal supraventricular tachycardia to normal sinus rhythm. Frequent side effects of the CCBs include peripheral edema, dizziness, lightheadedness, bradycardia, asthenia, and weakness.

Pharmacology of Nitrates for Angina

Nitrates were first introduced for the treatment of the chest pain of angina during the 19th century. Their affect on both oxygen supply and demand is rapid, hence the reason for their use in treating heart failure as nitrates are potent vasodilators.

Chronic stable angina, also known as **angina pectoris**, is a syndrome that occurs in people who have ischemic heart disease, which is approximately half of all patients with CAD. Its symptoms include a deep pressure pain in the sternum and a discomfort that radiates to the neck, jaw, left arm, or shoulder. It is usually brought on by exertion and is often relieved by rest or nitroglycerin. More women than men experience epigastric discomfort. Patients with diabetes may experience equivalent symptoms that are often mistaken for underlying ischemia. Angina is thought to be caused by the inability of the body to meet the demand for myocardial oxygen, particularly after exertion or exercise. Smoking, diabetes, stress, lack of exercise, hypertension, high levels of low-density lipoprotein (LDL), family history of atherosclerosis, previous peripheral vascular disease (PVD) or cerebral vascular disease (CVD), and being male are risk factors.

Exercise stress testing provides the clinician with functional information and helps set in motion risk stratification, which helps guide decision making for more testing and for selection of appropriate medications. Specific treatment is aimed at accomplishing four things: reducing myocardial oxygen demand, improving oxygen supply to myocardial tissue, treating the cardiac risk factors, and controlling any factors that could exacerbate or precipitate ischemia. To treat angina, a multipart approach is used, including the use of multiple drugs. This approach can be recalled by using the mnemonic ABCDE, the definition of which is as follows:

A = *aspirin and anticoagulant therapy*. Use of aspirin (ASA) in patients with stable angina has been shown to reduce cardiovascular incidents by 33% when using 325 mg ASA every other day (Physicians Health Study, 2010).

B = *beta-adrenergic antagonists and blood pressure control*. Any beta blocker is effective in controlling angina as it reduces heart rate (HR) and BP. Nitrates, either long-acting formulations for chronic use or sublingual tablets for acute angina, are adjuncts to baseline therapy. Sublingual tablets are to be used at first symptoms of angina or before engaging in any activities that may precipitate it. If angina fails to respond to the third sublingual dose, patients need to seek medical help. As more and more therapeutic options become available, clinicians need to also be aware of the lifestyle options available to aid in risk reduction such as:

C = *cholesterol-lowering agents*. Atherosclerosis is the most common risk factor for angina; the cholesterol reducing agents are commonly prescribed in an angina patient's therapy.

D = *cessation of smoking*. Produces a substantial risk reduction of all-cause mortality regardless of age, sex, and cardiac event.

E = *diet*. An individual should totally avoid the consumption of saturated fats and food stuffs that give rise to cholesterol. The individual's diet should include lots of fruits, cereals, rice, whole grain bread, vegetables, and fibrous foods. Oily fish (salmon, tuna, mackerel) are also important as sources of omega-3. Additionally patients should eat lean meat or chicken. Alcohol should be consumed in limited proportions, and the intake of chocolate, butter, red meat, sugar, and fried foods should be totally stopped.

F = *exercise*. Angina mostly occurs due to faulty eating habits; however, it can also happen to a person who is under lot of stress and tension. It is important for patients to learn important techniques that help in de-stressing, such as exercise, and that it be part of the patient's new lifestyle and habits.

A new agent, ranolazine (Ranexa), is being sold to treat chronic angina. It too is used in combination with amlodipine, beta blockers, and nitrates.

Conscientious Prescribing of Nitrates

■ Nitrates may aggravate angina caused by idiopathic hypertrophic cardiomyopathy.
■ Tolerance to the effects of nitrates frequently occurs.
■ Excessive dosage may produce severe headache.
■ Severe hypotension may occur in patients who are volume depleted or hypotensive.
■ Oral nitrates have a significant hepatic first-pass effect. Oral nitrates must be given in sufficiently high doses to sustain blood levels despite the first-pass effect.

Patient/Family Education for Nitrates

■ Instruct patients to take medication exactly as directed and at the same time each day. Inform the patient to take a missed dose as soon as remembered, unless the next scheduled dose of nitrate is scheduled to be taken within 2 hours.
■ Advise the patient to change positions slowly when getting up because orthostatic hypotension is possible.
■ Instruct the patient to take the first dose while in a reclining position until effects are known.
■ Inform the patient that headache is a common side effect of nitroglycerin, but it should stop as the therapy continues (ASA or acetaminophen can be used to treat the headache).
■ IF AN ACUTE ANGINAL ATTACK OCCURS: Instruct the patient to sit down and use the NTG as relief of first symptoms, which usually occurs within 5 minutes. If there is no relief within 5 minutes, repeat the dose. If no relief occurs after another 5 to 10 minutes, take a third tablet. If angina is not relieved after 15 minutes, the patient should go quickly to the nearest emergency room.

Nitroglycerin (NTG)

Nitroglycerin is available as an extended-release capsule (Nitrocot); extended-release tablet (Nitrong); extended-release buccal tablet (Nitrogard); IV preparation (Nitro-BID); translingual spray (Nitrolingual, Nitro-Mist); ointment (Nitro-Bid); sublingual tablet (Nitrostat); and a transdermal patch system (Nitro-Dur, Minitran, Transderm-Nitro).

Mechanism of Action

■ Increases coronary blood flow by dilating the coronary arteries and improving collateral flow to ischemic regions. This is accomplished by relaxing the cardiovascular smooth muscle by stimulation of the intracellular cycle guanosine monophosphate production.

- Reduces myocardial oxygen demand by decreasing preload and, to a lesser extent, decreasing afterload.
- Causes vasodilation that is greater in the veins than in the arteries, resulting in venous pooling and thereby decreasing left ventricular volume (preload) and reducing ventricular end diastolic volume.

Pharmacokinetics

- Absorption: Well absorbed by oral, buccal, sublingual, and transdermal routes. Sublingual absorption is dependent on salivary secretion.
- Distribution: Remains unknown.
- Metabolism and excretion: Undergoes rapid and almost complete metabolism in the liver and by enzymes in the bloodstream. In oral forms, it has a strong first-pass effect. Sublingual forms have no first-pass effect.
- Half-life: 1 to 4 minutes.

Dosage and Administration

Generic Name	Trade Name	Route	Dose
nitroglycerin	Nitrostat	Sublingual (0.3–0.6 mg tabs)	0.3–0.6 mg. May repeat every 5 min for 15 min for acute attack.
	Nitrolingual	Lingual spray (0.4 mg/spray)	1 or 2 sprays; may be repeated every 5 min for 15 min.
	Nitrogard	Buccal tablets Extended release	1 mg every 5 hr, dosage and frequency may be increased as necessary.
	Nitro-Bid, Nitrol	Ointment 2%	1 inch = 15 mg. Use 1–2 inches every 8 hr up to 5 doses in 24 hr.
	Nitro-Dur, Transderm Nitro, Deponit, Nitrek	Transderm patch system (0.1–0.6 mg/hr up to 0.8 mg/hr)	Patch should be worn 12–14 hr/day and then removed.
	Nitro-Bid IV, Tridil	Intravenous	5 mcg/min; increase by 5 mcg/min every 3–5 min to 20 mcg/min, then increase by 10–20 mcg/min every 3–5 minutes. Dosing is determined by hemodynamic parameters.

Clinical Uses

- For treating acute angina (translingual and sublingual dosage forms) and for long-term prophylaxis of angina pectoris (oral, buccal, and transdermal forms).
- When given in IV form, it is an adjunct in the treatment of acute MI and acute HF.

Adverse Reactions

CV: Tachycardia, hypotension, syncope, rebound hypertension, arrhythmia

DERM: Rash, contact dermatitis with ointment and patch forms, flushing
GI: Nausea, vomiting, diarrhea, abdominal pain
NEURO: Headache, lightheadedness, syncope, anxiety, nervousness, weakness

Interactions

- Antihypertensives, beta blockers, CCBs, Haldol, or phenothiazines: Additive hypotension effect.
- Drugs with anticholinergic effects: Decrease absorption of sublingual or buccal nitroglycerin.
- Aspirin: Increases nitrate serum concentrations and may potentiate their action.
- CONCURRENT USE OF NITRATES IN ANY FORM WITH SILDENAFIL (VIAGRA), TADALAFIL (CIALIS), AND VARDENAFIL (LEVITRA) INCREASES THE RISK OF A SERIOUS AND POTENTIALLY FATAL HYPOTENSIVE CRISIS.

Contraindications

- Hypersensitivity
- Severe anemia
- Closed-angle glaucoma
- Postural hypotension
- Early myocardial infarction
- Cerebral hemorrhage
- Pericardial tamponade

Conscientious Considerations

- Transdermal patches may be applied to any hairless site. Units are waterproof and do not fall off while showering.
- Patients with migraine headaches are at increased risk for the headaches caused by nitrates.

Patient/Family Education

- Instruct patients who are using sublingual tablets to accept tablets only in brown glass containers. They should be kept in these containers or in specially made metal containers. Tablets will lose potency in plastic or paper containers or in the presence of other tablets or capsules in the container. They will also absorb moisture, and exposure to air and heat will also cause their potency to decline.
- Instruct patients to avoid handling containers frequently, keeping them in a humid bathroom or hot glove compartment of the car, or carrying them in a pocket. They should also remember that after 6 months, tablets lose their potency; thus, keeping a large supply on hand is fruitless.
- Instruct patients who are using lingual spray to not shake the container or inhale the spray.
- Warn patients who are using ointment that they should not get it on their hands because it may be absorbed and cause side effects such as headache.
- Warn patients who are using the transdermal patch to stay away from microwave ovens because any leaking microwaves could heat one of the foil backing layers in the patch.

Isosorbide Dinitrate (Isordil) and Isosorbide Mononitrate (Imdur, Monoket)

Isosorbide dinitrate and mononitrate are used for the prevention of angina, not for the treatment of acute attacks of angina pectoris. They are also used to treat HF because they are able to produce vasodilation in which venous vasodilation is greater than arterial vasodilation.

Mechanism of Action

These drugs reduce myocardial oxygen consumption by increasing coronary blood flow, and because of the vasodilation, there is improved blood flow to ischemic regions.

Pharmacokinetics

■ Absorption: Isosorbide dinitrate undergoes extensive first-pass metabolism in the liver, resulting in 25% bioavailability; however, isosorbide mononitrate does not undergo first-pass metabolism, thus is 100% bioavailable.
■ Distribution: Unknown.
■ Metabolism: Isosorbide dinitrate is metabolized in the liver to two active metabolites, whereas isosorbide mononitrate is metabolized in the liver to inactive metabolites.
■ Excretion: All metabolites excrete in the urine.
■ Half-life: Isosorbide dinitrate: 1 hour; isosorbide mononitrate: 5 hours.

Dosage and Administration

Generic Name	Trade Name	Route	Dose
isosorbide dinitrate	Iso-Bid, Isordil, Sorbitrate, ISDN, ISOBID	Sublingual tablets, regular tablets Extended release	5–20 mg 2–3 times/day for prophylaxis of angina
isosorbide mononitrate	Imdur, Isotrate, Ismo, Monoket	Tablets Extended release	5–20 mg 2 times/day, given at least 7 hr apart

Clinical Uses

■ Relief and prevention of angina pectoris attacks

Adverse Reactions

CV: Hypotension, tachycardia, syncope
GI: Nausea, vomiting, abdominal pain
MISC: Flushing
NEURO: Dizziness, headache

Interactions

■ Concurrent use with any erectile dysfunction drug (sildenafil, tadalafil, vardenafil) may result in a fatal hypotension.
■ There is additive hypotension with beta blockers, alcohol, CCBs, and phenothiazines.

Contraindications

■ Anyone taking sildenafil, vardenafil, or tadalafil

Conscientious Considerations

■ Older patients may be more sensitive to these agents.

Patient/Family Education

■ Instruct the patient taking extended release tablets to not break or chew them, but rather to swallow them whole.
■ Inform patient that headache is a very common side effect that should discontinue with continued use.
■ Ask patient if he or she is taking any herbal, other prescribed, or OTC medications.
■ Instruct patient to avoid driving or any other activity requiring alertness until the effects of the drug are known.
■ Instruct the patient to not alter dosage to prevent a headache and to take last dose about 7 p.m. to prevent the development of tolerance.

Ranolazine (Ranexa)

In 2006 the Federal Drug Administration approved a new drug for the treatment of chronic angina. It is the first in a new class of antianginal drugs that differ from other agents. Chemically, it is a racemic mixture of a piperazine derivative, which as a novel metabolic/oxidation modulator is considered to be cytoprotective because it does not alter functions of the normal heart. Thus, ranolazine can be coadministered with beta blockers, nitrates, CCBs, antiplatelet therapy, ACE inhibitors, lipid-lowering agents, and ARBs.

Mechanism of Action

Ranolazine will not relieve acute anginal attacks. It is a partial fatty acid oxidation inhibitor that is designed to change myocardial energy metabolism from fatty acids to glucose. Thus, it increases the efficiency of adenosine triphosphate production under hypoxic conditions and exerts an antianginal and anti-ischemic effect without changing hemodynamics.

Pharmacokinetics

■ Absorption: Highly variable
■ Distribution: Distributed about two-thirds bound to protein
■ Metabolism: Hepatic using the cytochrome P40 system
■ Excretion: Primary in the urine as metabolites
■ Half-life: 7 hours

Dosage and Administration

Generic Name	Trade Name	Route	Dose
ranolazine	Ranexa	PO 500 mg, 100 mg tablets	500 mg 2 times/day

Clinical Uses

■ Treatment of chronic angina in patients who continue to be symptomatic while using beta blockers, calcium antagonists, or nitrates.

Adverse Reactions

CV: Syncope, bradycardia, palpitations, hypotension, orthostatic hypotension
EENT: Tinnitus, vertigo
GI: Constipation, abdominal pain, dry mouth
HEM: Hematocrit decreased

NEURO: Dizziness, headache, weakness
PUL: Dyspnea

Interactions

▪ Any CYP-3A4 inhibitor (diltiazem, ketoconazole, verapamil) will increase the effects of ranolazine.
▪ Because concurrent ingestion of grapefruit juice will increase the effects of ranolazine, it is contraindicated.
▪ Hypersensitivity.

Conscientious Considerations

▪ Use with caution in patients over 75 years of age; dosage may have to be adjusted if there is renal impairment.

Patient/Family Education

▪ DO NOT USE THIS DRUG FOR RELIEF OF ACUTE ANGINA ATTACKS.
▪ Instruct patients to not break, crush, or chew these tablets.

Direct-Acting Peripheral Arteriolar Vasodilators

Although these drugs are covered in detail in Chapter 7, Drugs Used to Regulate Blood Pressure, they are also discussed here because direct vasodilator therapy is a standard treatment for patients with HF. Arterial vasoconstriction (afterload) and venous vasoconstriction (preload) occur in patients with HF because the rennin-angiotensin-aldosterone matrix has been activated. It makes sense, therefore, that oral vasodilators should be part of the therapy given to patients with stabilized chronic HF, and parenteral vasodilators should be used in patients with acute HF. However, use of direct-acting vasodilators for HF is diminishing, except for hydralazine (Apresoline), a chemical derivative of phthalazine, and minoxidil (Loniten), a derivative of 2,4 pyrimidinediamine 3-oxide. Hydralazine acts directly on arterial smooth muscle to produce vasodilation and reduce afterload. Used in combination with nitrates, it improves the survival rate of HF patients. Hydralazine (37.5 mg) and isosorbide dinitrate (20 mg) in combination with beta blockers and ACEIs is standard therapy for African American patients, who have a highly disproportionate prevalence of hypertension when compared to other populations (Ghalia et al., 2007).

Hydralazine and minoxidil (are two direct-acting oral vasodilators used for their ability to provide vasodilating effects on peripheral arterioles. They decrease BP and peripheral resistance in cases of moderate to severe hypertension. They are often combined with a thiazide diuretic (chlorothiazide or hydrochlorothiazide) rather than used as monotherapy owing to significant reflex-mediated cardiac stimulation and water retention. Note that a drug-induced lupus syndrome is associated with hydralazine, and a drug-induced hypertrichosis is associated with minoxidil.

Implications for Special Populations

Pregnancy Implications

When prescribing for the pregnant female, clinicians should carefully consider their choice of drugs. A selected list of antianginal drugs, along with their assigned FDA Safety Category, follows.

CATEGORY	DRUGS
B	sotalol (Betapace), tocainide (Tonocard), flecainide (Tambocor)
C	digoxin, quinidine (Quinidex, Cardioquin), procainamide (Pronestyl, Procan SR), disopyramide (Norpace), lidocaine (Xylocaine), mexiletine (Mexitil), propafenone (Rythmol), nitroglycerin (NTG), isosorbide dinitrate (Isordril), isosorbide mononitrate (Monoket, IMDUR), hydralazine (Apresoline), minoxidil (Loniten), ranolazine (Ranexa)
D	amiodarone (Cordarone)
X	bretylium (Bretylol)
Unclassified	

Pediatric Implications

Although the safety of digoxin during pregnancy has never been established, it has been used safely during pregnancy. Digoxin has been around since 1775 and has never undergone the clinical trials and rigorous testing to pass FDA safety and efficacy testing. To do so today would require many pregnant women to submit to these trials, and no one wants to chance any kind of mishap using modern research. However, centuries of experience have told physicians that digoxin can be used in times of pregnancy on a case by case basis, especially when the mother's life is at risk.

Geriatric Implications

Geriatric patients are particularly susceptible to digoxin toxicity. Age-related changes due to lessened renal function require dosage adjustments.

LEARNING EXERCISES

Case 1

You are working in an urgent care center when an 82-year-old female is brought in by her granddaughter. The grandmother has lived alone for the last 3 years and has developed increased difficulty with driving and getting around town. Her granddaughter tells you that her grandmother just doesn't seem to be herself. When you ask the patient is wrong, she says that she just doesn't feel well. She is fatigued and short of breath when walking, but not at rest. She is taking multiple medications, but can't remember the names. Two are for blood pressure, one is for cholesterol, and one is to control her fast heart rate.

On examination, she appears to be thin and frail. Blood pressure is 110/60, pulse rate is 42, temperature is 99.0, BMI is 19, and clothes appear to be loose fitting. Her heart rate is slow and appears to be regular. She has no heart murmur, and no signs of pulmonary or peripheral edema.

What do you think is the cause of her fatigue and bradycardia? What are your next steps in the evaluation?

Case 2

You are taking care of a 64-year-old male who was recently admitted to the hospital with new onset of congestive heart failure. He has a long history of hypertension, smoking, obesity, and sedentary lifestyle. Prior to this hospitalization he was taking lisinopril, 10 mg daily, amlodipine, 10 mg daily, and atorvastatin, 20 mg daily. He presented to the hospital with shortness of breath over the last 6 months, which got to the point that he couldn't get through the morning without falling asleep due to fatigue. He was admitted to the hospital and placed on furosemide IV, 20 mg, 2 times per day. An echocardiogram showed systolic dysfunction, with an ejection fraction of 35%. By the third day of hospitalization, he was changed to furosemide, 20 mg by mouth twice daily. He was walking without difficulty, was feeling much better, and felt ready to go home. What should his home medications be?

References

The Criteria Committee of the New York Heart Association. (1994). *NYHA Nomenclature and criteria for diagnosis of diseases of the heart and great vessels* (9th ed., p. 253-256). Boston: Little, Brown & Co.

Curtis, L. H., Whellan, D. J., Hammill, B. G., Hernandez, A. F., Anstrom, K. J., Shea, A. M., et al. (2008). Incidence and prevalence of heart failure in elderly persons, 1994-2003. *Archives of Internal Medicine, 168*(4), 418-424.

Ghali, J. K., Tam, S. W., Ferdinand, K. C., Lindenfield, J., Sabolinski, M. L., Taylor, A. L., et al. (2007). Effects of ACE inhibitors or beta-blockers in patients treated with the fixed-dose combination of isosorbide dinitrate/hydralazine in the African-American Heart Failure Trial. *American Journal of Cardiovascular Drugs, 7*(5), 373-380.

Hunt, S. A., Abraham, W. T., Chin, M. H., Feldman, A. M., Francis, G. S., Ganiats, T. G., et al. ACC/AHA 2005 guideline update for the diagnosis and management of chronic heart failure in the adult: A report of the American College of Cardiology/American Heart Association Task Force on Practice Guidelines (Writing Committee to Update the 2001 Guidelines for the Evaluation and Management of Heart Failure). Retrieved May 20, 2013, from www.ncbi.nlm.nih.gov/pubmed/16160202

National Library of Medicine (NLM). Medline Plus. (June, 2010). *Heart failure.* Retrieved January 8, 2013, from www.nlm.nih.gov/medlineplus/ency/article/000158.htm

Physicians Health Study. (February, 2010). Retrieved January 8, 2013, from http://phs.bwh.harvard.edu

Sidney, S., Rosamond, W. D., Howard, V. J., Leupker, R. V., and American Heart Association. (2013). The "Heart Disease and Stroke Statistics—2013 Update" and the Need for a National Cardiovascular Surveillance System Circulation. 127:21-23.

Taylor, A. L., Ziesche, S., Yancy, C., Carson, P., D'Agostino, R., Ferdinand, K., et al. (2004). Combination of isosorbide dinitrate and hydralazine in blacks with heart failure. *The New England Journal of Medicine, 351,* 2049-2057.

chapter 7

Drugs Used to Regulate Blood Pressure

Dipesh Patel, Mona M. Sedrak, John M. Boltri

Key Terms

Adrenergic

Angiotensin

Angiotensin-
converting enzyme
inhibitors (ACEIs)

Angiotensin
II-receptor
blockers (ARBs)

Calcium channel
blockers (CCBs)

Diuresis

Edema

Extracellular fluid

Henle's loop

Hyperkalemia

Hypertension

Hypertensive
emergencies

Hypokalemia

Hyponatremia

Intrinsic
sympathomimetic
activity

Nephron

Prehypertension

Resorption

Torsade de pointes

CHAPTER FOCUS

This chapter helps the student develop a working knowledge of drugs used to regulate blood pressure (BP). Because blood pressure is a function of cardiac output (CO) and peripheral vascular resistance (PR), from a clinical standpoint alterations in BP can be achieved using drugs that either lower PR or slow CO. The agents discussed in this chapter include angiotensin-converting enzyme inhibitors (ACEIs); angiotensin II antagonists/blockers (ARBs); beta-adrenergic antagonists/blockers (beta blockers); calcium channel antagonists/blockers (CCBs); alpha-2 agonists; centrally acting arterial vasodilators, veno-vasodilators, and vasodilators; diuretics; and drugs used in hypertensive emergencies. Diuretic drugs are included in this chapter because they decrease cardiovascular and cerebral morbidity and mortality in mild to moderate hypertension. Finally, this chapter stresses the importance of patient education regarding adherence to medication regimen and lifestyle modifications.

OBJECTIVES

After reading and studying this chapter, the student should be able to:

1. Describe the etiology, prevalence, and pathophysiology of hypertension.
2. Define the treatment goals as established by the *Seventh Report of the Joint National Committee on Prevention, Detection, Evaluation, and Treatment of High Blood Pressure* (JNC 7).
3. Understand the mechanism of action of the functional classes of oral antihypertensive agents.
4. List the common adverse reactions and contraindications of oral hypertensive agents.
5. Analyze the precautions and advisories conscientious clinicians need to be mindful of when using antihypertensives.
6. Differentiate between the various classes of oral hypertensives and the advantages and disadvantages of one class over another.
7. Synthesize the pharmacodynamics and pharmacokinetics of drugs used in hypertensive emergencies.
8. Recall the rationale for drug selection for the various diuretics.
9. Describe the pharmacokinetic properties, contraindications, and major side effects of the various diuretics.
10. List the patient advisories conscientious clinicians should give to patients who are taking diuretics.

DRUGS USED TO TREAT HYPERTENSION

Functional Classes of Drugs Used as Antihypertensives

Direct-Acting Peripheral Vasodilators
- hydralazine (Apresoline)
- minoxidil (Loniten)

Beta Adrenergic Antagonists/Blockers (Beta Blockers)

Selective (beta-1 stimulation blocked)
- atenolol (Tenormin)
- betaxolol (Kerlone)
- bisoprolol (Zebeta)
- esmolol (Brevibloc)
- metoprolol (Lopressor)
- metoprolol succinate (Toprol XL)

Nonselective (Both BETa-1 and Beta-2 Stimulation Blocked)
- propranolol (Inderal)
- carvedilol (Coreg)
- nadolol (Corgard)
- timolol (Blocadren)
- sotalol (Betapace)

Combined Alpha/Beta Blockers
- carvedilol (Coreg)
- labetalol (Trandate; Normodyne)

Intrinsic Sympathomimetic Activity
- acebutolol (Sectral)
- carteolol (Cartrol, Ocupress)
- penbutolol (Levatol)
- pindolol (Visken)

Angiotensin-converting Enzyme Inhibitors (ACEIs)
- benazepril (Lotensin)
- captopril (Capoten)
- enalapril (Vasotec)
- fosinopril (Monopril)
- lisinopril (Prinivil, Zestril)
- moexipril (Univasc)
- quinapril (Accupril)
- ramipril (Altace)
- perindopril (Aceon)
- trandolapril (Mavik)

Angiotensin II Antagonists/Receptor Blockers (ARBs)
- candesartan (Atacand)
- irbesartan (Avapro)
- losartan (Cozaar)
- losartan and HCTZ (hydrochlorothiazide) (Hyzaar)
- olmesartan (Benicar)
- irbesartan (Avapro)
- telmisartan (Micardis)
- valsartan (Diovan)
- valsartan and HCTZ (Diovan-HCT)

Calcium Channel Antagonists/Blockers (CCBs)

Dihydropyridine
- isradipine (DynaCirc)
- nifedipine (Procardia, Adalat XL)
- nisoldipine (Sular)
- nicardipine (Cardene) SR

Nondihydropyridine
- amlodipine (Norvasc)
- diltiazem, SR, CD, XR (Cardizem; Dilacor; Tiazac)
- verapamil (Isoptin, Calan, Verelan)

Alpha-Adrenergic Antagonists
- doxazosin (Cardura)
- prazosin (Minipress)
- terazosin (Hytrin)

Agents Used in Hypertensive Emergencies

Direct-Acting Vasodilators
- nitroprusside Na (Nitride; Nitropress)

- hydralazine (Apresoline)
- minoxidil

Centrally Acting Adrenergic Agents
- clonidine (Catapres, Duraclon)
- methyldopa (Aldomet)

Oral Diuretics

Thiazides
- chlorothiazide (Diuril)
- hydrochlorothiazide (Esidrix, Hydrodiuril, Oretic, HCTZ)
- hydroflumethiazide
- methyclothiazide

Thiazide-like Diuretics
- chlorthalidone (Hygroton)
- indapamide (Lozol)
- metolazone (Zaroxolyn, Mykrox)

Loop Diuretics
- bumetanide (Bumex)
- furosemide (Lasix)
- torsemide (Demadex)

Potassium-Sparing Diuretics
- amiloride (Midamor)
- spironolactone (Aldactone)
- triamterene (Dyrenium)
- eplerenone (Inspra)

Parental (Osmotic) Diuretics
- mannitol (Osmitrol)

Special Use Diuretics

Carbonic Anhydrase Inhibitors
- acetazolamide (Diamox)
- dichlorphenamide (Daranide)
- methazolamide (Neptazane)

DRUGS USED IN THE TREATMENT OF HYPERTENSION

Hypertension (HTN) is a symptom that exists when blood pressure (BP) is elevated to a sustained level at which a patient is at increased risk for target organ damage. At least 50 million adult Americans have hypertension and are at risk for organ damage in one or more vascular beds of the retina, brain, heart, kidney, and the larger arteries. Hypertension becomes very significant for people over age 50 because systolic blood pressure (sBP) above 140 mm Hg causes a serious risk for coronary heart disease (CHD), a fourfold increase in risk for a cerebral vascular accident (CVA), and a sixfold increase in risk for congestive heart failure (CHF) or CHD when compared to normotensive people (NHLBI, 2011).

Hypertension is typically diagnosed when an asymptomatic patient undergoes a routine health screening, and it can be of two types: essential hypertension (also called primary hypertension) or secondary hypertension. Essential hypertension is usually symptom free, and although it makes up 90% of the cases of hypertension, the cause of it remains unknown. For this reason, the popular press often calls essential hypertension "the silent killer." Secondary hypertension may also be symptom free and is diagnosed in 10% of hypertension cases. It is so named because it is "secondary" to physiological causes such as renal disease, coarctation of the aorta, primary hyperaldosteronism, or problems with the adrenal-renal axis resulting in salt retention.

A physical examination of patients suspected of being hypertensive includes a thorough history, investigation for target organ damage using laboratory tests, and an assessment of cardiac function, especially for detection of left ventricular hypertrophy (LVH). Blood pressure measurements are typically performed several times, on multiple occasions, and under nonstressful conditions to obtain an accurate assessment. Home monitoring also helps assess a true average blood pressure, which in turn helps assess organ damage while ruling out other causes of blood pressure elevation, such as "white coat syndrome," prehypertension, drug resistance, and episodic hypertension.

The *Seventh Report of the Joint National Commission on Prevention, Detection, Evaluation, and Treatment of High Blood Pressure* (JNC 7) brought a significant shift to the diagnosis and treatment recommendations for hypertension, especially because it recognized the condition known as **prehypertension** and defined it as sBP of between 120 to 139 mm Hg and diastolic blood pressure (dBP) of between 80 to 89 mm Hg. This change is significant because JNC 7 recommends lifestyle modifications to reduce blood pressure *before* a state of hypertension exists. These lifestyle changes factors include the following:

■ Smoking cessation
■ Reduction in body weight if the patient is obese
■ Exercise in moderation
■ Reduction of alcohol use to very moderate levels
■ Low-sodium diet

In addition, JNC 7 recommends use of thiazide-type diuretics as the primary drug treatment for most cases of uncomplicated hypertension, either alone or in combination with drugs from other functional classes such as **angiotensin-converting enzyme inhibitors (ACEIs)** and calcium channel blockers (CCBs). The recommended target BP for medication therapy is a level below 140/90 mm Hg, or less than 130/80 mm Hg for those patients who have diabetes or chronic kidney disease. Finally, JNC 7 emphasizes the need for the clinician to motivate patients to be compliant and adhere to their medication regimen.

Hypertensive therapy should be a simple regimen to which a patient can easily commit and adhere. A majority of patients with mild hypertension can attain adequate control of their BP with single-drug therapy. Clinicians usually use monotherapy first and then multiple drug therapy if indicated. However, many clinicians use larger doses of the monotherapy before adding another agent. The well-known and accepted clinical trial, the Antihypertensive and Lipid-Lowering Treatment to Prevent Heart Attack Trial (ALLHAT) demonstrated that the initial drug choice for treating hypertension should be influenced by coexisting factors such as race, age, angina, any signs of CHF, renal insufficiency, obesity, left ventricular heart fraction, hyperlipidemia, gout, and bronchospasm. The ALLHAT hypertension study was a randomized, double-blind, practice-based clinical trial that sought to compare traditional antihypertensive medicines with newer classes of antihypertensives. It began in 1994 and lasted 8 years. One of its outcomes resulted in the withdrawal of preexisting diuretic therapy from many patients who were assigned to amlodipine or lisinopril (National Heart, Lung, and Blood Institute, 2005).

Conscientious Prescribing of Antihypertensives

■ Clinicians today typically initiate hypertensive therapy with ACEIs, angiotensin II-receptor blockers (ARBs), diuretics, and beta blockers because they reduce stroke morbidity and mortality and appear to be relatively safe.

■ Patients with a known history of coronary heart disease/chronic heart failure (CAD/CHF) should be treated with beta blockers and ACEIs.
■ Patients with a history of diabetes should be started on ACEIs or ARBs if not otherwise contraindicated.
■ Because BP response is usually consistent with the agent within a pharmaceutical class, if one agent fails to control BP, choosing another agent from within the same class will likely prove ineffective.
■ The lowest possible dose of any drug that is effective to control BP is the goal; however, every 1 to 3 months the effectiveness of the drug and dose needs to be assessed.
■ Should a second drug be needed, it can generally be chosen from among the other first-line agents. Adding a diuretic is usually a good option because doing so may enhance effectiveness of the first drug beyond more than a simple additive effect.
■ If the patient's response to the current therapy wanes or appears inadequate over time, the cause could be poor compliance; drug interactions (such as use of NSAIDS, antidepressants, steroids, caffeine, cocaine, thyroid hormones); high sodium in the diet; high alcohol consumption; or secondary hypertension.

Patient/Family Education for Antihypertensives

■ Patients taking hypertensive medication should have a thorough understanding of the overall treatment plan, the reasons why a specific drug has been prescribed, and why lifestyle modifications are just as important as the medication.
■ The importance of adherence to the medication regimen must be fully discussed to help prevent adverse events from a disease that has no symptoms until it's too late.
■ Patients should be taught to take their blood pressure at home.
■ Patients should involve their families and caregivers in their treatment plan.
■ Drug regimens should be integrated into routine activities of daily living because they are about to become a lifelong habit.
■ Patients should rise slowly to prevent dizziness until the effects of medication are known.
■ Patients should ask a clinician about any over-the-counter (OTC), cough, or allergy medication they may want to take.
■ Patients should tell their clinician they are on these drugs and being treated for high blood pressure if planning any surgery.

Angiotensin-Converting Enzyme Inhibitors (ACEIs)

Angiotensin-**converting enzyme** is a high molecular weight protein located in the membrane of endothelial cells throughout the body. It is especially active in the lungs. Once released, angiotensin-converting enzyme converts the inactive peptide **angiotensin** I to the active vasoconstrictor angiotensin II and inactivates the vasodilator bradykinin and other vasodilating prostaglandins.

Mechanism of Action

ACEIs block circulating and tissue levels of angiotensin II, blocking its potent vasoconstriction action. When levels of angiotensin II are lowered, there is an increase in plasma renin activity and a reduction in aldosterone secretion. ACEIs also act on the renin-angiotensin-aldosterone (RAA) system to help reduce blood pressure by decreasing sodium (Na) and water (H_2O) retention. ACEIs produce five therapeutic effects:

1. Lower BP in patients with hypertension
2. Decrease afterload in patients with heart failure (HF)
3. Decrease development of overt HF
4. Increase survival of patients with myocardial infarction (MI)
5. Decrease progression of diabetic nephropathy

Pharmacokinetics

■ Absorption: Fairly rapid from the intestine
■ Distribution: Well distributed
■ Metabolism: Rapidly and extensively to active metabolite, following extensive first-pass effects
■ Excretion: Hepatic clearance the main route of any unchanged drug, whereas metabolites found in feces and urine
■ Half-life: Varies among medications (see Dosage and Administration).

Dosage and Administration

Generic Name	Trade Name	Route	Usual Adult Daily Dose	Half-Life
benazepril*	Lotensin	PO	5–40 mg daily	22 hr
captopril	Capoten	PO	12.5–100 mg 2–3 times/day	1.9 hr if healthy; 20–40 hr if renal disease†
enalapril	Vasotec	PO	5–40 mg daily	2 hr if healthy; doubles if HF
fosinopril	Monopril	PO	10–40 mg 1–2 times/day	12 hr
lisinopril	Zestril, Prinivil	PO	2.5–40 mg daily	11–12 hr
moexipril	Univasc	PO	7.5–30 mg 1–2 day	1 hr
quinapril	Accupril	PO	10–80 mg daily	2 hr
ramipril	Altace	PO	2.5–20 mg 1–2 day	13-17 hr
trandolapril	Mavik	PO	1–4 mg daily	6 hr
perindopril	Aceon	PO	2–8 mg daily	11 hr, but rises to 30–120 hr due to slow disassociation of active and inactive metabolites from tissue-binding sites

*Note use of "pril" on end of each generic name.
†Dose adjustment is needed in patients with renal function impairment

Clinical Uses

■ Reduction of BP, either alone or in combination with other antihypertensive. ACEIs can be used as first-line treatment for hypertension in diabetics and in those with HF.

Adverse Reactions

CV: Postural (orthostatic) hypotension; first-dose hypotension is likely with ACEIs.
DERM: Rash.
GI: Nausea, vomiting, diarrhea.
GU: Impotence.
HEM: Leukopenia.
META: **Hyperkalemia** (serum potassium levels greater than 5.5 mEq/L).
NEURO: Headache, dizziness, fatigue, somnolence.
PUL: Persistent dry cough. The cough is thought to develop secondary to a hypersensitivity to bradykinins, which are inactivated by ACEIs, increases in prostaglandins, and accumulation of potent bronchoconstrictors.
RENAL: Increased serum creatinine, renal failure, oligohydramnios.

Interactions

■ Risk of hypotension is increased with diuretics (use lower doses), nitrates, excessive alcohol use, and anesthesia.
■ Potassium-sparing diuretics, salt substitutes, indomethacin may increase risk of hyperkalemia.
■ NSAIDs may decrease antihypertensive effects.
■ Absorption may be decreased by antacids.
■ ACEIs increase levels of digoxin and lithium and may induce toxicity.

Contraindications

■ Cross-sensitivity exists among ACEIs.
■ Pregnancy.
■ Hypersensitivity.
■ Renal artery stenosis.
■ Use cautiously in cases of renal impairment, hypovolemia, **hyponatremia** (low sodium in body fluids outside cells), and the elderly.
■ Contraindicated in African Americans with HTN.

Conscientious Considerations

■ Advise female patients to stop this medication if trying to conceive.
■ Watch for dry cough.
■ Watch for angioedema (it can happen even after years of taking this medication).
■ Monitor potassium and creatinine levels.

Patient/Family Education

■ Advise patient to take medicine at same time each day.
■ Advise patient not to discontinue the medication before talking to the clinician.
■ Advise patient to avoid salt substitutes and foods with high K or Na.
■ Advise patient to seek clinician's help when choosing any cold remedy.
■ Advise patient to change positions slowly to minimize hypotension.

■ Advise patient to watch for a change in taste, which can occur but will resolve within 8 to 12 weeks.

Angiotensin II Antagonists/Blockers

Angiotensin II antagonists or blockers are referred to as ARBs or *sartans*; hence, their generic names have suffix *-sartan* in them because they are able to moderate or modulate the renin-angiotensin-aldosterone system. Their main use is in treating hypertension, but they are also used in treating patients with diabetes who have had kidney damage and in treating heart failure (HF) (see Chapter 6).

Mechanism of Action

ARBs are **angiotensin II-receptor blockers** that competitively inhibit angiotensin II at its receptor sites, especially on smooth muscle and the adrenal glands, preventing it from exerting its vasoconstrictor effect. By reducing vasoconstriction, ARBs reduce peripheral resistance and lower BP. The main advantage of ARBs, compared to ACEIs, is that they do not produce the cough that is associated with ACEIs.

Pharmacokinetics

■ Absorption: From the intestinal wall giving 60% to 80% bioavailability
■ Distribution: Protein bound in plasma
■ Metabolism: Hepatic, CYP-2C9, and CYP-3A4 isoenzyme systems to active metabolites
■ Excretion: In feces (80%) and urine
■ Half-life: Differs with medications (see Dosage and Administration)

Dosage and Administration

Generic Name	Trade Name	Route	Dose	Half-Life
candesartan	Atacand	PO	4–32 mg daily	5–9 hr
irbesartan	Avapro	PO	75–300 mg daily	11–15 hr
losartan	Cozaar	PO	25–100 mg daily	6–9 hr
olmesartan	Benicar	PO	5–40 mg daily	13 hr
telmisartan	Micardis	PO	2–80 mg daily	24 hr
valsartan	Diovan	PO	80–320 mg daily	6 hr

Clinical Uses

■ ARBs are most effective when used to reduce blood pressure in special populations such as persons with diabetic nephropathy, patients with heart failure (especially with systolic dysfunction), and for cardiac protection in high-risk cardiac patients (including postmyocardial infarction and stroke patients).

Adverse Reactions

CV: Postural (orthostatic) hypotension, MI, palpitations, tachycardia
EENT (eye, ear, nose, and throat): Pharyngitis, rhinitis
DERM: RASH, pruritus
GI: NAUSEA, vomiting, diarrhea, abnormal hepatic function, hepatitis
GU: Impotence
HEM: Leukopenia, agranulocytosis, anemia, neutropenia

META: Hyponatremia
MS: Myalgia, paresthesia
NEURO: Headache, dizziness, fatigue, somnolence, vertigo, anxiety, depression, lightheadedness, drowsiness
RENAL: Renal failure, renal impairment

Interactions

■ ACEIs, diuretics, and other antihypertension medications may provide additive antihypertensive effects.
■ Herbs, lithium, monoamine oxidase inhibitors (MAOIs), NSAIDs, trimethoprim, potassium-sparing diuretics may increase the risk of hyperkalemia.

Contraindications

■ Do not use in cases of hypersensitivity, pregnancy, or lactation.
■ Use cautiously in HF because may they result in oliguria, acute renal failure, and/or death.
■ In African Americans, ARBs may not be effective as monotherapy; additional agents may be required.

Conscientious Considerations

■ Watch for hyperkalemia and hypernatremia.
■ This medication can cause increase in serum creatinine.
■ ARBs can be the first-line antihypertensive in patients with diabetes and/or CHF.
■ Pregnancy: Class D causing BIRTH DEFECTS: Neonatal skull hypoplasia, anuria, renal failure, oligohydramnios, death.
■ Lactation: Excretion mild or not determined, not recommended.

Patient/Family Education

■ Patients should be instructed that continuous treatment is necessary and not to stop the medication abruptly.
■ If a dose is missed, patients should be instructed to take the next dose as soon as it is remembered but not to double the dose if it is near time for the next dose.
■ Advise patients about possible postural hypotension and not to rise abruptly from a sitting or lying down position.
■ Advise women about the risks of becoming pregnant and why they should use a contraceptive.
■ Patients should be aware that these medications may cause dizziness.

Beta-Adrenergic Antagonists/Blockers (Beta Blockers)

Beta blockers may be used as single agents or combined with a diuretic. As a class, they all have names ending in *–olol*. Beta blockers have the affinity for antagonizing the effects of catecholamines at beta-adreno-receptors on myocardial tissue (beta-1) and uterine, vascular, and pulmonary tissue (beta-2). Most are pure antagonists, but some are partial antagonists causing only partial blocking of the receptors. Beta-1-receptor antagonists may have some advantage over the nonselective beta antagonists when blockade of beta-1 receptors is desired and beta-2-receptor blockade is undesirable. Currently no beta-1-selective antagonist is sufficiently specific to completely avoid interactions with beta-2 adrenoreceptors. Thus, it is helpful to place beta blockers into one of four groups:

1. Selective beta blockers (beta-1 stimulation blocked)
2. Nonselective beta blockers (both beta-1 and beta-2 stimulation blocked)
3. Combined alpha/beta blocker
4. Beta blockers having intrinsic sympathomimetic activity

These drugs have several clinical uses, such as treatment of cardiac arrhythmias, angina pectoris, and the treatment of hypertension. The mechanism for achieving a sustained BP reduction in primary hypertension is not well understood, but decreases in heart rate (HR) and cardiac output (CO) are obvious in the beginning of treatment, and later under chronic use the decrease in peripheral resistance is seen. Tolerance to the antihypertensive effects of beta blockers is not a problem as it is with other categories of drugs, nor is the orthostatic hypotension that occurs with other classes. What makes the beta blockers quite popular is that they are well tolerated, and serious side effects are seldom observed. Up to one-third of the patients who take them for mild to moderate hypertension achieve a significant drop in BP if the drug is used alone. When a thiazide diuretic is added as part of the regimen, up to 80% of patients respond well and achieve BP goals.

Mechanism of Action

NONSELECTIVE BETA BLOCKERS. Block stimulation of both beta-1 (myocardial) and beta-2 (pulmonary, vascular, uterine) **adrenergic** receptor sites. They also have some alpha-blocking activity, which can result in orthostatic hypotension. These drugs are also used to suppress arrhythmias.

SELECTIVE BETA-1 BLOCKERS. Selectively block stimulation of beta-1 (myocardial) adrenergic receptors but have little to no effect on beta-2 blockers at doses under 100 mg. They do not exhibit any alpha-blocking activity or intrinsic sympathomimetic activity.

BETA BLOCKERS WITH ALPHA-BLOCKING ACTIVITY. Also block stimulation of beta-1 (myocardial) receptors and beta-2 (pulmonary, vascular, and uterine) receptors and have some alpha-blocking activity, which can lead to orthostatic hypotension.

BETA BLOCKERS WITH INTRINSIC SYMPATHOMIMETIC ACTIVITY. Also block stimulation of beta-1 (myocardial) receptors, but do not usually affect beta-2 (pulmonary, vascular, uterine) receptors. However, they have some mild **intrinsic sympathomimetic activity** (ISA).

Therapeutic effects of all these drugs are a slowing of the heart rate, resulting in a drop of BP. This improved cardiac output slows progression of HF and decreases the risk of death.

Pharmacokinetics

■ Absorption: All are well absorbed after oral administration.
■ Distribution: Well distributed and crosses placenta; enters breast milk due to their high lipid solubility.

■ Metabolism: Extensive hepatic metabolism using cytochrome P450 (CYP) isoenzymes; also first-pass metabolism can be extensive.
■ Excretion: Sotalol, metoprolol elimination is mostly renal, carvedilol elimination is mostly feces, atenolol elimination is both feces and urine because metabolism is incomplete.

Dosage and Administration

	Generic Name	Trade Name	Route	Usual Adult Daily Dose	Half-Life
SELECTIVE BETA-BLOCKERS (Beta-1 Stimulation Blocked)	esmolol*	Brevibloc	IV	500 mcg/kg as loading IV dose over 1 min, then 50 mcg/kg infusion over 4 min	9 min
	atenolol	Tenormin	PO	25–100 mg daily	6–9 hr
	betaxolol	Kerlone	PO	5–40 mg/daily	14–22 hr
	bisoprolol	Zebeta	PO	2.5–20 mg daily	9–12 hr
	metoprolol	Lopressor Toprol XL	PO	50–450 mg daily	3–7 hr
NONSELECTIVE BETA BLOCKERS (Both beta-1 and beta-2 stimulation blocked)	propranolol	Inderal	PO	40–240 mg daily	3–5 hr
	propranolol LA	Inderal LA		60–240 mg daily	9–18 hr
	nadolol	Corgard	PO	20–240 mg	20–24 hr
	timolol	Blocadren	PO	20–40 mg daily	4 hr
	Sotalol	Betapace	PO	80 mg 2 times/day	12 hr
COMBINED ALPHA/BETA BLOCKER	labetalol	Trandate	PO	100–1,200 mg daily	6–8 hr
	carvedilol	Coreg	PO	12.5–50 mg daily	7–10 hr
BETA BLOCKERS HAVING INTRINSIC SYMPATHOMIMETIC ACTIVITY	pindolol	Visken	PO	5 mg 2 times/day, may increase every 2–3 weeks up to 45–60 mg/day	3–4 hr
	penbutolol	Levatol	PO	10–60 mg daily	5 hr
	acebutolol	Sectral	PO	100–1,200 mg daily	3–4 hr
	carteolol	Cartrol	PO	2.5–10 mg daily	7–10 hr

*Note how all generic names end with "olol".

Clinical Uses

■ Cardiac arrhythmias, prevention of MI, and decreased mortality in patients with recent MI
■ Angina pectoris
■ Hypertension
■ Management of stable, symptomatic HF due to ischemic hypertensive or cardiomyopathic origin
■ Migraine prophylaxis, tremors, aggressive behavior, anxiety

Adverse Reactions

CV: Postural hypotension, bradycardia, syncope, atrioventricular (AV) block
DERM: Pruritus, rash
GI: Nausea, vomiting
GU: Impotence
META: Hypertriglyceridemia, weight gain, weakness, bradycardia, syncope
NEURO: Dizziness, fatigue, headache, depression
PUL: Bronchospasm, asthma

Interactions

- Additive bradycardia may occur with digoxin.
- Other antihypertensive medications (alpha blocker, calcium channel blocker), alcohol, nitrates may result in additive hypotension.
- Thyroid administration may decrease effectiveness.
- May see altered effects of insulin and oral hypoglycemics.

Contraindications

- Hypersensitivities
- Uncompensated HF
- Cardiogenic shock
- Second- or third-degree block
- Severe sinus bradycardia
- Severe chronic obstructive pulmonary disease or asthma
- Severe hypotension

Conscientious Considerations

- Watch for effects on the lipid profile, especially increased triglyceride levels and decreased high-density lipoprotein levels with nonselective beta blockers.
- Watch for signs of abrupt withdrawal because it has been the precursor to an angina attack or an increase in BP as a result of an increase in adrenergic tone.

Patient/Family Education

- Patient instructions should be the same as those for patients taking ARBs.
- Patients may find they are more sensitive to cold.
- Patients with diabetes should closely monitor their blood sugar.
- Patients should report slow pulse, difficult breathing, wheezing, cold hands and feet, dizziness, light-headedness, confusion, depression, rash, fever, sore throat, and unusual bleeding or bruising.

Calcium Channel Antagonists/Blockers (CCBs)

Calcium channel antagonists or blockers (CCBs) are effective for treatment of hypertension and are used extensively because they generally produce no significant central nervous system (CNS) side effects. They are also used to treat diseases that co-exist with hypertension, such as angina. There are two types of calcium channel blockers: the shorter-acting dihydropyridine and the longer-acting nondihydropyridine. The nondihydropyridine is associated with a higher safety profile when used to reduce ischemic cardiac events. Calcium channel blockers vary in the extent to which they affect different calcium channels. This accounts for the differences seen clinically in the magnitude of their effect on heart muscle compared to blood vessels, their effects on conduction of electrical signals in the heart, and their use as a single agent or in combination with other drugs.

Mechanism of Action

Calcium Channel Blockers (CCBs) inhibit calcium ions from entering the slow channels or voltage-sensitive areas of vascular smooth muscle and myocardium during depolarization. This produces a relaxation of coronary vascular smooth muscle and coronary vasodilation, which results in increased myocardial oxygen delivery. They also reduce cardiac contractility, depress sinoatrial nodal activity, and slow AV conduction. Within this class, verapamil and diltiazem act on the heart and blood vessels, whereas nifedipine, amlodipine, nicardipine, and nisoldipine act primarily to cause vasodilation and hence lowering of blood pressure. All CCBs are metabolized in the liver, thus in patients with liver issues, such as cirrhosis, dosage adjustments are required. As expected, these drugs inhibit the metabolism of other drugs cleared through hepatic metabolism.

Pharmacokinetics

- Absorption: These oral agents are well absorbed.
- Distribution: All are well-distributed and bound almost 100% to serum protein.
- Metabolism: All are hepatically metabolized by CYP-3A4 isoenzymes.
- Excretion: See Dosage and Administration table.
- Half-life: See Dosage and Administration table.

Dosage and Administration

Generic Name	Trade Name	Route	Usual Adult Daily Dose	Half-Life/ Excretion Site
amlodipine	Norvasc	PO	2.5–10 mg/day	36 hr/renal
diltiazem	Cardizem	PO, IV	180–240 mg/day	3.5–9 hr/renal, feces
isradipine	DynaCirc	PO	2.5–10 mg 2 times/day	6 hr/renal, feces
nicardipine	Cardene	IV, PO	20–40 mg 3 times/day	4 hr/urine, feces
nifedipine	Procardia	PO	10–20 mg 3 times/day	2–4 hr/urine, feces
nisoldipine	Sular	PO	17–34 mg/day	9–18 hr/urine, feces
verapamil	Calan, Isoptin	PO	80–120 mg 3 times/day	4–7 hr/urine, feces

Clinical Uses

- Primarily used as antihypertensive agents.
- Diltiazem (Cardizem) is sometimes used to convert heart rhythm and control heart rate.
- Diltiazem and verapamil can be used to treat essential hypertension, chronic stable angina, angina from coronary artery spasm, atrial fibrillation, atrial flutter, and paroxysmal supraventricular tachycardia.

■ Amlodipine (Norvasc) can be used to treat hypertension, symptomatic chronic stable angina, vasospastic (Prinzmetal's angina), and diastolic heart failure.

Adverse Reactions

CV: Arrhythmias, peripheral **edema** (accumulation of excessive fluid), flushing, palpitations, dyspnea, bradycardia

DERM: Rash, pruritus

EENT: Amblyopia, rhinitis, pharyngitis

GI: Nausea, abdominal pain, dyspepsia, gingival hyperplasia, constipation, vomiting, diarrhea, anorexia, dry mouth, alkaline phosphatase increased, alanine aminotransferase increased, aspartate aminotransferase increased

GU: Male sexual dysfunction, impotence, gynecomastia

META: Weight gain

MS: Muscle cramps, dyspnea, gout, myalgia, neck rigidity

NEURO: Headache, dizziness, fatigue, somnolence

PUL: Pulmonary edema

RENAL: Crystalluria

Interactions

■ Additive hypotension may occur with use of fentanyl, other antihypertensives, nitrates, quinidine, and alcohol.
■ Antihypertensive effect may be decreased by use of NSAIDs.
■ Use with digoxin or phenytoin may lead to bradycardia.
■ Vitamin D and calcium compounds decrease effectiveness.

Contraindications

■ Hypersensitivity.
■ Diltiazem and verapamil are contraindicated in patients with second-degree and third-degree heart block, wide complex ventricular tachycardia.
■ Use cautiously when there is renal impairment, history of arrhythmias, pregnancy, lactation, and in geriatric patients.

Conscientious Considerations

■ Cost is a factor in prescribing these drugs because it can lead to nonadherence.
■ Consider alternatives to this drug if the patient has difficulty swallowing.
■ Clinician must monitor liver function.
■ Pregnancy and Lactation: Pregnancy Risk Factor C: Excretion into breast milk is unknown, thus use is not recommended.

Patient/Family Education

■ Inform patients that these agents can be taken with or without a meal.

Direct/Central Alpha-2 Adrenergic Agonists

These centrally acting agents are also called *centrally acting adrenergic inhibitors* or *central alpha-2 agonists*. Central alpha agonists, such as clonidine (Catapres) and methyldopa (Aldomet) are usually prescribed when all other medications have failed. When they are used, however, they are typically combined with a diuretic. Clinicians should keep in mind these agents are likely to produce nasal congestion, drying of nasal mucosa, and rebound hypertension, which limits their acceptance by patients.

Clonidine (Catapres)

Although prescribed historically as an antihypertensive, clonidine (Catapres) is finding use today in a number of venues, including relief of neuropathic pain, opioid detoxification, a treatment for insomnia, relief of menopausal symptoms, and as an adjunct in attention deficit hyperactivity disorder. Some clinicians use it as a mild sedative before surgery.

Mechanism of Action

Clonidine (Catapres) stimulates alpha-2-adrenoceptors in the brainstem, which activates an inhibitory neuron, reducing sympathetic outflow from the CNS and thus opening peripheral arteries. By decreasing peripheral as well as renal vascular resistance and reduction of HR, clonidine reduces blood pressure.

Pharmacokinetics

■ Absorption: Available as tablets, injection, and transdermal patches where absorption and bioavailability vary (i.e., injection = immediate, tablet = 0.5 hours, and patch = 2 to 3 days)
■ Distribution: As highly lipid soluble, distributes into extravascular sites
■ Metabolism: Hepatic to inactive metabolites
■ Excretion: Two-thirds in urine, one-third in feces
■ Half-life: 6 to 20 hours and longer in renal impairment

Dosage and Administration

Generic Name	Trade Name	Form/Route	Dosage
clonidine	Catapres	PO	0.1 mg–0.4 mg 2 times/day
		Transdermal patch	One transdermal patch per week (equivalent to 0.1 mg/day release)
		Epidural injection	

Clinical Uses

■ When used as a transdermal patch or oral tablet it, can be used to manage mild to moderate hypertension. Given as an epidural injection, it helps manage cancer pain unresponsive to opioids alone.

Adverse Reactions

CV: Angioneurotic edema

DERM: Alopecia, hives

EENT: Blurred vision

GI: Abdominal pain, anorexia, constipation, hepatitis

GU: Decreased sexual activity, erectile dysfunction, loss of libido, gynecomastia

HEM: Thrombocytopenia

MS: Leg cramps

NEURO: Fatigue, fever, headache, agitation, anxiety, delirium, delusional perception, hallucinations, insomnia, mental depression

Interactions

- Additive sedation may occur with other antihypertensives, antidepressants, alcohol, antihistamines, and hypnotics.
- There is an increased risk of adverse cardiovascular reactions with verapamil.
- MAOIs, beta blockers, amphetamines, and tricyclics may decrease antihypertensive effects.

Contraindications

- Hypersensitivity
- Hypotension

Conscientious Considerations

- Clinician will need to monitor intake and output ratios and daily weight and assess for edema on a daily basis, especially at the beginning of therapy.
- The transdermal system is to be applied once every 7 days to a hairless area, with absorption being greater when placed on chest or upper arm.
- Transdermal clonidine should not be interrupted during any surgery.

Patient/Family Education

- Remind patient this medication helps control blood pressure, but is not a cure.
- Teach patient to take blood pressure weekly and to report any significant changes.

Methyldopa (Aldomet)

Methyldopa is the second agent in the class of centrally acting adrenergic agonists that is used as an antihypertensive, especially in difficult-to-treat cases. It also continues to have a role in treating pregnancy-induced hypertension (gestational hypertension). However, the use of other safer and effective classes of drugs has led to a decline in its use.

Mechanism of Action

Stimulates central alpha-adrenergic receptors, resulting in a decrease in sympathetic outflow to the heart, peripheral vasculature, and kidneys. The result is a drop in blood pressure as cardiac output remains the same, but peripheral resistance and heart rate decrease.

Pharmacokinetics

- Absorption: Only 50% is absorbed from the GI tract.
- Distribution: Well distributed and crosses the blood-brain barrier.
- Metabolism: Intestinal and hepatic.
- Excretion: Metabolites and remaining active compound are excreted by the kidneys.
- Half-life: 60 to 90 minutes.

Dosage and Administration

Generic Name	Trade Name	Route	Dosage For Hypertension
methyldopa	Aldomet	PO	250 mg 3 times/day, max. 3 gm/day

Clinical Uses

- Hypertension in pregnancy
- Moderate to severe hypertension

Adverse Reactions

CV: Edema, myocarditis, bradycardia, ORTHOSTATIC HYPOTENSION

GI: Dry mouth, cholestasis or hepatitis, increased liver enzymes, jaundice, cirrhosis, SLE-like syndrome (systemic lupus erythematosus)

GU: Sexual dysfunction, gynecomastia

HEM: Hyperprolactinemia, thrombocytopenia, hemolytic anemia, positive Coombs' test, leukopenia

NEURO: Depression, headache, dizziness, sedation, decreased mental acuity

Interactions

- Additive hypertension with other antihypertensives, alcohol, nitrates
- Excessive sympathetic stimulation will occur with MAOIs, catechol-o-methyltransferase inhibitors
- Lithium toxicity may increase
- Additive CNS toxicity and hypotension with levodopa
- Antihypertensive effect of methyldopa decreased in presence of amphetamines, barbiturates, tricyclics, NSAIDs, and phenothiazines

Contraindications

- Hypersensitivity
- Hepatic disease (active)
- MAOIs

Conscientious Considerations

- Monitor the patient's temperature during therapy as a drug fever may occur shortly after initiation of therapy. If unexplained fever does occur, then hepatic function needs to be monitored.
- Patient's weight and intake and output ratios need daily monitoring to watch for development of edema, especially at the beginning of therapy. Diuretics will reverse this.
- BP and pulse need frequent monitoring during therapy.
- Patient's refills of prescriptions should be monitored to assess adherence.

Patient/Family Education

- Education is the same as other antihypertensives, especially the need to be compliant with the regimen and to implement lifestyle modifications.
- Advise patients of potential drowsiness but that it usually subsides after 7 to 10 days.
- Advise patients of dry mouth effect and that frequent oral rinsing and use of sugarless gum may minimize this effect, which usually lasts about 2 weeks.
- Caution patients to avoid use of alcohol and antidepressants.

Direct-Acting Peripheral Arterial and Venous Dilators

Direct-acting peripheral vasodilators in common use today are hydralazine (Apresoline), minoxidil (Loniten), and nitroprusside (Nitropress). Nesiritide (Natrecor), human natriuretic peptide, is administered intravenously for hemodynamic support of patients with acutely decompensated heart failure who are experiencing dyspnea at rest or with mild activity.

Hydralazine (Apresoline)

Although hydralazine is not commonly used to treat hypertension, it continues to be prescribed for certain patients. As a smooth muscle relaxing agent, it helps relax blood vessels so that blood can flow more freely through them.

Mechanism of Action

Hydralazine lowers blood pressure by exerting a peripheral vasodilating effect through direct relaxation of vascular smooth muscle. By altering cellular calcium metabolism, it interferes with the calcium movements within the vascular smooth muscle that are responsible for initiating or maintaining the contractile state. Thus, there is direct vasodilation of arterioles with little effect on veins, ending with a decrease in peripheral resistance and lower blood pressure.

Pharmacokinetics

- Absorption: Well absorbed orally with effects in 20 minutes. IV forms bring effects in 5 to 20 minutes.
- Distribution: Crosses placenta and enters breast milk.
- Metabolism: Extensive hepatic metabolism; extensive first-pass effect of the oral dosage form.
- Excretion: Excreted by kidneys.
- Half-life: 2 to 8 hours if normal renal function.

Dosage and Administration

Generic Name	Trade Name	Route	Dosage
hydralazine	Apresoline	Orally	10–25 mg 4 times/day

Clinical Uses

- Moderate to severe hypertension
- Hypertension secondary to preeclampsia
- Primary pulmonary hypertension

Adverse Reactions

CV: Palpitations, tachycardia, angina pectoris, hypotension, edema
DERM: Flushing, rash, urticaria, pruritus (**Note:** MAY CAUSE A LUPUS-LIKE SYNDROME when larger doses and longer durations are used.)
EENT: Lacrimation, nasal congestion
GI: Anorexia, nausea, vomiting, diarrhea, constipation
HEM: Blood dyscrasias
MS: Paresthesia, numbness, tingling, arthralgia
NEURO: Headache, dizziness

Interactions

- Additive hypotension with other antihypertensives and alcohol.
- MAOIs may exaggerate hypotension.
- NSAIDs may decrease hypertensive response.
- Beta blockers may decrease tachycardia from hydralazine therapy and thus are often combined for the benefit of this drug interaction.

Contraindications

- Some tablets contain tartrazine and should be avoided in people with known sensitivities.
- Hypersensitivity.

Conscientious Considerations

- If giving oral tablets, then administer with meals to permit enhanced absorption.
- Pharmacists often prepare oral solutions from hydralazine injection for patients who have difficulty swallowing.
- If administering IV, use solution as quickly as possible after drawing through needle into a syringe because contact with metal causes hydralazine to change color.
- Monitor pulse and BP frequently after injection.

Patient/Family Education

- Provide the same education as for other antihypertensives.
- Advise patient to notify clinician if general tiredness, fever, muscle or joint aching, chest pain, skin rash, sore throat, numbness, weakness, tingling or numbness in hands and feet occur. Vitamin B (pyridoxine) is useful for treating any peripheral neuritis.

Minoxidil (Loniten)

Minoxidil was originally used as an antihypertensive agent. Hirsutism was an observed side effect, which prompted the manufacturer to seek U.S. Federal Drug Administration (FDA) approval of minoxidil as a treatment for male pattern baldness under the name Rogaine.

Mechanism of Action

Minoxidil is a direct-acting peripheral vasodilator that reduces elevated systolic and diastolic blood pressure by decreasing peripheral vascular resistance.

Pharmacokinetics

- Absorption: Well absorbed; the drug's effect is seen in 30 minutes and peaks in 2 to 3 hours, with effects lasting 2 to 3 days.
- Distribution: Circulates in an unbound state.
- Metabolism: Conjugates with glucuronic acid in liver to an active metabolite.
- Excretion: Excreted by the kidneys.
- Half-life: Of drugs and metabolites 3 to 5 hours.

Dosage and Administration

Generic Name	Trade Name	Route	Dosage
minoxidil	Loniten	PO	10–40 mg single or divided doses, max. dose 100 mg/day.

Clinical Uses

■ Used only in the treatment of hypertension that is symptomatic or associated with target organ damage and is not manageable with maximum therapeutic doses of a diuretic plus two other antihypertensive drugs. Minoxidil is reserved for severe hypertension that is unresponsive to other agents.

Adverse Reactions

CV: Salt and water retention, pericarditis, pericardial effusion, pericardial tamponade, tachycardia, angina
DERM: Hypertrichosis (face, arms, back), red flushing of skin
GI: Nausea, vomiting, anorexia
HEM: Thrombocytopenia, leukopenia
MS: Breast tenderness
NEURO: Dizziness

Interactions

■ If given with antihypertensive, cyclosporine, herbs, or MAOIs may induce a severe hypotensive reaction.

Contraindications

■ Hypersensitivity reaction
■ Pheochromocytoma
■ Use with caution in patients with cerebral vascular disease and MI

Conscientious Considerations

■ No specific monitoring is required for minoxidil.

Patient/Family Education

■ Patients should be instructed to take the drug at the same time very day and to not miss a dose. If a dose is missed, they should not double up, but take the missed dose as soon as it is remembered.
■ Hypotensive reactions are the most troublesome and most common; patients should change positions slowly and should not exercise in hot weather.
■ Patients should be taught to take BP and pulse and should monitor them at home. They should report changes greater than 20 mm Hg or 20 beats per minute past baseline.
■ Minoxidil and hydralazine are pregnancy category C, so contraception should be started before they are prescribed.

Nitroprusside (Nitropress)

As a fast and direct-acting arterial and venous dilator, nitroprusside is the drug of choice for most **hypertensive emergencies**. It greatly relaxes both arterial and venous smooth muscle, but it is more active on veins. It reduces blood pressure almost immediately upon IV administration. Its action is short-lived (2 to 3 minutes) and it is titratable. Patients need close monitoring in an institutional setting to avoid a hypotensive crisis or hypersensitivity reaction. Therapy usually lasts no more than 24 to 72 hours because a renal insufficiency reaction can occur due to accumulation of a toxic metabolite (thiocyanate). Serum thiocyanate levels must be monitored after 48 hours in cases of renal impairment or after 5 days if there is no renal impairment.

If thiocyanate accumulates, signs of cyanide poisoning occur, which melds into metabolic acidosis, dyspnea, vomiting, dizziness, ataxia, and syncope.

Mechanism of Action

The principal pharmacological action of sodium nitroprusside is relaxation of vascular smooth muscle and consequent dilatation of peripheral arteries and veins, which reduces peripheral resistance. It increases cardiac output by decreasing afterload and reduces aortal and left ventricular impedance.

Pharmacokinetics

■ Absorption: Given by IV infusion, bioavailability is 100%, and its onset of action is within minutes. The duration of effect is between 1 to 10 minutes upon discontinuation of the IV infusion.
■ Distribution: How nitroprusside is distributed throughout the body remains unknown, but it is attached to red blood cells (RBCs) in hemoglobin (Hb).
■ Metabolism: Nitroprusside is converted to cyanide ions as it travels bound to Hb in RBCs starting about 2 minutes after IV infusion. It then quickly decomposes to prussic acid, which is neutralized by enzymatic action in the liver to thiocyanate. This metabolic by-product, thiocyanate, is a potentially toxic agent that has a half-life of 3 days.
■ Excretion: Thiocyanate is excreted by the kidneys.
■ Half-life: Less than 10 minutes, closer to 2 minutes.

Dosage and Administration

Depending on the desired concentration, a solution containing 50 mg of nitroprusside must be further diluted in 250 to 1,000 mL of sterile 5% dextrose injection to make an IV infusion. The solution must be freshly prepared and protected from light sources. It has a 24-hour life expectancy. The IV infusion dose is 0.3 mcg/kg/min, not to exceed 10 minutes of therapy.

Clinical Uses

■ It is indicated for the rapid reduction in blood pressure needed in hypertensive emergencies.
■ It is also used as adjunctive therapy in myocardial infarction, and in cases of valvular regurgitation.

Adverse Reactions

CV: Bradycardia, tachycardia
GI: Abdominal pain, palpitation, nausea, vomiting
HEM: Methemoglobinemia
META: Acidosis
MISC: Phlebitis at the injection site, thiocyanate toxicity (tinnitus, miosis, and hyperreflexia)
NEURO: Headache, dizziness, restlessness

Interactions

■ None are noted, but concurrent antihypertensive medication use can lead to severe hypotension.

Contraindications

■ Should not be used for treatment of compensatory hypertension

- Should not be used during surgery for patient with known inadequate cerebral circulation
- Should not be used for acute heart failure

Conscientious Considerations

- Nitroprusside overdose can be manifested as excessive hypotension or cyanide toxicity or thiocyanate toxicity.
- Use only for hypertensive emergency.
- Use with caution in patients with anemia, hyperthyroidism, fluid and electrolyte imbalances, and respiratory diseases.
- Pregnancy category C: Use is cautioned in anyone thinking of becoming pregnant. Caution must be used in nursing mothers because cyanide and thiocyanate metabolites are excreted into breast milk.
- Any patient taking nitroprusside by IV infusion must have plasma thiocyanate levels taken every day to monitor for symptoms of thiocyanate toxicity.
- Cyanide toxicity is also a danger and may manifest as lactic acidosis, hypoxemia, tachycardia, altered consciousness, and a breath odor similar to almonds (see Box 7-1).

Nesiritide (Natrecor)

Nesiritide is a biosynthesized medication that is manufactured from *Escherichia coli* using recombinant DNA technology. It is used to treat acutely decompensated HF with dyspnea that occurs at rest or with minimal exertion (such as talking, eating, or bathing). Nesiritide is the recombinant form of the 32-amino acid human B type natriuretic peptide, which is normally produced by the ventricular myocardium.

Mechanism of Action

Given IV, nesiritide is able to bind to guanylate cyclase receptors on vascular smooth muscle and endothelial cells. The result is an increase in intracellular cyclic GMP, which induces smooth muscle cell relaxation, producing a reduction in pulmonary capillary resistance and systemic arterial pressure.

Pharmacokinetics

- Absorption: IV bolus produces drop in blood pressure within 15 minutes because it is 100% bioavailable.

- Distribution: Distributes well throughout the plasma, but mechanism is unknown.
- Metabolism: Peptide enzymes at cellular binding sites and internal cell components render the agent inert.
- Excretion: Excreted by the kidneys.
- Half-life: 18 minutes.

Dosage and Administration

Adults' dosage is provided as a sterile lyophilized powder, given *only* by IV bolus at 2 mcg/kg and infused over 2 minutes through a port in IV tubing, followed by a continuous infusion of 0.01 mcg/kg.

Clinical Uses

- Quickly induced lowering of blood pressure in patients suffering decompensated HF and dyspnea at rest or under minimal exertion.

Adverse Reactions

CV: Hypotension, tachycardia, bradycardia, extra systoles, angina pectoris
DERM: Itching, rash, sweating
EENT: Amblyopia
GI: Abdominal pain, nausea, vomiting
HEM: Anemia
MS: Muscle pain, back pain
NEURO: Paresthesias, tremor, anxiety, confusion, dizziness, headache, insomnia

Interactions

- This agent is chemically and physically incompatible with most drugs given IV, such as heparin and insulin.

Contraindications

- Contraindicated for those who are hypersensitive, in cardiogenic shock, or have systolic BP less than 90 mm Hg, or have any condition where cardiac output is dependent upon venous return.

Conscientious Considerations

- Only administer in setting where BP can be continuously monitored.
- This product is to be kept away from light once it has been reconstituted from its lyophilized powder.

Patient/Family Education

- Explain to the patient the use and administration of this product and what can be expected once it has been administered.

Diuretics

Diuretic medications are those that increase the discharge/excretion of urine by the kidney or as it is commonly called "diuresis" as taken from the latin "diourein" meaning "to urinate". **Diuresis** is accomplished by altering how the kidney handles sodium. If the kidney increases its output of sodium, water excretion will also increase. Diuresis occurs by inhibiting the

---

BOX 7-1 Treatment for Cyanide Toxicity from Nitroprusside

1. Administer 4 to 6 mg/kg of a 3% solution of *sodium nitrite* over 2 to 4 minutes. This acts as a buffering solution for cyanide by converting hemoglobin to methemoglobin. If sodium nitrate administration is delayed or unavailable, have patient inhale a crushed ampoule of amyl nitrite every 15 to 30 seconds until the sodium nitrite begins.

2. Following the sodium nitrite infusion, administer 150 to 200 mcg/kg of a 25% or 50% solution of sodium thiosulfate. This will convert the cyanide to thiocyanate, which the kidneys can eliminate.

3. If necessary, repeat the entire regimen at 50% of the doses in 2 hours.

reabsorption of sodium at different segments along the renal tubular system (Figure 7-1). The ability of each diuretic to act at different segments has advantages. For example, diuretics can be given in combination because they can be more effective as multidrug therapy than when acting alone. This effect is called *synergism* as one **nephron** (i.e., the structural and functional units in the kidney that filter and excrete waste from blood and produce urine) segment compensates for altered sodium reabsorption at a different nephron segment. There are six classes of diuretics: loop diuretics, thiazide diuretics, thiazide-like diuretics, potassium-sparing diuretics, osmotic diuretics, and carbonic anhydrase inhibitors.

Renal Handling of Sodium and Water

To understand the action of diuretics, it is first necessary to review how the kidney filters fluid and forms urine. As blood flows through the kidney, it passes into glomerular capillaries located within the cortex. These capillaries are highly permeable to water and electrolytes. The glomerular capillary's hydrostatic pressure

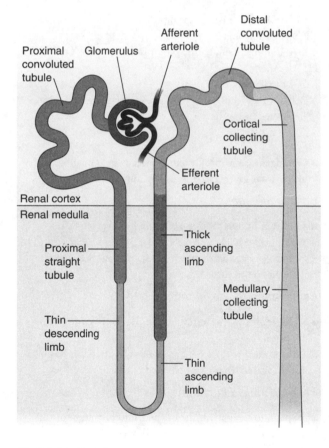

filters water and electrolytes into the Bowman's space and into the proximal convoluted tubule (PCT). The PCT is the site of sodium, water, and bicarbonate transport from the urine, across the tubule wall, and into the interstitium of the kidney cortex. About 65% to 70% of filtered sodium that is removed this way is then returned to the bloodstream. This is called *sodium reabsorption*; without it the body would soon be depleted of this valuable ion. Every sodium molecule that is reabsorbed is accompanied by a molecule of water. Because the interstitium of the medulla is very hyperosmotic and the **Henle's loop**. Named after the man who discovered it, F. G. J. Henle, this refers to the U-shaped portion of a nephron that creates a concentration gradient in a nephron making it permeable to water, so that water is reabsorbed from Henle's loop and into the medullary interstitium. This loss of water concentrates the urine within Henle's loop.

The thick ascending limb (TAL) is impermeable to water and has a coat transport system that reabsorbs sodium, potassium, and chloride at a ratio of 1:1:2. About 25% of the sodium load of the original filtrate is reabsorbed at the TAL. From the TAL, the urine flows into the distal convoluted tubule (DCT), which is another site of sodium transport. The DCT is also impermeable to water. The distal segment of the DCT and the upper collecting duct have a transporter that reabsorbs sodium in exchange for potassium and hydrogen ions that are excreted into the urine.

There are two important things to remember about this transporter. Its activity is dependent on the tubular concentration of sodium so that when sodium is high, more sodium is reabsorbed and more potassium and hydrogen ions are excreted. Also, this transporter is regulated by aldosterone. Increased aldosterone stimulates the **resorption** (the lysis and assimilation of a substance by biochemical activity) of sodium, which also increases the loss of potassium and hydrogen ion to the urine. Finally, water is reabsorbed in the collecting duct through special pores that are regulated by antidiuretic hormone, which is released by the posterior pituitary. Antidiuretic hormone increases the permeability of the collecting duct to water, which leads to increased reabsorption, a more concentrated urine, and reduced urine outflow.

Kidneys control the **extracellular fluid** volume by altering salt (NaCl) and water excretion. (Extracellular Fluid [ECF] is that clear liquid which contains proteins and electrolytes in blood plasma and in interstitial fluid. ECF is about 20% of a person's body weight and a normal body has about 15 quarts of it.) Blood pressure is maintained at the expense of extracellular fluid volume. Diuretics primarily prevent reabsorption of Na⁺ in the nephron.

Therapeutic Uses of Diuretics

There are several clinical uses for diuretics. Certain disease states may cause blood volume to increase outside of narrowly defined limits. These include hypertension, congestive heart failure, nephrotic syndrome, renal syndrome, liver cirrhosis, etc. (Table 7-1). Diuretics act to reduce extracellular fluid volume in different ways. The loop diuretics inhibit sodium reabsorption in the ascending Henle's loop whereas the thiazide-type

Site of diuretic action

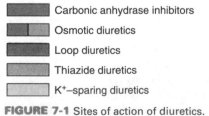

- Carbonic anhydrase inhibitors
- Osmotic diuretics
- Loop diuretics
- Thiazide diuretics
- K⁺–sparing diuretics

FIGURE 7-1 Sites of action of diuretics.

TABLE 7-1 Diuretics: Therapeutic Uses and Site of Action		
DIURETIC	**THERAPEUTIC USES**	**SITE OF ACTION**
Thiazide diuretics	1. Hypertension 2. Heart failure 3. Renal calculi 4. Nephrogenic diabetes insipidus 5. Chronic renal failure as an adjunct to loop diuretics 6. Osteoporosis	Distal convoluted tubule
Loop diuretics	1. Hypertension in patients with impaired renal failure 2. Heart failure (moderate to severe) 3. Acute pulmonary edema 4. Chronic or acute renal failure 5. Nephrotic syndrome 6. Hyperkalemia	Ascending limb of Henle's loop
Potassium-sparing diuretics	1. Chronic liver failure 2. Heart failure when hypokalemia is a problem	Collecting tubule
Osmotic diuretics	1. Acute or incipient renal failure 2. Reduce preoperative interocular or intracranial pressure 3. Reduce presurgical or post-trauma intracranial pressure	Proximal tubule, descending Henle's loop, collecting duct
Carbonic anhydrase inhibitors	1. Cystinuria (increase alkalinity of tubular urine) 2. Glaucoma (decrease ocular pressure) 3. Acute mountain sickness 4. Metabolic alkalosis	Proximal tubule

diuretics act on the distal renal tubule to inhibit sodium reabsorption. The potassium-sparing diuretics inhibit excretion of potassium distally (see Figure 7-1).

Antihypertensive management using diuretics is effective when coupled with reduced dietary sodium. However, first-line treatment of hypertension is with ACEIs, with the diuretics acting as adjuncts. Loop diuretics are the more effective for treating moderate congestive heart failure. Thiazide diuretics are have been proven to be most effective for mild to moderate HF and hypertension due to their ability to reduce cardiac output, blood volume, and eventually, systemic vascular resistance at doses of 12.5 or 25 mg and with a 3-days-per-week dosing schedule (i.e., 12.5 mg on Monday, Wednesday, Friday). Potassium-sparing, aldosterone-blocking diuretics are used in secondary hypertension caused by hyperaldosteronism. They are also sometimes used as an adjunct to thiazide treatment in primary hypertension to prevent **hypokalemia** (low potassium).

Diuretics are primarily used in heart failure to reduce pulmonary and/or systemic congestion and associated clinical symptoms such as shortness of breath. Heart failure leads to activation of the renin-angiotensin-aldosterone system, which causes increased sodium and water retention by the kidney and thus increases blood volume and contributes to the elevated venous pressures associated with heart failure. This leads to pulmonary and systemic edema.

Diuretics decrease blood volume in venous pressure through their effects on sodium and water balance. This decreases cardiac filling (preload) and decreases ventricular stroke volume and CO,

which leads to a fall in arterial pressure. Reduced capillary hydrostatic pressure is the result, causing less leakage from capillaries into the interstitium, which reduces edema.

Thiazide Diuretics

Thiazide diuretics such as chlorothiazide (Diuril), chlorthalidone (Hygroton, Thalitone), and hydrochlorothiazide (HCTZ) are most commonly used because they inhibit the sodium chloride transporter in the distal tubule. This transporter normally reabsorbs only about 5% of filtered sodium. Thus, thiazide diuretics are less effective than loop diuretics in producing diuresis. Because loop and thiazide diuretics increase sodium delivery to the distal segment of the distal tubule, the result will be potassium loss, which may lead to potentially fatal hypokalemia. Thiazide diuretics can also induce metabolic alkalosis, which accompanies an increase in tissue pH beyond normal, because hydrogen ions decrease and bicarbonate ions increase. The loss of potassium and hydrogen ions by loop and thiazide diuretics results partly from the activation of the renin-angiotensin-aldosterone system. This occurs because of reduced blood volume and arterial pressure. Increased levels of aldosterone stimulate sodium reabsorption and increase potassium and hydrogen ion excretion into the urine.

Mechanism of Action

Thiazide diuretics inhibit the sodium chloride transporter in the distal tubule and act fairly quickly once administered (Table 7-2). Their mechanism depends on renal prostaglandin production.

TABLE 7-2 Time-Action Profile of Diuretic Effect

DIURETIC	ONSET	PEAK	DURATION
chlorothiazide	2 hr	4 hr	6–12 hr
chlorthalidone	2 hr	2 hr	48–72 hr
hydrochlorothiazide	2 hr	3–6 hr	6–12 hr

Pharmacokinetics

- Absorption: All are rapidly absorbed after oral administration.
- Distribution: Well distributed into extracellular space. All cross the placenta and enter breast milk.
- Metabolism: All are excreted unchanged.
- Excretion: Excreted by the kidneys.
- Half-life: Chlorothiazide 1 to 2 hours, chlorthalidone 35 to 50 hours, hydrochlorothiazide 6 to 15 hours.

Dosage and Administration

	Generic Name	Trade Name	Route	Usual Adult Daily Dose
THIAZIDE DIURETICS	chlorothiazide	Diuril	PO, IV	250mg–500mg tabs 1–2 times/day
	hydrochloroth-iazide	Esedrix, HCTZ Microzide	PO	12.5mg–100 mg daily in 1-2 divided doses. Not to exceed 50mg/day in hypertesnsion as doses above 12.5mg/day are associated with electrolyte imbalances
	methycloth-iazide	Enduron	PO	2.5–5 mg daily
THIAZIDE-LIKE DIURETICS	chlorthalidone	Hygroton	PO	15–50 mg daily
	indapamide	Lozol	PO	1.25–5 mg daily
	metolazone	Zaroxolyn, Mykrox	PO	5–20 mg daily

Clinical Uses

- Mild to moderate hypertension
- Congestive heart failure
- Cirrhosis
- Renal insufficiency
- Nephrotic syndrome

Adverse Reactions

CV: Hypotension
ENDO: Hyperglycemia
GI: Anorexia, cramping, nausea, vomiting
GU: Erectile dysfunction
HEM: Blood dyscrasias
META: Hypokalemia, metabolic alkalosis, hyponatremia, dehydration leading to hypotension, hyperuricemia, hypercalcemia, hypomagnesemia, hypophosphatemia, hypovolemia
MS: Muscle cramps
NEURO: Dizziness, drowsiness, lethargy, weakness
RENAL: Azotemia

Interactions

- Hypokalemia potentiates digitalis toxicity.
- NSAIDs reduce diuretic efficacy.
- Beta blockers potentiate hyperglycemia, hyperlipidemia.
- Corticosteroids enhance hypokalemia.
- Concurrent use of allopurinol may increase incidence of hypersensitivity reactions.
- Bile acid-binding resins bind thiazide and reduce absorption by up to 85%.
- Synergistic diuresis and hypokalemia occur when used concurrently with loop diuretics.

Contraindications

- Anuria
- Renal decompensation
- Hypersensitivity to sulfonamide-derived drugs
- Hepatic coma or pre-coma

Conscientious Considerations

- The thiazides are extensively used in the treatment of hypertension, and it is always recommended that when any drug is added to a thiazide (or vice versa) a review for possible drug interactions be performed. Some interactions are important to remember. For example, the thiazide diuretics and/or the hypokalemia they produce increase the risk for **torsades de pointes**, a potentially life-threatening arrhythmia associated with sudden death.
- Given their ability to decrease glucose tolerance, insulin must be used with care.
- The thiazides may reduce the effectiveness of warfarin, lithium, loop diuretics, and vitamin D.
- Some drugs such as the NSAIDs and bile acid sequestrants may decrease the effectiveness of the thiazides. In addition, drugs that alkalinize the urine will decrease the effectiveness of thiazides.
- Thiazide diuretics are considered first-line agents for the treatment of hypertension.
- Thiazide diuretics produce a mild but sustained diuresis that tends to be limited by dehydration. They are useful for chronic diuretic therapy in heart failure in primary hypertension.
- Perform initial and periodic determinations of serum electrolytes, blood urea nitrogen (BUN), uric acid, and glucose.
- Observe patients for clinical signs of fluid or electrolyte imbalance.

Patient/Family Education

- Drug may cause GI upset; may be taken with food or milk.
- Drug will initially increase urination, which will subside after a few weeks.
- Take early during the day.
- Notify clinician if muscle pain, weakness or cramps, nausea, vomiting, restlessness, excessive thirst, tiredness, drowsiness, increased heart rate or pulse, diarrhea, or dizziness occurs.

- Drug may cause photosensitivity; avoid prolonged exposure to the sun and other ultraviolet light. Use sunscreen and wear protective clothing until tolerance is determined.
- Drug may increase blood sugar levels in patients with diabetes.
- Do not drink alcohol or take other medications without clinician's approval.
- Do not interrupt, discontinue, or adjust dose even if feeling well.

Thiazide-Like Diuretics

Indapamide (Lozol) and metaxalone (Zaroxolyn) are gaining in popularity for several reasons. Increasing glucose levels can be a problem for patients with diabetes. Hyperuricemia can be a problem for patients with gout, and metaxalone and indapamide are good choices for patients with this condition. If patients have a creatinine clearance (CCR) of less than 25 to 30 mL/min, then either of these agents are safe alternatives to other diuretics. Finally, metaxalone by itself is not a strong diuretic, but as an adjunct to a loop diuretic it works well to overcome situations in which HF is refractory and in cases in which its synergistic effect warrants a lowered dosage of a loop diuretic to avoid adverse effects.

Loop Diuretics

Loop diuretics such as bumetanide (Bumex), furosemide (Lasix), torsemide (Demadex), and ethacrynic acid (Edecrin) inhibit the sodium-potassium-chloride cotransporter in the ascending Henle's loop. This transporter system normally reabsorbs about 25% of sodium load. Loop diuretics are very similar to the thiazide diuretics in their pharmacology as well as their adverse effects (hyperglycemia, hyperuricemia, hypomagnesemia, and hypocalcemia).

Conscientious Prescribing of Loop Diuretics

- Loop diuretics produce a potent but short-lived diuresis that is not limited by dehydration.
- Excessive amounts of these drugs can lead to dire effects when water and electrolyte depletion is excessive.
- Loop diuretics are most useful for emergency reduction of fluid volume in congestive heart failure. Loop diuretics also appear to have a primary effect on prostaglandin production. They are associated with modest vasodilation, bronchodilation, and autoregulation of renal blood flow.
- Observe patients for blood dyscrasias, liver or kidney damage, or idiosyncratic reactions.
- Perform frequent serum electrolytes, renal and hepatic function, serum glucose, and uric acid levels, as well as CO_2, creatinine, and BUN determinations during the first few months of therapy and periodically thereafter.

Patient/Family Education for Loop Diuretics

- May cause GI upset. Can be taken with food or milk.
- Will increase urination, so take early in the day.
- May increase blood glucose levels, affecting urine glucose test.
- Photosensitivity may occur in some patients. Caution should be taken by wearing sunscreen and protective clothing.

- Hypertensive patients should avoid medications that may increase blood pressure, including OTC products for appetite suppression and cold symptoms.
- Notify a treating physician if muscle weakness, cramps, nausea, or dizziness occurs.
- Orthostatic hypotension may occur; get up slowly from a seated or sleeping position.
- Take as directed, do not double dose if one is missed.
- Use of alcohol, standing for a long time, exercise in hot weather may increase orthostatic hypertension.
- Consult a dietician if diet is high in vitamin K.
- Notify a clinician if taking any OTC drug or herbals.
- DO NOT CHANGE BRANDS when refilling prescriptions because bioavailability among brands is erratic.

Mechanism of Action

Loop diuretics inhibit reabsorption of sodium and chloride from Henle's loop and distal renal tubule, thus increasing renal excretion of water, sodium, chloride, magnesium, potassium, and calcium. The effects are seen as mobilization of excess fluid (edema) and a lowering of blood pressure, which persist even in cases of impaired renal function. These agents act on the thick ascending limb of Henle's loop and induce renal synthesis of prostaglandins, which contributes to their renal action, including the increase in the renal blood flow and redistribution of renal cortical blood flow.

Pharmacokinetics

- Absorption: About two-thirds is absorbed after oral administration; also absorbed from intramuscular (IM) sites.
- Distribution: Widely distributed because it is protein bound; crosses the placenta and enters breast milk.
- Metabolism: Partial metabolism by the liver for furosemide (30%-40%) and bumetanide (50%), but torsemide is 80% metabolized by liver.
- Excretion: The unchanged drug is mostly excreted by the kidney, but some is excreted in feces.
- Half-life: furosemide: 30 to 60 minutes; bumetanide: 60 to 90 minutes; torsemide: 3.5 hours.

Dosage and Administration

Generic Name	Trade Name	Route	Dosage
bumetanide	Bumex	PO, IV	0.5–2 mg daily
furosemide	Lasix	PO, IV	20–80 mg daily
torsemide	Demadex	PO, IV	10–20 mg daily
ethacrynic acid	Edecrin	PO, IV	50–200 mg daily

Clinical Uses

- Edema
- Renal insufficiency
- Ascites
- Nephrotic syndrome
- Pulmonary edema
- Congestive heart failure
- Hypertension
- Hypercalcemia

Adverse Reactions

NEURO: Dizziness, encephalopathy, headache, insomnia, and nervousness.

CV: Hypotension.

EENT: Dose-related hearing loss (ototoxicity). With bumetanide, ethacrynic acid, and furosemide, reversible and irreversible hearing loss has been reported, usually in persons with renal impairment and when an IV dosage has been given too rapidly.

GI: Constipation, dry mouth, dyspepsia, nausea, vomiting.

META: Hyponatremia, hypokalemia, metabolic alkalosis, hypomagnesemia, hypochloremia, dehydration leading to hypotension, metabolic acidosis, hyperuricemia, hyperglycemia.

HEM: Blood dyscrasias with furosemide.

MS: Arthralgia, myalgia.

MISC: Increased BUN.

Interactions

- Hypokalemia increases digoxin/digitalis toxicity.
- NSAIDs reduce diuretic efficacy.
- Beta blockers potentiate hyperglycemia and hyperlipidemia.
- Corticosteroids enhance hypokalemia.
- Aminoglycosides enhance ototoxicity and nephrotoxicity.
- Can increase the levels of lithium.

Contraindications

- Anuria
- Renal decompensation
- Hypersensitivity to sulfonamide-derived drugs
- Hepatic coma or pre-coma

Conscientious Considerations

- Assess fluid status throughout therapy.
- Assess patients receiving digitalis glycosides for anorexia, nausea, vomiting, muscle cramps, paresthesia, and confusion.
- Assess patients for tinnitus and hearing loss.
- Administer medication in the morning to avoid disruption of sleep cycle.

Patient/Family Education

- Teach patients about photosensitivity and how to best avoid it.
- Teach patients about the need for a diet high in potassium.

Potassium-Sparing Diuretics

Amiloride (Midamor), spironolactone (Aldactone), eplerenone (Inspra), and triamterene (Dyrenium) are called potassium-sparing diuretics because they do not produce hypokalemia as do the loop and thiazide diuretics. By inhibiting aldosterone-sensitive sodium reabsorption, potassium and hydrogen ion are exchanged for sodium by this transporter and therefore less potassium and hydrogen are lost to the urine. Because this class of diuretics had relatively weak effects on overall sodium balance, they are often used in conjunction with thiazides or loop diuretics to help prevent hypokalemia.

Conscientious Prescribing of Potassium-Sparing Diuretics

- Potassium-conserving agents may cause hyperkalemia, which, if uncorrected, may be fatal.
- The incidence of hyperkalemia is greater in patients with renal impairment, diabetes mellitus, and in the elderly.
- It is essential to monitor serum potassium levels carefully particularly when the drug is first introduced, at the time of diuretic dosage adjustments, and during any illness that could affect renal function.
- The use of potassium-conserving agents is often unnecessary in patients receiving diuretics for uncomplicated essential hypertension when such patients have a normal diet.
- Amiloride should rarely be used alone because it has a weak diuretic and antihypertensive effect when compared with thiazides.
- Spironolactone has been shown to be tumorigenic in chronic toxicity studies in rats. It should be used only in those conditions for which it is indicated and avoided otherwise.

Patient/Family Education for Potassium-Sparing Diuretics

- May cause GI upset; take with food.
- Notify clinician if muscle weakness, fatigue, or muscle cramps occur.
- May cause dizziness, headache, or visual disturbances; observe caution while driving or performing other tasks requiring alertness, coordination, or physical dexterity.
- Avoid potassium supplements and foods containing high levels of potassium, including salt substitutes.

Mechanism of Action

These agents inhibit sodium reabsorption in the kidney while saving potassium and hydrogen ions. Spironolactone does this by antagonizing aldosterone receptors. Although they are weak diuretics, they are often used as adjunctive therapy because they conserve potassium.

Pharmacokinetics

- Absorption: These agents have low (amiloride), moderate (triamterene), or good (spironolactone) absorption from the GI tract when given PO.
- Distribution: Amiloride and triamterene are widely distributed. All cross the placenta and enter breast milk; spironolactone is 90% protein bound.
- Metabolism: 50% of spironolactone and amiloride are metabolized in the liver. Spironolactone is converted by the liver to its active compound (canrenone); 80% of triamterene is metabolized by the liver.
- Excretion: 50% of amiloride and spironolactone are excreted unchanged by the kidney; triamterene is excreted in the bile.
- Half-life: Amiloride: 6 to 9 hours; spironolactone: 78 to 84 minutes; triamterene: 1.7 to 2.5 hours.

Dosage and Administration

Generic Name	Trade Name	Route	Dose
amiloride	Midamor	PO	5–20 mg a day
spironolactone	Aldactone	PO, IV	100–400 mg a day
triamterene	Dyrenium	PO	100–300 mg a day
eplerenone	Inspra	PO	50–100 mg daily

Clinical Uses

- Help restore normal serum potassium levels in patients who develop hypokalemia when taking other diuretics.
- Prevent development of hypokalemia in patients who would be exposed to particular risk if hypokalemia were to develop.
- Spironolactone is effective in lowering systolic and diastolic blood pressure in both primary hyperaldosteronism and essential hypertension.
- Cirrhosis.
- Nephrotic syndrome.
- Heart failure.

Adverse Reactions

CV: Arrhythmias
ENDO: Gynecomastia
GI: Gastric problems, including peptic ulcer
GU: Impotence (triamterene: blue-colored urine)
HEM: Thrombocytopenia, blood dyscrasias (spironolactone and triamterene)
META: Hyperkalemia, hyponatremia, metabolic acidosis
NEURO: Weakness, fatigue, dizziness, headache, dry mouth
RENAL: Azotemia, elevated BUN and creatinine, renal stones

Interactions

- ACEIs: Potentiate hyperkalemia
- NSAIDs: Reduce diuretic efficacy

Contraindications

- Should not be used in the presence of elevated serum potassium levels
- Renal impairment

Conscientious Considerations

- Monitor intake/output ratios, weight, BP, and responses.
- Periodic ECG if patient is on prolonged therapy.
- Discontinue at least 3 days before a glucose tolerance test because of severe hyperkalemia.
- Administer in the morning to avoid disrupting sleep cycle.

Patient/Family Education

- Caution patients about use of salt substitutes and foods with high levels of potassium and sodium.
- Advise against OTC decongestants, cough or cold preparations, and appetite suppressants taken concurrently because of potential for increased BP.
- If patient is on triamterene, advise about possible photosensitivity and what to do about it. Also advise patients that triamterene will discolor their urine.

Osmotic Diuretics

Three chemically inert agents are used as osmotic diuretics: mannitol (Osmitrol) and urea (Ureaphil) plus anhydrous glycerin (Osmoglyn). They are administered parenterally. Anhydrous glycerin is used as a topical application on the cornea to reduce corneal edema. Mannitol, an inert chemical osmotic, is the focus of this discussion.

Mechanism of Action

Mannitol induces diuresis by adding to the solutes already present in the renal tubular fluid. Thus, more water is pulled from the circulation into the tubular fluid, which allows less sodium chloride and water to be reabsorbed by the kidneys. Mannitol is used to treat cerebral edema in emergencies and is used with other agents in treatment of acute renal failure.

Pharmacokinetics

- Absorption: Very little is absorbed because IV administration completes the bioavailability.
- Distribution: None, confined to the extracellular space.
- Metabolism: Very little mannitol is metabolized in the liver. Urea is metabolized in the GI tract to ammonia and CO_2, which may then be resynthesized into urea.
- Excretion: Mannitol is excreted by the kidney.
- Half-life: Mannitol 100 minutes (onset of action as IV is 30 to 60 minutes).

Dosage and Administration of Mannitol

Generic Name	Trade Name	Route	Dosage
Mannitol	Osmitrol	IV Solution Available As 5%, 10%, 15%, And 30% Solution	Administer 0.25 Gm/Kg To 2.0 Gm/Kg Over 30–60 Min

Clinical Uses

- Acute renal failure
- Glaucoma
- Cerebral edema

Adverse Reactions

CV: Chest pain, tachycardia
DERM: Rash
EENT: Dry mouth
GI: Nausea, vomiting, dry mouth, diarrhea, thirst
GU: Renal failure
META: Hyperkalemia, hypernatremia, hypokalemia, hyponatremia, dehydration
NEURO: Headache, visual disturbances, confusion

Interactions

When mannitol is given with digitalis, hypokalemia may develop and result in digitalis toxicity.

Contraindications

- Hypersensitivities
- Severe cardiopulmonary impairment
- Severe kidney impairment

Conscientious Considerations

■ Osmotic diuretics are used primarily to reduce tissue edema and to expand circulatory volume. This ability is depends on intact blood vessels.

■ Use with caution in those with hypovolemia, hyperkalemia, and hyponatremia.

■ All vital signs, urinary output, pulmonary pressure, and electrolytes must be monitored throughout administration (before and hourly during administration) of the drug. Patients must also be monitored for signs of intracranial pressure if IV use is to reduce cerebral edema.

Patient/Family Education

■ Patients will not be self-administering the drug, but they and their families should be taught why the drug is being used and what they can expect.

Carbonic Anhydrase Inhibitors

Carbonic anhydrase inhibitors are the weakest of the diuretics and are seldom used in cardiovascular disease today. Their main use is in the treatment of glaucoma, and they are described more fully in Chapter 5.

Mechanism of Action

As a class of drugs, they have been supplanted by the thiazide diuretics, which were discovered during the 1960s. However, acetazolamide (Diamox), dichlorphenamide (Daranide), and methazolamide (Neptazane), all sulfonamide derivatives, remain in use today. Renal excretion of sodium, potassium, and sodium bicarbonate is increased by carbonic anhydrase inhibition. Diuresis is a result primarily of sodium and bicarbonate excretion and only a small amount of chloride excretion. Interestingly, the fractional increase in sodium is generally limited to about 5% because d most of the sodium is reabsorbed downstream. However, fractional potassium loss can be as much as 70%. The elevated bicarbonate due to consumption of these drugs leads to an alkaline urine and, in many cases, metabolic acidosis. Today, these agents are used primarily as an adjunctive treatment for chronic simple (open-angle) glaucoma. They are also used preoperatively in acute-angle-closure glaucoma where delay of surgery is desired to lower intraocular pressure. Carbonic anhydrase inhibitors reduce intraocular pressure (IOP) by partially suppressing the secretion of aqueous humor (inflow). The mechanism by which they do this in the eye is not fully understood, but it is believed that HCO_3^- ions are produced in the ciliary body by hydration of carbon dioxide under the influence of carbonic anhydrase, and it then diffuses into the posterior chamber. The posterior chamber of the eye contains more Na^+ and HCO_3^- ions than plasma, and consequently, it is hypertonic, allowing water to be drawn into the posterior chamber by osmosis and resulting in a drop in intraocular pressure.

Pharmacokinetics

■ Absorption: Both are well absorbed into tissue: acetazolamide 2 to 4 hours, methazolamide 6 to 8 hours; absorption is slow.

■ Distribution: Distributed throughout the body including the plasma, cerebrospinal fluid, aqueous humor of the eye, red blood cells, bile, and extracellular fluid, with about half bound to proteins.

■ Metabolism: Slowly in the GI tract.

■ Excretion: Excreted by the kidney.

■ Half-life: Unknown.

Dosage and Administration

Generic Name	Trade Name	Route	Dosage
Acetazo-lamide	Diamox	PO	Take 500 mg every 12 h for glaucoma Take 100–125 mg caps up to 4 times/day for glaucoma
Dichlor-phenamide	Daranide	PO	Take 25–50 mg, 2 or 3 times/day for glaucoma
Methazo-lamide	Neptazane	PO	Take 25–50 mg, 2 or 3 times a day for glaucoma use

Clinical Uses

■ Chronic simple, open-angle glaucoma (tablets)
■ Epilepsy
■ Motion sickness
■ Drug-induced edema, edema due to congestive heart failure (IV use)
■ Symptoms associated with mountain sickness

Adverse Reactions

DERM: Rash (including erythema multiforme, Stevens-Johnson syndrome, toxic epidermal necrolysis)

HEM: Bone marrow depression; thrombocytopenic purpura, hemolytic anemia, leukopenia, pancytopenia, and agranulocytosis

META: Hypokalemia, metabolic acidosis

MISC: Anaphylaxis, fever

NEURO: Sedation, paresthesia

RENAL: Crystalluria, renal calculus

Interactions

■ Caution is advised in patients receiving concomitant high-dose aspirin and carbonic anhydrase inhibitors because anorexia, tachypnea, lethargy, and coma have been rarely reported due to a possible drug interaction.

Contraindications

■ Caution is advised for patients receiving high-dose aspirin and these agents concomitantly.

Conscientious Considerations

■ Cautions are advised for early detection of any sulfonamide reactions to these drugs, and if so warranted, the drug should be discontinued and alternative therapy instituted.

Patient/Family Education

■ Patients need education on why and when these drugs are to be used. They will not be self-administering the IV drug under acute HF use, however tablet use or extended release capsule use under glaucoma conditions should be explained, especially the odds of adverse effects.

SPOTLIGHT ON DIURETIC RESISTANCE AND ADAPTION

To be effective, diuretic drugs must establish a negative sodium ion gradient so that they may mobilize edema or extracellular fluid. Restriction of dietary sodium is an essential part of diuretic therapy. It therefore follows that one cause of diuretic failure could be the patient's continued ingestion of salt in the diet. Some of the older diuretics, however, appear to be self-limiting; that is, their diuretic effect diminishes over time. This effect is minimized through the use of intermittent diuretic therapy to prevent excessive disturbances in body electrolytes. It is fairly common to see drugs such as the thiazides dosed on a Monday, Wednesday, Friday regimen.

Diuretics such as the thiazides and loop diuretics must reach the tubular lumen before they become effective. They reach the kidney's distal tubule or ascending Henle's loop through secretion because they are organic acids bound to plasma proteins. Any disease, drug, or condition that impairs this secretion will result in diuretic failure or an altered response. Compensatory proximal reabsorption of sodium may also contribute to the resistance seen with loop diuretics.

The dilemma of diuretic resistance is often resolved by prescribing smaller doses of combined diuretics. To help with patient compliance and pill load, some commercial products are a combination of two diuretics. Once the initial correction of fluid and electrolyte balance has been achieved, maintenance of homeostasis is the goal of treatment. Thus, drug dosage and frequency, along with sodium intake in the diet, need to be monitored.

Although the mechanism of action of diuretics seems straightforward, it is important to remember that the body adapts to repeated administration of many drugs, and diuretics are no exception. The adaptation to diuretics is most likely caused by the simple fact that diuresis only happens for a short period of time, after which compensatory changes in the body may occur. In acute, short-term adaptation, sodium excretion during a 24-hour period is essentially unchanged, but an increase in sodium excretion as a result of taking a diuretic drug is reversed by the body's compensatory mechanisms over the course of 1 day. The compensatory action may be the result of salt intake in the diet during the day, or it may be due to a change in the sodium transporters that have been modified by the diuretics. The sodium transporters are suppressed when the diuretic is ingested, but once a diuretic's effective concentration falls, ion transporters become enhanced and sodium retention increases. Thus, a decline in sodium excretion occurs with long-term use of diuretics and with it a reduction in natriuresis. This effect is called *long-term adaptation* or the *diuretic braking phenomenon* because the body's compensatory processes are engaged. Included in these compensatory processes is the renin-angiotensin-aldosterone system. Triggered by decreased sodium chloride in the macula densa or a reduction in extracellular fluid volume, renin is released, activating the renin-angiotensin-aldosterone system. The activation of the renin system is important because the ACEIs act in synergy with diuretics by blocking this activation.

IMPLICATIONS FOR SPECIAL POPULATIONS

Pregnancy Implications

When prescribing for the pregnant female, clinicians should carefully consider their choice of drugs.

Hypertension in a pregnant patient is of special concern because of the potential for fetal and maternal morbidity and mortality associated with an elevated blood pressure and the resultant syndromes of preeclampsia and eclampsia. Teratogenic effects on fetal development is also a possibility. Because of the risks, treatment for hypertension in pregnancy needs to be considered if diastolic BP is greater than 100 mm HG. First-line therapy of hypertension in pregnancy is methyldopa because of its proven safety. Other agents used as alternatives are hydralazine and labetalol because of their IV dosage forms. ACEIs also have a role. However, any patient suspected of having preeclampsia or eclampsia is in dire need of an obstetrician who specializes in high-risk pregnancy.

FDA PREGNANCY SAFETY CATEGORY	DRUGS
B	chlorthalidone, hydrochlorothiazide, indapamide, metolazone, ethacrynic acid
C	minoxidil, Aldomet, chlorothiazide, furosemide, bumetanide
	All CCBs, such as amlodipine (Norvasc); diltiazem, SR, CD, XR (Cardizem; Dilacor; Tiazac); isradipine (DynaCirc); nicardipine (Cardene); nifedipine (Procardia; Adalat, XL); nisoldipine (Sular); and verapamil (Isoptin; Calan; Verelan)
D	All ACEIs: benazepril (Lotensin), captopril (Capoton), enalapril (Vasotec), fosinopril (Monopril), lisinopril (Prinivil, Zestril), moexipril (Univasc), perindopril (Aceon), quinapril (Accupril), ramipril (Altace), trandolapril (Mavik). All ARBs: candesartan (Atacand), irbesartan (Avapro), losartan (Cozaar), losartan and HCTZ (Hyzaar), olmesartan (Benicar), irbesartan (Avapro), telmisartan (Micardis), valsartan (Diovan), and the combination of valsartan and hydrochlorothiazide (Diovan-HCT). All beta blockers, such as propranolol (Inderal), carvedilol (Coreg), metoprolol (Lopressor), atenolol (Tenormin), metoprolol succinate (Toprol XL)
X	Unclassified

Pediatric Implications

- Safety and efficacy of chlorthalidone, hydrochlorothiazide, and methyclothiazide have not been established in children.
- Metolazone is not recommended for use in children.

Geriatric Implications

It is important that the elderly have a functioning renal system because they may be more sensitive to diuretic-induced hypotension and the accompanying disturbances in electrolytes. It is a well-accepted axiom that the elderly start on doses that are one-half of the lowest recommended adult dose, then slow upward titration should follow as necessary.

Many older adults refer to diuretics as water pills and believe they must restrict their fluid intake when taking them. All adults must be advised that normal fluid intake is necessary. Any diuretic will increase urinary incontinence and contribute to erectile dysfunction. Should an elderly person require discontinuance of a diuretic, it must be done slowly to avoid a rebound effect of fluid retention and edema.

LEARNING EXERCISES

Case 1

The patient is a 67-year-old male who says his blood pressure had been running high lately. When his BP was taken at a health fair, it was 150/90; when it was taken at a nearby health center his BP was 152/90 and 150/94 mm Hg. You check his BP in the office, and it is 160/90 mm Hg.

The patient's BMI is 30. You do a complete physical exam, which is normal.

1. Write the prescription for the medication you will prescribe.

   Rx: _____

   #: _____

   Sig: _____

2. Why did you choose that medication and what advice will you give him?

3. What side effects will you monitor and discuss with the patient?

Case 2

JC is a 72-year-old female with a history of hypertension, diabetes, and hypercholesterolemia. This is her first visit with you. JC is on lisinopril, 10 mg once a day; Norvasc, 5 mg PO once a day; and lovastatin, 20 mg once a day. She complains of constipation and swelling in her legs, which concerns her. JC brought her echocardiogram report, which shows normal ejection fraction and mild Left Ventricular Hypertrophy (LVH) . Today, her BP is 120/70 mm Hg in right arm and 122/70 mm Hg in the left arm.

1. What will you do next?
   A. Stop the lisinopril and increase the Norvasc.
   B. Stop the Norvasc and increase Lisinopril dose.
   C. Add Hydrochlorothiazide.
   D. Add Lasix and give laxative.

References

JNC 7 guidelines for treatment of hypertension are being updated to JNC 8. Retrieved January 19, 2013, from www.nhlbi.nih.gov/guidelines/hypertension/jnc8/index.htm

National Heart, Lung, and Blood Institute (NHLBI). (2005). ALLHAT Information for Health Professionals. U.S. Dept. of Health and Human Services, National Institutes of Health, NHLBI. Retrieved April 20, 2011, from www.nhlbi.nih.gov/health/allhat/qckref.htm

National Heart Lung and Blood Institute (NHLBI). Diseases and Conditions Index. High Blood Pressure Risk Factors. U.S. Dept. of Health and Human Services. Retrieved January 18, 2012, www.nhlbi.nih.gov/health//dci/Diseases/Hbp/HBP_WhoIsAtRisk.html

Drugs Used in the Treatment of Hyperlipidemias

chapter 8

Mona M. Sedrak, John M. Boltri, William N. Tindall

CHAPTER FOCUS

This chapter focuses on the relationship between hyperlipidemia and atherosclerosis. Atherosclerosis is one of the major causes of coronary artery disease (CAD). Lowering of plasma lipid levels (management of hyperlipidemia) is essential to preventing many of the half million deaths that occur each year in the United States due to CAD. This chapter also focuses on the management of hyperlipidemia as based on the National Cholesterol Education Program (NCEO), which provides specifics for each of the drugs used to lower plasma lipids.

OBJECTIVES

After reading and studying this chapter, the student should be able to:

1. Describe the relationship between plasma lipids and coronary heart disease.
2. Describe how cholesterol is formed and the various medications that are used to inhibit its formation.
3. Explain the rationale for drug selection among the various classes of drugs used to reduce triglycerides and cholesterol.
4. Describe the relevant pharmacodynamics and pharmacokinetics of the agents used to lower cholesterol.
5. List the patient advisories for patients receiving hyperlipidemia therapy.
6. List the types of combination therapies and their rationales.
7. Define rhabdomyolysis and its association with lipid-lowering agents.
8. Restate the rule of 6 and explain why it is important in statin therapy.
9. List the common side effects associated with each class of lipid-lowering agents.
10. Recall the optimal levels for high-density lipoprotein (HDL) and low-density lipoprotein LDL in the 10-step process of the National Cholesterol Education Program (NCEP) treatment guidelines.

Key Terms

Atherosclerosis

Bile acid sequestrants

Chylomicrons

High-density lipoprotein (HDL)

Lipoproteins

Low-density lipoprotein (LDL)

Rhabdomyolysis

Triglycerides

Very low-density lipoprotein (VLDL)

DRUGS USED TO TREATMENT HYPERLIPIDEMIAS

HMG-CoA Reductase Inhibitors (Statins)
  lovastatin (Mevacor)
  pravastatin (Pravachol)
  simvastatin (Zocor)
  fluvastatin (Lescol)
  atorvastatin (Lipitor)
  rosuvastatin (Crestor)

Bile Acid Sequestrants
  cholestyramine (Questran, Prevalite)

  colestipol (Colestid)
  colesevelam (Welchol)

Nicotinic Acid
  immediate-release (crystalline)
    nicotinic acid
  extended-release nicotinic acid
    (Niaspan)
  sustained-release nicotinic acid

Fibric Acids
  gemfibrozil (Lopid)

  fenofibrate (TriCor)
  clofibrate (Atromid-S)

Cholesterol Absorption Inhibitor
  ezetimibe (Zetia)

Combinations
  ezetimibe/simvastatin (Vytorin)
  niacin/simvastatin (Simcor)
  niacin/lovastatin (Advicor)
  amlodipine/simvastatin (Caduet)

Dyslipidemia and other abnormalities of serum lipids play a major role in plaque formation, which in turn leads to coronary heart disease (CHD) and other forms of atherosclerosis. Also known as hyperlipidemia, dyslipidemia is a metabolic disorder characterized by increasing levels of two serum lipids, cholesterol and triglycerides. **Atherosclerosis** is a condition in which large-sized and medium-sized arteries develop lipid deposits in their inner linings, which eventually restrict blood flow and cause degenerative changes. These changes produce coronary artery disease (CAD) and coronary heart disease, which may manifest as angina, heart failure, hypertension, myocardial infarction (MI), cerebral vascular accidents (CVA), peripheral arterial disease (PAD), and insufficient blood flow to renal arteries.

CHD is a leading cause of death in both men and women in the United States and in many industrialized countries. Heart disease has been a leading cause of death in the United States for the past 80 years (CDC, 2011). Although heart disease is sometimes thought of as a man's disease, it is the leading cause of death for both women and men in the United States, and women account for nearly 50% of heart disease deaths. In 2012, heart disease was the leading cause of death (Hoyert, 2012). The development of coronary heart disease is a lifelong process. Clinical trials have consistently demonstrated that lowering serum cholesterol reduces atherosclerosis progression and mortality from CHD. Whereas genetics contribute to an individual's lipid profile, years of poor dietary habits, sedentary lifestyle, obesity, and smoking significantly impact the development of atherosclerosis. Many individuals at risk for CHD do not receive lipid-lowering medications or are not optimally treated.

UNDERSTANDING SERUM LIPID CONTROL

Cholesterol is an essential substance that is manufactured by most cells in the body. Other major lipids in the body are triglycerides and phospholipids. Because cholesterol is a water-insoluble molecule, it does not circulate through the blood alone; cholesterol, along with **triglycerides, lipoproteins,** and **phospholipids,** are packaged in larger carrier proteins referred to as apolipoproteins. Lipoproteins are water-soluble and allow transportation of major lipids in the blood. Lipoproteins vary in size and density, as does the amount of cholesterol and triglycerides carried by the lipoprotein. There are five major groups of lipoproteins which in order of size the larges is **chylomicrons,** followed by **very low-density lipoprotein (VLDL), intermediate-density lipoprotein (IDL), low-density lipoprotein (LDL),** and **high-density lipoprotein (HDL).** They all enable cholesterol and triglycerides to be transported throughout the water-based blood stream of a healthy person. In fact 30% of blood cholesterol is carried by HDL. Thus HDL particles are also able to remove cholesterol out of arteries and transport it back to the liver for excretion. This is why HDL is called the "good cholesterol" as people with higher numbers of HDL/Dl have fewer heart problems. Clinical laboratories measure and report serum total cholesterol, but what they are actually measuring and reporting are total cholesterol molecules and all the

major proteins. The estimated value of LDL cholesterol is found using the following equation:

$$\text{LDL cholesterol} = \text{total cholesterol} - (\text{HDL cholesterol} + \text{triglycerides}/5)$$

The LDLs contain the major portion (60% to 70%) of cholesterol in the blood, and it is the LDLs that are considered the most harmful when they are elevated. **Very low-density lipoproteins** carry fat from the liver to the adipose tissue. Intermediate-density lipoproteins are usually not detectable in the blood. Low-density lipoproteins carry cholesterol from the liver to the cells of the body and are sometimes referred to as the "bad cholesterol" lipoprotein. **High-density lipoproteins** collect cholesterol from the body's tissues and bring it back to the liver; repetitive.

In the United States, prevention and treatment of CHD is based primarily on guidelines issued in 2001 and updated in 2004 by the National Cholesterol Education Program (NCEP) Expert Panel on Detection, Evaluation, and Treatment of High Blood Cholesterol in Adults (adult treatment panel III or ATP III). Low-density lipoprotein cholesterol is the primary diagnostic and therapeutic target. In fact, the NCEP ATP III guidelines have set the optimal level for LDL cholesterol for all patients as less than 100 mg/dL. In 2004 the NCEP panel issued an update to the ATP III guidelines that outlined additional treatment options for certain patient populations, specifically those who are at high risk for recurrent CHD events (Table 8-1). The treatment options emphasize the benefits of diet, exercise, and weight control as well as the use of 3-hydroxy-3-methylglutaryl coenzyme A (HMG-CoA) reductase inhibitors or statins as first-line drugs. Other drugs that can be used in the treatment of hyperlipidemia include bile acid sequestrants, nicotinic acid, and fibric acids. It is recommended that if statins or other drugs are used to treat hyperlipidemia, doses that reduce LDL cholesterol by at least 30% to 40% should be used. The NCEP guidelines provide clinicians with a 10-step process for evaluating and treating patients with hyperlipidemia. These 10 steps are discussed in the Spotlight on Hyperlipidemia later in the chapter.

HMG-CoA Reductase Inhibitors

Statins are very effective LDL-lowering medications that are proven to reduce the risk of CHD, stroke, and death. The NCEP ATP III considers these medications the preferred drugs for lowering LDL. In fact, data concerning the efficacy and safety of these medications go back nearly 25 years. Statins are effective in reducing myocardial infarction, stroke, cardiovascular death, and in some cases, total mortality. The effectiveness of these medications has been demonstrated in both genders, the elderly, patients with diabetes, and hypertension, as well as those with preexisting CHD.

Conscientious Prescribing of HMG-CoA Reductase Inhibitors

- Before starting therapy with statins, clinicians should rule out secondary causes of hyperlipidemia such as poorly controlled hypothyroidism, nephrotic syndrome, and obstructive liver disease.
- A substantial reduction in LDL cholesterol occurs at the usual starting dose, and each doubling of the daily dose

TABLE 8-1 ATP III Classification of LDL, Total, and HDL Cholesterol (mg/dL)

	TOTAL AND HDL CHOLESTEROL (MG/DL)	CLASSIFICATION
LDL CHOLESTEROL—PRIMARY	<100	Optimal
TARGET OF THERAPY	100–129	Near optimal/above optimal
	130–159	Borderline high
	160–189	High
	≥190	Very high
TOTAL CHOLESTEROL	<200	Desirable
	200–239	Borderline high
	≥240	High
HDL CHOLESTEROL	<40	Low
	≥60	High

Source: National Heart Blood and Lung Institute, ATP III. (2001). At-A-Glance: Quick Desk Reference. Retrieved January 13, 2013, from www.nhlbi.nih.gov/guidelines/cholesterol/atglance.htm

produces only an additional 6% average reduction (known as the *rule of 6*). This is important when considering dose escalation vs. adding an additional LDL-lowering drug.

■ Obtain liver function tests at baseline and 6 to 12 weeks after starting therapy or any dose escalation.

■ Annual monitoring of liver function tests (LFTs) is usually sufficient.

■ Because of the risk of **rhabdomyolysis,** the breakdown of muscle fibers resulting in the release of muscle fiber contents (myoglobin) into the bloodstream, baseline creatine kinase (CK) should be obtained for patients who develop persistent muscle discomfort or weakness or brown urine while taking a statin. Follow-up CK should be attained only in patients complaining of muscle pain, weakness, tenderness, or brown urine. Routine monitoring of CK is of little value in the absence of clinical signs or symptoms.

■ Clinicians should assess patients for symptoms of myopathy 6 to 12 weeks after starting therapy and at each visit.

Patient/Family Education for HMG-CoA Reductase Inhibitors

■ Patients should be educated on the signs and symptoms of myopathy. Risk factors for myopathy include small body frame, multisystem diseases, and multiple medication regimens.

■ Patients should limit grapefruit juice intake while on some statins because it may result in increased plasma levels of statins, which increases risk of myopathy. Suggested ingestion of grapefruit juice is 200 mL/day or about 6 ounces taken 2 hours before ingestion of the statin. The interaction of the statins and grapefruit juice is more significant with atorvastatin (Lipitor), lovastatin (Mevacor), and simvastatin (Zocor).

■ Advise patients that these drugs may cause photosensitivity. Patients should avoid prolonged exposure to the sun, use sunscreens, and wear protective clothing.

■ Advise patients that these medications should be used in conjunction with diet restrictions (fat, carbohydrates,

cholesterol, and alcohol), exercise, and cessation of smoking.

■ Any unexplained muscle pain, tenderness, or weakness should be reported to the clinician, especially if fever or malaise is present as well.

■ Pregnancy should be reported to the clinician.

Mechanism of Action

Statins inhibit conversion of 3-hydroxy-3 methylglutaryl coenzyme A, the enzyme that catalyzes early steps in cholesterol synthesis. Subsequently, total cholesterol and LDL cholesterol, as well as triglycerides, are lowered, and a slight elevation in HDL occurs. Their peak effects take place usually after about 4 weeks of use.

Pharmacokinetics

■ Absorption: Most agents are rapidly absorbed, but undergo rapid first-pass metabolism such that only about 14% to 24% is bioavailable.

■ Distribution: Statins are highly protein bound, can enter breast milk, and can cross the blood–brain barrier and placenta.

■ Metabolism: All of these agents are extensively metabolized in the liver.

■ Excretion: Minimal in urine.

■ Half-life: Atorvastatin: 14 hours; fluvastatin: 1.2 hours; lovastatin: 3 hours; pravastatin: 2 hours; rosuvastatin: 19 hours; simvastatin: 2 hours. **Note:** Medications with a shorter half-life should be taken at bedtime.

Dosage and Administration

Generic Name	Trade Name	Route	Usual Adult Daily Dose
atorvastatin	Lipitor	PO	20–80 mg daily
fluvastatin	Lescol	PO	20–80 mg 1–2/day, at night
lovastatin	Mevacor	PO	20–80 mg daily, at night
pravastatin	Pravachol	PO	20–40 mg daily, at night
rosuvastatin	Crestor	PO	20–80 mg daily
simvastatin	Zocor	PO	20–80 mg* daily, at night

*The U.S. Food and Drug Administration announced safety label changes for simvastatin because its highest approved dose—80 mg—has been associated with an elevated risk of muscle injury, or myopathy, particularly during the first 12 months of use (FDA, 2011).

Clinical Uses

Indica-tion	Atorvas-tatin	Fluvas-tatin	Lovas-tatin	Pravas-tatin	Rosuvas-tatin	Simvas-tatin
Heterozy-gous familial hyperc-holes-terolemia and ado-lescents	X		X	X		X
Homozy-gous familial hyperlipi-demia	X				X	X
Hyper-triglyc-eridemia	X			X	X	X
Mixed dys-lipidemia	X	X	X	X	X	X
Primary dysbetal-ipopro-teinemia	X			X		X
Primary hyperc-holes-terolemia	X	X	X	X	X	X
Primary preven-tion of coronary events			X	X		X
Secondary preven-tion of cardio-vascular events		X	X	X		X

Adverse Reactions

CV: Chest pain, peripheral edema

DERM: Rash

EENT: Rhinitis

GI: Abdominal cramps, constipation, flatus, diarrhea, heart-burn, altered taste, SERIOUS elevation in liver function tests indicating liver toxicity

MS: SERIOUS myopathy, including rhabdomyolysis, depletion of coenzyme Q-10, and development of myalgias

NEURO: Dizziness, insomnia, headache, weakness

Interactions

■ Statins undergo biotransformation by the cytochrome P-450 system. Therefore, drugs known to inhibit CYP-450 enzymes should be used cautiously, otherwise statin metab-olism could be impaired, leading to elevated serum levels and risk of rhabdomyolysis. Use with extreme caution in the presence of gemfibrozil, protease inhibitors, niacin,

cyclosporine, amiodarone, erythromycin, or a rise in the incidence of rhabdomyolysis may be seen.

■ Coadministration of statins with bile acid sequestrants will reduce bioavailability and effectiveness of the statins. Thus, statins must be given 1 hour before or 4 hours after bile acid resins.

■ St John's wort may reduce serum levels and effectiveness.

■ Large quantities of grapefruit juice (1 quart) increase blood levels of statins and hence risk of myopathies and rhabdomyolysis.

■ Coadministration with coenzyme Q-10 may decrease muscle-related symptoms.

Contraindications

■ Liver disease and history of alcoholism.

■ Unexplained, persistent elevated LFTs.

■ Pregnancy.

■ Hypersensitivities.

■ USE STATINS CAUTIOUSLY IN PATIENTS OF ASIAN ANCESTRY because pharmacokinetic studies have found higher blood levels of statins occur in Asians because of their dietary intake of red rice yeast as a basic food staple. Red Rice Yeast, and Chinese red barbecued pork contain the active ingredient lovastatin, which, when isolated, became the first statin drug Mevacor.

Bile Acid Sequestrants

The **bile acid resins** available today are cholestyramine (Questran, Prevalite), colestipol (Colestid), and colesevelam (Welchol). Also known as **bile acid sequestrants**, they are moderately effective in lowering LDL cholesterol, but do not lower triglycerides. These agents are resins, which as highly charged molecules are able to bind to bile acids in the intes-tines, forming an insoluble complex. The resin-bile acid complex is then excreted in the feces. Resins have been shown to reduce CHD events in patients. However, in patients with elevated triglycerides, the use of a resin may worsen the condition.

Conscientious Prescribing of Bile Sequestrants

■ Before instituting therapy, vigorously attempt to control serum cholesterol with appropriate dietary regimen and weight reduction.

■ A large number of patients stop this medication due to GI side effects.

■ Resins should be started at the lowest dose and escalated slowly over weeks to months as tolerated until the desired response is attained.

■ Resins reduce LDL cholesterol from 15% to 30%, with a modest increase in HDL cholesterol.

■ Resins are often used as adjuncts to statins in patients who require additional lowering of LDL cholesterol.

■ Bile acid sequestering is not recommended as monotherapy in patients with triglyceride levels higher than 400 mg/dL or in patients with familial dysbetalipoproteinemia. They may be used as monotherapy in patients with triglyceride levels less than 200 mg/dL.

■ Combined cholesterol-lowering effects of bile sequestrants and statins are additive. Additive effects on LDL cholesterol are also seen with combined cholestyramine and nicotinic therapy.

■ Determine serum cholesterol levels at baseline, then frequently during the first few months of therapy, and periodically thereafter.

■ Periodic measurement of serum triglyceride levels to detect significant changes is also recommended.

Patient/Family Education for Bile Sequestrants

■ Instruct patients to prepare the powder formulation with 6 to 8 ounces of noncarbonated fluid, usually juice or water.

■ Instruct patients to swallow, not chew or crush, tablets.

■ Increasing fluid and dietary fiber intake may relieve constipation and bloating symptoms.

■ For maximal efficiency, these drugs should be taken before each meal and at bedtime, except colesevelam (WelChol), which can be taken once (6 tabs) or twice (3 tabs) a day.

Mechanism of Action

Bile acid sequestering resins bind to bile acids in the intestine to form an insoluble complex that is excreted in the feces. The increased fecal loss of bile acids leads to an increased oxidation of cholesterol to bile acids. This results in an increased number of LDL receptors, increased hepatic uptake of LDL, decreased beta lipoprotein or LDL serum levels, and decreased serum cholesterol levels. Plasma cholesterol levels fall secondary to an increased rate of clearance of cholesterol-rich lipoproteins from the plasma.

Pharmacokinetics

■ Absorption: Bile acid sequestering resins are hydrophilic, but water insoluble. They are not hydrolyzed by digestive enzymes and not absorbed; thus, because their action takes place in the GI tract, no absorption occurs.

■ Distribution: No distribution.

■ Metabolism: After binding, the bile acid insoluble complex is eliminated in the feces.

■ Excretion: In the feces.

■ Half-life: Unknown for all three.

Dosage and Administration

Generic Name	Trade Name	Route	Usual Adult Daily Dose
colestipol	Colestid	PO	5.0 gm of granules 1-2 times a day, may be increased up to 30 gm/day in 1 or 2 doses
cholestyramine	Questran	PO	4–24 gm/ twice a day, as tolerated
colesevelam	Welchol	PO	3 tabs (625mg) twice a day or 6 tabs once/day

Clinical Uses

■ *Treatment of* Hyperlipidemia: Adjunctive therapy to diet for the reduction of elevated serum cholesterol in patients with primary hypercholesterolemia who do not respond adequately to diet.

Adverse Reactions

DERM: Pruritus (cholestyramine only): Associated with excessive levels of bile acids in the bloodstream and the resultant deposit of bile acids in the skin

EENT: Irritation of the tongue

GI: Nausea, constipation, bloating, flatulence, fecal obstruction and constipation, anal irritation, increase in LFTs

META: Vitamin A, D, E, and K deficiency

NEURO: Insomnia, lightheadedness, weakness

Interactions

■ All resins have the potential to prevent the absorption of other drugs such as digoxin, warfarin, thyroxine, thiazide, beta blockers, fat-soluble vitamins (A, D, E, and K), and folic acid.

■ Potential drug interactions can be avoided by taking a resin either 1 hour before or 4 hours after these other agents are taken.

Contraindications

■ Those with liver disease or any biliary obstruction.

■ Use cautiously in those with any history of constipation or bowel obstruction.

Nicotinic Acid/Niacin

Niacin (vitamin B_3) has broad use in the treatment of lipid disorders when used at higher doses than those used for nutritional supplements. It is indicated for patients with elevated triglycerides, low HDL cholesterol, and elevated LDL cholesterol. There are several different formulations available on the market: niacin controlled release (CR), niacin sustained release (SR), and niacin extended release (ER). Niacin has been shown to reduce CHD events in total mortality as well as the progression of atherosclerosis when combined with a statin.

Conscientious Prescribing of Niacin

■ Niacin should be started at the lowest dose and gradually titrated to a maximum dose of 2 mg daily for the ER and SR product and no more than 5 gm daily for immediate-release products. As a dietary supplement 10-20 mg/day is adequate but in cases if dietary deficiencies up to 500 mg/day in divided doses. In cases of hyperlipidemias it is not uncommon to see 100-500 mg/day to start that is slowly titrated up to 1-2 grams three times a day.

■ Less flushing occurs with the sustained-release (SR) formulations.

■ Niacin ER was developed as a once-a-day formulation to be taken with the goal of reducing the incidence of flushing without increasing the risk of hepatotoxicity. It is the only long-acting niacin product approved by the U.S. Food and

Drug Administration (FDA) for dyslipidemia. It has an absorption rate of 8 to 12 hours and therefore balances metabolism more evenly.

■ Niacin lowers LDL cholesterol by 5% to 25%, increases HDL cholesterol by 5% to 35%, and decreases triglycerides by 20% to 50%.

■ Liver function tests should be performed on all patients during therapy with niacin: before treatment begins, every 6 to 8 weeks after reaching a daily dose of 1,500 mg, then again 6 to 8 weeks after reaching the maximum daily dose prescribed for that patient, then annually thereafter.

Patient/Family Education for Niacin

■ Taking niacin at bedtime can minimize the impact of flushing. The flushing episode usually occurs within the first 2 hours of taking the drug. The flushing is usually transitory and subsides with continuous therapy.

■ The use of 300 mg aspirin or a NSAID 30 minutes prior to taking niacin can help control the cutaneous reactions of flushing and pruritus of the face and body.

■ Taking niacin with food and avoiding hot liquids at the time niacin is taken is helpful in minimizing flushing and pruritus.

■ Concomitant alcohol or hot drinks may increase the side effects of flushing and pruritus and should be avoided around the time of the nicotinic acid ingestion.

■ Patients should be told that niacin products that are labeled as "no flush" don't contain nicotinic acid and therefore have no therapeutic role in the treatment of lipid disorders.

■ Timed-release capsules and tablets should not be crushed, broken, or chewed.

■ Rise from sitting position SLOWLY, so as to minimize the effect of orthostatic hypotension.

■ INSTRUCT PATIENTS TAKING ANY LONG-TERM DOSAGE FORMS TO REPORT ANY DARKENING OF URINE, LIGHT GRAY-COLORED STOOL, LOSS OF APPETITE, SEVERE STOMACH PAIN, or YELLOW EYES OR SKIN, all of which may be signs of hepatotoxicity.

Mechanism of Action

Niacin, in large doses, inhibits fatty acid release from adipose tissue and inhibits fatty acid and triglyceride synthesis in the liver. This results in an increased intracellular degradation of apolipoprotein B, and in turn a reduction in the number of LDL particles secreted. Thus, niacin reduces triglyceride synthesis, which in turn leads to lower levels of VLDL, lower levels of LDL, and higher levels of HDL

Pharmacokinetics

■ Absorption: Rapidly and extensively absorbed when administered orally.

■ Distribution: Widely distributed following its conversion to niacinamide.

■ Metabolism: Amounts required for metabolic processes are converted to niacinamide. These metabolites concentrate in the liver, kidney, and adipose tissue.

■ Excretion: Niacin and its metabolites are rapidly eliminated in the urine.

■ Half-life: 45 minutes.

Dosage and Administration

Generic Name	Trade Name	Route	Dosage
nicotinic acid	Niacin Niacor	PO	50 mg, 100 mg, 250 mg, 500 mg daily
nicotinic acid SR	Niacin SR	PO	125 mg, 500 mg daily
nicotinic acid CR	Slo-Niacin	PO	250 mg, 500 mg, 750 mg daily
nicotinic acid ER	Niaspan	PO	500 mg, 750 mg, 1,000 mg daily

Clinical Uses

■ Decreased blood lipids in states of hypercholesterolemia and hypertriglyceridemia.

■ Prevention of recurring myocardial infarction in patients with a history of MI and hypercholesterolemia. It is indicated to reduce the risk of recurrent, nonfatal MI.

■ Atherosclerotic disease.

Adverse Reactions

CV: Orthostatic hypotension, cardiac arrhythmias, palpitations, syncope.

DERM: Flushing of the face and neck, pruritus.

EENT: Blurry vision.

GI: Upper GI distress, **hepatotoxicity with extended-release form only.**

HEM: Niaspan ER has been associated with small but significant dose-related reductions of platelet count.

META: Interference with glucose control in diabetics, exacerbation of gout.

NEURO: Nervousness, panic.

Interactions

■ HMG-CoA reductase inhibitors: Rare cases of rhabdomyolysis have been associated with concomitant administration of lipid-altering doses of niacin and statins.

■ Anticoagulants: Interactions with anticoagulants results in prolonged prothrombin times.

■ Antihypertensive therapy: Potentiate the effects of ganglionic-blocking agents and vasoactive drugs, resulting in postural hypotension.

■ Aspirin: Concomitant use of aspirin may decrease the metabolic clearance of nicotinic acid.

Contraindications

■ Chronic liver disease.

■ Use with caution in patients with diabetes, peptic ulcer disease, and hyperuricemia.

Cholesterol Absorption Inhibitor

Ezetimibe (Zetia, Estetrol)

Mechanism of Action

Ezetimibe has a mechanism of action that differs from those of other classes of cholesterol-reducing compounds. It does not inhibit cholesterol synthesis in the liver or increase bile acid in excretion; rather, it acts at the small intestine and inhibits the absorption of cholesterol, causing a decrease in intestinal cholesterol available to the liver. Thus, in turn it causes a reduction in hepatic cholesterol stores and a decrease in cholesterol circulating in the blood, a known risk factor for atherosclerosis.

Pharmacokinetics

- Absorption: Following its absorption, it is extensively conjugated to a pharmacologically active phenolic complex, ezetimibe-glucuronide.
- Distribution: Highly bound to human plasma protein.
- Metabolism: Metabolized primarily in the small intestine and liver.
- Excretion: Mostly biliary/feces elimination and minimal renal excretion.
- Half-life: 22 hours.

Dosage and Administration

- Dosage: 10 mg once a day with or without food.
- Coadministration with statins or fenofibrate: The daily dose of ezetimibe may be taken at the same time as the other medications.
- Coadministration with bile acid sequestrants: Dosing of ezetimibe should occur at least 2 hours before or at least 4 hours after administration of a bile acid sequestrant.

Clinical Uses

- Use alone or in combination with other agents, especially HMG-CoA reductase inhibitors.
- Homozygous familial hypercholesterolemia.
- Homozygous sitosterolemia.
- Mixed hyperlipidemia in combination with fenofibrate.
- Primary hypercholesterolemia in combination with statins.

Adverse Reactions

DERM: Rash
GI: Elevated liver function tests (increased transaminases when combined with statins), abdominal pain, diarrhea, cholecystitis, cholelithiasis, nausea
HEM: Angioedema
META: Fatigue
MS: Arthralgia, back pain

Interactions

- Antacids
- cholestyramine
- Cyclosporin

Contraindications

- The combination of ezetimibe with a statin is contraindicated in patients with active liver disease or unexplained persistent elevations in serum transaminase.

Conscientious Considerations

- Ezetimibe reduces total cholesterol, LDL cholesterol, apolipoprotein B, and triglycerides and increases HDL cholesterol in patients with hypercholesterolemia. When administered with statins, it is effective in improving serum total cholesterol, LDL cholesterol, triglycerides, and HDL cholesterol beyond either treatment alone.
- Administration with fenofibrate is effective in improving serum total cholesterol, LDL cholesterol, and HDL cholesterol in patients with mixed hyperlipidemia as compared with either treatment alone.
- Prior to starting therapy, exclude, or if appropriate treat, secondary causes of dyslipidemia. Perform a fasting lipid profile to measure total cholesterol, LDL, HDL, and triglycerides.
- Studies are mixed; although ezetimibe improved lipid profiles, some studies suggest that it does not improve clinical outcomes.

Fibric Acid Derivatives

Hypertriglyceridemia denotes elevated blood levels of triglycerides and is the most common dyslipidemia, characterized by high amounts of fatty molecules circulating in the human body. Hypertriglyceridemia may result in an increased risk of premature atherosclerosis, or it may lead to pancreatitis. If the triglyceride level is markedly raised, the fibric acid derivatives (fibrates) are indicated for use in therapy. It is of note that dietary fish oils are also used to lower elevated triglycerides with good effect (Mattar & Obeid, 2009). The predominant effects of the fibric acid derivatives, gemfibrozil (Lopid), fenofibrate (TriCor), clofibrate (Atromid-S), which are synthetic drugs, are a decrease in triglyceride levels by 20% to 50% and an increase in HDL cholesterol by 9% to 30%. Fibrates achieve these effects by increasing the size and reducing the density of LDL particles, similar to the effects of niacin. Their effect on LDL cholesterol is less predictable than niacin, and in patients with high triglycerides, LDL cholesterol may increase. They are the most effective triglyceride-lowering drugs and are used primarily in patients with very high elevated triglycerides and low HDL and in those with a risk of pancreatitis. There is no evidence that fibrates decrease total mortality or rates of fatal MI. Fibrates may be appropriate in the prevention of CHD events for patients with low HDL cholesterol and triglycerides above 200 mg/dL. However, LDL-lowering therapy should be the primary target if LDL cholesterol is elevated; therefore, statins are first-line therapy.

Conscientious Prescribing of Fibric Acid Derivatives

- The risk of myopathy and rhabdomyolysis appears to increase with renal insufficiency or concurrent statin therapy.
- If using a statin concurrently with a fibrate, fenofibrate is preferred because it appears to inhibit the glucuronidation of the statin hydroxy and moiety less than gemfibrozil does, allowing greater renal clearance of the statin. However, clinicians tend to avoid concurrent use of any fibrate with a statin.
- ALFT should be done before therapy is started and when symptoms occur. CK levels should be checked for a patient reporting myalgias.
- These drugs increase cholesterol and can cause gallbladder and bile duct disorders.

Patient/Family Education for Fibric Acid Derivatives

Patients should be advised to promptly report unexplained muscle pain, tenderness, or weakness, particularly if accompanied by malaise or fever.

Mechanism of Action

These medications work by regulating gene transcription of enzymes involved in VLDL and fatty acid breakdown and facilitate reverse cholesterol transport. They also facilitate uptake of LDL by the liver.

Pharmacokinetics

■ Absorption: All are well absorbed (60%) after oral administration.
■ Distribution: Remains unknown; protein binding is up to 99%.
■ Metabolism: Rapidly converted to fenofibric acid, which is an active metabolite. Fenofibric acid is metabolized in the liver.
■ Excretion: Fenofibric acid and its metabolites are excreted in the urine.
■ Half-life: Fenofibrate: about 20 hours; gemfibrozil: about 1.5 hours; clofibrate 12 to 35 hours.

Dosage and Administration

Generic Name	Trade Name	Route	Usual Adult Daily Dose
gemfibrozil	Lopid	PO	1,200 mg 2 times/day
fenofibrate	TriCor	PO	48–145 mg daily
	Triglide	PO	50–160 mg daily
	Antara	PO	43–130 mg daily
clofibrate	Atromid-S	PO	1.0–1.5 gm/day

Clinical Uses

■ With dietary restrictions to be used in hypertriglyceridemia or hypercholesterolemia to reduce LDL, cholesterol, total cholesterol, and triglycerides in adult patients.
■ For prevention of cardiovascular disease, gemfibrozil is indicated as an adjunctive therapy to diet for reducing the risk of developing coronary heart disease in those without a history of existing CHD symptoms and in those who have had inadequate response to weight loss, dietary therapy, exercise, and other pharmacological agents.

Adverse Reactions

CV: Arrhythmias.
DERM: Rash.
GI: Dyspepsia, abdominal pain, diarrhea, flatulence, liver dysfunction gallbladder disease, such as cholelithiasis, pancreatitis. GI complaints usually result when fibrates are combined with statins.
MS: Muscle pain, myopathy, rhabdomyolysis.
MISC: Hypersensitivities.
NEURO: Fatigue, weakness, headache.

Interactions

■ There is an increased risk of bleeding in patients taking both warfarin and a fibrate.

■ Concurrent use with a HMG-CoA reductase inhibitor will increase risk of rhabdomyolysis.
■ Absorption of all fibrates is reduced by presence of bile acid sequestrants.

Contraindications

■ Patients with gallbladder disease, liver dysfunction, or severe kidney dysfunction.
■ Safety in pregnancy not established, use only if risks to a fetus are outweighed by the benefits.
■ Avoid use in breastfeeding women.

Combination Therapy

Many individuals will not achieve the NCEP cholesterol targets for a variety of reasons, including inadequate patient adherence, adverse events, inadequate starting doses, lack of dose increasing, and low treatment target goals. Those patients who have concomitant elevations and triglycerides and or HDL cholesterol may need combination drug therapy to normalize their lipid profile. Combination drug therapy is an effective means to achieve greater reductions in LDL cholesterol as well as raise HDL cholesterol and lower serum triglycerides. However, one clinical trial, the Simvastatin and Ezetimibe in Aortic Stenosis study, sponsored by the drug's manufacturer, reported an increase in cancer rates without any decrease in cardiovascular mortality with combined use of ezetimibe and simvastatin (Rossebø et al., 2008). The FDA has asked clinicians to report any side effects noticed in patients taking these drugs by using its MedWatch Adverse Event Reporting System.

AIM-HIGH, sponsored by the National Heart Lung and Blood Institute of the NIH, was stopped 18 months early because early data showed that adding high-dose extended-release niacin to a statin drug among people with heart and vascular disease did not reduce their risk of cardiovascular events (NHLBI, n.d.).

Dosage and Administration

Generic Name	Trade Name	Route	Usual Adult Daily Dose
amlodipine besylate/ atorvastatin calcium	Caduet	PO	2.5/10 mg–10 mg/80 mg daily
niacin/ lovastatin	Advicor	PO	500 mg ER/20 mg–1,000 mg ER/40 mg at night
ezetimibe/ simvastatin	Vytorin	PO	10 mg/10 mg–10 mg/80 mg at night
niacin/ simvastatin	Simcor	PO	500 mg ER/20 mg–1,000 mg ER/40 mg at night

For patients who do not achieve their LDL or non-HDL cholesterol goals with statin monotherapy and lifestyle modifications, combination therapy may be appropriate. Although statins and resins or ezetimibe combine effectively to augment LDL cholesterol reduction, whether combination therapy reduces mortality is poorly understood.

Ezetimibe/Simvastatin (Vytorin)

Ezetimibe/simvastatin drug is used as adjunctive therapy to diet for the reduction of elevated total cholesterol, LDL cholesterol, apolipoprotein B, triglycerides, and non-HDL cholesterol, and increased HDL cholesterol. The usual starting dose is 10 mg/20 mg and the maximum dose is 10 mg/80 mg. Adverse events are similar to those of each product taken separately; however, the percentage of patients with Liver Function Test (LFT) elevations greater than three times normal is slightly higher than among those using a statin alone, and thus there is a slightly higher risk of myopathy and rhabdomyolysis when statins and ezetimibe are combined as Vytorin. However when added to a statin, ezetimibe can reduce LDL cholesterol levels by an additional 18% to 21% or up to 65% total reduction with maximum doses of the more potent statins. However, it is not clear whether using this combination reduces mortality.

Niacin/simvastatin (Simcor)

Niacin/simvastatin is used for hypercholesterolemia to reduce total cholesterol, low-density lipoprotein cholesterol, apolipoprotein B, high-density lipoprotein cholesterol, or triglycerides, or to increase high-density lipoprotein cholesterol in patients with hypercholesterolemia and mixed dyslipidemia when treatment with simvastatin and monotherapy or niacin monotherapy is considered inadequate. This medication should be taken as a single 500 mg/20 mg dose daily with a low-fat snack at bedtime. The dosage of niacin extended-release should not be increased by more than 500 mg daily every 4 weeks. As with other niacin medications, flushing may be reduced in frequency or severity by pretreatment with aspirin or other NSAIDs approximately 30 minutes prior to taking the medication. Flushing, pruritus, and GI distress can also be reduced by gradually increasing the dose of niacin and avoiding administration on an empty stomach.

SPOTLIGHT ON HYPERLIPIDEMIA: GUIDELINES BY NCEP

In the United States, prevention and treatment of coronary heart disease is based on the guidelines issued by the National Cholesterol Education Program Expert Panel on Detection and Evaluation and Treatment of High Blood Cholesterol in Adults (NCEP ATP III). These guidelines were updated in 2004 based on recent clinical trial evidence. The treatment options emphasized in the guidelines stress the benefits of diet, exercise, and weight control, and the use of statins as first-line drugs. The American Heart Association and American College of Cardiology issued guidelines for secondary prevention in patients with CHD or other atherosclerotic vascular disease based on the results of two additional trials published after the 2004 NCEP update. These guidelines suggest it is reasonable to set an LDL cholesterol goal of less than 70 mg/dL in all patients with CHD or other forms of atherosclerotic vascular disease. To help clinicians diagnose and treat patients with hyperlipidemia, the NCEP guidelines offer a 10-step systematic process for treatment:

STEP 1: Determine Lipoprotein Levels–Obtain Complete Lipoprotein Profile After 9- to 12-Hour Fast. The NCEP guidelines recommend that all adults older than 20 years of age be screened at least every 5 years using a fasting blood sample to obtain a lipid profile consisting of a total cholesterol, LDL cholesterol, HDL cholesterol, and triglycerides. A fasting lipid profile is preferred so that an accurate assessment of LDL cholesterol can be made. Children between the ages of 2 and 20 should also be screened for high cholesterol if their parents have premature CHD or if one of their parents has a total cholesterol greater than 240 mg/dL.

STEP 2: Rule Out Secondary Causes of Dyslipidemia. Certain diseases and drugs can cause abnormalities in serum lipids and should be evaluated before starting treatment for hyperlipidemia (Table 8-2). Efforts to correct and control underlying diseases such as renal disease should be made. Strong consideration should be given to reducing or stopping medications known to induce lipid abnormalities prior to initiating long-term lipid-lowering therapy.

STEP 3: Identify Presence of Clinical Atherosclerotic Disease That Confers High Risk for Coronary Heart Disease (CHD) Events (CHD Risk Equivalent). Individuals with established CHD, other clinical atherosclerotic disease, or diabetes have a greater than 20% risk over a 10-year period of developing CHD (Box 8-1). For high-risk patients who have a history of one of the

TABLE 8-2	Secondary Conditions and Drugs That May Cause Hyperlipidemia	
MEDICAL CONDITIONS	**MEDICATIONS**
Diabetes	Estrogen
Hypothyroidism	Progestin
Obstructive liver disease	Protease inhibitors
Renal disease	Anabolic steroids
Hemodialysis	Beta blockers
Obesity	Atypical antipsychotics

BOX 8-1 Diseases That Confer High Risk for CHD Events

- Myocardial infarction
- Unstable angina
- Chronic stable angina
- Peripheral artery disease
- Symptomatic carotid artery disease
- Diabetes, type 1 and 2
- Multiple risk factors with a Framingham calculated risk greater than 20%

following or more diseases, the NCEP ATP III guidelines set the target LDL cholesterol level at less than 100 mg/dL. The benefits of lowering LDL cholesterol to as low as 70 mg/dL have been demonstrated in clinical trials. In patients who are considered very high risk, an LDL cholesterol goal of less than 70 mg/dL is a therapeutic goal. These individuals are those that have an established CHD diagnosis plus multiple other major risk factors, such as diabetes, cigarette smoking, metabolic syndrome, and acute coronary syndromes.

STEP 4: Determine Presence of Major Risk Factors (Other Than LDL). For those patients who do not have an established CHD or CHD equivalent risk, the next step for clinicians is to count

Continued

SPOTLIGHT ON HYPERLIPIDEMIA: GUIDELINES BY NCEP—cont'd

major risk factors for CHD (Table 8-3). These risk factors are considered independent predictors of CHD. However, for those patients that have an HDL cholesterol of greater than or equal to 60 mg/dL, one risk factor can be subtracted because this is considered a negative risk factor.

STEP 5: If Two Or More Risk Factors (Other Than LDL) Are Present Without CHD or CHD Risk Equivalent, Assess 10-Year (Short-Term) CHD Risk. The Framingham Risk Calculator is used to estimate a 10-year risk by assigning points to risk factors such as age, total cholesterol level, smoking status, HDL cholesterol level, and systolic blood pressure. The score is then used to determine the patient's risk category and the intensity of the treatment necessary to lower LDL cholesterol. There are three levels of 10-year risk: greater than 20% (CHD risk equivalent), 10% to 20%, and less than 10%. Individuals with less than or equal to one risk factor have less than a 10% 10-year risk for CHD and do not require Framingham calculation. Because individuals with two or more risk factors may carry a risk equivalent to individuals with established CHD, the Framingham Coronary Heart Disease Study is used to estimate their

10-year risk, which is 0 to 20%. To calculate a Framingham score for yourself or someone else go to http://framinghamriskscore.com/framingham-risk-calculator/. Updates as of January 22, 2013.

STEP 6: Determine Treatment Goals and Therapy. Determining treatment goals for LDL cholesterol and threshold for starting lifestyle changes in pharmacotherapy is an important next step (Table 8-4).

STEP 7: Initiate Therapeutic Lifestyle Changes If LDL Is Above Goal. Therapeutic lifestyle changes (TLC) should be the first approach tried in all patients, but pharmacotherapy should be instituted concurrently in high-risk patients. Dietary restrictions of cholesterol and saturated fats, as well as exercise and weight reduction, make up the plan (Table 8-5).

STEP 8: Consider Adding Drug Therapy If LDL Exceeds Levels Shown in Table 8-5. Patients who are unable or unlikely to achieve their LDL cholesterol goals following a 12-week trial of TLC (for those without CHD and sooner for those at high risk or with LDL greater than 190 mg/dL) should be started on drug therapy.

STEP 9: Identify Metabolic Syndrome and Treat, If Present, After 3 Months of TLC. (See Table 8-6.) Patients with metabolic syndrome are twice as likely to develop type 2 diabetes and four times more likely to develop CHD. Treatment of metabolic syndrome and underlying causes (overweight/obesity and physical inactivity) begins with intensifying weight management and increasing physical activity. Also, it is important to treat lipid and nonlipid risk factors if they persist, despite these lifestyle therapies:

■ Treat hypertension.
■ Use aspirin for CHD patients to reduce prothrombotic state.
■ Treat elevated triglycerides and/or low HDL (as shown in Step 10 below).

Patients with metabolic syndrome have an additional lipid parameter that needs to be assessed: non-HDL cholesterol. The target for non-HDL cholesterol is less than the patient's LDL cholesterol

TABLE 8-3 Risk Factors for Coronary Heart Disease

RISK FACTOR	EXPLANATION
Cigarette smoking	Within the past month
Hypertension	Blood pressure ≥140/90 mm Hg or on antihypertensive medication
Low HDL cholesterol	<40 mg/dL
Age	Men ≥ 45 years; women ≥ 55 years
Family history of premature CHD	CHD in male first-degree relative <55 years; CHD in female first-degree relative <65 years

TABLE 8-4 NCEP ATP III Treatment Goals for LDL Cholesterol and Threshold for Starting Therapeutic Lifestyle Changes in Pharmacotherapy

RISK CATEGORY	LDL GOAL	LDL LEVEL AT WHICH TO INITIATE THERAPEUTIC LIFESTYLE CHANGES	LDL LEVEL AT WHICH TO CONSIDER DRUG THERAPY
CHD or CHD risk equivalents (10-year risk >20%)	<100 mg/dL	≥100 mg/dL	≥130 mg/dL (100–129 mg/dL: drug optional)*
2+ risk factors (10-year risk ≥20%)	<130 mg/dL	≥130 mg/dL	10-year risk 10%–20%: ≥130 mg/dL 10-year risk <10%: ≥160 mg/dL
0–1 risk factor†	<160 mg/dL	≥160 mg/dL	≥190 mg/dL (160–189 mg/dL: LDL-lowering drug optional)

* *Some authorities recommend use of LDL-lowering drugs in this category if an LDL cholesterol <100 mg/dL cannot be achieved by therapeutic lifestyle changes. Others prefer use of drugs that primarily modify triglycerides and HDL, e.g., nicotinic acid or fibrate. Clinical judgment also may call for deferring drug therapy in this subcategory.*

† *Almost all people with 0–1 risk factor have a 10-year risk <10%, thus 10-year risk assessment in people with 0–1 risk factor is not necessary.*

Source: National Cholesterol Education Program: Third Report of the Expert Panel on Detection, Evaluation, and Treatment of High Blood Cholesterol in Adults (Adult Treatment Panel III) by National Heart, Lung, and Blood Institute, National Institutes of Health, and Public Health Service. (2001). Retrieved January 12, 2013, from www.nhlbi.nih.gov/guidelines/cholesterol/atglance.htm#Step5

SPOTLIGHT ON HYPERLIPIDEMIA: GUIDELINES BY NCEP—cont'd

TABLE 8-5   Nutrient Composition of the TLC Diet

NUTRIENT	RECOMMENDED INTAKE
Saturated fat*	Less than 7% of total calories
Polyunsaturated fat	Up to 10% of total calories
Monounsaturated fat	Up to 20% of total calories
Total fat	25%–35% of total calories
Carbohydrate†	50%-60% of total calories
Fiber	20–30 gm/day
Protein	Approximately 15% of calories
Cholesterol	Less than 200 mg/day
Total calories (energy)‡	Balance energy intake and expenditure to maintain desirable body weight and prevent weight gain

*Trans fatty acids are another LDL-raising fat that should be kept at a low intake.

†Carbohydrate should be derived predominantly from foods rich in complex carbohydrates, including grains, especially whole grains, fruits, and vegetables.

‡Daily energy expenditure should include at least moderate physical activity (contributing approximately 200 Kcal per day).

Source: National Heart, Lung, and Blood Institute, National Institutes of Health, and Public Health Service. ATP III Guidelines: Therapeutic Lifestyle Changes (TLC.) Retrieved January 12, 2013, from hp2010.nhlbihin.net/ncep_slds/atpiii/download/part4.pdf

TABLE 8-6   Clinical Identification of the Metabolic Syndrome (any three of the following)

RISK FACTOR	DEFINING LEVEL
Abdominal obesity*	Waist circumference†
Men	>102 cm (>40 in)
Women	>88 cm (>35 in)
Triglycerides	≥150 mg/dL
HDL cholesterol	
Men	<40 mg/dL
Women	<50 mg/dL
Blood pressure	130/ ≥85 mm Hg
Fasting glucose	≥110 mg/dL

*Overweight and obesity are associated with insulin resistance and the metabolic syndrome. However, the presence of abdominal obesity is more highly correlated with the metabolic risk factors than is an elevated body mass index (BMI). Therefore, the simple measure of waist circumference is recommended to identify the body weight component of the metabolic syndrome.

†Some male patients can develop multiple metabolic risk factors when the waist circumference is only marginally increased, for example, 94–102 cm (37–39 in). Such patients may have a strong genetic contribution to insulin resistance. They should benefit from changes in life habits, similarly to men with categorical increases in waist circumference.

Source: National Heart, Lung, and Blood Institute, National Institutes of Health, and Public Health Service. National Cholesterol Education Program: Third Report of the Expert Panel on Detection, Evaluation, and Treatment of High Blood Cholesterol in Adults (Adult Treatment Panel III) Retrieved January 12, 2013, from www.nhlbi.nih.gov/guidelines/cholesterol/atglance.htm#Step5

target plus 30 mg/dl. After assessment and control of LDL cholesterol, patients with serum triglycerides between 200 and 499 mg/dl should be assessed for atherogenic dyslipidemia.

STEP 10: Treat Elevated Triglycerides. Elevated triglycerides are an independent CHD risk factor. Factors contributing to elevated triglycerides in the general population include: obesity and overweight, physical inactivity, cigarette smoking, excess alcohol intake, high-carbohydrate diets, and diseases such as type 2 diabetes and chronic renal failure. Certain drugs such as corticosteroids, estrogens, retinoids, and higher doses of beta-adrenergic blocking agents have also been implicated. Treatment for elevated triglycerides depends on the causes of the elevation and its severity. The primary aim of therapy is to achieve the target goal for LDL cholesterol for all patients with elevated triglycerides (Table 8-7). For patients with *borderline high* (150–199 mg/dL) cholesterol, emphasis should be placed on weight reduction and increased physical activity. If triglycerides are greater than or equal to 200 mg/dL after LDL goal is reached, set secondary goal for non-HDL cholesterol (total − HDL) 30 mg/dL higher than LDL goal.

For patients with *high triglycerides* (200–499 mg/dL) after LDL goal is reached, consider adding drug, if needed, to reach non-HDL goal, intensifying therapy with LDL-lowering drug, or adding nicotinic acid or fibrate to further lower VLDL. If triglycerides are 500 mg/dL, first lower triglycerides to prevent pancreatitis and start patients on very low-fat diet (greater than or equal to 15% of calories from fat) and a weight management and a physical activity program. When triglycerides are less than 500 mg/dL,

TABLE 8-7   ATP III Classification of Serum Triglycerides (mg/dL)

<150	Normal
150–199	Borderline high
200–499	High
≥ 500	Very high

Source: National Heart, Lung, and Blood Institute, National Institutes of Health, and Public Health Service. National Cholesterol Education Program: Third Report of the Expert Panel on Detection, Evaluation, and Treatment of High Blood Cholesterol in Adults (Adult Treatment Panel III). Retrieved January 12, 2013, from www.nhlbi.nih.gov/guidelines/cholesterol/atglance.htm#Step5

turn to LDL-lowering therapy. Treatment of low HDL cholesterol (less than 40 mg/dL) consists of intensifying weight management and increasing physical activity. If triglycerides are 200–499 mg/dL, achieve non-HDL goal. If triglycerides are less than 200 mg/dL (isolated low HDL) in CHD or CHD equivalent, consider nicotinic acid or fibrate.

Implications for Special Populations

Pregnancy Implications

When prescribing for the pregnant female, clinicians should carefully consider their choice of drugs.

Below is a selected list of drugs along with their assigned FDA Safety Category.

FDA PREGNANCY SAFETY CATEGORY	DRUGS
B	Bile acid sequestrants
C	ezetimibe, fibrates, niacin
D	
X	All statins
Unclassified	

Pediatric Implications

Only four of the statins have been approved for use in older children, otherwise they should not be used in children under 8 years of age. The four FDA-approved statins for children are simvastatin (Zocor), lovastatin (Mevacor), atorvastatin (Lipitor) for ages 10 to 17 boys and postmenarchal girls, and pravastatin (Pravachol) for ages 8 to 13, all at reduced adult dosages however (Belay, Belamarich, & Revzon, 2007).

Geriatric Implications

The existing evidence suggests, that there is not any benefit from using statin drugs in those who are over 65 years of age, especially any benefit as it pertains to the prevention of cardiovascular disease. In addition, tolerance for and adherence to long-term therapies is always a consideration when dealing with older adults. Statins have been shown to affect survivability in long-term use among middle-aged men (35–70) and those at risk for cardiovascular disease (Pederson et al., 2000). However muscle problems from statins and rhabdomyolysis take on a variety of symptoms, most notably, shortness of breath as the "respiratory exchange ratio" (ratio of carbon dioxide exhales to oxygen inhaled) is altered in people with statin myotoxicity. Although the issue of muscle problems has been found to be of higher prevalence in the older adult, it especially affects women over 80 who are of small frame and who are on multiple drug therapy (Pasternek et al., 2002). Another issue with statins is cognitive decline, which by itself is more prevalent among the elderly but is not explainable by lipid lowering nor anti-inflammatory effects (Anderson, 2007). In fact, no clinical studies exist to demonstrate harm on cognition in older adults, and the definitive/relevant work on the subject shows mixed results (Katz & Gilbert, 2009).

LEARNING EXERCISES

Case 1

A 65-year-old male comes to see you 3 months after a four-vessel coronary artery bypass graft (CABG). He feels great but was told by his surgeon to follow up with you regarding his cholesterol and triglycerides. His medical history is significant for hypertension, benign prostatic hyperplasia, erectile dysfunction, mild osteoarthritis (OA). Current medications are aspirin; metoprolol, 50 mg by mouth 2 times a day; simvastatin, 40 mg by mouth at bedtime. On physical exam his pulse = 68, blood pressure = 130/78, and his examination is normal. Laboratory results are as follows:

Total cholesterol: 180

HDL: 42

Triglycerides: 100

LDL: 118

1. From a pharmacological perspective, what is your next step?

2. What lifestyle changes would you recommend?

3. When would you schedule follow-up?

Case 2

At his follow-up visit 6 weeks later, the patient from case 1 has the following laboratory results:

Total Cholesterol (TC): 170

triglycerides (TG) : 105

HDL: 42

LDL: 107

1. What is your next step? Give three options.

References

Anderson, P. (November, 2007). Link between cognition and statins gets more complicated. *Neurology, 69*:1873-1880. Cited in Medscape Medical News, www.medscape.com/viewarticle/565920

Belay, B., Belamarich, P. F., & Revzon, T. C. (2007). The use of statins in pediatrics: Knowledge base, limitations, future directions. *Pediatrics, 119*(2), 37–380.

Centers for Disease Control and Prevention (CDC). February is American Heart Month. Retrieved January 31, 2013, from www.cdc.gov/Features/HeartMonth

Hoyert, D. L., Xu J. Death: Preliminary Data for 2012, vol 61, no 6. Hyattsville MD, October 10, 2012. National Center for Health Statistics. Accessed on January 22, 2013, www.cdc.gov/nchs/data/nvsr61-06.pdf

Katz, P., & Gilbert, J. (2008). Diabetes and cardiovascular disease among older adults: Dyslipidemia. *Geriatrics in Aging, 11*(9), 509–514.

Mattar, M., & Obeid, O. (2009). Fish oil and the management of hypertriglyceridemia. Nutrition and Health, *20*(1):41–49.

The National Heart, Lung, and Blood Institute (NHLBI) of the National Institutes of Health. (n.d.). AIM-HIGH Clinical Trial. Retrieved October 11, 2011, from www.aimhigh-heart.com

Pasternak, R. C., Smith, S. C. Jr., Bairey-Merz, C. N., Grundy, S. M., Cleeman, J. I., Lenfant, C., et al. (2002). ACC/AHA/NHLBI clinical advisory on the use and safety of statins. *Circulation, 106*:1024–1028.

Pedersen, T. R., Wilhelmsen, L., Faergeman, O., Strandberg, T. E., Thorgeirsson, G., Troedsson, L., et al. (2000). Follow-up study of patients randomized in the Scandinavian Simvastatin Survival Study (4S) of cholesterol lowering. *American Journal of Cardiology, 86*:257–262.

Rossebø, A. B., Pedersen, T. R., Boman, K., Brudi, P., Chambers, J. B., Egstrup, K., et al. for the SEAS Investigators. (2008). Intensive lipid lowering with simvastatin and ezetimibe in aortic stenosis. *New England Journal of Medicine, 359*:1343–1356.

U.S. Food and Drug Administration (FDA). (2011). *FDA drug safety communication: New restrictions, contraindications, and dose limitations for Zocor (simvastatin) to reduce the risk of muscle injury.* Retrieved January 12, 2013, from www.fda.gov/Drugs/DrugSafety/ucm256581.htm

Drugs Used in the Treatment of Blood Disorders

chapter 9

Richard Ackermann

CHAPTER FOCUS

This chapter provides an introduction to selecting drugs used to treat common blood disorders, such as drugs to treat anemia, anticoagulants to prevent and treat venous thromboembolism and other diseases, antiplatelet drugs to prevent cardiovascular events, and fibrinolytic drugs to manage acute coronary syndrome. These are high-risk drugs and are an essential part of outpatient and hospital practice. It behooves all clinicians to have a good working knowledge of these agents if they are to truly help people.

OBJECTIVES

After reading and studying this chapter, the student should be able to:

1. Evaluate and treat nutritional causes of anemia with iron, folic acid, and vitamin B_{12}.
2. Prescribe recombinant erythropoietin for selected patients with chronic renal failure, HIV disease, and those receiving chemotherapy.
3. Explain the use of acute anticoagulants, including heparin and the newer low molecular weight heparins.
4. Prescribe and carefully monitor the high-risk drug warfarin, with attention to side effects and drug interactions.
5. Advocate for appropriate use of antiplatelet drugs to prevent cardiovascular events.
6. Understand the rationale for prompt treatment of patients with acute coronary fibrinolytic therapy to establish reperfusion.

Key Terms

Acute coronary syndrome

Anemia

Anticoagulation

Erythropoietin

International normalized ratio (INR)

Partial thromboplastin time (PTT)

Prothrombin time (PT)

Venous thromboembolism

DRUGS USED TO TREAT BLOOD DISORDERS

Drugs Used to Treat Anemia
Iron Supplementation

oral ferrous sulfate (Feosol, Fer-in-sol, Feratab)

oral ferrous fumarate (Feostat, Femiron, Hemocyte, Ferrocite, Iron Fumarate

oral ferrous gluconate (Femiron, Fergon, Simron)

oral carbonyl iron (Feosol, Icar)

iron dextran (Dextran, Dexferrum, INFeD)

iron polysaccharide complex (Hytinic, Niferex)

iron sucrose (Venofer)

sodium ferric gluconate (Ferrlecit)

Folic Acid Supplements (A type of Vitamin B) folic acid (Folvite, Folate)
Vitamin B_{12}

cyanocobalamin (Ancobon, Cobex, Primabalt, Cyanoject)

erythropoietin (Epoetin alfa, Darbepoetin alfa)

Anticoagulants: Heparins warfarin (Coumadin) dabigatran (Pradaxa)

heparin (Calcilean, Heparin Leo, Hep-Lock)

Anticoagulants: Low Molecular Weight Heparin (LMWH)

danaparoid injection (Orgaran)

enoxaparin (Lovenox)

dalteparin (Fragmin)

fondaparinux (Arixtra)

tinzaparin (Innohep)

Antiplatelet Agents

aspirin

clopidogrel (Plavix)

prasugrel (Effient)

dipyridamole (Persantine)

Fibrinolytic Agents

alteplase (Activase, Cathflo Activase)

reteplase (Retavase)

tenecteplase (TNKase)

DRUGS USED IN THE TREATMENT OF BLOOD DISORDERS

Drugs Used to Treat Anemia

Iron, the oxygen carrier of hemoglobin and myoglobin (transport proteins for tissue, enzyme, and respiratory reactions), is essential for the normal functioning of many organs. Elemental iron is stored in the liver, spleen, and bone marrow. Healthy people need to ingest 8 to 18 mg of iron per day in their diet or they develop anemia with its symptoms of fatigue and impaired immune function. The World Health Organization (WHO) defines **anemia** as a state in which one's hemoglobin level is less than 13 gm/dL in men, less than 12 gm/dL in menstruating women, and less than 11 gm/dL in pregnant women (WHO, 2008). The Centers for Disease Control and Prevention (CDC) defines anemia in children as hemoglobin less than 11 g/dL for infants 6 months to 5 years old and less than 11.5 g/dL for children 5 to 12 years old (CDC, 1998). The lack of circulating iron can be reversed through consumption of lean red meats or iron supplements. Ingested iron is converted to its ferrous state by gastric juices, making it more readily absorbed.

Iron Supplements

One common classification of anemia is by size of resultant red blood cells—microcytic, normocytic, or macrocytic. The differential diagnosis of microcytic anemia includes iron deficiency, thalassemia trait, sideroblastic anemias, the anemia of chronic disease, and lead poisoning. Iron deficiency itself is not a primary diagnosis; it is caused by something else such as decreased iron intake (poor diet, gastrectomy, celiac disease, achlorhydria); increased iron loss (GI infection, peptic ulcer, malignancy, atrioventricular (AV) malformations, excessive menstruation, blood donation); or increased requirements for iron, as in infants or pregnant and lactating women. Patients with chronic renal failure often become iron deficient for multiple reasons, including loss of iron associated with dialysis as well as blood lost from diagnostic tests, and gastrointestinal (GI) bleeding from telangiectasia.

Iron products should only be used to treat iron deficiency, not just as a general tonic or to treat nonspecific anemia. Iron deficiency is generally straightforward to diagnose. As iron deficiency develops, the patient is initially asymptomatic, and serum iron stores gradually fall, which is reflected in low iron saturation and ferritin levels. Eventually, when iron stores in the bone marrow are depleted, the patient becomes anemic, usually with microcytic, hypochromic indices, unless there is a second cause of anemia also present. Thus, iron deficiency anemia, which affects 1% to 4% of Americans, is the end-stage of iron deficiency.

Symptoms of iron deficiency include fatigue, lethargy, dyspnea on exertion and in infants, abnormal behavior, and impaired development.

Healthy full-term infants are born with 75 mg/kg of iron. These stores are depleted during the rapid growth of the first 6 months of life, after which iron requirements decrease. By adulthood, the average man has 50 mg/kg of iron, whereas women have approximately 35 mg/kg because of periodic menstruation. Almost all of the iron in the body is found in hemoglobin and myoglobin, the major protein in muscle.

Mechanism of Action

Iron is an essential ingredient in the production of hemoglobin. Hemoglobin is produced when one molecule of iron becomes incorporated into a protoporphyrin ring called heme, and one heme unit attaches to a globin protein. Then four heme-globin subunits combine to make one unit of hemoglobin.

Pharmacokinetics

- *Absorption:* The metabolism of most drugs is controlled by excretion, but for iron, absorption is the major control point. Iron is only lost from the body through bleeding or loss of cells, such that men and nonmenstruating women lose only about 1 mg of iron per day. Menstruating women lose 10 to 40 mg per menstrual cycle and approximately 700 mg of iron during pregnancy. One unit of transfused blood provides 250 mg of iron. Iron absorption occurs mainly in the jejunum and is only about 5% to 10% of oral intake, although this amount can double or triple in states of iron deficiency. The typical American diet provides about 6 mg of elemental iron per 1,000 kcal, thus dietary deficiency is common. Heme iron (iron as part of animal blood) is well absorbed regardless of other dietary factors, whereas non-heme iron is absorbed better in the presence of vitamin C or meat and worse in the presence of calcium, fiber, tea, coffee, or wine. Ferrous iron (Fe^{+++}) is better absorbed than is the ferric (Fe^{++}) form.
- Iron deficiency is caused by inadequate intake, poor absorption, or loss of blood. Iron deficiency is not a diagnosis by itself; rather, it is a precipitating factor. In the United States, risk factors for iron deficiency include being African American or of Mexican ethnicity, blood donation, low socioeconomic status, pregnancy and the postpartum state, child and adolescent obesity, and a vegetarian diet.
- *Distribution:* Iron remains in the body for many months and will cross the placenta and enter breast milk. It circulates at about 90% or more protein bound.
- *Metabolism/Excretion:* Iron is mostly recycled with small daily losses occurring through desquamation, sweat, urine, and bile.
- *Dosage:* Adults should receive at least 3 to 6 months of oral therapy to replace depleted stores. Repeat therapy is often necessary, but should not continue iron indefinitely unless there is documented evidence of iron deficiency.

Dosage and Administration

Generic Name	Trade Name	Adult Dosage*	Administration Notes
oral ferrous sulfate	Feosol, Fer-In-Sol, Feratab	325 mg/day for prophylaxis, 325 mg 2–4 times/day for therapeutic use	Ferrous sulfate provides 20% elemental iron, thus one 325-mg tab provides 65 mg of elemental iron
oral ferrous fumarate	Feostat, Femiron, Fumasorb	200 mg/day for prophylaxis, 200 mg 3–4 times a day for therapeutic use	Ferrous fumarate provides 33% elemental iron, thus one 325-mg tab provides 108 mg of elemental iron
oral ferrous gluconate	Femiron, Fergon, Simron	325 mg/day prophylactic; 325 mg 4 times/day for therapeutic use	Oral iron gluconate contains 12% elemental iron or 35 mg of elemental iron in a 325-mg tab
oral carbonyl iron	Feosol, Icar	50 mg tabs, oral suspension, 15 mg/1.25 mL	Carbonyl iron contains 100% elemental iron but is less toxic than iron salts. It is available as tabs, chewable tabs, and liquid.
iron dextran	Iron dextran IV and IM Dexferrum, INFeD	Adults >15 kg (dose in mL) 0.0442 (desired Hb – observed Hb) × lean body wt + (0.26 + wt) – dose in mL	A test dose of 0.25 mL should be given first. Note: Max daily dose is not more than (NMT) 100 mg iron (2 mL) IM dose is via Z-track dose deep into outer quadrant of buttock; IV dose is gradual over 5 min
iron polysaccharide complex	Hytinic, Niferex, Nu-Iron	50–100 mg 2/day of elixir or tabs	Available as 150-mg capsules, 50-mg tabs, and 100 mg/5 mL of elixir.
iron sucrose	Venofer	1 IV 100 mg (5 mL) administer 1–3/week during dialysis as a 15-min event over 10 sessions	Used for iron deficiency anemia in hemodialysis-dependent cases and for other cases in which oral therapy is ineffective or not well tolerated. Available as 20 mg/mL in 5-mL single-use vial.
sodium ferric gluconate	Ferrlecit	62.5 mg elemental Fe/5 mL	For use in peritoneal dialysis. Generally dosed as 10 mL (125 mg) infused over 60 min, and repeated during 8 sequential dialysis treatments to a total dose of 1,000 mg.

*Maximal oral absorption of iron in adults occurs with a daily dose of 200 mg of elemental iron. There is no advantage to higher doses, which only cause more GI intolerance. In fact, some patients may be able to tolerate only 100 mg or even less per day of elemental iron.

Clinical Uses

■ Prevention and treatment of iron-deficiency anemia.

Adverse Reactions

DERM: Flushing, urticaria.

GI: Heartburn, nausea, abdominal cramps, diarrhea, or constipation. Tolerance is improved when patients start with small doses and gradually work up to the full dose over several days to weeks. A polysaccharide-iron complex marketed as Niferex may cause fewer side effects, but there is some question regarding whether this product is well absorbed.

MISC: Pain at IM site (iron dextran), phlebitis at IV site, strong metallic taste.

NEURO: Seizures, dizziness, headache, syncope.

OTHER DELAYED REACTIONS: Hemosiderosis, lymphadenopathy, myalgia, fatigue, arthralgia and fever, anaphylactoid reaction.

Interactions

■ All metals, including iron, need to be taken separately from thyroxine because it decreases metals' efficacy.
■ Avoid coadministration with drugs that raise the gastric pH, such as antacids, H_2 blockers, or proton pump inhibitors.
■ Iron absorption is also reduced in the presence of coffee, tea, and fiber/bran products.
■ Iron supplements increase the absorption of tetracyclines, fluoroquinolones, and penicillamine.

Contraindications

■ Iron should not be given to patients with iron overload syndromes such as hemosiderosis or hemochromatosis.
■ Iron is also not indicated for patients who are not iron deficient. Do not prescribe empiric iron for a nonspecific anemia.
■ Long-term (multiple years) iron is also not necessary unless there is a continued problem with absorption or blood loss.

Conscientious Considerations

■ High-risk infants (those living in poverty, African American/Native American ethnicity, immigrants, preterm or low birth weight, or if the primary dietary intake is regular cow's milk) should receive routine iron supplementation between ages 6 and 12 months.
■ Men or women over about age 50 years with iron deficiency anemia should be evaluated for GI cancers. For younger patients, use judgment in deciding whether to pursue a cancer workup.
■ If iron therapy does not resolve the anemia, consider these explanations: incorrect diagnosis, complicating illness, noncompliance, inadequate dose, continuing iron loss, or iron malabsorption.
■ Iron therapy should cause rapid improvement of iron-deficiency anemia symptoms. First will be an increase in reticulocytes, followed by the red cell count, the hemoglobin, and later the red cell indices. Hemoglobin should be normal by 2 months after oral replacement begins.
■ All iron products should be kept in childproof containers.
■ Infants and children with iron deficiency anemia are generally treated with 1.5 to 2.0 mg/kg of elemental iron, divided

into three daily doses. Use elixirs and syrups, although they can stain the teeth. Children can generally take iron on an empty stomach.

■ In some cases, patients cannot tolerate oral iron supplementation or replacement needs to be more rapid. In these cases, red cell transfusion or intravenous iron can be useful.

■ Until recently, there was only one product available for intravenous replacement—iron dextran, which had a substantial risk of anaphylactic reactions. Due to the anaphylactic risk, give a test dose of 25 mg. If this is tolerated, then the entire replacement dose may be given at once, using an online calculator (iron dextran injection calculator, or INFeD –). Although this is the only intravenous iron product that allows complete treatment in a single setting, most clinicians use one of the newer products, which have less risk of anaphylaxis.

■ Iron sucrose is also used for patients on peritoneal dialysis. A suggested schedule is 300 mg over 90 minutes, 300 mg 2 weeks later, 400 mg 2 weeks after that. For patients with chronic renal disease who are not yet on dialysis, a suggested schedule is 200 mg over 15 minutes on five different occasions over a 2-week period.

■ Oral iron supplementation is routine in pregnancy, because the developing fetus requires more iron than the stores that many mothers can provide. Iron supplementation is also routine for infants. In no other circumstance should oral iron be prescribed without a specific diagnosis of iron deficiency.

■ Nutritional iron deficiency is common in menstruating girls and women because these patients may be unable to ingest enough iron in their diet to keep up with periodic blood loss. For other patients, such as men or older adults, in addition to prescribing iron, be sure to investigate why the patient is iron deficient. Up to 10% of patients over age 65 years with iron deficiency will have a GI malignancy.

■ The single most accurate laboratory test is the serum ferritin test; a level less than 25 mcg/L is highly specific for iron deficiency, whereas a level greater than 100 mcg/L reliably rules this out. Patients with chronic inflammatory disease such as rheumatoid arthritis or chronic liver disease may have higher ferritin levels because ferritin is an acute phase reactant. Other tests suggesting iron deficiency are a reduced transferrin saturation (TSAT = Fe/total iron binding [TIBC]) or an increased serum transferrin receptor assay. The gold standard for diagnosis of iron deficiency is the lack of stainable iron on bone marrow biopsy, but this test is rarely necessary. A reasonable strategy is get an initial serum ferritin result, and if the result is intermediate (25 to 100 mcg/L), pursue other testing.

■ Ingesting iron with ascorbic acid (500 mg) will keep the iron in the ferrous state and enhance absorption. Advise patients to place one 325-mg iron tablet and one 500-mg vitamin C tablet on the edge of their plate during the largest meal of the day, and ingest both pills in the middle of the meal to avoid any GI upset.

■ Adults should receive at least 3 to 6 months of oral therapy to replace depleted stores. Repeat therapy is often necessary, but do not continue iron indefinitely, unless there is documented evidence of iron deficiency.

Patient/Family Education

■ Encourage patients to comply with the medication regimen and to try not to miss a dose. If a dose is remembered within 12 hours of not taking it, they should take it as soon as remembered, otherwise return to their regular dosing schedule and do not double the doses.

■ Remind patients that iron will turn their stools black or dark green and that this is a harmless coloration.

■ If children are involved, instruct caregivers on what it means to eat a high iron diet.

■ Patients will know they are back to good health not by just feeling less fatigued but by a lab test used to retest their hemoglobin levels.

■ Avoid foods and medications that reduce iron absorption, including tea, bran, cereal, antacid, H_2 blockers, and proton pump inhibitors.

Folic Acid

Folic acid (folate) is a water-soluble cofactor for many enzymatic reactions of metabolism, particularly those involved in the production of purines and pyrimidines. Folic acid is essential in the production of all hematologic cell lines. Folate is present is nearly all foods; particularly rich sources are leafy green vegetables, meats, yeast, nuts, beans, organ juice, dairy products, grains, and cereals. American grain and cereal products are routinely fortified with folate, but large losses of folate can occur with cooking. The recommended daily intake, expressed in dietary folate equivalents, varies from 400 to 600 mcg per day. Women of reproductive age should take an additional 400-mcg folic acid supplement, because this has been shown to reduce the risk of neural tube defects in subsequent pregnancies (IOM, 1998, U.S. Department of Health and Human Services, 2010).

Folate deficiency causes a macrocytic anemia and may also infrequently cause neurological dysfunction in adults. Deficiency is diagnosed by a serum folate level below 2.5 mcg/L, although some experts use 5.0 mcg/L in older adults. Serum folate level does depend on recent folate intake: There is another test, red blood cell (RBC) folate, which is thought to be a truer indication of folate stores.

Folate deficiency is usually multifactorial in that its causes include dietary insufficiency, malabsorption, alcohol use, inborn errors of metabolism, and increased folate demand, as in pregnancy, lactation, and chronic hemolytic anemias.

Mechanism of Action

Folate stimulates the production of protein synthesis necessary for red blood cells, white blood cells, and platelet formation.

Pharmacokinetics

■ Absorption: With an oral dose, folic acid is well absorbed within 30 to 60 minutes in the proximal small intestine.

■ Distribution: Half of all folic acid cycles through the enterohepatic circulation; the rest circulates bound to serum protein.

■ Metabolism: Converted by the liver to an active metabolite, dihydrofolate reductase.

- Excretion: Excess amounts are excreted unchanged by the kidney.
- Half-life: Unknown.

Dosage and Administration

Generic Name	Trade Name	Dosage	Usual Adult Dose
folic acid	Folvite, vitamin B, folate	PO, IM, SC, IV	1 mg/day (therapeutic) for about a month 0.4 mg/day (maintenance)

Clinical Uses

- Folic acid is used to treat folate deficiency, and it is also used to prevent folate deficiency in certain situations, such as with drugs that inhibit folate synthesis, absorption, or metabolism, and in patients with chronic hemolysis with an enhanced need for folic acid (e.g., sickle cell anemia). Folic acid is also recommended for all pregnant women and all women considering pregnancy because supplementation of 400 mcg per day markedly reduces the incidence of neural tube defects in their offspring.

Adverse Reactions

DERM: Rashes
MISC: Fevers

Interactions

- Folic acid may decrease the serum concentration of phenytoin, and phenytoin itself is associated with folate deficiency.

Contraindications

- There are no clear contraindications, but do not prescribe folic acid without ensuring that B_{12} stores are adequate.

Conscientious Considerations

- Remember to check a vitamin B_{12} level before administering folic acid.
- In patients with anemia caused by folate deficiency, administration of folic acid should cause a reticulocytosis in 5 to 10 days, and the hemoglobin should rise after that.
- Drugs associated with folate deficiency include sulfasalazine, phenytoin, and other anticonvulsants. Folate deficiency is strongly associated with methotrexate, which is used not only for malignancies, but also for diseases such as rheumatoid arthritis. The predictable folate deficiency in these patients can be bypassed by administering a special reduced form of folic acid called *leucovorin*.
- Elevated serum homocysteine levels are linked to an increase in the risk of cardiovascular outcomes such as myocardial infarction and vascular death. Although folic acid, along with other B vitamins, can clearly reduce the serum homocysteine level, randomized trials have unfortunately concluded that this does *not* translate into a reduction in vascular events.
- In patients with macrocytic anemia due to folate deficiency, be sure that there is not also a simultaneous vitamin B_{12} deficiency. Folate replacement in this setting may improve hematological parameters, whereas the neurological damage

from B_{12} deficiency progresses. It is possible that routine folate supplementation in food may be exacerbating the problem of B_{12} deficiency in older adults.

Patient/Family Education

- Educate patients about diet, that is, the best source of vitamin B is a well-balanced diet with food from the four basic food groups. Foods high in folic acid include vegetables, fruits, and organ meats.
- Let patients know that cooking heat can destroy folic acid in foods.
- Caution patients who are self-medicating about exceeding U.S. Food and Drug Administration (FDA) Required Daily Allowances (RDA) because the effectiveness of megadoses is unproven and unsafe.
- Explain that doses of folic acid may turn urine yellow.
- Explain that follow-up visitations are the only way to check on effectiveness and progress.
- Ask patients to return to their clinicians should they notice a rash.

Vitamin B_{12}

Vitamin B_{12}, or cobalamin, is a cofactor in only two human enzymatic reactions: in the conversion of homocysteine to methionine and in the conversion of methylmalonic acid to succinyl-coenzyme A. Because humans cannot produce vitamin B_{12}, it must be supplied from either animal or bacterial sources or by supplementation. In the past, pernicious anemia, where the body produces antibodies to intrinsic factor, thus interfering with active absorption of the vitamin, was thought to be the common cause of B_{12} deficiency. However, this is clearly not the case; the most common cause is inability of the patient to split the R factor from B_{12} in foods. As gastric acidity is required for this function, patients with achlorhydria or those taking drugs that reduce or eliminate gastric acidity (e.g., H_2-blockers or proton pump inhibitors), are at risk for B_{12} deficiency. Other more unusual causes of B_{12} deficiency are surgical resection of the stomach (no production of intrinsic factor), surgical resection of the ileum (no active absorption), or a vegan diet.

Vitamin B_{12} is bound to an "R factor" in animal proteins; once this R factor–vitamin B_{12} complex is ingested, the R factor is split off by low gastric pH, and then intrinsic factor (IF), produced by the gastric parietal cells, attaches to the B_{12}. This B_{12}-IF complex travels to the distal ileum, where specific receptors facilitate absorption. After absorption, B_{12} binds to the transport protein transcobalamin II and is converted at the tissue level to active forms of the vitamin. B_{12} is principally stored in the liver.

Vitamin B_{12} is a water-soluble vitamin, and most patients have several years' worth stored in their liver. The minimum daily requirement of vitamin B_{12} is 1 to 3 mcg. The normal range of serum vitamin B_{12} varies by laboratory. Generally, levels of less than 100 pg/mL are diagnostic of B_{12} deficiency, and levels greater than 400 pg/dL exclude the diagnosis. For intermediate levels of 100 to 400 pg/dL, you have two major choices: treat empirically (low risk and low cost) or verify the diagnosis by documenting elevation of either serum homocysteine or methylmalonic acid.

Mechanism of Action

Acts as a coenzyme for many metabolic processes, including fat and carbohydrate metabolism and protein synthesis.

Pharmacokinetics

- Absorption: Absorption from the GI tract requires the presence of intrinsic factor and calcium, well absorbed after IM and IV administration.
- Distribution: Stored in the liver.
- Metabolism and Excretion: Any excess amounts are eliminated unchanged in the urine.
- Half-life: 6 days (400 days in liver)

Traditionally, vitamin B_{12} was replaced by intramuscular injections. For example, in a patient with macrocytic anemia caused by vitamin B_{12} deficiency, one can prescribe vitamin B_{12} 1 mg IM every week for 4 weeks, and then monthly, usually for life. However, studies clearly document that oral B_{12} is absorbed, even in patients without intrinsic factor or without an ileum. Up to 1% of oral B_{12} is directly absorbed outside the intrinsic factor pathway. In almost all cases of B_{12} deficiency, including those cases caused by pernicious anemia, oral administration will work well. However, there seems to be a substantial placebo effect of the characteristic deep red IM preparation, and there is no harm in giving the drug IM.

Dosage and Administration

Generic Name	Trade Name	Route	Typical Adult Dose
cyanocobalamin	Anacobin, Cobex, Primabalt	PO	1 mg daily, indefinitely
cyanocobalamin	Cyanoject	IM, SC	30–50 mcg/day for 6–7 days, then 100 mcg/day for a month
		Nasal spray	500 mcg (1 spray in 1 nostril) once a week

Note: If concerned about compliance, start with weekly injections of vitamin B_{12} (1 mg), followed by monthly shots of the same dose.

Clinical Use

- Vitamin B_{12} deficiency

Adverse Reactions

CV: Peripheral vascular thrombosis.
DERM: Itching, urticaria, swelling.
GI: Diarrhea, nausea, vomiting.
META: Hypokalemia can occur under heavy dosing due to intracellular shift of the potassium ion.
MISC: Pain at injection site, hypersensitivity reactions, including anaphylaxis.
NEURO: Headache, anxiety.

Interactions

- Oral absorption of B_{12} is decreased with neomycin, colchicine, anticonvulsants, metformin, and heavy alcohol use.

Contraindications

- Patients with Leber's optic nerve atrophy may suffer rapid progression of their eye disease when treated with vitamin B_{12}.

Conscientious Considerations

- Clinicians should consider vitamin B_{12} deficiency in patients with dementia, peripheral neuropathy, or macrocytic anemias because, if vitamin B_{12} deficiency goes undiagnosed, it can lead to irreversible neurological damage.
- Before replacing vitamin B_{12}, check not only the serum B_{12} level, but also the hematocrit, reticulocyte count, and folate and iron levels. The reticulocyte count should rise within a few days, and the anemia and other symptoms should resolve in weeks. For severe megaloblastic anemia, monitor the serum potassium and platelet count.
- In many cases, patients who have been taking IM B_{12} can be safely switched to the oral route. If a patient is unable to eat for several days or even weeks because of surgery, for example, there is no need to immediately convert to the IM form, because B_{12} stores usually last for several months or years.
- In a patient with documented vitamin B_{12} deficiency (by low serum levels), it is reasonable to check a serum B_{12} level again after several month, to ensure that the deficiency has resolved.

Patient/Family Education

- Educate patients who are self-medicating about the dangers of exceeding daily RDA requirements.
- Explain that meats, seafood, egg yolk, and fermented cheese are high in vitamin B_{12}, and that little vitamin B_{12} is lost with cooking.
- Solitary vitamin B_{12} deficiency is rare, thus patients are usually administered this vitamin in concert with others.
- If taken orally, vitamin B_{12} absorption is enhanced with meals.
- The IV route is not recommended.

Erythropoietin/Epoetin

Erythropoietin is a glycoprotein produced by the kidney; it is the major regulator of red blood cell synthesis by the bone marrow. This glycosylated 165-amino acid polypeptide is coded by the *EPO* gene on chromosome seven. The two available products, epoetin and darbepoetin, are equivalent in both efficacy and side effects. A recombinant form synthesized by mammalian cells is commercially available.

With anemia or hypoxemia, erythropoietin synthesis may increase 100-fold. Levels of erythropoietin can be detected by serum assays (serum EPO level), with normal levels ranging from 5 to 30 mU/mL. Consider other correctable causes of anemia before using erythropoietic stimulants; review the drug list and consider checking iron, folate, B_{12}, fecal occult blood, and serum creatinine.

Mechanism of Action

Erythropoietin induces red blood cell production by stimulating division and differentiation of erythroid precursor cells in the bone marrow. It also induces the release of reticulocytes from the marrow into the bloodstream. This effect is dose-dependent and can be measured first by a rise in the reticulocyte count, followed by improvement in the hemoglobin and hematocrit levels.

Pharmacokinetics

- Absorption: The drug is rapidly absorbed from subcutaneous injection sites (bioavailability about 20% to 30%) and taken up by the bone marrow, liver, and kidneys.
- Distribution: Remains unknown.
- Metabolism and excretion: Metabolized mainly by the liver to inactive metabolites; small amounts are excreted unchanged in the urine.
- Half-life: 4 to 13 hours.

Dosage and Administration

Dose	Epoetin Alfa			Darbepoetin Alfa
CHRONIC RENAL FAILURE				
Initial	500–100 units/kg three times/week IV or SC (pediatric dose 50 units/kg) Note: Epogen comes packaged as 2,000 units/ml up to 20,000 units per ml.			For patients on dialysis, 0.45 mcg/kg IV weekly For patients not on dialysis, 0.75 mcg/mL SC every 2 weeks.
Increase dose by 25% if	Hemoglobin (Hb) < 10 g/dL and has not increased by 1 g/dL after 4 weeks, or Hb decreases < 10 g/dL			The increase in Hb is < 1 g/dL over 4 weeks.
Reduce dose by 25% if	Hb approaches 12 g/dL or Hb increases > 1 g/dL in any 2-week period			
ZIDOVUDINE-TREATED PATIENTS WITH HIV INFECTION				
Initial	100 units/kg 3 times/week IV or SC for 8 weeks			Not FDA-approved for this use.
Titrate	By 50–100 units/kg 3 times/week to a maximum dose of 300 units/kg 3 times/week			
CANCER/CANCER CHEMOTHERAPY-ASSOCIATED ANEMIA				
Initial	150 units/kg 3 times/week SC	40,000 units SC weekly (pediatric dose 600 units/kg weekly)	500 mcg SC every 3 weeks	2.25 mcg/kg SC weekly
Withhold dose	If Hb > 12 g/dL, and restart at 25% below the previous dose when Hb falls		Hb exceeds 12 g/dL, until Hb ≤ 11 g/dl, restart at 40% below the previous dose	
Reduce dose	By 25% when Hb reaches target Hb or increases > 1 g/dL in any 2-week period		By 40% of previous dose when Hb > 11 g/dl or Hb increases > 1 g/dl in 2 weeks	
Increase dose	To 300 units/kg 3 times/week SC if response is not satisfactory after 8 weeks	To 60,000 units SC weekly (pediatric dose to 900 units/kg weekly) if response is not satisfactory after 8 weeks	To 4.5 mcg/kg if there is < 1 g/dL increase in Hb after 6 weeks	

SC = subcutaneously, IV = intravenously

The optimal hemoglobin goal is still controversial. National Kidney Foundation guidelines suggest a target Hb range of 11 to 13 g/dL, while the FDA has a long-standing recommendation that Hb should not exceed 12 g/dL (NKF, 2007).

Epoetin alfa is produced by two companies, first as Epogen, produced by Amgen, and also as Procrit, produced by Ortho Biotech. These drugs come in vials for IV or SC injection. In a preservative-free form, it comes as 2,000 units/mL, 3,000 units/mL, 4,000 units/mL, 10,000 units/mL and 40,000 units/mL. It also comes with a benzyl alcohol preservative as 10,000 units/mL and 20,000 units/mL.

Darbepoetin alfa is marketed as Aranesp by Amgen. It comes in a wide range of concentrations: 25, 40, 60, 100, 150, 200, 300, and 500 mcg/mL.

Before and during treatment with erythropoietin, iron stores should be evaluated. If there are inadequate iron stores in the bone marrow, treatment of erythropoietin will be ineffective. Patients with low ferritin or transferrin saturation should receive iron supplementation.

For patients with chronic renal failure, the initial intravenous or subcutaneous dose is generally 50 to 100 units/kg three times per week. For patients on dialysis, the dose may be given intravenously after a dialysis session. The dose is reduced when the hemoglobin approaches 12 g/dL or when the hemoglobin increases by 1 g/dL or more in any 2-week period. The usual target hemoglobin is 10 to 12 g/dL. Maintenance doses are individualized but are usually about 75 units/kg three times per week for patients on dialysis and 75 to 150 units/kg three times per week in non-dialysis patients.

For HIV patients with zidovudine-associated anemia, patients with erythropoietin levels greater than 500 mU/mL will not likely respond. For appropriate patients, the initial IV or SC dose is 100 units/kg three times per week for 8 weeks, with titration as needed.

For patients receiving chemotherapy, erythropoietin should be limited to patients whose serum erythropoietin level is less than 200 mU/mL. Typical starting doses are 150 units/kg three times per week or 40,000 units once weekly, with titration as needed.

For patients who are to undergo elective surgery, first ensure that the hemoglobin is between 10 and 13 g/dL. Typical doses of erythropoietin are 300 units/kg/day for 10 days before surgery, on the day of surgery, and for 4 days postoperatively.

For the non-FDA approved indication of anemia associated with critical illness, a typical dose is 40,000 units SC weekly.

Clinical Uses

- Primarily used to treat the anemia associated with renal failure, including both patients on dialysis (peritoneal or hemodialysis) and patients not on dialysis. Before using erythropoietin in these patients, the hematocrit should be less than 30%, the ferritin should be greater than 100 ng/dL, and the transferrin saturation (Fe/TIBC) should be greater than 20% to 30%.
- Indicated to treat the anemia associated with zidovudine therapy in HIV patents, when the endogenous erythropoietin

level is low (less than equal to 500 mU/mL) and the dose of zidovudine is less than or equal to 4,200 mg/week.

■ Indicated for some cancer patients and for those with other hematological diseases undergoing chemotherapy, when that therapy causes anemia, to reduce the need for red blood cell transfusion.

■ Indicated in patients with mild anemia (Hg 10 to 13 g/dL) who are scheduled to undergo elective, noncardiac, nonvascular surgery to reduce the need for red blood cell transfusions.

■ Clinicians also use this drug in conditions that have not been approved by the FDA. These include anemia associated with chronic disease, rheumatic disease, Rh hemolytic disease, sickle cell disease, acute renal failure, Gaucher's disease, Castleman's disease, paroxysmal nocturnal hemoglobinuria, anemia in the critical care setting, and others. In these settings, some experts suggest that a serum erythropoietin level greater than 100 mU/mL predicts lack of response to erythropoietin treatment.

Adverse Reactions

CV: Can precipitate hypertensive crisis, especially if blood pressure is poorly controlled. Hypertension and seizures may be more common if the hematocrit rises excessively fast. Myocardial infarction (MI), chest pain, vascular thrombosis, especially in hemodialysis patients.

DERM: Transient rashes.

ENDO: Restored fertility, resumption of menses.

GI: Nausea, diarrhea.

HEM: Thromboembolism is more likely in patients taking erythropoietin, especially in those with a prior venous thrombosis or prolonged immobilization. It is unknown if concomitant use with aspirin or anticoagulants could lower this risk of deep vein thrombosis (DVT). Rarely, patients on erythropoietin will develop neutralizing antibodies to erythropoietin.

ONCOLOGY: Cancer patients taking erythropoietin may have lower survival times and other adverse effects on cancer prognosis. The risks and benefits need to be individualized by the patient's oncologist.

MS: Paresthesias.

NEURO: Seizures, headache.

PUL: Upper respiratory infection.

Interactions

■ No drug interactions have been reported.

Contraindications

■ Do not give erythropoietin for nonspecific anemia.

■ Patients with allergies to albumin cannot take erythropoietin.

■ Patients with uncontrolled hypertension should have their blood pressure condition controlled before using erythropoietin, and blood pressure should be carefully monitored while on this treatment.

Conscientious Considerations

■ Do not use erythropoietin as an alternative to transfusion in patients with severe anemia. There should never be an emergency or STAT order for erythropoietin.

■ Erythropoietin may have limited effectiveness if there is concomitant iron, folic acid, or vitamin B_{12} deficiency, blood loss, infection or inflammation, aluminum overload (this inhibits iron incorporation into heme), neoplastic bone marrow replacement, or poor compliance. Consider these if you don't get the expected response in the hematocrit.

■ Erythropoietin is very expensive, with annual costs sometimes exceeding $10,000. Its use should strictly follow guidelines and be prescribed by an expert.

■ Erythropoietin has been promoted directly to consumers, promising renewed energy, increased work capacity, and athletic enhancement. None of these uses is appropriate.

Patient/Family Education

■ Patients and families need to know the rationale behind the use of this medication and why it may be used concurrently with iron therapy.

■ Discuss possible return to menses and fertility in women of childbearing age, adding contraceptive options if appropriate.

■ Discuss the importance of dietary restrictions and compliance with other medications and dialysis. When home dialysis patients are determined to administer their own epoetin, they need instruction on dosage and administration techniques.

Anticoagulants

Drugs used for **anticoagulation** (stopping or preventing blood from clotting through antagonizing the effects of vitamin K) include heparin, low molecular weight heparins, and warfarin. They are used to treat deep vein thrombosis (DVT), pulmonary embolism (PE), stroke, transient ischemic attacks (TIA), **acute coronary syndrome** (ACS), and other conditions such as those induced by medical prosthetic heart devices or in cases of atrial fibrillation where anticoagulation therapy helps prevent blood clot formation resulting from the arrhythmia and for which the clot leads to an embolism or a cerebrovascular accident (CVA) (Rubboli, 2011).

Heparin

Heparin, sometimes called unfractionated heparin, is a mixture of glycosaminoglycan chains over a molecular weight range of 4,000 to 30,000 daltons. Heparins are produced by human mast cells. Low molecular weight heparins (LMWHs) are also mixtures, but the average chain lengths are much smaller. The low molecular weight heparins have a longer half-life and can be used in once or twice daily dosing, whereas unfractionated heparin is usually given either as a continuous intravenous infusion or as multiple daily subcutaneous injections.

Mechanism of Action

Antithrombin (AT), formerly called antithrombin III, is a native anticoagulant that slowly binds to thrombin and other coagulants. However, its full action requires a cofactor, heparin. When heparin binds to AT, it induces a conformational change that converts AT to a rapid and powerful anticoagulant. With heparin attached, AT binds to a variety of clotting enzymes, especially thrombin (factor II) and activated factor X (Xa). This prevents the conversion of fibrinogen to fibrin. To bind to factor II, the heparin chain must be at least 18 saccharide units long. However, the binding site for factor Xa is a small pentasaccharide unit. The synthetic LMWH fondaparinux (Arixtra) contains only this active pentasaccharide; therefore, this drug does not inactivate factor II, but it remains a powerful activator of Xa. To summarize, in low doses AT prevents the conversion of prothrombin to thrombin by its effect on factor Xa, in higher doses it neutralizes thrombin by its effect on factor Xa.

Pharmacokinetics

■ Absorption: Heparin is not absorbed orally and must be administered either by continuous IV infusion or subcutaneously. When heparin is given SC, the dose should be higher than the IV dose to compensate for the reduced bioavailability of the SC route. Heparin has an immediate onset of action when given intravenously; SC absorption is very good and is the preferred method of administration.

■ Distribution: In the bloodstream, heparin binds very well to a variety of plasma proteins, especially low-density lipoproteins (LDLPs; globulins and fibrinogens), which reduces its anticoagulant activity.

■ Metabolism and Excretion: Heparin is cleared by two methods: rapid saturable binding to endothelial receptors and macrophages and nonsaturable renal clearance. Its complex kinetics make the anticoagulant response to heparin nonlinear. It thus requires continuous monitoring by the partial thromboplastin time (PTT) because heparin probably is reabsorbed by the reticuloendothelial system (lymph nodes, spleen).

■ Half-life: Half-hour.

Dosage and Administration

Generic Name	Trade Name	Dosage Form	Dvt/ Prophy-laxis	Dvt/ Pretreat-ment	Acute Coronary Syndrome
heparin	Calcilean, Heparin Leo, Hep-Lock	Solution for injection: 10 units/mL, 100 units/mL, 1,000 units/mL, 5,000 units/mL, 7,500 units/mL	Heparin 5,000 units SC every 8–12 hr	Heparin, 80 units/kg IV bolus, then 18 units/kg/hr, titrated by periodic PTT measurements*	A bolus of 60-70 units/kg (maximum of 5000 units), followed by an infusion of 12-15 units/kg/hr (maximum 1000 units/hr). For patients who are treated with fibrinolytic drugs for ST-segment elevation MI, the dose is even lower: an initial bolus of 60 units/kg (maximum 4000 units), with an infusion of 12 units/kg/hr (maximum 1000 units/hr)

*PTT is generally checked every 6 hr while patients are on intravenous heparin.

The following table can be used to adjust the heparin dose.

While on IV Heparin, if the PTT is	Change The Heparin Dose:
<35 sec	Give another 80 units/kg IV bolus and increase the drip by 4 units/kg/hr.
35–45 sec	Give another 40 units/kg IV bolus and increase the drip by 2 units/kg/hr.
46–70 sec (desired)	No change
71–90 sec	Reduce the drip by 2 units/kg/hr.
>90 sec	Stop the IV infusion for 1 hr, then reduce drip by 3 units/kg/hr.

It is standard practice to monitor heparin activity with the activated partial thromboplastin time (aPTT), although the level of evidence of activity is weak. In special circumstances, such as with percutaneous coronary interventions or cardiac surgery, the activated clotting time (ACT) may be used instead. With the aPTT, the therapeutic range for heparin is thought to be about 1.5 to 2.5 times the control.

Clinical Uses

■ To prevent venous thromboembolism, formation in a blood vessel of a clot (thrombus) that breaks loose and is carried by the bloodstream to plug another vessel (VTE) and to treat either venous or arterial thromboembolism.

■ Immediately following the institution of heparin/low molecular weight heparin, long-term anticoagulation with warfarin can begin (see warfarin section below).

Adverse Reactions

GI. Drug-induced hepatitis.
DERM: Long term use may induce alopecia, rashes, urticaria.
HEM: Bleeding, sometimes trivial and sometimes life-threatening, especially when it is into sites like the brain, bowel, or retroperitoneal space. Heparin-associated bleeding is increased with higher drug doses, when coadministered with fibrinolytics or glycoprotein IIb/IIIa inhibitors, and in patients with recent surgery, trauma, invasive procedures, or underlying coagulopathies. All heparins, including low molecular weight heparins, can cause thrombocytopenia.
MS: Osteoporosis, by binding to osteoblasts, which then release factors that activate osteoclasts. This is only a problem in patients who require long-term treatment.

Interactions

■ Heparin will enhance the effect of other anticoagulants. Be careful in combining these drugs with antiplatelet drugs such as aspirin, clopidogrel, aspirin-extended release dipyridamole (Aggrenox), or thrombolytic agents.

Contraindications

■ Use heparin with caution in patients with a history of peptic ulceration or gastrointestinal angiodysplasia, patients with poorly controlled hypertension, or those with diabetic retinopathy.

■ If a patient has ever had heparin-induced thrombocytopenia, they can never again be exposed to any heparin products, including LMWHs.

Conscientious Considerations

■ *Never* administer heparin to a patient until the *dose* has been checked by a second licensed person.

■ Coadministration with warfarin requires monitoring of the international normalized ratio (INR).

■ Avoid NSAIDs in patients on these drugs because these may also enhance bleeding. Pain relief in patients prescribed heparin can generally be accomplished with either acetaminophen or opioids.

■ Patients on prescribed anticoagulants should avoid over-the-counter products that have bleeding side effects; these include gingko, garlic, ginseng, vitamin E, and fish oil supplementation.

■ With heparin, obtain a baseline PT/PTT, hemoglobin/hematocrit (Hb/Hct), and a platelet count. Follow the PTT, get a periodic platelet count, and monitor for signs of bleeding.

Patient/Family Education

■ Patients and families need knowledge of what these drugs are and what is going to be happening to them. If they are going to be on long-term therapy and started on oral anticoagulant therapy, they should know that the SC heparin injections will continue for another 4 to 5 days.

■ Patients will have to take a role in looking for any unusual signs of bruising or bleeding and to report it immediately.

■ It is often helpful to many patients to learn that they should use a soft toothbrush during therapy to prevent gum bleeding and to use an electric razor to avoid cuts or nicks.

■ Encourage heparin therapy patients to wear a medical alert ID bracelet or carry an ID card at all times.

Low Molecular Weight Heparins (LMWH)

Low molecular weight heparins (LMWHs) are similar to heparin in that they are also mixtures, but they differ in that their average chain lengths are much smaller (in daltons) when compared to heparin. Examples of LMWHs are danaparoid (Orgaran), enoxaparin (Lovenox), dalteparin (Fragmin), fondaparinux (Arixtra), and tinzaparin (Innohep). Because they are anticoagulants like heparin, their lower molecular weight gives them an advantage of having a longer half-life, which translates into once-a-day dosing. Additionally, they can be synthesized in a laboratory; for example, enoxaparin (Lovenox) is produced by chemically altering porcine heparin to produce a shorter molecule, with an average molecular weight of 4,500 daltons. Dalteparin's averagemolecular weight is 5,000 daltons. Fondaparinux is totally synthetic.

Mechanism of Action

These agents potentiate the effect of antithrombin on factor Xa and thrombin, but compared to unfractionated heparin, LMWHs preferentially inhibit factor Xa more than does thrombin.

Pharmacokinetics

■ Absorption: All LMWHs are destroyed by enzymes in the bowels, necessitating parenteral administration. Once administered, the LMWH have higher bioavailability (90%) than does heparin, which makes their anticoagulant effects more predictable than heparin.

■ Distribution: Remains unknown.

■ Metabolism/Excretion: Some are partially metabolized or not at all, but these agents are excreted renally.

■ Half-life: Enoxaparin: 3 to 6 hours, which allows once- or twice-daily dosing. Dalteparin: 2 hours; danaparoid: 24 hours; tinzaparin: 4 hours; fondaparinux: 17 hours in younger adult, up to 21 hours in the elderly, which allows for once-daily safe and effective therapy without monitoring in a large range of patients.

Dosage and Administration

Generic Name	Trade Name	Dosage For Dvt Prophylaxis of Abdominal Surgery	Preparation
danaparoid	Orgaran	SC 750 IU SC every 12 hr, starting 1–4 hr preoperatively and 2 hr postoperatively for 7–10 days	750 antifactor Xa IU/0.6 mL in prefilled syringes
enoxaparin	Lovenox	40 mg SC once daily, starting with 24 hr postoperatively, then continuing for 7–10 days or ambulatory	30 mg/0.3mL, 20 mg/0.4 mL, 40 mg/0.4 mL, 60 mg/0.6 mL, 80 mg/0.8 mL, 100 mg/mL, in prefilled syringes
dalteparin	Fragmin	2,500 IU SC, 2–3 hr before surgery, then once daily for 5–10 days	2,500 IU/2-mL syringe
fondaparinux	Arixtra	2.5 mg/day SC for DVT prophylaxis without adjustment for weight	2.5 mg/0.5 ml, 0.5 mg/0.4 mL, 7.5 mg/0.6 mL, and 10 mg in prefilled syringes
tinzaparin	Innohep	Treatment of DVT; 175 IU/kg SC once daily for 6 days until adequate anticoagulation	20,000 anti XA units/mL in 2-mL vial

Clinical Use

■ LMWHs are used in a wide range of conditions, including the prevention and treatment of DVT and PE. Compared with unfractionated heparin, LMWHs are safer and more effective in the treatment of acute coronary syndrome.

Adverse Reactions

DERM: Local skin reactions.

GI: Nausea, and diarrhea.

HEM: Bleeding is the most common adverse reaction with LMWHs and can occur at any site. The most serious bleeding sites are the central nervous system, GI tract, and retroperitoneal space.

META: Elevation of transaminases.

MS: Long-term use of LMWHs may cause osteoporosis.

Interactions

■ There are no important drug interactions with LMWHs, but remember that concomitant use of oral anticoagulants or antiplatelet agents may enhance bleeding side effects.

Contraindications

■ LMWHs carry a black box FDA warning that they should not be given to patients who have spinal or epidural catheters. Administration of these drugs to patients with these catheters, or immediately after they have been withdrawn, has rarely been associated with spinal and epidural hematomas, some of which caused permanent paralysis. To be safe, wait at least 4 hours after the catheter has been removed.

Conscientious Considerations

■ These drugs must be given subcutaneously, not intramuscularly.
■ Heparin, the LMWHs, and fondaparinux are not interchangeable. Each has its own indications for use and doses.
■ These drugs may be cautiously used in older adults, taking into account the renal insufficiency that frequently accompanies aging.
■ Although the drugs are expensive ($20 to $100 per day), treating DVT with LMWH or fondaparinux is often cheaper because there is no heparin drip or PTT monitoring, and sometimes hospitalization can be avoided.
■ The prefilled syringes of the low molecular weight heparins come with an air bubble, which should *not* be expelled before injection.
■ Several commonly used herbals should also be avoided: dong quai, evening primrose, garlic, ginger, gingko, ginseng, and green tea.
■ Thrombocytopenia can occur with enoxaparin, dalteparin, and fondaparinux. Heparin-induced thrombocytopenia (HIT) is much less common with LMWHs than with unfractionated heparin, and the risk of osteoporosis is also lower. To date, there are no reported cases of HIT with fondaparinux. Discontinue any of these drugs if the platelet count falls below 100,000/mm³.
■ There is no proven method to reverse the anticoagulant effects of LMWHs or fondaparinux.

Patient/Family Education

■ Same as heparin, especially to advise patients against use of aspirin and NSAIDs.
■ Teach patients to watch for signs of internal bleeding and to report any unusual bruising.

Warfarin (Coumadin)

Warfarin (Coumadin) is the most commonly used anticoagulant because it can be administered as a tablet. It has a wide range of indications, the most common being chronic atrial fibrillation and the prevention and treatment of deep venous thrombosis and pulmonary embolism. Warfarin is *not* a treatment for these conditions, but rather it is used to prevent the complications that can arise from DVT and PE.

Warfarin use is monitored by measuring the **prothrombin time (PT)**, or more specifically, the **international normalized ratio (INR)**. The PT is very dependent on the specific thromboplastin reagent used by the laboratory. To standardize for this, and to allow anticoagulation to be compared between laboratories, the INR measurement was developed: INR = (patient's PT/reference PT)^{ISI}, where the ISI (International Sensitivity Index) is a measurement of the thromboplastin sensitivity. Although PTs may vary between two laboratories, the INRs should be identical.

For most clinical conditions, the therapeutic range for the INR is 2 to 3, with a goal of 2.5. Warfarin is one of the most dangerous drugs in clinical use because it has extensive variability between patients, because it has numerous drug interactions, and most importantly, because it can cause serious, even fatal bleeding. Oral direct thrombin inhibitors may replace warfarin over the next decade; one of these (dabigatran) is now approved by the FDA.

Mechanism of Action

Warfarin works by interfering with the hepatic synthesis of the vitamin-K dependent clotting factors (factors II, VII, IX, and X). Warfarin inhibits vitamin K epoxide reductase, the enzyme that recycles vitamin K to its reduced form after it has carboxylated blood coagulation proteins, especially factors II and VII. Anticoagulation effects generally start within 1 to 2 days, but it often takes 5 to 6 days for a stable effect. A typical daily dose to maintain an INR of 2 to 3 is 2 to 5 mg/day, but there is wide variation. Older adults generally need lower warfarin doses to reach a therapeutic INR.

Pharmacokinetics

■ Absorption: Warfarin is only given orally because it has nearly 100% bioavailability when it is absorbed from the GI tract.
■ Distribution: It crosses the placenta but does not enter breast milk because it is 99% protein bound.
■ Metabolism and Excretion: Hepatic metabolism.
■ Half-life: One-half day to 3 days because half-life varies widely among individuals, and this necessitates the need for careful monitoring of its anticoagulant effect (using INR).

Dosage and Administration

Warfarin is available only as an oral preparation, but there is a wide range of available dosage forms: that is, 1-, 2-, 2.5-, 3-, 4-, 5-, 6-, 7.5-, and 10-mg tablets. Rather than prescribe different tablet sizes to patients as the clinician titrates the dose, consider starting with the 5-mg tablet. With this practice, patients are less likely to become confused with several different doses of warfarin. Patients who need less than 5 mg per day can be prescribed half a tablet once daily or even less often. Warfarin (Coumdain) dosing is guided by clinical factors and pharmacogenomics despite the availability of dosage calculators. Thus, dosing of oral Warfarin is achieved using the availability of many tablet strengths that allow for needed titration of dosage strength but still allow continuance of the original administration schedule in order to avoid issues with patient adherence.

Weekly Dosing Schedule for Warfarin (Coumadin) Tablets

Weekly Warfarin Dose (MG)	Daily Dose (5-MG Tablets)
7.5	0.5 tab 3 days/week
10	0.5 tab 4 days/week
12.5	0.5 tab 5 days/week
15	0.5 tab 6 days/week
17.5	1.5 tab daily
20	1 tab, 1 day/week, 0.5 tab 5 days/week
25	1 tab, 3 days/week, 0.5 tab 4 days/week
30	1 tab, 5 days/week, 0.5 tab 2 days/week
35	1 tab daily
40	1 tab, 5 days/week, 1.5 tabs 2 days/week
45	1 tab 3 days/week, 1.5 tabs 4 days/week
50	1 ta, 1 day/week, 1.5 tabs 6 days/ week
57.5	1.5 tabs daily
and so on.	

When starting warfarin, obtain a baseline INR. If the patient is already on heparin or an LMWH (for example, for a patient with acute DVT), start the warfarin (usually 5 mg) immediately after the heparin/LMWH has begun. Check the INR daily. Generally, it will take about 5 days for the INR to become therapeutic. Continue the heparin/LMWH until the warfarin has produced the desired INR for at least 2 consecutive days.

If the patient is not on heparin/LMWH (for example, in a patient with atrial fibrillation), the process is easier. Start with a low dose of warfarin (generally 2.5 to 5 mg/day) and monitor the INR twice weekly, adjusting the warfarin dose as the INR rises.

Once the INR is in the therapeutic range, space out the INR monitoring interval, perhaps initially to once weekly for 2 to 4 weeks, and then monthly if the INR remains consistently in the therapeutic range.

Most patients with chronic nonvalvular atrial fibrillation should take chronic warfarin, which has been shown to reduce subsequent stroke by 40% to 80%. Patients under age 65 years with no clinical or echocardiographic evidence of coronary disease can consider aspirin instead of warfarin because their risk of stroke is quite low. Patients at high risk of stroke should go on warfarin; these patients include those over age 75 years and those with a prior nondisabling stroke/TIA, hypertension, low ejection fraction, or prosthetic heart valve. However, many of these older adults have serious comorbidities and functional limitations, and many are at serious risk of falls and bleeding. Individualize the decision to use an anticoagulation agent in patients such as these.

For patients with atrial fibrillation, lifelong warfarin may be indicated. However, as patients age and develop comorbidities, reassess the benefit/risk ratio; for many patients, the duration of warfarin anticoagulation should be limited. When warfarin is used solely as prophylaxis for DVT/PE, such as in patients who have undergone total hip replacement, stop the drug in 1 month or when the patient's mobility has been regained.

In the treatment of DVT and PE, old guidelines suggested duration of 3 months for DVT and 6 months for PE. However, more recent studies suggest that clinicians should individualize the duration, depending on the patient's risk of recurrent thromboembolism. At one extreme, if a 35-year-old patient has a minor popliteal DVT because of a long-leg cast, the warfarin can safely be discontinued 6 weeks after the cast has been removed, as long as the patient has returned to baseline. Another low-risk patient would be a woman who had a DVT induced by oral contraception. Again, 6 weeks of treatment would be sufficient.

At the other extreme, consider a frail 80-year-old woman who has a serious pulmonary embolism because she is relatively immobile from multiple chronic diseases. Her mobility is not likely to improve, so her risk of recurrence is much higher, and experts now recommend that she be treated with warfarin for at least 1 to 2 years, and perhaps even for life.

Many patients will have an intermittent risk of recurrence. Clinicians should use their best judgment, but should not continue to give patients warfarin forever simply because they are on the drug. Ask why the patient was prescribed the drug and whether the patient still meets criteria for continued use.

There are important ethical issues related to prescribing the drug for some patients on chronic warfarin. For example, if a patient with mild dementia develops atrial fibrillation, chronic warfarin anticoagulation is often indicated. As the patient progresses to severe and end-stage dementia, it is appropriate to reassess whether prevention of stroke is still a reasonable goal of care. In patients such as these, the goal of care changes to relief of symptoms and comfort care, and preventive drugs such as warfarin can be discontinued.

Clinical Uses

- Reduce the risk of stroke and peripheral embolism in patients with chronic nonvalvular atrial fibrillation.
- Patients who develop thromboembolism are first treated with either heparin or LMWHs, then transitioned to long-term warfarin use.
- In patients with metal cardiac valves used short term after receiving bioprosthetic cardiac valves.

Adverse Reactions

DERM: Skin necrosis and gangrene, due to a paradoxical local thrombosis, is a well-recognized but rare complication. This is usually seen in the first week of therapy; is often localized to the limbs, penis, or breast; and is more common in patients with protein C or S deficiency. There is also a "purple toes syndrome," due to microembolization of cholesterol, which occurs after several weeks to months of therapy.

HEM: The major adverse effect is bleeding, a direct consequence of the drug's mechanism of action.

MS: Other side effects are rare and idiosyncratic. Long-term warfarin is associated with osteoporosis.

Interactions

■ Drug interactions are common and potentially serious (Table 9-1). Most of these interactions occur with drugs that are substrates, inducers, or inhibitors of a variety of the cytochrome P-450 enzymes. Other drugs can interfere with the oral absorption of warfarin or can displace warfarin from protein binding. Still other drugs may cause enhanced bleeding, not from these effects, but because the drug itself causes bleeding or peptic ulceration.

■ The most commonly used drugs that decrease the anticoagulant effects of warfarin (either by induction of enzymes or by decreasing drug absorption) are antithyroid drugs, barbiturates, carbamazepine, phenytoin, rifampin, and cholestyramine. For example, patients taking barbiturates for a seizure disorder may need substantially higher than average warfarin doses to bring the INR to 2 to 3 because barbiturates are potent inducers of the CYP2C8/9 system.

■ The list of drugs than can enhance the anticoagulant effects of warfarin is much larger, including drugs that decrease absorption, displace warfarin, inhibit its metabolism, or other effects. Note that many commonly used drugs are in this table, including many oral antibiotics and even acetaminophen. These interactions are not always predictable, and there is no clear guidance on how to alter dosing or monitoring. The clinician should be aware that higher doses of warfarin may be needed, that more frequent INR monitoring is indicated, and that the dose of warfarin may need to be reduced as postoperative pain abates and less pain medicine is used.

■ To make things even more difficult, many nutritional and over-the-counter supplements may interact with warfarin. Binge alcohol intake decreases the metabolism of warfarin (increases the INR), whereas chronic alcohol use does just the opposite; it increases the metabolism (decreases the INR). Foods that are rich in natural vitamin K are directly antagonistic to warfarin. However, these foods are also generally very healthy (e.g., leafy green vegetables); clinicians need not routinely restrict access to high-vitamin K foods in patients taking warfarin, but the vitamin K intake does need to be consistent. Patients on warfarin should not take vitamin preparations that contain vitamin K. Clinicians will often need to read the labels themselves to ensure that these preparations are vitamin K-free. Some natural supplements are high in vitamin K, such as alfalfa. St. John's wort may decrease the serum level of warfarin, and coenzyme Q may decrease response to warfarin (a pharmacodynamic effect). Other herbal products for patients to avoid while taking warfarin include dong quai, evening primrose, feverfew, garlic, green tea, ginseng, and gingko.

Contraindications

■ Contraindications include any active bleeding or history of recent important bleeding. Cautious use is recommended in patients who are malnourished or in patients with severe hypertension, severe liver disease, or malignancies. Patients who have trouble with compliance for any reason may be poor candidates for this drug, which requires assiduous monitoring.

■ Warfarin is contraindicated in pregnancy.

Conscientious Considerations

■ Errors with warfarin dosing may be life threatening. To avoid confusion, consider prescribing all patients the 5-mg tablet.

■ Do not prescribe a large loading dose of warfarin to patients new to the drug. This does not reliably hasten a therapeutic INR and is more likely to cause bleeding. Generally, prescribe 5 or 10 mg daily to most patients and titrate based on the INR. For malnourished patients (they may be vitamin K depleted) or patients with hepatic disease, CHF, and those at higher risk of bleeding, start with lower doses.

■ Patients at highest risk of warfarin-induced bleeding include older adults, those on higher doses, and those who require higher INR targets, although most serious bleeding occurs in patients with therapeutic INRs (e.g., 2 to 3). When a patient bleeds while taking warfarin, in addition to rescuing the patient from that bleeding episode, consider conducting a workup for the patient for abnormal bleeding sites.

■ Treatment of warfarin toxicity depends on the level of the INR and whether there is associated bleeding. For INRs

TABLE 9-1 Selected Drugs, Foods, and Dietary Supplements that Interact with Warfarin

DRUGS THAT ↑ INR	DRUGS THAT ↑ INR
Anti-infectives: amoxicillin, azithromycin, ciprofloxacin, clarithromycin, cotrimoxazole, erythromycin, fluconazole, isoniazid, itraconazole, levofloxacin, metronidazole, tetracycline	Anti-infectives: dicloxacillin, griseofulvin, nafcillin, ribavirin, rifampin, ritonavir
Cardiovascular: amiodarone, aspirin, diltiazem, fluvastatin, gemfibrozil, metolazone, propafenone, propranolol, simvastatin	Cardiovascular: cholestyramine
CNS: alcohol, citalopram, disulfiram, entacapone, fluvoxamine, phenytoin (in both lists), sertraline	CNS: barbiturates, carbamazepine, chlordiazepoxide, phenytoin (in both lists)
GI: cimetidine, fish foil, grapefruit, mango, omeprazole	GI: avocado, soy milk, sucralfate
Herbals: don quai, fenugreek, PC-SPES	Herbals: ginseng
Others: acetaminophen, anabolic steroids, fluorouracil, gemcitabine, paclitaxel, tamoxifen, tolterodine	Others: antithyroid drugs, azathioprine, influenza vaccine, mercaptopurine, raloxifene

under 5 without bleeding, simply omit one or two doses of warfarin and restart at a lower dose. For INRs between 5 and 10 without bleeding, this strategy of withholding the dose and restarting at a lower dose is also appropriate. Another option is to give 1 to 2.5 mg of oral vitamin K. If the INR is between 10 and 20 without bleeding, stop the warfarin, give 3 to 5 mg of oral vitamin K, and closely monitor the INR. Repeated doses of vitamin K may be necessary.

■ If rapid reversal of warfarin is needed, for example if the INR is greater than 20 or if there is serious bleeding or a deliberate warfarin overdose, stop the warfarin and give 10 to 20 mg of vitamin K by slow intravenous infusion. Doses of vitamin K may need to repeated, depending on the follow-up INR. In life-threatening cases such as intracranial hemorrhage, clinicians may also need to provide immediate anticoagulant proteins, either by fresh frozen plasma or by more specific products such as thrombin complex concentrates. With elevated INRs, be careful not to give too much vitamin K, unless the bleeding is life threatening, because it may take several days for the patient to become responsive to warfarin once again.

■ Before deciding on chronic warfarin in the older adult, consider the risk of bleeding, drug interactions, compliance, cognitive status, living situation, and the risk of falls.

■ Many drugs directly interfere with warfarin absorption or metabolism, and other drugs may directly cause bleeding. Clinicians need to take a drug history for patients taking warfarin to ensure they are avoiding aspirin, clopidogrel, dipyridamole, NSAIDs, ticlopidine, and corticosteroids. However, in some cases, combinations of warfarin with one or more of these drugs may be indicated, causing these patients to need more frequent monitoring of INR and bleeding.

Patient/Family Education

■ Clinicians should instruct patients to immediately report any bleeding and to consider wearing a MedicAlert bracelet indicating that they take an oral anticoagulant.

■ Patients should ask their clinician before starting any new medications, vitamins, herbs, or supplements.

■ Insist that patients receive regular INR monitoring–for chronic stable patients, at least monthly. For initial titration and when patients are unstable or taking potentially interacting drugs, clinicians should check the INR more frequently.

Dabigatran (Pradaxa)

Dabigatran is the first in a new class of direct oral thrombin inhibitors, a class that in some circumstances may replace warfarin. To date, the FDA has approved its use only in the prevention of stroke and systemic embolism in patients with atrial fibrillation, but other uses, including prevention and treatment of venous thromboembolism or in the treatment of acute coronary syndrome, may come in the future. Advantages of dabigatran over warfarin include predictable anticoagulation without routine laboratory monitoring, rapid onset of action (no need to administer heparin or LMWH first), and low food or drug interactions. Its major disadvantages include being more expensive (dabigatran cost about $8 per day in 2011), having no antidote, having limited role in patients with chronic kidney disease, and having unknown long-term safety.

Mechanisms of Action

Dabigatran prevents the development of clots by directly inhibiting the production of thrombin, which is the final step in the clotting cascade. Intravenous forms have been available for several years, but dabigatran is the first oral drug in the class.

Pharmacokinetics

■ Absorption/Distribution: only about 3% to 7% of orally administered drug is absorbed into the systemic circulation, but it is rapidly absorbed, reaching peak serum concentrations within 2 hours.

■ Metabolism/Excretion: Dabigatran's half-life is 12 to 17 hours, allowing for twice daily dosing. The parent drug is a prodrug and is metabolized to its active metabolite in the liver. Elimination is mainly by the kidneys, and dose reduction is necessary in patients with chronic renal disease. The drug is not recommended in patients with severe renal insufficiency.

Dosage and Administration

There are two dosage formulation for dabigatran (Pradaxa) available, 75-mg and 150-mg capsules, which contain specially prepared beads. The capsules must be swallowed whole and cannot be chewed or emptied into liquids or food.

Dosage depends upon the estimated creatinine clearance:

CrCl > 30 mL/min	dabigatran 150 mg PO twice daily
CrCl 15–30 mL/min	dabigatran 75 mg PO twice daily
CrCb < 15 mL/min	Not recommended

There are details to consider when converting to and from other anticoagulants and when surgical procedures are planned. When converting from *warfarin to dabigatran*, the clinician should discontinue the warfarin and start dabigatran when the INR falls below 2. Conversely, when converting from *dabigatran to warfarin*, for patients with a CrCl greater than 50 mL/min, start the warfarin 3 days before stopping dabigatran. For patients with CrCl 31 to 50 mL/min, start the warfarin 2 days before stopping dabigatran, and for patients with CrCl 15 to 30 mL/min, start the warfarin 1 day before stopping dabigatran.

When converting from *heparin or LMWH to dabigatran*, the clinician should start the dabigatran 0 to 2 hours before the next dose of heparin/LMWH is due.

For patients who are to undergo surgical interventions while taking dabigatran, the clinician should discontinue dabigatran 1 to 2 days before surgery (if the CrC is greater than 50 mL/min) or 3 to 5 days before the procedure (if the CrCl is less than 50 mL/min). Dabigatran should be promptly restarted after surgery, as long as bleeding (or a high risk of bleeding) is not present.

Clinical Uses

■ Currently, dabigatran is FDA approved only for the prevention of stroke and systemic embolism in patients with chronic atrial fibrillation. In addition, these patients should not have prosthetic heart valves, hemodynamically significant valvular dysfunction, CrCl less than 15 mL/min, or advanced liver disease. Researchers are investigating other uses, such as prevention and treatment of venous thromboembolism and acute coronary syndrome.

Adverse Reactions

GI: Dyspepsia and abdominal pain.

HEM: Major risk is bleeding, especially serious bleeding into spaces such as the brain, gut, or retroperitoneum. In the seminal clinical trial known as the Randomized Evaluation of Long-Term Anticoagulant TherapY (or RE-LY trial,) in which dabigatran was compared with standard warfarin in patients with chronic nonvalvular atrial fibrillation, major bleeding rates were about the same in the two groups (about 3% to 4% per year). However, compared with warfarin, dabigatran caused fewer intracranial bleedings but more GI bleeds.

Interactions

■ The only drug that must be avoided in patients taking dabigatran is the P-450 inducer rifampin, which would reduce the serum concentration of this drug.

Contraindications

■ The only clear contraindication is the presence of active bleeding, but this would also be true for other anticoagulant drugs

Conscientious Considerations

■ Prescribe the drug only in highly selected patients with chronic non-valvular atrial fibrillation, until more clinical evidence accumulates in other clinical conditions.
■ An initial assessment would include complete blood count (CBC), PTT, and INR, as well as baseline renal functions. No routine coagulation monitoring (such as with INR) is required; the drug causes reliable anticoagulation without monitoring.
■ The clinician should periodically measure the serum creatinine to detect the presence of renal impairment, which would require either dose reduction or discontinuation of the drug.
■ A major disadvantage of dabigatran is its cost, at least $8 per day, compared with pennies per day for warfarin. However, there are no routine coagulation laboratory tests are needed to monitor dabigatran, and clinician visits may not be required as frequently, which would offset costs.
■ If bleeding does occur, there is no specific antidote, unlike for warfarin or heparin. For mild bleeding, simply delay the next dose or discontinue the drug after reassessing risks and benefits. For moderate to severe bleeding, provide general resuscitation and consider oral charcoal and/or hemodialysis. For life-threatening bleeding, experts recommend administering either recombinant factor VIIa or prothrombin complex concentrate, but evidence for these is weak.
■ A major advantage of dabigatran over warfarin is that are no other substantial drug interactions and essentially no food interactions (the patient need not restrict leafy green vegetables).

Patient/Family Education

■ The patient must take the drug faithfully.
■ The capsule must be swallowed whole, not chewed or sprinkled onto any liquid or food.
■ The patient should be taught signs of subtle bleeding, such as darkening of the stool or urine, and of nosebleeds or enhanced mucosal/skin bleeding, and report these promptly to the clinician.
■ No dietary restrictions are necessary, unlike the situation with chronic warfarin.

Antiplatelet Agents

Antiplatelet therapy is indicated in the prevention and treatment of a wide range of cardiovascular diseases. Nearly 800,000 people in the United States suffer a stroke each year, resulting in significant morbidity and mortality, with roughly 90% of all strokes being ischemic in nature, and the remaining 10% resulting from intracerebral hemorrhage or subarachnoid hemorrhage. Stroke, defined as abrupt-onset neurological dysfunction lasting more than 24 hours, is the third leading cause of death and the leading cause of serious, long-term disability in this country (Rosamond & Flegel, 2008). In many patients with acute coronary syndromes and/or after coronary stent deployment, dual antiplatelet therapy (for example, aspirin and clopidogrel) is important. In addition, some of these patients may also have a compelling reason for oral anticoagulation with warfarin, for example, atrial fibrillation or a prosthetic valve replacement. Thus, it is common to see patients prescribed triple antithrombotic therapy—dual antiplatelet therapy plus warfarin (Vande Griende, 2008). Although an individual patient may have indications for all three therapies, the risk of serious bleeding is clearly increased with the triple regimen. Consider carefully whether all three agents are truly needed and whether strategies can be deployed to reduce bleeding risks in patients who require such treatment. Table 9-2 lists the American College of Chest Physicians' recommendations for antiplatelet therapy for the prevention of cardiovascular disease (Sobel & Verhaeghe, 2008).

Aspirin as an Antiplatelet Agent

Platelets are anucleate cells continuously formed by marrow megakaryocytes; they circulate in the blood and have about a 10-day lifespan. Activated platelets produce many prostaglandins, particularly thromboxane A_2 (TXA_2); this chemical induces platelet aggregation and vasoconstriction. On the other hand, the major prostaglandin produced by vascular endothelium is prostacyclin (PGI_2). This chemical does just the opposite; it inhibits platelet aggregation and is a potent vasodilator. Platelets are vital components of hemostasis because they can adhere to injured blood vessels and accumulate at sites of injury. If this process is uncontrolled, it can lead to pathological vascular occlusion, ischemia, and infarction. Available antiplatelet drugs can interfere with a variety of steps in platelet activation, including adhesion, release, and aggregation.

TABLE 9-2 Recommendations of the American College of Chest Physicians for Use of Antiplatelet Drugs in the Prevention of Cardiovascular Disease

CONDITION	RECOMMENDATION
FOR ALL ACUTE CORONARY SYNDROMES	Aspirin 162–325 mg immediately, then 75–100 mg/day indefinitely or clopidogrel, 300 mg immediately, then 75 mg/day if aspirin is not tolerated. Plus clopidogrel 300 mg, then 75 mg/day for a year, whether or not PCI occurs. If no stent, discontinue clopidogrel after 1 year. If stent, consider clopidogrel indefinitely if no bleeding or cost issues
AFTER NONCARDIOEMBOLIC STROKE/TIA	Aspirin 50–100 mg/day, indefinitely or aspirin/dipyridamole extended-release 25/200 two times/day or clopidogrel 75 mg/day (the latter two may be slightly more effective). Avoid combining aspirin and clopidogrel in these patients.
PATIENTS WITH PAD, OR AFTER CABG OR CAROTID ENDARTERECTOMY	Aspirin 75–100 mg/day indefinitely (or clopidogrel 75 mg/day if aspirin is not tolerated)
PRIMARY PREVENTION (TREATMENT OF MULTIPLE RISK FACTORS, NO ESTABLISHED DISEASE)	Consider aspirin 75–100 mg/day if 10-year risk of cardiac events >10%. Do not use clopidogrel unless there is an allergy to aspirin AND moderate to high risk of cardiovascular disease.

Source: American College of Chest Physicians.

Mechanism of Action

Aspirin is a potent irreversible inhibitor of cyclooxygenase (COX-1), the rate-limiting enzyme in the production of prostaglandins. A single dose of aspirin efficiently eliminates TXA_2 production by the platelet, and because this cell has no nucleus, it cannot produce more enzyme. However, the vascular endothelium can regenerate prostacyclin (PGI_2) through transcription and then translation of more protein. Therefore, low-dose aspirin may tip the balance of (thromboxane) TXA_2, a powerful yet unstable vasoconstrictor and inducer of platelet aggregation and PGI_2 (prostacyclin) which is also unstable but is a powerful vasoconstrictor and i8nhibitor of platelet aggregation. Thus these two agents are opposite poles of a homeostatic equation that regulates platelet aggregation *in vivo*.

Pharmacokinetics

■ Absorption: Aspirin is rapidly absorbed in the stomach and upper bowel; peak plasma concentrations are reached within 30 to 40 minutes, and platelet inhibition is detectable by 1 hour. By contrast, enteric-coated aspirin products take up to 3 to 4 hours to reach peak plasma levels. Therefore, if an acute effect is needed, such as in acute coronary syndrome, plain aspirin should be used (it should be chewed), not enteric-coated preparations. The bioavailability of the plain product is between 50% and 75% whereas the bioavailability of enteric-coated products is much less.
■ Distribution: Although the plasma level rapidly declines after a single oral dose of aspirin, platelet cyclooxygenase remains irreversibly acetylated. The optimal dose of aspirin seems to be 50 to 100 mg/day, perhaps as low as 30 mg/day, when used for chronic conditions such as the prevention of myocardial infarction or stroke. On the other hand, for

acute conditions such as acute coronary syndrome or acute ischemic stroke, a higher initial dose (160 to 325 mg) is indicated to cause quick and complete platelet inhibition. For chronic use, there is no reason to exceed 81 mg as the daily dose. Higher doses are not more effective, but they do place the patient at a higher risk for bleeding.

■ Metabolism: Aspirin is hydrolyzed to its active metabolite, salicylate, by esterases in GI mucosa, red blood cells, synovial fluid, and blood. Metabolism of the salicylate occurs by hepatic conjugation.
■ Excretion: 75% is excreted as salicyluric acid in the urine, with 10% as salicylic acid.
■ Half-life: 2 to 3 hours for low doses, up to 15 to 30 hours with large doses because of saturation of the hepatic metabolism.

Dosage and Administration

See Table 9-2. A full-dose of 325 mg of aspirin is only indicated in the acute treatment of myocardial infarction and perhaps in stroke. For virtually all other indications, prescribe 81 mg daily.

Clinical Uses

■ Aspirin has been shown in to be highly effective in reducing vascular endpoints in a wide range of clinical conditions. The endpoint reduction is generally about 25%. Chronic conditions for which there is unequivocal evidence for a benefit in aspirin include patients with previous myocardial infarction, stable coronary artery disease, carotid stenosis, prior TIA or stroke, and peripheral arterial disease.
■ Patients who have undergone coronary artery bypass grafting or carotid endarterectomy are also excellent candidates for aspirin treatment.
■ It is unclear whether aspirin will benefit patients at intermediate or low risk of vascular disease. In healthy middle-aged

men and women with cardiovascular risk factors but no history of heart disease or stroke, aspirin may reduce the risk of nonfatal myocardial infarction, but it does not reduce cardiovascular or total mortality rates. These benefits are weighed against an increase in bleeding events, including a small increase in the risk of hemorrhagic stroke. For healthy patients without cardiovascular risk factors, aspirin prophylaxis does more harm than good.

Adverse Reactions

GI: The major risk of low-dose aspirin is gastrointestinal toxicity, particularly ulcer bleeding, gastric perforation, and gastric outlet obstruction. The risk of GI bleeding is dose-related, with the risk of major GI bleeding with doses of 75 to 100 mg daily about one to two episodes per 1,000 patient-years. This GI risk does not depend on the baseline cardiovascular risk of the patient. There is no clear evidence that prescribing enteric-coated or buffered aspirin will reduce this GI complication rate. Coadministration of aspirin with a proton pump inhibitor may reduce GI complications by 50%.

HEM: There is also a small increase in the risk of very serious bleeding, such as intracranial hemorrhage, but with low-dose aspirin, this risk is very low, less than 1/1,000 patient-years.

PUL: A minority may experience bronchospasm or other hypersensitivity.

Interactions

■ Use of aspirin with a traditional NSAID not only increases the risk of GI toxicity, but also may negate aspirin's cardioprotective effect.

Contraindications

■ There is a contraindication for aspirin use in patients with previous GI bleeding, but some of these patients also have a compelling vascular indication for aspirin. How should a clinician manage a patient with cardiovascular disease who has ulcer bleeding when taking low-dose aspirin? A common strategy, after taking care of the bleeding and healing the ulcer, was to convert the patient to clopidogrel. But two independent, randomized controlled trials now suggest this is not a good choice. In these studies, a combination of daily esomeprazole, 20 mg, and low-dose aspirin, 75 mg, caused markedly less recurrent bleeding than did daily clopidogrel (Siemens et al., 2009).

■ Patients who are allergic to aspirin can consider cardiovascular prophylaxis with clopidogrel.

Conscientious Considerations

■ Aspirin is probably the most underused drug in medicine. One way to consider the benefit-risk ratio for an individual patient is to realize that aspirin reduces cardiovascular events about 25% (the risk reduction may be as high as 50% in patients with unstable coronary syndromes). If the baseline risk of cardiovascular events is low, for example at 1 to 2/1,000 patient-years, as in a patient with isolated hypertension or isolated hyperlipidemia but no known heart disease, then a 25% reduction reduces the cardiovascular risk by 0.25 to 0.5/1,000 patient-years. As a rate of GI bleeding of 1 to 2/1,000 patient-years can be expected, this patient probably has more risk than benefit from aspirin prophylaxis.

■ Now consider patients at higher risk of cardiovascular events. Patients with stable angina have cardiovascular events about 10/1,000 patient-years, those with prior MI about 30/1,000 patient-years. The 25% reduction in cardiovascular events is now clearly more than the 1 to 2/1,000 risk of major GI bleeding. Long-term aspirin prophylaxis benefits patients with angina, prior MI, unstable angina, and prior TIA/stroke.

■ Rarely, children are prescribed aspirin for rheumatic diseases. In general, avoid using aspirin in infants and children because this drug has been strongly linked to the development of Reye's syndrome.

■ There is a condition called *aspirin resistance* in which some patients do not have the expected inhibition of platelet aggregation with standard doses of aspirin. There is no way to test for this at present and no clinical recommendations on dealing with this. Also, just because a patient has a vascular event while taking aspirin does not mean that he or she is aspirin resistant: Atherothrombotic events are multifactorial. At present, if a patient has a vascular event while on aspirin, there is no clear rationale to simply increase the dose of the aspirin.

Patient/Family Education

■ Advise patients to take aspirin with a full glass of water.

■ Advise patients that more than three glasses of alcohol per day may increase the risk of GI bleeding.

■ Teach patients to monitor for side effects such as tinnitus, unusual bleeding of gums, black/tarry stools, bruising, or fever lasting more than 3 days.

■ Patients on a sodium-restricted diet should avoid effervescent tablets or buffered aspirin.

■ Patients undergoing surgery should not miss a single dose of aspirin unless the surgery is intracranial, posterior eye chamber, cardiac, or associated with heavy bleeding. This is a new recommendation. Physicians previously recommended aspirin be routinely held for 1 week prior to surgery: This is now rarely recommended.

■ Remind patients that if they are taking aspirin (81 mg) to avoid transient ischemic attacks (TIA) or MI, then increasing the dose will not provide additional protection.

■ Caution patients against taking acetaminophen or NSAIDs at the same time.

■ Remind patients they should buy aspirin in smaller packages. If the tablets emit an odor of vinegar, it is a sign of deterioration.

Clopidogrel (Plavix)

Clopidogrel (Plavix) is the first in a new class of drugs that inhibit platelet action in a manner different from aspirin. It can reduce vascular events such as myocardial infarction, stroke, and vascular death, particularly in patients who have undergone coronary angioplasty with stents. Clopidogrel has replaced ticlopidine, because it has greater effects on thrombosis and because it is safer, causing less neutropenia. This drug dramatically reduces the risk of stent thrombosis, and it has rapidly become standard of care in many settings.

Mechanism of Action

Clopidogrel is a thienopyridine that blocks platelet activation by selectively and irreversibly blocking the binding of adenosine diphosphate (ADP) to the platelet. This prevents ADP-dependent activation of the GpIIb-IIIa complex, which is the major platelet surface receptor for fibrinogen.

Pharmacokinetics

- Absorption: The drug is well absorbed after oral administration and is quickly metabolized in the liver to its active metabolite. Some patients do not metabolize the drug well and therefore receive less benefit; there is no widely available way to detect this as yet in clinical practice. Platelet inhibition is detectable 2 hours after a loading dose, or during the second day of routine oral use, although peak platelet effect may take up to a week.
- Distribution: Unknown.
- Metabolism: Rapidly converted in the liver to its active metabolite.
- Excretion: 50% in urine, 45% in feces.
- Half-Life: Active metabolite 8 hours.

Dosage and Administration

Generic Name	Trade Name	Availability	Dosage For AcuteCoronary Syndrome (Acs)*	Long-Term Use
clopidogrel	Plavix	75-mg, 300-mg tabs	Loading dose of 300 mg, followed with 75 mg/day	75 mg/day

*Some clinicians use a higher loading dose of 600 mg, but not in older patients. No adjustment is necessary for renal impairment, but the dose may need to be reduced in patients with severe liver disease.

Clinical Uses

- Clopidogrel, along with aspirin, should be routinely used in the management of acute coronary syndrome, including unstable angina pectoris and acute myocardial infarction, as well as in patients undergoing acute coronary angioplasty with either bare metal or drug-eluting stents, unless there is a clear contraindication. After a year has passed since the ACS or angioplasty, should the clopidogrel be continued? The benefit after this time is less, whereas the risk of bleeding continues. Most experts recommend that aspirin plus clopidogrel should be continued indefinitely in patients with coronary stents if the drug is well tolerated, it is affordable to the patient, and the patient is not at high risk of bleeding. If the ACS was treated without coronary stenting, it is reasonable to discontinue clopidogrel after 1 year, and continuing aspirin indefinitely.

- A second, larger group of patients include those with vascular disease who have not yet had a myocardial infarction or a coronary stent. These patients include those with stable coronary artery disease, prior TIA or stroke, or peripheral arterial disease. In these patients, randomized trials suggest that aspirin alone is sufficient and that the combination of aspirin and clopidogrel should generally be avoided, because there is no additional benefit, but a definite increase in bleeding. If the patient with vascular disease is allergic to aspirin, then clopidogrel alone is a reasonable choice.
- There is an even larger group of patients who have no established vascular disease but who have cardiovascular risk factors such as hypertension, cigarette smoking, hyperlipidemia, or a strong family history of vascular disease. There is evidence to suggest that these patients should take aspirin alone; these patients should not take the combination of aspirin and clopidogrel. If patients with CV risk factors but without established disease are allergic to aspirin, then clopidogrel alone is an appropriate choice.

Adverse Reactions

CV: Chest pain, edema, hypertension

DERM: Pruritus, purpurea, rash

HEM: The major serious complication of clopidogrel, like all drugs that affect hemostasis, is bleeding. Risk depends not only on the drug, but also on other medical conditions, the use of other medications, and probably advanced age. Very rarely, clopidogrel can cause thrombotic thrombocytopenic purpura (TTP).

GI: Abdominal pain, nausea, vomiting, and constipation.

NEURO: Headache, dizziness, depression, fatigue, and generalized pain.

Interactions

- Clopidogrel is a minor substrate of CYP1A2 and CYP3A4, and it weakly inhibits CYP2A8/9. Atorvastatin, clarithromycin, and erythromycin may decrease the effectiveness of clopidogrel, whereas rifampin has the opposite effect. Use of clopidogrel with other platelet-active drugs such as aspirin, as well as with drugs such as warfarin, heparin, or thrombolytics, may increase the risk of bleeding.
- There is recent concern that proton pump inhibitors may interfere with the antiplatelet effects of clopidogrel, particularly in patients with certain genetic polymorphisms for the cytochrome P450 enzyme CYP2C19. This combination should be avoided until more information is available.

Contraindications

- Do not use clopidogrel with patients with active bleeding, such as gastrointestinal or intracranial hemorrhage, or in those with coagulopathies.
- Use caution in patients who have had prior episodes of bleeding.

Conscientious Considerations

■ Clopidogrel has a clear but limited use in cardiovascular disease, the most compelling indications of which are in patients with acute coronary syndrome and those with coronary angioplasty. All of these patients should take low-dose aspirin and clopidogrel 75 mg/day for at least a year. After 1 year, if there was a stent and the patient has no bleeding or cost issues, consider continuing both. After 1 year, if there was no stent, discontinue the clopidogrel.

■ Clopidogrel can also be used after noncardioembolic stroke/TIA to prevent another episode. Choices in this setting are aspirin alone, clopidogrel alone, or the combination of aspirin and extended-release dipyridamole. Do not combine aspirin and clopidogrel in these patients. Efficacy doesn't increase, there is just more bleeding (Connolly, Pogue, & Hart, 2009).

■ For patients with stable coronary artery disease, peripheral arterial disease, or patients who have had either coronary artery bypass graft (CABG) or carotid endarterectomy, prescribe low-dose aspirin alone. If aspirin is not tolerated, then clopidogrel alone at 75 mg/day is reasonable.

■ Do not prescribe clopidogrel for the primary prevention of cardiovascular disease unless both of these conditions occur in your patient: allergy to aspirin and moderate to high risk of cardiovascular disease.

Patient/Family Education

■ Discontinue this drug 7 days before planned elective surgery.
■ Patients should immediately report any bruising or bleeding to their clinician
■ Do not use other medications without the approval of a clinician.

Prasugrel (Effient)

Prasugrel (Effient), approved in 2009 by the FDA, is the second thienopyridine approved as an antiplatelet drug. The major clinical trial that led to its FDA approval was the Triton-Timi 38 study, which demonstrated the higher inhibition of platelet activity by prasugrel resulted in a significant reduction in the combined endpoint of cardiovascular death, MI, and stroke. A significant reduction in stent thrombosis, urgent target vessel revascularization, and myocardial infarction was also observed. However, this benefit was offset by a significant increase in serious bleeding complications. Thus, the drug appears to have both greater efficacy and more side effects, but until this issue is more clearly resolved, prasugrel should probably not be routinely used (Pride et al., 2010), then only to prevent blood clots in patients undergoing angioplasty.

Mechanism of Action

Prasugrel itself is a prodrug in that it undergoes metabolic activation by intestinal esterases and then through the liver's CYPA34 and CYPA2B6 systems. This active metabolite then binds to the ADP receptor on the platelet surface, which leads to an irreversible inhibition of platelet activity for the 7- to 10-day life of that cell.

Pharmacokinetics

■ Absorption: It is rapidly absorbed within 30 minutes of oral administration.
■ Distribution: Plasma proteins.
■ Metabolism: Hepatic cytochrome P450 isoenzymes (CYP3A4, CYP2C9, CYP2C19, CYP2B6).
■ Excretion: Mostly in urine, some in feces.
■ Half-Life: 7 hours. Onset of antiplatelet activity is 30 minutes, and steady state is reached in 3 days.

Dosage and Administration

Prasugrel is available in 5- and 10-mg tablets. The loading dose for acute coronary syndromes or coronary angioplasty is 60 mg, and the maintenance dose is 10 mg per day. For patients who weigh less than 60 kg, the maintenance dose should be reduced to 5 mg daily. There is no dose adjustment for patients with mild to moderate liver or renal dysfunction, but there is not yet enough information about patients with severe liver or renal disease.

Patients taking long-term prasugrel should also take a daily low dose of aspirin: 81 mg would be appropriate. There are currently no long-term indications for prasugrel alone.

Clinical Uses

■ Indicated for patients with an acute coronary syndrome who are undergoing primary coronary interventions (angioplasty and stent).

Adverse Reactions

ITEM: Bleeding is the most important adverse effect; it is more common in patients over the age of 75 years. Because of this effect, most experts would advise against the use of this drug in the very elderly (Medline Plus, 2009).

Interactions

■ Coadministration of prasugrel with NSAIDs or other antiplatelet or anticoagulant drugs will increase the risk of bleeding.
■ To date, there does not seem to be an interaction with the CYP3A4 inhibitor ketoconazole or the CYP3A4 inducer rifampin.
■ And unlike clopidogrel, there does not appear to be an interaction with proton pump inhibitors.

Contraindications

■ Avoid this drug in the elderly, particularly those over age 75 years or under 60 kg in weight.
■ Do not use this drug in patients who have a history of bleeding or in patients with a history of stroke or TIA.

Conscientious Considerations

■ Discontinue this drug at least 7 days before any planned elective surgery.
■ Do not use this drug in patients who are likely to need urgent CABG surgery.

Patient/Family Education

■ The same instructions as those listed for clopidogrel should be given.

Dipyridamole (Persantine)

Dipyridamole (Persantine) is an antiplatelet agent with limited use in the prevention of cardiovascular disease. It is prescribed in a fixed combination with aspirin for specific patient populations. The drug is further used in an intravenous formulation to dilate the coronary arteries during noninvasive testing for atherosclerotic coronary artery disease (stress testing).

Mechanism of Action

The mechanism of this drug is not entirely clear, but it inhibits platelet adenosine deaminase and phosphodiesterase, which causes an accumulation of adenosine, adenine nucleotides, and cyclic AMP. These mediators in turn inhibit platelet aggregation by their effect on phosphodiesterases, which in turn cause vasodilation of normal coronary arteries, and by reducing flow to vessels that are narrowed.

Pharmacokinetics

■ Absorption: With oral dosing, dipyridamole is moderately (30% to 60%) absorbed.
■ Distribution: Widely distributed, crossing placenta and breast milk.
■ Metabolized: By the liver into a glucuronide conjugate.
■ Excretion: By the bile into feces.
■ Half-life: 10 to 12 hours

Dosage and Administration

For oral use, the only recommended product is a fixed combination with aspirin (a tablet that contains 50 mg of aspirin and 200 mg of extended-release dipyridamole, marketed as Aggrenox), and this tablet is dosed twice daily for prevention of vascular events. Although generic dipyridamole is available, experts recommend against creating a cheaper version of Aggrenox by combining aspirin with generic dipyridamole because it is possible that clinical effectiveness depends on the extended-release formulation.

For intravenous use, cardiologists use 0.14 mg/kg/min for 4 minutes to cause maximal coronary vasodilation (maximum dose 60 mg); this should only be used in cardiac stress-testing facilities that are accustomed to its use.

Clinical Use

■ The most common use of dipyridamole is to prevent stroke. The PRoFESS trial compared clopidogrel (Plavix) with the combination of aspirin and extended-release dipyridamole (Aggrenox) in patients with a recent ischemic stroke. The primary outcome, recurrent stroke, was equivalent in the two groups, but moderate bleeding was marginally more common in the Aggrenox group. Clopidogrel may be preferable in situations or patients with recent ischemic stroke because it causes less bleeding, is slightly less expensive, and is equally as effective as dipyridamole. However, dipyridamole remains useful as a brief intravenous infusion to cause maximal coronary vasodilation in cardiac stress testing for patients who are unable to exercise because the vasodilation causes a reflex tachycardia and thus simulates exercise.

Adverse Reactions

CV: When given IV only, hypotension, flushing, arrhythmia
DERM: Rash
GI: Nausea, vomiting, diarrhea
NEURO: Dizziness, headache, rash, and abdominal distress
PUL: When given IV only, bronchospasm

Interactions

■ Dipyridamole will increase serum levels of the drug adenosine. It may also counteract the effects of cholinesterase inhibitors and worsen myasthenia gravis. Furthermore, xanthines (e.g., caffeine, theophylline) reduced the effect of dipyridamole: Patients on theophylline should not take that drug for 2 days prior to cardiac stress testing.
■ Avoid this drug if the patient is taking other platelet active agents such as clopidogrel or herbs such as dong quai, garlic, ginger, gingko, ginseng, or green tea.

Contraindications

■ The drug should be used cautiously or not at all in patients with bronchospasm, either asthma or chronic obstructive lung disease.

Conscientious Considerations

■ In primary care, the only common use of dipyridamole (as Aggrenox) is to prevent recurrent stroke, and in this group of patients, aspirin alone or clopidogrel alone is usually as effective and safer.
■ For patients with established coronary artery disease or peripheral arterial disease, aspirin alone is clearly preferable to Aggrenox.
■ For patients who do not have established cardiovascular disease but do have risk factors such as hypertension, hyperlipidemia, cigarette smoking, or a family history of vascular disease, do not prescribe Aggrenox. Rather, prescribe aspirin alone, based on the risk of subsequent vascular events.

Fibrinolytic (Thrombolytic) Agents

Drugs that lyse blood clots are called fibrinolytic or thrombolytic drugs. Alteplase (Activase, Cathflo Activase), reteplase (Retavase), and tenecteplase (TNKase) are examples of fibrinolytic drugs. Streptokinase was the first fibrinolytic approved for use in the United States, but it is no longer marketed here.

Mechanism of Action

Alteplase, reteplase, and tenecteplase are all modified forms of tissue plasminogen activator (tPA), produced by recombinant DNA technology. When given intravenously, tPAs bind to fibrin and convert plasminogen to plasmin. Locally, this causes local fibrinolysis, dissolving clots, such as the culprit in acute myocardial infarction. About 80% of patients with acute myocardial infarction have thrombus in the infarct-related coronary artery.

Pharmacokinetics

- Absorption: All three drugs are used only intravenously.
- Distribution: The initial volume of distribution approximates plasma volume.
- Metabolism/Excretion: Alteplase and tenecteplase are mainly metabolized by the liver, whereas reteplase has both liver and renal excretion.
- Half-Life: All three drugs have short half-lives, from 20 to 60 minutes.

Dosage and Administration

Generic Name	Trade Name	Availability	Typical Adult Dose For Myocardial Infarction (Mi)*	Typical Adult Dose For An Occluded Device	Typical Adult Dose For Pulmonary Embolism
alteplase*	Activase, Cathflo	2 mg/vial, 20 mg/vial, or 50 mg/vial powder for injection. Use depends on indication	If >65 kg, 6–10 mg as bolus in first 1–2 min, then 60 mg over first hr, 20 mg over second hr, then 20 mg over third hr	2 mg/2 mL instilled in occluded catheter. If unsuccessful, repeat once after 2 hr	100 mg over 2 hr. Follow with heparin
reteplase	Retavase	10.8 units/vial	n/a	10 units STAT bolus followed 30 min later by additional 10 units	n/a
tenecteplase†	TNKase	50 mg/vial with 10-mL syringe	IV for > 65 kg Give 30 mg	n/a	440 IU/kg loading dose, followed by 4,400 IU/kg/hr for 12 hr

*Alteplase can be given by two different methods to patients with acute myocardial infarction, an accelerated infusion or a 3-hour infusion. In the accelerated method, give an initial 15 mg intravenous bolus, followed by 0.75 mg/kg (maximum 50 mg) over 30 minutes, followed by 0.5 mg/kg (maximum 35 mg) over 60 minutes. In the 3-hour infusions, a total of 100 mg is given, 60 mg in the first hour (of which 6 to 10 mg is usually given as an initial bolus), and 40 mg in the second and third hours.

†Tenecteplase is dosed by weight. Give 30 mg IV for weights under 60 kg, 35 mg for weights 60 to 69.9 kg, 40 mg for weights 70 to 79.9 kg, 45 mg for weights 80 to 89.9 kg, and 50 kg for patients weighing 90 kg or more. It comes as a 50-mg vial, which is reconstituted with sterile water.

Clinical Uses

- All three drugs are indicated for the treatment of ST-segment elevation myocardial infarction (STEMI).
- Alteplase is indicated for acute massive pulmonary embolism to either relieve obstruction of blood flow to multiple lobes or to help with hemodynamic instability.
- Alteplase is indicated for the treatment of acute ischemic stroke, but it should be used only within 3 hours of initial symptoms and after exclusion of intracranial hemorrhage.

- Alteplase is used in a special reduced dose to open clotted central venous access devices.

Adverse Reactions

CV: Reperfusion arrhythmias (sinus bradycardia, accelerated idioventricular rhythm, PVCs, or ventricular tachycardia hypotension).
DERM: Flushing, urticaria, ecchymoses.
GI: GI bleed, retroperitoneal bleeding.
GU: GU tract bleeding.
HEM: Serious bleeding is the most common and dreaded complication of fibrinolysis, especially intracranial hemorrhage (ICH), which is fatal in up to two thirds of cases; the risk is probably higher in patients with prior cerebrovascular disease. Major bleeding occurs in about 1.1% of patients receiving fibrinolysis, and this translates to an excess of seven major bleeds for every 1,000 treated patients. Risk factors for major bleeding include advanced age, low body weight, and female gender. It is possible that the more fibrin-specific agent tenecteplase may cause less major bleeding.
MISC: Cholesterol embolization, which is mainly seen in patients who undergo invasive vascular procedures.

Interactions

- There are no specific drug interactions, but patients also taking anticoagulants (heparin, LMWH, warfarin) or antiplatelet drugs are more likely to have bleeding.

Contraindications

- There is a long list of contraindications and cautions for using fibrinolytic drugs in the setting of STEMI. Emergency departments generally place these contraindications on a checklist as part of a comprehensive order set for these patients (Box 9-1).

Conscientious Considerations

- All patients with STEMI (without contraindications) who see a clinician within 12 hours of onset of symptoms should undergo reperfusion therapy promptly. This recommendation is based on dozens of randomized controlled trials with a total of over 150,000 randomized patients. The reperfusion strategy should be either primary percutaneous coronary intervention (PCI) or fibrinolysis. In a meta-analysis of fibrinolysis vs. controls, there were 18 fewer deaths for every 1,000 patients treated, with the highest benefit seen in among patients at highest risk of death.
- In some settings, administration of fibrinolytic therapy can occur before hospitalization, administered by qualified emergency medical technicians who have sent an electrocardiogram and clinical information to a supervising physician in a hospital emergency department.
- Choices of fibrinolytic therapy include alteplase, reteplase, or tenecteplase. The original fibrinolytic drug, streptokinase, is longer marketed in the United States.

BOX 9-1 **Checklist of Contraindications When Using Fibrinolytic Drugs in Patients with STEMI**

__Any prior intracranial hemorrhage

__Known structural cerebrovascular lesion, e.g., arteriovenous malformation

__Known malignant intracranial neoplasm, primary or metastatic

__Ischemic stroke within 3 months (not including ischemic stroke within the last 3 hours)

__Suspected aortic dissection

__Active bleeding or bleeding diathesis (not including menses)

__Significant closed head or facial trauma within 3 months

__History of chronic, severe, poorly controlled hypertension

__Severe uncontrolled hypertension on presentation (systolic BP greater than 180 mm Hg or diastolic BP greater than 110 mm Hg

__Traumatic or prolonged (greater than 10 minutes) CPR

__Major surgery within 3 weeks

__Recent (less than or equal to 2 to 4 weeks) internal bleeding

__Pregnancy

__Active peptic ulcer

__Noncompressible vascular punctures

__Current use of warfarin: the higher the INR, the higher the risk of bleeding

FDA PREGNANCY RISK FACTOR CATEGORY	DRUGS
A	oral iron supplementation (ferrous sulfate, fumarate gluconate carbonyl iron, dextran polysaccharide complex, iron sucrose sodium ferric gluconate) folic acid (Folvite, Folate)
B	vitamin B_{12} (Cyanocobalamin) low molecular weight heparins (danaparoid, enoxaparin, dalteparin, fondaparinux, tinzaparin) clopidogrel (Plavix), prasugrel (Effient), dipyridamole (Persantine)
C	erythropoietin (Epoetin alfa, Darbepoetin) heparin dabigatran (Pradaxa) Aspirin fibrinolytic agents: alteplase, reteplase, tenecteplase
X	warfarin (Coumadin)
Unclassified	

Patient/Family Education

■ It is unclear whether there is a survival benefit for patients over age 75 with STEMI who are treated with fibrinolysis. If there is a benefit, it is much smaller than for younger adults. It is also unclear whether fibrinolysis is helpful in patients with EKGs that are normal, show nonspecific findings, or are ST-segment depression only.

■ The cost of one course of fibrinolytic therapy is about $2,500 to $3,000.

Implications for Special Populations

Pregnancy Implications

When prescribing drugs for the pregnant female, clinicians should carefully consider their choice of drugs. Below is a selected list of drugs along with the assigned FDA Safety Category. Please note that most of these topically applied agents have not had adequate animal studies done to indicate use during human pregnancy.

Pediatric Implications

Accidental overdosing of iron-containing products is one of the leading causes of fatal accidental poisoning among children; thus, there is a burden on clinicians to warn parents of this danger.

Safety and efficacy of folic acid use in pediatrics has not been established by the FDA, but pernicious anemia should always be ruled out before using folic acid in children because the folic acid can hide symptoms of this anemia.

Clopidogrel has been used for decades in pediatrics to prevent thrombosis in children with cardiac diseases that predispose them to clot formation. However, it was not until 2010 that the FDA issued a black box warning calling attention to studies that showed a reduced efficacy of this drug when used in pediatric cases and when the patient is a poor metabolizer.

Fibrinolytics such as alteplase (Activase) are indicated in adult and pediatric patients for the restoration of function to central venous access devices that have become occluded due to a blood clot.

Geriatric Implications

Studies have not been done on adults over age 65 to determine if they respond to iron products and folic acid differently from younger cohorts. When using these products, it is prudent to lower starting doses to reflect the greater incidence of reduced renal, hepatic, and cardiac function as well as the prevalence of concomitant disease(s) in the older adult. The American College of Chest Physicians recommends that patients over the age of 75 should not take this drug for more than 28 days at a dose of 75 mg per day.

Anticoagulants are one of the most common medications implicated in preventable adverse drug reactions (ADRs) in the geriatric population. These drug interactions may be of a pharmacokinetic nature, resulting in changes in serum concentrations, or they may be of a pharmacodynamic nature, resulting in changes in homeostasis or platelet function. Thus, clinicians must have a strong working knowledge of anticoagulant drug interactions, especially the risk factors for bleeding that increase with age.

LEARNING EXERCISES

Case 1

In a family medicine clinic, you see an 80-kg 70-year-old man who has noticed acute swelling of his left leg over the 3 days since he was discharged from the hospital. He had been hospitalized for 10 days for reversal of a colostomy, which was complicated by an intra-abdominal abscess that responded to percutaneous drainage and intravenous antibiotics. His wound is well healed. You suspect deep venous thrombosis. He has no symptoms to suggest pulmonary embolism (dyspnea, chest pain), and he is anxious not to return to the hospital if at all possible. You order a duplex venous ultrasound scan of the legs for the following morning.

1. Write orders for his anticoagulation.

2. How long should he be treated with oral warfarin?

Case 2

You admit an otherwise healthy 58-year-old man to the hospital with fever, cough, dyspnea, and weakness. He is dehydrated and has purulent sputum. His temperature is 38.2°C, respiration 24/min, blood pressure 136/88 mm Hg. You find crackles in the left upper lung field, and chest x-ray confirms a left upper lobe consolidation consistent with pneumonia.

1. In addition to treating the infection, should you prescribe a regimen to prevent venous thromboembolism?

2. What would you do if he had evidence of GI bleeding or was at high risk of intracranial hemorrhage?

References

Centers for Disease Control and Prevention (CDC). (1998). Recommendations to prevent and control iron deficiency in the United States. *MMWR, 47*(RR-3), 1-36.

Connolly, S. J., Pogue J., Hart, R. G., Hohnloser S. H., Pfeiffer M., et al. (2009). The effect of clopidogrel added to aspirin in patients with atrial fibrillation. *New England Journal of Medicine, 360,* 2066-2078. Accessed January 21, 2013, http://columbiamedicine. org/education/r/Cardiology/Arrhythmia/A-Fib/Active-A.pdf

Institute of Medicine (IOM). National Academy of Sciences. (1998). *Dietary reference intakes for thiamin, riboflavin, niacin, vitamin B₆, folate, vitamin B₁₂, pantothenic acid, biotin, and choline.* Washington DC: National Academy Press.

Medline Plus. U.S. National Library of Medicine, National Institutes of Health. (2009). Prasurgel. Retrieved January 20, 2012, from www.nlm.nih.gov/medlineplus/druginfo/meds/a609027.html

National Kidney Foundation (NKF). (2007). *KDOQI clinical practice guidelines and clinical practice recommendations for anemia in chronic kidney disease: 2007.* Retrieved January 20, 2012, from www.kidney. org/professionals/kdoqi/guidelines_anemia/cpr21.htm

Pride, Y. B., Tung, P., Mohanavelu, S., Zorkun, C., Wivilott, D., Antman, E. M., et al. (2010). Angiographic and clinical outcomes among patients with acute coronary syndromes presenting with isolated anterior ST-segment depression: A TRITON-TIMI 38 (Trial to Assess Improvement in Therapeutic Outcomes by Optimizing Platelet Inhibition With Prasugrel-Thrombolysis in Myocardial Infarction 38) substudy. *JACC Cardiovascular Interventions, 3*(8), 806-811.

Rosamond, W., Flegal, K., Furie, K., Go, A., Greenlund, K., Haase, N., et al. (2008). Heart disease and stroke statistics—2008 update: a report from the American Heart Association statistics committee and stroke statistics subcommittee. *Circulation, 117*(4), e25-146.

Rubboli, A., Kovacic, J. C., Mehran, R., Lip, G. H. Y. (2011). Coronary stent implantation in patients committed to long-term oral anticoagulation therapy: Successfully navigating the treatment options. *Chest, 139*(5), 981-987; doi:10.1378/chest.10-2719.

Sobel M., Verhaeghe, R. (2008, June). *Antithrombotic therapy for peripheral artery occlusive disease: American College of Chest Physicians evidence-based clinical practice guidelines* (8th edition). *Chest, 133*(6 Suppl), 815S-843S. Available from Pub Med, retrieved January 22, 2013, from www.ncbi.nlm.nih.gov/pubmed/18574279

U.S. Dept. of Health and Human Services Office on Women's Health. (2010). Womenshealth.gov. *Folic acid fact sheet.* Retrieved January 20, 2012, from www.womenshealth.gov/publications/our-publications/fact-sheet/folic-acid.cfm

Vande Griende, J. P. (2008). Combination antiplatelet agents for secondary prevention of ischemic stroke. *Pharmacotherapy, 28*(10), 1233-1243.

World Health Organization. (2008). *Worldwide prevalence of anaemia 1993–2005. WHO global database on anaemis.* Geneva: World Health Organization. Retrieved June 25, 2011, from http://whqlibdoc.who.int/publications/2008/9789241596657_eng.pdf

chapter 10

Drugs Used in the Treatment of Pulmonary Diseases and Disorders

William N. Tindall, John M. Boltri, Mona M. Sedrak

Key Terms

Adrenomimetic

Allergic rhinitis

Asthma

Beta-2 receptor agonist

Bronchospasm

Chronic obstructive pulmonary disease (COPD)

Hyperresponsiveness

Leukotriene receptor antagonists (LTRA)

Mast Cell Stabilizers

Metered dose inhaler (MDI)

Sodium Cromoglycates

Sympathomimetic

Xanthines

CHAPTER FOCUS

This chapter focuses on drugs used to treat asthma and how they work on bronchial smooth muscle to reduce bronchospasms. This chapter also introduces the learner to some characteristics of how the lungs handle drugs. The chapter introduces inhaled corticosteroids (ICS) and leukotriene receptor agents, which act to reduce inflammation in patients with asthma. Beta-2 receptor agonists, xanthine derivatives, and anticholinergics used to treat asthma and COPD are also discussed. Inhaled anti-inflammatory agents, such as **cromoglycates, leukotriene receptor agonists (LTRA), lipoxygenase inhibitors, and monoclonal antibodies** are introduced as agents to treat chronic obstructive pulmonary disease (COPD). Finally this chapter presents antihistamine and antitussive agents for treatment of allergic and seasonal rhinitis.

OBJECTIVES

After reading and studying this chapter, the student should be able to:

1. Describe and discuss the drugs used in the treatment of pulmonary disorders.
2. Discuss the stepwise approach in classifying and treating patients with asthma.
3. Described the use of steroids, inhaled and systemic, for pulmonary disorders.
4. Describe and discuss the drugs used in the treatment of COPD.
5. Understand the use of antihistamines, antitussives, and intranasal agents in the treatment of seasonal allergic rhinitis.

DRUGS USED IN THE TREATMENT OF PULMONARY DISEASES AND DISORDERS

Bronchodilators

Adrenomimetic Agents
epinephrine (Primatene)
isoproterenol (Isuprel)

Long-Acting Beta Agonists (LABA)
formoterol (Foradil)
salmeterol (Serevent)
bitolterol (Tornalate)

Short-Acting Beta Agonists (SABA)
albuterol (Ventolin, Proventil)
metaproterenol (Alupent)
pirbuterol (Maxair)
terbutaline (Brethine)

Xanthine Derivatives
theophylline
aminophylline

Mast Cell Stabilizers (Sodium Chromoglycates)
cromolyn (NasalCrom)
nedcromil (Tilade)

Anticholinergics
ipratropium (Atrovent)
tiotropium (Spiriva)
Sodium Chromoglycates

Steroids

Inhaled corticosteroids (Long-Term Anti-Inflammatory Agents)
beclomethasone (QVAR)
budesonide (Pulmicort)
flunisolide (AeroBid)
fluticasone (Flovent)
triamcinolone (Azmacort)

Systemic/Oral Steroids (Short-Term "Burst" Therapy)
methylprednisolone
prednisolone
prednisone

Anti-inflammatory Agents

Leukotriene Receptor Antagonists (Inhibitors)/Mast Cell Inhibitors
zafirlukast (Accolate)
montelukast (Singulair)

Inhibitors
zileuton (Zyflo CR)

Combination Products
albuterol/ipratropium (Combivent)
salmeterol/fluticasone (Advair)
formoterol/budesonide (Symbicort)
formoterol/mometasone (Dulera)

DRUGS USED IN THE TREATMENT OF PULMONARY DISEASES AND DISORDERS—cont'd

Monoclonal Antibodies
   omalizumab (Xolair)
Antihistamines
   azelastine (Astelin)
   brompheniramine (Dimetane, Dimetapp),
   cetirizine (Zyrtec)
   clemastine (Tavist OTC)
   chlorpheniramine (Chlortrimeton-otc,
      Chlor-Phen Rx)

desloratadine (Clarinex)
diphenhydramine (Benadryl)
fexofenadine (Allegra)
loratadine (Claritin)
levocetirizine (Xyzal)
Decongestants
   pseudoephedrine (Sudafed)
Antitussives
   dextromethorphan

Intranasal Products
   flunisolide (Nasarel)
   beclomethasone (Beconase AQ)
   triamcinolone (Nasacort AQ)
   budesonide (Rhinocort Aqua)
   fluticasone (Flonase, Veramyst)
   ciclesonide (Omnaris)
   mometasone (Nasonex)

To properly care for patients with pulmonary disorders such as asthma and chronic obstructive pulmonary disorders (COPD) and make appropriate drug choices, clinicians must be knowledgeable about the pathophysiology of lung disorders and the pulmonary system structures used in the exchange of oxygen and carbon dioxide. The efficiency of the lung airways is determined by several factors:

- Shape and size of each of the anatomical structures of the respiratory tract, such as the nasal cavity, pharynx, larynx, trachea, bronchi, bronchioles, and alveolar sacs
- Presence of ciliated mucus-secreting epithelial lining that covers much of the respiratory tract
- Character of the respiratory tract secretion
- Pressure gradients and traction of the airway walls
- Absence of foreign substances in the respiratory tract

Changes in any of the preceding factors affect airflow and air clearance, with injuries, allergics, or diseases, in particular, leading to airway resistance. A number of diseases or events such as acute respiratory failure, asthma, bronchitis, COPD, allergic or seasonal rhinitis, pleurisy, or pneumonia present distinct challenges for the clinician as well as the patient because there is a delicate balance between healthy and unhealthy lung functioning. Most pharmacological treatments are designed to either open up the airways (bronchodilators) or reduce the inflammation that prevents the maintenance of adequate oxygenation. Furthermore, clinicians must also be aware that drugs used to treat pulmonary disorders are categorized into those for acute exacerbations or those for long-term maintenance therapy.

The three main respiratory disorders that are responsive to drug treatment are asthma, allergic rhinitis, and cough. Other disorders that are less responsive to treatment are COPD and chronic bronchitis. **Asthma** is an inflammatory disorder of the tracheobronchial tree characterized by attacks of wheezing, shortness of breath, chest tightness, and coughing (Medline Plus, 2010). The bronchial **hyperresponsiveness** may induce mild to severe airway obstruction, which restricts or limits airflow. **Chronic obstructive pulmonary disease** is the leading pulmonary disorder and is responsible for the death of 10% to 15% of smokers (PubMed Health, 2009). The airflow obstruction seen in COPD is caused by emphysema and/or chronic bronchitis in which the airflow obstruction is progressive, may be accompanied

by airway hyper-reactivity, and may be partially reversible. Like asthma and COPD, acute bronchitis is an inflammation of the large airways; however, in this condition the causative agent is not a hyper-reactive airway but rather a viral or bacterial infection (Mayo Clinic, 2010). Acute and chronic **allergic rhinitis** (hay fever) are two of the most common diseases of modern society and to a great extent are the major causes of illness, loss of productivity, hospitalization, and even death. Because the relative incidence of allergic rhinitis is 43%, nonallergic rhinitis 23%, and mixed rhinitis 34%, it is imperative that underlying triggers be identified and either eliminated or modified (World Allergy Organization, 2006).

BRONCHODILATORS

Bronchodilating agents, also known as **beta-2 receptor agonists** or beta-agonists, are the main drugs used to treat the reversible bronchoconstriction seen in asthma patients of all ages. Asthma, often referred to as restrictive airway disease, responds to a variety of prescription medications that are readily available in a variety of formulations. At one time the only two drugs available were the **adrenomimetic** agents epinephrine (Primatene) and isoproterenol (Isuprel), but today the most commonly used agent is the beta agonist albuterol (Ventolin, Proventil). Others, such as metaproterenol (Alupent), terbutaline (Brethine), bitolterol (Tornalate), pirbuterol (Maxair), levalbuterol (Xopenex), and salmeterol (Serevent), are used in modern bronchodilator therapy because, besides reversing acute episodes of **bronchospasm**, these agents are effective for long-term treatment by keeping open otherwise constricted airways. Unfortunately, by stimulating beta-adrenergic receptors long-term, they can also induce tachycardia, anxiety, and tremor depending on how selective each agent is for beta receptors throughout the body.

One of the first adrenomimetic agents for asthma treatment was adrenaline (epinephrine). Its bronchodilating effect is achieved by formulating it in a **metered dose inhaler (MDI)** (Fig. 10-1), which is sold under the brand name of Primatene. In 2008 the FDA announced that sales of this OTC product must cease as of December 31, 2011, as part of an international ban (the Montreal Protocol of Substances that Deplete the Ozone Layer) against its chlorofluorocarbon propellant. Adrenaline has a rapid onset of action as a bronchodilator and is still useful in emergency situations for asthma. It also has many side effects, and improper

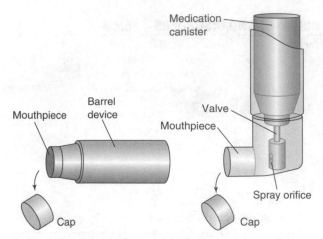

FIGURE 10-1 The components of a typical metered dose inhaler include canister with valve, propellent, and drug substance. **Note:** Per the U.S. agreement to the 1987 Montreal Protocol on Substances that Deplete the Ozone Layer, since 2008 all metered dose inhalers use hydrofluoroalkane propellants, effectively removing chlorofluorocarbons from these devices at the manufacturer level.

use can increase mortality. The bronchodilating agents used today are much safer, effective, and are easy to use.

Beta receptor agonists have differing selectivity as sympathomimetic agents or adrenergic agonists. They stimulate *both* beta-1 adrenergic receptors, causing some cardiac stimulation, and beta-2 adrenergic receptors, causing vasodilation and bronchial dilation. In addition, they also stimulate alpha-1 adrenergic receptors, causing relaxation of the bronchial smooth muscle (bronchodilation), as well as vasoconstriction and some pressor effects. The net result is increased cardiac contractility, stroke volume, and cardiac output. Bronchodilators are used to treat bronchospasm associated with acute and chronic bronchial asthma, exercise-induced bronchospasm, bronchitis, emphysema, or other obstructive pulmonary diseases.

Conscientious Prescribing of Bronchodilators

■ Ventricular arrhythmias may occur if the heart rate (HR) exceeds 130 beats per minute.
■ Prolonged administration or excessive dosing may result in metabolic acidosis due to increased serum lactic acid concentrations.
■ Blood pressure (BP), HR, and intraocular pressure (IOP) should all be monitored in patients using these drugs.
■ Patients using the metered-dose inhalation formulation should be told to wait 3 to 5 minutes between inhalations and to *shake* the inhaler before use.
■ Patients should be observed using their inhalation techniques to be sure they are doing it correct.

Patient/Family Education for Bronchodilators

■ Patients should be informed that beta blockers may decrease effects of long-acting beta-2 agonists (LABAs).

■ Patients should be informed that caffeine can increase stimulant effect.
■ Patients should be observed using their inhalation techniques ensure they are doing it correctly.
■ Patients using the metered-dose inhalation (MDI) formulation should be told to wait 3 to 5 minutes between inhalations and to *shake* the inhaler before use.
■ To avoid rebound congestion, advise patients not to use common cold preparations containing decongestants for more than 3 to 5 days.
■ Patients should never be prescribed inhaling devices without proper instruction in their use.
■ Patients should also be made aware that overuse of these agents may lead to their being ineffective and cause severe paradoxical bronchoconstriction.
■ Patients using short-acting beta-2 agonists (SABA) should be informed that if they use the drug on a regular daily basis, they need to be reevaluated by their clinician. Patients using more than one 15-mL canister in 8 weeks (i.e., 200 inhalations over 2 months) should also see their clinician.

Long-Acting Beta-2 Agonists (LABAs)

The long-acting beta-2 agonists, or LABAs, are most commonly used to treat the bronchospasm associated with asthma, bronchitis (acute and chronic), and COPD. Long-acting beta-2 agonists have a sustained duration of effect of 12 hours. Metered dose inhalers can be administered twice a day. They are best taken along with inhaled corticosteroids because there are data to suggest that there is an increased incidence of asthma-related deaths if only one drug is used.

Mechanism of Action

Long-acting beta-2 agonists stimulate an intracellular enzyme that catalyzes adenosine triphosphate (ATP) to cyclic adenosine monophosphate (cAMP). When cAMP levels increase, it causes relaxation of bronchial, uterine, and vascular smooth muscle through stimulation of beta-2 adrenergic receptors. Thus, this adrenergic agonist stimulates beta-2 adrenergic receptors in the lungs, resulting in a relaxation of bronchial smooth muscle.

Pharmacokinetics

■ Absorption: Low systemic absorption with effect primarily in the lungs. Formoterol onset is 1 to 3 minutes; salmeterol onset is 20 minutes. Duration (all agents) is 12 hours.
■ Distribution: Protein binding is 90%.
■ Metabolism: Even though their action is primarily local, any minimal systemic absorption of salmeterol and formoterol are hydroxylated in the liver.
■ Excretion: Salmeterol metabolites are eliminated primarily by feces; formoterol is excreted mostly in urine; bitolterol is eliminated in both feces and urine.
■ Half-life: Salmeterol: 3 to 4 hours; formoterol: 10 hours; bitolterol: 3 hours.

Dosage and Administration

Generic Name	Trade Name	Route	Dosage
salmeterol	Serevent Diskus	Inhalation	Adults, elderly, and children age >4: for prevention and maintenance treatment of asthma, 50 mcg/puff (1 inhalation) every 12 hr. To prevent exercise-induced bronchospasm, 1 inhalation 30 min before exercise
bitolterol	Tornalate	Inhalation	To prevent bronchospasm, 2 inhalations every 8 hr
formoterol	Foradil	Inhalation	For prevention of exercised-induced bronchospasm, one 12-mcg capsule at least 15 min before exercise

Because they are long-acting beta agonists, formoterol (Foradil) and salmeterol (Serevent) are dosed every 12 hours; they can be dosed 15 minutes before exercising to prevent exercise-induced bronchospasm because their onset of effect is 15 minutes. The short-acting beta agonists, such as albuterol (Ventolin, Proventil) and metaproterenol (Alupent), are generally dosed using inhalation devices three to four times a day and can be used as a "rescue" medication if an attack seems imminent.

Clinical Uses

■ Control of reversible airway obstruction
■ Prevention of exercise-induced asthma
■ Prevention of bronchospasm in COPD
■ Emphysema

Adverse Reactions

CV: Palpitations, tachycardia. Salmeterol and formoterol may, through excessive sympathomimetic stimulation, prolong the QT interval, resulting in venous tachycardia, palpitations, extrasystole, and chest pain.
GI: Nausea, heartburn, GI distress, diarrhea.
META: Hypoglycemia and hypokalemia
NEURO: Headache, tremor, dizziness, vertigo.
PUL: Cough, dry throat, pharyngitis.

Interactions

■ Beta blockers used for hypertension or as eyedrops can cause a decreased action of salmeterol and formoterol. Beta blockers taken with furosemide may cause increased hypokalemia.

Contraindications

■ These drugs should not be used in acute asthma attacks.
■ Preexisting arrhythmias, angina, palpitations, chest pain, narrow-angle glaucoma, or sensitivity to any component in the formulation are contraindications.

Conscientious Considerations

■ Use with caution in patients with CVD, diabetes, glaucoma, hyperthyroid, pregnancy, and in children younger than 4 years.
■ Excessive use leads to tolerance.

■ The beneficial effects of LABAs in combination therapy should be weighed against the increased risk of severe exacerbations, although uncommon.
■ LABAs do *not* eliminate the need for a patient to be treated concurrently with an inhaled corticosteroid (ICS), nor should they be considered as monotherapy for long-term control of asthma.
■ These medications should not be used for patients whose asthma can be managed by occasional use of short-acting inhaled beta-2 agonists.
■ Of all the adjunctive therapies available, LABAs remain the agents most commonly combined with ICS in youths 12 years of age or older as well as in adults.
■ For patients 5 years of age or older who have moderate persistent asthma or asthma inadequately controlled on low-dose ICS, the option to increase the ICS dose should be given equal weight with the option of adding an LABA.
■ For patients 5 years of age or older who have severe persistent asthma or asthma inadequately controlled on step 3 care, the combination of an LABA and an ICS is the therapeutic recommendation of the Expert Panel Report 3 of the National Heart, Lung, and Blood Institute (2007).
■ In addition, clinicians must be aware of the important considerations that apply to all bronchodilators (see page 160, Conscientious Prescribing of Bronchodilators).

Short-Acting Beta-2 Agonists (SABAs)

SABAs are the mainstays of treatment for acute symptoms of bronchospasm. This is true whether asthma is being treated through routine outpatient management or in a hospital emergency department. SABAs are quite effective as bronchodilators and have few negative cardiovascular effects. By way of contrast, in the past, two SABAs (isoprenaline and fenoterol), which were less selective or used at higher doses, were associated with severe and fatal attacks of asthma. However, albuterol (Ventolin, Proventil) is regularly prescribed for patients with mild or moderate asthma on an as-needed basis; however, like the LABAs, these agents can produce serious drug interactions when they are coadministered with tricyclic antidepressants, furosemide, and beta blockers.

Mechanism of Action

These agents are **sympathomimetics** in that they stimulate beta-2 adrenergic receptors in the lung, giving rise to a relaxation of bronchial smooth muscle.

Pharmacokinetics

■ Absorption: Inhaled: Gradually absorbed from the bronchi, with onset of action in 5 to 15 minutes. Oral forms: Rapidly absorbed from the GI tract, with onset of bronchodilation effects in 15 to 30 minutes.
■ Metabolism: Metabolized by the liver
■ Excretion: Excreted in the urine
■ Half-life: When inhaled, 2.7 to 5 hr; tablets, 2 to 3.8 hr
■ Of the adjunctive therapies available, LABAs remain the preferred agents to combine with ICS in youths 12 years of age or older, as well as in adults.

Dosage and Administration

Generic Name	Trade Name	Route	Dosage For Bronchodilation
albuterol	Ventolin, Proventil	PO, inhalation	PO 2–4 mg, 3–4 times a day. Inhalation 4 yr of age: MDI inhaler, 2 inhalations every 4–6 hr or 2 inhalations 15 min before exercise
metaproterenol	Alupent	Inhalation	Adults >12: MDI 2–3 inhalations every 3–4 hr, not to exceed 12 inhalations/day
pirbuterol	Maxair	Inhalation	MDIs: 1 or 2 inhalations every 6 hr; to prevent exercise-induced bronchospasm, 1 or 2 puffs 15 min before exercise
terbutaline	Brethine	PO, SC, Inhalation	PO (adults and youths >15): 2.5 mg–5 mg every 6 hr; inhalation (adults and youths >12): 2 inhalations every 4–6 hr SC: 250 mcg, may repeat in 15–30 min
levalbuterol	Xopenex	Inhalation	0.63 mcg–1.25 mcg via nebulization every 6–8 hr

Clinical Uses

■ Acute asthma
■ Exercise-induced bronchospasm
■ COPD

Adverse Reactions

CV: Hypertension and tachycardia. Excessive sympathomimetic stimulation may produce palpitations, arrhythmias, chest pain, myocardial infarction, and elevated BP, followed by decreased BP, diaphoresis, chills, and skin blanching.
GI: Nausea, vomiting.
NEURO: Headache, nervousness, tremor, dizziness.

Interactions

■ Furosemides, beta blockers, monoamine oxidase inhibitors (MAOIs), and tricyclic antidepressants. As do the LABAs, the SABAs have serious drug-drug interactions when coadministered with these agents. To avoid potentiating SABAs' actions, MAOIs should not be coadministered for at least 2 weeks.

Contraindications

■ Sensitivity to sympathomimetics
■ Preexisting arrhythmias, angina, palpitations, chest pain, narrow-angle glaucoma, or sensitivity to any component in the formulation

Conscientious Considerations

■ Use with caution in patients with hyperthyroidism, diabetes mellitus, and cardiovascular disorders.
■ Regularly scheduled, daily, chronic use of SABA is not recommended.

■ Use of more than one SABA in a metered dose inhaler canister every 1 or 2 months placed patients at an increased risk of initiating an acute exacerbation of their asthma. This usually results in a visit to the emergency department of a hospital and a stay in the institution. One canister of albuterol provides 200 "puffs," enough for 1 month of treatment (2 puffs per inhalation administered four times a day). If used more frequently, the patient is likely over-relying on the medication, and the usage suggests inadequate control of the asthma or no lessening of the life-style factors that act as triggers.

■ The frequency of SABA use can be clinically useful as a barometer of disease activity because increasing use of SABA has been associated with increased risk for death or near death in patients who have asthma.

■ Another indication of poor asthma control occurs when the patient is using a SABA more than twice a week to control bronchospasms; this is a sign that anti-inflammatory corticosteroids are to be initiated or intensified.

■ Every patient also should be considered a candidate for a "spacer" device.

■ Albuterol is used extensively in children as young as 2 years old and has become the first-choice medication in asthma because it is only minimally a cause of adverse effects.

■ Metaproterenol and levalbuterol may be used in children age 6 and older.

■ The safety of pirbuterol and bitolterol in children aged 12 and under has not been established because serious cardiac adverse events are an issue.

Xanthine Derivatives

Xanthines, including theophylline and aminophylline, are older drugs that are infrequently used today as antiasthmatic bronchodilators. In addition to having an anti-inflammatory and bronchodilator effect, theophylline improves respiratory muscle function and stimulates the respiratory center. Both are used in asthma and COPD.

Mechanism of Action

These derivatives of xanthine act as bronchodilators by directly relaxing smooth muscle in the bronchial airways and by relaxing pulmonary blood vessels. Their exact mechanism of action is not known; however, it *is* known that these drugs increase the force of contraction of diaphragmatic muscles by enhancing calcium uptake through adenosine-mediated channels and that they suppress the response of airways to stimuli.

Pharmacokinetics

■ The pharmacokinetics of theophylline is such that it varies widely among similar patients and cannot be predicted with any certainty by using age, sex, body weight, or other demographic parameters.

■ Absorption: Rapid and completely absorbed from oral dosage forms, XR dosage is slow but complete.

■ Distribution: Distributed freely in fat-free tissues, crosses placenta, enters breast milk.

- Metabolism: Aminophylline is converted to theophylline, and then converted again in the liver to caffeine; this metabolite is excreted renally.
- Excretion: 10% is excreted unchanged.
- Half-life: 4 to 8 hours (decreased in smokers).

Dosage and Administration

- Titrate dose using theophylline serum level monitoring (want steady state serum 5 to 12 mcg/mL); however, serum theophylline levels as measured by a clinical pharmacist is a practice that is waning in favor of continuous albuterol nebulization.

Clinical Uses

- Today, use of theophylline in chronic asthma or other lung diseases is limited because it is considered a drug to be held in reserve for patients who are on maximal therapy with safer medications.
- Although theophylline is a weak bronchodilator, it does have some mild anti-inflammatory properties. Some clinicians discourage its use because of its slow onset of action, its side effects profile, its variable efficacy and response rate, and its high risk of drug interactions.

Adverse Reactions

Toxicities are dose-related and occur near the usual therapeutic dose.

CV: Arrhythmia, angina, palpitations, TACHYCARDIA
GI: Nausea, vomiting, anorexia, cramps, increased GI acid
NEURO: Seizures, anxiety, headache, restlessness, tremors, central nervous system (CNS) stimulation

Interactions

- Caffeine, herbals, St. John's wort, and ephedra will increase xanthine levels.
- Any patient on beta blockers may see a reduced effect.

Contraindications

- Hyperthyroidism
- Geriatric patients
- Obesity (dose is based on body weight)
- Preexisting arrhythmias, angina, palpitations, chest pain, narrow-angle glaucoma, or sensitivity to any component in the formulation
- Contraindicated for smokers, because smoking increases their clearance rate and thus reduces their overall effects

Conscientious Considerations

- The clinician should be mindful that serious side effects can occur without any preceding signs of less serious toxicity, thus these drugs are reserved for patients with severe asthma who are maximized on other therapies.
- Monitoring of serum concentration levels is required due to significant toxicities, narrow therapeutic range, and individual differences in metabolic clearance.
- Once the drug is titrated, ongoing serum levels are needed to determine therapeutic levels every 6 to 12 months or at

any time the patient's status changes to avoid toxicity. For example, with aminophylline, a therapeutic level is between 10 and 15 mcg/mL, with toxicity occurring at 24 mcg/mL for adults and 15 mcg/mL for neonates.

- Monitoring serum concentration with oral theophylline is a complex task. For example there is a diurnal variation in absorption of sustained release (SR) products; that is, absorption is faster in the morning and slower at night. Thus, with a SR product given every 12 hours, drawing serum samples can lead to confusing monitoring parameters if serum concentrations are used to adjust doses.
- When dosing different sources of xanthine derivatives, the clinician must take into account the percentage of anhydrous theophylline available from various salts used to make the manufacturer's preparation. For example, if a manufacturer uses theophylline monohydrate, it releases 91% anhydrous theophylline. If the manufacturer's product uses theophylline ethylenediamine, the patient gets 79% anhydrous theophylline, thus different salt forms of a drug do make a difference in how much of an active ingredient a patient will get from a fixed dose.

Patient/Family Education

- Encourage the patient to drink 1,000 mL water per day to minimize airway secretions.
- Advise patient to avoid over-the-counter (OTC) cough and cold preparations because they may cause arrhythmia.
- The patient should contact clinician if drug's effect seems to wane.
- If GI upset occurs, patient should take tablets with 8 ounces of water.

Anticholinergics

Anticholinergic agents inhibit muscarinic cholinergic receptors and reduce intrinsic vagal tone of the airway. Ipratropium bromide provides additive benefit to SABA in moderate-to-severe asthma exacerbations and in COPD. These drugs may be used as an alternative bronchodilator for patients who do not tolerate SABA. Ipratropium (Atrovent) and tiotropium (Spiriva) are the two agents used today, with Spiriva being a longer acting agent.

Mechanism of Action

These agents are competitive inhibitors of acetylcholine at parasympathetic sites in bronchial smooth muscle, or put another way, they are cholinergic blocking agents or anticholinergics, thus they cause bronchodilation and inhibit nasal secretions. They are less potent as bronchodilators than are inhaled beta-2 agonists, and therefore their use as a single agent is in question because more potent agents are available. But because these drugs have a slow onset of action, some clinicians find them useful in patients who are intolerant of beta-2 agonists or find they are useful to generate an additive effect when using a beta-2 agonist.

Pharmacokinetics

- Absorption: Minimal systemic absorption after inhalation. With Spiriva, the amount reaching the lungs is 19%; the rest finds its way into the GI tract.

■ Metabolism: Ipratropium, if absorbed, is metabolized in the liver. Tiotropium, if absorbed, is largely unchanged and excreted in urine; if it is not absorbed, it goes unchanged into feces.

■ Excretion: Ipratropium: primarily in the feces; tiotropium: primarily in urine.

■ Half-life: Ipratropium: 1.5 to 4 hours; tiotropium: 5 to 6 days.

Dosage and Administration

Generic Name	Trade Name	Route	Dosage
ipratropium	Atrovent	Inhalation, intranasal	For acute treatment of bronchospasm: 4–8 puffs as needed; for maintenance treatment of bronchospasm: 2–3 puffs every 6 hr
tiotropium	Spiriva	Inhalation	For COPD: 18 mcg once a day (24-hr maintenance therapy; 1 capsule offers 2 inhalations)

Clinical Use

■ To prevent acute bronchospasm in patients with bronchitis, emphysema, rhinorrhea, or COPD

Adverse Reactions

EENT: Worsen angle-closure glaucoma, causing severe eye pain and blurred vision.
GI: Nausea
GU: Will worsen enlarged prostates and bladder neck issues such as blockages
NEURO: Headache
PUL: Cough, dry mouth, dry nose and mouth, nasal irritation

Interactions

■ Ipratropium (Spiriva) has a potential for creating additive anticholinergic effects.

Contraindications

■ Narrow-angle glaucoma, enlarged prostate, bladder blockages, or any history of sensitivity to atropine.

Conscientious Considerations

■ Clinicians should assess respiratory rate, breath sounds, and pulse before administration and at the time of peak effect.

■ A thorough history of prescribed, OTC, and herbal medications, especially eyedrops, is important before prescribing.

■ A combination of ipratropium and albuterol is sold as Combivent.

Patient/Family Education

■ Patients should be observed using their inhalation techniques to ensure they are doing it correctly.

■ Advise patients not to use common cold preparations with decongestants for 3 to 5 days to avoid rebound congestion.

■ Patients should be instructed not to use Spiriva to treat a bronchospasm attack. It will not work fast enough.

■ Patients should be instructed to contact their clinician if the medication does not seem to work well in treating or preventing bronchospasm.

■ Patients should be instructed never to use these drugs in larger doses or for longer than recommended.

■ Patients using the metered-dose inhalation formulation should be told to wait 3 to 5 minutes between inhalations and to *shake* the inhaler before each and every use.

■ Patients need instruction on use of the Spiriva Handihaler. They should be instructed never to take Spiriva capsules by mouth and to use only one capsule at a time.

■ Serious allergic reactions such as itching, rash, swelling of the lips, tongue, or throat (trouble swallowing), blurry vision, or halos may occur after taking Spiriva as a result of conjunctival and cornea congestion. Patients who experience these symptoms need to stop taking the medication and seek emergency help.

SPOTLIGHT ON ASTHMA

Asthma is a chronic or intermittent obstructive airway disease caused by inflammation of the airways. This narrowing of the airway is caused by contraction of bronchial smooth muscle triggered by agonists, such as histamine, **leukotrienes**, and prostaglandins, released from inflammatory cells. The inflammation extends from the large airways to the small airways and can be found even at the first presentation of symptoms, with its histological characteristic being infiltration of airway walls by eosinophils. Bronchial smooth muscle contraction is worsened by thickening of the airway caused by acute edema, cellular infiltration, remodeling, and other secretions, which in turn further limits breathing, causes fatigue, and creates a situation of possible respiratory failure. Although what causes the airway to be hyperresponsive to so many triggers (exercise, cold, dry air, etc.) remains a mystery; when it does occur, it typically moves forward in four distinct physiological phases
■ Thickening of the basement membranes in the airways
■ Edema and infiltration in bronchial walls

■ Increased size of the submucosal glands
■ Airway wall hypertrophies under prolonged bronchoconstriction
The clinical presentation of asthma varies widely, which is one reason its wheezing, production of mucus, and cough are commonly misdiagnosed as symptoms of recurrent pneumonia or chronic bronchitis. Conversely, young children often suffer viral infections that mimic symptoms of asthma. An asthma diagnosis is based on patient history and tests such as spirometry and peak expiratory flow (PEV), which test pulmonary function. Asthma is a common respiratory complaint; it affects 20 million Americans, the majority of whom are children. Asthma is twice as common in males during childhood, but its incidence equalizes between the sexes during adulthood (American Academy Allergy, Asthma & Immunology, 2010).

Medical Management of Asthma
The goals for successful management of asthma are outlined in the National Heart, Lung, and Blood Institute (2007) publication

Guidelines for the Diagnosis and Management of Asthma (EPR-3).
The guidelines address these goals of asthma management:
■ Achieve and maintain control of symptoms
■ Prevent asthma exacerbations
■ Maintain pulmonary function as close to normal levels as possible
■ Maintain normal activity levels, including exercise
■ Avoid adverse effects from asthma medications
■ Prevent the development of irreversible airflow limitation
■ Prevent asthma mortality

Based on the Expert Panel Report (EPR-3), long-term outpatient management of asthma should follow a stepwise model incorporating four treatment components:
■ Objective measures of lung function
■ Environmental control measures and avoidance of risk factors
■ Comprehensive pharmacological therapy
■ Patient education

The *Guidelines for the Diagnosis and Management of Asthma (EPR-3)* also put forth a classification system for asthma and their recommendations for drug treatment for people in four age groups: children 0 to 4 years, children 5 to 11 years, youths greater than 12 years, and adults. However, it makes a strong recommendation that all patients who have asthma must be monitored continuously because the processes underlying asthma can vary in intensity over time, and treatment should be adjusted accordingly. Thus today the pharmacological treatment of asthma is based on dependent factors, such as the following:
■ severity of the disease
■ pharmacological properties of the drug, their ease of use, and cost
■ patient's age, because young patients tend to metabolize glucocorticoid, theophylline, and beta-2 agonists *faster* than do adults)

Medications for asthma are categorized into two general classes: long-term control medications used to achieve and maintain control of persistent asthma and quick-relief medications used to treat acute symptoms and exacerbations.

Long-term control medications (listed in alphabetical order) are as follows:
■ Corticosteroids
■ Sodium Chromoglycates (Cromolyn sodium and nedocromil)
■ Immunomodulators
■ Leukotriene
■ LABAs
■ Xanthine derivatives

Quick-relief medications (listed in alphabetical order) are as follows:
■ Anticholinergics
■ SABAs
■ Systemic corticosteroids

Finally, it is best to always recommend use of a spacer with any MDI.

Emergency Care of the Asthmatic Patient

From time to time, both adults and children may require emergency care for an exacerbation of asthma that is life threatening. If the patient presents with diminished oxygen saturation, supplemental administration of O_2 will be required. Short-acting bronchodilators may be given, but the likelihood of oral or intravenous glucocorticoids being given is dependent on the severity of the exacerbation. Of course, close monitoring of the patient is essential during this time of crisis because any exacerbation can be life threatening. The systemic corticosteroids commonly used in cases of asthma emergencies are hydrocortisone (Solu-Cortef), prednisone (Deltasone), and methylprednisolone (Solu-Medrol) because they all work quickly and effectively. It is suggested that hospitalized patients receiving these medications do so up to the point that acute symptoms are relieved and the patient reaches 80% saturation as measured using a peak flow meter (AAAI, 2010).

Prevention of Asthma Attacks

In addition to medication therapy, there is a role for the clinician team to help prevent and control patient risk factors and exposure to triggers. Patients should be counseled regarding self-management skills and how to recognize signs and symptoms of an impending attack. Much has been written about the benefits of having the patient help with the development of a written plan to help avoid exacerbations (Mayo Clinic, 2010).

Training patients to monitor their asthma, whether moderate to severe, is a good idea, especially training to monitor peak flow and inhaler technique. There are no specific monitoring guidelines for bronchodilators; however, response to these agents should be monitored using a peak flow meter.

Steroids

Steroids block late-phase reaction to allergens, reduce airway hyperresponsiveness, and inhibit inflammatory cell migration and activation. They are the most potent and effective anti-inflammatory medications currently available. Inhaled corticosteroids are used in the long-term control of asthma. Short courses of oral systemic corticosteroids are often used to gain prompt control of the disease prior to initiating long-term therapy; long-term oral systemic corticosteroid is used for severe persistent asthma.

Inhaled Corticosteroids

Inhaled corticosteroids are the most effective drugs for long-term control, suppression, and reversal of asthma. Inhaled corticosteroids are accepted as the most useful medications for the control of persistent asthma symptoms. The beneficial effects relate to the basic pathophysiology of the disease and by what is known about the pharmacological effects of this class of drugs. Because asthma is, after all, an inflammatory airway disease, inhaled corticosteroids help prevent asthma attacks by exerting nonspecific effects on several of the inflammatory cells implicated in the pathogenesis of asthma and COPD.

Mechanism of Action

The methods by which steroids exert their effects in the treatment of asthma and allergic rhinitis are primarily anti-inflammatory and are not entirely understood, but experts believe their effects are mediated through glucocorticoid receptors widely expressed in most cell types throughout the body. It is believed that corticosteroid use results in the following:

■ Reduction in the number of circulating eosinophils, by either a direct action at the bone marrow or by reducing the number of cytokines known to be required for eosinophil survival.

■ Inhibition of release of inflammation mediator cells from lymphocytes, alveolar macrophages, and airway epithelial cells.

■ Reduction of mucosal mast cells in epithelium by reducing cytokines and growth factors necessary for cell survival.

■ Reduction vascular/capillary permeability so that smooth muscle relaxation of bronchial tree occurs.

Pharmacokinetics

Upon inhalation, a significant portion of the drug is deposited in the mouth and pharynx, where it can exert local side effects. If this portion of the dose is not promptly rinsed from the mouth with water or spit out, and thus is swallowed, it will be absorbed from the GI tract. Once absorbed, it escapes first-pass metabolism in the liver (and inactivation). It will enter the general circulation in an active form, potentially systemic side effects. In addition, much of the dose that enters the airways can be absorbed into the general circulation through the changing pulmonary vasculature, again giving rise to the potential for systemic side effects. Thus, clinicians need to consider the impact of various pharmacokinetic parameters such as bioavailability, receptor binding, and drug half-life because they contribute to the safety and efficacy of each medication chosen.

Metabolism and excretion are critical factors in the systemic side effect profile of corticosteroids. As a general rule, faster metabolism leads to lower concentrations and reductions in systemic side effects. It is generally agreed (although the numbers are controversial) that an inhaled corticosteroid with a long half-life that is present in low concentrations likely has a better safety profile than an inhaled corticosteroid with a short half-life in higher concentrations.

■ Absorption: Readily and completely absorbed from pulmonary, nasal, and GI tissue.

■ Distribution: 87% is protein bound

■ Metabolism: Undergoes extensive first-pass metabolism in the liver

■ Excretion: Inhaled corticosteroids are rapidly cleared by multiple organs following systemic absorption. Beclomethasone: excreted primarily in the feces; dexamethasone, fluocinolone: excreted in urine; mometasone: excreted in bile; ciclesonide: excreted in multiple organs.

■ Half-life: Beclomethasone: 15 hr; dexamethasone: 3.5 to 4 hr; fluocinolone: 1.3 to 1.7 hr; mometasone: 5.8 hr; ciclesonide: 0.7 hr.

Dosage and Administration

ICSs are well tolerated and safe at the recommended dosages. The preferred route of administration of a corticosteroid for treatment of asthma is inhalation. This delivers the drug directly to the lung tissue where it can act locally and minimize the opportunity for systemic side effects associated with oral or parenteral administration.

Dosage and Administration of Inhaled Corticosteroids Used in Asthma

Generic Name	Trade Name	Dosing* Adults	Dosing Children < 12 Years
beclomethasone	QVAR	42 mcg/inhaler: 2 inhalations, 34 times a day, no more than (NMT) 20 per day	42 mcg/inhaler: 2 inhalations, 3–4 times a day, NMT 10 per day
budesonide	Pulmicort	200 mcg/inhaler: 12 inhalations twice a day	12 mo–8 yr, use Pulmicort Respules dose form 0.25 mg/day as single dose
flunisolide	AeroBid	250 mcg/dose, MDI, 2 inhalations twice a day	250 mcg/dose MDI 2 inhalations twice a day if >4 years
fluticasone†	Flovent	Dry powder inhaler 100 mcg twice a day	Dry powder inhaler 50 mcg twice a day if age 4–11 yr
mometasone	Asmanex	Dry powder inhaler, 220 mcg/inhalation, 1 inhalation daily	Dry powder inhaler, 220 mcg/per inhalation; 1 inhalation daily if older than age 12
triamcinolone	Azmacort	100 mcg/ inhalation MDI with 240 inhalation; 2 MDI inhalation, 3-4 times a day	100 mcg/ inhalation MDI with 240 inhalations; 1-2 MDI inhalation, 3-4 times a day if 6–12 years old

*These doses are the daily doses and are to be given in divided schedules of 2, 3, or 4 times/day

†Doses listed for fluticasone are for the metered dose inhaler (MDI). The product is also available in a combination product, Advair Diskus, which combines fluticasone with salmeterol 50 mcg/puff.

Dosage and Administration: Intranasal Aerosol Steroids Used in Allergic Rhinitis

Generic Name	Trade Name	Dosage And Children >12
beclomethasone	Beconase	1 spray/nostril, 2–4 times a day (50 mcg/spray)
ciclesonide	Omnaris	2 sprays/nostril, once a day 150 MDI doses per can (50 mcg/spray)
triamcinolone	Nasacort	2 sprays each nostril, twice a day 55 mcg/spray in 100-spray MDI can
budesonide	Rhinocort	2 sprays each nostril, twice daily 32 mcg/MDI spray, 200 sprays/can
flunisolide	Nasarel	2 sprays/nostril 2–3 times/day, not to exceed 16 sprays/day 29 mcg/MDI spray, 200 sprays/can
mometasone furoate	Nasonex	2 sprays in each nostril once a day 50 mcg/MDI spray, 120 sprays/can
fluticasone propionate	Flonase	2 sprays in each nostril once a day 50 mcg/MDI spray 120 doses per can

Clinical Uses

■ Prophylactic treatment of asthma
■ Allergic rhinitis

Adverse Reactions

EENT: Intranasal: nasal burning, mucosal dryness, localized fungal infections, sore throat, ulceration of nasal mucosa, nasal epistaxis, nasal candidiasis, eye pain.

MISC: Note an acute hypersensitivity reaction can occur that manifests itself as urticaria, bronchospasm, and angioedema.

PUL: Inhalation: throat irritation, dry mouth, hoarseness, cough, transient bronchospasm, esophageal candidiasis.

SYSTEMIC: Systemic side effects associated with inhaled or intranasal corticosteroids may include osteoporosis, reduced growth in children, thinning of the skin, and cataracts. These effects occur if the corticosteroid is able to suppress the hypothalamus-pituitary-adrenal system.

Interactions

■ Any medication that is a cytochrome P450 (CYP3A4) inhibitor will increase the levels and effects of these agents.

Contraindications

■ Hypersensitivity to the agent or any component in its formulation

Conscientious Considerations

■ These medications have no role in treatment of acute asthma, but they are indicated for long-term use in preventing the exacerbations of mild, moderate, or persistent asthma.
■ Although local side effects associated with inhaled corticosteroids do not lead to significant morbidity, these side effects do diminish patient adherence to the prescribed regimen.
■ To reduce the potential for adverse effects, the following measures are recommended:
  ■ Spacers or valved holding chambers (VHCs) used with non-breath-activated MDIs reduce local side effects, but there are no data on use of spacers with ultrafine-particle hydrofluoroalkane (HFA) MDIs.
  ■ Advise patients to rinse their mouths (rinse and spit) after inhalation.
  ■ Use the lowest dose of ICS that maintains asthma control. Evaluate patient adherence and inhaler technique as well as environmental factors that may contribute to asthma severity before increasing the dose of ICS.
  ■ To achieve or maintain control of asthma, consider adding an LABA to a low or medium dose of ICS rather than using a higher dose of ICS.
  ■ For children, monitor growth (see Special Case: Inhaled Corticosteroid Use in Children).
  ■ In adult patients, consider supplements of calcium (1,000–1,500 mg/day) and vitamin D (400–800 units/day), particularly in perimenopausal women. Bone-sparing therapy (e.g., bisphosphonate), where appropriate, may be considered for patients on medium or high doses of ICS, particularly for those who are at risk of osteoporosis or who have low bone mineral density (BMD) scores as determined by dual energy x-ray absorptiometry (or DEXA) scan. In children, age-appropriate dietary intake of calcium and exercise should be reviewed with the child's caregivers.

SPECIAL CASE: Inhaled Corticosteroid Use in Children

Over the decades, reports of children having their growth stunted by inhaled corticosteroids have flourished. However, evidence indicates that although these agents may slow bone growth, a child's overall growth is not affected, nor have rates of osteoporosis increased. Thus inhaled corticosteroids are considered to be fairly safe (Allen, 2002). Should oral steroids be used in an asthmatic young patients, however, they should be reserved only for short bursts.

Patient/Family Education

■ Rinse mouth with water following inhalation to decrease the possibility of developing fungal infections. Rinsing and using spacer devices can also reduce the likelihood of adverse reaction.
■ Always review with patients on a regular basis their technique for using the inhaler.
■ Let the patient know that the response to nasal and inhaled steroids appear in 3 days to 2 weeks. If there is no improvement in 3 weeks, the medication should be discontinued.

Systemic–Oral Corticosteroids

Although many systemic corticosteroids exist, the three that are commonly used in asthma are hydrocortisone (Solu-Cortef), prednisone (Deltasone), and methylprednisolone (Solu-Medrol). Although not short acting, oral systemic corticosteroids are used for moderate and severe exacerbations as adjuncts to SABAs to speed recovery and prevent recurrence of exacerbations.

Mechanism of Action

These adrenocortical steroids inhibit accumulations of anti-inflammatory cells at inflammation sites. They also inhibit phagocytosis, lysomal enzyme release, and synthesis and release of mediators of inflammation. Their mechanism of action allows them to be used to suppress or prevent cell-mediated immune reactions and decrease or prevent tissue responses to the inflammatory process. This means corticosteroids suppress inflammation and the normal immune response system, and for this reason they are used in conditions such as shock, acute adrenal insufficiency, and status asthmaticus.

Pharmacokinetics

■ Absorption: Rapid from any site.
■ Distribution: 65% to 91% are protein bound in serum.
■ Metabolism: Drugs such as prednisone are hepatically converted from its inactive state to its active state (prednisolone). This may be impaired if there is hepatic dysfunction or end-stage renal disease.
■ Excretion: Excreted through the urine.
■ Half-life: Prednisone: 2.5 to 3.5 hours; prednisolone: 3.5 hours; methylprednisolone: 3 to 3.5 hours; hydrocortisone: 1.5 to 2 hours.

Dosage and Administration

Oral steroids should be given in the lowest dose possible; interestingly the best time of day for administrating them to achieve their maximum effect is 3:00 p.m.

Generic Name	Trade Name	Route	Dosage
hydrocortisone	Solu-Cortef	PO	Adults 20–240 mg/day in 1–4 divided doses
prednisone	Deltasone	PO	Adults 5–60 mg/day as a single dose or as divided doses
methylprednisolone	Solu-Medrol	PO	Adults 120–180 mg/day in divided doses 3–4 times/day for 48 hr, then 60–80mg/day in 2 divided doses

Clinical Uses

■ Asthma (as short-term burst therapy); COPD; replacement therapy in adrenal insufficiency; Crohn's disease

Adverse Reactions

DERM (dermatological): Acne, facial flushing, delayed wound healing

ENDO (endocrinological): Suppress growth in adolescents and cause development of Cushing's syndrome; induced diabetes mellitus

GI: heartburn, abdominal distention, increased appetite, diarrhea, constipation

MISC: High-dose systemic corticosteroids can be immuno-suppressive; if such treatment is used, appropriate steps should be taken to monitor and prevent infection.

NEURO: Insomnia, nervousness, mood swings, psychoses
  (See Special Case: Adverse Effects Associated with Short Courses of Systemic Corticosteroids.)

SPECIAL CASE: Adverse Effects Associated with Short Courses of Systemic Corticosteroids

Little information is available regarding the risk of adverse effects related to short courses of systemic corticosteroids, and available studies used different products at varying doses. One epidemiological study suggests that children 4 to 17 years of age, who require more than four courses of oral corticosteroids per year (with an average duration 6.4 days) as treatment for underlying disease have an increased risk of fracture (van Staa et al., 2003). Another landmark study demonstrated and recommended that multiple short courses of oral corticosteroids (median four courses in the preceding year) in the treatment of asthma in children 2 to 17 years of age were not associated with any lasting effect on bone metabolism, bone mineralization, or adrenal function (Ducharme et al., 2003).

SPOTLIGHT ON COPD

COPD is a progressive lung disease characterized by the presence of airflow obstruction due to chronic bronchitis or emphysema. The airflow obstruction may be accompanied by airway hyperreactivity, and it may be partially reversible. Chronic bronchitis is defined clinically as the presence of a chronic productive cough for 3 months during each of 2 consecutive years, other causes of cough being excluded (Yawn and Keenan, 2007). Emphysema is defined as an abnormal, permanent enlargement of the air spaces distal to the terminal bronchioles, accompanied by destruction of their walls and without obvious fibrosis. Approximately 14.2 million people have COPD, approximately 12.5 million have chronic bronchitis, and 1.7 million have emphysema (Yawn and Keenan, 2007). The primary cause of COPD is cigarette smoking because it develops in 15% of cigarette smokers who have smoked at least 20 cigarettes per day for 20 or more years before COPD's common symptoms of cough, sputum, and dyspnea develop (Roeland, Sachs, and Verheij, 2007). Patients with more severe COPD display tachypnea and respiratory distress upon undertaking any activities requiring simple exertion.

Interactions

■ Insulin and oral hypoglycemics. Increased circulating levels of glucose may be seen with these agents, and thus adjustments to insulin or oral hypoglycemics would be warranted.
■ Ethanol should be avoided because it may increase gastric mucosal secretions.

Contraindications

■ Any condition in which there are serious fungal, viral, or tubercle skin infections.

Conscientious Considerations

■ In asthma patients, oral corticosteroids should only be used for short-term burst therapy of 3 to 10 days to gain control over inadequately controlled persistent asthma.
■ Long-term use will likely lead to adrenal suppression.
■ Dosing adjustment may be necessary in patients suffering from unusual stress, because stress may induce production of cortisol.
■ Because high-dose systemic corticosteroids can be immunosuppressive, if such treatment is used appropriate steps should be taken to monitor and prevent infection.
■ Today, the benefits of every-other-day dosing have been shown to be effective because the prevalence of side effects has dropped. However, inhaled costicosteroids do remain more effective than the oral alternate-day therapy.
■ Serum potassium and glucose maybe monitored.
■ Monitor patient for edema, weight change, BP, CHF, and mental status changes.

Patient/Family Education

■ Let patients know that if they experience GI upset, they may take medication with meals.
■ Instruct patients to minimize any side effects and prevent hoarseness and candidiasis by rinsing the mouth with water after each dose.

Medical Management of COPD
The goal of management is to improve daily living and quality of life by preventing symptoms and limiting the recurrence of exacerbations by preserving optimal lung function. Once the diagnosis of COPD is established, educate the patient about the disease. Encourage the patient to participate actively in therapy. Smoking cessation continues to be the most important therapeutic intervention.

Oral and inhaled medications are used for patients with stable disease to reduce dyspnea and improve exercise tolerance. Most of the medications employed are directed at four potentially reversible causes of airflow limitation in a disease state that has largely fixed obstruction: (1) bronchial smooth muscle contraction, (2) bronchial mucosal congestion and edema, (3) airway inflammation, and (4) increased airway secretion.

COPD patients who have no measurable increase in expiratory flow benefit from use of short-acting beta-2 agonists. However, beta-2 agonists produce less bronchodilatation in patients with COPD than in patients without it. Furthermore, spirometric changes may be insignificant despite symptomatic benefit; inhaled beta-2 agonists are commonly used for their effectiveness against acute exacerbations of COPD.

Long-Acting Bronchodilators Adding theophylline to use of a bronchodilator can result in further benefit in stable COPD. The response to theophylline therapy may vary among patients with severe COPD.

Anticholinergic Agents: Aerosolized anticholinergic agents (e.g., ipratropium bromide, Atrovent) are used primarily to treat COPD and not asthma, and in many cases it may be more effective than a beta-2 agonist. These agents are quaternary amines with a structure similar to atropine. Ipratropium is available as a single agent or combined with albuterol and packaged as Combivent.

Oral Steroids The use of corticosteroids requires a careful evaluation for individual patients who are on adequate bronchodilator therapy but who do not improve sufficiently or who develop an exacerbation. Experts suggest that long-term treatment of COPD patients with oral steroid therapy is not recommended (GOLD, 2005).

Inhaled Steroids Minority of COPD patients who respond to oral corticosteroids can be maintained on long-term inhaled steroids. Despite a lack of conclusive evidence to support the role of inhaled corticosteroids in the management of COPD, the use of these agents is widespread in spite of conflicting evidence of whether or not COPD patients' lung function benefits from either inhaled or oral corticosteroids (Kerstjens et al., 2005). As a result, inhaled corticosteroids are added much later in the therapy of COPD than they are in asthma. The anticholinergic bronchodilators, such as ipratropium (Atrovent), are started sooner in COPD than in asthma because of the greater responsiveness rate seen in COPD. Inhaled corticosteroids have fewer adverse effects than do oral corticosteroids. Although effective, these agents improve expiratory flows less

effectively than oral preparations, even at high doses. These agents may be beneficial in slowing the rate of progression in a subset of patients with COPD who have rapid decline.

Phosphodiesterase-4 Inhibitors Cilomilast and roflumilast are systemically available, second-generation, selective phosphodiesterase-4 inhibitors. They cause a reduction of the inflammatory process (macrophages and CD8+ lymphocytes) in patients with COPD.

Antibiotics In patients with COPD, chronic infections or colonizations with *Streptococcus pneumoniae, Haemophilus influenzae*, and *Moraxella catarrhalis* are common in the lower airways. Empiric antimicrobial therapy must be comprehensive and should cover all likely pathogens in the context of the clinical setting. The goal of antibiotic therapy in COPD is not to eliminate organisms, but rather to treat acute exacerbations.

Mucolytic Agents These agents reduce sputum viscosity and improve secretion clearance. Viscous lung secretions in patients with COPD consist of mucus-derived glycoproteins and leukocyte-derived DNA.

Oxygen Therapy COPD is commonly associated with progressive hypoxemia. Oxygen administration (therapy) reduces mortality rates in patients with advanced COPD because of the favorable effects on pulmonary hemodynamics. However, too much supplemental oxygen can reduce respiratory drive and cause additional harm to the patient. Thus, using a pulse oximeter or drawing arterial blood for an arterial blood gas (ABG) measurement is a fairly standard procedure to monitor for oxygen levels below 88%.

Emergency Care

Emergency department and hospital management of COPD is essentially the same as for asthma, but responses are often slower and less dramatic in the patient with COPD. (See Special Case: Differences Between the Treatment of Asthma and COPD.)

SPECIAL CASE: Differences Between the Treatment of Asthma and COPD

In the COPD patient there is *no* reversible asthma component, except during an acute exacerbation. This means the use of bronchodilators is likely to be unpredictable.

Theophylline may be more useful in COPD patients than in asthma patients, even though both asthma and COPD are inflammatory conditions. The use of cromolyn, nedocromil, and leukotriene inhibitors in COPD is not warranted.

Inhaled Anti-Inflammatory Agents: Mast Cell Stabilizers

These anti-inflammatory agents are synthetic compounds that inhibit antigen-induced bronchospasm. Although cromolyn was originally produced to be a bronchodilator, it has *no* bronchodilating activity; nevertheless, it does have activity as a mast cell stabilizer and antihistamine and thus is useful as an adjunct in the long-term control of allergic disorders, including rhinitis and asthma.

Conscientious Prescribing of Inhaled Anti-Inflammatory Agents (Mast Cell Stabilizers)

■ Reduction in dosage of other asthma medications may be possible after 2 to 4 weeks of therapy, thus patients need monitoring from the start of therapy.

■ Because these drugs are given prophylactically, it must be stressed and remembered that these medications are not used clinically for acute attacks.

■ To increase the effectiveness of these agents as an inhaled product, the clinician should consider pretreatment with bronchodilators as well.

Patient/Family Education for Inhaled Anti-Inflammatory Agents

■ Patients should be advised that they are to use the prescribed agents exactly as indicated and not to take them any more frequently than prescribed.

■ Missed doses should be taken as soon as remembered, and other doses should be spaced at regular intervals.

■ Patients should be told that the capsules containing these agents for inhalation should only be used with the proper inhalation devices.

■ Patients will need instruction on how to properly use their inhalation devices.

■ Patients should be advised that gargling and rinsing the mouth after each dose helps to decrease dryness of the mouth, hoarseness, and throat irritation.

■ Patients also should be advised that if their asthma begins to worsen, they need professional help.

Sodium Cromoglycates

Cromolyn (Intal) and nedocromil (Tilade) are chemically related drugs, **sodium chromoglycates,** that are administered by inhalation for the prophylaxis of mild or moderate asthma and allergic rhinitis. They have good safety profiles and thus are useful in treating children. Remember that neither drug has any bronchodilator effect, nor do they have any effect on inflammatory mediators already released into the body. Nedocromil appears to be more effective than cromolyn, but both drugs are used for prophylactic treatment, with nedocromil (Tilade) approved for asthma patients not controlled with beta agonists alone. **Note:** Both of these drugs were removed from the market in 2010 because they contained propellants that were depleting the ozone layer. Newer medicines, such as the leukotriene receptor agonists, have proven to be as effective without causing environmental harm.

Leukotriene Modifiers

Leukotriene modifiers were the first new class of agents approved by the U.S. Food and Drug Administration (FDA) for treatment of persistent asthma; by 2007 nearly one-third of all patients with persistent asthma were taking one of these agents (Scow, Luttermoser, & Dickerson, 2007). They are synthetic agents, developed from the metabolism of arachidonic acid in leukocytes. Also known as slow-reacting substances of inflammation, they help reverse the ability of leukotriene to constrict airway smooth muscle through inflammatory processes of asthma and allergy, including airway edema, smooth broncial-muscle constriction, and cellular changes.

There are two kinds of leukotriene modifiers available for the treatment of asthma: the leukotriene receptor agonists montelukast (Singulair) and zafirlukast (Accolate), and the 5-lipoxygenase (5-LO) inhibitor zileuton (Zyflo). Although there is little doubt there are advantages to their efficacy and once-a-day dosing, people's diverse response to them raise some questions.

Leukotriene Receptor Agonists (LTRAs)

There are two LTRAs currently available:

■ montelukast (Singulair), for patients 12 months of age and older

■ zafirlukast (Accolate), for patients 5 to 11 years of age, and adults (older than12 years of age)

Leukotriene receptor agonists are not the preferred drugs for treating mild persistent asthma, but when zafirlukast is used in chronic asthma in adults and children older than 5 years of age, it provides a dual benefit by being *both* an anti-inflammatory drug and a bronchodilator. Montelukast is used in the treatment of asthma, but unlike zafirlukast, it is approved for use in children 12 months and older. Both drugs have found some favor in

inhibiting bronchoconstriction in cases in which it is caused by specific antigens such as grass, cat dander, and ragweed.

Mechanism of Action

Montelukast is a selective competitive antagonist of the cysteinyl-leukotriene receptor and another receptor, D4, whereas zafirlukast is a synthetic, selective, and competitive inhibitor of leukotriene receptors D4 and E4. They are receptors associated with airway edema, smooth muscle constriction, and altered cellular activity involved in inflammatory processes where both agents demonstrate they can antagonize the contractile activity in the conducting airway smooth muscle. Montelukast may also inhibit symptoms of allergic rhinitis because leukotrienes are released into nasal mucosa under exposure to allergens causing allergic rhinitis. To put it more simply, montelukast and zafirlukast inhibit an enzyme responsible for producing the inflammatory response to leukotrienes by blocking the leukotrienes' receptor, which would make broncho constriction possible.

Pharmacokinetics

■ Absorption: Rapid absorption after taking orally, but food reduces absorption; thus, it must be taken on an empty stomach.

■ Distribution: Protein binding is 90% to 99%, with peak concentration occurring in 3 hours.

■ Metabolism: Metabolized extensively by the liver's cytochrome P450 pathway with metabolites being almost inactive.

■ Excretion: If metabolized, excreted in urine, if not excreted in the feces.

■ Half-life: Zafirlukast: 10 hours; montelukast: 2.5 to 5.5 hours.

Dosage and Administration

Generic Name	Trade Name	Dosage
zafirlukast	Accolate	20 mg, 2 times/day both in children and adults over 12 and 10 mg 2 times/day if the child is between age 5 and 11
montelukast	Singulair	10 mg once a day for both adults and children over 15 years of age. If child is 12 months to 5 years old, give 4 mg/day; if 6 to 14 years old, give 5 mg once a day

Clinical Uses

■ For long-term control and prevention of symptoms in mild persistent asthma.

■ Zafirlukast is used in chronic asthma in children age 5 or older, whereas montelukast can be used in children 12 months and older.

■ For moderate persistent asthma, it may also be used with inhaled corticosteroids as combination therapy.

■ Some prescribers like to use these drugs in children and adults who demonstrate a great deal of nocturnal symptoms of asthma.

Adverse Reactions

EENT: Pharyngitis, rhinitis

GI: Gastritis, GI upset; rare but serious liver dysfunction can occur.

HEM: Eosinophil conditions

NEURO: Headache, weakness

PUL: Cough, may cause CHURG-STRAUSS syndrome (a rare pulmonary vasculitis).

Interactions

■ Zafirlukast has a high drug interaction potential. The clinician should always order a patient drug screen before using these medications because any agent metabolized by CYP2C9, a cytochrome P450 enzyme, will interact. For example, coadministration of a drug metabolized in the liver's CYP450 system with zafirlukast results in about a 45% increase in plasma zafirlukast. Coadministration of zafirlukast with aspirin increases plasma concentration of zafirlukast, and coadministration of zafirlukast with erythromycin decreases plasma levels of zafirlukast.

Contraindications

■ Active liver disease or any impaired liver function

Conscientious Considerations

■ These drugs should not be used to treat acute asthma.
■ Use of either drug must be used with caution in any patients who are suspected of heavy alcohol use.
■ Because increased incidences of infection can occur, especially in patients over age 55, the use of these agents in these patients must be evaluated.

Patient/Family Education

■ Instruct the patient that these drugs should be taken regularly, even during symptom-free periods, and that routine pulmonary function tests will be required.
■ Remind patients not to use these drugs to treat acute episodes of asthma.

Oxygenase Inhibitors (5-Lipoxygenase Inhibitors)

Zileuton (Zyflo, Zyflo CR) is used in the long-term management of asthma, but its mechanism of action is different from the other two leukotriene receptor agonists because it is a leukotriene synthesis inhibitor. However, it is only approved for use in those over 12 years of age because it is metabolized in the liver by the cytochrome P450 system, and it is likely to have associated drug interactions.

Mechanism of Action

Zileuton blocks the production of leukotriene B4, another arachidonic acid metabolite with proinflammatory activity. It suppresses synthesis of the leukotrienes by inhibiting 5-lipoxygenase, a key enzyme in the conversion of arachidonic acid to leukotrienes. Thus, it is an agent that is often considered along with zafirlukast and montelukast as a "mast cell stabilizer" because it has the same issues and side effects as do the other two drugs in the LTRA category.

Pharmacokinetics

■ Absorption: Rapid
■ Distribution: Well with 93% protein binding
■ Metabolism: Metabolized in liver spilling several metabolites back into plasma and urine

■ Excretion: Better than 95% in urine as metabolites.
■ Half-life: 2.5 hours

Dosage and Administration

Generic Name	Trade Name	Dosage in Those Over 12 Years of Age
zileuton	Zyflo CR*	600 mg Zyflo CR twice a day and within 1 hr of morning and evening meals

*CR means "controlled release."

Clinical Uses

■ For long-term control of mild persistent asthma in those older than 12 years of age.
■ For moderate persistent asthma in patients older than 12 years old, it may be used with inhaled corticosteroids as combination therapy.

Adverse Reactions

■ It is associated with elevation of liver enzymes (see Conscientious Considerations, p. 172, for monitoring).

Interactions

■ Any drug that is CP450 metabolized.
■ Theophylline interacting with zileuton will cause a doubling in serum concentration.

Conscientious Considerations

■ These drugs should not be used to treat acute asthma.
■ Liver dysfunction occurs rarely and may manifest as right upper-quadrant pain, nausea, fatigue, lethargy, pruritus, jaundice, and flu-like symptoms.
■ Transaminase levels must be monitored periodically during the first year of prolonged therapy to monitor for liver damage. Monitor alanine aminotransferase (ALT) every 3 months for first year, then periodically thereafter, due to the association of this drug with elevation of liver enzymes.

Patient/Family Education

■ Instruct patients not to use the drug in acute episodes of asthma.
■ Instruct patient that the drug must be taken regularly, even if there are no symptoms.

Monoclonal Antibodies

Monoclonal antibodies are antibodies produced by a single clone of cells; therefore, they are a single, pure, homogenous type of antibody. Because they can be produced in large amounts in a laboratory using a modified fermentation process, they have become the cornerstone of immunology because they have allowed long-lived cell lines to make antibodies of a single kind. Thus, given almost any substance, it is possible to create monoclonal antibodies that specifically bind to that substance; they can then serve to detect or purify that substance. This has become an important tool in biochemistry, molecular biology, and medicine. When used as medications, by convention their generic names end in "-mab"; for example, omalizumab.

Omalizumab (Xolair)

Omalizumab was the first monoclonal antibody approved for use in patients over age 12 with moderate to severe allergic asthma caused by year-round allergens in the air. It will reduce the number of asthma attacks per year, even though the patient is taking inhaled corticosteroids that may not appear to be controlling the asthma.

Mechanism of Action

This monoclonal antibody selectively binds to human immunoglobulin E (IgE) receptors on mast cells and eosinophils, preventing release of mediators to the allergic response. Its effect, then, is to prevent or reduce the number of exacerbations of asthma.

Pharmacokinetics

- Absorption: Given as a SC injection, the drug is slowly absorbed from its site.
- Distribution: Circulating protein in serum.
- Metabolism: Hepatic degradation.
- Excretion: Hepatic as well as reticuloendothelial system.
- Half-Life: 26 days, but time to peak effect is 7 to 8 days.

Dosage and Administration

Adults, elderly, and children 12 years and older: 150 to 375 mg SC, every 2 to 4 weeks, with the dosing and frequency individualized based on weight and pretreatment immunoglobulin levels.

Clinical Use

- Moderate to severe persistent asthma in those patients who are reactive to a perennial allergen and in whom asthma symptoms are not controlled by inhaled corticosteroids.

Adverse Reactions

DERM: Urticaria around injection site
EENT: Sinusitis, pharyngitis
MISC: Malignant neoplasms, viral infections, ANAPHYLAXIS
NEURO: Headache

Interactions

- None have been noted.

Contraindications

- Hypersensitivities to the monoclonal antibody are rare, but use them cautiously in those under 12 years of age because safety has not been established.

Conscientious Considerations

- This drug should not be used to control acute episodes of asthma.
- If dosing a patient after a year has lapsed, do not retest serum IgE levels; rather, use the initial levels to determine dosing.

Patient/Family Education

- Instruct patients not to use the medication in acute episodes of asthma.
- Inform the patient who is starting on omalizumab that systemic or inhaled corticosteroids should not be stopped abruptly.
- Advise patients not to change the dose of or discontinue any other medication because they are on omalizumab.
- Let patients know that immediate improvements may not be noticeable after beginning therapy.
- Inform patients that because the solution is slightly viscous it may take 5 to 10 seconds to administer.
- Instruct patients that, once it is reconstituted, this is one medication that needs to be stored in the refrigerator (36° to 46°F).

Combination Products

Some manufacturers prepare fixed doses of two active ingredients and offer them as one product. The rationale for these products is that the clinician is assured the patient is getting the right dose of each medication at the right time and that adherence rates will climb. On the other hand, many clinicians believe this offers little in the way of specialization of a therapeutic regimen on a patient-by-patient basis. The rationale that the combination product saves the patient money over buying two single products does not always prove to be true. But combining a bronchodilator and an anti-inflammatory for adherence reasons has some merit, especially among adolescents. Salmeterol/fluticasone (Advair) is one example of a popular product combining a bronchodilator and an anti-inflammatory, as is albuterol/ipratropium (Combivent).

Combivent combination product is approved for use in COPD, as well as asthma, as a long-term controller medication. This combination product provides 90 mcg of albuterol per activation. The patient is to use 1 to 2 inhalations every 4 to 6 hours. Contraindications include heart disease, high blood pressure, congestive heart failure, and seizure disorders. Patients who are allergic to soybeans, peanuts, or any other food containing soy lethica should not use Combivent. The canister of any metered dose inhaler should be stored away from heat because even the heat of the sun on a closed car can raise the temperature and cause the canister to burst.

Combination Products Using Inhaled Steroids

These combination steroid products have clinical differences in potency; consequently, equal doses of these products should not be expected to produce clinically equivalent effects. Thus, dosing regimens must be adjusted when switching from one inhaled corticosteroid to another. Furthermore, the delivery device used for these corticosteroids influences their effect. They are available as metered dose inhalers, dry powder inhalers, or both, or they may be packaged for intranasal use. The inhalers' propellants were traditional chlorofluorocarbons (CFCs), but in keeping with a worldwide ban on such propellants, they have been reformulated using non-CFC propellants, requiring that each manufacturer apply for FDA approval. A recent example of a drug approved for use in the United States is Dulera, a combination of formoterol and mometasone. Dulera has been advertised to reduce the wheezing of asthma, but it is not approved as a rescue inhaler nor for use in children under age 12.

AGENTS USED TO TREAT CHRONIC AND SEASONAL ALLERGIC RHINITIS

Asthma and allergic rhinitis are two of the most common diseases of modern society and to a great extent a major cause of illness, loss of productivity, hospitalization, and even death. The inhaled and intranasal corticosteroids such as beclomethasone, fluticasone, and mometasone remain the drug of choice for these conditions because these newer corticosteroids have better pharmacokinetic properties that provide target-specific delivery, especially in intranasal form. With higher concentrations working at sites of action, they minimize systemic exposure and subsequent side effects. The oral steroids can be effective in severe cases and if they are used infrequently. For example, some clinicians use 40 mg prednisone to start and then taper it down over 10 days. Other agents used in allergic rhinitis are antihistamines and antitussives for cough.

Antihistamines

There are three classes of histamine antagonists: H1, H2, and H3. The H1 group was introduced during the 1930s at a time when the classification of histamine receptors was not known. Today the term *antihistamine* refers, by convention, to the H1 receptors because they affect various anti-inflammatory and allergic mechanisms. The more recently developed H2 receptor antagonists have their main clinical effect on gastric secretions. Several H3 receptor agonists have been developed for use in CNS conditions.

The list of antihistamines used in allergic rhinitis is long. It may include single formulations of one antihistamine such as azelastine (Astelin), brompheniramine (Dimetane, Dimetapp), cetirizine (Zyrtec), and clemastine (Tavist OTC). The number of formulations with two or more ingredients is lengthy and beyond the scope of this work, with most being OTC and some being prescription medications. The prescription antihistamines tend to be less sedating but are more expensive.

Mechanism of Action

The H1 receptor antagonists decrease histamine-mediated contraction of the smooth muscle of the bronchi, intestine, and uterus. As chemicals, they are piperidine derivatives, for example, fexofenadine, desloratadine, or ethanolamine (diphenhydramine), and are structurally similar to histamine, thus competing with histamine for H1 receptor sites on affected cells.

Pharmacokinetics

■ Absorption: Rapidly absorbed after oral administration (13 to 30 minutes).
■ Distribution: About 60% to 70% is protein bound.
■ Metabolism: Minimal for all, but exception is desloratadine, which is extensively metabolized by first-pass mechanism into an active metabolite.
■ Excretion: Fexofenadine, desloratadine, and loratadine are eliminated in both feces and urine, whereas the others are primarily excreted in the urine.
■ Half-Life: Wide ranging. Fexofenadine: 14.4 hours; desloratadine: 27 hours; cetirizine: 6.5 to 10 hours; brompheniramine: 25 hours; diphenhydramine: 1-4 hours. Clemastine half-life is unknown.

Dosage and Administration

	Generic Name	Trade Name	Dosage*	Special Instructions
FIRST GENERA-TION	brompheniramine	Dimetane	Adults: 4 mg PO, every 4–6 hr	With or without food
	clemastine	Tavist	Adults: 1 mg, 2 times/day	Dose without regard to meals
	chlorpheniramine	Chlor-Trimeton	Adults: 4 mg, every 4–6 hr	Dose without regard to meals
	diphenhydramine	Benadryl	25–50 mg, every 4–6 hr	Dose without regard to meals; may cause drowsiness
SECOND GENERA-TION	cetirizine	Zyrtec	5–10 mg once a day	Food may delay absorption
	desloratadine	Clarinex	5 mg once a day	Use cautiously in renal impairment, geriatrics, children <12 yr.
	fexofenadine	Allegra	60 mg, 2 times/day	Dose without regard to meals
	loratadine	Claritin	10 mg once a day	Dose without regard to meals
	levocetirizine	Xyzal	5 mg once a day in the evening	Avoid alcohol or sedatives and do not use in children <12 yr

*Note: Dosage for adults applies to children over age 12.

Clinical Uses

■ Prevents allergic responses mediated by histamine, such as rhinitis and urticaria

Adverse Reactions

CV: Some potential for QT prolongation
GI: Nausea, vomiting, abdominal distress
GYN: Dysmenorrhea
NEURO: Somnolence, headache, fatigue

Interactions

■ Antacids with Ca and Mg will decrease absorption

Contraindications

None known

Conscientious Considerations

■ No one antihistamine has an advantage over another, and most are available OTC.
■ Antihistamines such as chlorpheniramine have a higher incidence of sedation but are less expensive.
■ Antihistamines such as diphenhydramine are quite sedating and are often used as sleep aids, but the elderly are very susceptible to their drug reactions and anticholinergic effects, such as delirium, acute confusion, dizziness, dry mouth, blurry vision, tachycardia, urinary retention, and constipation.

Patient/Family Education

■ Advise patients that despite some antihistamines being promoted as "nondrowsy," all antihistamines are capable of producing drowsiness to a certain degree.

Antitussives

The primary agents that affect the cough center are codeine and dextromethorphan. However, use of codeine has diminished because it is a controlled substance with more potential for abuse, and one of its side effects is constipation. The antitussive most commonly used today is dextromethorphan bromide. It is sold in many OTC combination products such as Vicks and Robitussin. The label of these OTC products should be read carefully because in many cases the dosage is likely too small to produce cough suppression.

Mechanism of Action

Dextromethorphan is a chemical in the morphine family, that is, a D-isomer of levorphanol, but it has none of the addicting properties of morphine. It acts on the cough center in the medulla oblongata by elevating its threshold for the cough reflex. It is one-half as effective as codeine.

Pharmacokinetics

- Absorption: Rapidly absorbed from the GI tract.
- Distribution: Into the cerebrospinal fluid.
- Metabolism: In the liver, it is metabolized to dextrorphan, an active metabolite.
- Excretion: Both unmetabolized dextromethorphan and the metabolite dextrorphan are excreted renally.
- Half-life: Parent compound: 1.2 to 3.9 hours; with metabolites, 5 hours.

Dosage and Administration

Category	Generic	Trade	Route	Dosage
Pain reducer/ antihistamine	acetamino-phen 325 mg/ chlorpheni-ramine 4 mg	Coricidin	PO	Do not give to child under 4 y/o
Antitussives antihistamine/ antitussive	dextromethor-phan/ diphenhy-dramine	Delsym	PO	1 tsp every 12 hr*
		Duratuss DM	PO	1 tsp every 5 hr†
Antitussives/ expectorant	guaifenesin/ hydrocodone bitartrate (RX only)	Hycotuss	PO	1 tsp not less than 4 hr apart‡ **Note:** Can be habit forming
Antitussives/ Antihistamine	hydrocodone 10 mg/ chlorpheni-ramine 8 mg/ 5 mL	Tussionex	PO extended-release suspension	1 tsp every 12 hr, but not for children under age 6§
Antitussive	Benzonatate	Tessalon	PO 100-mg capsules	100 mg three times/ day for adults and children over 10
Antitussive	Hydrocodone‖	Hycodan	PO 5-mg tabs and 5-mg/ tsp syrup	5 mg every 4–6 hr as needed

*Delsym is different from other formulations in that it is a 12-hour extended-release formulation. Delsym is 30-mg dextromethorphan/5 mL tsp and needs dosage adjustments for any child under 5 years of age

†Duratuss is not recommended for children under age 4.

‡Hycotuss DM is not recommended for children under age 2.

§Tussionex Children 6 to 12 maybe given one-half teaspoon.

‖U.S. formulations of hydrocodone also contain homatropine. Hydrocodone is believed to be 8 to 10 times more potent than codeine.

Clinical Uses

- Cough suppression, throat irritation. As a cough suppressant, it is one-half as effective as codeine. It is less constipating than codeine, but some literature states this is only marginally so.
- It is often combined with benzocaine (a local anesthetic) in throat lozenges to block the pain from throat irritation when coughing.

Adverse Reactions

GI: Abdominal discomfort, constipation, GI upset, nausea
NEURO: Dizziness, drowsiness

Interactions

- MAOIs. Antitussives potentiate the activity of MAOIs by increasing the risk of toxicity, which manifests as hypotension and coma.
- Phenelzine
- Antitussives and alcohol potentiate each other and can lead to respiratory distress.

Contraindications

- Concurrent MAOI use.
- Hypersensitivity to these agents is especially common in children.

Conscientious Considerations

- Overdose may manifest as muscle spasticity, increase or decrease in BP, blurry vision, blue lips, hallucinations, and respiratory depression.
- Because dextromethorphan is the D-isomer of levorphanol, it lacks CNS activity, but it does act at the cough center in the medulla. Its chemistry, however, makes the substance easily manipulated by "bathtub chemists" for substance abuse users.
- Dextromethorphan is often combined with benzocaine in a lozenge. The benzocaine is used to block pain from coughing. However, the effective strength of either drug in an OTC product is highly controversial because, as a cough suppressant, it is one-half as effective as codeine (thus it is less constipating than codeine).

Patient/Family Education

- Advise patients not to drink alcohol when taking these drugs because they potentiate each other and can lead to respiratory distress.
- Advise patients of the dangers of any of these drugs to children and why, if they are used in children, a significant dosage change is needed.

INTRANASAL PRODUCTS

It has been increasingly popular to supply active ingredients directly to the rich blood supply in the nasal passages. Following are some such products made available because of new technologies in drug delivery systems.

Category	Generic Name	Trade Name	Usual Adult Daily Dose (Mg)
antihistamine	azelastine	Astelin	2 sprays, 2 times/day
anticholinergic	ipratropium bromide	Atrovent	2 sprays, 3 times/day
sympathomimetic	oxymetazoline	Afrin	2 sprays, 2 times/day
steroid	beclomethasone	Beconase AQ	2 sprays, 2 times/day
steroid	triamcinolone	Nasacort AQ	2 sprays, daily
steroid	budesonide	Rhinocort Aqua	2 sprays, daily
steroid	fluticasone	Flonase, Veramyst	2 sprays, daily
steroid	mometasone	Nasonex	2 sprays, daily
steroid	ciclesonide (see Special Case: Ciclesonide [Omnaris])	Omnaris	2 sprays, daily

SPECIAL CASE: Ciclesonide (Omnaris)

This drug is a nonhalogenated glucocorticoid prodrug that is hydrolyzed, following intranasal administration, to an active metabolite, des-ciclesonide by the cytochrome p450 system in the liver. However, these drugs are also metabolized in the nasal mucosa or lungs by local esterases before systemic routes take the drug to be metabolized in the liver. This causes it to have a high affinity for the glucocorticoid receptors. As an agent in allergic rhinitis, its exact mechanism of action is unknown, but it is believed to be the combination of three important characteristics: an anti-inflammatory action, and immunosuppressive action, and an antiproliferation property. Its activity begins in 24 to 48 hours, with improvement seen in 1 to 2 weeks if treating seasonal rhinitis, or in 5 weeks if treating perennial allergic rhinitis.

SPOTLIGHT ON SEASONAL ALLERGIC RHINITIS

Rhinitis, like asthma, is an inflammatory condition, but of the nasal mucous membranes. It is characterized by nasal discharge, congestion, and sneezing. The vasodilatation that occurs owing to the inflammation causes mucosal congestion and edema to appear. When rhinitis is triggered as a result of allergens (allergic rhinitis) conjunctivitis and itching of the nose, eyes, ears, and palate are commonly seen.

Medical Management
Drug therapy for allergic rhinitis rests on using antihistamines, but often decongestants are combined with antihistamines because antihistamines have no decongestant effect. Should no relief occur from use of antihistamine, intranasal cromolyn (NasalCrom 4%) can be used for mild to moderate cases, intranasal corticosteroids for severe symptoms, and antitussives if a dry cough is keeping the patient awake. A patient experiencing a productive cough (one with active mucus) should never be told to suppress this natural defense system of the body to rid itself of invading organisms.

Nonpharmacological treatment (humidifiers, drinking hot liquids, saline irrigation) also provides relief. The common comorbidities of asthma and allergic rhinitis have led to the concept of "one airway-one disease" and the need for one common approach. Because of the need for optimal treatment, the Allergic Rhinitis and Its Impact on Asthma (ARIA) group, in collaboration with the World Health Organization (WHO), is recommending that patients who are treated for allergic rhinitis should also be evaluated for asthma, and vice versa (Chul et al., 2007). This approach gives the best opportunity for drug treatment strategies to be optimal in terms of efficacy and safety.

Implications for Special Populations

Pregnancy Implications

When prescribing drugs affecting the respiratory system for the pregnant female, clinicians should carefully consider their choice of drugs. Following is a selected list of drugs, along with the assigned FDA Safety Category.

FDA PREGNANCY RISK FACTOR CATEGORY	DRUGS
B	cromolyn, ipratropium, nedocromil, zafirlukast, omalizumab
C	albuterol, steroids (beclomethasone, flunisolide triamcinolone), isoproterenol, theophylline, zileuton, antihistamines (azelastine, etc.) dextromethorphan, metaproterenol, salmeterol, formoterol
D	None

Pediatric Implications

■ Periodic pulmonary function tests are indicated.
■ Many products are not approved for use in children under 2 years of age. Special dosing is needed for children under 12 years of age.

Geriatric Implications

Therapeutic recommendations for treatment of COPD are not age specific but rather age modified according to the patient's overall health assessment. A host of age-related changes can occur in the respiratory system, such as loss of respiratory reserve capacity in the lung, which makes for inadequate responsiveness to stressors. A loss of height (osteoporosis) due to aging can lead to a decrease in lung volume. Neurological conditions can lead to loss of the swallowing reflex.

Among older adults, COPD is more prevalent than asthma, but polypharmacy must be assessed as a potential contributor affecting treatment outcomes for both diseases because it can lead to many adverse drug interactions, especially with inhaled agents. Additionally, bronchodilator response to inhaled beta-2 antagonists does decline with age. Because asthma and COPD are characterized by airflow obstruction, distinguishing between these diseases is difficult in the older adult, and many clinicians undertreat, misdiagnose, and misperceive asthma as it being a disease of young people.

LEARNING EXERCISES

Case 1

JO is a 62-year-old black male with chronic asthma. He has been experiencing frequent shaving cuts that bleed quite a bit. The patient reveals that he has been on Coumadin for 5 years initiated as a result of a stroke and that he has had asthma since childhood. You also learn that the patient recently had oral theophylline added to his decades' old asthma regimen of an inhaled corticosteroid and beta-2 adrenoreceptor agonist salmeterol (Serevent). He reports that this new regimen has considerably cut down on the frequency and severity of any asthma episodes. What do you think is the reason for the patient's bleeding problems?

Case 2

A group of health professions students are working in a clinic. Their preceptor calls them together and introduces them to a teenage girl who has just been diagnosed with moderate asthma. He turns to the first student and says, "What would be the standard of care for treating her asthma?" Student A replies, "I think she should be started on theophylline, an older but safer drug, but she also needs an exercise regimen." Student B student interrupts the conversation and says, "I think a better therapy to start a teenager on would be an inhaled bronchodilators and avoid all steroids." Student C chimes in and says, "I think she needs to get her inflammation under control first by starting on inhaled corticosteroids." Student D responds, "You are all wrong. She needs to start out with a combination regimen that includes inhaled bronchodilators and inhaled corticosteroids." Which of these students is correct?

References

Allen, D. B. (2002). Safety of inhaled corticosteroids in children. *Pediatric Pulmonology, 33*(3), 208-220.

American Academy of Allergy, Asthma, and Immunization (AAAI). (2010). Tips to Remember: Peak Flow Meter. Retrieved January 23, 2012, from www.aaaai.org/patients/publicedmat/tips/whatispeakflowmeter.stm

Chul, H. L., Jeong, H. J., Hyun, J. L., Kim, I. T., Kim, C. D., Won, Y. S., et al. (2008). Clinical characteristics of allergic rhinitis according to allergic rhinitis and its impact on asthma guidelines. *Clinical & Experimental Otorhinolaryngology, 1*(4), 196–200. Retrieved January 23, 2013, from www.ncbi.nlm.nih.gov/pmc/articles/PMC2671762/

Ducharme, F. M., Chabot, G., Polychronakos, D., Glorieux, F., & Mazer, B. (2003). Safety profile of frequent short courses of oral glucocorticoids in the acute pediatric asthma, *Pediatrics, 111*(2), 376-384.

Global Initiative for Chronic Obstructive Lung Disease (GOLD). (December, 2011). Executive summary. In *Global Strategy for the Diagnosis, Management, and Prevention of Chronic Obstructive Pulmonary Disease* (GOLD). Retrieved January 28, 2013, from www.goldcopd.org/guidelines-global-strategy-for-diagnosis-management.html

Kerstjens, H. A. M., Postma, D. S., ten Hacken n., Rabe, K. F., Kiri, V., Visick, G. T., et al. (2005). Chronic obstructive pulmonary disease. *Clinical Evidence, *(13), 1923-1947.

Mayo Clinic. (2010). Childhood Asthma: Creating an Asthma Action Plan. Retrieved January 23, 2013, from www.mayoclinic.com/health/asthma/HQ00273

Medline Plus. (2010). U.S. National Library of Medicine, National Institutes of Health. Asthma. Retrieved January 23, 2013, from www.nlm.nih.gov/medlineplus/ency/article/000141.htm

National Heart Lung and Blood Institute, (2007). *Expert Panel Report (EPR-3): Guidelines for the Diagnosis and Management of Asthma. Clinical Practice Guidelines.* Retrieved January 23, 2013, from www.ncbi.nlm.nih.gov/books/NBK7232

PubMed Health (May, 2011). Chronic Obstructive Pulmonary Disease. Retrieved January 28, 2013, from www.ncbi.nlm.nih.gov/pubmedhealth/PMH0001153

Roeland, M. M., Sachs, A. P. E., & Verheij, T. J. M. (2006). Incidence and determinants of COPD in male smokers aged 40–65 years, a 5 year study. *The British Journal of General Practice, 56*(530), 656-661. Retrieved January 23, 2013, from www.ncbi.nlm.nih.gov/pmc/articles/PMC1876630

Scow, D. T., Luttermoser, G. K., & Dickerson, K. S. (2007). Leukotriene inhibitors in the treatment of allergy and asthma. *American Family Physician, 75*(1), 65-67.

Van Staa, T. P., Cooper, M. A., Leufkens, H. G. M., & Bishop, N. (2003). Children and the risk of fractures caused by oral corticosteroids. *Journal of Bone and Mineral Research, 18*(5), 913-918.

World Allergy Organization (WAO), Scarupa, M. D., & Kaliner, M. A. (2006). In-Depth Review of Allergic Rhinitis. Retrieved January 23, 2013, from www.worldallergy.org/professional/allergic_diseases_center/rhinitis/rhinitis_indepth.php

Yawn, B. P., & Keenan, J. M. (2007). COPD: The primary care perspective; addressing epidemiology, pathology, diagnosis, treatment of smoking's multiple morbidities and the patient's perspective. *COPD 4*, 67–83.

Drugs Used in the Treatment of Common Disorders of the Gastrointestinal System

chapter 11

Mona M. Sedrak, Dipesh Patel

CHAPTER FOCUS

This chapter is designed to assist the learner in developing a working knowledge of pharmacological agents commonly used to treat gastrointestinal diseases and disorders. The therapeutic options for the treatment of gastroesophageal reflux disease (GERD) and peptic ulcers are discussed, including antacids, histamine-2 blockers, proton pump inhibitors, and cytoprotective agents. Agents used as antidiarrheals, laxatives, and antiemetics are also discussed. Finally, this chapter presents the drugs used to treat inflammatory bowel disease, the 5-aminosalicylate (5-ASA) products, and the anticholinergics and antispasmodics used for treating irritable bowel disease.

OBJECTIVES

After reading and studying this chapter, the student should be able to:

1. Define dyspepsia and gastroesophageal reflux disease.
2. Describe the therapeutic options in the treatment of gastroesophageal reflux disease.
3. State the pharmacological interventions involved in the treatment of *Helicobacter pylori*.
4. Recall the mechanism of action, clinical uses, adverse reactions, and contraindications of antacids, histamine-2 (H2) blockers, cytoprotective agents, and proton pump inhibitors.
5. List the causes of chronic constipation and the different types of laxatives, their mechanism of action, and adverse effects.
6. Differentiate between irritable bowel disease and inflammatory bowel disease.
7. Explain the difference between step-up therapy and step-down therapy in the treatment of gastroesophageal reflux disease and inflammatory bowel disease.
8. Discuss the drugs used in the treatment of nausea and vomiting and their mechanism of action, adverse effects, and contraindications.
9. Explain the use of orlistat in the treatment of obesity.

Key Terms

Anticholinergic
Constipation
Diarrhea
Dyspepsia
Emesis
Fecal impaction
Helicobacter pylori
Inflammatory bowel disease
Irritable bowel syndrome
Laxatives
Step-down therapy
Step-up therapy

KEY DRUGS IN THIS CHAPTER

Drugs Used as Antiemetics
dimenhydrinate (Dramamine, Gravol)
meclizine (Antivert, Bonine)
odansetron (Zofran)
promethazine (Phenergan)
prochlorperazine (Compazine)
scopolamine (Scopace)

Drugs Used to Alleviate Diarrhea
bismuth subsalicylate (Kaopectate)
difenoxin hydrochloride with atropine sulfate (Motofen)

diphenoxylate hydrochloride with atropine sulfate (Lomotil)
loperamide hydrochloride (Imodium)

Drugs Used in the Treatment of Gastroesophageal Reflux Disease (GERD) and Peptic Ulcer Disease (PUD)
Antacids
magnesium hydroxide (Dulcolax Milk of Magnesia)
aluminum hydroxide (Alu-Tab, Amphojel)

calcium carbonate (Rolaids, Tums)
sodium citrate (Citra pH)
sodium bicarbonate
Histamine-2 Receptor Antagonists/Blockers
cimetidine (Tagamet)
ranitidine (Zantac)
famotidine (Pepcid)
nizatidine (Axid)
Proton Pump Inhibitors
dexlansoprol (Dexilant)
omeprazole (Losec, Prilosec)

continued

A broad ranging and wide variety of drugs are available for treating disorders within the gastrointestinal tract. Some drugs are simple, such as the cholinergic drugs that increase gastric acid secretion and increase peristalsis or the **anticholinergic** drugs that inhibit acid production (antacids) and inhibit peristalsis (antidiarrheals). Some agents, such as polyethylene glycol (PEG), bismuth subsalicylate, and stool softeners, are inert chemicals that change the environment inside the gastrointestinal (GI) tract. Several groups of drugs are exclusive to the GI tract, such as the histamine-2 (H2) blockers and the proton pump inhibitors (PPI), which are acid-suppressive agents rather than acid neutralizers. The GI tract can also become inflamed and there are agents specific for this problem (5-aminosalicylates). This chapter introduces the learner to a wide variety of agents used to treat nausea, vomiting, and diarrhea, the three most common complaints of GI disorders. These symptoms are also the most commonly reported adverse reactions to most agents. Therefore, the clinician is challenged to make an accurate diagnosis of GI disorders, the key to effective prescribing.

DRUGS USED AS ANTIEMETICS

Nausea and vomiting (**emesis**), which have many causes, are common complaints in primary care medicine. Treatment is often nonpharmacological, but antiemetics may be used to provide some symptom relief and prevent fluid and electrolyte disturbances. Drug classes with antihistamine properties that are used for nausea and vomiting include antihistamines, phenothiazines, and sedative hypnotics. The drugs most commonly used for antiemetic properties include prochlorperazine (Compazine), promethazine (Phenergan), and ondansetron (Zofran). For the nausea associated with motion sickness, the antihistamine meclizine (Antivert, Bonine) and the anticholinergic scopolamine (hyoscine) are often used (Box 11-1). Scopolamine, which is available as a transdermal patch, is also used to prevent motion sickness. It can also be given intramuscularly, subcutaneously, and intravenously to manage nausea associated with opioid use or general anesthesia.

Conscientious Prescribing of Antiemetics

■ For short-term treatment of nausea and vomiting caused by drugs' adverse effects, metabolic disorders, and gastroenteritis, the phenothiazines are a good choice as a single dose or for short-term use. The phenothiazines are available in a variety

---

BOX 11-1 Treatment of Motion Sickness

For treatment of nausea associated with motion sickness, the antihistamine meclizine (Bonine) is popular as an OTC choice as well as in its prescription-strength format, Antivert. Bonine and Antivert differ in their dosages: Bonine is given 25 mg once a day, and Antivert is given as 12.5 mg or 25 mg up to three times a day. As an antihistamine, it should be avoided in individuals with narrow-angle glaucoma.

For short trips, the most widely used agent is dimenhydrinate (Dramamine). Available without a prescription, Dramamine is usually dosed as 50 or 100 mg every 4 hours, but no more than 400 mg in 24 hours.

The scopolamine patch (Transderm-Scop), which is applied to the skin behind the ear every 3 days, is a preferable choice for many who have longer trips. For longer periods of motion (boat rides, cruises), the patch should be applied 4 to 8 hours before the trip.

The side effects of these medications include blurry vision, dry mouth, and drowsiness. Caution should be used when prescribing these medications for the elderly, because they can cause confusion and hallucination in this age group.

Finally, there is growing interest in using ginger tea as an herbal remedy for motion sickness.

of dosage forms, including suppositories, which can be useful for the patient who is nauseated.

■ Nausea and vomiting are usually self-limiting.

■ Before drug therapy begins, there should be a clear indication for their use and for correction of fluid and electrolyte imbalances.

■ If treatment with phenothiazines is to last several days, a complete blood count (CBC) count before and during therapy is needed to monitor for blood dyscrasias that tend to occur from week 4 to 10 of therapy.

Patient/Family Education for Patients Using Antiemetics

■ Advise the patient that these agents are for short-term use only and that they usually work on the first dose.

■ Resting the GI tract is usually a good option, done by taking clear fluids in small amounts for about 8 hours.

■ Instruct the patient that the phenothiazines will turn the urine a red or pink color, but this is harmless.

■ Prochlorperazine can be given with food, milk, or a full glass of water to minimize GI distress. If using the syrup dosage form, dilute in citrus- or chocolate-flavored drinks.

■ If a patient has difficulty swallowing, promethazine and prochlorperazine tablets may be crushed and given with food, but *do not* crush or chew extended release capsules.

Mechanism of Action

The 5-HT3 receptor antagonists ondansetron (Zofran), palonosetron (Aloxi), dolasetron (Anzamet), and granistetron (Kytril) selectively block serotonin 3 receptors located in vagal nerve terminals and central nervous system (CNS) chemoreceptor trigger zones, thus they are used to control severe nausea and vomiting associated with chemotherapy and radiation therapy. However, ondansetron (Zofran) in its intravenous and intramuscular formulations is most widely used to prevent and treat postoperative nausea and vomiting.

The phenothiazines (prochlorperazine and promethazine) also act on the chemoreceptors in the brain but by blocking dopaminergic D1 and D2 receptors. They also block alpha-1, cholinergic, adrenergic, and histamine receptors, which accounts for their many side effects and makes a drug such as ondansetron (Zofran) much preferable.

Pharmacokinetics: The Phenothiazines

■ Absorption: The phenothiazines are quickly absorbed, with an onset of action of their oral dosage forms in 30 to 40 minutes.

■ Distribution: Well absorbed and crosses both placenta and blood-brain barrier.

■ Metabolism: Primarily hepatic to active metabolite.

■ Excretion: Half in kidney, half through enterohepatic circulation.

■ Half-life: Promethazine: 9 to 16 hr; prochlorperazine: 3 to 5 hr.

Pharmacokinetics: Ondansetron

■ Absorption: 100% if IM or IV, 50% if oral

■ Distribution: Unknown

■ Metabolism: Extensively metabolized in the liver

■ Excretion: 95% as a metabolite in the kidneys, 5% excreted unchanged

■ Half-life: Ondansetron: 3 to 6 hr

Dosage and Administration

Generic Name	Trade Name	Route	Usual Adult Daily Dose
ondansetron	Zofran	PO, IM	24 mg, 30 min for chemotherapy
promethazine	Phenergan	PO, IM, by rectum (PR)	25 mg every 4 hr
prochlorperazine	Compazine	PO, IM	5–10 mg 3–4 times/day

Clinical Uses

■ Ondansetron is indicated for the prevention of nausea and vomiting associated with cancer chemotherapy and radiotherapy.

■ Promethazine and perchlorperazine are used for milder cases of nausea.

Adverse Drug Reactions for the Phenothiazines

CV (cardiovascular): Cardiac arrest, hypotension, cardiac edema

DERM (dermatological): Contact dermatitis, photosensitivity, urticaria

EENT (eye, ear, nose, and throat): Blurred vision, cornea and lens changes

ENDO (endocrine): Amenorrhea, breast enlargement, galactorrhea, changes in libido and menstruation

GI (gastrointestinal): Appetite increased, constipation, nausea, weight gain, xerostomia, biliary jaundice

GU (genitourinary): Ejaculatory dysfunction, impotence, priapism

HEM (hematological): Aplastic anemia, agranulocytosis, leukopenia

NEURO (neurological): Agitation, catatonia, cough reflex suppressed, drowsiness, headache, impairment of temperature regulation, neuroleptic malignant syndrome, restlessness, seizure, extrapyramidal symptoms

PUL (pulmonary): Asthma, nasal congestion

Contraindications

■ People with hypersensitivities or other selective serotonin antagonists.

■ The phenothiazines are contraindicated in children under 2 years of age and in people with severe depression.

Patient/Family Education

■ Advise patients taking ondansetron to notify their clinician if they experience any involuntary movement of eyes, face, or limbs.

■ Dosage schedule needs to be reviewed regularly, and drugs should be taken exactly as ordered.

■ Advise patients they may experience dizziness.

■ Patients should notify their clinician if dry mouth persists beyond 2 weeks.

■ Geriatric patients are at increased risk for orthostatic hypotension, thus they should be taught to change positions slowly.

■ Strongly advise against concurrent use of alcohol and other CNS suppressants.

■ When used as a prophylaxis for motion sickness, patients should take the drug at least 30 minutes, and preferably 1 to 2 hours, before departure.

■ Advise patients to ask for professional help if they experience sore throat, fever, jaundice, or uncontrolled movements.

PRACTICAL PHARMACOLOGY OF ANTIDIARRHEALS

Diarrhea is a common complaint. Patients often attempt to treat themselves with over-the-counter (OTC) medications before seeking help from their clinician. Diarrhea seen in the primary care setting is often food or drug induced, due to infectious etiology, or resulting from inflammatory bowel disease or irritable bowel disease. Diarrhea that lasts less than 2 weeks is considered to be acute whereas cases that last more than 2 weeks are considered to be chronic. Most cases of diarrhea are acute and self-limiting, with few serious consequences. The exceptions are diarrhea in children and the elderly because both populations can quickly experience dehydration due to diarrhea. Chronic diarrhea may result in poor nutrition and weight loss as well as dehydration. Food-induced diarrhea can result from food poisoning, or diarrhea may be infectious and may require antimicrobial therapy. Diarrhea that is drug induced may be easily treated by removing the causative agent. In this chapter we will focus on drugs used for the symptomatic relief of diarrhea.

Three main classes of drugs are used in the treatment of diarrhea: absorbent preparations such as bismuth subsalicylate (Pepto-Bismol, Kaopectate); opiates such as diphenoxylate with atropine (Lomotil), difenoxin with atropine (Motofen), loperamide (Imodium); and anticholinergics used for inflammatory bowel disease.

Conscientious Prescribing for Patients Using Antidiarrheals

■ Use all antidiarrheal agents with caution in older adults. The elderly are especially sensitive to diphenoxylate or difenoxin because of the atropine content and anticholinergic properties.

■ None of the antidiarrheals have established safety for children younger than age 2 years.

■ Patients should be instructed to take antidiarrheal medications as directed. Do not double the dose once it is missed, do not exceed the maximum number of doses permitted.

■ If diarrhea continues beyond 48 hours or if abdominal pain, fever, or distention occurs, contact clinician.

■ Patients taking digoxin, cephalosporins, warfarin, or heparin, or central nervous system depressants should first contact their clinician before taking any over-the-counter antidiarrheals.

■ Adding fiber to the diet and using oral rehydrating solutions may be advised.

■ Stress the importance of handwashing after each bowel movement to avoid infectious spread of diarrhea.

■ Educate patients about maintaining nutritional intake.

■ The bananas, rice, applesauce, and toast (BRAT) diet can assist in maintaining nutrition and is also helpful in reducing diarrhea.

■ Stop milk and other lactose-based food products for a few days.

Mechanism of Action

■ Kaolin and pectin decrease stool fluid content by absorbing moisture in the stool, although they do not affect total water loss.

■ Bismuth subsalicylate has an antisecretory and antimicrobial effect in vitro against bacterial and viral enteral pathogens. It may have some anti-inflammatory effects.

■ Diphenoxylate with atropine is a constipating meperidine congener that lacks analgesic activity. Atropine provides anticholinergic effects that decrease secretion in the bowel and slow peristalsis.

■ Loperamide inhibits peristalsis by a direct effect on the circular and longitudinal muscles of the intestinal wall. It also reduces fecal volume, increases viscosity and bulk, and diminishes the loss of fluid and electrolytes. Although it has opioid-like properties, it does not have an opioid effect.

Pharmacokinetics

Generic Name	Absorption & Distribution	Metabolism	Excretion	Half-Life
bismuth subsalicylate	Undergoes chemical dissociation in the GI tract; salicylate is absorbed with plasma levels reaching those of a similar dose of aspirin	Salicylate metabolized in liver	> 90% in urine	2–3 hr for low doses; 15–30 hr for larger doses
difenoxin with atropine	Well absorbed from GI tract. Unknown distribution. Atropine crosses blood-brain barrier and produces anticholinergic effect	Rapidly metabolized to an inactive hydroxylase metabolite	In urine and feces	24–72 hr
diphenoxylate with atropine	Well absorbed from GI tract. Unknown distribution. Atropine crosses blood-brain barrier and produces anticholinergic effect	Rapidly and extensively metabolized to diphenoxylic acid	14% of drug and metabolites in urine; 49% in feces	2.5 hr
loperamide	40% absorbed after oral administration; does not cross the blood-brain barrier	Partially metabolized by liver and undergoes enterohepatic recirculation until 70% completely metabolized	30% excreted unchanged in feces as free drug; minimal excretion in urine	10.8 hr

Dosage and Administration

Generic Name	Trade Name	Route	Usual Adult Daily Dose
difenoxin hydrochloride with atropine sulfate	Motofen	PO	1 mg difenoxin and 0–5 mg atropine sulfate; 2 tablets starting dose, then 1 tablet after each loose stool; 1 tablet every 3–4 hr as needed
diphenoxylate hydrochloride with atropine sulfate	Lomotil	PO	2.5 mg diphenoxylate hydrochloride and 0.025 mg atropine sulfate; initial dose is 5 mg 4 times/day
loperamide hydrochloride	Imodium	PO	2 mg; 4 mg initially, followed by 2 mg after each loose stool.
bismuth subsalicylate	Kaopectate Pepto-Bismol	PO	2 tablets or 30 mL; repeat dose every 30 min–1 hr as needed.

Clinical Uses

■ Simple, acute diarrhea
■ Chronic diarrhea associated with pancreatic insufficiency
■ Chronic infantile diarrhea
■ Loperamide: Traveler's diarrhea, chronic diarrhea associated with inflammatory bowel disease

Adverse Reactions

GI: Rebound constipation. Bismuth subsalicylate can turn the tongue and stools gray-black. Diphenoxylate and difenoxin (both with atropine) can cause dry mouth and mucous membranes. Flushing, tachycardia, and urinary retention may also occur with this drug. These drugs may also cause central nervous system reactions of dizziness and drowsiness.

Interactions

Drug Name	Interacting Drug	Possible Effect
bismuth subsalicylate	Aspirin	May potentiate salicylate toxicity
	Tetracycline	May decrease the GI absorption
	warfarin or heparin	May increase risk for bleeding
diphenoxylate with atropine	CNS depressants, alcohol, antihistamines, opioids, hypnotics	Additive CNS depression
kaolin/pectin	Digoxin	Decreases GI absorption
loperamide	CNS depressants, alcohol, antihistamine, opioids, hypnotics	Additive CNS depression

Contraindications

■ The atropine component of diphenoxylate and difenoxin contraindicates their use in patients with narrow-angle glaucoma and requires these agents be used with caution in patients with prosthetic hyperplasia.
■ Children with Down syndrome have increased sensitivity to atropine. Therefore, this drug should be avoided or used with extreme caution in children.

■ Diphenoxylate and difenoxin with atropine may prolong or aggravate diarrhea with organisms that penetrate the intestinal mucosa such as *Escherichia coli*, *Salmonella*, and *Shigella* or in pseudomembranous colitis associated with broad-spectrum antimicrobial therapy.
■ The salicylate component of bismuth subsalicylate contraindicates its use in children or teenagers during or after recovery from chickenpox or flulike illness.

THERAPEUTIC OPTIONS FOR GASTROESOPHAGEAL REFLUX DISEASE (GERD) AND PEPTIC ULCER DISEASE (PUD)

Dyspepsia is chronic or recurring epigastric pain or discomfort when stomach contents and acids move from the stomach into the esophagus. Patients with frequent heartburn or acid regurgitation are considered to have gastroesophageal reflux disease (GERD) until proven otherwise. GERD is so common that a globally accepted definition of it, the Montreal definition, was written in 2006 and is widely accepted by physicians, patients, and researchers (Vakil et al., 2006). GERD can be diagnosed in primary care on the basis of symptoms alone without additional diagnostic testing. This approach is appropriate for most patients and does not use unnecessary resources. Symptoms reach a threshold where they constitute disease when they are troublesome to patients and affect their functioning during usual activities of living. This patient-centered approach to diagnosis includes asking patients how their symptoms affect their everyday lives. Ten percent of patients complain they are affected by their symptoms on a daily basis. The true incidence of GERD may never be known and its incidence is understated because a large number of individuals self-treat by buying OTC treatments.

Patients with GERD complain of a variety of symptoms including upper abdominal pain, bloating, belching, nausea, and early satiety. Patients may also complain of a burning sensation in the middle of the chest that is sometimes sharp or feels like pressure on the chest. This pain may mimic the pain of a heart attack and can radiate to the back. It is aggravated by meals and by lying down and is relieved by sitting up. Patients may also complain of a sore throat, hoarseness, laryngitis, chronic dry cough (especially at night), and halitosis. The severity of the disease varies from mild postprandial discomfort to severe esophageal inflammation, stricture, bleeding, and esophageal carcinoma. GERD can precipitate an asthma attack because the nerves that are stimulated by the acid reflux can also stimulate nerves in the lungs, which in turn constrict the narrow breathing tubes and precipitate an asthma incident. GERD may also interfere with restful sleep.

GERD results from the reflux of chyme flowing from the stomach into the esophagus. The lower esophageal sphincter plays an important part in maintaining a pressure barrier between the stomach and the esophagus. In patients with GERD, the resting tone of the lower esophageal sphincter is less than normal, thus permitting transient relaxation of the lower esophageal sphincter 1 to 2 hours after eating. This relaxation then allows gastric contents to regurgitate into the esophagus. There are certain foods that decrease the lower esophageal sphincter tone such as alcohol, peppermint, chocolate, and other foods that have a high concentration of fat. Tobacco will also decrease the sphincter tone.

When symptoms of GERD are acute and self-limiting, the patient requires no testing and no further treatment. However, when the symptoms are continuous, patients require pharmacological intervention and lifestyle changes. The evaluation and management of esophageal reflux disease is best carried out using a stepwise approach. Much of the time the evaluation and treatment of patients with ongoing symptoms can be managed by primary clinicians, with only a few patients having to be referred to a gastroenterologist. To aid in the diagnosis of gastroesophageal reflux disease patients may undergo endoscopy and testing for *Helicobacter pylori*.

There are a variety of drug classes that can be used in the treatment of GERD that will help increase the tone of the lower esophageal sphincter, reduce the amount of acid in the chyme, improve peristalsis and thereby decrease the time chyme is available to produce reflux, and decrease the exposure of the mucosa to the highly acidic material. These classes of drugs include antacids, H2 blockers, cytoprotective agents, and proton pump inhibitors. Patients with gastroesophageal reflux disease are often treated with a step-up approach. The steps are based on symptom relief and degree of esophageal damage (Zagaria, 2007).

Step 1: Lifestyle modifications (see Box 11-2).

Step 2: If symptoms continue, patients are then usually started on H2 blockers if there is no erosive disease. Some patients may require a prokinetic agent before each meal and at bedtime.

Step 3: If symptoms are refractory after 6 weeks of step 2 therapy, or if the endoscopy shows evidence of erosive disease, PPIs may be used. PPIs are central to the management of this step. They are either used with or replace H2 blockers.

Step 4: If symptoms do not improve with over-the-counter or prescription H2 blockers and PPIs, patients are referred to a gastroenterologist. While waiting for referral, step 3 interventions are continued. At this point, if the patient is not already on a prokinetic agent, then these agents should be added.

The step-up approach is appropriate for patients with mild disease. However, some clinicians may use a step-down approach. In this approach, step 1, lifestyle modifications, and a standard dose of PPIs are used initially. If the symptoms do not improve, step 2 involves increasing the dose of the PPI for another trial period. Step 3 involves H2 blockers or prokinetic agents added to the PPI dose. Step 4 involves decreasing the PPI dose once the initial symptoms are resolved. Also, the patient may be stepped down to an H2 blocker. This approach is more appropriate for those patients with moderate to severe disease or daily symptoms for which quick action is necessary. Whether clinicians use a step-up or step-down approach, failure to achieve symptom relief within a 3-month span suggests a more complicated disease pattern, and a referral to a gastroenterologist for further evaluation is required.

Pharmacology of Antacids Used to Neutralize Gastric Acid

Antacids are weak bases that react with the GI system's output of excessive hydrochloric acid to form salt and water. They are primarily used to reduce gastric acidity in the treatment of gastroesophageal reflux disease and peptic ulcer disease. They come in a variety of combinations such sodium bicarbonate, magnesium hydroxide, and calcium carbonate. These agents neutralize gastric acidity, which subsequently causes an increase in the pH of the stomach. They also inhibit the activity of pepsin and increase the lower esophageal sphincter tone. Aluminum-based antacids inhibit smooth muscle contraction thereby slowing gastric emptying. Calcium-based and aluminum-based antacids also play a role in the treatment of calcium deficiency states, whereas magnesium-based antacids are used to treat magnesium deficiencies from malnutrition and alcoholism.

It is important when selecting an antacid that clinicians consider the acid-neutralizing capacity (ANC) of the agent. The ANC varies for commercial antacid preparations and is expressed as milliequivalents (mEq). Antacids must neutralize at least 5 mEq per dose. Those that have higher ANC values are more likely to be effective. Sodium bicarbonate and calcium carbonate have the greatest neutralizing capacity but are not suitable for chronic therapy because of their systemic effects. Suspensions have a greater neutralizing capacity than powders or tablets. For maximum effectiveness, tablets should be thoroughly chewed. If ingested in the fasting state, antacids reduce acidity for approximately 20 to 40 minutes because of rapid gastric emptying. If they are ingested 1 hour after meals, they reduce acidity for at least 3 hours.

Conscientious Prescribing of Antacids

■ Sodium content: The sodium content of antacids may be a significant consideration in patients with hypertension, congestive heart failure, marked renal failure, and those on restricted or low-sodium diets. These patients should use low-sodium preparations.

■ Acid rebound: Antacids may cause dose-related rebound hyperactivity because they may increase the gastric secretion or serum gastrin level.

BOX 11-2 Lifestyle Modifications for the Management of GERD

■ Sleep with the head of the bed elevated 6 to 8 inches by using extra pillows or wedges.

■ Avoid lying down within 3 hours after eating.

■ Avoid bending down within 3 hours after eating.

■ Avoid strenuous exercise within 3 hours after eating.

■ Achieve and maintain appropriate body weight.

■ Avoid spicy, acidic, or fatty foods.

■ Avoid chocolate, peppermint, and citrus fruits and juices.

■ Limit intake of coffee, tea, and alcohol.

■ Avoid overeating.

■ Avoid eating meals at bedtime or snacks within 3 hours of going to bed.

■ Stop smoking.

■ Milk-alkali syndrome: This can be an acute illness with symptoms of headache, nausea, irritability, and weakness or a chronic illness with alkalosis, hypercalcemia, and, possibly, renal impairment. It can occur following the concurrent use of high-dose calcium carbonate and sodium bicarbonate.

■ Hypophosphatemia: Prolonged use of aluminum-containing antacids may result in hypophosphatemia in patients with normal phosphate levels if phosphate intake is not adequate.

■ Gastrointestinal hemorrhage: Aluminum hydroxide should be used with caution in patients who have recently experienced a massive upper GI bleed.

■ Absorption: Systemic antacids such as sodium bicarbonate are readily absorbed and are capable of producing systemic electrolyte disturbances. Nonsystemic antacids form compounds that are not absorbed to a significant extent and thus do not exert appreciable systemic effects unless their usage is chronic, in high doses, or the patient has other pathology.

Patient/Family Education for Patients Taking Antacids

■ If taking a chewable antacid, thoroughly chew before swallowing and follow with a glass of water.

■ If using effervescent tablets, allow the tablet to completely dissolve in water and stop bubbling before drinking.

■ Be aware that antacids may interact with certain prescription medications.

■ Notify clinician of any symptoms of bleeding such as black tarry stools or coffee-ground vomitus.

■ Taking too much of these products can cause the stomach to secrete excess stomach acid.

■ Do not use for more than 2 weeks unless otherwise instructed by a clinician.

■ Calcium-based antacids should not be administered with food containing large amounts of oxalic acid, such as spinach, or phytic acid, such as bran or cereals, because these foods decrease the absorption of calcium.

■ Aluminum and calcium-based antacids may cause constipation. Increase the bulk in the diet and increase fluid intake to prevent constipation.

■ Magnesium-based antacids may cause diarrhea. Increasing fiber in the diet may alleviate this problem.

Mechanism of Action

■ Antacids neutralize gastric acidity resulting in an increase in the pH of the stomach and duodenal bulb. By increasing the gastric pH above 4, these agents inhibit the activity of pepsin.

■ Antacids increase the lower esophageal sphincter tone.

■ Products that contain aluminum inhibit smooth muscle contraction, thus inhibiting gastric emptying.

Pharmacokinetics

■ Absorption: Aluminum-based and magnesium-based antacids are not absorbable with routine use; calcium-based antacids require the presence of vitamin D for any to be absorbed.

■ Distribution: None, unless a small amount is absorbed.

■ Metabolism: Because their action occurs locally inside the GI tract, there is no metabolism.

■ Excretion: Magnesium-based antacids are excreted in the urine. Aluminum-based antacids bind with phosphates to form an insoluble aluminum phosphate complex that passes into the feces. Most of the calcium-based antacids are eliminated in the feces, but 20% may pass through urine.

■ Half-life: Not relevant because these agents are not absorbed. However, antacids' peak effect occurs in 30 minutes and lasts about an hour.

Dosage and Administration for Various Indications

Generic Name	Trade Name	Route	Usual Adult Daily Dose	Indications
magnesium hydroxide	Milk of Magnesia, Dulcolax Philips chewable	PO	Chewable tablets: 2–4 tablets 4 times/day Liquid: 30–60 mL in single or divided doses	Constipation, dyspepsia, and evacuation of the colon or rectal and bowel examinations
aluminum hydroxide	Alu-tab, Amphojel	PO	Tablets/capsules: 500–1,500 mg 3–6 times daily 320-960 mg PO qid as 1-3 hrs AFTER MEALS AND BEDTIME	Uncomplicated peptic ulcer disease, gastric hyperacidity CHILDREN, hyperacidity
calcium carbonate	Rolaids, Tums	PO	2–4 tablets as needed, not to exceed 12 tablets in a 24-hr period	Gastric hyperacidity
sodium citrate	Citra pH	PO	30 mL daily	Quick relief of acid indigestion or dyspepsia
magaldrate	Riopan Lowsium	PO	Suspension: Adults: 5–20 mL, 20 min–1 hr after meals and at bedtime. Chewable tablets: Adults: 1–4 tablets, 20 min–1 hr after meals and at bedtime.	Used for upset stomach, ulcers hiatal hernia, esophagitis, GERD, but has many drug interactions
aluminum hydroxide/ magnesium hydroxide	Alamag, Kudrox, MAH, Maalox, RuLox	PO	Chew tab thoroughly and take with full glass of water, mix liquid with milk or water. Dose is 1–4 tablets at a time but no more than 15 in a day, oral dose is 5-10 ml 4-6 times a day	Take only as directed; they neutralize acid only for 30–60 min
aluminum hydroxide/ magnesium hydroxide, simethicone,* sorbitol	Maalox Mylanta Gelusil	PO	10–20 mL or 2–4 tablets, but no more than 4–6 doses/day	Temporary relief of hyperacidity
Aluminum hydroxide and magnesium trisilicate	Gaviscon	PO	Chew 2–4 tablets 4 times/day	Temporary relief of hyperacidity

*Simethicone is a defoaming agent that allows air bubbles in stomach to break up, thus easily allowing swallowed air to be released via belching.

Clinical Uses

- Relief of GI symptoms associated with hyperacidity: heartburn, gastroesophageal reflux, peptic ulcer disease
- Hyperphosphatemia
- Calcium deficiency

Adverse Reactions

GI: Magnesium-containing antacids: Laxative effect as saline cathartic may cause diarrhea, hypermagnesemia, and renal failure in patients. Aluminum-containing antacids: Constipation, aluminum intoxication, osteomalacia and hypophosphatemia, accumulation of aluminum in serum, bone, and CNS.

META: Aluminum-containing antacids: Osteomalacia and hypophosphatemia, accumulation of aluminum in serum, bone, and CNS.

MISC: Milk-alkali syndrome.

NEURO: Dose-dependent rebound hyperactivity.

Interactions

- Antacids may increase the gastric pH and alter disintegration, dissolution, solubility, and gastric emptying time. Absorption of weak acidic drugs is decreased, resulting in decreased drug effect: digoxin, phenytoin, and isoniazid.
- They may bind drugs such as tetracycline to their surface, resulting in decreased bioavailability.
- Antacids may increase urinary pH and affect the rate of drug elimination, thus inhibiting the excretion of basic drugs: amphetamines, quinidine. May also cause enhanced excretion of acidic drugs such as salicylates.

Contraindications

- Renal function impairment: Magnesium-containing products should be used with caution, particularly when more than 50 mEq of magnesium is given daily. Hypermagnesemia and toxicity may occur. Prolonged use of aluminum-containing antacids in patients with renal failure may result in or worsen dialysis osteomalacia.
- All antacids are contraindicated in the presence of severe abdominal pain of unknown cause, especially if it is accompanied by fever.
- Calcium-based antacids are contraindicated in the presence of hypercalcemia and renal calculi.

Pharmacology of Histamine-2 Receptor Blockers/Antagonists

Histamine-2 receptor blockers are also known as H2 antagonists because they inhibit acid secretion by gastric parietal cells through a reversible blockade of histamine at histamine-2 receptors. Gastric parietal cells have three receptors that can be stimulated to cause the parietal cells to produce H+, acetylcholine, and histamine-2. They are highly selective and do not affect histamine-1 receptors. They are not anticholinergic agents. These agents are potent inhibitors of all phases of gastric acid secretion, including that caused by muscarinic agonists and gastrin. The drugs in this class affect gastric juice concentration, gastric emptying, and the lower esophageal sphincter pressure. Thus, these agents are used to reduce gastric acid in patients with duodenal and gastric ulcers as well as gastroesophageal reflux disease.

Conscientious Prescribing of H2 Receptor Antagonists

- Ranitidine is 5 to 12 times more potent than cimetidine. Potency is not to be confused with efficacy; because ranitidine is more potent, it can produce its clinical effect with a lesser amount of medication than can cimetidine.
- Famotidine is 30 to 60 times more potent than cimetidine in controlling gastric acid secretion.
- Cimetidine seems to cause the most problems in patients with decreased renal clearance whereas ranitidine causes the least problems.
- Due to the potential for hepatocellular damage, patients who require higher doses or more than short-term use of this class of drugs should have laboratory testing of liver function prior to initiation of therapy and at regular intervals throughout therapy.

Patient/Family Education for Patients Taking H2 Receptor Antagonists

- Patients should be instructed to take the drug as prescribed for the full course of therapy, even if they are feeling better.
- If a dose is missed, patients should be instructed not to double the dose.
- These agents should be taken with meals or immediately afterward and at bedtime to achieve the best effects.
- If also taking antacids or other drugs whose interaction with histamine blockers produces interference with absorption, drug administration should be separated by at least 30 minutes to an hour.
- Histamine blockers may cause drowsiness or dizziness; patients should be warned to avoid driving until they know their response to the drug.
- Patients should be advised to report the onset of black, tarry stools and other adverse reactions that may indicate gastrointestinal bleeding.
- Smoking interferes with the absorption of histamine blockers and increases gastric acid secretion. Thus, patients must be advised to stop smoking.
- Alcohol and products containing aspirin or NSAIDs and some acidic foods may also increase gastric acid secretion. **Note:** Acidic foods (citrus fruits, high protein meat, and especially highly processed foods) add hydrogen ions to the body and thus turn its pH acidic; likewise, alkaline foods (spinach, raisins, soybeans, carrots) decrease hydrogen ions, leaving the body more alkaline. The American diet with all its processed food is a source of acid stomach for too many people.

Mechanism of Action

These agents inhibit acid secretion by gastric parietal cells through a reversible blockade of histamine at histamine-2 receptors.

Pharmacokinetics

- Absorption: All agents in the class are well absorbed.
- Distribution: Well distributed, but not highly bound to protein.
- Metabolism: All agents are metabolized to differing degrees by the cytochrome P450 enzymes system of the liver.
- Excretion: These agents are excreted in differing percentages as unchanged drug in the urine.
- Half-Life: All agents have a half-life of 2 to 3 hours.

Dosage and Administration of H2 Blockers

Generic	Trade Name	Route	Dosage
cimetidine	Tagamet	PO	800 mg at night or 300 mg 4 times/day with meals and at bedtime
ranitidine	Zantac	PO	100–150 mg 2 times/day or 300 mg at night
famotidine	Pepcid	PO	40 mg/day at night or 20 mg 2 times/day
nizatidine	Axid	PO	300 mg at night or 150 mg 2 times/day

Clinical Use

- These agents are used in the treatment of duodenal and gastric ulcers as well as gastroesophageal reflux disease.

Adverse Reactions

CV: Arrhythmia, vasculitis
DERM: Erythema, rash
ENDO: Gynecomastia and possibly impotence
GI: Constipation, diarrhea, nausea, pancreatitis
HEM: Agranulocytosis, granulocyte leukemia, thrombocytopenia, aplastic anemia
NEURO: Mental confusion, agitation, psychosis, depression, disorientation

Interactions

- Drug reactions in this class of drugs are related to their metabolism by the cytochrome P450 enzymes system of the liver.
- Cimetidine is the most problematic because it uses several isoenzymes, whereas famotidine, nizatidine, and ranitidine have less effect on the cytochrome P450 system and fewer isoenzymes in their metabolism.
- May increase blood alcohol levels.
- Antacids and anticholinergics may decrease absorption of cimetidine.

Contraindications

- These agents should be used with caution in patients with renal impairment because they are more subject to central nervous system adverse reactions.

- These drugs are contraindicated in patients with liver failure or liver disease.

Patient/Family Education for H2 Blockers

- Remind patients that alcohol consumption will increase acidity.
- Advise patients to take their medication as a full-course of therapy and not to stop even if feeling better.
- Advise patients that smoking interferes with the action of their histamine antagonists.
- Advise that these medications may cause drowsiness.
- Advise patients that increasing fiber, fluid intake, and exercise will help minimize constipation.
- Advise patient to report any signs of a black tarry stool, fever, sore throat, diarrhea, rash, confusion, or hallucinations.

Pharmacology of Proton Pump Inhibitors (PPI)

Proton pump inhibitors (PPI) are antisecretory agents used to treat gastric conditions characterized by hyperacidity. These agents do not exhibit anticholinergic or histamine blockade properties, but they do suppress gastric acid secretion. They do this by inhibition of the $H^+/K^+/ATPase$ enzyme system at the secretory surface of the parietal cell itself to block the final steps in H^+ secretion. These agents are so effective that they reduce gastric acid by more than 90% and frequently produce achlorhydria. The decrease in acid secretion caused by these agents lasts for up to 72 hours after each dose. Three to 5 days after the drug is discontinued gastric acid secretion begins again, and it returns to the pretreatment levels within 2 weeks to 3 months depending on which drug is used.

Conscientious Prescribing of Proton Pump Inhibitors

- Patients taking proton pump inhibitors to treat ulcers may be tested for *H. pylori* infection by urea breath testing. However, patients should stop the agent 2 weeks prior to testing.
- Proton pump inhibitors alone rarely eradicate *H. pylori* infections, but they can suppress it; thus testing during antisecretory therapy may lead to false negative.

Patient/Family Education for Proton Pump Inhibitors

- Agents in this class should be taken before meals, preferably in the morning.
- These drugs may be taken safely with antacids.

Mechanism of Action

The agents in this class are antisecretory compounds that do not exhibit anticholinergic or histamine antagonistic properties, but they suppress gastric acid secretion by specific inhibition of the $H^+/K^+/ATPase$ enzyme system at the secretory surface of the gastric parietal cell.

Pharmacokinetics

- Absorption: Absorption is rapid and begins only after the granules leave the stomach.
- Distribution: 95% protein bound.

- Metabolism: These agents are extensively metabolized by the liver to inactive metabolites.
- Excretion: Little unchanged drug is excreted in the urine, with the remainder of the metabolites excreted in the feces.
- Half-life: Less than 2 hours.

Dosage and Administration

Generic Name	Trade Name	Route	Daily Dose/Indication
dexlanosoprole	Dexilant	PO	30–60 mg once a day for up to 8 weeks for healing esophageal ulcers, up to 4 weeks for GERD
omeprazole	Prilosec, Losec	PO	20 mg daily for GERD
lansoprazole	Prevacid	PO	15 mg daily for up to 8 weeks for GERD
esomeprazole	Nexium	PO	20–40 mg daily for 4–8 weeks for healing esophageal ulcers, 20 mg once a day for 4 weeks for GERD
pantoprazole	Protonix	PO	20–40 mg daily for 4–8 weeks for healing esophageal ulcers, 20 mg once a day for 4 weeks for GERD
rabeprazole	Aciphex	PO	20 mg daily for up to 4 weeks for GERD

Clinical Uses

- Erosive gastritis
- Gastroesophageal reflux disease

- Zollinger-Ellison syndrome
- Short-term treatment of active peptic ulcer disease to treat ulcers caused by *H. pylori*

Adverse Reactions

DERM: Rash.

GI: Atrophic gastritis, abdominal pain, constipation, diarrhea, flatulence.

MS: Weakness.

NEURO: Dizziness, drowsiness, headache.

LONG-TERM USE: The U.S. Food and Drug Administration (FDA) has determined there is an increased risk of fractures of the wrist, hip, and spine in people who take high doses of PPI or take them for more than 1 year. Researchers believe that the reduction in stomach acid by the PPI also has an effect on the amount of calcium dissolved in the stomach available for absorption, or the PPIs interfere with the acid production of osteoclasts (Seppa, 2007).

Interactions

- Drug interactions related to their use of the cytochrome P450 system have occurred.
- All drugs in this class interfere with the absorption of drugs given orally that depend on gastric acid pH to be effective, for example, ketoconazole, ampicillin, and digoxin.

Contraindications

- These agents should be used with caution in older adults and patients with hepatic insufficiency or renal impairment.

SPOTLIGHT ON *H. PYLORI*

H. pylori is a common pathogen that plays an important role in the pathogenesis of peptic ulcer disease (PUD), gastric malignancy, and chronic gastritis. Successful eradication of *H. pylori* reduces the risk of ulcer reoccurrence. The prevalence of *H. pylori* is closely tied to socioeconomic conditions because the infection is more common in developing countries than in developed countries such as the United States. However, it has been estimated that 30% to 40% of the U.S. population is infected with *H. pylori*. The presence of this bacterium causes chronic low-level inflammation of the stomach lining, but over 80% of people with the bacteria are asymptomatic (Porter et al., 2010).

Controversy exists regarding testing for *H. pylori* in the presence of dyspepsia, gastroesophageal reflux disease, NSAID use, iron deficiency anemia, or risk factors for developing gastric cancer. Testing is indicated in those patients with active peptic ulcer disease, a past history of documented ulcer, and mucosa-associated lymphoid/lyphatic tissue lymphoma. In patients who have not been receiving a proton pump inhibitor within 1 to 2 weeks or an antibiotic or bismuth within 4 weeks of endoscopy, the rapid urease test is inexpensive and accurate. For those who have been treated, testing should include biopsy from the gastric body and antrum for histological examination.

The test-and-treat strategy is recommended for patients younger than age 55 years with uninvestigated dyspepsia who have no warning features such as bleeding. In the United States, the recommended primary therapies for *H. pylori* infection include the following:

- Clarithromycin-based triple therapy: A proton pump inhibitor, clarithromycin, and amoxicillin or metronidazole for 14 days.
- Bismuth quadruple therapy: a proton pump inhibitor or histamine blocker, bismuth, metronidazole, and tetracycline for 10 to 14 days.

Recent studies suggest that eradication rates achieved by first-line treatment with a proton pump inhibitor, clarithromycin, and amoxicillin have decreased to 70% to 85%, in part due to increasing clarithromycin resistance (Gatta et al., 2009). Eradication rates may also be lower with 7-day vs. 14-day regimens. Bismuth-containing quadruple regimens for 7 to 14 days are another first-line treatment option. The most commonly used salvage regimen in patients with persistent *H. pylori* is bismuth quadruple therapy. Recent data suggest that a PPI, levofloxacin, and amoxicillin given for 10 days is more effective and better tolerated than bismuth quadruple therapy for persistent *H. pylori* infection, although this needs to be validated in the United States (Gatta et al., 2009). There are treatment regimens for eradication of *H. pylori* that have been approved by the FDA, and they have a success rate of 70% to 90% (Box 11-3).

SPOTLIGHT ON *H. PYLORI*—cont'd

Treatment failure following *H. pylori* therapy is due to poor compliance and antibiotic resistance. Thus, it is critical for clinicians to stress the importance of taking the medications as prescribed to minimize treatment failure. Limited evidence suggests that smoking, alcohol consumption, and diet may also adversely affect the likelihood of successful eradication.

BOX 11-3 FDA Approved Regimens for Eradication of H. Pylori*

Omeprazole 40 mg daily + clarithromycin 500 mg 3 times/day for 2 wks, then omeprazole 20 mg daily for 2 wks
OR
Ranitidine bismuth citrate (RBC) 400 mg 2 times/day + clarithromycin 500 mg 3 times/day for 2 wks, then RBC 400 mg 2 times/day for 2 wks
OR
Bismuth subsalicylate (Pepto-Bismol) 525 mg 4 times/day + metronidazole 250 mg 4 times/day + tetracycline 500 mg 4 times/day* for 2 wks + H2 receptor antagonist therapy as directed for 4 wks
OR
Lansoprazole 30 mg 2 times/day + amoxicillin 1 g 2 times/day + clarithromycin 500 mg 3 times/day for 10 days
OR
Lansoprazole 30 mg 3 times/day + amoxicillin 1 g 3 times/day for 2 wks†

OR
RBC 400 mg 2 times/day + clarithromycin 500 mg 2 times/day for 2 wks, then RBC 400 mg 2 times/day for 2 wks
OR
Omeprazole 20 mg 2 times/day + clarithromycin 500 mg 2 times/day + amoxicillin 1 g 2 times/day for 10 days
OR
Lansoprazole 30 mg 2 times/day + clarithromycin 500 mg 2 times/day + amoxicillin 1 g 2 times/day for 10 days

*Although not FDA approved, amoxicillin has been substituted for tetracycline for patients for whom tetracycline is not recommended.
†This dual therapy regimen has restrictive labeling. It is indicated for patients who are either allergic or intolerant to clarithromycin or for infections with known or suspected resistance to clarithromycin.
Source: Centers for Disease Control and Prevention (CDC). (2006). Helicobacter pylori *and peptic ulcer disease: The key to cure.* H. pylori Fact Sheet for Health Care Providers. www.cdc.gov/ulcer/keytocure.htm

---

Pharmacology of Cytoprotective Agents

Peptic ulcer disease can be caused by a variety of conditions. The administration of NSAIDs has been associated with gastric mucosal damage and ulcer formation. There are two agents in this class of drugs that are commonly used to treat or prevent ulcer formation: sucralfate and misoprostol.

Conscientious Prescribing of Cytoprotective Agents

■ Drug selection is based on indications. Sucralfate is preferred over misoprostol for treatment of active duodenal ulcers not caused by NSAIDs.
■ Sucralfate is also the drug of choice in women of childbearing age.

Patient/Family Education for Cytoprotective Agents

■ Increased fluid intake, dietary bulk, and exercise may reduce the incidence of constipation associated with sucralfate.
■ Patients should report to their clinician any onset of black, tarry stools or severe abdominal pain, which may indicate treatment failure and the onset of GI bleeding.
■ Women of childbearing age should be informed that misoprostol will cause spontaneous abortion and the drug should not be prescribed until contraceptive therapy is established (see Special Case: Misoprostol and Pregnancy).
■ Patients should be advised to take the drug as prescribed.

■ Sucralfate is taken on an empty stomach whereas misoprostol should be taken with food.

Special Case: Misoprostol and Pregnancy

Misoprostol is pregnancy category X. It is been associated with altered fertility and may cause abortion, premature birth, or birth defects based on its action on the uterus. Uterine rupture has been reported in pregnant women. This drug should not be prescribed to women of childbearing age unless the patient is at high risk of complications from gastric ulcers associated with the use of NSAIDs. In such cases, before the drug is prescribed, the patient must have a negative serum pregnancy test within 2 weeks prior to the beginning of therapy and be capable of complying with effective contraceptive measures. Also, the patient should receive both oral and written warnings of the hazards of misoprostol, the risk of possible contraception failure, and the danger to other women of childbearing potential should the drug be taken by mistake.

Mechanism of Action

Sucralfate is a basic aluminum salt that acts by polymerization and selective binding to necrotic ulcer tissue. It covers the ulcer site and acts as a barrier to acid, pepsin, and bile salts. It has no acid-neutralizing activity and little of it is absorbed.

Misoprostol is a methyl analogue of prostaglandin E, and its mechanism of action is to inhibit gastric secretion through inhibition of histamine-stimulated cyclic AMP production. It has mucosa-protective qualities.

Pharmacokinetics

- Absorption: Sucralfate is minimally absorbed and its actions are largely topical; misoprostol is rapidly and extensively absorbed after oral administration.
- Distribution: Well distributed, bound to protein.
- Metabolism: Hepatic metabolism is a de-esterification to an active metabolite.
- Excretion: 15% of sucralfate is excreted in the feces. The active metabolite misoprostol acid is excreted in the urine.
- Half-life: 20 to 40 minutes.

Dosage and Administration

Generic Name	Trade Name	Route	Usual Adult Daily Dose
sucralfate	Carafate	PO	1 g, 4 times/day, 1 hr before meals and at bedtime
misoprostol	Cytotec	PO	100–200 mcg, 4 times/day with food

Clinical Uses

- Prophylaxis and treatment of duodenal ulcers associated with NSAID use
- Treatment of duodenal ulcers from other causes

Adverse Reactions

GI: Constipation, diarrhea, abdominal pain, flatulence
NEURO: Dizziness, insomnia, sleeplessness, vertigo

Interactions

- Misoprostol: When taken with magnesium-based antacids, there is an increased risk for diarrhea.
- Sucralfate: When taken with aluminum-based antacids, there is an increased risk for constipation. When taken with anticoagulants, there is a decrease in the effect of warfarin. When taken with digoxin, there is a reduced serum level of digoxin. Absorption of hydantoins may be decreased.

Contraindications

- Misoprostol must be used with caution in patients with renal impairment.

DRUGS USED IN THE TREATMENT OF IRRITABLE BOWEL SYNDROME (IBS)

Irritable bowel syndrome (IBS) is a common chronic functional bowel disorder characterized by abdominal pain and altered bowel habits in the absence of specific and unique organic pathology. IBS is a diagnosis of exclusion because no specific motility or structural problems have been consistently demonstrated. Women are two to three times more likely to develop irritable bowel syndrome then are men, with approximately 50% of people reporting symptoms beginning before the age of 35. The Rome III criteria for diagnosing irritable bowel syndrome requires that patients must have recurrent abdominal pain or discomfort at least 3 days per month during the previous 3 months that is associated with two or more of the following problems:

- Abdominal pain or discomfort relieved by defecation
- Abdominal pain or discomfort associated with a change in stool frequency
- Abdominal pain or discomfort associated with a change in stool form or appearance

Other symptoms include the following: altered stool frequency, altered stool form, altered stool passage with straining or urgency, and abdominal loading. Four different bowel patterns may be seen with irritable bowel syndrome (Dorn et al., 2009):

- IBS-D (diarrhea predominant)
- IBS-C (constipation predominant)
- IBS-M (mixed diarrhea and constipation)
- IBS-A (alternating diarrhea and constipation)

Pharmacology of Anticholinergics/Antispasmodics

Treatment of patients with IBS includes diet and lifestyle modification as well as pharmacological interventions. Pharmacological treatment of patients with IBS includes the use of antispasmodic agents, anticholinergic drugs, antidiarrheals, prokinetic agents, bulk-forming laxatives, the chloride channel activator lubiprostone (Amitiza), and tricyclic antidepressants.

Antispasmodics and anticholinergic drugs are generally used in the treatment of IBS and as adjunctive therapy for peptic ulcer disease. They are also used in functional gastrointestinal disorders such as spastic colon, ulcerative colitis, and diverticulitis. They can be used for spastic disorders of the biliary tract in conjunction with narcotic analgesics. Atropine and scopolamine are also used as preanesthetic medications to control bronchial, nasal, pharyngeal, and salivary secretions and to block cardiac vagal inhibitory reflexes during induction of anesthesiology and incubation period. Scopolamine can also be used for motion sickness. Gastrointestinal anticholinergic drugs are used primarily to decrease motility in the gastrointestinal, biliary, and urinary tracts and for antisecretory effect. Antispasmodic-related compounds decrease gastrointestinal motility by acting on smooth muscle.

Conscientious Prescribing of Anticholinergics/Antispasmodics

- Lower doses of antispasmodic drugs should be prescribed to geriatric patients because this population may react with increased adverse effects such as agitation, excitement, confusion, or delusions.

■ Patients should be monitored for anticholinergic effects such as increased heart rate and blood pressure, dry mouth, constipation, blurred vision, or urinary retention.

Patient/Family Education for Anticholinergics/Antispasmodics

■ Patients should use caution when driving or performing other tasks requiring alertness, coordination, or physical dexterity.
■ Patients should be told that these medications may cause dry mouth, difficulty in urination, constipation, and increased sensitivity to light.
■ Patients taking antispasmodic medications should be told to stay out of hot and humid environments while taking these medications and notify clinician of side effects, especially eye pain, rash, or flushing.

Mechanism of Action

■ Belladonna alkaloids inhibit the muscarinic actions of acetylcholine at postganglionic parasympathetic neuroeffector sites, including smooth muscle, secretory glands, and central nervous system sites.
■ The antispasmodic dicyclomine (Bentyl) is also used in IBS because it has indirect and direct effects on the smooth muscle of the gastrointestinal tract. It indirectly blocks the acetylcholine receptor site and directly antagonizes bradykinin and histamine in the GI tract smooth muscle. Both of these actions relieve smooth muscle spasm.

Pharmacokinetics

■ Absorption: Belladonna alkaloids are rapidly absorbed after oral use and readily cross the blood-brain barrier and affect the central nervous system. The major difference between these agents is that atropine at the usual therapeutic dose is a stimulant, whereas scopolamine is a central nervous system depressant. Quaternary anticholinergics are poorly and unreliably absorbed orally. Propantheline and the other quaternary anticholinergics are incompletely absorbed from the GI tract; their distribution remains unknown.
■ Distribution: Because they do not cross the blood-brain barrier, central nervous system effects are slight. They are also less likely to affect the pupil or ciliary muscles of the eye. Their duration of action is more prolonged than alkaloids. Antispasmodics have little or no antimuscarinic activity and thus no significant effect on gastric acid secretion. They do exhibit a nonspecific direct relaxing effect on smooth muscle. For propantheline and the other quaternary anticholinergics distribution remains unknown.
■ Metabolism: Scopolamine, atropine, hyoscine, belladonna are metabolized by the liver.
■ Excretion: Propantheline and the other quaternary anticholinergics are inactivated in the upper small intestine and excreted in the feces.

Dosage and Administration

	Generic Name	Trade Name	Route	Usual Adult Daily Dose
ANTICHOLINERGICS BELLADONNA ALKALOIDS	atropine sulfate	Donnatal	PO, SC, IM	0.4 mg, PO every 6–8 hr
	scopolamine	Scopace	PO, SC, IV	0.4–0.8 mg, 4 times/day
	L-hyoscyamine sulfate	Anaspaz, Levsin, Levbid	PO, IV,	Adults: 1–2 tabs PO every 4 hr
	belladonna		PO	0.6–1 mL, 3–4 times a day
QUATERNARY ANTICHOLINERGICS	glycopyrrolate	Robinul	PO	1 mg, 3 times/day
	methscopolamine bromide	Pamine	PO	2.5 mg before meals; 2.5–5 mg/day at bedtime
	clidinium bromide	Librax	PO	2.5–5 mg, 3–4 times/day
	mepenzolate bromide	Cantil	PO	25 or 50 mg, 4 times a day with meals and at bedtime
	propantheline bromide	Pro-Banthine	PO	15 mg, 30 min before each meal and 30 mg at night
ANTISPASMODICS	dicyclomine hydrochloride	Bentyl	PO, IM, IV	80–160 mg/day PO in 4 equal doses

Clinical Uses

■ Irritable bowel syndrome
■ Peptic ulcer disease
■ Diarrhea
■ Spastic colon
■ Ulcerative colitis
■ Diverticulitis

Adverse Reactions

CV: Palpitations, bradycardia, tachycardia.
DERM: Severe allergic reactions including anaphylaxis, urticaria.
EENT: Blurred vision, mydriasis, and photophobia.
GI: Diarrhea may be an early symptom of incomplete intestinal obstruction. Altered taste perception, nausea, vomiting, bloated feeling.
GU: Urinary hesitancy and retention, impotence.
MISC: Heat prostration can occur with anticholinergic drugs due to decreased sweating in the presence of high environmental temperature.
NEURO: Anticholinergic psychosis has been reported in patients sensitive to anticholinergic drugs. Signs and symptoms of this psychosis include confusion, disorientation, short-term memory loss, hallucinations, ataxia, fatigue, agitation, and coma. Headache, flushing, nervousness, drowsiness, weakness, dizziness, and confusion.

Interactions

■ Amantadine: Coadministration of anticholinergics may result in an increase in the anticholinergic side effects.
■ Atenolol: Effects of atenolol may be increased by concurrent anticholinergic administration.

■ Digoxin: Effects of digoxin may be increased by anticholinergic coadministration.

■ Phenothiazines: The antipsychotic effectiveness may be decreased by cholinergic coadministration.

■ Tricyclic antidepressants: Anticholinergic coadministration may increase side effects such as dry mouth, constipation, and urinary retention because of an additive effect.

Contraindications

■ Narrow-angle glaucoma

■ Unstable cardiovascular problems such as myocardial ischemia

■ Gastrointestinal obstructive disease such as achalasia and pyloric obstruction

■ Obstructive neuropathy, renal disease

■ Myasthenia gravis

Pharmacology of Drugs Used for Constipation

Constipation is a common symptom that many patients experience. It is defined as a change in bowel habits that result in acute or chronic symptoms that would be resolved with the relief of the constipation. It involves infrequent bowel movements, typically less than three times per week; difficulty during defecation; straining during more than 25% of bowel movements, or subjective sensation of hard stools, or the sensation of incomplete bowel evacuation. There are many causes of constipation, and the problem can be divided into metabolic, neurogenic, and idiopathic causes (Table 11-1). In addition, there are numerous drugs that are associated with constipation (Box 11-4).

Management of patients with constipation symptoms should include counseling regarding adequate fiber intake, deficient fluid intake, and physical activity. Often with attention to fiber, water, and physical activity, the symptoms of constipation will improve. There are a number of medications to treat constipation on the market today, and these include bulk-forming agents, emollient stool softeners, and rapidly acting lubricants and **laxatives**. Use of these agents should be monitored carefully because many patients will self-prescribe and misuse them. If long-term laxative use is required, bulk-forming agents such as psyllium; hyperosmolar laxatives such as polyethylene glycol, lactulose, and sorbitol; and saline laxatives such as magnesium sulfate, magnesium citrate, and

---

BOX 11-4 Drug Classes Associated with Constipation

Narcotic analgesics/opiates

Anticholinergic drugs

Antidepressants (cyclic antidepressants)

Antihypertensives

Antihistamine

Phenothiazines

Diuretics

NSAID medications

Antacids containing aluminum or calcium salts

Antihistamines

Anti-Parkinson agents

---

magnesium phosphate are preferred to stimulant laxatives. Stimulant laxatives are not recommended for long-term use because they may cause degeneration of the nerve plexus, thus exacerbating the symptoms of constipation.

Conscientious Prescribing of Laxatives

■ Prior to prescribing laxatives, consider living habits affecting bowel function, including disease state and drug history.

■ Excessive laxative use may lead to significant fluid and electrolyte imbalance. Monitor patients periodically.

■ Preparations containing sodium should be used cautiously by individuals on a sodium-restricted diet and in the presence of edema, congestive heart failure, renal failure, or borderline hypertension.

■ Use sodium phosphate and sodium biphosphate with caution; hyperphosphatemia, hypernatremia, acidosis, and hypocalcemia may occur.

■ Chronic use of laxatives may result in fluid and electrolyte imbalances, osteomalacia, diarrhea, and liver disease.

■ Laxative abuse syndrome is often seen in women with depression, personality disorders, or anorexia nervosa.

■ Lipid pneumonitis may result from oral ingestion and aspiration of mineral oil, especially when the patient reclines.

■ Impaction or obstruction may be caused by bulk-forming agents.

TABLE 11-1 Causes of Constipation			
METABOLIC- ENDOCRINE DISORDERS	**NEUROGENIC DISORDERS**	**CENTRAL NERVOUS SYSTEM DISORDERS**	**IDIOPATHIC CAUSES**
Hypothyroidism	Peripheral neuropathy	Multiple sclerosis	Colonic inertia
Diabetes mellitus	Hirschsprung's disease	Parkinson's disease	Pelvic floor dyssynergia
Pregnancy	Neurofibromatosis	Cerebral vascular accident	Irritable bowel syndrome meta
Hypercalcemia	Intestinal pseudo-obstruction	Spinal cord injury	
Hypocalcemia			
Uremia			

Patient/Family Education for Laxatives

- Treatment and prevention of constipation include adequate fluid intake; proper dietary habits, including increasing fiber intake; responding to the urge to defecate; and daily exercise.
- Restrict self-medication to short-term therapy of constipation, and educate patients that chronic use of laxatives may lead to dependence.
- Laxative use is only a temporary measure; do not use more than 1 week unless otherwise prescribed. Prolonged or frequent use may result in dependence or electrolyte imbalance.
- Pink-red, red-violet, violet, red-brown, yellow-brown, or black discoloration of urine may occur with cascara sagrada or senna.

Mechanism of Action and Pharmacokinetics

Laxatives function differently to produce their effect, either by promoting active electrolyte secretion, decreasing water and electrolyte absorption, increasing water in intestinal lumen, or increasing hydrostatic pressure in the gut.

Laxatives		Onset of Action	Site of Action	Mechanism of Action
Saline	Magnesium citrate Magnesium hydroxide Magnesium sulfate Sodium biphosphate	0.5–3 hr	Small and large intestine	Attract/retain water in intestinal lumen, increasing intraluminal pressure
Stimulant/ irritant	Bisacodyl tabs Senna Bisacodyl suppository	0.25–1 hr	Colon	Direct action on intestinal mucosa or nerve plexus; alters water and electrolyte secretion
Bulk producing	Methylcellulose Polycarbophil Psyllium	12–72 hr	Small and large intestine	Holds water in stool to increase bulk-stimulating peristalsis; forms emollient gel
Emollient	Mineral oil	6–8 hr	Colon	Retards colonic absorption of fecal water; softens stool
Fecal softeners/ surfactants	Docusate	12–72 hr	Small and large intestine	Facilitates admixture of fat and water to soften stool
Hyperosmotic	Glycerin suppository	0.25–1 hr	Colon	Local irritation; hyperosmotic action
	Lactulose	24–48 hr		Osmotic effect retains fluid in the colon, lowering the pH and increasing colonic peristalsis
Osmotic	Polyethylene glycol* (MiraLax) GoLYTELY	Depends on dosage, but usually 30–60 min	Small and large intestine	Facilitates stool evacuation without modifying stool weight

*Polyethylene glycol is the basis for a number of laxatives and is commonly used (with electrolyte additives) as a bowel preparation prior to surgery or colonoscopy. There is some consensus that this can be taken chronically to treat constipation (DiPalma et al., 2007).

Dosage and Administration

	Generic Name	Trade Name	Route	Usual Adult Dose
SALINE LAXATIVES	magnesium citrate	Evac-Q-Mag	PO	1.75 g/30 mL (½–1 bottle)
	magnesium hydroxide	Dulcolax Milk of Magnesia	PO	400 mg/5 mL; 30–16 mL/day
IRRITANT/ STIMULANT LAXATIVES	sennosides	Senokot, Ex-Lax	PO PO	8.6 mg (2 tablets)/day 15 mg (2 tablets) 1–2 times/day
	bisacodyl	Dulcolax, Correctol	PO Rectal suppository	5–15 mg as a single dose 1 suppository
BULK-PRODUCING LAXATIVES	psyllium	Metamucil,	PO	0.52 g (2–6 capsules)/day
		Fiberall	PO	3.5 g (1 tsp) in 6 oz of water or juice/day
	polycarbophil	Fiber-Lax, FiberCon	PO	625 mg (2 tablets) 1–4 times/day
	methylcellulose	Citrucel	PO	1 heaping tbsp (19 g) or 1 packet (10.7 g) and 8 oz of water, 1–3 times/day
EMOLLIENTS	mineral oil	mineral oil, Kondremul plain		15–45 mL (1–3 tbsp)
FECAL SOFTENERS/ SURFACTANTS	docusate sodium	Colace	PO	50–300 mg/day
HYPEROSMOTIC AGENTS	lactulose	Cephulac, Lactulose	PO	30–45 mL containing 20–30 g of lactulose 3–4 times/day
OSMOTIC	polyethylene glycol	MiraLax	PO	240 mL every 10 min up to 4 L or until stool is dislodged and discharge is clear and free of solids

Clinical Uses

- Constipation.
- Rectal/bowel examination: Certain stimulants, lubricant, and saline laxatives are useful for evacuation of the colon or for rectal and bowel examination.
- Prophylaxis: Fecal softeners or mineral oil are useful prophylactically in patients who should not strain during defecation; for example, patients who have had rectal surgery or have suffered a myocardial infarction.
- Psyllium: Useful in patients with irritable bowel syndrome and diverticular disease.
- Polycarbophil: For constipation or diarrhea associated with conditions such as irritable bowel syndrome and diverticulosis; acute nonspecific diarrhea.
- Mineral oil (enema): Relief of **fecal impaction,** or when a solid piece of dry hard stool becomes stuck in the rectum as a result of chronic constipation. **Note:** When a patient is on long-term narcotics for relief of chronic pain, the regular

scheduled use of laxatives may be warranted, otherwise consider laxatives as short-term therapy.

Adverse Reactions

GI: nausea, diarrhea, vomiting, perianal irritation, flatulence, obstruction of the esophagus, stomach, small intestine, and cecum

Interactions

■ Surfactants when concomitantly administered with mineral oil may increase mineral oil absorption. Nonabsorbable antacids, like those listed above, when they are given concurrently with lactulose, may inhibit the desired drop in colonic pH.

Contraindications

■ Nausea, vomiting, or other symptoms of appendicitis
■ Fecal impaction
■ Intestinal obstruction
■ Undiagnosed abdominal pain

Lubiprostone (Amitiza)

This drug was approved by the FDA on January 31, 2006, and is commonly used for idiopathic constipation and to treat irritable bowel syndrome with constipation. Lubiprostone is a locally acting chloride channel activator, a bicyclic fatty acid derived from prostoglandinE1 that enhances chloride-intestinal fluid secretion without altering sodium and potassium concentrations in the serum. It acts by specifically activating CIC-2 chloride channels thereby creating a chloride rich intestinal fluid secretion. C1C-2 chloride channels are involved in transepithelial solute transport and neuronal chloride homeostatis. These CIC channels are present in all cells and in this case, by their increasing of intestinal fluid secretion, they cause a softening of the stool and an increase in GI motility in the intestine, thereby increasing the passage of stool and alleviating symptoms associated with chronic idiopathic constipation. This medication is usually well tolerated, but it may cause nausea. Patients who experience nausea should be instructed to eat before taking the drug to reduce the symptoms. This drug should not be administered to patients who have severe diarrhea or symptoms that suggest mechanical gastrointestinal obstruction. Clinicians who prescribe this medication should periodically assess their patients to determine if they need continuing therapy.

PHARMACOLOGY OF DRUGS USED IN THE TREATMENT OF INFLAMMATORY BOWEL DISEASE (IBD)

Inflammatory bowel disease (IBD) is an idiopathic disease involving a group of disorders in which there is an inflammation of the intestines, likely as a result of the body's immune system reacting to its own intestinal tract. There are two major types of IBD: ulcerative colitis (UC) and Crohn's disease (CD). Because researchers have never found the cause of IBD, it remains idiopathic. Because the intestinal wall is damaged, it presents as bloody diarrhea and intestinal pain. The clinical course of both diseases can differ from a mild form in which the patient reaches long-term remission without taking permanent medications, to a chronic active form, in which remission is only reached by taking immunosuppressive and biological medications permanently or by taking them for extended periods of time. Whereas ulcerative colitis is limited to the colon, Crohn's disease can involve any segment of the gastrointestinal tract from the mouth to the anus. Both diseases usually have a waxing and waning intensity and severity. The disease causes inflammation of the mucosal lining of the intestinal tract causing ulceration, edema, bleeding, and fluid and electrolyte loss. In the United States, it is estimated that 1 to 2 million people have ulcerative colitis or Crohn's disease. The male–to–female ratio is approximately equal for both diseases, and both are commonly diagnosed in young adults, during late adolescence, and during the third decade of life.

Patients with Crohn's disease involving the small intestine frequently have abdominal pain, bloody diarrhea, and occasionally have symptoms of intestinal obstruction. Patients sometimes complain of fatigue, which is related to the inflammation and anemia that accompanies disease activity. The medical approach to treating patients with IBD that is symptomatic or "flaring" follows a stepwise approach to medication therapy, with the progression of the medical regimen until a response is achieved. Drugs used in the treatment of inflammatory bowel disease include 5-aminosalicylates (5-ASAs), antibiotics such as metronidazole, corticosteroids, immunosuppressives, methotrexate and cyclosporine, and biological therapies. Also used are antidiarrheal agents. A **step-down therapy** entails using the most effective biological or immunosuppressive treatments on the market, even without prior use of therapeutics such as steroids, to reach an effective remission as soon as possible. Conversely, a **step-up therapy** means using a classical treatment approach by, for example, starting with an aminosalicylate and ending with an immunosuppressive or biological medication. In this chapter, the focus will be on 5-ASAs and antidiarrheal agents for the treatment of patients with IBD.

5-Aminosalicylates (5-ASAs)

Sulfasalazine is split into sulfapyridine and mesalamine (5-ASAs) by bacteria in the colon. Mesalamine is thought to be the active component and is an aminosalicylate. The mechanism of action of sulfasalazine and mesalamine is unknown, but it is thought to be topical rather than systemic. These agents act by blocking cyclooxygenase and inhibiting prostaglandin production in the colon. The 5-ASAs are bowel-specific drugs that are metabolized in the gut where the predominant action occurs. These drugs are derivatives of salicylic acid and are also antioxidants that trap free radicals that are potentially damaging by-products of metabolism. In the treatment of ulcerative colitis, these drugs function as free radical traps as well as anti-inflammatory drugs.

The six oral aminosalicylate preparations available for use in the United States are sulfasalazine (Azulfidine), mesalamine

(Asacol, Lialda, Pentasa), balsalazide (Colazal), and olsalazine (Dipentum). Enema and suppository formulations are also available. The major differences are in the mechanism of delivery. Some of these drugs also have unique adverse effects that other agents of this class lack. All of the aminosalicylates are useful for treating flares of IBD and for maintaining remission. None of the aminosalicylates have been proven to have greater efficacy for the treatment of ulcerative colitis or Crohn's disease over any of the others. All of them are more effective in persons with ulcerative colitis than in persons with Crohn's disease; in persons with Crohn's disease, the primary utility is for colonic disease.

Dosage and Administration of 5-ASAs

Generic Name	Trade Name	Route	Usual Adult Daily Dose
sulfasalazine	Azulfidine	PO	500 mg PO 2 times/day, may increase to 1,000 mg PO 4 times/day
mesalamine	Asacol Lialda Pentasa	PO	Active disease: TWO 400-mg tablets PO 3 times/day for 6 weeks using delayed release capsules or dose with 2 to 4 tablets of 1.2 gm tablets once /day for 6 weeks
olsalazine sodium	Dipentum	PO	1 g/day in 2 divided doses
balsalazide disodium	Colazal	PO	3 capsules 3 times/day (6.75 g per day)

Sulfasalazine (Azulfidine)

Sulfasalazine is a 5-ASA connected to sulfapyridine by an azo bond; colonic bacteria break the azo bond, releasing the active 5-ASA. It is used for the treatment of acute disease and for maintenance of remission. When taken with iron, digoxin, and folic acid, sulfasalazine decreases their effects. Conversely, it increases the effect of oral anticoagulants, oral hypoglycemic agents, and methotrexate. Adverse reactions include cyanosis, anorexia, vomiting, gastric distress, hepatotoxicity, elevated liver function tests, hemolytic anemia, leukopenia, thrombocytopenia, headache, and dizziness. Clinicians should perform a complete blood count test, including differential white cell counts and liver function tests, before starting this drug and every second week during the first 3 months of therapy. Also, urine analysis and assessment of renal function should be done periodically during treatment with this drug. This medication should be used with caution in patients with hepatic or renal damage. This drug is contraindicated for patients who are allergic to sulfonamides or salicylates.

Mesalamine (Asacol, Lialda, Pentasa)

The oral mesalamine products currently approved in the United States differ only in the mechanism of drug delivery. Asacol has mesalamine within a coating that dissolves and releases the mesalamine at pH 7, which typically occurs in the terminal ileum. Pentasa is 5-ASA in ethylcellulose and has a time-release coating. Release of mesalamine from Pentasa begins at the pylorus; because of this, the drug is often used when proximal

intestinal Crohn's disease is suggested. Lialda is indicated to induce remission in active ulcerative colitis. It has a proprietary release mechanism that is referred to as MMX technology. This is actually a combination of the release mechanisms of Asacol (with a pH-dependent coating) and Pentasa (a water-soluble matrix). Rectal dosage forms deliver high concentrations of mesalamine to the left colon as high as the splenic flexure (enema with 30-minute retention) or to the rectum for use in proctitis (suppository). Although these drugs are effective, they are associated with a relatively high relapse rate upon discontinuation.

The most common adverse effects are rash, occasional fever, and flulike syndrome. Clinicians should use this drug with caution in patients with renal or hepatic impairment. Elderly patients may have difficulty administering and retaining a rectal suppository. These drugs decrease the effects of iron, digoxin, and folic acid. They increase the effects of oral anticoagulants, methotrexate, and oral hypoglycemic agents.

Biological Therapies (Monoclonal Antibodies) for Treating IBD

The goal of medical treatment is to suppress IBD's abnormal inflammation to allow intestinal tissue to heal and to decrease the frequency of flare-ups while maintaining remission; thus, taking a stepwise approach to the use of medications is appropriate. The most benign drugs are used first; if they fail to provide relief, drugs from a second or higher step are used. In this case, the aminosalicylates and symptomatic agents are step 1 drugs, as are antibiotics. These agents are helpful in persons with Crohn's disease who have perianal disease or an inflammatory mass.

Corticosteroids constitute step 2 drugs and can be used if step 1 drugs fail to provide adequate response and control. They are considered successful if they provide rapid relief of symptoms as well as a significant decrease in inflammation.

The immune modifying agents, or biologicals, are step 3 drugs, which come into play if the corticosteroids fail or if the corticosteroids are required for prolonged periods. These agents are not used in acute flare-ups because the time from initiation of treatment to the onset of significant action may be as long as 2 to 3 months. An agent such as infliximab (Remicade) is a step 3 drug to be used in persons with moderate to severely active Crohn's disease. Its pharmacology is discussed at length in the Chapter 4, Drugs Used in the Treatment of Bone and Joint Disorders, because it is a monoclonal antibody used in treating rheumatoid arthritis. Infliximab is administered intravenously, which affords complete bioavailability. The drug is distributed throughout the vascular compartment, but its metabolism and excretion remain unknown. When administered as an intravenous infusion over 2 hours, it is dosed at 5 mg/kg and repeated 2 and 6 weeks after the initial infusion. Patients should be advised to watch for fatigue, headache, upper respiratory tract infections, abdominal pain, nausea and vomiting, fever, and a large host of adverse effects, all of which may occur 3 to 12 days after treatment. However, adverse events usually resolve in 1 to 3 days once they appear.

In practice, drugs from all steps may be used additively; however, the goal is to remove corticosteroids from the regimen as soon as possible to prevent long-term side effects.

PROKINETIC AGENTS/GASTROINTESTINAL STIMULANTS

Prokinetic agents are also known as gastrointestinal stimulants. These drugs stimulate the motility of the gastrointestinal tract without stimulating gastric, biliary, or pancreatic secretions. They are used in the management of a wide variety of disorders of the gastrointestinal tract in which GI motility is a problem. These disorders include gastroparesis, often associated with diabetes mellitus, emesis associated with cancer chemotherapy, and gastrointestinal reflux disease. There are two drugs in this class: metoclopramide and dexpanthenol, which is used prophylactically after major abdominal surgery to minimize the possibility of a paralytic ileus.

Metoclopramide (Reglan)

Metoclopramide was approved by the FDA in 1985. It is the most commonly used drug in this class.

Conscientious Prescribing of Metoclopramide

- Patients with a history of depression should be given metoclopramide only if the expected benefits outweigh the potential risk.
- Patients with Parkinson's disease should be treated cautiously if at all with this drug because they may experience exacerbation of the Parkinsonian symptoms.
- Metoclopramide should not be used for long-term treatment or management of gastroesophageal reflux disease. It should not be used for more than 8 weeks because there is a much higher risk for adverse reactions, including extrapyramidal symptoms.
- This drug should be used cautiously for patients with diseases that place them at higher risk for extrapyramidal symptoms.
- Because there is a need to adjust the dose in the presence of renal impairment, renal function should be assessed before therapy is begun.

Patient/Family Education for Metoclopramide

- Patients should be advised that this drug may impair their mental or physical ability to perform hazardous tasks such as operating machinery or driving a motor vehicle.
- Patients should be advised to take the drug exactly as prescribed: 30 minutes before each meal and at bedtime. Patients should be advised that if they miss a dose, it should be taken as soon as they remember unless it is time for the next dose. They should also be advised that they cannot double the dose or exceed the recommended dose.
- Patients should be warned to notify their clinician immediately if involuntary movements of the eyes, face, or limbs occur.

- Lifestyle modifications should be tried before any drug in the management of both gastroesophageal reflux disease and diabetic gastroparesis. Patients should avoid alcohol and NSAIDs. They should be encouraged to stop smoking, follow a weight loss plan, sleep with the head of the bed elevated, and avoid caffeine and citrus foods as well as large meals consisting of fatty foods.

Mechanism of Action

This drug stimulates motility of the upper gastrointestinal tract. Mode of action is unclear, but it seems to sensitize tissues to the action of acetylcholine. Metoclopramide increases the tone and amplitude of gastric contractions, relaxes the pyloric sphincter and the duodenal bulb, and increases peristalsis of the duodenum and jejunum, resulting in accelerated gastric emptying and intestinal transit. It increases the resting tone of the lower esophageal sphincter but has little effect on the motility of the colon or gallbladder.

Pharmacokinetics

- Absorption: Rapidly and well absorbed
- Distribution: Widely distributed throughout the body tissues, crosses the blood-brain barrier and the placenta, and enters breast milk in concentrations greater than in plasma
- Metabolism: Metabolized by the liver
- Excretion: Excretion is principally through the kidneys
- Half-life: 4 to 6 hours under normal renal functioning

Dosage and Administration

Generic Name	Trade Name	Route	Usual Adult Daily Dose
metoclopramide	Reglan	PO, IM, IV	10–15 mg by mouth 4 times/day, 30 min before each meal and at bedtime

Clinical Uses

- Short-term therapy for adults with symptomatic, documented gastroesophageal reflux who failed to respond to other conventional therapies
- For the relief of symptoms associated with acute and recurrent diabetic gastric stasis (gastroparesis)

Adverse Reactions

CV: Hypotension, hypertension, super ventricular tachycardia, bradycardia, fluid retention, acute congestive heart failure.
ENDO: Galactorrhea, amenorrhea, gynecomastia.
GI: Nausea and bowel disturbances such as diarrhea.
HEM: Neutropenia, leukopenia, agranulocytosis.
NEURO: Restlessness, drowsiness, fatigue, insomnia, headache, confusion, dizziness, mental depression. **Mental depression** has occurred in patients with and without a history of depression where symptoms have ranged from mild to severe and have included suicidal ideation and suicide. **Extrapyramidal symptoms** are manifested as acute dysthymic reactions that occur in approximately 1 in 500 patients. These effects are usually seen during the first 24 to 48 hours of treatment with metoclopramide and occur more frequently in pediatric patients and adult patients younger than 30 years of age.

Symptoms include involuntary movements of limbs and facial grimacing, torticollis, rhythmic protrusion of tongue, and dysthymic reactions resembling tetanus. **Parkinson-like symptoms** occur more frequently within the first 6 months after beginning treatment with metoclopramide. Symptoms generally subside within 2 to 3 months following discontinuation of the drug. **Tardive dyskinesia** is a syndrome that consists of potentially irreversible and involuntary dyskinetic movements that may develop in patients treated with metoclopramide. Although the prevalence of this syndrome appears to be highest among the elderly, especially elderly women, it is impossible to predict which patients are likely to develop the syndrome. The risk of developing the syndrome and the likelihood that it will become irreversible increases with the duration of treatment and the total cumulative dose.

Interactions

- The effects of metoclopramide on gastrointestinal motility are antagonized by anticholinergic drugs and narcotic analgesics. Additive sedative effects can occur when this agent is given with alcohol, sedatives, hypnotics, narcotics, or tranquilizers.
- Absorption of drugs from the stomach may be diminished by metoclopramide in such drugs as digoxin. The rate or extent of absorption of drugs from the small bowel may be increased in drugs such as acetaminophen, tetracycline, and levodopa.

Contraindications

- This drug is contraindicated whenever stimulation of the GI motility might be dangerous, such as in the presence of a gastrointestinal hemorrhage, mechanical obstruction, or perforation.
- It is also contraindicated in patients with pheochromocytoma because the drug may cause hypertensive crisis due to the release of catecholamines from the tumor.
- It is contraindicated in patients with known sensitivity or intolerance to the drug.
- Because this drug is mainly excreted through the kidneys, it should be used with caution for patients with renal impairment.
- Metoclopramide should not be used in patients with epilepsy or those receiving other drugs that are likely to cause extrapyramidal reactions because the frequency and severity of seizures or extrapyramidal reactions may be increased.

Lipase Inhibitors

Orlistat (Alli, Xenical)

Orlistat (Alli, Xenical) is the only drug in this class and was approved by the FDA in 1999. It is commonly used for obesity management, including weight loss and weight maintenance, in conjunction with a reduced-calorie diet. It is also indicated to reduce the risk for weight regain after prior weight loss. This drug is indicated for obese patients who have an initial body mass index of 30 kg/m^2 or more or 27 kg/m^2 in the presence of other risk factors such as hypertension, diabetes, or dyslipidemia. Orlistat is a reversible inhibitor of lipase. It exerts its therapeutic activity in the lumen of the stomach and small intestine by forming a covalent bond with the active serine residues site of gastric and pancreatic lipases. The inactivated enzymes are unavailable to hydrolyze dietary fat into undigested triglycerides. Thus, as undigested triglycerides are not absorbed, the resulting caloric deficit may have a positive effect on weight control.

Orlistat can be found and bought over the counter by adults 18 years or older. The recommended dose of over-the-counter orlistat is a 60-mg capsule taken three times a day with each main meal containing fat. Because orlistat has been shown to reduce absorption of some fat-soluble vitamins and beta carotene, patients should be counseled to take a multivitamin containing fat-soluble vitamins to ensure adequate nutrition while taking this medication. This drug should be taken with a reduced calorie low-fat diet and exercise program until the patient's weight loss goal is reached. Most weight loss occurs in the first 6 months. The most commonly observed adverse reactions are fatty/oily stools, fecal urgency and incontinence, flatulence with discharge, oily spitting on evacuation, and increased defecation. This drug is contraindicated in patients with chronic malabsorption syndrome or cholestasis.

Implications for Special Populations

Pregnancy Implications

When prescribing for the pregnant female, clinicians should carefully consider their choice of drugs. Following is a selected list of drugs used in treating GI disorders, along with their assigned FDA Safety Category.

FDA PREGNANCY SAFETY CATEGORY	DRUGS
B	cimetidine (Tagamet)
	ranitidine (Zantac)
	famotidine (Pepcid)
	nizatidine (Axid)
	sulfasalazine (Azulfidine)
	mesalamine (Asacol, Lialda, Pentasa)
	olsalazine sodium (Dipentum)
	balsalazide Disodium (Colazal)
	sucralfate (Carafate)
	ondansetron (Zofran)
	promethazine (Phenergan)
	prochlorperazine (Compazine)
	metoclopramide (Reglan)
	orlistat (Alli, Xenical)
C	omeprazole (Nexium, Prilosec)
	lansoprazole (Prevacid)
	esomeprazole (Protonix)
	rabeprazole (Aciphex)
D	
X	misoprostol (Cytotec)
Unclassified	

Geriatric Implications

■ GI issues are quite common in the elderly and every symptom needs to be evaluated before treating them because secondary causes are frequent.

■ Acid secretion in the GI tract reaches its peak during the night, thus the elderly who are being prescribed the histamine 2 blockers should take them at bedtime. In addition, the side effects of these drugs occur more in the elderly than they do in younger adults.

■ Should mental issues appear in the elderly while on histamine 2 blockers, it is usually a sign that the dose is too high.

■ Any elderly person who smokes is likely to find that it increases the amount of acid pouring into the stomach, thus older adults should quit smoking.

LEARNING EXERCISES

Case 1

JS is a 62-year-old male who is taking several cardiac medications that are known to cause constipation. The results of a physical exam and colonoscopy are normal. He tried Metamucil, a bulking agent, to "get regular," but it is not working.

1. Along with medication, what lifestyle issues should you discuss with the patient?

2. What treatment options are available for this patient?

Case 2

BJ is a 19-year-old college student who has been complaining of diarrhea that has lasted for 3 weeks. His symptoms include frequent loose stools, abdominal pain and cramping, fever, chills, some weight loss, and feeling thirsty. Up to now, he has not been treating himself, thinking every day that this is the day it will all go away.

1. What might be BJ's problem?

2. What can you do to help BJ?

References

Centers for Disease Control and Prevention (CDC). (2006). *Helicobacter pylori* and peptic ulcer disease: The key to cure. *H. pylori* Fact Sheet for Health Care Providers. Retrieved January 24, 2013, from www.cdc.gov/ulcer/keytocure.htm

Di Palma, J. A., Cleveland, M. B., McGowan, J., & Herrera, J. L. (2007). A randomized, multicenter comparison of polyethylene glycol laxative and tegaserod in treatment of patients with chronic constipation. *The American Journal of Gastroenterology, 102*(9), 1964–1971.

Dorn S. D., Morris, C. B., Hu, Y., et al. (2009). Irritable bowel syndrome subtypes defined by Rome II and Rome III criteria are similar. *Journal of Clinical Gastroenterology, 43*(3), 214-220.

Gatta, L., Vakil, L., Leandro, G., Di Mario, F., & Vaira, D. (2009). Sequential therapy or triple therapy for *Helicobacter pylori* infection: Systematic review and meta-analysis of randomized controlled trials in adults and children. *The American Journal of Gastroenterology, 104*, 3069-3079.

Porter, C. K., Gormley, R., Tribble, D. R., Brooks, D. C., & Riddle, M. S. (2011). The incidence and gastrointestinal infectious risk of functional gastrointestinal disorders in a healthy US adult population. *American Journal of Gastroenterology, 106*, 130–138.

Seppa, N. (2007). Bad to the bone: Acid stoppers appear to have a downside. *Science News, 171*(1): 3.

Vakil, N., van Zanten, S., Kahrilas, P., Dent, J., Jones, R., & Global Consensus Group. (2006). The Montreal definition and classification of gastro-esophageal reflux disease (GERD)—A global evidence-based consensus. *American Journal of Gastroenterology, 101*(8), 1900–1920.

Zagaria, M. A. E. (2007). GERD update: The refractory patient, *U.S. Pharmacist, 2007*(32), 20-23.

Drugs Used to Treat Endocrine Gland Disorders

chapter 12

Alice A. House, William N. Tindall, Mona M. Sedrak

CHAPTER FOCUS

The role of endocrinologists is expanding, both in responsibility and complexity. In this chapter we briefly discuss hormones, both agonists and antagonists, that have become available for therapeutic use. Thus, this chapter focuses on how a few synthesized hormones can be used to fight disorders of the endocrine system as either substitutes or replacements in hormone deficiencies, as modifiers of malfunctioning endocrine organs, or as adjuncts to normally functioning endocrine organs. With this objective in mind, this chapter discusses drugs for thyroid, parathyroid, adrenal, and pituitary disorders, leaving the pancreatic hormone disease of diabetes to be discussed in Chapter 13.

OBJECTIVES

After reading and studying this chapter, the student should be able to:

1. Identify the major hormones, how they are produced, and their function in the body.
2. Describe the signs and symptoms associated with hypothyroidism, hyperthyroidism, hypoparathyroidism, and hyperparathyroidism.
3. Discuss the primary agents used in the treatment of hypothyroidism, their mechanism of action, clinical use, side effect profile, drug interactions, and patient advisories.
4. Explain the effects of iodine, radioactive iodine, and thioamide drugs in the treatment of hyperthyroidism.
5. Describe the use and dosage of calcium and vitamin D products in the treatment of hypoparathyroidism.
6. Describe the indications for and mechanism of action of vasopressin and oxytocin.
7. Discuss the use of corticosteroids, their mechanism of action, clinical use, side effect profile, drug interactions, and patient advisories.

Key Terms

Addison's disease
Adrenal insufficiency
Agranulocytosis
Androgens
Cretinism
Cushing's syndrome
Diabetes insipidus
Estrogen replacement therapy
Goiter
Graves' disease
Hashimoto's thyroiditis
Hormone
Hyperparathyroidism
Hyperthyroidism
Hypoparathyroidism
Hypothyroidism
Myxedema
Negative feedback
Resorption
Thyroid storm
Thyrotoxicosis
United States Pharmacopeia Convention (USP)

KEY DRUGS IN THIS CHAPTER

Drugs Affecting the Thyroid Gland

Drugs Used in the Treatment of Hypothyroidism
levothyroxine sodium (Synthroid, Levoxyl)
liothyronine (Cytomel, Triostat)
liothyronine (T3)/levothyroxine (T4) combination (Euthroid).
liotrix (Thyrolar)
thyroid extract USP (generic)

Drugs Used in the Treatment of Hyperthyroidism
propylthiouracil (PTU)
methimazole (Tapazole)

Drugs Affecting the Parathyroid Glands
Drugs Used in the Treatment of Hyperparathyroidism
cinacalcet (Sensipar)

Drugs Used in the Treatment of Hypoparathyroidism
calcitriol (Rocaltrol)

Drugs Affecting the Pituitary Gland
Drugs Affecting the Posterior Pituitary Gland
vasopressin (Pitressin)
oxytocin (Pitocin)

continued

The endocrine system consists of more than a dozen glands. These specialized glands secrete about 50 naturally occurring substances into the bloodstream, and they initiate and/or regulate the activity of an organ or group of cells. The sex glands and adrenal glands secrete substances known as steroids whereas the rest of the endocrine glands secrete hormones. By definition, a **hormone** is a chemical substance produced in the body to control and regulate the activity of certain cells or organs essential for activities of daily living, including the processes of digestion, metabolism, growth, reproduction, and mood control. Many of these hormones, such as the neurotransmitters, are active in more than one physical process. Hormones have well-defined effects on metabolism. The major hormones include the following:

■ Products of secretion from anterior and posterior pituitary glands
■ Thyroid hormones
■ Parathyroid hormones
■ Pancreatic insulin and glucagon
■ Epinephrine and norepinephrine from the adrenal medulla
■ Several steroids from the adrenal cortex
■ Gonadal hormones of both sexes

Hormones from the various endocrine glands work in harmony to regulate various functions:

■ Secretory and motor activities of the digestive tract
■ Energy production and regulation
■ Internal homeostasis (composition and volume of extracellular fluid)
■ Reproduction and lactation
■ Growth and development
■ Adaptation (acclimatization and immunity)

The study of hormones has revealed there are three kinds of hormones: protein hormones, amine hormones, and steroid hormones. Protein hormones exert their effect on receptors within the membrane and bind to the receptors on the outside of membrane. Their effects occur the most rapidly of all the hormones. Amine hormones show relatively the same fast receptor response because they are protein hormones. Finally, steroid hormones bind to the intercellular receptors and have slow action.

To maintain the internal environment, hormone secretion is regulated and controlled by a self-regulating series of events known as negative feedback. In **negative feedback**, a hormone produces a physiological effect that, when strong enough, inhibits further secretion of that hormone, thus inhibiting the physiological effect. Increased hormone secretion may be evoked

in response to stimuli from the external environment such as our emotions and perceptions or our behaviors.

In exerting their physiological effects, hormones are not used up but rather must be inactivated or excreted. While inactivation occurs enzymatically in the blood or intercellular spaces, liver, kidney, or target tissues, excretion occurs primarily via the urine and the bile. Although most hormones are destroyed rapidly, with a half-life of 10 to 30 minutes, thyroid hormones have a half-life measured in days. Catecholamines, by contrast, have a half-life that is measured in seconds. The endocrine system is so flexible that some hormones exert a physiological effect immediately, whereas others require minutes to hours before their effect is felt. Some effects end immediately when the hormone disappears, and others may persist for hours to days after hormone concentrations have returned to basal levels. Alterations in either hormone secretion or receptor responses may lead to endocrine disease states.

A hormone is broadly defined as any chemical, irrespective of whether it is produced by a special gland or not, that controls and regulates the activity of certain cells or organs. The word *hormao* was used in ancient Greek to mean, "I set in motion" or "I stir up." The term *hormone* came into modern use in 1902 when the English physiologists William M. Bayliss and Ernest H. Starling reported their discovery of a substance made by glands in the small intestine that stimulated secretion from the pancreas. They called that substance *secretin* and dubbed it a *hormone*, making this the first reference to a hormone. This chapter focuses on some of the common medications used to correct the secretion of either too much or too little of specific hormones.

DRUGS AFFECTING THE THYROID GLAND

Thyroid diseases are among the most frequent and most challenging endocrine disorders. The thyroid is one of the largest endocrine glands in the body (normal weight is 15 to 25 g). It is a butterfly-shaped structure located below and to the sides of the trachea. Its rich blood supply is derived from the external carotids via the superior thyroid arteries and from the subclavian arteries via the inferior thyroid arteries. The rate of blood flow through it is greater than 500 mL/100 g of tissue per minute.

The thyroid gland secretes three hormones essential for the regulation of metabolism: L-thyroxine (T4), L-triiodothyronine (T3) and calcitonin. To make T3 and T4, the thyroid does the following:

■ Transports iodide into the thyroid gland via a specific iodide pump.

■ Extracts iodide from plasma proteins circulating through the gland.

■ Oxidizes the iodide to iodine and couples it to tyrosine. The iodine can couple with either one molecule of an amino acid, monoiodotyrosine (MIT; contains 1 iodine), or it can couple with two molecules of tyrosine, diiodotyrosine (DIT; contains 2 iodines) (Fig. 12-1).

■ T4 secretion is stimulated by thyroid-stimulating hormone (TSH), and in turn TSH secretion is inhibited by a negative feed-back loop that keeps the T4 levels at the biological level of a very narrow range.

If a one-molecule monoiodotyrosine couples with one molecule of diiodotyrosine, then T3 is produced. If two molecules of diiodotyrosine couple together, T4 is produced (Fig. 12-2). A coupling reaction then allows synthesis of the hormones:

$$MIT + DIT = T3 \text{ (3 iodines) and } DIT + DIT = T4$$
$$\text{(4 iodines)}$$

MIT and DIT are stored in association with a thyroid protein molecule called thyroglobulin within the thyroid gland. Proteolysis of thyroglobulin releases T3 and T4 from thyroglobulin, and these hormones are secreted in a ratio of 5:1 (T4/T3). Once secreted, L-thyroxine (T4) stimulates metabolism (body heat rises), and T3 and T4 are highly bound to specific plasma proteins. However, only unbound T3 and T4 are able to enter body cells to exert an effect. Only 0.4% of T3 and 0.04% of T4 exist in the free form with any metabolic activity. The pituitary, liver, kidneys, heart, skeletal muscle, lungs, and intestines have high-affinity binding sites for T3 and T4 in the nucleus of a hormone-responsive cell. T4 receptor affinity is 10 times lower than T3 affinity. Thus, T3 is more potent than T4 and is responsible for most systemic effects.

All thyroid preparations undergo metabolism in the liver and other tissues. They also undergo enterohepatic recirculation and excretion in the feces in the bile.

Drugs Used in the Treatment of Hypothyroidism

Hypothyroidism refers to the clinical manifestations of thyroid hormone deficiency. It can be seen as a consequence of three different processes:

1. Defective synthesis of thyroid hormone with compensatory development of **goiter**
2. Inadequate function of thyroid parenchyma as a result of thyroiditis or surgical resection of the gland
3. Inadequate secretion of TSH by the pituitary or of thyroid-releasing hormone (TRH) by the hypothalamus.

About 90% of all problems involving the thyroid are due to dysfunction of the thyroid itself, such as primary hypothyroidism. Secondary hypothyroidism can be the result of Hashimoto's disease, iatrogenic causes, and drugs that contain iodine, such as lithium.

Primary hypothyroidism is most often seen in the fifth and sixth decade and is more common in women than in men. Most patients have circulating antibodies to thyroid antigens. Non-goitrous hypothyroidism may also result from antibodies that block TSH receptors without deactivating the thyroid. Patients with primary hypothyroidism have decreased T3 and T4 levels and an elevated TSH. Those with pituitary (secondary) hypothyroidism and hypothalamic (tertiary) hypothyroidism have decreased T3, T4, and TSH. Thus, a logical approach to treating hypothyroidism is to replace either the T4 or T3 with a preparation containing the missing substances. Interestingly, these supplements do produce the same effects on the body as do naturally occurring hormones. They also exert their same effect on the negative feedback loop to reduce secretion of TSH and further thyroid hormone production.

Thyroid hormones are indicated as replacement or supplemental therapy for hypothyroidism of any etiology except transient hypothyroidism during the recovery phase of subacute thyroiditis. Thyroid hormones are also indicated in the treatment or prevention of various types of euthyroid goiters including thyroid nodules, subacute or chronic lymphocyte thyroiditis, and multinodular goiter, and in the management of thyroid cancer. In the past, desiccated thyroid from animal sources such as pork was the major source of thyroid hormone, but today the most frequently used thyroid preparations are synthetics, which has assured the public of uniform content and bioavailability from dose to dose. It is also popular to use a combination of T3 and T4 in the same preparation; liotrix (Thyrolar) is a popular 4:1 mixture of T3 and T4.

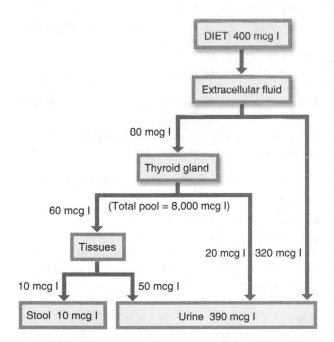

Iodine trap:
● Active transport
● Energy dependent
● Synthesis stimulated by TSH
● Maintains thyroid/plasma ratio of 30:1

FIGURE 12-1 Iodide turnover in humans.

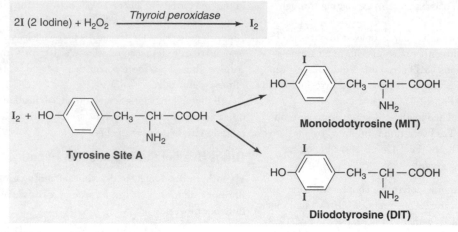

FIGURE 12-2 Synthesis of thyroid hormones.

Conscientious Prescribing of Thyroid Hormones

■ Long-term therapy has been associated with decreased bone density in the hip and spine, and this has happened in both premenopausal and postmenopausal women.

■ If dosage is excessive, signs of **hyperthyroidism** may be seen (weight loss, palpitations, increased appetite, tremors, nervousness, tachycardia, headache, hypertension, menstrual irregularities).

■ In primary hypothyroidism, the goal of therapy is to maintain TSH plasma within normal limits. Thus, plasma TSH is to be measured every 2 to 3 months and the dosage adjusted in small increments of 10 to 25 mcg at 6- to 8-week intervals until normal plasma TSH is reached.

■ Periodic assessment of thyroid status by the appropriate laboratory tests should be performed, as well as a full clinical evaluation.

■ Drugs with thyroid hormone activity, alone or together with other therapeutic agents, have been used for the treatment of obesity. In euthyroid patients, doses within the range of daily hormonal requirements are ineffective for weight reduction.

Patient/Family Education Regarding Thyroid Hormones

■ Make sure that patients understand that replacement therapy is to be taken for a lifetime, with the exception of cases of transient hypothyroidism and in those patients receiving a therapeutic trial of the drug.

■ Patients with concomitant diabetes mellitus should be informed that the daily dosage of antidiabetic medication may need readjustment once the therapeutic goal of thyroid hormone replacement is achieved. If thyroid medication is stopped, a downward readjustment of the dosage of insulin or oral hypoglycemic agents may be necessary.

■ Patients should be instructed to take the medication at the same time each day. Patients should follow a routine of taking the drug in the morning, preferably 30 minutes before breakfast. If a dose is missed, take as soon as remembered unless it is near time for the next dose. If more than 2 to 3 doses are missed, contact the clinician.

■ Ask patients to monitor their pulse. Dose should be withheld if pulse is greater than 100 beats per minute (bpm).

■ Instruct patients to make certain the pharmacist does *not* change brands, because bioavailability may be affected.

■ Tell patients to inform all caregivers that they are on thyroid therapy.

■ Instruct patients to report any signs or symptoms of thyroid hormone toxicity such as chest pain and increased pulse or any other unusual signs.

■ Ask patients to recite possible side effects and to call the clinician if these side effects occur:
  ■ If the dose is too LOW you may see bradycardia, constipation, fatigue, lethargy.
  ■ If the dose is too HIGH, you may see diarrhea, dysrhythmia, heat intolerance, hyperthermia, irritability, or tachycardia.

■ Patients should be told that this drug takes about 1 month before its full effects can be seen.

■ Exposing the medication to heat can inactivate the medication, thereby affecting absorption.

Levothyroxine sodium/thyroxine/L-thyroxine (T4) (Synthroid, Levoxyl, Unithroid)

Levothyroxine (T4) is used as a replacement for thyroid hormone or as a supplemental therapy in cases of hypothroidism. The body does not differentiate between natural sources or synthetic sources of thyroid hormone. It is administered as the sodium salt of the naturally occuring levorotating isomer of T4 as the preparation of choice for maintaining plasma T4 and T3 levels.

Mechanism of Action

How T3 and T4 work to control body metabolic processes is still a mystery, but it is believed they play a role in DNA and protein synthesis.

Pharmacokinetics

■ Absorption: Levothyroxine is variably (50% to 80%) absorbed from gastrointestinal (GI) tract, whereas liothyronine (T3) is 95% absorbed within 4 hours.

■ Distribution: 99% of both circulating hormones are bound to serum proteins. They flow to most body tissues, do not cross placenta, have minimal amount in milk. T3 and T4 exist in the body in equilibrium between bound and free drug, but only the free drug produces the hormone's effects.
■ Metabolism: Metabolized by liver and other target tissues
■ Excretion: Hormones undergo enterohepatic recirculation and are excreted in feces via bile.
■ Half-life: T4, 6 to 7 days.

Dosage and Administration

Generic Name	Trade Name	Route	Usual Adult Daily Dose
levothyroxine sodium/thyroxine/ L-thyroxine (T4)	Synthroid, Levoxyl, Unithroid	PO, IM, IV	50 mcg as a single dose initially, which may be increased every 2–3 weeks (see Fig. 12-3)

Clinical Uses

■ Increases basal metabolism
■ Enhances gluconeogenesis
■ Stimulates protein synthesis

Adverse Reactions

CV: Tachycardia
DERM: Urticaria
META: Heat intolerance
NEURO: Tremors, rash

Interactions

■ Bile acid sequestrants, iron salts, antacids, decrease thyroid hormone absorption.
■ Estrogens may decrease the response to thyroid hormone.
■ Beta blockers, digoxin, and warfarin find decreased effectiveness in the presence of thyroid hormones.

Contraindications

■ Recent myocardial infarction
■ Thyrotoxicosis if uncomplicated by hypothyroidism

Mrs. I. M. Sick
123 Main Street   Date: _____
Hometown, USA

RX: Levothyroxine – 50 mcg generic
Mitte: c
Sig: I tab daily for thyroid

Dr. I M Smart: _____

Refill x 4 – (Have patient call in
2 wks to adjust dose)

Cost: $24/100 tabs.

FIGURE 12-3 Sample prescription for a thyroid patient.

Conscientious Considerations

■ Thyroxine (T4) is the drug of choice because of its consistent potency, good absorption, and prolonged duration of action.
■ Because of its long half-life, it allows for convenient once-a-day dosing.
■ In addition, clinicians must be aware of the important considerations that apply to all thyroid hormone preparations (see p. 200, Conscientious Prescribing of Thyroid Hormones).

Patient/Family Education

■ The advisories for patients who are taking levothyroxine are the same as those for patients taking any other thyroid preparation (see p. 200, Patient/Family Education Regarding Thyroid Hormones).

liothyronine (Cytomel, Triostat)

Liothyronine is the sodium salt of the naturally occurring levorotatory isomer of T3. Liothyronine (T3) in synthetic form is four times as potent as nonsynthetic T3.

Mechanism of Action

These hormones enhance oxygen consumption by most tissues of the body and increase the basal metabolic rate and the metabolism of carbohydrates, lipids, and proteins. They exert a profound influence on every organ system in the body and are of particular importance in the development of the central nervous system.

Pharmacokinetics

■ Absorption: Absorption of orally administered T4 varies from 40% to 80% of the administered dose. Absorption is increased by fasting and decreased by malabsorption syndrome.
■ Distribution: More than 99% of circulating hormones are bound to serum proteins, including pyroxene-binding globulin and pyroxene-binding prealbumin and albumin, whose capacities and affinities vary for the hormones.
■ Metabolism: In the liver to a conjugated form.
■ Excretion: From hepatic circulation they are excreted in the feces once entered into bile.
■ Half-life: Because of its short half-life, liothyronine is not generally used alone for maintenance thyroid hormone replacement therapy.

Dosage and Administration

Generic Name	Trade Name	Route	Usual Adult Daily Dose
liothyronine	Cytomel, Triostat	PO, IM	5 mcg/day and increase 5–10 mcg/week. Maintenance dose for myxedema, goiter, is about 75 mcg/day.

Clinical Uses

■ Treatment of myxedema (in combination with Synthroid)
■ Short-term suppression of TSH in patients undergoing surgery for thyroid cancer

Adverse Reactions

CV: Arrhythmias, tachycardia
DERM: Hair loss (reversible) in children at start of therapy, dry skin, rash, hives
GI: GI Intolerance
NEURO: Headaches

Interactions

■ Oral anticoagulants (e.g., warfarin): Thyroid preparations increase the catabolism of vitamin K-dependent clotting factor.

■ Insulin and oral hypoglycemic: Initiating thyroid replacement therapy may cause increases in necessary doses of the oral hypoglycemics.

■ Bile acid sequestrants (cholestyramine): These agents impair absorption of both T3 and T4 in the intestine.

■ Tricyclic preparations (imipramine, Tofranil): Use of thyroid preparations increases the activity of tricyclic antidepressants and enhances their antidepressant effects as receptors are made more sensitive.

■ Digitalis and thyroid hormone potentiate each other to the extent that digitalis toxic effects occur. Because thyroid replacement increases metabolic rates, reduced dosages of digitalis may be needed.

Contraindications

■ Diagnosed but yet uncorrected adrenal cortical insufficiency

■ Untreated thyrotoxicosis

■ Apparent hypersensitivity

Conscientious Considerations

■ Other thyroid products have *longer* half-lives, so this must be considered if switching from those products to liothyronine.

■ Patients with hepatic impairment require a dosage adjustment. This agent is more cardiotoxic than is Synthroid.

■ It is usually given as a single oral dose before breakfast.

■ In addition, clinicians must be aware of the important considerations that apply to all thyroid hormone preparations (see p. 200, Conscientious Prescribing of Thyroid Hormones).

Patient/Family Education

The advisories for patients who are taking liothyronine are the same as those for patients taking any other thyroid preparation (see p. 200, Patient/Family Education Regarding Thyroid Hormones).

Liotrix (T₃/T₄ Thyrolar) (Liothyronine [T3] and Levothyroxine [T4] Combination)

When the body functions normally, the ratio of T4 to T3 released from the thyroid gland is 20:1. However, manufacturers have created several combinations of both hormones, such as liotrix or Euthroid tablets, containing a combination of sodium levothyroxine (T4) and sodium L-triiodothyronine (T3) in a ratio of 4:1 by weight.

Mechanism of Action

The principal effect of these agents is to increase the metabolic rate of body tissues by promoting gluconeogenesis and increasing the utilization of glycogen stores. In addition, they promote protein synthesis, cell growth and differentiation, and development of the brain and central nervous system (CNS).

Pharmacokinetics

■ Metabolism and distribution: This drug is not firmly bound to serum protein; it is readily available to body tissues. The onset of activity is rapid, occurring within a few hours. Maximum pharmacological response occurs within 2 or 3 days.

■ Absorption: Almost totally absorbed, 95% in 4 hours.

■ Excretion: In feces.

■ Half-life: 2 1/2 days.

Dosage and Administration

Generic Name	Trade Name	Form	Usual Adult Dosage
liotrix liothyronine (T3)/ levothyroxine (T4) combination	Thyrolar Euthroid	Tablet PO	The dosage of thyroid hormones is determined by the indication and must in every case be individualized according to patient response and laboratory findings. For example, start with 50 mcg levothyroxine/12.5 mcg liothyronine (Liotrix) for 1 month, and then double it every month until desired effect is observed.

Clinical Uses

■ Hypothyroidism of any etiology except transient hypothyroidism during the recovery phase of subacute thyroiditis

■ Treatment or prevention of various types of euthyroid goiters, including thyroid nodules, subacute or acute chronic lymphocytic thyroiditis, and nodular goiter

■ Suppression testing to differentiate suspected mild hyperthyroidism or thyroid gland autonomy

Adverse Reactions

CV: CARDIOVASCULAR COLLAPSE, arrhythmia, tachycardia, increased blood pressure (BP)
DERM: Increased sweating
ENDO: Hyperthyroidism, menstrual irregularities
GI: Nausea, vomiting, cramps
META: Weight loss, heat intolerance
MISC: In children, accelerates bone maturation
NEURO: Insomnia, irritability, nervousness, headache

Interactions

■ Oral Anticoagulants (e.g., warfarin): Thyroid preparations increase the catabolism of vitamin K-dependent clotting factor.

■ Insulin and oral hypoglycemics: Initiating thyroid replacement therapy may cause increases in necessary doses of the oral hypoglycemics.

- Bile acid sequestrants (cholestyramine): These agents impair absorption of both T3 and T4 in the intestine.
- Tricyclic preparations (imipramine [Tofranil]): Use of thyroid preparations increases the activity of tricyclic antidepressants and enhances their antidepressant effects because receptors are made more sensitive.
- Digitalis: Digitalis and thyroid hormone potentiate each other to the extent that digitalis toxic effects occur. Because thyroid replacement increases metabolic rates, reduced dosages of digitalis may be needed.
- Mineral supplements (iron, calcium, aluminum), soy-containing foods, sucralfate, and cholestyramine can bind with and hinder thyroxine absorption. It is advisable that dosing of thyroxine be separated from ingestion of these items by at least 4 hours.

Contraindications

- Thyrotoxicosis
- Myocardial infarction without hypothyroidism
- Hypersensitivity
- The older patient with a cardiac problem

Conscientious Considerations

- Although combining T4 and T3 as replacement therapy to mimic the normal ratio secreted by the thyroid gland seems like a good idea, experience has proven it offers no therapeutic advantage over levothyroxine alone.
- In addition, clinicians must be aware of the important considerations that apply to all thyroid hormone preparations

(see p. 200, Conscientious Prescribing of Thyroid Hormones).

Patient/Family Education

The advisories for patients who are taking liotrix are the same as for patients taking any other thyroid preparation (see p. 200, Patient/Family Education Regarding Thyroid Hormones).

BOX 12-1 Thyroid U.S. Pharmacopeia (USP)

Thyroid USP is the natural thyroid derived from dried and defatted thyroid glands of domesticated animals. Slaughterhouses send these glands from bovine or porcine sources to a manufacturer for processing. Such preparations are rarely used in the United States because total thyroid hormone can vary from batch to batch. Patients with hepatic impairment require dosage adjustments to be standardized according to their iodine content. This is not a complete assay because, while an assay may satisfy USP content for iodine, a batch-to-batch comparison of T3 and T4 content may show variation. Note: USP means it meets the standards of the United States Pharmacopeia Convention which is a scientific/private/government agency that sets standards for around the world safety, identity, manufacture, quality purity, and benefit of agents used in pharmaceuticals. Its recommendations are enforced by the U.S. Food and Drug Administration (FDA) and are relied upon in more than 140 countries.

SPOTLIGHT ON HYPOTHYROIDISM

Hypothyroidism is a clinical syndrome resulting from a deficiency of thyroid hormones, which in turn results in a generalized slowing down of metabolic processes. Hypothyroidism may also be secondary to inadequate stimulation by TSH, either due to insufficient or ineffective pituitary production or hypothalamic disorders. Primary hypothyroidism is common and is present in almost 5% of individuals. It is more common in women, in those of advancing age, in whites, and in Latinos. The causes vary and include dietary iodine insufficiency (chief cause in underdeveloped countries), surgical thyroid resection, thyroid gland agenesis, infiltrative thyroid disorders, and functional disturbance to the pituitary or hypothalamic tracts. In the United States, autoimmune causes (**Hashimoto's thyroiditis**) prevail, with specific measurable circulating autoantibodies.

Hypothyroidism with onset in adulthood causes a generalized decrease in metabolism, with slowed heart rate, diminished oxygen consumption, and deposition of glycosaminoglycans in intracellular spaces, particularly in skin and muscle, producing in extreme cases the clinical picture of myxedema. **Myxedema** is severe, long-lasting, inadequately treated or untreated hypothyroidism. The development is insidious and causes a gradual retardation of physical and mental functions.

The synthesis of thyroid hormones depends on an adequate intake of iodine. Prolonged iodine deficiency in the diet results in enlargement of the thyroid gland known as a simple goiter. When thyroid hormones fail to synthesize because of a lack of iodine, the anterior lobe of the pituitary is stimulated to increase the secretion of thyrotropic hormone, which in turn causes hypertrophy and hyperplasia of the gland. This type of goiter can be prevented by providing adequate amounts of iodine.

Hypothyroidism in infants and children is called **cretinism** and results in marked slowing of growth and development, with serious permanent consequences, including mental retardation, when it occurs in infancy.

Suspected primary hypothyroidism is confirmed by an elevated TSH level. Established reference ranges for TSH levels typically extend from 0.5 to 4.5 mIU/L with a mean TSH level estimated to be 1.5 mIU/L. Measurement of the free T4 level confirms the diagnosis of primary hypothyroidism and characterizes its severity. A low free T4 level in conjunction with a persistently elevated TSH level establishes the diagnosis of overt primary hypothyroidism, whereas a low-normal free T4 level with an elevated TSH level is termed mild primary hypothyroidism.

Medical Management

Medical management is focused on replacing endogenous thyroid hormone while avoiding thyrotoxicosis. Levothyroxine sodium (thyroxine) is the preparation of choice for both primary and secondary hypothyroidism. Thyroxine has a narrow therapeutic index drug range, and doses that differ by as little as 12% can have clinical consequences. Adherence to one manufacturer's single

Continued

thyroxine formulation is advisable because of fluctuations in bioavailability among differing manufacturers. Optimal dosing for replacement therapy is related to lean body weight, with most adults requiring a daily dose of 1.25 mcg/kg. The dose requirement for elderly adults is typically lower (e.g., 1 mcg/kg/day) because of reduced metabolic clearance.

Various conditions alter replacement values. Patients with nephrotic syndrome and other systemic illnesses that may lead to rapid clearance of thyroid hormone require higher daily doses. Dose requirements increase by an average of 50% to 75% in most pregnant women. One-third of postmenopausal women beginning estrogen replacement therapy have increased dose requirements. In patients with underlying coronary artery disease, the positive chronotropic and inotropic effects of thyroxine may exacerbate myocardial ischemia. Adults with known or suspected ischemic heart disease should be started on a low dose that is titrated upward in small increments once tolerance is ensured (e.g., starting with 25 mcg daily, then increasing the dose by 12.5 to 25 mcg every 4 to 6 weeks).

Follow-up and Monitoring

Adequacy of thyroxine therapy can be assessed by TSH measurement 4 to 6 weeks after the dose is started or adjusted. The target TSH level for most individuals should be the lower half of the reference range (i.e., 1 to 2 mIU/L). Once an adequate dose has been established, a TSH level should be checked annually.

Drugs Used in the Treatment of Hyperthyroidism (Thyrotoxicosis)

Antithyroid drugs are used to decrease the levels of T3 and T4 in cases in which the gland produces too much of these hormones (hyperthyroidism/**thyrotoxicosis**). There are essentially two agents used in the treatment of hyperthyroidism: propylthiouracil (PTU), which inhibits peripheral T4 to T3 conversion, and methimazole (Tapazole), which has an easier dosing schedule. The cause of most (60% to 90%) excessive secretion of thyroid hormones is an autoimmune disorder known as **Graves' disease**, in which thyroid hyperfunction leads to TSH suppression because the feedback loop from elevated levels of thyroid hormone are not being controlled by the immune system.

Neither of these drugs treats any underlying pathology, and only about 20% of patients on therapy for a year experience any kind of remission.

Conscientious Prescribing of Drugs Used to Treat Hyperthyroidism

■ During the initial 3 months of therapy, TSH levels and CBCs should be monitored for **agranulocytosis**.
■ Monitor weight two to three times per week.
■ Drugs for treating hyperthyroidism may cause goiter and cretinism in fetus.
■ Correction of hyperthyroidism may alter the disposition of beta blockers, digoxin, and theophylline, necessitating dosage adjustments downward.

Patient/Family Education Regarding Drugs Used to Treat Hyperthyroidism

■ Patients should be aware they need to contact their clinician if they experience fever, sore throat, unusual bleeding, rash, skin yellowing, nausea and vomiting.
■ Consult professional on dietary sources of iodine (salt, shellfish).
■ Carry Medic Alert bracelet or ID notifying authorities of medication regime.
■ Patients should be taught to take doses evenly spaced throughout the day.

Propylthiouracil (PTU)

Propylthiouracil (PTU) is a timed-release thiourea derivative used to lower the amount of thyroid hormone released by the thyroid gland. At the time of publication of this text, there are no brand named products on the market and it is sold as PTU or propylthiouracil.

Mechanism of Action

Propylthiouracil inhibits oxidation of iodine in the thyroid gland and thus blocks synthesis of both thyroxine and triiodothyronine.

Pharmacokinetics

■ Absorption: Onset of action is 24 to 36 hours despite rapid absorption to peak concentration in about 1 hour.
■ Distribution: Concentrated in the thyroid gland after being highly serum protein bound.
■ Metabolism: Completely metabolized by the liver, having a significant first-pass effect.
■ Excretion: 35% excreted in urine.
■ Half-life: 1.5 to 5 hours.

Dosage and Administration

Generic Name	Trade Name	Form	Usual Adult Daily Dosage
propylthiouracil	propylthiouracil	50-mg, 100-mg tablets; 270 tablets (50 mg/tab)	300–900 mg/ day, initially in approximately three divided doses/day for 2 months, then 50–600 mg/day, 1 tab daily or divided doses, if symptoms persist. Maintenance dose is set by patient response.

Clinical Uses

■ Palliative treatment of hyperthyroidism
■ Adjunct in preparation for thyroidectomy or radioactive iodine therapy
■ To control hyperthyroidism while awaiting spontaneous remission
■ Treatment of thyrotoxicosis (**thyroid storm**)

Adverse Reactions

DERM: Hair loss, pruritus, rash, skin pigmentation, urticaria.

GI: Nausea.

HEM: Agranulocytosis can occur as long as 4 months after therapy, and it can lead to a fatal hepatitis.

MISC: A lupus-like syndrome, drug fever.

NEURO: Headache, paresthesia.

Interactions

■ Warfarin. Propylthiouracil may increase the anticoagulant effect of warfarin.

■ Correction of hyperthyroidism may alter the disposition of beta blockers, digoxin, and theophylline, necessitating a dosage reduction in these agents.

Contraindications

■ Pregnancy and breastfeeding. May cause goiter in fetus and nursing infants.

Conscientious Considerations

■ Instruct patients to take PTU at the same time in relation to meals every day; that is, always with meals or always between meals.

■ PTU is preferred over methimazole in cases of thyroid storm because it is a better inhibiter of peripheral conversion as well as synthesis of thyroid hormone.

■ In addition, clinicians must be aware of the important considerations that apply to all drugs used to treat hyperparathyroidism (see p. 204, Conscientious Prescribing of Drugs Used to Treat Hyperparathyroidism).

Patient/Family Education

■ The advisories for patients who are taking PTU are the same as those for patients taking any other thyroid preparation (see p. 204, Patient/Family Education Regarding of Drugs Used to Treat Hyperparathyroidism).

Methimazole (Tapazole)

Methimazole is an antithyroid drug and part of the thioamide group of chemicals. Its major use is to treat hyperthyroidism. It is effective in dosages administered once a day, which give it an advantage over PTU when it comes to adherence to the regimen.

Mechanism of Action

Methimazole (Tapazole) works in the same way as PTU, by inhibiting synthesis of thyroid hormone. It does this by blocking the oxidation of iodine in the thyroid gland. Specifically, it interferes with iodine's ability to combine with tyrosine to form thyroxine and triiodothyronine (T3) without destroying circulating T4 and T3 thyroid.

Pharmacokinetics

■ Absorption: Well absorbed but at variable rates, with onset of action in 12 to 18 hours

■ Distribution: Concentrated in thyroid gland but does cross placental barrier; it is not protein bound

■ Metabolism: Mostly metabolized by the liver

■ Excretion: 80% metabolites in urine, some unchanged in urine

■ Half-life: 4 to 13 hours

Dosage and Administration

Generic Name	Trade Name	Form	Usual Adult Dosage
methimazole	Tapazole	5-mg and 10-mg tablets, 100 tablets	15–60 mg/day as a single dose or divided dose for 6–8 weeks; thereafter, maintenance dose for up to 2 years. Peak effect in 4–10 weeks.

Clinical Uses

■ Palliative treatment of hyperthyroidism

■ Adjunct in preparation for thyroidectomy or radioactive iodine therapy

■ Thyrotoxicosis (thyroid storm)

Adverse Reactions

DERM: Rash, pruritus

GI: Loss of taste, nausea, vomiting

HEM: AGRANULOCYTOSIS, unusual bleeding or bruising

NEURO: Dizziness, peripheral paresthesia (numbness in fingers, toes, face)

Interactions

■ Anticoagulant effects of warfarin may be decreased.

■ Methimazole may decrease the effects of codeine, hydrocodone, oxycodone, tramadol.

■ Seafood that is high in iodine (shellfish, shrimp) and other iodine-containing foods (spinach) may cause an increase in thyroid hormone because they stimulate the thyroid gland.

Contraindications

■ Hypersensitivity

Conscientious Considerations

■ This is the drug of choice for the treatment of hyperthyroidism based on patient adherence and improved outcomes.

■ In addition, clinicians must be aware of the important considerations that apply to all drugs used to treat hyperparathyroidism (see p. 204, Conscientious Prescribing of Drugs Used to Treat Hyperparathyroidism).

Patient/Family Education

■ The advisories for patients who are taking methimazole are the same as those for patients taking any other thyroid preparation (see p. 204, Patient/Family Education Regarding of Drugs Used to Treat Hyperparathyroidism).

SPOTLIGHT ON THYROTOXICOSIS AND THYROID STORM

Thyrotoxicosis is a clinical syndrome that results when tissues are exposed to high levels of circulating thyroid hormones. It results in a generalized acceleration of metabolic processes. In most instances, thyrotoxicosis is due to hyperactivity of the thyroid gland, or hyperthyroidism. Occasionally, thyrotoxicosis may be due to other causes such as excessive ingestion of thyroid hormone or nonthyroid tissue hormone production. It presents in 1 of every 2,000 adults, affecting 1% of all individuals during the course of a lifetime. Females are involved about five times more commonly than males. The disease may occur at any age, with a peak incidence in the 20- to 40-year age group. It develops when there is excessive synthesis and secretion of thyroid hormone caused by thyrotropic stimulus or autonomous function of thyroid tissue.

The combination of an elevated free T4 and a suppressed TSH makes the diagnosis of hyperthyroidism. Approximately 5% of patients have normal free T4 levels, but elevated serum T3 levels, a situation termed "T3" thyrotoxicosis. Sensitive TSH immunoassays with a detection limit less than 0.02 mIU/L can accurately discriminate between clearly suppressed TSH levels characteristic of all common forms of thyrotoxicosis and mildly suppressed levels that fall just beneath the reference range, as may occur in otherwise sick and elderly euthyroid individuals. Measurements of serum free T4 and total or free T3 levels will confirm a diagnosis of thyrotoxicosis, define its severity, and occasionally provide a clue to its underlying etiology. Overt thyrotoxicosis is characterized by free T4 or T3 levels above the upper limit of the reference range, whereas mild or subclinical thyrotoxicosis is characterized by a suppressed TSH level with free T4 and T3 levels within the normal reference range.

What is Thyroid Storm?

Thyrotoxic crisis, also known as **thyroid storm**, is a potentially life-threatening syndrome that is usually the end result of severe and sustained thyrotoxicosis. It can affect patients with other medical conditions that render them vulnerable to the cardiovascular, neuropsychiatric, and gastrointestinal effects of exposure to excessive amounts of thyroid hormone. Thyrotoxic crisis typically develops in the setting of inadequately treated Graves' disease and may be precipitated by underlying illness, surgery, myocardial infarction, uncontrolled diabetes, severe infection, or treatment with radioactive iodine. Affected individuals present with fever out of proportion to other findings, atrial tachyarrhythmia, congestive heart failure, nausea and vomiting, diarrhea, and seizures. Mental status changes can include agitation, delirium, psychosis, and coma. Prompt recognition and treatment in a monitored setting is crucial.

Medical Management of Thyrotoxicosis and Thyroid Storm

Before the advent of the antithyroid drugs, PTU and methimazole (Tapazole), treatment was limited to gradual resection of the thyroid gland. Today, PTU is the more common agent. Middle-aged and elderly patients often respond well to radioactive therapy.

A multifaceted treatment regimen should incorporate antipyretics, beta blockers, thionamides, iodinated contrast agents, and glucocorticoids, as well as aggressive evaluation and management of underlying medical problems.

DRUGS AFFECTING THE PARATHYROID GLANDS

The parathyroid glands lie just above and behind the thyroid gland. Humans have two pairs of parathyroid glands, and their primary function is to maintain adequate levels of calcium in the extracellular fluid. The parathyroid gland has multiple effects, leading ultimately to the mobilization of calcium from the bone and reducing phosphate concentrations, which in turn allows more calcium to be mobilized. Cholesterol-derived provitamin D is converted to vitamin D3 by the action of sunlight on the skin. Then parathyroid hormone (PTH), along with vitamin D3, is converted to its active form in the kidney where it is made ready for its involvement in calcium, phosphate, and magnesium metabolism in bone and the GI tract. Parathyroid hormone is a polypeptide whose active component has a half-life of 30 minutes, and the inactive component has 7 to 10 days. The mechanism of PTH action on bone or kidney is not completely understood, although it has been suggested that PTH-receptor binding and adenylate cyclase activity are coupled events that are subjected to downregulation of the receptors.

In patients with hyperplastic parathyroid glands, PTH circulates in elevated concentrations as a result of diminished calcium levels. This can be seen in patients with impaired renal function or intestinal malabsorption. Elevated PTH levels may lead to metabolic bone diseases such as osteoporosis or osteomalacia.

Drugs Used in the Treatment of Hyperparathyroidism

Primary **hyperparathyroidism** is the most common parathyroid disorder, most often caused by adenomas, chief cell hyperplasia, or hypertrophy. Elevations of PTH cause changes in the functions of renal tubular cells, bone cells, and gastrointestinal tract mucosa, leading to elevated levels of calcium and increased bone **resorption**, which results in the development of renal calculi.

Secondary hyperparathyroidism is a disease that occurs in patients with chronic kidney failure who are on dialysis. In secondary hyperparathyroidism, the parathyroid gland has become overactive in response to low blood calcium. Failing kidneys do not convert vitamin D to its active form, and they do not excrete as much phosphorus. When this happens, insoluble calcium phosphate forms in the body and removes calcium from the circulation. Both processes then lead to hypocalcemia, and hence this can cause serious problems with the bones, heart, blood vessels, and lungs. Unlike patients with *primary* hyperparathyroidism, these patients do *not* get parathyroid tumors.

Drugs for treating primary hyperparathyroidism can be divided into two main groups:

- Antiresorptive drugs that inhibit the increased bone turnover. These can be further divided into:
  - Estrogen-like compounds, estrogen, oral contraceptives, and selective estrogen receptor modulators (SERMs).
  - Bisphosphonates and calcitonin.

■ Drugs that interfere with PTH secretion. (At the time of publication of this text only cinacalcet is available. No drugs that interfere with PTH action are available.)

All of the preceding classes of drugs are able to lower serum calcium levels. However, calcitonin does so only temporarily. Estrogen-containing compounds (hormone replacement therapy) may be less attractive because of the potential risk of breast cancer, cardiovascular disease, and deep vein thromboembolism. Oral contraceptives have not been shown to prevent fractures in the general population, and no data are available on their effect in women with primary hyperparathyroidism. The only SERM marketed for hyperparathyroidism is raloxifene (Evista); this has not been associated with an increased risk of breast cancer and cardiovascular diseases and has been shown to be able to prevent vertebral fractures in postmenopausal women with osteoporosis.

Bisphosphonates have been shown to decrease serum calcium and increase BMD in patients with primary hyperparathyroidism, but PTH levels may increase. This leaves cinacalcet as the only drug that effectively induces a sustained decrease in serum calcium and PTH for up to 1 year.

Cinacalcet (Sensipar)

Cinacalcet belongs to a class of medications called calcimimetics, a group of drugs that work by signaling the body to produce less parathyroid hormone to decrease the amount of calcium in the blood.

Mechanism of Action

Cinacalcet increases the sensitivity of the calcium-sensing receptors on the parathyroid gland. Activation of the calcium-sensing receptors is expressed in various human organ tissues.

Pharmacokinetics

■ Absorption: Oral administration provides readily available blood levels in 2 to 6 hours. High-fat meals lower absorption.
■ Distribution: Over 90% is distributed bound to protein.
■ Metabolism: Metabolized by the multiple enzymes in the cytochrome P450 system.
■ Excretion: Metabolites are excreted 85% in urine, 15% in feces.
■ Half-life: 30 to 40 hours.

Dosage and Administration

Generic Name	Trade Name	Route	Usual Adult Daily Dosage
cinacalcet	Sensipar	PO	Dosing is highly individualized, usually starting with 30 mg once daily and titrated once a week depending on serum intact PTH (iPTH) levels.

Clinical Uses

■ Treatment of secondary hyperparathyroidism in dialysis patients

■ Treatment of hypercalcemia in patients with parathyroid carcinoma

Adverse Reactions

CV: Arrhythmias, chest pain
GI: Vomiting, diarrhea
MS: Muscle aches or cramps, sudden tightening of the muscles in the hands, feet, face, or throat
NEURO: Dizziness; weakness; burning; tingling; unusual feelings of the lips, tongue, fingers, or feet, seizure

Interactions

■ Amitriptyline and nortriptyline levels will increase in the presence of cinacalcet.

Contraindications

■ Hypersensitivity

Conscientious Considerations

■ Because cinacalcet lowers serum calcium, patients should be monitored for signs of hypocalcemia, such as paresthesias, myalgia, tetany, cramping, and convulsions.
■ Sensipar (cinacalcet) is *not* approved by the FDA for treating patients with *primary* hyperparathyroidism and can be problematic if given to these patients.
■ Patients with *secondary* hyperparathyroidism are usually treated with a combination of medications and dialysis to control all of the problems they have with the chemical balance of their blood (due to the lack of kidney function).

Patient/Family Education

■ Patients should be instructed to take this drug with food.

Drugs Used in the Treatment of Hypoparathyroidism

The natural history of mild **hypoparathyroidism** is characterized by decreased levels of PTH that lead to hypocalcemia. In many patients, the disorder has a benign course with little change in findings or serum levels of calcium, but severe or progressive loss of bone mass. Although it can lead to increased fractures, the risk seems low. The drugs used in the treatment of hypoparathyroidism are therefore oral supplements of calcium or synthetic vitamin D. To normalize the levels of calcium and phosphorus, either or both are administered.

Calcitriol (Rocaltrol, Calcijex)

Calcitriol is an analogue of fat-soluble vitamin D, which is essential for absorption and utilization of calcium phosphate and normal calcification of bone. Vitamin D deficiency causes rickets in children and osteomalacia in adults, but less dramatic deficiencies contribute to osteoporosis.

Mechanism of Action

Calcitriol works by stimulating calcium and phosphate absorption from the small intestine, promoting secretion of calcium from bone to blood, promoting renal tubule phosphate resorption, acting on bone cells to promote skeletal growth, and acting on the parathyroid gland to suppress hormone synthesis and secretion.

Pharmacokinetics

- Absorption: Rapidly absorbed from the small intestine and widely distributed
- Metabolism: Metabolized extensively in the kidney
- Excretion: Primarily in feces, minimal in kidney
- Half-life: 5 to 8 hours

Dosage and Administration

Generic Name	Trade Name	Form	Usual Adult Dosage For Hypoparathyroidism
calcitriol	Calcijex	IV	0.5–4 mcg every other day
	Rocaltrol	PO	0.25–1 mcg/day

Clinical Uses

- Calcijex (calcitrol injection): Hypocalcemia; patients undergoing chronic renal dialysis; reducing elevated parathyroid hormone levels, which results in an improvement of renal osteodystrophy
- Rocaltrol: Treatment for postmenopausal women who have osteoporosis (however, it is not licensed for the prevention of osteoporosis)

Adverse Reactions

CV: Arrhythmias
GI: Constipation, metallic taste, nausea
META: Hypercalcemia, polyuria
NEURO: Headache, irritability

Conscientious Considerations

- Caution should be taken in prescribing these medications for patients who take calcium channel blockers for cardiac disorders.
- Excessive dosage of Rocaltrol induces hypocalcemia and in some instances hypercalciuria; therefore, early in treatment during dosage adjustment, serum calcium should be determined twice weekly.
- SERIOUS: **Early signs of overdose** manifest as weakness, headache, nausea, vomiting, constipation, muscle and bone pain, metallic taste sensations.
- **Later signs of overdose** manifest as polyuria, polydipsia, anorexia, somnolence, weight loss, photophobia, rhinorrhea, pruritus, hallucinations, hyperthermia, hypertension, and cardiac arrhythmias.
- Patients with hepatic impairment require a dosage adjustment.
- In dialysis patients, a fall in serum alkaline phosphatase levels usually antedates the appearance of hypocalcaemia. An abrupt increase in calcium intake as a result of changes in diet (e.g., increased consumption of dairy products) or uncontrolled intake of calcium preparations may trigger hypocalcemia. Should hypocalcemia develop, treatment with Rocaltrol should be stopped immediately. During periods of hypocalcemia, serum calcium and phosphate levels must be determined daily. Blood calcium and phosphate determinations are to be made weekly until the patient is stable.

Patient/Family Education

- Calcium supplements can cause gastrointestinal side effects such as constipation in some people; therefore, they should be taken only under the guidance of a clinician.
- Patients should consult with a dietitian to learn about a diet that is rich in calcium. This includes dairy products, nuts, green leafy vegetables, and fortified orange juice and breakfast cereals. Foods that contain high amounts of phosphorus in the form of phosphoric acid, such as carbonated soft drinks and some nuts, should be avoided.

SPOTLIGHT ON HYPOPARATHYROIDISM

Hypoparathyroidism represents a loss of homeostasis resulting from removal of the parathyroid gland resulting in loss of hormone (PTH) secretion. It is usually caused by a deficiency in parathyroid hormone or removal of the parathyroid hormone under surgery, or it may be idiopathic. The symptoms include the following:

- Muscle spasms
- Convulsions
- Gradual paralysis with dyspnea
  Death from exhaustion may also result.

Medical Management

In choosing a treatment for hypoparathyroidism, factors such as symptoms, including their severity, and overall health are considered. The goal of treatment is to normalize the levels of calcium and phosphorus. A treatment regimen typically includes oral calcium carbonate tablets and vitamin D analogues.

In some cases, when immediate relief of symptoms is needed, hospitalization is preferred to administer calcium by intravenous (IV) infusion. These IV infusions may be important if severe spasms occur. After hospital discharge, continuance of calcium and vitamin D as an oral supplement is resumed.

Because hypoparathyroidism is a chronic disorder, and treatment strategies are generally lifelong. Regular blood tests determine whether calcium in particular is at normal levels and if doses of supplemental calcium are needed if blood calcium levels fall.

When blood calcium remains low, despite treatment, a prescription diuretic, a thiazide such as hydrochlorothiazide or metolazone, is indicated. Whereas other types of diuretics (loop diuretics) decrease calcium levels, the thiazides can increase them. Even though thiazide drugs raise blood calcium levels in some people, their effectiveness is not universal. However, people who are treated for hypoparathyroidism often keep their symptoms under good control if they continue to receive treatment long term. This is particularly true with an early diagnosis.

DRUGS AFFECTING THE PITUITARY GLAND

The pituitary is located at the base of the brain and exerts important effects in regulating the secretion of hormones. It consists of the anterior lobe (adenohypophysis), the posterior lobe (neurohypophysis), and smaller pars intermedia. The pituitary and its target glands have a negative feedback relationship.

The number of hormones that are secreted by the anterior pituitary gland is unknown, although there are seven that are established and have specific actions:

■ Growth hormone (somatotropin, somatropin) promotes skeletal, visceral, and general growth. Disorders such as acromegaly, gigantism, and dwarfism are associated with pathological conditions of the anterior lobe of the pituitary.
■ Follicle-stimulating hormone (FSH) stimulates the growth and maturation of the ovarian follicle and also stimulates spermatogenesis in males.
■ Luteinizing hormone, together with FSH, causes maturation of the graafian follicles, ovulation, formation of the corpus luteum, and the secretion of estrogen in females. It also causes spermatogenesis, androgen formation, and growth of intestinal tissue in males.
■ Thyroid-stimulating hormone (TSH) is necessary for the normal development and function of the thyroid gland.
■ Lactogenic factor (prolactin) is active in the proliferation and secretion of the mammary glands in mammals.
■ Adrenocorticotropic hormone (ACTH) stimulates the cortex of the adrenal gland.
■ Melanocyte-stimulating hormones' physiological role is unknown, but when injected in humans, it darkens the skin.

The posterior pituitary is derived from nervous tissue, and from it two protein hormones are released that synthesize hormones in the hypothalamus: oxytocin and vasopressin. Hormones released from the anterior pituitary are dormant unless directed to be released and synthesized in the hypothalamus by releasing factors.

Drugs Affecting the Posterior Pituitary Gland

Hormones known classically as posterior pituitary hormones are synthesized by the hypothalamus. They are then stored and secreted by the posterior pituitary into the bloodstream as oxytocin and vasopressin. Insufficient secretion of vasopressin is central to **diabetes insipidus**, in which the body loses the capacity to concentrate urine. Affected individuals excrete as much as 20 L of dilute urine per day. Oversecretion of vasopressin causes the syndrome of inappropriate antidiuretic hormone.

Drugs used to correct these conditions include vasopressin (Pitressin), oxytocin (Pitocin, Syntocinon), desmopressin (DVAPP, Stimate), and lypressin (DIADD).

Conscientious Prescribing for Drugs Affecting the Posterior Pituitary Gland

■ Clinicians should monitor urine osmolality and volume during therapy.
■ ECG should also be monitored by clinicians during therapy.

Patient/Family Education for Drugs Affecting the Posterior Pituitary Gland

■ Instruct patients that directions for administration are to be followed exactly.
■ Caution patients to avoid concurrent use of alcohol.
■ Advise patients that side effects are not severe and usually subside in a few minutes.
■ Advise patients that identification programs such as MedicAlert are good ways to help identify them in case of a crisis.
■ Advise patients of signs and symptoms of diabetes insipidus.

Vasopressin (Pitressin)

Vasopressin is a posterior pituitary hormone that is also called antidiuretic hormone.

Mechanism of Action

Vasopressin increases the reabsorption of water by the renal tubules through its action on a receptor in the collecting tubules of the nephron. It also directly stimulates smooth muscle receptors in the GI tract and in arterioles causing peristalsis and vasoconstriction. It has a minor third effect of mediating secretion of ACTH.

Pharmacokinetics

■ Absorption: Rapidly absorbed from IV/subcutaneous (SC) injection sites. SC onset in 1 to 2 hours with 2 to 8 hours duration. IV administration is immediate, with a 0.5- to 1-hour duration.
■ Distribution: Distributed throughout extracellular fluid.
■ Metabolism: Metabolized by liver and kidney.
■ Excretion: Primarily excreted in urine.
■ Half-life: 10 to 20 minutes.

Dosage and Administration

When used in diabetes insipidus, vasopressin solution that is ordinarily used for injection is instead often administered intranasally on cotton pledgets, by nasal spray, or by a nasal dropper.

Generic Name	Trade Name	Form	Usual Adult Dosage
vasopressin	Pitressin	Solution as an injection (given IM, SC, or as an IV infusion)	Dosages must be carefully individualized. Example: IV infusion: 0.5 mU/kg/hr. May double every hr to max dose of 10 mU/kg/hr

Clinical Uses

■ Treatment of diabetes insipidus
■ Prevention of abdominal distention following surgery
■ GI hemorrhage
■ Vasodilatory shock

Adverse Reactions

CV: Myocardial infarction, diaphoresis
DERM: Rash, skin blanching, pallor
GI: Nausea, vomiting, diarrhea

NEURO: Dizziness
MISC: Anaphylaxis, causes pain at the injection site, water intoxication

Interactions

■ None known

Contraindications

■ Hypersensitivity

Conscientious Considerations

■ Clinicians should monitor ECG, fluid and electrolyte status, because extravasation may occur; necrosis may also occur.

Patient/Family Education

■ Patients should be aware that a number of legal cases have erupted when vasopressin, branded as "Pitressin," has been prescribed and "Pitocin" was dispensed because of the confusion caused by their soundalike–look-alike nomenclature.

Oxytocin (Pitocin, Syntocinon)

Another agent released by the posterior pituitary is oxytocin.

Mechanism of Action

Oxytocin stimulates contractions of uterine smooth muscle as well as enhances lactation.

Pharmacokinetics

■ Absorption: Intramuscularly (IM): Uterine contractions occur within 3 to 5 minutes, with a duration of 2 to 3 hours. IV: Uterine contractions occur within 1 minute, with a duration of approximately 1 hour. Oxytocin is rapidly absorbed through nasal membranes and is sometimes given in that form.
■ Distribution: Widely distributed in extracellular fluid. Small amounts reach fetal circulation.
■ Metabolism: Rapidly metabolized by the liver and kidneys.
■ Excretion: Excreted in the urine.
■ Half-life: 3 to 9 minutes.

Dosage and Administration

Generic Name	Trade Name	Form	Usual Adult Dosage
oxytocin	Pitocin, Syntocinon	IV, IM, intranasally	For induction or stimulation of labor: 0.5–1 mU/min IV. To *control postpartum bleeding:* 10–40 units in a liter of fluid administered IV at a rate sufficient to control bleeding or as 10 units IV after delivery.

Clinical Uses

■ Dosing is particularly sensitive whether used to induce or stimulate labor, induce abortion, or control postpartum bleeding.

Adverse Reactions

CV: Tachycardia, premature ventricular contractions, hypotension in *both* mother and neonate.
EENT: Neonatal retinal hemorrhage.

GI: Nausea and vomiting in *both* mother and neonate.
MISC: Prolonged IV infusion of oxytocin has caused severe water intoxication with seizures, coma, and death resulting.
OB/GYN: Postpartum hemorrhage in the mother.

Interactions

■ Dinoprostone and misoprostol increase the effect of oxytocin.

Contraindications

■ Hypersensitivities
■ Anticipation of a nonvaginal delivery

Conscientious Considerations

■ Always monitor fluid intake and output during administration as well as monitor the fetus.
■ A host of conditions ranging from adequate uterine activity that fails to progress, to hypertonic or hypoactive uterus, to obstetrical emergencies, fetal positioning, or active genital herpes, placenta previa require the exercise of extreme caution in using this drug, necessitating that it be administered only by experts with a thorough history of the patient.
■ Although it is used routinely for induction of labor at term and for the control of uterine bleeding postpartum, oxytocin is not the drug of choice for induction of labor for abortion.

Desmopressin (DDAVP, Stimate)

Desmopressin is a synthetic posterior pituitary hormone.

Mechanism of Action

Desmopressin increases reabsorption of water by increasing the permeability of collecting ducts in the kidney, thus decreasing urinary output. This agent also works as a plasminogen activator increasing plasma factor VIII (antihemophiliac factor).

Pharmacokinetics

■ Absorption: Given PO, IV, or intranasally, it is poorly absorbed.
■ Distribution: Although its distribution remains unknown, it is known to enter breast milk.
■ Metabolism: Unknown.
■ Excretion: Unknown.
■ Half-life: Oral: 1.2 to 2.5 hours; intranasal: 3.5 hours; IV, 0.4 to 4 hours.

Dosage and Administration

Generic Name	Trade Name	Form	Usual Adult Dosage
desmopressin	DDAVP Stimate	Intranasal spray or inhalation: 0.1 mg/mL or 10 mcg/inhalation spray; IV solution for SC injection (4 mcg/mL); and 0.1 mg oral tablets.	For nocturnal enuresis: Intranasal spray (children): 0.2 mL at bedtime, using ½ dose in each nostril before bedtime. For diabetes insipidus: (adults and children over 12) 0.05 mg, 2 times/day is sufficient to start.

Clinical Uses

- Primary nocturnal enuresis in both children and adults
- Diabetes insipidus
- Hemophilia and von Willebrand's disease (owing to its impact on plasma factor VIII)

Adverse Reactions

CV: Acute MI, thrombosis, facial flushing, edema, increased BP, palpitations
EENT: From intranasal spray rhinorrhea, nasal congestion
GI: Abdominal cramps, nausea
GU: Decreased urination
META: Water intoxication, rapid weight gain
NEURO: Agitation, coma, headache, insomnia, confusion, seizures

Interactions

- Chlorpropamide and ethanol may increase the effect of desmopressin.
- Demeclocycline and lithium may decrease the effect of desmopressin.

Contraindications

- Hypersensitivity
- Mild to moderate renal impairment

Conscientious Considerations

- Although useful in treating children with enuresis, relapse following discontinuance is common.
- Desmopressin is best used conservatively and sparingly (e.g., if the child has an overnight trip staying with a friend).

Patient/Family Education

- Advise patient to drink only enough water to satisfy thirst.
- Teach patients to use the nasal tube delivery system. (The nasal spray, however, works like any other spray.)

Lypressin (Diapid)

Lypressin is a lysine derivative of vasopressin hormone. It is initially harvested from the pituitary glands of swine, then stabilized for use in humans.

Mechanism of Action

Lypressin promotes the reabsorption of water by increasing the cellular permeability of the collecting ducts in the kidney, thus decreasing urine output by increasing urine osmolality.

Pharmacokinetics

- Absorption: Rapidly absorbed from the nasal cavity with peak effects in 30 to 120 minutes
- Distribution: Widely distributed
- Metabolism: Undergoes both renal and hepatic biotransformation
- Excretion: Renal, with a small amount being unchanged
- Half-life: About 15 minutes

Dosage and Administration

Generic Name	Trade Name	Form	Usual Adult Dosage
lypressin	Diapid	Nasal spray	Adults and children >12 years: Spray once or twice in each nostril 4 times/day.

Clinical Uses

- Used as an antidiuretic and vasopressor to control diabetes insipidus symptoms (frequent urination, increased thirst, and loss of water).

Adverse Reactions

CV: Feeling of tightness in chest, shortness of breath, or troubled breathing
EENT: Irritation or pain in the eye; itching, irritation, or sores inside nose; runny or stuffy nose
GI: Abdominal or stomach cramps, heartburn; increased bowel movements
NEURO: Coma, confusion; convulsions (seizures), drowsiness, headache (continuing), problems with urination, weight gain

Interactions

- Carbamazepine, chlorpropamide, and clofibrate may potentiate the antidiuretic effect of lypressin when used concurrently.
- Demeclocycline, lithium, and norepinephrine may decrease the antidiuretic effect of lypressin when used concurrently.

Contraindications

- None known

Conscientious Considerations

- Patients sensitive to vasopressin may also be sensitive to lypressin.
- Risk-benefit should be considered when the following medical problems exist; allergic rhinitis, nasal congestion, or upper respiratory infection, because these may interfere with absorption of lypressin through the nasal mucosa; hypertensive cardiovascular disease (although pressor effects of lypressin are minimal); and sensitivity to lypressin.
- Although the usual dosage is 1 to 2 sprays in each nostril four times a day, in actual practice the dosage has ranged from 1 spray per day at bedtime to 10 sprays in each nostril every 3 to 4 hours.
- Whenever the frequency of urination increases or increased thirst develops, the patient may be told to administer 1 or 2 sprays to control these symptoms.
- If the regular daily dosage of lypressin does not control nocturia, an additional dose may be given at bedtime.

Patient/Family Education

- Patients should be instructed to use this medicine only as directed because not to do so may increase the chance of unwanted effects.

- Patients should be instructed to rinse the tip of the bottle with hot water, taking care not to suck water into the bottle, dry it with a clean tissue, then replace the cap right after use to keep the spray tip clean.
- The patient should be instructed to first gently blow his/her nose, hold the bottle upright, then with the bottle held upright, gently but firmly squeeze the bottle and spray into the nostril.

SPOTLIGHT ON DIABETES INSIPIDUS

Diabetes insipidus (DI) is a syndrome of polyuria resulting from the inability to concentrate urine and, therefore, to conserve water as a result of lack of vasopressin action. Central diabetes insipidus can be either permanent or transient, reflecting the natural history of the underlying disorder. The initial clinical presentation of diabetes insipidus is polyuria (urine output of 10 to 20 L/day) that will continue despite conditions that would normally decrease urine output such as dehydration. The other prominent symptom is great thirst. Adults may complain of frequent urination at night (nocturia), and children may present with bed-wetting (enuresis). If the patient is unable to maintain a water intake commensurate with water loss, dehydration can develop and may rapidly progress to coma. Most cases of DI are inherited, but nephrogenic diabetes insipidus may also be acquired during life as a result of drug use, kidney disease, obstruction of the tubes that carry urine from the kidneys to the bladder (ureters), and prolonged metabolic imbalances such as low levels of potassium in the blood (hypokalemia) or low levels of calcium in the blood (hypocalcemia).

Medical Management
The pharmacological treatment of diabetes insipidus is established by knowing the cause. The patient is subjected to a water deprivation test in a controlled environment, and water intake and output are measured. To determine the etiology, plasma vasopressin levels are measured and a desmopressin stimulation test is conducted. If the patient has a high plasma vasopressin level and does not respond well to the desmopressin challenge, a condition of nephrogenic diabetes insipidus is determined. The goal of therapy then is to replace the defective hormones.

Drugs Affecting the Anterior Pituitary Gland

Unlike the posterior lobe, the anterior lobe is genuinely glandular. Under the influence of the hypothalamus, the anterior pituitary produces and secretes several peptide hormones that regulate many physiological processes, including stress, growth, and reproduction.

Conscientious Prescribing for Drugs Affecting the Anterior Pituitary Gland

- Laboratory tests are required for periodic assessment. If the patient is hypothyroid, then thyroid hormone replacement will be necessary for growth hormones to be effective.
- Prescribers will need to monitor for development of neutralizing antibodies.
- Prescribers will monitor for bone age and growth rates every 3 to 6 months during therapy.

Patient/Family Education for Drugs Affecting the Anterior Pituitary Gland

- Patients will need instruction on correct procedures for reconstituting the medication, site selection for rotating injections, and disposal of needles. Dosage schedule will also need review.
- Patients need to be reminded of the importance of follow-up with their endocrinologist to ensure that appropriate laboratory tests, growth rate, and bone age is occurring.
- Patients need assurances that these drugs are totally synthetic and safe.

Somatrem (Protropin) and Recombinant Somatropin (Genotropin, Humatrope, Norditropin, Nutropin, Serostim)

These drugs are a biosynthesized chain of 192 polypeptide amino acids. They are produced by recombinant DNA processes using *Escherichia coli* as a carrier.

Mechanism of Action

Somatrem and recombinant somatropin mimic human growth hormone produced by the anterior pituitary and are mediated by insulin-like growth factor-I (IGF-I), which is synthesized in the liver and other tissues in response to growth hormone stimulation. IGF-I concentrations are low in children with growth hormone deficiency but normalize in response to administration of exogenous growth hormone.

Growth hormone stimulates linear growth by doing the following:

- Affecting cartilaginous growth areas of long bones
- Increasing the number and size of skeletal muscle cells
- Influencing the size of organs
- Increasing red cell mass through erythropoietin stimulation
- Influencing metabolism of carbohydrates by decreasing insulin sensitivity and possibly by affecting glucose transport of fats by causing mobilization of fatty acids
- Influencing metabolism of minerals by causing the retention of phosphorus, sodium, and potassium through promotion of cellular growth
- Influencing metabolism of proteins by increasing protein synthesis, which results in nitrogen retention
- Influencing metabolism of connective tissue by stimulating synthesis of chondroitin sulfate and collagen and by increasing urinary excretion of hydroxyproline

Somatrem is a synthetic agent able to stimulate these biological processes.

Pharmacokinetics

- Absorption: Highly absorbed from injection sites, whether SC or IM
- Distribution: Localizes to highly perfused organs such as kidney and liver
- Metabolism: Mostly metabolized in renal cells, it is cleaved to its constituent amino acids and returned to the circulation

■ Excretion: Mainly biliary
■ Half-life: IV: 20 minutes; SC, IM: 3 to 5 hours

Dosage and Administration

This is one medication that requires very careful training by those who give it and careful monitoring of the patient using it. The specific activity of growth hormone is defined as International Units (IU) per milligram of protein. In October 1994, a new standard was developed that changed the conversion amount from 2.6 IU per milligram of growth hormone to 3 IU per milligram of growth hormone. This change did not affect the milligram per kilogram dosing or the quantity (mg) of growth hormone per vial. The only change was the increase in the number of IUs per milligram.

Generic Name	Trade Name	Form	Usual Dosage
somatrem	Protropin	SC, IM	Pediatric dose for growth hormone deficiency is intramuscular or subcutaneous, up to 0.3 mg (0.9 IU)/kg of body weight a week, with dosing and dosing regimen individualized according to the patient's needs. It is recommended that this dose be divided into the appropriate dose for daily injection (6 or 7 times/week). The SC route of administration is preferred to the IM route.
somatropin, recombinant	Genotropin, Humatrope, Norditropin, Nutropin, Serostim	The drug is packaged in a two-part vial, one part being the lyophilized dry powder, the second being a diluent provided by the manufacturer. At the time of administration, the diluent of sterile (bacteriostatic) water is added to reconstitute the powder using aseptic technique. Once reconstituted, the solution is good for 14 days, if refrigerated.	

Clinical Uses

■ Somatrem and recombinant somatropin are indicated in children for long-term treatment of growth failure caused by pituitary growth hormone deficiency (pituitary dwarfism), including growth hormone deficiency caused by cranial irradiation.
■ Recombinant somatropin is indicated in adults for treatment of growth failure caused by growth hormone deficiency when any one of the following is present:
   ■ Adult Growth Hormone Deficiency (GHD) alone or with multiple hormone deficiencies, such as hypopituitarism, as a result of hypothalamic or pituitary disease, radiation therapy, surgery, or trauma
   ■ Growth hormone deficiency of childhood onset that was not confirmed until adulthood
   ■ Turner syndrome
   ■ Idiopathic short stature
   ■ Negative response to a standard growth hormone stimulation test

Adverse Reactions

CV: Edema of hands and feet
ENDO: Hypoglycemia, hypothyroidism, insulin resistance
MISC: Pain at injection site

Interactions

■ Combinations containing any of the following medications, depending on the amount present, may interact with this medication:
   ■ Anabolic steroids. Because of the great differences in individual responses to steroids, it is recommended that no more than half the usual doses be used and that they only be used in extenuating circumstances, such as stress during acute febrile illness.
   ■ Thyroid hormones. These may accelerate epiphyseal closure.

Contraindications

■ Contraindicated in closure of the epiphyses or active neoplasms

Concientious Considerations

■ Prolonged use of this product in someone without acromegaly is likely to induce acromegaly features and other organ issues such as organ enlargement, diabetes mellitus, arteriosclerosis, hypertension, and carpal tunnel syndrome.
■ The importance of regular visits to the clinician cannot be overemphasized.
■ Before placing a patient on this medication, conditions affecting its use must be determined, especially sensitivity to any component of the growth hormone product, concomitant use of other medications, especially corticosteroids or corticotropin (ACTH). Other medical problems, especially untreated hypothyroidism, must be determined.
■ Clinicians must monitor growth curves, monitor periodic thyroid function tests and tests for glucose and IGF-1 levels, and monitor for Prader-Willi syndrome (sleep apnea, reparatory infections, snoring) and Turner's syndrome (ear and cardiovascular disorders).
■ Generally, after 2 years of treatment with growth hormone, growth rate declines. Giving growth hormone therapy to adults results in increases in lean body mass, total body water, and physical performance, and decreases in body fat and waist circumference.

Octreotide (Sandostatin)

Octreotide is used to achieve normalization of growth hormone in patients with acromegaly by reducing blood levels of growth hormone and IGF-1. It is used when patients have not responded to the other treatments of surgical resection, radiation of the pituitary, or bromocriptine. It has a record of working about 50% of the time in these patients and in some cases is used as an adjuvant to radiation therapy because the outcomes of radiation are not fully seen for several years.

Mechanism of Action

Octreotide gets its name from being an eight-sided protein salt that, as a long-acting peptide, has a pharmacological action that mimics the action of the natural hormone somatostatin.

Pharmacokinetics

- Absorption: SC injection is completely absorbed in about one-half hour.
- Distribution: Rapidly distributed bound to plasma lipoprotein and albumin.
- Metabolism: Metabolized by the liver by cytochrome P450 system of enzymes.
- Excretion: About half is excreted unchanged in the urine.
- Half-life: 1.7 to 1.9 hours (the natural hormone has a half-life of 3 minutes).

Dosage and Administration

Clinicians should always use the smallest volume of drug to deliver the desired dose, and if multiple injections are to be given within short periods, then the injection sites should be rotated in a systematic manner.

Generic Name	Trade Name	Form	Usual Dosage
octreotide	Sandostatin	Routes: IV, SC (most often administered SC). Because it is a peptide salt, it is provided in buffered solutions of 50, 100, and 500 mcg/mL ampoules for IV or SC injection.	For acromegaly: The initial dosing found to be most effective is 100 mcg. However, age, gender, weight, disease state, and other disease factors influence a wide range of dosing regimens from 50 mcg to 500 mcg. There is little benefit at doses higher than 300 mcg.

Clinical Uses

- Acromegaly
- To suppress the severe diarrhea and flushing episodes associated with metastatic cancer

Adverse Reactions

CV: Sinus bradycardia, arrhythmias
ENDO: Hypothyroidism
GI: Gallbladder abnormalities, especially gallbladder stones and biliary sludge, diarrhea, loose stools, nausea, abdominal discomfort, vomiting, flatulence, distention, and constipation
META: Hypoglycemia or hyperglycemia can develop in acromegaly patients

Interactions

- Octreotide has been linked to altering absorption of nutrients and orally administered drugs.
- Insulin, oral hypoglycemics, beta blockers, calcium channel blockers, or any drug affecting fluid and electrolyte balance may need dosage adjustments if taken with octreotide.
- Because metabolic clearance is by cytochrome P450 enzymes, any other drug with a low therapeutic index should be used with caution.

Contraindications

- Hypersensitivities

Conscientious Considerations

- Patients with acromegaly are at an increased risk for development of diabetes, hypothyroidism, and cardiovascular disease. Octreotide may hasten development of these conditions.
- As little as a single dose is capable of inhibiting gallbladder contractility and decreasing bile secretions. If the patient uses this medication for up to a year, then he or she must be monitored for development of gallbladder stones or sludge.

Patient/Family Education

- Inform patients that this drug alters the balance of regulatory hormones in the body (insulin, glucagons, and growth hormone) and therefore has several side effects.

DRUGS AFFECTING THE ADRENAL GLANDS

The adrenal glands are located on the top of each kidney. The inner part secretes epinephrine and norepinephrine, and the outer part secretes aldosterone and cortisol. The adrenal glands maintain salt levels in the blood, maintain blood pressure, help control kidney function, and control overall fluid concentrations in the body.

The adrenal cortex (outer) produces about 50 different chemicals, including some that are useful as medications:

- Mineralocorticoids (outer layer)
- Glucocorticoids, cortisol (middle layer)
- Androgens (innermost layer), primarily dehydroepiandrosterone

The adrenal medulla (inner core) produces epinephrine, norepinephrine, and dopamine.

Glucocorticoids

Glucocorticoids are hormones that predominantly affect the metabolism of carbohydrates and, to a lesser extent, fats and proteins. Glucocorticoids are made in the outside portion (the cortex) of the adrenal gland and are chemically classed as steroids, with cortisol being the major natural glucocorticoid. The term *glucocorticoid* also applies to equivalent hormones synthesized in the laboratory and available in many commercial preparations as cortisol or hydrocortisone. In contrast to loss of mineralocorticoids, failure to produce glucocorticoids is not acutely life threatening. Nevertheless, loss or profound diminishment of glucocorticoid secretion leads to a state of deranged metabolism and an inability to deal with stressors, which, if untreated, is fatal.

In addition to their physiological importance, glucocorticoids are also among the most frequently used drugs and are often prescribed for their anti-inflammatory and immunosuppressive properties.

One example of a commercial glucocorticoid is dexamethasone; a fluorinated glucocorticoid that is more potent and longer acting than cortisol (and also possesses all of the adverse effects of cortisol). Because it lacks mineralocorticoid activity, dexamethasone is not used in replacement therapy but instead is used for its anti-inflammatory properties.

Conscientious Prescribing of Glucocorticoids

■ Use cautiously because chronic treatment will lead to adrenal suppression.

■ Use the lowest possible doses for the shortest duration of time.

■ During times of stress (surgery, infections, etc.) supplemental dosing may be required.

■ Signs of infection (fever, inflammation, etc.) may be masked.

■ When a dose is ordered daily or every other day, administer it in the morning to coincide with the body's normal secretion of cortisol.

■ If administering PO, give with meals to minimize GI irritation.

■ If giving IM or SC, shake suspension well before drawing up.

■ Patients on prolonged therapy need hematological values, serum electrolytes, and serum and glucose levels evaluated.

Patient/Family Education for Glucocorticoids

■ Instruct patients on correct administration regimens and techniques. They should not double doses, and if a dose is missed, it should be taken as soon as it is remembered, but not if the next dose is due soon.

■ Instruct patients to avoid others with contagious diseases because these drugs may mask signs of infections.

■ Caution patients to avoid vaccines while on therapy.

■ Review side effects with patients and be sure they understand they are to contact their prescriber if abdominal pain or tarry stools appear.

■ Patients should not have surgery while on these drugs.

■ While on these drugs, a medical history card or alert system should be carried in the event of an emergency in which the patient is unable to relate his or her medical history.

■ For patients who are taking these drugs long term, it should be emphasized that their diet should be high in protein, calcium, and potassium and low in sodium and carbohydrates.

■ Alcohol should also be avoided.

■ Warn patients about abrupt withdrawals.

Mechanism of Action

GLUCOSE METABOLISM. The name *glucocorticoid* derives from early observations that these hormones are involved in glucose metabolism. In the fasting state, cortisol stimulates several processes that collectively serve to increase and maintain normal concentrations of glucose in blood. These effects include the following:

■ Stimulation of gluconeogenesis, particularly in the liver: This pathway results in the synthesis of glucose from nonhexose substrates such as amino acids and lipids and is particularly important in carnivores and certain herbivores.

Enhancing the expression of enzymes involved in gluconeogenesis is probably the best-known metabolic function of glucocorticoids.

■ Mobilization of amino acids from extra hepatic tissues: These serve as substrates for gluconeogenesis.

■ Inhibition of glucose uptake in muscle and adipose tissue: This inhibition is a mechanism to conserve glucose.

■ Stimulation of fat breakdown in adipose tissue: The fatty acids released by lipolysis are used for production of energy in tissues such as muscle, and the released glycerol provide another substrate for gluconeogenesis.

INFLAMMATION AND IMMUNE FUNCTION. Glucocorticoids have potent anti-inflammatory and immunosuppressive properties. This is particularly evident when they are administered in pharmacological doses, but they are also important in normal immune responses. As a consequence, glucocorticoids are widely used as drugs to treat inflammatory conditions such as arthritis or dermatitis and as adjunct therapy for conditions such as autoimmune diseases.

OTHER EFFECTS OF GLUCOCORTICOIDS. Glucocorticoids have multiple effects on **fetal development**. An important example is their role in promoting maturation of the lung and production of the surfactant necessary for extrauterine lung function.

Several aspects of **cognitive function** are known to both stimulate glucocorticoid secretion and be influenced by glucocorticoids. Fear provides an interesting example of this. Excessive glucocorticoid levels resulting from administration as a drug or hyperadrenocorticism have effects on many systems. Some examples include inhibition of bone formation, suppression of calcium absorption, and delayed wound healing. These observations suggest a multitude of less dramatic physiological roles for glucocorticoids.

Pharmacokinetics

■ Absorption: Well absorbed after oral administration. Sodium succinate and sodium phosphate salts are best absorbed by IM.

■ Distribution: Widely distributed to all tissues.

■ Metabolism: Metabolized by the liver. Cortisone is converted by the liver to hydrocortisone. Prednisone is converted by the liver to prednisolone, which is then metabolized by the liver.

■ Excretion: Excreted in urine as 17-hydroxysteroids and 17-ketsteroids.

■ Half-life: Plasma half-lives range from 0.5 to a few hours; tissue half-lives range from half a day to a few days, allowing placement in these three categories:
  ■ Short acting: Cortisone (Cortone), hydrocortisone (Cortef)
  ■ Intermediate acting: Methylprednisolone (Medrol), prednisolone (Delta-Cortef), prednisone (Cordal, Meticorten), triamcinolone (Aristocort)
  ■ Long-acting: Betamethasone (Celestone), budesonide (Entocort), dexamethasone (Decadrol)

Dosage and Administration

Generic Name	Trade Name	Form	Usual Dosage
glucocorticoids or corticosteroids	Topical preparations are usually insoluble steroids that produce little to no absorptions and thus few side effects There are a number of OTC glucocorticoids sold in strengths that meet FDA guidelines for OTC products (e.g., CortAid)	Tablet form; solutions for IV, IM, SC; topical creams, ointments, gels, and powders The oral route is preferred for long-term use. IV route is used in emergencies, because peak plasma levels usually occur within 1 hr	For anti-inflammation and immunosuppression effects: Dosages range from 25,300 mg/day in divided doses every 12–24 hr Dosage is dependent on the patient's response to the medication

Clinical Uses

Uses include, but are not limited to the following:

- Addison's disease (hormone replacement)
- Cancer therapy
- Decreasing the inflammation of systemic lupus erythematosus
- Rheumatoid arthritis
- Inflammatory bowel disease
- Asthma
- Chronic obstructive pulmonary disease
- Respiratory distress syndrome in infants
- Suppressing rejection of skin grafts
- Acute renal insufficiency
- Shock
- Simple inflammatory rashes

Adverse Reactions

CV: Tachycardia

DERM: Acne, delayed wound healing, facial flushing

ENDO: Hyperglycemia, **Cushing's syndrome** (The signs and symptoms [round face, obesity] of prolonged exposure to high levels of cortisol, as when people prolong exposure to steroids or most likely when tumors of the pituitary release excessive ACTH which causes the adrenal glands to up production of cortisol)

GI: Abdominal distention, diarrhea, constipation, heartburn, increased appetite, peptic ulcers, and GI bleeds

MISC: Increased susceptibility to infection, allergic reactions

NEURO: Anxiety, insomnia, mood swings, hallucinations, depression

Interactions

- Oral anticoagulants. Hydrocortisone in combination with oral anticoagulants may increase prothrombin time.
- Potassium-depleting diuretics. With potassium-depleting diuretics there is risk of hypokalemia.

- Cardiac glycosides. With cardiac glycosides there is increased risk of cardiac toxicity and arrhythmia.
- Calcium. Hydrocortisone interferes with calcium absorption in food.
- St. John's wort. In presence of St. John's wort the absorption of glucocorticoids is decreased.

Contraindications

- Fungal disease or suspected fungal disease
- Live virus vaccine
- Hypertension
- Heart failure
- Renal impairment
- Presence of any infection that appears resistant to antibiotic treatment

Conscientious Considerations

- Serious effects of long-term use to watch for are hypocalcemia, osteoporosis, edema, muscle wasting in arms and legs, fluid and electrolyte disturbances, spontaneous fractures, amenorrhea, cataracts, glaucoma, peptic ulcer disease, and congestive heart failure. Serious effects of abrupt withdrawal from long-term therapy are anorexia, nausea, fever, headache, joint pain, rebound inflammation, fatigue, weakness, lethargy, dizziness, and orthostatic hypotension. Gradual systemic withdrawal is paramount as these conditions can exist for up to 1 year after discontinuation.
- Occasionally check fluid balance, potassium, and glucose levels.
- Make sure the patient is compliant to the prescribed dose regimen and does not stop suddenly.
- Assess any underlying infection or delays in wound healing.
- Assess for Cushing's syndrome.
- Check stools for occult blood.
- Check for additional stress in the patient's life, which may cause dosage changes.
- Consider treatment with steroids as being palliative, not curative. Only in a few cases (leukemia, nephrotoxic syndrome) do steroids alter prognosis.
- The benefits of treatment must be weighed against the side effects of the steroids.
- Patient's age is an important factor because toxic effects are more apt to occur in the old, infirm, and those with a CV condition.
- Once steroid therapy is initiated, use the lowest possible dose and stop therapy as soon as possible using a step-down process.
- Monitor the patient for serum K, glucose, edema, blood pressure, congestive heart failure, mental status, weight gain.
- For asthma: Inhaled steroids, such as beclomethasone and betamethasone, are effective alternates to systemic steroids because they can be delivered directly to the target site in relatively low doses. They are useful in asthma treatment because they have the potential for more frequent administration (see Chapter 10, Drugs Used in the Treatment of Pulmonary Diseases and Disorders).

Drugs Used in the Treatment of Adrenal Insufficiency

Aldosterone regulates sodium and potassium balance in the blood and promotes sodium reabsorption in the kidney to preserve extracellular fluid volume. Its production in normal patients is maintained by the renin-angiotensin system and the concentration of potassium in the blood. Aldosterone secretion is stimulated by increased potassium levels and a decrease in aldosterone circulating volume owing to such things as loss of blood, excessive diuresis, and low salt intake. Aldosterone secretion is suppressed by elevated sodium levels in the blood.

Tertiary adrenal insufficiency due to exogenous corticosteroid administration is the most common problem encountered. In **adrenal insufficiency**, aldosterone deficits occur, sodium reabsorption is inhibited, and potassium excretion decreases. Also, hyperkalemia occurs and is accompanied by a mild acidosis. The dose and duration of corticosteroids used to reverse adrenal insufficiency is highly variable. There are some regimens that, if followed, should not lead to significant adrenal suppression, for example, daily therapy of 5 mg or less of prednisone or its equivalent, or alternate-day therapy, or any given dose for no longer than 3 weeks. Three drugs used to treat the sodium loss and hypotension associated with adrenal insufficiency are fludrocortisone (Florinef), aminoglutethimide (Cytadren), and arimidex (Anastrozole).

Fludrocortisone (Florinef)

Fludrocortisone is a synthetic corticosteroid. It displays moderate potency as a glucocorticoid but much greater potency as a mineralocorticoid.

Mechanism of Action

Chemically, the structure of fludrocortisone is identical to cortisone except there is the substitution of a fluorine moiety in place of one hydrogen. In low doses it acts on the distal tubules to increase potassium and hydrogen ion secretion, thereby replacing sodium. In higher doses it inhibits exogenous adrenal cortical secretion, thymic activity, and secretion of corticotropin in the pituitary gland. Fludrocortisone is used to replace aldosterone.

Pharmacokinetics

- Absorption: Well absorbed from the GI tract. It is 42% protein bound.
- Distribution: Widely distributed throughout bloodstream.
- Metabolism: Metabolized by liver and kidney.
- Excretion: Primarily excreted in urine.
- Half-life: 3.5 hours.

Dosage and Administration

Generic Name	Trade Name	Form	Usual Dosage
fludrocortisone	Florinef	Formulated as a 0.1-mg tablet.	For mineralocorticoid replacement (children): typical daily dose is between 0.05 mg and 0.1 mg/day; (adults): 0.05 mg–0.2 mg/day dosed 3 times/week.

Clinical Uses

- Various forms of adrenal insufficiency (i.e., **Addison's disease,** a rare condition when adrenals fail to produce sufficient glucocorticoids marked by weight loss, muscle weakness, fatigue, low BP, and skin color changes which can result in abdominal pain, loss of BP, and coma)
- Congenital adrenal insufficiency (a salt-wasting disease)

Adverse Reactions

DERM: Acne
GI: Ulcers, increased appetite, abdominal distention, upset stomach, vomiting
META: Cold, unusual hair growth
MISC: Potential for decreases in inflammatory and immune responses, weight gain, swollen limbs
NEURO: Dizziness, headaches, exaggerated sense of well-being, insomnia, mood swings, depression, anxiety

Interactions

- Rifampin, barbiturates, and hydantoins will decrease the effect of fludrocortisone.
- Amphotericin induces excessive potassium depletion.
- Loop diuretics induce excessive potassium loss.
- Thiazide diuretics induce excessive potassium depletion.
- Heart medicine digitalis taken concurrently can induce digitalis toxicity and hypokalemia.
- Contraceptives taken orally and other corticosteroids, because serious side effects can result.

Contraindications

- Those with hypersensitivity
- Those with concurrent fungal infections

Conscientious Considerations

- This medication may become addictive, and a course of therapy should last no longer than a few weeks.
- Long-term use may result in muscle wasting (especially arms and legs), osteoporosis, spontaneous fractures, amenorrhea, cataracts, glaucoma, fever, peptic ulcer disease, and congestive heart failure.
- Overdose constitutes a medical emergency requiring immediate attention. Signs of overdose are the following: weakness in the muscles, high blood pressure, unusual weight gain, hypokalemia, water retention.
- It is of paramount importance to strictly follow the dosing directions and never exceed the dose prescribed.
- Abrupt withdrawal can cause anorexia, nausea, fever, headache, joint pain, rebound inflammation, fatigue, weakness, lethargy, dizziness, and orthostatic hypertension.
- Ask if the patient is pregnant or if she is breastfeeding because handling this drug can lead to absorption of the drug to an infant or fetus where suppression of the hypothalamic-pituitary-adrenal axis can occur from minute doses over a prolonged period.

■ Renin plasma, sodium, and potassium levels must be checked through blood tests to verify that an effective dosage has been reached.

■ It is usually taken in the morning with food or milk.

Patient/Family Education

■ Fludrocortisone is not a simple medication. Even though administered in pill form, it is one of those medications with serious side effects and precautions. The clinician should teach all patients and their caregivers the long list of precautions (see Conscientious Considerations).

■ The patient should be advised to avoid any skin tests or vaccinations during the treatment.

■ The patient may be restricted to a high-protein, low-salt and sodium, potassium-rich diet during the treatment.

■ The patient should be told to avoid drinking alcohol beverages during treatment.

■ The patient should be advised against abrupt withdrawal of this medication.

Aminoglutethimide (Cytadren)

Aminoglutethimide is an adrenal androgen inhibitor.

Mechanism of Action

As an adrenal androgen blocker, aminoglutethimide blocks corticosteroids from being made, which in turn stops them from signaling the body to produce other hormones, such as estrogens, androgens, glucocorticoids, and mineralocorticoids. In cases of cancer (breast, prostrate), the resulting decrease of estrogen and androgens interferes with the stimulation of cancer growth in tumors sensitive to these hormones.

Pharmacokinetics

■ Absorption: Rapid and complete after oral administration
■ Distribution: Well distributed
■ Metabolism: Some drug converted in liver to acetylated form
■ Excretion: 34% to 54% excreted in urine as unchanged drug
■ Half-life: 12.5 hours

Dosage and Administration

Generic Name	Trade Name	Form	Usual Dosage
aminoglutethimide	Cytadren	PO	250 mg every 6 hr for adrenal suppression. Increase every 1–2 weeks to 2 g/day.

Clinical Uses

■ Suppression of adrenal function in selected patients with Cushing's syndrome
■ Adrenal carcinoma and ectopic ACTH-producing tumors
■ Treatment of breast cancer in postmenopausal women
■ Treatment of metastatic prostate cancer

Adverse Reactions

GI: Nausea or loss of appetite (during the first few weeks of treatment)
NEURO: Drowsiness, dizziness, headache, weakness

Interactions

■ Corticosteroids. Aminoglutethimide has drug interactions with all the corticosteroids.

Contraindications

■ Hypersensitivities.
■ Aminoglutethimide is not recommended for use during pregnancy nor should the drug be allowed to pass into breast milk.

Conscientious Considerations

■ Because this medication must be used under close medical supervision, the following laboratory tests will be needed: thyroid function, baseline hematological, serum glutamic-oxaloacetic transaminase, alkaline phosphatase, bilirubin.

■ The patient's medical history should be screened for chicken pox, shingles (herpes zoster), infection, kidney or liver disease, and an underactive thyroid.

■ Steroid tablets must also be prescribed along with aminoglutethimide because aminoglutethimide itself stops steroid production.

■ Aminoglutethimide has gained notoriety because of its misuse by weight-training athletes and bodybuilders, who have used it for a chemical muscle enhancement despite its severe risks as an anabolic steroid.

■ Because Cytadren does not affect any underlying disease, it is used primarily as an interim measure until more definitive therapy such as surgery can be undertaken. Only a small number of patients have been treated for longer than 3 months because a decreased effect or "escape phenomenon" seems to occur in patients with pituitary-dependent Cushing's syndrome, probably because of increasing ACTH levels in response to the decreases in glucocorticoid. Upon withdrawal of aminoglutethimide, the ability of the adrenals to synthesize steroid usually returns within 72 hours.

■ Use of aminoglutethimide is limited because of its lack of selectivity for aromatase and its toxicity profile. Studies show drugs such as aminoglutethimide can lower aromatase activity between 74% and 91%, with falls in estradiol levels of 58% to 76%.

Patient/Family Education

■ Patients should be advised to contact their clinician or seek medical help if fainting, rapid heartbeat, itching, skin rashes, yellowing of the eyes or skin, any difficulty with walking, coordination and balance, or breathing difficulties develop.

■ If patients are on any anticoagulants, clotting times need to be checked and dosage of anticoagulants may need to be changed.

■ Let the patient know that a rash is common during the first week of treatment and most often disappears in 5 to 8 days. If the rash does not clear, the drug may be stopped.

■ Because of potential dizziness, the patient should be advised to use caution when driving or performing other tasks requiring alertness.

■ The use of alcohol while on this medication is prohibited because of its potentiation of dizziness and drowsiness.

Anastrozole (Arimidex)

Although tamoxifen has been the mainstay of endocrine treatment for over 20 years, other agents have superior activity and better safety profiles. The first of these orally active, potent, selective, third-line aromatase inhibitors in the management of hormone-sensitive breast cancer is anastrozole (Arimidex).

Mechanism of Action

Many breast cancers have estrogen receptors, and once stimulated by estrogens, the tumors grow. Thus, one goal of breast cancer treatment is to decrease estrogen levels by using antiestrogen drugs. In postmenopausal women, one source of estrogens is the conversion of adrenal-generated androstenedione by an enzyme, aromatase, found in peripheral tissues, especially adipose tissue. Furthermore, androstenedione is converted to estradiol. A selective, potent nonsteroidal aromatase inhibitor, anastrozole can decrease tumor mass or delay progression of tumor growth.

Pharmacokinetics

■ Absorption: With oral administration, absorption quickly rises to 85% of the administered dose, even in the presence of food.
■ Distribution: Well distributed with 40% bound to plasma proteins.
■ Metabolism: Liver metabolism accounts for about 85% of elimination.
■ Excretion: Excreted in the urine as 60% metabolites, 10% as unchanged.
■ Half-life: About 50 hours.

Dosage and Administration

Generic Name	Trade Name	Form	Usual Dosage
anastrozole	Arimidex	1 mg tablet	1 mg/day for as long as there is tumor progression. In some cases this has been as long as 5 years. In some cases women have tolerated doses up to 10 mg/day very well.

Clinical Uses

■ Breast cancer in postmenopausal women
■ Adjuvant therapy for early estrogen receptor–positive breast cancer
■ First-line therapy for metastatic breast cancer
■ Advanced therapy if treatment with tamoxifen fails and disease progression continues

Adverse Reactions

CV: Peripheral edema
GI: Nausea/vomiting
GYN: Vaginal bleeding, hot flashes
MISC: Flu syndrome, cataracts
MS: Fractures, sore muscles, fatigue, accidental injuries
NEURO: Mood disturbances

Interactions

■ Any patient taking **estrogen replacement therapy (ERT)** is likely to find the effect of anastrozole diminished.
■ It is unlikely that the coadministration of a 1-mg dose of anastrozole (Arimidex) with other drugs will result in clinically significant drug inhibition of cytochrome P450-mediated metabolism of the other drugs.
■ No significant interaction with warfarin has been reported.

Contraindications

■ Pregnancy (harm may result to the fetus)

Conscientious Considerations

■ Anastrozole is not to be used in premenopausal women because safety profiles have not been established.
■ Anastrozole may cause a decrease in bone mineral density.
■ Because total cholesterol and LDL-cholesterol increase in patients receiving anastrozole, it should be used with caution in patients with hyperlipidemia.
■ Women with renal insufficiency will find diminished clearance requiring dosage adjustment.

Patient/Family Education

■ Patient should be advised that this medication must be taken regularly to get the most benefit from it, preferably the same time each day, with or without food.
■ Patients should not increase or decrease their dosages without clinician approval because it will not hasten recovery or lessen side effects.
■ Because this drug can be absorbed through the skin, women who are pregnant or breastfeeding should not handle nor break tablets.

Implications for Special Populations

Pregnancy Implications

When prescribing drugs affecting the endocrine system for the pregnant female, clinicians should carefully consider their choice of drugs. Following is a selected list of drugs along with the assigned FDA Safety Category.

CATEGORY	DRUGS
C	corticotropin, fludrocortisone
D	aminoglutethimide, propylthiouracil, methimazole
X	trilostane
Unclassified	Strong iodine solution (Lugol's solution), potassium iodide

Glucocorticoids

■ Do not use in patients who are breastfeeding because steroids are excreted in breast milk. Don't use in those who are pregnant because it can interfere with infant growth and endogenous steroid production.

Pediatric Implications

■ Pituitary hormone. Somatrem is indicated for the treatment of growth failure in children caused by growth hormone deficiency.

■ Glucocorticoids. Do not use in pediatric patients.

Geriatric Implications

Thyroid Hormones

■ Because the elderly are more sensitive to and experience more adverse reactions to thyroid hormones, it is recommended that dosing be individualized. In some patients, doses may need to be 25% lower than the usual adult dose.

■ Hypothyroidism is the second most common endocrine disease in the elderly and is often misdiagnosed because only about a third of geriatric patients present with the typical signs and symptoms. Most often geriatric patients have nonspecific symptoms such as failure to thrive, stumbling and falling episodes, incontinence, and neurological involvement. Thus, patients are often misdiagnosed with dementia or depression.

LEARNING EXERCISES

Case 1

A 25-year-old male college student, otherwise in good health, was brought to University Campus Hospital (UCH) after being found lying down in his dormitory unresponsive to his roommate's shaking him and shouting at him. He exhibited some "moaning," "thrashing," and "yelling," and the ambulance attendants administered Ativan to calm him down. Once at the UCH, he presented with a rectal temperature of 104.8°F, but showed no signs of infection. His skin was warm and sweaty, he had some sinus tachycardia, his lungs showed clear upon X-ray, and his pupils were dilated. His medical records indicated he was not on any medications, but his roommate stated he smoked a "joint" from time to time. Laboratory studies revealed higher than normal levels of free T4, triiodothyronine, thyroid-stimulating immunoglobulin, and thyroglobulin antibody.

1. What is the diagnosis for this patient?

2. How would you treat him?

Case 2

JB and BL are happy and well-adjusted boys who go to the same school and have the same friends. JB is a little short and has been found to have growth-hormone deficiency (GH) without growth hormone treatment, and he is predicted to grown no taller than 5'2". His parents are insisting that JB be given growth hormone therapy (GHT) so that he can be "tall" like his mom (5'4") and his dad (5'10"). BL is also short and at the urging of JB's family was tested for growth hormone deficiency. It was found that BL will likely grow to be no more than 5'2" even though his parents are both 6' but he does not demonstrate any growth hormone deficiency.

1. Is it unjust to provide treatment to JB but not his friend BL, just because JB has an identifiable medical deficiency?

2. Is this a situation of applying Aristotle's dictum "equal cases must be treated equally"?

Drugs Used in the Treatment of Diabetes Mellitus

chapter 13

Mona A. Sedrak, Alice A. House, William N. Tindall

CHAPTER FOCUS

Diabetes mellitus (DM) is a complex, heterogeneous group of metabolic disorders characterized by alterations in glucose metabolism (hyperglycemia). Because it results from defects in insulin secretion, insulin activity, or both, medications are used to regain glycemic control, alleviate symptoms, and prevent acute and long-term complications. The agents in this chapter are specific diabetic medications taken orally, such as insulin secretagogues, alpha-glucosidase inhibitors, and thiazolidinediones, as well as the self-injection insulin replacement products that are rapid acting, intermediate acting, and long acting.

Dietary modifications, exercise, and patient education are integral to the management of diabetes. To ensure success, clinicians must instruct patients to self-monitor, adjust medications, and maintain glycemia in a target range.

OBJECTIVES

After reading and studying this chapter, the student should be able to:

1. Describe the etiology, prevalence, and pathophysiology of type 1 and type 2 diabetes.
2. Define the treatment goals for type 1 and type 2 diabetes established by the American Diabetes Association and the American Association of Clinical Endocrinologists.
3. Compare and contrast the mechanism of action of the oral hypoglycemic agents involved in the treatment of type 2 diabetes.
4. Summarize the treatment algorithms set by the American Diabetes Association for type 2 diabetes.
5. List common adverse reactions and contraindications of oral hypoglycemic agents as well as insulin.
6. Compare and contrast the various types and administration of insulin used in type 1 and type 2 diabetes.
7. Differentiate between the various insulin preparations and their use in type 2 diabetes.

Key Terms

Biguanide
Gastroparesis
Glycemic control
Hemoglobin A1c (HbA1c)
Hyperglycemia
Hypoglycemia
Insulin
Insulin pump
Ketoacidosis (DKA)
Monotherapy
Nephropathy
Neutral Protamine Hagedorn (NPH)
Prandial
Prediabetes
Secretagogue
Sulfonylurea
Titrate
Type 1 diabetes mellitus (T1DM)
Type 2 diabetes mellitus (T2DM)

DRUGS USED IN THE TREATMENT OF DIABETES MELLITUS

Oral Hypoglycemic Agents	glyburide (DiaBeta, Glynase, Micronase)	**Alpha-Glucosidase Inhibitors**
Insulin Secretagogues	glimepiride (Amaryl)	acarbose (Precose)
(Sulfonylureas)	**Biguanides**	miglitol (Glyset)
First Generation	metformin (Glucophage)	**Amylin Agonists**
acetohexamide (Dymelor)	**Meglitinides (Glinides)**	exenatide (Byetta)
chlorpropamide (Diabinese)	repaglinide (Prandin)	pramlintide (Symlin)
tolazamide (Tolinase)	nateglinide (Starlix)	**Incretin Mimetics (Glucagon-Like**
tolbutamide (Orinase)	**Thiazolidinediones ([TZDs] or Glitazones)**	**Peptide-1 Agonists [GLP-1])**
Second Generation	pioglitazone (Actos)	exenatide (Byetta)
glipizide (Glucotrol)	rosiglitazone (Avandia)	liraglutide (Victoza)

continued

DRUGS USED IN THE TREATMENT OF DIABETES MELLITUS—cont'd

Dipeptidyl Peptidase-4 Inhibitors (DPP-4)	Short Acting	(HumulinL,NovulinL, Iletin II Lente)
sitagliptin (Januvia)	Regular Insulin (Humulin-R, Novolin-R)	*NPH (Neutral Protamine Hagadorn)
Glucagon	**Intermediate Acting**	**Long Acting, Basal**
Injectable Insulins	NPH* Insulins	insulin glargine (Lantus)
Rapid Acting	Insulin Zinc Suspension	insulin detemir (Levemir)
insulin aspart (NovoLog)	(HumulinN, NovulinN, Iletin II NPH)	extended zinc insulin suspension
insulin glulisine (Apidra)	Lente Insulins	(Ultralente)
lispro (Humalog)	Isophane Insulin Suspension	protamine zinc insulin suspension (PZI)

Diabetes mellitus (DM) affects 26.9% of Americans over the age of 65. Approximately 215,000 people younger than age 20 have either type 1 diabetes mellitus (T1DM) or type 2 diabetes mellitus (T2DM). Unfortunately, 35.8% of adults over the age of 20 have **prediabetes** (also called "borderline diabetes" where blood glucose levels are higher than normal but not quite high enough to be called diabetes), putting 79 million Americans at risk for diabetic complications. It is unfortunate that 70 million people in the United States remain undiagnosed (National Diabetes Information Clearinghouse [NDIC], 2011). Diabetes, both type 1 and type 2, directly or indirectly causes at least 230,000 deaths per year (ADA, 2011), making diabetes the leading cause of kidney failure, nontraumatic lower-limb amputations, and new cases of blindness among adults in the United States as well as being a major contributor to hyperlipidemia, hypertension, coronary heart disease (CAD), and stroke. Fortunately, because diabetes mellitus is now being treated aggressively and at an earlier stage, the number of diabetes-treated patients with visual impairment is increasing, but the percentage/prevalence of diabetes-induced visual impairment is decreasing among all groups except blacks and those who had diabetes for 3 or more years before treatment (CDC, 2011).

THE PATHOPHYSIOLOGY OF DIABETES

The pancreas secretes a fluid that digests fats, proteins, and carbohydrates as well as insulin and glucagon. From the islet of Langerhans, insulin is secreted from its beta cells in response to high levels of glucose in the blood. **Insulin** is a hormone made up of several polypeptide chains and 48 amino acids, which are chemically linked to zinc, cobalt, cadmium, and nickel. Insulin is stored in the pancreas as proinsulin, a larger protein, and when released in relatively small amounts, it acts as a catalyst of cell metabolism in body tissue.

Carbohydrate metabolism is a mix of several factors including insulin, adrenal, anterior pituitary, and thyroid hormones, but the exact role of insulin is not completely understood. Glucagon is produced by the alpha cells of the islets of Langerhans. Glucagon acts by mobilizing liver glucagons and converting it to glucose, which in turn elevates glucose concentration in the blood.

Type 1 Diabetes Mellitus

Type 1 diabetes mellitus (T1DM), accounts for 5% to 10% of all diabetes mellitus cases in the United States (ADA, 2011). T1DM results from a deficiency of insulin secretion induced by a cellular-mediated, autoimmune destruction of insulin-producing pancreatic beta cells in the islet of Langerhans. This beta cell destruction can be initiated by viruses, including rubella, coxsackie B virus, cytomegalovirus, adenovirus, and mumps, as well as physical injury. Beta cell autoantigens, macrophages, dendrite cells, B lymphocytes, and T lymphocytes have been shown to be involved in the pathogenesis of autoimmune diabetes. There are two subtypes of T1DM: immune mediated and nonimmune mediated. Nonimmune-mediated T1DM is the result of secondary diseases, such as pancreatitis. Immune-mediated T1DM occurs when beta-cell autoantigens are released from beta cells by cellular turnover or damage and are processed and presented to helper T cells by antigen-presenting cells. A majority of patients (86% to 90%) who are seen with the immune-related subtype of diabetes present with tyrosine phosphatase 1A-2 and IA-2 beta antibodies. In the few remaining cases, patients present with no known etiology and are classified as idiopathic T1DM. Most of these patients are African Americans or Asian Americans.

The rate of beta-cell destruction varies; infants and children often experience rapid beta-cell destruction, whereas in adults it is usually slower. Individuals who are at increased risk for T1DM can often be identified by serological evidence of an autoimmune pathological process occurring in the pancreatic islet cells and genetic markers (Yoon, 2007).

Type 2 Diabetes Mellitus

Type 2 diabetes mellitus (T2DM) accounts for 90% to 95% of all DM cases; however, prevalence does vary among ethnic groups, with it being more prevalent among native Americans, Hispanics, African Americans, and ethnic immigrants. T2DM is caused by a combination of complex metabolic disorders that result from coexisting effects of multiple organ sites such as insulin resistance in the muscle and subsequent to increased adipose tissue, a progressive decline in pancreatic insulin secretion, unrestrained hepatic glucose production, and other hormonal deficiencies such as a genetic defect in insulin secretion or action, exocrine pancreatic disease, Cushing's syndrome, acromegaly, drugs, or pancreatectomy. Interestingly, the autoimmune destruction appearing in T1DM does not appear here; however, there is a strong genetic disposition. For example, the siblings of a diabetic person are at a 7% to 14% risk for developing it, and children and young adults with T1DM have a 50% chance of transmitting the disease to their offspring.

Plasma insulin levels in T2DM may be low, medium, or high, because the main physiological alteration is insulin resistance, a suboptimal response of insulin-sensitive tissues. Prior to the appearance of clinical symptoms of T2DM, patients may experience hyperglycemia, which causes pathological and functional changes in target tissues. Most affected individuals are obese and have variable degrees of this insulin resistance, especially in liver, muscle, and visceral fat, to the extent that there is an increase in endogenous glucose production secondary to glucagon levels being increased because the liver cells are not receiving feedback messages about the amount of glucose already in the bloodstream. Those patients who are not obese may have an increased percentage of visceral fat, which can also cause insulin resistance. Thus, if the pancreas is the major organ involved in T1DM, it must be remembered that it is the liver that is the major organ involved in causing T2DM. Thus, the body may survive well with many years of compensatory hyperinsulinemia, but over time the beta-cell responsiveness to glucose diminishes, and the clinical symptoms of diabetes start and hyperglycemia prevails. Risk factors for T2DM include the following:

- A family history of diabetes
- A family history of cardiovascular disease
- Overweight/obese
- Sedentary lifestyle
- Latino/Hispanic, non-Hispanic black, Asian American, Native American, or Pacific Islander ethnicity
- Diagnosis of impaired glucose tolerance or impaired fasting glucose
- Diagnosis of hypertension
- Increased levels of triglycerides or low concentrations of high-density lipoproteins
- History of gestational diabetes
- History of delivering an infant over 9 lbs
- History of polycystic ovary syndrome
- History of psychiatric illness (Handelsman et al., 2011)

DIAGNOSIS AND TREATMENT GOALS

Diagnosis of DM is based on demonstration of its classic symptoms of excess glucose excreted in the kidney (glycosuria), excessive urination (polyuria), increased appetite (polyphasia), increased thirst (polydipsia), unexplained weight loss, weakness (fatigue), itching (pruritis vulvae as a candida yeast infection, or just generalized pruritus), and abnormal plasma glucose concentrations (Table 13-1). Early and aggressive **glycemic control** (people are advised to keep their blood glucose under control to typical levels in order to prevent microvascular and cardiovascular disease). Doing so in patients with DM (Table 13-2) lowers the

TABLE 13-1 Clinical Interpretations of Plasma Glucose Concentrations

GLUCOSE CONCENTRATION (MG/DL)	CLINICAL INTERPRETATION
Fasting	
<100	Within the reference range
100–125	Impaired fasting glucose/ prediabetes mellitus
≥126	Overt diabetes mellitus
Two-hour postchallenge load (75 g oral glucose tolerance test)	
<140	Within the reference range
140–199	Impaired glucose tolerance/ prediabetes mellitus
≥200	Overt diabetes mellitus

From Handelsman, et al. (2011).

TABLE 13-2 Guidelines for Normalization of Blood Glucose Targets*

SOURCE	HBA1C TARGET
American Association of Clinical Endocrinologists (AACE)	<6.5%
American Diabetes Association	<7.0 %
American Geriatrics Society (frail elderly)	8.0%
National Institutes of Health	6.5%–7.0%
Canadian Diabetes Association	<7.0%

*To prevent risk of macrovascular and microvascular complications

risk for cardiovascular disease by at least 42% (Narayan, 2005). Regarding complications of DM, there is no specific glycemic threshold for the reduction of these complications; however, the better the glycemic control, the lower the risk of complications. Patients with poor glycemic control are at an increased risk for retinopathy and **nephropathy** as well as myocardial infarction and other morbidities.

Pharmacological Management of Diabetes

A wide variety of pharmacological therapies exist that can safely and effectively lower glycemia to near normal levels. For example, new rapid-acting and long-acting insulin analogues address specific pancreatic hormone and incretin-hormone deficiencies to better control and lower **hemoglobin A1c (HbA1c)** levels, thereby reducing glycemic variability and reducing weight. To help patients adjust insulin dosing, "smart" **insulin pumps** are available to adjust insulin injections on an individualized need. Additionally, prefilled syringes of insulin have dramatically increased the accuracy and consistency of insulin dosing. However, the cornerstones of both T1DM and T2DM care remains nonpharmacological. Lifestyle changes such as weight control, proper nutrition, and exercise have a strong positive impact on the overall health of the patient with diabetes, not only improving glycemic control, but also improving cardiovascular disease risk factors such as blood pressure and atherosclerosis. Thus, patients must be educated and motivated to take an active role in management of their disease.

SPECIAL CASE: Insulin Pumps

Continuous subcutaneous (SC) insulin infusion is indicated for the following:

- Patients who are unable to achieve acceptable control using a regimen of multiple daily injections
- Patients with a history of frequent hypoglycemia or hypoglycemia unawareness
- Patients who are pregnant
- Patients with extreme insulin sensitivity
- Patients with a history of dawn phenomenon
- Patients who require more intensive diabetes management because of complications, including neuropathy, nephropathy, and or retinopathy
- Patients taking multiple daily injections who have demonstrated the willingness and ability to comply with prescribed diabetes self-care behavior, including frequent glucose monitoring, carbohydrate counting, and insulin adjustment

Various types of electromechanical devices (infusion pumps) have been developed to reduce fluctuations in blood glucose levels associated with conventional insulin therapy (subcutaneous injections). Insulin pumps are inserted into a vein much like an injection or catheter system, but the insertion needle is changed every 3 days. Patients using an insulin pump must continue monitoring their blood glucose and continue with their diet and exercise plan.

ORAL HYPOGLYCEMIC AGENTS FOR TREATMENT OF TYPE 2 DIABETES MELLITUS

Consideration of oral hypoglycemic agents for the treatment of T2DM is based on the patient's HbA1c profile (Table 13-2). Most guidelines for a target HbA1c place that target near 7% and also suggest that the clinician should tailor that target guideline as he or she assesses a patient's risk for microvascular and macrovascular complications and comorbidities. Thus, all guidelines are just that—guidelines— and as a "guide" they should be tempered by individualizing recommendations to the patient. For instance, patients with an HbA1c between 6% and 7% will typically be started on monotherapy with persistent monitoring and titrating of medications over 2 to 3 months until glycemic goals are achieved. Additional oral agents that are tailored to meet the patient's specific disease process may be added. However, oral hypoglycemic medications are most effective when they are part of a comprehensive approach that involves diet and exercise.

Patients who are not obese are less likely to be insulin resistant and more likely to benefit from sulfonylureas. Obese patients are more likely to benefit from metformin because it acts more on glucose utilization and hepatic glucose storage and production. Both sulfonylureas and metformin are considered first-line therapy and should be used as the main agents in treatment, with other drugs being adjunctive therapy.

Several pharmacological regimens are available for monotherapy as well as for combination therapy (Table 13-3) (American College of Clinical Endocrinologists [ACCE] Diabetes Care Plan Guidelines, 2011). Clinicians using monotherapy typically start with metformin and move up through the other oral hypoglycemics. If glycemic control is not achieved at the end of 2 to 3 months, clinicians can initiate a more intensive regimen and persistently monitor and **titrate** therapy over the next 2 to 3 months until glycemic control is achieved. Patients who are currently treated with monotherapy or combination therapy who have not achieved glycemic goals may require either increased dosages of their current medication or the addition of a second or third medication.

Patients with a high risk for hypoglycemia benefit most from a drug, such as metformin, that is less likely to produce it. Patients with high postprandial blood glucose levels benefit most from the addition of a glucosidase inhibitor or a meglitinide. Additionally, patients may need insulin therapy if their HbA1c is greater than 8% or if they are experiencing symptomatic hyperglycemia. **Hyperglycemia** is usually transient and nonsymptomatic, but chronic hyperglycemia presents with any number of symptoms, including polyphagia, polydipsia, polyuria, blurry vision, sleeplessness, weight loss, dry mouth, itching skin, erectile dysfunction, cardiac arrhythmia, and stupor. It can result in death.

The American Diabetes Association (ADA) has a T2DM treatment algorithm that takes into account the characteristics of the individual interventions, their synergies, and expense (Figure 13-1). The algorithm is the basis for the ADA's stepwise approach to drug treatment of patients with T2DM, which follows.

STEP ONE: LIFESTYLE INTERVENTION AND METFORMIN. Lifestyle interventions should be initiated as the first step in treating new-onset T2DM. Metformin is recommended as the initial pharmacological therapy in the absence of its specific contraindication, renal insufficiency. Metformin should be titrated to its maximally effective dose over 1 to 2 months.

STEP TWO: ADDITIONAL MEDICATIONS. If lifestyle intervention and maximal tolerated dose of metformin fail to achieve or sustain glycemic goals, another medication should be added within 2 to 3 months of the initiation of therapy or at any time when HbA1c goals are not achieved. Clinicians can choose among insulin, sulfonylureas, or thiazolidinediones (TZDs).

STEP THREE: GLYCEMIC CONTROL. If lifestyle interventions, metformin, and a second medication do not result in glycemic control,

TABLE 13-3 Considerations for Oral Therapy in Patients With Type 2 Diabetes Mellitus

DRUG CLASS	PRIMARY MECHANISM	POSSIBLE ADVERSE EFFECTS	MONITORING	COMMENTS
Sulfonylureas acetohexamide (Dymelor) chlorpropamide (Diabinese) tolazamide (Tolinase) tolbutamide (Orinase) glipizide (Glucotrol) glyburide (DiaBeta, Glynase, Micronase) glimepiride (Amaryl)	Stimulates insulin release	Hypoglycemia Weight gain	Fasting plasma glucose at 2 weeks HbA1c at 3 months	Response plateaus after half maximum dose Glipizide and glimepiride may be preferred in elderly patients
Biguanides metformin (Glucophage)	Inhibits hepatic glucose output	Dose-related diarrhea (usually self-limiting in 7–10 days) Lactic acidosis in patients with renal compromise	Serum creatinine at initiation Fasting plasma glucose at 2 weeks HbA1c at 3 months	Less associated weight gain than with sulfonylureas and thiazolidinediones; weight loss may occur; helps limit weight gain in combination therapy Maximum effective dosage is 2 gm/day Contraindications: Serum creatinine >1.5 mg/dL (men); >1.4 mg/dL (women) Congestive heart failure drug therapy Hepatic disease Alcohol abuse
Alpha-glucosidase inhibitors acarbose (Precose) miglitol (Glyset)	Delays carbohydrate absorption to decrease postprandial hyperglycemia	Dose-related diarrhea, abdominal pain, flatulence	PPG at initiation HbA1c at 3 months	Administer with first bite of each meal Use slow titration to avoid GI adverse effects (e.g., 25 mg 1 time/day for 2 weeks; then 25 mg 2 times/day for 2 weeks; then 25 mg 3 times/day for 8 weeks; maximum dosage is 100 mg 3 times/day). Must use glucose if hypoglycemia occurs
Thiazolidinediones pioglitazone (Actos) rosiglitazone (Avandia)	Enhances insulin sensitivity	Edema Weight gain Congestive heart failure	aspartate aminotransferase (AST) and alanine aminotransferase (ALT) at baseline Monitor for signs of fluid overload	Decrease in glucose may not be apparent for 4 weeks Maximum efficacy of dose may not be observed for 4–6 months Contraindications: ALT >2.5 times the upper limit of normal Hepatic disease Alcohol abuse NYHA class III or IV
Meglitinides repaglinide (Prandin) nateglinide (Starlix)	Stimulates insulin secretion	Hypoglycemia	Fasting plasma glucose at 2 weeks HbA1c at 3 months PPG at initiation	Commonly used for basal-bolus dosing schedules
DPP-4 inhibitors sitagliptin (Januvia)	Restores GLP-1 and gastric-inhibitory polypeptide levels	Not clinically significant	PPG at initiation Fasting plasma glucose at 2 weeks HbA1c at 3 months	Reduce dosage in patients with renal insufficiency No weight gain or markedly reduced incidence of hypoglycemia

Source: Handelsman et al. (2011).

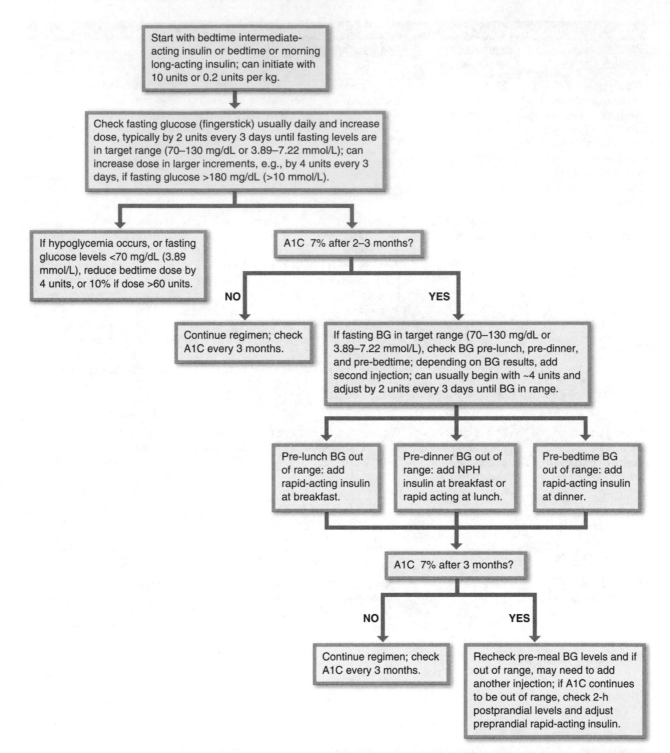

FIGURE 13-1 American Diabetes Association algorithm for the initiation and adjustment of insulin regimens for patients with type 2 diabetes. *Source: Nathan, D. M., Buse, J. B., Davidson, M. B., et al. (2006). Management of hyperglycemia in type 2 diabetes: A consensus statement from the American Diabetes Association and the European Association for the Study of Diabetes. Diabetes Care, 29(8), 1963-1972. Available at http://care.diabetesjournals.org/content/29/8/1963.full*

the next step is to start or intensify insulin therapy. When HbA1c is close to the goal (less than 8%), addition of a third oral agent could be considered. However, this approach is not as effective in controlling and lowering glycemia as adding or intensifying insulin.

Sulfonylureas

Sulfonylureas were the first class of drugs used to treat T2DM. They are still an important class of drugs, but because of the risk for **hypoglycemia** and limited action on insulin resistance there is controversy regarding whether or not they should be given first-line status. Sulfonylureas enhance the release of insulin from the beta cells in the pancreas, decrease the breakdown of glycogen stored in the liver (glycogenolysis), decrease the conversion of excess glucose to glucagon for storage in skeletal muscle and the liver (gluconeogenesis), and increase the cellular sensitivity to insulin in body tissue. The net hypoglycemic effect of these agents is to reduce circulating blood glucose in persons with a functioning pancreas.

Conscientious Prescribing of Sulfonylureas

■ The toxicity profile of some of these agents may preclude their use in patients with preexisting conditions.

■ These agents should be taken 30 to 40 minutes before food and never be given to a fasting patient.

■ Therapy should be started with the lowest dose and titrated upward over several weeks.

■ Hypoglycemia occurs more often with the long-acting agents.

■ Patients newly diagnosed with T2DM who have mild to moderate fasting hyperglycemia respond best to sulfonylureas.

■ Chlorpropamide and glyburide are metabolized to active metabolites having significant renal secretion, thus they should be avoided in the elderly and those with impaired renal function.

■ Metformin is the only agent useful in those in whom weight gain is *not* desirable.

■ Thiazolidinediones are associated with increases in heart failure among patients with diabetes who take them and especially patients with a heart failure who are in borderline compensation.

■ Combination therapy using a **secretagogue** (name for a substance that causes another substance to be excreted, two example are: sulfonylureas which trigger insulin release by direct action on pancreatic beta cells, and angiotensin II which releases aldosterone from adrenal glands) and an insulin sensitizer should be considered a first-line approach in patients having HbA1c levels greater than 9. Widely used regimens include a sulfonylurea plus metformin or a TZD plus a sulfonylurea.

Patient/Family Education for Patients Taking Sulfonylureas

■ Sulfonylureas should be taken 30 to 40 minutes before meals, but at the same time each day.

■ Weight gain, hypoglycemia, gastrointestinal (GI) intolerance, dizziness, and flatulence are common side effects.

■ Inform patients these drugs are not a cure and that therapy will be long term.

■ Instruct patient in proper testing of serum glucose and ketones.

■ Caution patient to avoid aspirin and alcohol while on these medications.

Mechanism of Action

Sulfonylureas lower blood glucose by increasing insulin secretion from the pancreatic beta cell. These drugs bind to sulfonylurea receptors on the surface of the pancreatic beta cell. By doing this, these agents close the potassium adenosine triphosphate channels, which facilitates cell membrane depolarization, calcium entry into the cell, and insulin secretion out of the cell. Sulfonylurea medications reduce HbA1c levels by 1% to 2%, and all are equally effective in controlling hyperglycemia at equivalent doses.

Pharmacokinetics

	Generic Drug Name (Trade Name)	Onset of Action	Peak Effect	Duration of Action	Half-Life	Metabolism/Excretion
SULFONYLUREAS FIRST GENERATION	acetohexamide (Dymelor)	1 hr	1.5–6 hr	8–24 hr	6 hr	Metabolized in liver. Metabolite potency is equal to or greater than parent; renally eliminated
	chlorpropamide (Diabinese)	1 hr	2–4 hr	24–72 hr	35+ hr	Metabolized in liver, excreted unchanged in urine
	tolazamide (Olinase) Tolinase	4–6 hr	3–4 hr	12–24 hr	7 hr	Metabolized in liver to weaker compound than parent; renally eliminated
	tolbutamide (Orinase)	1 hr	3–4 hr	6–12 hr	7 hr	Metabolized in liver to inactive metabolite; renally excreted
SECOND GENERATION	glimepiride (Amaryl)	1 hr	2–3 hr	18–28 hr	4–6 hr	Metabolized in liver to inactive metabolites; renally eliminated
	glipizide (Glucotrol)	1–1.5 hr	1–3 hr	10–24 hr	3 hr	Metabolized in liver to inactive metabolites; renally excreted
	glyburide (DiaBeta, Micronase)	2–4 hr	4 hr	24 hr		Metabolized in liver; 50% excreted in feces, 50% excreted in urine

Clinical Uses

■ Sulfonylureas are approved for use as monotherapy and in combination with other drug classes including insulin. However, they should not be used in combination with meglitinides.

Dosage and Administration

	Generic Drug Name (Trade Name)	Initial Dosage	Maximum Dosage	Comment
				Sulfonylureas are mostly administered at or near meal-time to minimize gastric irritation. They also are not given after the last meal of the day.
FIRST GENERATION	acetohexamide (Dymelor)	250–1,000 mg/day	1,000 mg/day	Use with caution in elderly and those with renal insufficiency.
	chlorpropamide (Diabinese)	250–500 mg/day	500 mg/day	The longest acting; produces more side effects.
	tolazamide, (Tolinase)	100–500 mg at breakfast	500 mg/day	Active metabolites may increase if renal impairment
	tolbutamide (Orinase)	250–2,000 mg/day in divided doses	2,000 mg/day	Short acting; rapidly metabolized to inactive forms
SECOND GENERATION	glyburide (DiaBeta, Micronase)	1.25 to 5 mg 1 time/day	20 mg in 1 or 2 divided doses 1 or 2 times/day	Administer 1 time/day with breakfast or first main meal Doses >10 mg/day should be divided and given 2 times/day
	glipizide (Glucotrol)	5 mg 1 time/day; 2.5 mg 1 time/day in elderly patients	40 mg in 2 divided doses	Administer 1 time/day 30 min before breakfast or after first main meal of day(to minimize gastric irritation Doses >15 mg/day should be divided and given 1 time/day
	glimepiride (Amaryl)	1 to 2 mg 1 time/day	8 mg 1 time/day	Administer 30 min before breakfast or first main meal

Adverse Reactions

CV: Edema, syncope
DERM: Rash, urticaria, pruritus, photosensitivity
EENT: Blurry vision
ENDO: Hypoglycemia, hyponatremia
GI: Anorexia, nausea, vomiting, diarrhea, flatulence, heartburn, constipation

HEM: Aplastic anemia, hemolytic anemia, bone marrow depression, thrombocytopenia, agranulocytosis
MISC: Disulfiram-like reaction (due to the sulfa moiety), especially if patient ingests alcohol
MS: Arthralgia, leg cramps, myalgia, tremor
NEURO: Anxiety, depression, dizziness, headache, insomnia
RENAL: Minor diuretic effect

Interactions

■ May see an increased effect with cytochrome P450 inhibitors such as the azoles, NSAIDs, sulfonamides, antidepressants, monoamine oxidase inhibitors (MAOIs), and digitalis
■ May see a decreased effect with cytochrome P450 inducers such as phenobarbital, beta blockers, and hydantoins

Contraindications

■ There is a cross-sensitivity with sulfonamides, including thiazide diuretics.
■ Severe renal, hepatic, thyroid, or other endocrine disorder.
■ Uncontrolled infection, burns, and trauma.

Biguanides: Metformin (Glucophage)

Biquanide refers to a class of drugs based upon the molecule guanidine extracted from a plant source during the 1920s. Because of the discovery of insulin about the same time the quanidine lanquised until about 1950 when it was introduced as phenformin for the use of type 2 diabetes. However phenformin had a high incidence of fatal lactic acidoses and was withdrawn from the market to be replaced with metformin, an agent with a better safety profile and which is now used around the world. Metformin, which was first released in the United States in December 1994, is still the only **biguanide** available. It is considered first-line therapy and has been shown to lower HbA1c levels by 1% to 2%. Its major effect is to decrease hepatic production of glucose as well as decrease intestinal absorption of glucose, however this mechanism of action is still not well understood. Unlike sulfonylureas, metformin does not stimulate insulin release from the pancreatic beta cells; therefore, there is minimal risk for hypoglycemia. Most patients tolerate this medication well, although there are some common gastrointestinal adverse effects, and monotherapy with metformin is associated with weight loss. Lactic acidosis (state of decreasing low pH in body tissues and blood accompanied by the buildup of lactate as the end point of glucose breakdown) rarely occurs, but patients should be cautioned about it. Signs of lactic acidosis include chills, diarrhea, dizziness, low blood pressure, muscle pain, sleepiness, slow pulse, dyspnea, and weakness.

Conscientious Prescribing of Biguanides

■ Metformin decreases low-density lipoprotein cholesterol levels, triglyceride levels, and the antifibrinolytic factor plasminogen activator inhibitor-1 levels.
■ The combination of glyburide and metformin is more effective than glyburide or metformin alone.

- Adding repaglinide to metformin therapy produces additional lowering of fasting blood glucose levels and HbA1c levels.
- Monitor renal function and for **ketoacidosis** and metabolic acidosis.
- Discontinue the drug in times of hypoxic states (e.g., heart failure, shock, acute myocardial infarction [MI]), loss of blood glucose control due to stress (give insulin), acidosis, dehydration, sepsis.
- Temporarily discontinue prior to surgery (due to restricted food intake) and procedures requiring intravascular iodinated contrast materials.
- May decrease serum vitamin B_{12} levels.
- Increased risk of hypoglycemia in elderly, debilitated/malnourished, adrenal or pituitary insufficiency, or alcohol intoxication.
- Assess patient health using fasting plasma glucose (FPG) test, hemoglobin A1c (HbA1c), renal function tests (plasma creatinine, blood urea nitrogen [BUN], electrolytes, and urinalysis), liver function test (LFT), and complete blood count (CBC).
- Assess for heart failure (HF), septicemia, acute or chronic metabolic acidosis, adrenal or pituitary insufficiency, alcoholism, pregnancy status.
- Evaluate for other medical/surgical conditions and for possible drug interactions.

Patient/Family Education for Patients Taking Biguanides

- Inform patients that the drug is an adjunct to diet and exercise, which must be followed carefully to prevent hypoglycemic and hyperglycemic episodes, because these drugs do not cure their condition.
- Advise that excessive alcohol intake increases hypoglycemia risk.
- Report unexplained hyperventilation, myalgia, malaise, nausea, vomiting, and somnolence.
- Instruct patient in proper testing of blood glucose and urine ketones.
- Regular follow-up is needed and patient should know this is required.
- Advise patient to take this medication exactly as prescribed, especially if a dose is missed. Missed dose should be taken within an hour of the scheduled time; if this cannot be done, then the patient should wait and take the next scheduled dose. Patients should not double dose.

Mechanism of Action

The precise mechanism of action is not fully understood. Its primary effect is to reduce hepatic glucose production in the presence of insulin.

Pharmacokinetics

- Absorption: Absolute bioavailability (50%–60%) with onset of action within days and peak effects in up to 2 weeks.
- Distribution: Protein binding is negligible because metformin partitions into erythrocytes.

- Metabolism: Not metabolized.
- Excretion: 90% or more is excreted unchanged in the urine.
- Half-life: Plasma: 6.2 hours; blood: 17.6 hours.

Clinical Use

- Metformin is approved for use as **monotherapy** or in combination with other hypoglycemic agents.

Dosage and Administration

Generic Drug Name, (Trade Name)	Initial Dosage	Maximum Dosage	Comments
metformin (Glucophage)	500 mg 2 times/day or 850 mg 1 time/day in the morning	2,550 mg in 3 divided doses	Administer with meals Maximum effective dose is 2,000 mg/day
metformin extended release (Glucophage XR)	500 mg 1 time/day in the evening	2,000 mg 1 time/day	Increase dosage by 500 mg/day weekly If glycemic control not tightened, switch to 2 times/day regimen May have better gastrointestinal tolerance than immediate-release metformin
glyburide + metformin (Glucovance)	1.25 mg/250 mg 1 or 2 times/day	20 mg/2,000 mg divided/day	Starting doses should not exceed daily doses of glyburide or metformin already taken; dose increases can be made at 2-wk intervals
sitagliptin + metformin (Janumet)	50 mg sitagliptin/ 500 mg metformin 2 times/day with meals	50 mg sitagliptin/ 1,000 mg metformin 2 times/day	Increase doses slowly to reduce any gastric side effects associated with the metformin

Adverse Reactions

GI: GI distress such as abdominal pain, nausea, diarrhea, bloating, unpleasant metallic taste.

META: Hypoglycemia; lactic acidosis has been reported (rare), but is of increased risk with renal dysfunction, increased age, DM, HF, and other conditions having risks for hypoperfusion and hypoxemia.

MISC: Decreased vitamin B_{12} levels.

Interactions

- Furosemide, nifedipine, cimetidine, cationic drugs (e.g., digoxin, amiloride, procainamide, quinidine, quinine, ranitidine, trimethoprim, vancomycin, triamterene, morphine) may increase metformin levels.
- Thiazides, other diuretics, corticosteroids, phenothiazines, thyroid products, estrogens, oral contraceptives, phenytoin, nicotinic acid, sympathomimetics, calcium channel blockers,

and isoniazid may increase the risk of hyperglycemia when administered concurrently with metformin because these drugs can also cause hyperglycemia on their own.

■ Risk of hypoglycemia with alcohol. Excess alcohol may increase potential for lactic acidosis.

Contraindications

■ Do not use in patients who are at increased risk for lactic acidosis because of renal impairment.

■ Do not use in patients with hepatic dysfunction, heart failure, metabolic acidosis, dehydration, or alcoholism.

Meglitinides

Repaglinide (Prandin) and nateglinide (Starlix) were first released in April 1988. These drugs close ATP-dependent potassium channels in the beta cell membrane by binding at specific receptor sites. Like sulfonylureas, the meglitinides stimulate insulin secretion, although they bind to a different site within the sulfonylurea's receptor. Because they have a shorter half-life than do sulfonylureas, meglitinides must be administered more frequently. Of the two meglitinides currently available in the United States, repaglinide is almost as effective as metformin in decreasing HbA1c. These drugs have a similar risk for weight gain as the sulfonylureas; however, the incidence of hypoglycemia may be less frequent than with some of the sulfonylureas. These drugs do not directly affect fasting blood glucose levels or any of the other defects in metabolism seen in T2DM. They are most useful in patients with postprandial hyperglycemia.

Conscientious Prescribing of Meglitinides

■ In patients previously treated with diet and exercise, repaglinide and nateglinide can be used as a single agent and produce the same postprandial glycemic effects, but repaglinide monotherapy has better long-term effects of reducing fasting blood glucose and HbA1c.

■ Patients who are stabilized on a diabetic regimen but who may experience stress, trauma, infection, or surgery, may require administration of insulin; thus, withhold these agents until resolution of these acute episodes.

■ There is no fixed dose requirement for these agents because the dose is based on long-term monitoring of glycosylated hemoglobin levels.

Patient/Family Education for Patients Taking Meglitinides

■ Repaglinide (Prandin) is taken with meals two to four times a day and should be taken 30 minutes before meals; if no meal is planned, the dose should be skipped. Nateglinide (Starlix) should be taken 10 minutes before meals.

■ Patients on repaglinide should watch for weight gain and hypoglycemia.

■ Nateglinide is usually well tolerated, and risk of hypoglycemia seems minimal.

Mechanism of Action

Repaglinide and nateglinide produce more insulin release after a meal and more postprandial blood glucose lowering than do the sulfonylureas. Repaglinide and nateglinide are meglitinide analogues having similar mechanisms of action as sulfonylureas, but these secretagogues bind to a different site, albeit adjacent to the sulfonylurea site, to stimulate pancreatic insulin secretion. Unlike the sulfonylureas, the meglitinides have a very short-acting onset of action and a short half-life. Their short-lived release of insulin from pancreatic beta cells has an effect that lasts for 1 to 2 hours. Their overall effect is to lower HbA1c 0.6% to 1%.

Pharmacokinetics

■ Absorption: A single dose is rapidly absorbed.
■ Distribution: About 98% protein bound, so effect is seen in less than 1 hour.
■ Metabolism: Metabolized by the liver's CYP-450 system to inactive metabolites.
■ Excretion: Repaglinide in bile; nateglinide in urine.
■ Half-life: Repaglinide: 1 to 2 hours; nateglinide: 1.5 hours.

Clinical Use

■ Postprandial hyperglycemia
■ T2DM

Dosage and Administration

Generic Drug Name (Trade Name)	Initial Dosage	Maximum Dosage	Comments
repaglinide (Prandin)	Elderly patients and patients not previously treated with hypoglycemic agents or patients with hemoglobin A1c <8%: Give 0.5 mg 3 times/day Patients previously treated with hypoglycemic agents or those with hemoglobin A1c >8%: Give 1–2 mg 3 times/day	16 mg/day	Administer 15–30 min before each meal.
nateglinide (Starlix)	120 mg 3 times/day; 60 mg 3 times/day in elderly patients	120 mg 3 times/day	Administer 15–30 min before each meal

Source: Handelsman, et al. (2011).

Adverse Reactions

CV: Ischemia, chest pain
EENT: Sinusitis
ENDO: Hypoglycemia
GI: Constipation, diarrhea, tooth pain
GU: Genitourinary infections
MS: Muscle pain, back pain
NEURO: Headache
PUL: Upper respiratory infections

Drug Interactions

■ Increased effects of these drugs may occur in the presence of any drug affected by the CYP-450 system and its substrates.
■ Gemfibrozil, macrolide antibiotics, and many herbals such as St. John's wort, ethanol, and garlic may increase serum concentrations leading to hypoglycemia.

Contraindications

- Use with caution in any patient with mild to severe hepatic impairment.
- Hypersensitivity can also be an issue.

Thiazolidinediones (TZDs)

TZDs are oral antihypoglycemic drugs, which were first released in March 1997. The first drug in this class, troglitazone (Rezulin), was removed from the market in 1999 as a result of the number of patients who developed liver damage while taking it. Two other TZDs were approved by the U.S. Food and Drug Administration (FDA) in 1999, pioglitazone and rosiglitazone, because of their lower risk of causing liver damage. However, rosiglitazone (Avandia) use has declined since the FDA released its notice in 2010 restricting its use to only those type 2 diabetics who cannot control their diabetes using any other medication. This warning was issued due to concerns about rosiglitazone's relationship to elevated risk of cardiovascular events such as myocardial infarction and stroke. These drugs increase the sensitivity of muscle, fat, and liver, as well as endogenous and exogenous insulin. They lower HbA1c levels the same degree as metformin and sulfonylureas. Unlike sulfonylureas, these drugs do not produce hypoglycemia in diabetic or nondiabetic patients except in special situations. They do not cause hyperinsulinemia because they do not stimulate insulin release from the pancreatic beta cells. Similar to metformin, TZDs have a modest effect on lipids because of their action in the liver. The most common adverse effects are weight gain and fluid retention.

Conscientious Prescribing of Thiazolidinediones

- The risk of drug-induced hepatotoxicity when using these agents mandates that liver function be closely monitored for at least 12 months.
- Edema and cytopenia occur with these agents and need to be monitored for as well.
- The TZDs increase insulin sensitivity in muscle, adipose tissue, and liver, thus patients who have a considerable exogenous insulin secretion respond best to these agents.
- These medications increase high-density lipoprotein cholesterol concentrations and decrease triglyceride concentrations.
- Combining hypoglycemic agents from different drug classes produces an additive effect.
- TZDs are known to precipitate heart failure in patients with borderline congestive heart failure.
- Women of premenopausal age having intercourse should use a form of contraception other than oral forms, or higher doses of oral forms could be used, because ovulation may resume when using TZDs. Thus, alternative contraception should be advised to avoid unwanted pregnancies.

Patient/Family Education for Patients Taking Thiazolidinediones

The risk of heart failure increases when there has been a history of coronary artery disease, hypertension, edema, renal failure, or heart valve disease, or the patient is elderly; thus, the patient needs to know the importance of providing the clinician a full medical history before starting these drugs.

Mechanism of Action

Although the mechanism of action is not fully understood, TZDs are known to directly affect target cells and lower blood glucose by improving the cellular response to insulin without increasing the output of insulin from the pancreas. The mechanism of action is dependent on the presence of insulin.

Pharmacokinetics

- Absorption: TZDs are well absorbed (99% bioavailability), but it may take up to 12 weeks to see their peak effect. Absorption is decreased in the presence of food.
- Distribution: 99% protein bound to albumin.
- Metabolism: Cytochrome P450 metabolism in the liver.
- Excretion: Inactive metabolites about two-thirds in urine, one-third in feces.
- Half-life: Pioglitazone: parent drug, 3 to 7 hours, metabolites 16 to 24 hours; rosiglitazone: 3 to 4 hours.

Clinical Use

- TZDs are indicated as monotherapy and in combination with metformin, sulfonylureas, and insulin.

Dosage and Administration

Generic Drug Name (Trade Name)	Initial Dosage	Maximum Dosage	Comments
pioglitazone (Actos)	15 or 30 mg 1 time/day	45 mg 1 time/day	Administer with or without food
pioglitazone + metformin (ActoPlus Met)	If inadequately controlled on metformin monotherapy: Either 15 mg/500 mg or 15 mg/850 mg 1 or 2 times/day. If initially responsive to pioglitazone monotherapy or switching from combination therapy of pioglitazone + metformin as separate tablets: Either 15 mg/500 mg 2 times/day or 15 mg/850 mg 1 or time/day	If taking the 15mg/500mg combination the dose is one tablet twice a day; if taking the 15mg/850 mg combination the dose is once tablet once a day. Indicated for patients: (a) with type 2 diabetes mellitus treated with combination pioglitazone + metformin, (b) with glycemia not adequately controlled with metformin alone, (c) initially responsive to pioglitazone alone but require additional glycemic control. Dosage schedule based on current dose of each component Consider administering in divided daily doses with meals to reduce the gastrointestinal adverse effects associated with metformin
rosiglitazone (Avandia)	4 mg 1 time/day or 2 mg 2 times/day	8 mg 1 time/day or 4 mg 2 times/day	Administer with or without food
rosiglitazone + metformin (Avandamet)	2 mg/500 mg 2 times/day	4 mg/1000 mg 2 times/day	Dosage schedule based on current dose of each component Administer with meals
rosiglitazone + glimepiride (Avandaryl)	4 mg/1 mg or 4 mg/2 mg 1 time/day	8 mg rosiglitazone and 4 mg glimepiride	Administer with first meal of the day

Source: Handelsman, et al. (2011).

Adverse Reactions

CV: Edema and risk of cardiovascular events (myocardial infarction, stroke)
ENDO: Hypoglycemia, weight gain, increased total cholesterol, low-density lipoprotein (LDL), and high-density lipoprotein (HDL)
GI: Diarrhea
HEM: Anemia
MS: Back pain
NEURO: Headache, fatigue
PUL: Upper respiratory infections

Interactions

■ Potential drug interactions occur with phenobarbital, amiodarone, rifampin, and fluconazole.
■ Because pioglitazone alters the levels of medications metabolized by the cytochrome P450 isomer CYP 3A4, drug interactions with carbamazepine, cyclosporine, felodipine, and some oral contraceptives are possible.

Contraindications

■ These drugs should not be used in patients with congestive heart failure or hepatic impairment.

Alpha-Glucosidase Inhibitors

Medications in the alpha-glucosidase inhibitor class were first released in January 1996. Alpha-glucosidase inhibitors (Acarbose, Miglitol) reduce the rate of digestion of polysaccharides in the proximal small intestine by lowering postprandial glucose levels without causing hypoglycemia. These agents reduce HbA1c levels by approximately 1% compared with HbA1c levels of placebo-treated patients. They are less effective in lowering glycemia than metformin or the sulfonylureas. Because carbohydrates are absorbed more distantly, malabsorption and weight loss do not occur as often with these drugs. These drugs do cause increased gas production and gastrointestinal symptoms; Because of these side effects, as many as 25% to 45% of participants in clinical trials have stopped the medication. These drugs have a limited role as adjunct therapy.

Conscientious Prescribing of Alpha-Glucosidase Inhibitors

■ Each drug should be initiated at low doses (25 mg two to three times per day with food), and doses should be increased slowly over several weeks in increments of 2.5 mg to minimize GI upset.
■ Monotherapy with these agents seldom gives satisfactory results.
■ Acarbose has been associated with raised liver enzymes, thus periodic monitoring is necessary.
■ Patients who show signs of mild to moderate hypoglycemia should be treated with glucose, not sucrose (cane sugar).
■ Temporary insulin therapy may be necessary at times of stress, such as fever, trauma, infection, or surgery. Not recommended with renal impairment (SrCr greater than 2 mg/dL).

■ Assess for diabetic ketoacidosis, inflammatory bowel disease, colonic ulceration, partial intestinal obstruction, chronic intestinal disease, renal function, and pregnancy status.
■ Intestinal absorbents (e.g., charcoal) and digestive enzyme preparations (e.g., amylase, pancreatin) may reduce effects.
■ Monitor for hypoglycemia, FPG, HbA$_{1c}$, renal function, diabetic ketoacidosis, GI symptoms, skin rash, and serum iron.

Patient/Family Education for Patients Taking Alpha-Glucosidase Inhibitors

■ Inform the patient that the drug is adjunct to diet and exercise.
■ Counsel the patient about adverse effects that are dose related, such as diarrhea, bloating, abdominal cramping, and flatulence.
■ Advise the patient to take drug as prescribed and schedule regular follow-ups.
■ Medication requirements may change during periods of stress (fever, trauma, infection, or surgery); patients should seek medical advice promptly.

Mechanism of Action

These drugs produce postprandial glucose control by decreasing the absorption of carbohydrates from the GI tract. They work by inhibiting alpha-glucosidase, an enzyme located in the proximal small intestine epithelium that breaks down saccharides and more complex carbohydrates. Thus, these complex oligosaccharides delay intestinal carbohydrate absorption, thereby lowering a rise in blood glucose following a meal and making it possible for people with T2DM to enjoy reduced levels of glycosylated hemoglobin.

Pharmacokinetics

■ Absorption: Less than 2% gets absorbed as the active site is the GI tract.
■ Distribution: Not an issue because it acts in the GI tract.
■ Metabolism: Exclusively by GI bacteria and digestive enzymes into 13 metabolites.
■ Excretion: In the urine.
■ Half-life: Miglitol: 2 hours; acarbose: unknown.

Clinical Use

■ These drugs are approved for use as monotherapy and in combination with sulfonylureas.

Dosage and Administration

Generic Drug Name (Trade Name)	Initial Dosage	Maximum Dosage	Comments
acarbose (Precose)	25 mg 3 times/day	100 mg 3 times/day	Administer with first bite of each main meal Dosage should be gradually increased as tolerated over several weeks
miglitol (Glyset)	25 mg 3 times/day	100 mg 3 times/day	Administer with first bite of each main meal Dosage may be gradually increased as tolerated over several weeks

Source: Handelsman, et al. (2011).

Adverse Reactions

DERM: Rash

GI: Flatulence, diarrhea, abdominal discomfort

Interactions

- Miglitol: May decrease absorption of digoxin, propranolol, and ranitidine.
- Acarbose: May decrease effects of digoxin, thiazide diuretics, thyroids, estrogens, oral contraceptives, and calcium channel blockers.

Contraindications

- Inflammatory bowel disease
- GI obstruction
- Colonic ulceration
- Cirrhosis
- Malabsorption syndrome

Amylin Analogue (Pramlintide [Symlin])

There is only one drug in the amylin analogue class, pramlintide, which is a synthetic analogue of human amylin, a naturally occurring hormone that is cosecreted with insulin by the pancreatic beta cells. Although pramlintide was the first drug approved for adjunctive therapy with insulin, a second drug, exenatide (Byetta), was approved in the fall of 2011. Byetta was first approved as a single agent in 2005, but it is now is approved as an add-on therapy for use with insulin glargine with or without metformin and/or a thiazolidinedione in conjunction with diet and exercise for adults not achieving glycolic control on insulin glargine alone. These agents are administered subcutaneously before meals and slow gastric emptying, thus inhibiting glucagon production in a glucose-dependent fashion, and predominantly decreasing postprandial glucose excursions. After a few months of treatment, they have been found to decrease HbA1c by an additional 0.5% to 0.7% over use of insulin alone. Nausea remains the most common side effect and is an issue with almost 40% of patients.

Conscientious Prescribing of Pramlintide and Exenatide

- This drug is used as an adjunct therapy in patients with diabetes mellitus who use **prandial** insulin and who have not achieved desired glycemic control.
- Before initiating therapy, reduce the insulin dose by 50%. Monitor blood glucose frequently.
- Adjust the insulin dose once target dose of pramlintide is maintained.
- Ensure that the patient does not have a confirmed diagnosis of **gastroparesis (delayed gastric emptying)** or hypoglycemia unawareness.
- Assess if the patient has failed to achieve proper glycemic control despite individualized insulin management.
- Assess use in patients with visual or dexterity impairment.
- Assess patient health using fasting plasma glucose (FPG) test; HbA1c; renal function tests (plasma creatinine, BUN, electrolytes, and urinalysis); LFT; and CBC.
- Assess also for signs of hypoglycemia, especially if using a combination drug regimen.

Patient/Family Education for Patients Taking Pramlintide

- Patients taking this medication should reduce rapid-acting or short-acting insulin dosages by 50%.
- Frequent monitoring of blood glucose levels is needed and the dosage must be titrated.
- Do not mix with insulin; administer as separate injections.
- Do not transfer from pen-injector to syringe.
- If a dose is missed, wait until the next scheduled dose and administer the usual amount. Instruct the patient to administer immediately prior to each major meal (greater than or equal to 250 calories or greater than or equal to 30 g of carbohydrates).
- Instruct the patient that insulin dose adjustments should be made only by the clinician.
- Patients should have fast-acting sugar (e.g., hard candy, glucose tablet, juice) at all times. Self-glucose monitoring should be done on a daily basis.
- Counsel about signs and symptoms of hypoglycemia (e.g., hunger, headache, sweating, tremor, irritability).
- Instruct the patient regarding the critical importance of maintaining proper glucose control, especially when operating heavy machinery (e.g., motor vehicles).

Mechanism of Action

Amylin has a neuroendocrine action that regulates glucose influx including suppression of glucagon, slowing of gastric emptying, and a potential effect on feeding behavior and weight control.

Pharmacokinetics

- Absorption: Absolute bioavailability due to subcutaneous (SC) administration.
- Distribution: Protein bound to plasma.
- Metabolism: Not extensively bound to blood cells or albumin (40% unbound).
- Excretion: Kidneys (primarily). Des-lys pramlintide (primary active metabolite).
- Half-life: 48 minutes

Clinical Uses

- Adjunct treatment in patients with T1DM or T2DM who use mealtime insulin therapy and who have failed to achieve desired glucose control despite optimal insulin therapy.
- May be used with or without sulfonylurea and/or metformin in T2DM.

Dosage and Administration

Generic Name	Trade Name	Route	Usual Adult Daily Dose
pramlintide	Symlin	SC	T2DM: Initial: 60 mcg SC immediately prior to meals. Titrate: 120 mcg as tolerated. T1DM: Initial: 15 mcg SC immediately prior to meals. Titrate: Increase by 15 mcg increments to 30 mcg or 60 mcg as tolerated.

Adverse Reactions

BLACK BOX WARNING: Use with insulin. Risk of insulin-induced severe hypoglycemia, particularly with T1DM. Severe hypoglycemia usually occurs within 3 hours of injection. Serious injuries may occur if severe hypoglycemia occurs while operating a motor vehicle, heavy machinery, or other high-risk activities. Appropriate patient selection, careful patient instruction, and insulin dose adjustments are necessary to reduce this risk.

EENT: Pharyngitis
ENDO: Severe hypoglycemia
GI: Nausea, vomiting, anorexia, abdominal pain
MS: Arthralgia
NEURO: Headache, fatigue, dizziness
PUL: Coughing

Interactions

■ Do not administer with agents that alter gastrointestinal motility (e.g., anticholinergic agents such as atropine), or agents that slow intestinal absorption of nutrients (e.g., alpha-glucosidase inhibitors).
■ Administer analgesics and other oral agents that require rapid onset 1 hour before or 2 hours after injection.

Contraindications

■ This medication is contraindicated in patients with hypoglycemia unawareness or a diagnosis of gastroparesis.

Glucagon-Like Peptide-1 (GLP-1) Agonists

Exenatide (Byetta), is administered subcutaneously twice a day, and appears to lower HbA1c by lowering postprandial blood glucose levels. Byetta mimics the antidiabetic or glucose-lowering actions of incretins, naturally occurring human hormones. It stimulates insulin production and the response to elevated levels of blood glucose, inhibits the release of glucagon after meals, slows the rate at which nutrients are absorbed, and increases satiety. It is not associated with hypoglycemia, but it has a relatively high frequency of gastrointestinal side effects; 30% to 45% of patients treated with the drug experience one or more episodes of nausea, vomiting, or diarrhea. Currently, it is approved for use with sulfonylureas and or metformin.

Conscientious Prescribing of Exenatide

■ Exenatide should not be used as a substitute for insulin.
■ Monitor for symptoms of acute pancreatitis (severe abdominal pain, vomiting), renal function, fasting blood glucose, HbA1c hypoglycemia, and body weight.
■ Assess for T1DM, pancreatitis, renal function test, gastroparesis, and HbA1c.

Patient/Family Education for Patients Taking Exenatide

■ Take exenatide within 60 min of eating the morning and evening meals.
■ Do not administer after a meal.
■ If a dose is missed, resume treatment regimen as prescribed with the next scheduled dose.

■ Report side effects.
■ Protect drug from light.
■ Discard pen 30 days after the first use, even if some drug remains.

Mechanism of Action

Exenatide is an analogue of the hormone incretin, which increases insulin secretion. It exhibits many of the same effects as human incretin hormone (glucagon-like peptide 1), which is secreted in response to food and which regulates postprandial glycemia. Glucagon-like peptide-1 (GLP-1) also protects and induces proliferation of beta-1 cells; thus, it has multiple effects on the stomach, liver, pancreas, and brain, which decrease postprandial hyperglycemia, reduce glucagon secretion, and induce weight loss.

Pharmacokinetics

■ Absorption: Minimal if any.
■ Distribution: Acts in intestine.
■ Metabolism: Because systemic absorption is minimal, degradation may occur following glomerular filtration.
■ Excretion: In the urine.
■ Half-life: 2.4 hours.

Clinical Uses

■ Approved for the treatment of T2DM in patients who have not achieved glycemic goals using metformin, a sulfonylurea, or both.
■ Combination therapy with a sulfonylurea, metformin, sulfonylurea plus metformin, and thiazolidinedione with or without metformin.

Dosage and Administration

Generic Name	Trade Name	Route	Usual Adult Daily Dose
exenatide	Byetta, Victoza	SC	5 mcg SC 2 times/day, 60 min before breakfast and dinner. Titrate: May increase to 10 mcg 2 times/day after 1 mo.

Adverse Reactions

DERM: Generalized pruritus and/or urticaria, macular or papular rash, angioedema, rare reports of anaphylactic reaction
GI: Nausea, vomiting, diarrhea, feeling jittery, dyspepsia, abdominal pain, acute pancreatitis
META: Increased incidence of hypoglycemia with sulfonylureas
MISC: Injection-site reactions; when used with thiazolidinediones, possible injection site nodules (77%) or injection site reaction (17%) and/or chronic hypersensitivity pneumonitis
NEURO: Dizziness, headache, somnolence

Interactions

■ Caution with drugs that require rapid GI absorption.
■ Drugs dependent on threshold concentrations for efficacy (e.g., contraceptives, antibiotics) should be taken 1 hour before taking exenatide.
■ Caution with concomitant use of warfarin; may lead to increased international normalized ratio (INR) and possible bleeding.

Contraindications

- Avoid with T1DM, treatment of diabetic ketoacidosis, severe renal impairment (estimated creatinine clearance [CrCl] less than 30 mL/min), or severe GI disease.

Dipeptidyl-Peptidase-4 Inhibitors (DPP-IV)

Sitagliptin (Januvia) and saxagliptin (Onglyza) inhibit dipeptidyl-peptidase 4 (DPP-IV), an enzyme that rapidly inactivates and prolongs incretin hormone. Under normal circumstances, incretin hormones are released by the intestine during the day and levels are increased in response to food. Because incretin hormones are rapidly inactivated by the DPP-IV enzyme, administering sitagliptin inhibits the DPP-IV enzyme, resulting in prolonged active incretin levels. Increasing the levels of active incretin or prolonging their activity increases insulin productivity in response to meals and decreases the amount of glucose that is produced by the liver.

Conscientious Prescribing of Sitagliptin and Saxagliptin

- Patients who take these agents have significant weight loss, in contrast to the weight gain associated with glipizide treatment.
- Assess renal function prior to initiation of treatment.
- May cause hypoglycemia when used in combination with a sulfonylurea.
- Assess FPG, HbA1a renal function, pregnancy status, T1DM. Evaluate for other medical/surgical conditions and for possible drug interactions.
- Monitor for hypoglycemia, FPG, HbA1a renal function, diabetic ketoacidosis, nasopharyngitis, and hypersensitivity reactions (e.g., anaphylaxis, angioedema, and exfoliative skin conditions, including Stevens-Johnson syndrome).

Patient/Family Education for Patients Taking Sitagliptin

- Inform the patient that the drug is to be taken as an adjunct to diet and exercise.
- Counsel the patient about adverse effects, and advise the patient to seek medical attention if any develop.
- The medication should be taken as prescribed and regular follow-up visits should be scheduled.
- During periods of stress (e.g., fever, trauma, infection, surgery), medication requirements may change; seek medical advice promptly.

Mechanism of Action

This drug exerts its action in part by slowing the inactivation of incretin hormones GLP-1 and glucose-dependent insulinotropic polypeptide by DPP-IV, which increases the concentration of these intestinally produced hormones that are decreased in patients with T2DM.

Pharmacokinetics

- Absorption: Rapidly absorbed providing high bioavailability.
- Distribution: Plasma protein binding.
- Metabolism: Not excessively, but some via CYP3A4 and CYP2C8 (minor).

- Excretion: Feces, urine.
- Half-life: 12.4 hours.

Clinical Uses

- Targets postprandial blood glucose and has been shown to decrease fasting plasma glucose levels.
- Approved for use as monotherapy and in combination with metformin or a thiazolidinedione.

Dosage and Administration

Generic Name	Trade Name	Route	Usual Adult Daily Dose
sitagliptin	Januvia	PO	Adults: 100 mg/day. CrCl ≥30 to <50 mL/min: 50 mg/day. CrCl <30 mL/min: 25 mg/day.
saxagliptin	Onglyza	PO	Adults: 2.5 mg or 5 mg suppresses DPP-4 activity for 24 hr.
saxagliptin + metformin	Kombiglyze	PO	5 mg saxagliptin/100 mg metformin extended release in a once-a-day formulation taken at the evening meal.
sitagliptin + metformin	Janumet	PO	50 mg sitagliptin/500 mg metformin taken 2 times/day.

Adverse Reactions

EENT: Nasopharyngitis
META: (Combination therapy) hypoglycemia
NEURO: Headache
PUL: Upper respiratory tract infection

Interactions

- May slightly increase digoxin levels; monitor appropriately.
- May require lower dose of sulfonylurea to reduce risk of hypoglycemia.

Contraindications

- Anaphylaxis or angioedema.

Glucagon

Glucagon is a polypeptide hormone secreted by the alpha cells in the islets of Langerhans in the pancreas. Although it has several actions, its use in medicine today is to elevate blood glucose levels in diabetic patients who have hypoglycemia or insulin overdose. The drug is administered intramuscularly (IM), intravenously (IV), or subcutaneously (SC), and it is often kept in primary care offices or emergency rooms in its IV or IM form for emergencies.

Conscientious Prescribing of Glucagon

- Use with caution in patients with a history suggestive of insulinoma and/or pheochromocytoma. Glucagon can cause pheochromocytoma tumor to release catecholamines, which may result in a sudden and marked increase in blood pressure (BP).
- Effective in treating hypoglycemia only if sufficient liver glycogen is present.
- Glucagon is not effective in states of starvation, adrenal insufficiency, or chronic hypoglycemia; use glucose to treat instead.

Patient/Family Education for Patients Taking Glucagon

■ In the event of an emergency, instruct the patient how to properly prepare and administer glucagon. Inform patients about measures to prevent hypoglycemia. This includes following a uniform regimen on a regular basis, careful adjustment of insulin program, frequent testing of blood or urine for glucose, and routine carrying of hyperglycemic agents that will quickly elevate blood glucose levels (sugar, candy, or readily absorbed carbohydrates).

■ Inform the patient about symptoms of hypoglycemia and how to treat it appropriately.

■ Advise the patient to inform the clinician when hypoglycemia occurs.

Mechanism of Action

This drug works to accelerate glycogenolysis by stimulating cyclic adenosine monophosphate (cAMP) synthesis and increasing phosphorylase activity, resulting in increased breakdown of liver glycogen and its conversion to glucose. The result is an increase in blood glucose levels. It also acts to relax smooth muscle of the GI tract.

Pharmacokinetics

■ Absorption: Given IV, its effect is seen in 5 to 20 minutes; given IM, its effect is seen in 30 minutes; given SC, its effect is seen in 30 to 45 minutes.

■ Distribution: Found in breast milk, but its distribution remains unknown.

■ Metabolism: Extensively metabolized in the liver and kidneys and degraded in the plasma.

■ Excretion: Urine.

■ Half-life: 3 to 6 minutes.

Clinical Uses

■ Treatment for severe hypoglycemia.

■ Diagnostic aid for radiological examination of the stomach, duodenum, small bowel, and colon.

Dosage and Administration

Generic Name	Trade Name	Route	Usual Adult Daily Dose
glucagon	generic	SC/IM/IV	Adults: Severe hypoglycemia: 1 mg (1 unit) SC/IM/IV. May give another dose after 15 min if patient does not respond, but IV glucose would be a better alternative. Diagnostic aid: Duodenum/small bowel: 0.25–0.5 mg (0.25–0.5 units) IV, or 1 mg (1 unit) IM, or 2 mg (2 units) IV/IM before procedure. Stomach: 0.5 mg (0.5 unit) IV or 2 mg (2 units) IM before procedure. Colon: 2 mg (2 units) IM 10 min before procedure.

Adverse Reactions

CV: Hypotension
DERM: Urticaria
GI: Nausea, vomiting
PUL: Respiratory distress

Interactions

■ The effects of oral anticoagulants may be increased, and bleeding is possible after several days. This is dose dependent, but it is not associated with a single dose used to resolve hypoglycemia.

Contraindications

■ Pheochromocytoma

INJECTABLE INSULINS

Insulin is the oldest of the currently available medications for treating T1DM and has had the most clinical use. Although insulin was initially developed to treat patients with insulin-deficient type 1 diabetes, it is also used to treat the insulin-resistant form of diabetes. Of the diabetes medications, it is the most effective at lowering glycemia. When used in adequate doses, insulin decreases any level of elevated HbA1c to either the therapeutic goal or close to it. Unlike other blood glucose–lowering medications, there is no maximum dose of insulin. Naturally occurring insulin promotes the storage of fat as well as glucose and influences cell growth and metabolic functions in a wide variety of tissues. These receptors open to allow glucose to enter the cells. The number of insulin receptors, however, can be downregulated by factors such as obesity and long-standing hyperglycemia. This may explain why weight loss can be a significant factor in diabetes management. Insulin lowers blood glucose levels by stimulating peripheral glucose uptake by skeletal muscle and fat and by inhibiting hepatic glucose production.

Insulin acts on the liver to increase storage of the glucose as glycogen and resets the liver after food intake by reversing the amount of catabolic activity. Furthermore, insulin decreases urea production and protein metabolism and promotes triglyceride synthesis. It also increases potassium and phosphate uptake by the liver. Increasing amino acid transport and stimulating insulin promotes protein synthesis. Finally, insulin reduces the circulation of free fatty acids and promotes the storage of triglycerides in adipose tissue. Thus, administration of the drug insulin produces the same effect as the naturally occurring hormone.

Insulin preparations are derived from animals (extracted from beef or pork pancreas) or are synthesized using recombinant DNA technology using strains of *Escherichia coli*. Beef insulin differs from human insulin by three amino acids, and pork insulin differs from human insulin by only one amino acid. Recombinant insulin is identical to human insulin. Most patients do well using the beef-pork combination insulins, if they have no allergies or are not able to take the pork insulin for religious reasons. The pork insulin, because it is closer in chemistry to human insulin, often results in lower doses being used and in improvement of local allergies and prurituss at the injection sites. A fast-acting insulin analogue (insulin lispro or Humalog) uses regular human insulin but reverses the sequence of two amino acids, giving it a rapid onset of action. Thus, it can be used 15 minutes before a meal and be effective. People using it, however, also take a long-acting insulin product. Insulins by convention are divided into categories based on onset, duration, and intensity of action following subcutaneous injection.

Conscientious Prescribing of Insulin for Patients with T2DM

- Many patients are reluctant to begin insulin therapy, and thus much patient education has to be given.
- Common initial insulin regimens include the following:
  - Long-acting insulin analogue
  - Long-acting insulin analogue with rapid-acting insulin analogue or inhaled insulin at largest meal of the day
  - Once-daily premixed insulin analogue (intermediate-acting/rapid-acting insulin analogue) at largest meal of the day
  - Long-acting insulin analogue with rapid-acting insulin analogue or inhaled insulin twice daily at breakfast and supper
- Initial dose of 10 units per injection is a safe starting dose for once-daily and twice-daily subcutaneously administered insulin regimens.
- Because more than 90% of patients with T2DM are insulin resistant, much higher doses are often required to achieve glycemic targets.
- When initiating insulin therapy, patients should be advised to measure their blood glucose levels at least twice daily and provide self-monitoring of blood glucose to the clinician on a weekly basis.
- Stepwise adjustments to insulin regimens are made in response to glucose levels.
- For those patients on intermediate-acting insulin, adjustments can be made in prebreakfast dosages based on presupper glucose levels. Adjustments in presupper dosage adjustments are made based on prebreakfast glucose levels.
- Two-hour postprandial glucose should be measured and addressed if the HbA1c level is elevated but premeal glucose levels are at target.
- Consider changing the regimen if glycemic goals are not met after 2 to 3 months of therapy or if the patient experiences recurrent hypoglycemia.
- Patients who require a more intensive insulin regimen should transition from a long-acting insulin analogue to a premixed insulin analogue twice daily. The patient can also transition from a once-a-day premix of insulin analogue to a premixed insulin analogue twice daily. Furthermore, transitions can be made from a long-acting insulin analogue to a rapid-acting insulin analogue at the largest meal.
- Insulin is the therapy of choice in patients with advanced chronic kidney disease.

Glucagon

Conscientious Prescribing of Insulin for Patients with T1DM

- Instruct patients to administer preprandial rapid-acting analogue insulin 20 to 30 minutes before the meal when the premeal blood glucose level is high and after the meal has begun when the premeal blood glucose level is below the reference range.
- Patients should measure 2 a.m. to 3 a.m. blood glucose periodically to check for nocturnal hypoglycemia, especially when the morning blood glucose level is elevated.
- Consider using regular insulin instead of rapid-acting insulin analogues to obtain better control of postprandial and premeal glucose levels in patients with gastroparesis. Insulin pumps may also be advantageous in these patients.
- Some patients with T1DM may require daily injections of basal insulin to achieve greater stability.
- Assess postprandial glucose levels when the HbA1c level is elevated and the premeal glucose measurements are at target levels.
- Patients should test postprandial glucose levels periodically to detect unrecognized exaggerated postprandial glucose excursions, even when the HbA1c level is at or near target.
- Patients with T1DM should have continuous glucose monitoring if they have unstable glucose control or if they are unable to achieve an acceptable HbA1c.
- Some patients who use pramlintide may achieve better postprandial and premeal glucose control by combining it with regular insulin rather than with rapid-acting analogues.

Patient/Family Education for Patients Using Insulin

- Each insulin has its own unique characteristics; therefore, patients need to be aware that they are *not* to switch brands, syringes, or needles without the supervision of their clinician.
- Hypoglycemia can result from excessive insulin dosing, excessive work or exercise, not eating at mealtime, or from food that is not absorbed because of diarrhea or vomiting. It may also be induced by concomitant use of another drug such as alcohol that increases the hypoglycemic effect of insulin. Thus, every clinician and patient should know the signs and symptoms of hypoglycemia, which are decreased level of consciousness, hunger, diaphoresis, weakness, dizziness, and tachycardia.

Mechanism of Action

As expected, the stabilized form of exogenous insulin acts in the same way as the endogenous insulin released from pancreatic basal cells, which are at a constant low basal rate with intermittent responses that correlate to increased stimuli, such as stress, vagal activity, and high blood glucose. Once insulin has arrived at a sensitive cell, it is bound to cell receptors found on the cell membrane. These receptors foster changes within the cell membrane that move glucose transporters from sequestered sites to the cell surface. Once on the cell surface, the transporter eases the intake of glucose into the cell where it influences cell metabolism, cell growth in a wide variety of tissues, and the storage of fat. Thus, insulin has four effects:

1. It acts on glucose cell membrane transporters that regulate insulin release and glucose homeostasis. The total number of insulin receptors can be downregulated by obesity, which explains why it is so hard to induce weight loss as part of a diabetes management regimen.
2. It acts on the liver where glucose increases storage of glucose as glycogen and resets the liver's catabolic activity after ingesting food.
3. It acts on adipose tissue where insulin reduces circulating free fatty acids (FFAs) and promotes storage of triglycerides in adipose tissues.
4. It acts on muscle cell growth where insulin promotes protein synthesis by increasing amino acid activity and

glycogen synthesis to replace glycogen that has been depleted during work or exercise.

Pharmacokinetics

■ Absorption: If given orally, insulin would be destroyed by enzymes in the stomach, so it is given IM or IV where absorption is determined by the injection rate and injection site. Human insulin has a more rapid onset and shorter duration of action than does pork or beef insulin. Injection sites in the abdomen have as much as 50% more absorption than does the arm, followed by the thighs, then the buttocks.
■ Distribution: To receptor sites sensitive to insulin.
■ Metabolism: Metabolized by the liver, kidney, and muscle cells.
■ Excretion: Nearly all of it is metabolized, but a small amount goes unchanged and is excreted in the urine.

Drug	Onset	Peak	Duration	Source* and Use In Glucose Management
RAPID-ACTING INSULIN				Rapid-acting insulin covers insulin needs when meals are eaten at the same time as the injection. This type of insulin is used with longer-acting insulin.
insulin aspartate (NovoLog)	10–20 min	40–50 min	3–5 hr	
insulin glulisine (Apidra)	20–30 min	30–90 min	<5 hr	
lispro (Humalog)	15–30 min	30–90 min	<5 hr	
SHORT-ACTING INSULIN				Short-acting insulin covers insulin needs when meals are eaten within 30–60 min.
regular (Humulin-R)	30–60 min	2–5 hr	5–8 hr	
Velosulin	30–60 min	2–3 hr	2–3hr	For use in insulin pumps
INTERMEDIATE-ACTING INSULIN				Covers insulin needs for about half the day or overnight. This type of insulin is often combined with rapid- or short-acting insulin.
NPH (Neutral Protamine Hagedorn) (Humulin-N)**	1–1.5 hr	4–12 hr	<24 hr	
Lente	1–2 hr	7–15 hr	<24 hr	
LONG-ACTING INSULIN				Long-acting insulin covers insulin needs for about 1 full day. This type of insulin is often combined, when needed, with rapid- or short-acting insulin.
insulin glargine (Lantus)	1.1 hr	<5hr	<20–24 hr	
protamine zinc insulin (PZI)	4–8 hr	14–24 hr	<36 hr	
insulin detemir (Levemir)	1–2 hr	6–8 hr	24 hr	Modified human recombinant DNA
ultralente	4–8 hr	18–24 hr	<36 hr	
PREMIXED INSULINS				These products are usually taken 2 times/day before mealtime and are a combination of specific proportions of intermediate-acting and short-acting insulin in either 1 bottle or a 1-dose insulin pen. The numbers following the brand name indicate the percentage of each type of insulin.
75% lispro prota-mine suspension/ 25% lispro injection (Humalog 75/25)	15 min	30 min– 2.5 hr	16–20 hr	
50% insulin lispro protamine suspension/50% lispro injection (Humulin Mix 50/50)	30 min	2–5 hr	18–24 hr	
70% insulin aspart protamine suspension/30% insulin aspart (NovoLog 70/30)	20–30 min	1–4 hr	<24hr	
70% NPH/30% regular Novolin)	30 min	2–4 hr	14–24 hr	

*Since January 2006, the FDA has required all insulin varieties to be manufactured by recombinant DNA processes to help reduce impurities present when insulin were made with bovine, pork, horse, or fish pancreases. These sources were effective in humans because of the similar structures of human-sourced insulin and that of other species. Today, insulin is usually made by injecting human DNA into an E. coli culture/broth and adding nutrients to increase yield.

** NPH stands for Neutral Protamine Haggedorn, an insulin named after the man who acquired the rights to make insulin in Sweden in 1926. Haggedorn formed the company Novo Nordisk and in 1936 formulated a suspension of crystalline zinc insulin with a positively charged polypeptide (protamine). The result was an injectable insulin that had longer duration of action than regular insulin. Today NPH insulin is all made by recombinate human DNA synthesis and marketed at Humulin and Novolin.

Dosage and Administration

The success of insulin therapy depends on sufficient doses of insulin. A general rule is 0.6 to greater than 1 units of insulin per kilogram of body weight per day to achieve normal glycemia rather than any specific pattern of administration. Optimal glycemic control usually occurs when the patient is getting more than 100 units of insulin per day, but weight gain in populations using this dosage can be considerable without a diet and exercise program. The number and types of insulins available in the United States are constantly changing, and clinicians should consult the most current drug references for a current list of products. Insulins are grouped into four categories: regular, protamine, lente, and modified (insulin lispro or insulin aspart). Lente insulins are modified by a fish protein and protamine insulins by a zinc moiety, which causes in both a prolongation of their insulin action. Insulin detemir (Levemir), another long-acting insulin, is a human insulin analogue produced by binding a fatty acid (myristic acid) to one of the amino acids when manufacturing basal insulin using recombinant DNA technology.

Adverse Reactions

META: Hypoglycemia: The peak time for an attack of hypoglycemia is the peak time of effect of the insulin. Mild attacks of hypoglycemia can be treated with an oral dose of glucose; adjustments in dosage, meal patterns, or exercise are also needed. Severe attacks that lead to coma or unconsciousness need IM or IV injections of glucagon or concentrated IV glucose.

Diabetic ketoacidosis (DKA) is usually the result of undue stress, illness, or infections, but in many cases it is because of missed doses of insulin. Symptoms include drowsiness, dim vision, and labored breathing, preceded by a lengthy episode of polyuria, polydipsia, polyphagia, weight loss, vomiting, dehydration, and a distinct ketone odor to the breath (like musty apples). Treatment requires hospitalization and a correction of acid-base and fluid imbalances, as well as blood glucose. Low-dose regular insulin given SC or IV is usually part of the therapy.

Interactions

■ Many drugs either decrease or increase the effects of insulin because they influence blood glucose (Table 13-4). Beta

TABLE 13-4 Partial List of Common Drugs That Interact with Insulin

DRUGS THAT DECREASE THE HYPOGLYCEMIC EFFECTS OF INSULIN	DRUGS THAT INCREASE THE HYPOGLYCEMIC EFFECTS OF INSULIN
• acetazolamide	• alcohol
• antiretrovirals	• anabolics
• corticosteroids	• beta blockers
• estrogens	• lithium
• morphine	• MAOIs
• niacin	• sulfonamides
• phenothiazines	• sulfonylureas
• nicotine (smoking)	• salicylates
• thiazides	• tetracyclines
• thyroids	

blockers are the most problematic, because they increase insulin resistance and can mask signs of hypoglycemia. Patients taking beta blockers need to check their blood sugar more often and especially when they feel any sign of diaphoresis.

Implications for Special Populations

Pregnancy Implications

Gestational diabetes, which occurs in 4% of pregnancies, usually resolves after delivery. However, most women who have gestational diabetes develop type 2 diabetes later in life. Insulins are used to control gestational diabetes. The FDA Safety Categories for Diabetic Drugs follow.

FDA Category	Drugs
B	All sulfonylureas acetohexamide (Dymelor, generic) chlorpropamide (Diabinese, generic) tolazamide (Tolinase) tolbutamide (Orinase) glipizide (Glucotrol) glyburide (DiaBeta, Glynase, Micronase) glimepiride (Amaryl) sitagliptin (Januvia) Acarbose, Miglitol glucagon insulin (Regular, Lispro)
C	metformin, pramlintide, exenatide, repaglinide nateglinide (Starlix), ploglitazone (Actos), rosiglitazone (Avandia) The insulins (aspart, detemir, glargine, glulisine, inhalation, NPH)
D	
X	
Unclassified	

Pediatric Implications

The pediatric population is experiencing a rising incidence of type 2 diabetes due to poor lifestyle habits. Although sulfonylureas are not currently approved for use in children, pediatric endocrinologists do use sulfonylureas with metformin when monotherapy with metformin has been unsuccessful. All practitioners should refer children and adolescents to a pediatric endocrinologist when multiple drugs are needed. Chlorpropamide has been successful in pediatrics when there is no renal dysfunction, no other drugs are being used, and there is no evidence of alcohol use. Metformin has been used in children ages 10 to 16 years when strategies to control weight and increase exercise have failed.

Geriatric Implications

Chlorpropamide and glyburide should be avoided in older adults because they are associated with causing higher incidences of hypoglycemia and more severe hypoglycemia. The older adult does well on a short-acting agent such as glipizide.

Less stringent glycemic controls are usually set in older adults due to the considerable risk of older adults developing hypoglycemia and the probable risk of long-term microvascular complications. Shorter-acting secretagogues or sulfonylureas may be tried for thin older adults. In the older adult, those over age 80, the risk for lactic acidosis is higher, making the use of metformin in this age group risky unless renal function is very normal; thus, in these populations simple insulin regimens are often used.

LEARNING EXERCISES

Case 1

JM is a 55-year-old African American who presents complaining of fatigue. JM states he had been in good health until approximately 6 to 8 weeks ago when he started to feel "weak and tired" more than usual. On further questioning, he has been getting up two or three times a night to urinate, has been more thirsty than usual during the day, and drinks a couple of glasses of water or juice every 1 to 3 hours.

During the last 5 years, he has steadily been gaining weight, but during the last 2 months he has been losing weight in spite of a robust appetite. He also notes that he no longer exercises because he has pain in both feet, which is worse at night and sometimes keeps him awake. It is burning in character, and sometimes his toes feel numb. At times his vision is blurry, especially in the afternoon. His father died at age 71 from a massive stroke. His mother died at age 66 from end-stage kidney disease and suffered from diabetes since age 45. His physical exam is essentially normal except for a body mass index (BMI) of 30. BP is 128/82; pulse is 82; and temperature is 98.8.

Laboratory results:
Urinalysis: 4+ glucose, negative for ketones and protein.
Random blood glucose: 450 mg/dL.
Hemoglobin A1c (HbA1c): 9.2.
Total cholesterol: 254 mg/dL; HDL: 21 mg/dL; triglycerides: 434 mg/dL.

1. What is your diagnosis?

2. What pharmacological and nonpharmacological treatment options would you recommend?

3. What patient education would you give this patient?

Case 2

AJ is a 69-year-old plumber with a 7-year history of type 2 diabetes. Although he was diagnosed in 2002, he had intermittent symptoms that were likely due to hyperglycemia for 2 years prior to diagnosis that went unrecognized. He states that initially he was told he had "borderline diabetes." He was told he had to lose weight and change his eating habits or he would have to take medications. He attempted weight loss without much success and was afraid to return to his doctor. A year ago he finally went back to his doctor complaining of foot pain and nocturia and was started on glyburide (DiaBeta), 2.5 mg every morning. He states he stayed on the medication for 4 months and then stopped taking it because of dizziness,

often accompanied by sweating and a feeling of mild agitation in the late afternoon. He also takes atorvastatin (Lipitor), 10 mg daily, for hypercholesterolemia. He does not test his blood glucose levels at home. Both his mother and father had type 2 diabetes. Mr. AJ's diet history reveals excessive carbohydrate intake in the form of bread and pasta. On exam his BP is 166/94; BMI is 28, with no other significant findings.

Laboratory results:
Hemoglobin A1c (HbA1C): 12.
Total cholesterol: 230 mg/dL; HDL: 19 mg/dL
Triglycerides: 500 mg/dL
Urinalysis: 4+ glucose, positive protein.
Random blood glucose: 377

1. What are your diagnoses?

2. What pharmacological and nonpharmacological recommendations would you suggest for this patient?

References

American College of Clinical Endocrinologists: Diabetes Care Plan Guidelines, Endocrine Practice, 2011;17(suppl 2) March/April 2011. Retrieved February 5, 2013, from www.aace.com/files/dm-guidelines-ccp.pdf

American Diabetes Association (ADA). (2011). Diabetes Statistics. Data from the 2011 National Diabetes Fact Sheet (released January 26, 2011). Retrieved February 3, 2013, from www.diabetes.org/diabetes-basics/diabetes-statistics/?utm_source=WWW&utm_medium=DropDownDB&utm_content=Statistics&utm_campaign=CON

Centers for Disease Control and Prevention (CDC). (2011). Self-reported visual impairment among persons with diagnosed diabetes–United States, 1997–2010. *Morbidity and Mortality Weekly Report, 60*(45), 1549-1553. Retrieved February 3, 2013, from www.cdc.gov/mmwr/preview/mmwrhtml/mm6045a2.htm

Handelsman, Y., Blonde, L., Bloomgarden, Z., Dagogo-Jack, S., Einhorn, D., Garber, A. J., et al. (2011). American Association of Clinical Endocrinologists Medical Guidelines for Clinical Practice for Developing a Diabetes Mellitus Comprehensive Care Plan. *Journal of Endocrine Practice, 17*(Suppl. 2), 1-53. Retrieved February 3, 2013, from http://aace.metapress.com/content/t7g5335740165v13/fulltext.pdf

Narayan K. M. V. (2005). Glycemic control and cardiovascular disease in patients with type 1 diabetes. *New England Journal of Medicine, 353*; 2643-2645.

Nathan, D. M., Buse, J. B., Davidson, M. B., Heine, R. J., Holman, R. R., Sherwin, R., et al. (2006). Management of Hyperglycemia in Type 2 Diabetes: A Consensus Algorithm for the Initiation and Adjustment of Therapy: A Consensus Statement From the American Diabetes Association and the European Association for the Study of Diabetes. *Diabetes Care, 29*(8), 1963-1972. Retrieved February 3, 2013, from http://care.diabetesjournals.org/content/29/8/1963

National Diabetes Information Clearinghouse (NDIC). (2011). National Institutes of Health. National diabetes statistics. Retrieved February 3, 2013, from www.diabetes.niddk.nih.gov/dm/pubs/statistics/#fast

Yoon, J. W. & Jun, H.S. (2005). Autoimmune destruction of pancreatic beta cells. *American Journal of Therapeutics, 12*(6), 580-591.

Drugs Used to Treat Common Neurological Conditions

William N. Tindall, Kathy Kemle, Mona A. Sedrak

CHAPTER FOCUS

This chapter focuses on drugs used to treat neurological conditions or disorders of the body's three nervous systems (central, peripheral, and autonomic) resulting from structural, biochemical, and electrical abnormalities. Epilepsy, migraine headaches, Parkinson's disease (PD), multiple sclerosis (MS), and neuropathies are discussed. Alzheimer's disease is discussed in this chapter (as well as in Chapter 22, Prescribing for the Geriatric Patient). Sleep disorders are included in this chapter because drugs are commonly prescribed in the United States to treat them. Drugs used to treat psychiatric disorders are discussed in Chapter 15, but some crossover exists between these drugs and drugs used to treat neurological disorders, both in their application and in adverse effects. Finally, anorexiants (appetite suppressants) are discussed in this chapter because they increase the sensation of fullness or decrease the sense of appetite through their ability to increase serotonin or catecholamine.

LEARNING OBJECTIVES

After reading and studying this chapter, the student should be able to:

1. Describe the major neurotransmitters, how they are produced, and what their functions are in the body.
2. Explain why so many drugs used to treat central nervous system disorders have other uses as well (e.g., antipsychotic agents).
3. Explain why the body responds differently to nerve impulses and hormones.
4. Describe the mechanism of action, pharmacokinetics, and adverse effects of drugs used for appetite suppression, insomnia, epilepsy, Alzheimer's disease, Parkinson's disease, and migraine headaches.
5. Describe the international classification of seizures and the importance of its role in identifying and classifying seizures before choosing drug treatment protocols.
6. Differentiate between the neurotransmitters that cause Alzheimer's disease and Parkinson's disease and the rationale for drugs used to correct "imbalances" in both.
7. Differentiate between the classes of agents used to treat Parkinson's disease and explain why one class may be used rather than another.
8. Differentiate between the classes of drugs used to treat Alzheimer's disease and explain the rationale for why one is chosen rather than another.
9. Briefly describe how over-the-counter sleep aids such as melatonin and antihistamines help a patient to fall asleep.
10. Compare and contrast the various medications used to treat multiple sclerosis and why the U.S. Food and Drug Administration has approved their use in the marketplace.
11. Describe the various agents used to allay peripheral neuropathies.

Key Terms

Absence seizures

Acetylcholinesterase

Alzheimer's disease (AD)

Catechol-O-methyltransferase (COMT) inhibitors

Complex partial seizures

Epilepsy

Gamma-aminobutyric acid (GABA) enhancers

Hydantoin

Iminostilbenes

Insomnia

Lipophilic

MAOB inhibitors

Migraine

Parkinson's disease (PD)

Seizure threshold

Simple partial seizures

Status epilepticus

Tonic-clonic (grand mal) seizures

KEY DRUGS IN THIS CHAPTER

Anorexiants
- benzphetamine (Didrex)
- diethylproprio (Tenuate)
- mazindol (Mazanor)
- phendimetrazine (Bontril)
- phentermine (Adipex)

Anticonvulsants

Hydantoins
- phenytoin (Dilantin)
- fosphenytoin (Cerebyx)

Iminostilbenes
- carbamazepine (Tegretol)
- oxcarbazepine (Trileptal)

Succinimides
- ethosuximide (Zarontin)

GABA Analogue
- gabapentin (Neurontin)
- pregabalin (Lyrica)

Miscellaneous Anticonvulsants
- valproate (Depakote)
- topiramate (Topamax)
- lamotrigine (Lamictal)
- levetiracetam (Keppra)
- lacosamide (Vimpat)

Sleep Aids

Over the Counter
- diphenhydramine (Benadryl, Excedrin PM, Sominex, Tylenol PM, Nytol)
- doxylamine (Unisom)
- melatonin

Prescription
- eszopiclone (Lunesta)
- zolpidem (Ambien)
- zalepon (Sonata)

Antimigraine Drugs

Abortives

Serotonin Receptor Agonists
- almotriptan (Axert)
- eletriptan (Relpax)
- frovotriptan (Frova)
- sumatriptan (Imitrex)
- sumatriptan + naproxen (Treximet)
- naratriptan (Amerge)
- rizatriptan (Maxalt)
- zolmitriptan (Zomig)

Ergotmines
- ergotamine (Ergostat)
- ergot with caffeine (Cafergot)
- dihydroergotamine (DHE 45, Migranol)

Prophylactic Medications
- topiramate (Topamax)
- propranolol (Inderal)
- timolol (Blocadren)
- divalproex (Depakote)
- Botox

Antiparkinson Agents

Anticholinergic Agents
- benztropine (Cogentin)
- trihexyphenidyl (Artane)

Dopamine Replacement Drugs (Dopamine Precursors)
- carbidopa-levodopa (Sinemet)

Dopamine Agonists
- bromocriptine (Parlodel)
- pergolide (Permax)
- pramipexole (Mirapex)
- ropinirole (Requip)
- apomorphine (Apokyn)

Catechol-O-Methyltransferase (COMT) Inhibitors
- entacapone (Comtan)
- tolcapone (Tasmar)

MAOB Inhibitor
- selegiline (Eldepryl, Zelapar)
- rasagiline (Azilect)

Alzheimer's Agents
- donepezil (Aricept)
- tacrine (Cognex)
- galantamine (Razadyne)
- rivastigmine (Exelon)
- memantine (Namenda)
- caprylic tryglycerides (Axona)

Multiple Sclerosis Agents
- interferon beta-1a (Avonex, Rebif)
- interferon beta-1b (Betaseron, Extavia)
- glatiramer acetate (Copaxone)
- mitoxantrone (Novantrone)
- natalizumab (Tysabri)
- fingolimod (Gilenya)

THE IMPORTANCE OF NEUROTRANSMITTERS

Drugs used to treat neurological conditions are classified broadly in two ways: drugs used to treat behavioral/psychiatric disorders and drugs used to treat other neurological conditions. The assessment of a neurological patient can be difficult. Finding the right drug to treat a diagnosed neurological disorder requires thorough knowledge of neurotransmitters and neuroreceptors and how drugs can enhance, emulate, or diminish the effect of the relevant neurotransmitter(s) residing in synaptic clefts (Fig. 14-1).

Neurotransmitters respond through the stimulation of connector sites called *synapses*. Once stimulated by any sensory stimulus, neurotransmitters are released from the axon of a neuron into the synapse's cleft (i.e., gap), transverse it, then bind to receptors on the postsynaptic membrane, whereupon ion channels can be either excited or inhibited. The neurotransmitters (e.g., acetylcholine) depolarize postsynaptic membranes by opening sodium channels and allow sodium (Na^{++}) to flow inward. The neurotransmitters at the inhibitory synapses hyperpolarize postsynaptic membranes (e.g., gamma-aminobutyric acid, or GABA), affect synapses in the brain by binding to GABA-specific receptors, and thereby open up chloride ($Cl-$) and potassium (K) channels, allowing specific proteins to

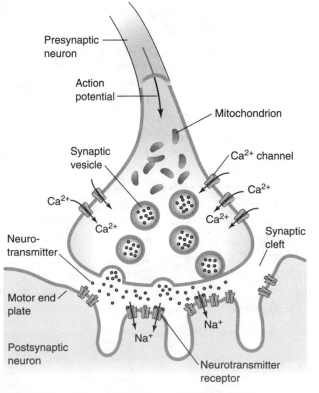

FIGURE 14-1 The pharmacology of nerve transmission.

outflow. This string of events takes only about 1 millisecond to occur. In both situations, the resulting flow of ions (chloride *in*; potassium *out*) *increases* the membrane potential to the point that it counteracts any excitatory signals that may arrive at that neuron. Thus, neurotransmitters are chemicals that allow the transmission of nerve impulses across synapses. They are also found at the axon ending of nerve fibers connected to muscle tissue, where they stimulate muscle fibers and help with such things as muscle coordination, walking, and gait.

SEVEN IMPORTANT NEUROTRANSMITTERS

Seven important neurotransmitters in the human body are acetylcholine (ACh), norepinephrine, dopamine, gamma-aminobutyric acid (GABA), glutamate, serotonin, and endorphins.

Acetylcholine

Acetylcholine, or ACh, was discovered in 1921, and it has many functions. It is released at the terminals of all motor neurons and is responsible for stimulation of muscles, especially muscles of the gastrointestinal tract (GIT), and movement. In sensory neurons and in the autonomic nervous system, acetylcholine plays a role in rapid eye movement (REM), or dreaming sleep. Acetylcholine is released at preganglionic neurons of the autonomic nervous system, postganglionic neurons of the parasympathetic branch (PNS) of the autonomic nervous system, and at synapses in the brain that enhance short-term memory. Drugs that enhance release of acetylcholine or inhibit its destruction (such as **acetylcholinesterase** inhibitors) are useful in the treatment of diseases such as Alzheimer's disease (AD) because acetylcholine levels are low in the brains of patients with Alzheimer's. Blocking or antagonizing acetylcholine causes muscles to relax. Thus, an ACH agent derived from botulinum toxin, Botox, is used to temporarily remove wrinkles in the forehead by relaxing underlying muscle, treat movement disorders such as dystonia, and treat migraine headache.

Dopamine (DA)

Dopamine was discovered in 1958 and is manufactured inside dopamine neurons from an amino acid precursor, L-tyrosine. People obtain L-tyrosine through their diet. Once created from its precursor L-tyrosine, dopamine is then stored in vesicles within nerve terminals from which it can be released into the synapse. The release of dopamine affects postsynaptic receptors that influence behavior. The actions of dopamine are terminated by the reuptake of the neurotransmitter into the presynaptic terminal by means of an active dopamine transporter. Dopamine may then reenter the synaptic vesicles for re-release later or be degraded by the enzyme monoamine oxidase.

Several distinct dopamine neuronal systems exist within the hypothalamus, pituitary gland, midbrain, basal ganglia, retina, and olfactory system. In this chapter, we are interested in midbrain dopamine and its receptors as they are involved in behavior, attention and arousal, and disorders such as Parkinson's disease, which involve a degeneration of midbrain dopamine neurons. Treatment of Parkinson's disease provides the patient with

levodopa (L-dopa), which is readily converted to dopamine in the brain and replaces the deficit dopamine. In Chapter 15, Practical Pharmacotherapy of Drugs Used to Treat Psychiatric Disorders, dopamine is discussed in relation to attention deficit disorder and schizophrenia.

Endorphin

In 1973 the neurotransmitter endorphin, a combination of the words *endogenous* and *morphine,* was discovered. The chemical structure of endorphins is very similar to the opioids, but endorphins are peptides, amino acid chains that are shorter than proteins. They are rapidly inactivated by enzymes called *peptidases*. Endorphins are manufactured in the brain, spinal cord, and many other parts of the body. They are released in response to neurotransmitters and bind to certain neuron receptors, the same receptors that bind opiate medicines. Endorphins act as analgesics by diminishing the perception of pain and as sedatives, and endorphins are the reason humans feel pleasure. They are released following a sexual orgasm. Endorphins also slow heart rate, respiration, and metabolism like an opioid.

Gamma-Aminobutyric Acid (GABA)

Gamma-aminobutyric acid was synthesized in 1883 and was known then only as a plant and microbe metabolic product. It came to prominence as the basis for monosodium glutamate (MSG), the flavoring agent. In 1950, however, GABA was discovered to be an integral part of the human central nervous system as an inhibitory neurotransmitter, slowing or stopping the excitatory neurotransmitters that give rise to anxiety. GABA is the most abundant inhibitory neurotransmitter in the brain. Although GABA is an amino acid, it is classified as a neurotransmitter because it helps induce relaxation and sleep by inhibiting overexcitation. GABA contributes to motor control, vision, and many other cortical functions. Some drugs that increase the level of GABA in the brain are gamma-aminobutyric acid enhancers such as gabapentin, tiagabine, and valproate. Drugs such as lamotrigine, felbamate, and clonazepam are used to treat epilepsy, but their mechanism of action is essentially unknown. It is believed that they stabilize neuronal membranes by inhibiting sodium transport. These agents are also used to relieve trembling associated with Huntington's disease (HD). Drugs such as alcohol, sedatives, narcotics, and other anti-anxiety drugs such as the barbiturates and diazepam all work by influencing GABA.

Glutamate

Glutamate is an excitatory relative of GABA and was discovered as a neurotransmitter in 1994. Although known as a chemical since 1907, it was not recognized until 90 years later as a neurotransmitter, even though it is the most common neurotransmitter in the central nervous system (CNS). As many as one-half of all neurons in the brain are affected by glutamate, and the agent has a large role in memory processes. Physical brain damage or death of brain cells (e.g., from a stroke) initiates an excess of glutamate accumulating in the extracellular fluid, which in turn triggers the death of many more brain cells than the original trauma.

Norepinephrine and Epinephrine

Known since the late 1940s, norepinephrine (noradrenalin) and epinephrine (adrenalin) are neurotransmitters prevalent in the sympathetic nervous system where they have an impact on heart rate and blood pressure. They are also important in memory formation. They are released from the adrenal glands as part of the "fight or flight" reflex at times of stress. Thus, stress tends to deplete stores of these neurotransmitters and exercise tends to raise them, as well as levels of other neurotransmitters such as dopamine and serotonin.

Serotonin

Serotonin (5-hydroxytryptamine or 5HT) is an inhibitory neurotransmitter (antagonist) found in the late 1940s to be involved in emotion and mood. The name 5-HT is commonly used among technical and professionals because the part of its popular name "sero" means blood, and this has proven to be false even though serotonin, or 5-HT, is a vasoconstrictor. Too little serotonin leads to depression, problems with anger control, obsessive-compulsive disorder, and suicidal ideation. Too little serotonin also leads to an increased appetite for carbohydrates (starchy foods) and trouble sleeping, which are also associated with depression and other emotional disorders. Serotonin deficiency has also been tied to migraines, irritable bowel syndrome, and fibromyalgia.

Widely distributed in animals, plants, vertebrates, fruits, nuts, and venoms, a number of congeners of serotonin have been shown to possess a variety of peripheral and central nervous system activities. Although serotonin may be obtained from a variety of dietary sources, endogenous 5-HT is synthesized in situ from tryptophan, an amino acid, through the actions of the enzymes tryptophan hydroxylase and aromatic L-amino acid decarboxylase. Both dietary and endogenous 5-HT are rapidly metabolized and inactivated by monoamine oxidase and aldehyde dehydrogenase to its major metabolite, 5-hydroxyindoleacetic acid (5-HIAA). Among all the neurotransmitter substances, serotonin is perhaps the most implicated in the etiology or treatment of various disorders, including anxiety, depression, obsessive-compulsive disorder, schizophrenia, stroke, obesity, pain, hypertension, vascular disorders, migraine, and nausea.

First isolated from blood in 1948, serotonin has a relatively simple chemical structure, but its pharmacological characteristics are complicated. Serotonin's chemical structure is similar to that of norepinephrine and dopamine. Therefore, it is not surprising that serotonin, like its catecholamine counterparts, possesses a wide range of complex effects that are difficult to systematize, but they include both peripheral effects and central effects (Table 14-1).

As it is with all the central neurotransmitters, 5-HT is synthesized in brain neurons and stored in vesicles. On activation by nerve impulse, 5-HT is released into the synaptic cleft, where it diffuses over a much larger area than just postsynaptic receptors and in effect activates 5-HT receptors of nearby neurons. Its action is then terminated by one of three means: diffusion, metabolism, or uptake back into the synaptic cleft through the actions of specific amine membrane transporter systems. Thus, the actions of 5-HT can be modulated by agents that do one of the following: stimulate or inhibit its biosynthesis, block its storage, stimulate or inhibit its release, mimic or inhibit its actions at its various postsynaptic receptors, inhibit its uptake back into the nerve terminal, or affect its metabolism.

Anything that affects the behavior of a neurotransmitter will also affect the function of the organs with which it is associated. Understanding how neurotransmitters function helps clinicians understand the cause of some diseases and the effects of certain agents, illicit and/or recreational substances, and prescribed medicinals. For example, deficiencies or excessive intake of dietary minerals and vitamins can disrupt 5-HT levels either by disrupting its production or its reuptake system. If serotonin levels are

TABLE 14-1 Effects of 5-HT (serotonin)			
	CARDIOVASCULAR ACTION	**VASOCONSTRICTION, ESPECIALLY RENAL VESSELS**	
PERIPHERAL EFFECTS		Vasoconstriction when coronary vessels are damaged, vasodilation when they are not	
	Action on heart	Positive chronotropic action on rhythm of heart	
	Blood pressure	It's a complex action of either hypertension, hypotension, or nothing	
	Smooth muscle	Contractions of intestine, bronchia, and uterus	
	Other actions	Migraine (from vasodilation of brain vessels)	
		Myocardial ischemia	
CENTRAL EFFECTS		Regulation of sleep, mood (antidepressant action), sexual and hallucinogenic behavior, temperature, and appetite suppression	
		Overstimulation of 5-HT receptors could induce psychotic disorders	
		Modulates other neurotransmitters and plays a role in adaptation	

increased through medicinal substances, it can lead to serotonin syndrome. Additionally, some drugs may block the reuptake of serotonin to its presynaptic source and thus increase extracellular serotonin available to its postsynaptic receptor(s) downstream. Thus, some drugs are very specific at blocking current levels of serotonin and preventing it from reentering its presynaptic releasing points.

The seven neurotransmitters described here are not a complete list because more than 50 neurotransmitters are known to exist and more are being discovered all the time.

DRUGS USED TO SUPPRESS APPETITE

Anorexiants have a long history of use as appetite suppressants, but their long history of abuse has also made their use controversial. As a result of their misuse and abuse, they are placed into the Schedule IV Category of Controlled Substances by the federal government and should only be used as short-term adjuncts in a regimen of weight reduction. Agents used as anorexiants include benzphetamine (Didrex), diethylpropion (Tenuate), mazindol (Mazinor), phendimetrazine (Bontril), and phentermine (Adipex).

Mechanism of Action

These agents are sympathomimetic amines and are believed to act like amphetamines in that they stimulate centers in the hypothalamus and limbic regions of the brain that tell the body it is satiated and needs no further caloric intake.

Pharmacokinetics

- Absorption: Absorbed by both stomach and small intestine, depending on whether or not they are administered as regular tablets or sustained release tablets.
- Distribution: Well distributed as lipid soluble agents and will cross the blood-brain barrier.
- Metabolism: In the liver.
- Excretion: All are excreted through the kidneys into the urine.
- Half-life: 2 to 20 hours, depending on the agent; their duration of action is typically 4 to 6 hours in regular dosage form and 8 to 10 hours in extended dosage form.

Dosage and Administration of Agents for Appetite Suppression

Generic Name	Trade Name	Route	Usual Adult Daily Dose
benzphetamine	Didrex	PO	25–50 mg/day
diethylpropion	Tenuate	PO	25 mg 3 times/day
phendimetrazine	Bontril	PO	35 mg 2 times/day
mazindol	Mazinor	PO	1 mg 2 times/day before meals or 2 mg/day taken 1 hr before lunch
phentermine	Adipex	PO	8 mg 3 times/day before meals or 15 mg/day before breakfast

Clinical Use

- Short-term adjunctive treatment as a part of weight loss program (e.g., including caloric limitations and behavioral/cognitive conditioning)

Adverse Reactions

CV: Hypertension, palpitations, arrhythmias, TACHYCARDIA, pulmonary hypertension, HEART VALVE INSUFFICIENCY.
EENT: Mydriasis, blurred vision.
GI: Dry mouth, constipation, vomiting, diarrhea, unpleasant taste.
GU: Impotence, urinary urgency increases, gynecomastia, changes in libido.
META: Diabetics may experience altered insulin or oral hypoglycemic dosage adjustments.
MISC: Dizziness, fatigue, depression when the drug is suddenly withdrawn.
NEURO: Overstimulation, agitation, convulsions, confusion, psychosis.

Interactions

- COADMINISTRATION OF MONOAMINE OXIDASE INHIBITORS (MAOIS) MAY CAUSE A LIFE-THREATENING HYPERTENSIVE CRISIS.
- Taken with alcohol, these agents can induce depression.
- Phenothiazines coadministered with anorexiants may cause an increase in psychoses.
- Insulin/sulfonylureas used with anorexiants may alter requirements in patients with diabetes.

Contraindications

- Substance abuse (e.g., cocaine, phencyclidine, and methamphetamine) because of the potential for excessive adrenergic stimulation.

Conscientious Considerations

- These agents should be prescribed for severely obese patients only as short-term adjuncts to other weight-loss measures such as diet, exercise, and behavioral modification therapy.
- The significant risks associated with these agents cannot be overemphasized.
- These drugs are effective in the short term, but weight gain occurs almost universally upon stopping them.
- Due to their high risk of tolerance development as well as physical and psychological dependence, these drugs should not be used in people with a history of drug addiction or alcoholism.
- Significant increases in blood pressure can occur and need to be monitored. Use in hypertensive patients is therefore inadvisable.
- One advisable course of therapy is to use the drugs for no longer than 6 months, where the drug is dosed for 1 or 2 weeks, a 2-week drug holiday is taken, and then another 2-week cycle is started again. This 2-week off-and-on cycle is fairly common and usually lasts for less than 3 months.

Patient/Family Education

- Patients should avoid an evening dose because of resultant **insomnia or sleeplessness**.

- Watch for overstimulation of CNS (agitation, anxiety, sleeplessness).
- Avoid alcohol while using these drugs.
- Monitor pulse rate and heart rate, either by the clinician or by teaching the patient at home.
- Patients should be made aware that regular medical monitoring will take place to counsel them on lifestyle modifications and their nutritional needs.

DRUGS USED IN THE TREATMENT OF SEIZURES

Anticonvulsants are drugs used to control or inhibit seizures by prolonging the time between which they occur. Anticonvulsants are not a cure, but rather they suppress the rapid firing of neurons that start a seizure. Seizures result when an abnormal discharge of neurons disrupts the stability of the neurons and the message it sends is garbled. Many factors, including sleep deprivation, hormonal changes, alcohol withdrawal, and emotional stress have been known to cause seizures. There are three major classes of antiseizure medications: the hydantoins, the iminostilbenes, and the succinimides. In addition, some anticonvulsant drugs are increasingly being used to treat mood disorders. For example, lamotrigine (Lamictal), carbamazepine (Tegretol), oxcarbazepine (Trileptal), and valproate (Depakote) are used to treat bipolar disorder. Finally, because there are a great number of agents already on the market for treating epilepsy and their use also produces good outcomes, the newer agents, such as levetiracetam (Keppra) and pregabalin (Lyrica), are being approved as adjunct therapies. These adjunct therapies are not a distinct class of medications, although they are distinct chemicals and have unique and differing mechanisms of action. However, these adjuncts are likely to lead to more and more patients taking more than just one medication to control their seizures.

Conscientious Prescribing of Anticonvulsants

- In general, the exact mechanism of action of all these drugs is complex. They do appear to stabilize the neuron cell membrane by altering transport of the cations (sodium, potassium, and calcium), thus suppressing excitability and spread of seizure discharge.
- It is possible for patients with epilepsy to be weaned from the use of anticonvulsants after being seizure free for 2 years and having three normal EEGs separated by at least 1 year. There is approximately a 95% chance that the seizures will not recur if the patient is slowly weaned off the anticonvulsant.
- Baseline liver function, urinalysis, and blood counts need to be taken as well as periodic plasma levels for hydantoins before starting treatment because many drugs, especially ibuprofen, can either raise or lower plasma hydantoins.

Patient/Family Education Regarding Use of Anticonvulsants

- Advise the patient to wear a MedicAlert-type bracelet that identifies him or her as having a seizure disorder.

- Advise the patient to report frequent or increased drowsiness while on these on medications.
- Care should be taken when using these drugs because sedation could be a danger if mental and physical alertness is necessary.
- Patients should report symptoms such as skin lesions, bruising on skin, fever, or sore throat.
- Patients should take these medications exactly as directed. In the event that a dose is missed, the missed dose should be taken as soon as possible; however, if it is time for the next dose, do not double the dose to make up for the missed dose.
- Patients need to be cautioned that abrupt withdrawal or discontinuance of these medications could lead to status epilepticus, a medical emergency.
- Warn patients to avoid alcohol use.
- Patients should be cautioned to not take any over-the-counter (OTC) medications with these drugs before checking with their clinician because drug interactions may occur with many OTC medications.

SPOTLIGHT ON CONVULSIVE STATUS EPILEPTICUS

Convulsive **status epilepticus** is a medical emergency that has high mortality and morbidity. Significant physiological changes accompany convulsive status epilepticus because of the catecholamine surge that accompanies the seizures. Because the cortical neurons require ATP for energy and the brain's supply of ATP is rapidly used during status epilepticus, the end point is the death of thousands of brain cells. As these brain cells die, systemic effects include hypertension, tachycardia, cardiac arrhythmias, and hyperglycemia with up to a 20% mortality rate if there is a 30-minute or more state of unconsciousness from anoxia.

Many situations, including toxins, alcohol withdrawal, cerebral infarction, CNS tumor, infections, trauma, or metabolic causes such as low blood concentrations of calcium or glucose, may precipitate status epilepticus; however, the most common cause of status epilepticus is sudden discontinuation of anticonvulsant medication.

Emergency care of status epilepticus is a complex regimen that includes confirming the presence of status epilepticus and that repetitive seizures have occurred, assessing the patient's airway and oxygen, and evaluating vital signs. Administer lorazepam (Ativan), diazepam (Valium), or midazolam (Versed) as an intravenous infusion and monitor the patient for hemodynamic instability. Diazepam is administered because of its high lipid solubility, which allows it to rapidly enter the brain. The infusion is given as 5 or 10 mg per minute, which will terminate most seizures. Lorazepam is less lipid soluble than is diazepam, thus its effects are longer (6 to 12 hours) than diazepam when 4 to 8 mg/min is given. When appropriate, fosphenytoin may be administered as an IV infusion in a dose of 15 to 20 mg/kg at a rate of 150 mg/min.

The Hydantoins

The prototype **hydantoin** drug is phenytoin (Dilantin), which was discovered as researchers looked for a drug with less sedation than phenobarbitol. It is the drug of choice for all types of seizures except absence seizures (petit mal). It is especially useful in treating tonic-clonic (grand mal) and partial complex seizures. Another hydantoin available today is fosphenytoin (Cerebyx). It is only used in hospitals because it is a prodrug of phenytoin and formulated to be administered intravenously.

Mechanism of Action

All of the hydantoins inhibit and stabilize electric discharges from neurons in the cortex of the brain by affecting ion exchanges (sodium, calcium, potassium) during polarization and repolarization. They also affect the brainstem's role in contributing to the tonic phase of tonic-clonic seizures.

Pharmacokinetics

- Absorption: Oral absorption is slow from the intestine.
- Distribution: Once absorbed, hydantoins quickly enter the brain and are later redistributed throughout the body. Plasma levels range from 10 to 20 mcg/mL and relate to treatment effect.
- Metabolism: Takes place in the liver.
- Excretion: Via the kidneys.
- Half-life: Ranges from 6 to 24 hr; phenytoin: 24 hr.

Dosage and Administration

Generic Name	Trade Name	Route	Usual Adult Daily Dose
fosphenytoin	Cerebyx	IV	IV loading dose 15–20 mg/PE*/kg for status epilepticus note: Doses of fosphenytoin are expressed as "phenytoin sodium equivalents"
phenytoin	Dilantin	PO	Initial 1 gm in 3 divided doses, then after 24 hr 300 mg/day in 1 dose (extended release) or 3 times/day regular dose Children: 4–8 mg/kg/day in divided doses

Clinical Use

- First-line treatment of choice for generalized tonic-clonic (grand mal) and simple complex and simple partial seizures.

Adverse Reactions

CV: Hypotension, tachycardia
DERM: Skin rashes, photophobia, hypertrichosis
EENT: Diplopia, nystagmus
GI: Nausea, vomiting, anorexia, altered taste, constipation, dry mouth, gingival hyperplasia (the latter is very common)
GU: Urinary retention, reddish-brown color
HEM: Life-threatening hematopoietic changes such as AGRANULOCYTOSIS and APLASTIC ANEMIA
META: Hyperglycemia
MS: Polyarthropathy
MISC: Coarseness of facial features, enlargement of lips, allergic reactions including STEVENS-JOHNSON SYNDROME

NEURO: Agitation, ataxia, confusion, dizziness, drowsiness, headache, nystagmus, decreased coordination

Interactions

- Drugs that lower serum levels of hydantoins and decrease their effect are many and include carbamazepine, chronic alcohol use, barbiturates, rifampin, antacids, and influenza virus vaccines.
- Drug interactions are believed to occur between influenza vaccines and four drugs: phenytoin, aminopyrine, theophylline, and warfarin. The vaccine inhibits the cytochrome P-450 system and thus the resultant decrease in drug metabolism leads to increased circulating drug. However, such interactions are rare, so rare that clinicians still give influenza vaccine to the elderly but monitor the patient because these reactions can occur up to 28 days postvaccination. Manufacturers of flu vaccine (Fluzone, Fluarix, Fluvirin) still ask that patients report to their clinician their drug history, especially use of phenytoin and warfarin.
- Drugs that increase the serum levels of phenytoin and hence its effects are many and include acute alcohol intake, amiodarone, chloramphenicol, chlordiazepoxide, diazepam, isoniazid, methylphenidate, phenothiazines, phenylbutazone, salicylates, succinimides, sulfonamides, tolbutamide, trazodone.
- Drugs that may increase or decrease serum levels of hydantoins include phenobarbitol, valproate, valproic acid.
- Drugs whose efficacy is impaired by hydantoins include: corticosteroids, coumarin anticoagulants, digoxin, doxycycline, estrogens, furosemide, oral contraceptives, quinidine, rifampin, sulfonylureas, theophylline, and vitamin D.
- Although not a true drug interaction, tricyclic antidepressants have been known to precipitate seizures and thus phenytoin dosages need adjusting.

Contraindications

- Hypersensitivities
- Patients with any kind of bradycardia or sinoatrial block

Conscientious Considerations

- Clinicians need to watch for phenytoin hypersensitivities, a syndrome that may develop in 3 to 8 weeks (fever, skin rash, lymphadenopathies).
- Plasma levels of hydantoins need to be monitored, especially because many drugs can affect its levels.
- Pregnancy risk is category D. Clinicians must consider other options should a woman desire pregnancy, because some fetal abnormalities have been associated with hydantoin use.
- Use cautiously in patients with myocardial insufficiency and hypotension.
- In patients with diabetes, blood glucose must be carefully monitored.

- Older adults may show signs of toxicity at lower than usual doses.
- Phenytoin-induced hepatitis is a common hypersensitivity reaction.
- Phenytoin administered too rapidly by IV has been associated with cardiac problems such as hypotension. However, when administered over a slower time frame, it is associated with hyperglycemia and induced diabetic ketoacidosis (DKA).
- A potential side effect of phenytoin is suicide ideation.
- **In addition, clinicians must be aware of the important considerations that apply to *all* anticonvulsants (see p. 246, Conscientious Prescribing of Anticonvulsants).**

Patient/Family Education

- Because of gingival hyperplasia, the patient must practice good oral hygiene to prevent tenderness, bleeding, and gum recession.
- Patients must be made aware the urine may change to a reddish-brown color but that this is no cause for alarm.
- In addition, the clinician must be aware of the advisories that apply to patients taking *any* anticonvulsant (see p. 246, Patient/Family Education).

The Iminostilbenes

The two primary agents in the class of **iminostilbenes** are carbamazepine (Tegretol) and oxcarbazepine (Trileptal). These medications are chemically related to tricyclic antidepressants. Because carbamazepine can be used in the treatment of all types of seizures, with the exception of absence seizures, it is considered an equivalent to phenytoin in efficacy and side effects. Oxcarbazepine can be used alone or in combination with other agents to treat partial seizures in adults and in children between the ages of 4 to 16. By being chemically related to tricyclic antidepressants, these medications can also be used to treat bipolar affective disorder (BAD).

Mechanism of Action

The area of the brain associated with the spread of seizure discharge is the thalamus.

Carbamazepine (Tegretol) and oxcarbazepine (Trileptal) exert their effect in the thalamus, where they inhibit voltage-gated sodium channels in neurons. By doing so they stabilize hyperexcitability states, inhibit repetitive neuronal firing, and decrease propagation of synaptic impulses.

Pharmacokinetics

- Absorption: Absorption from the stomach in immediate release tablets is slow and erratic because of the drugs' low water solubility (high **lipophilic** property).
- Distribution: Because these drugs are highly lipophilic, they result in high body tissue binding.
- Metabolism: In the liver, where it induces metabolism of many CYP-450 substrates.
- Excretion: Through urine and feces.
- Half-life: Can be as long as 25 to 65 hours, but as dosing continues, it decreases to 12 to 17 hours.

Dosage and Administration

Generic Name	Trade Name	Route	Usual Adult Dose
carbamazepine	Tegretol	PO	200 mg 2 times/day; increase by 200 mg/day weekly to max of 1,000 mg
oxcarbazepine	Trileptal	PO	300 mg 2 times/day; increase by 600 mg/day weekly to max of 1,200 mg 2 times/day

Clinical Use

- Used as monotherapy or adjunctive therapy for partial complex seizures; also used in trigeminal neuralgia and bipolar affective disorder.

Adverse Reactions

EENT: Blurry vision, tinnitus, diplopia, nystagmus

DERM: Rash, acne

GI: Nausea, vomiting, dry mouth, hepatic damage, abnormal pain, dyspepsia, thirst

GU: Impotence, incontinence, renal failure, azotemia

HEM: Leucopenia, agranulocytosis, aplastic anemia, thrombocytopenia, a transient increase in white blood cell (WBC) count. CARBAMAZEPINE HAS AN FDA BLACK BOX WARNING OWING TO ITS POTENTIAL TO CAUSE BLOOD DYSCRASIAS, SOME FATAL

META: Hyponatremia, impaired antidiuretic hormone release (ADH) leading to water retention

NEURO: Ataxia, gait disturbances, tremor, headache

Interactions

- Drugs that increase the plasma levels of carbamazepine and oxcarbazepine are acetaminophen, hydantoins, cimetidine, erythromycin, and verapamil.
- Drugs that decrease plasma levels are phenobarbital, phenytoin, rifampin, theophylline.
- Concomitant use with ethanol should be avoided, because CNS depression may result.
- Grapefruit juice will interact with these drugs, causing serum drug levels of these drugs to increase.
- Evening primrose tea, St. John's wort, valerian, and kava kava have all reduced the **seizure threshold** (that genetically determined point in an individual where a stimulation causes the brain to produce a convulsive state) when used as supplements with these drugs.

Contraindications

- Hypersensitivities to drug itself or to tricyclic antidepressants.
- Use with MAOIs.
- Coadministration with nefazodone.
- Any history of blood disorders, especially bone marrow suppression.
- Pregnancy (teratogenic effects have occurred).

Conscientious Considerations

- Plasma drug levels should be monitored on a regular basis (therapeutic range is 4 to 12 mcg/mL, whereas higher levels lead to toxicities). Children can develop toxicities below 12 mcg/mL.
- Although a transient increase in WBC count can occur, it is manageable.
- Due to the potential for increased intraocular pressure (IOP) resulting from the mild anticholinergic effects of these agents, patients should be checked for a baseline and monitored.
- Doses are adjusted according to serum concentrations and responses; however, most often twice-a-day dosing is used for oxcarbazepine and twice-a-day or four-times-a-day dosing is used for carbamazepine.
- **In addition, clinicians must be aware of the important considerations that apply to *all* anticonvulsants (see p. 246, Conscientious Prescribing of Anticonvulsants).**

Patient/Family Education

- If taken with food or GRAPEFRUIT JUICE, serum levels of these drugs can be increased and hence the effect of these drugs as well.
- **In addition, the clinician must be aware of the advisories that apply to patients taking *any* anticonvulsant (see p. 246, Patient/Family Education Regarding Use of Anticonvulsants).**

The Succinimides

The succinimide ethosuximide is used for the treatment of absence seizures (petit mal) in children and adults. It is considered a first-choice drug because it lacks the idiosyncratic hepatotoxicity of the alternate absence seizure drug, valproic acid. Because the patent on the branded product Zarontin has expired, generic equivalents are available.

Mechanism of Action

This agent acts by decreasing nerve impulses and transmission in the motor cortex, resulting in an increase in the seizure threshold, specifically by blocking T-type voltage-gated calcium channels in thalamic neurones.

Pharmacokinetics

- Absorption: Administered orally and well absorbed from the GI tract
- Distribution: Well distributed
- Metabolism: In the liver
- Excretion: In the urine
- Half-life: Ethosuximide 30 to 60 hours

Dosage and Administration

Generic Name	Trade Name	Route	Usual Adult Daily Dose
ethosuximide	Zarontin	PO	250–500 mg daily; may increase to a max of 1.5 gm/day

Clinical Use

- Control of absence (petit mal) seizures in children and adults that are refractory to other drugs

Adverse Reactions

CV: None.
DERM: Rash, pruritus.
GI: Upset and distress.
GU: Phensuximide will color the urine a reddish-brown.
HEM: The succinimides have been associated with BLOOD DYSCRASIAS.
NEURO: Depression, headache, mood changes, lethargy.

Interactions

- When coadministered with tricyclic antidepressants, phenothiazines, antihistamines, or alcohol, CNS depression is likely to be increased.
- Ethosuximide crosses the placental barrier, and thus the risk of women having teratogenicities is higher than if they were not taking any antiepileptic drug (AED). This risk is higher for women on two or more AEDs.

Contraindications

- History of hypersensitivity

Conscientious Considerations

- Use cautiously in patients who have liver or kidney issues or any kind of blood dyscrasia.
- Plasma levels, as well as periodic liver, renal, and heme studies, need to be monitored for adverse effects.
- Ethosuximide crosses into breast milk.
- (See p. 246, Conscientious Prescribing of Anticonvulsants).

Patient/Family Education

- Any GI distress can usually be relieved by taking with a glass of milk.
- Patients who are using oral contraceptives should use a backup form of birth control.
- In addition, the clinician must be aware of the advisories that apply to patients taking *any* anticonvulsant (see p. 246, Patient/Family Education Regarding the Use of Anticonvulsants).

Miscellaneous Anticonvulsants

A number of agents are used as miscellaneous anticonvulsants and serve as alternatives and adjuncts to the use of hydantoins, iminostilbenes, and succinimides. In many cases, their exact mechanism of action remains unknown. One such example is primidone (Mysoline), a member of the barbiturate family that raises seizure thresholds similar to phenobarbitol. Use today is mostly confined to relief of essential tremor.

The gamma-aminobutyric acid (GABA) enhancers are also called miscellaneous anticonvulsants because of their high affinity for GABA binding sites in the brain where voltage-gated calcium ion channels are modified to modulate release of excitatory neurotransmitters. How zonisamide (Zonegran) and lamotrigine (Lamictal) act as anticonvulsants remains unknown, but it is believed they stabilize neuronal membranes and suppress excitatory activity at sodium and calcium channels. Agents such as felbamate (Felbatol) and clonazepam (Klonopin) are also miscellaneous anticonvulsants, but they are chemically similar to the barbiturates and thus are believed to act like them.

To enhance the activity of GABA and suppress some of the discharge in absence seizures by decreasing nerve transmission in the motor cortex, agents such as clonazepam (Klonopin), diazepam (Valium), and lorazepam (Ativan) make abnormal electrical activity less likely by their ability to slow CNS activity. Diazepam and lorazepam are usually administered intravenously for the treatment of prolonged seizures (status epilepticus). Diazepam is also available in a gel that can be administered rectally during a cluster of seizures. If administered within 15 minutes of seizure onset, the diazepam gel is quite effective at ending the seizure activity. Clonazepam is the most common benzodiazepine because it is administered in tablet form and can be used for long-term treatment or for short-term treatment in people taking other AEDs. However, most patients do not respond well to clonazepam over the long run.

The gamma-aminobutyric acid enhancers are gabapentin (Neurontin), tiagabine (Gabitril), valproate (Depakote), and vigabatrin (Sabril). These are oral agents used in the treatment of refractory **complex partial seizures** (CPS) in adults. Partial seizures start on one side of the brain as opposed to both sides. Vigabatrin is often prescribed with other medications. Vigabatrin (Sabril) is recommended for use after other options have proven ineffective in treating the seizures of a particular patient as one side effects of vigabatrin is loss of vision and its use is typically confined to late teens or adults.

Gabapentin (Neurontin, Nupentin) is a GABA analogue that is available in tablets, capsules, and oral solutions. It is used for restless leg syndrome, postherpetic neuralgia (PHN), and seizures. It shifts the way the body perceives pain for PHN, and it decreases normal excitatory nerve impulses in the brain to affect seizures. How it treats restless leg syndrome is still unknown. Tiagabine (Gabitril) is primarily used as adjunctive therapy for epilepsy because it is a selective gamma-aminobutyric acid reuptake inhibitor, which in turn increases synaptic availability of GABA and reduction of partial seizures. Its other use is in the treatment of panic disorder.

Valproic acid (VPA) is a liquid at room temperature, but when mixed with sodium hydroxide, it becomes sodium valproate. The mixture of the two is marketed as Depakote, Depacon, or Depakene. These medications are used in control of complex partial seizures and absence seizures. Patients may experience significant weight gain while taking this medication. Additionally, high plasma drug levels may induce severe tremors as well as liver damage, which has been fatal in children. Routine blood tests and careful monitoring will reduce this risk. Valproate

affects GABA in the brain by blocking voltage-gated sodium channels and T-type calcium channels, and enhancing GABA transmission by inhibiting GABA transaminase, thus making it a broad spectrum anticonvulsant. It is also used in the treatment of the manic phases of bipolar disorder and prophylaxis of migraine headaches.

Dosage and Administration of Miscellaneous Anticonvulsants Used to Treat Seizures

Class	Generic Name	Trade Name	Route	Usual Adult Daily Dose
SULFONAMIDE DERIVATIVE	zonisamide	Zonegran	PO	100 mg/day for 2 weeks; may increase to 200 mg/day, then up to 400 or 600 mg/day after 2-week increments, if needed
GAMMA-AMINOBU-TYRIC ACID ENHANCERS	gabapentin	Neurontin	PO	300 mg 3 times/day; if necessary, increase up to 1,800 mg/day
	tiagabine	Gabitril	PO	4 mg once a day for a week; may increase by 4–8 mg/week depending on response
	valproate	Depakote	PO	Up to 2,500 mg/day in divided doses
UNKNOWN MECHANISM	lamotrigine	Lamictal	PO	25 mg 2 times/day; may increase weekly up to max of 200 mg 2 times/day
	felbamate	Felbatol	PO	100 mg/day in 3–4 divided doses
	clonazepam	Klonopin	PO	1.5 mg in 3 divided doses; increase by 0.5 mg–1 mg every 3 days until seizures are controlled
MISCELLA-NEOUS	pregabalin	Lyrica	PO	
	levetiracetam	Keppra Keppra SR	PO, IV	Initial dose is 500 mg 2 times/day; increase dose every 2 weeks up to max dosage of 3,000 mg/day.
	topiramate	Topamax	PO	For adults and children over 10, give 400 mg/day in divided doses.
				If between age 2 and 10, start with 25 mg/day and titrate up based on child's weight.
	lacosamide	Vimpat	PO	Start with 50 mg 2 times/day, then increase every week up to 200–400 mg/day given 2 times/day

SPOTLIGHT ON TREATMENT OF SEIZURE DISORDERS

Characterization of seizures

Epilepsy is a term used to describe a group of chronic neurological disorders characterized by sporadic but recurrent episodes of seizures. Epilepsy is and has been classified in many ways: by symptoms, cause, area of the brain from which the abnormal

electrical discharges originate, or by the changes observed on an EEG. A common international classification that takes into account both the symptoms during a seizure and the localization of abnormal electrical activity in the brain is used today. This classification divides seizures into the following groups.

SPOTLIGHT ON TREATMENT OF SEIZURE DISORDERS—cont'd

Tonic-clonic seizures are generalized convulsions also known as *grand mal* seizures. During tonic-clonic seizures the person falls to the ground, often with a scream, breathing stops, and the arms and legs become rigid (tonic phase). Then the person starts to shake and jerk (clonic phase) and may foam (mixture of blood and saliva) at the mouth and bite his/her tongue.

Absence seizures are known also as *petit mal* or minor seizures, and they occur mostly in childhood epilepsy. The seizure starts without warning and consists of short intervals of loss of consciousness, during which the person temporarily blacks out. In nearly all cases, they last such a short time that muscular tension (tonus) is preserved, and the person does not fall over. Sometimes tonus can be lost in a hand, and the person will drop what he or she was holding. If the seizure is prolonged, tonus may be lost in the whole body, and the person falls to the floor. During seizures, one may observe rapid blinking, rolling up of the eyes, and/or face pulling or twitching. These symptoms are not very common. Many times the seizures stop as suddenly as they started, and the child immediately regains normal consciousness and is able to continue with what he/she was doing, unaware of what just happened. Some children can have this type of seizure up to 100 times a day and not remember the missing parts of their day.

Simple partial seizures are defined as seizures caused by localized abnormal discharges of neurons that do not affect consciousness. Simple partial seizures can develop into complex partial seizures, if consciousness is impaired. Simple partial seizures are often the precursor to a larger seizure. As the larger seizure manifests, it is often preceded by an aura that should be taken as a warning that a larger seizure is on the way. This aura manifests as a simple visual disturbance, a feeling of déjà vu, or some type of depersonalization rising from the stomach to the head. It can also involve light, sound, smell, or other sensation. This aura can differ widely from person to person, but it will usually be the same each time if the abnormal electrical discharges occur in the same area of the brain each time.

Partial seizures are those caused by a localized abnormal discharge in the brain, which leads to an impairment of consciousness. Partial seizures can occur as simple partial seizures, or they can develop into complex partial seizures. In complex partial seizures, abnormal brain discharges are localized in the temporal lobes, and during the seizure, automatic movements such as pulling at clothing, lip smacking, chewing, face pulling, or other aimless repeated movements are often seen. If the seizure lasts for a long period of time, these automatisms can become more complicated; in fact many people carry out complicated tasks, of which they have no memory.

Conscientiously choosing an anticonvulsant medication requires an accurate diagnosis and subsequent classification of the seizure type (Table 14-2). Indications and dosage schedules are tailored to seizure type. For example, the succinimides remain first-line agents for treating children diagnosed with absence seizure disorders. Clinicians need to monitor serum (plasma) levels of some anticonvulsant drugs in addition to helping monitor seizure activity in case dosage adjustments are necessary. Renal, liver, and hematological studies need to be done because of the adverse effects that some of these drugs have on those systems. Finally, patient education programs are a must with these drugs because patients must be cognizant of and committed to avoiding alcohol, watching for mood changes, avoiding hazardous activities if sedation occurs, and avoiding GI distress.

TABLE 14-2 Types of Epilepsy and Use of Medication

AGENT	USE IN SEIZURE TYPE OF EPILEPSY	SIGNIFICANT AND CAUTIONARY NOTES
valproate (Depakote)	All types of epilepsy First line for generalized tonic-clonic seizures	Avoid in women of childbearing potential Less sedating than others
carbamazepine (Tegretol)	First line for partial complex seizures Also used in tonic-clonic and mixed seizures	A good drug of choice if patient seeking pregnancy Slow-release preparations work better May worsen absence or myoclonic seizures
lamotrigine (Lamictal)	Use in most forms of epilepsy, especially as alternate for partial epilepsies	Start low and go slow to avoid rash Avoid doses over 200 mg in women of childbearing potential
phenytoin (Hydantoin)	Treatment/prevention of tonic-clonic (grand mal) and complex partial seizures. May worsen myoclonic or absence seizures	Therapeutic monitoring is necessary due to erratic pharmacokinetics. Use is waning because of its narrow therapeutic index
gabapentin (Neurontin)	Adjunctive treatment of partial seizures with or without secondary generalized tonic-clonic seizures	Use is more for neuropathy pain
topiramate (Topamax)	Adjunctive therapy of partial onset seizures and generalized tonic-clonic seizures	Can decrease serum digoxin and serum levels of oral contraceptives by 30%. Often used as adjunctive therapy
ethosuximide (Zarontin)	Only effective for absence (petit mal) seizures.	Not widely used today
vigabatrin (Sabril)	Use when refractory complex partial seizures occurs	Use is limited by irreversible visual field defects. Perform visual field testing every 6 months.
pregabalin (Lyrica)	Effective as adjunctive treatment of partial-onset seizures in adults	Use as adjunctive therapy

Continued

SPOTLIGHT ON TREATMENT OF SEIZURE DISORDERS—cont'd

TABLE 14-2   Types of Epilepsy and Use of Medication—cont'd

AGENT	USE IN SEIZURE TYPE OF EPILEPSY	SIGNIFICANT AND CAUTIONARY NOTES
levetiracetam (Keppra)	Limited use, but effective in partial onset seizures and myoclonic seizures	Psychotic symptoms may occur
oxcarbazepine (Trileptal)	Monotherapy or adjunctive therapy of partial seizures in adults	May inhibit CYP-450 enzymes and thus alter other drugs metabolized by this system

DRUGS USED TO AID SLEEP

Nonprescription melatonin and several prescription medications, including eszopiclone (Lunesta), zolpidem (Ambien and Ambien CR), ramelteon (Rozerem), and zalepon (Sonata), are able to induce sleep. The prescription medications are classified as non-benzodiazepine hypnotics because they act on benzodiazepine receptors in the brain and appear to be safe and effective for initiating sleep. They can be habit-forming, which is why they should not be used for more than 7 to 10 days. Prescription sleep aids should be used with caution in the elderly and in patients with respiratory dysfunction.

Mechanism of Action

Prescription sleep aids act on GABA receptors by binding to them and producing CNS depression. They are also known as the *nonbenzodiazepine GABAergics.* Although structurally similar to the benzodiazepines, these agents are quite selective for the GABA-1 receptor complex, where they enhance chloride conductance on the neuronal membrane. Thus, these drugs reduce excitability and responsiveness to stimulating signals, such as anxiety, stress, and physical discomfort (cold feet in bed). Because they are benzodiazepine-like, they have been classified as Schedule IV drugs under the Controlled Substances Act. Although these aids were designed for induction of sleep, zolpidem has developed a controlled release form, sold as Ambien CR, which offers 6.25 mg of zolpidem at onset (30 minutes) and another 6.25 mg over 6 to 8 hours.

Pharmacokinetics

- Absorption: All are rapidly absorbed through oral administration.
- Distribution: Zaleplon is minimally bound, zolpidem is 92% protein bound.
- Metabolism: All three are metabolized by the CYP-3A4 isoenzymes in the liver.
- Excretion: All excreted in the kidney.
- Half-life: Zalepon: 1 hour; eszopiclone: 5.8 hours; zolpidem: 2.5 hours.

Dosage and Administration

Generic Name	Trade Name	Route	Usual Adult Daily Dose
zolpidem	Ambien	PO	5- or 10-mg capsule at bedtime
eszopiclone	Lunesta	PO	1-, 2-, or 3- mg tablet at bedtime
zalepon	Sonata	PO	5- or 10-mg capsule at bedtime

Clinical Use

- To provide sedation during episodes of insomnia

Adverse Reactions

CNS: Abnormal dreams, sleepwalking, speech problems, vertigo
CV: Increased blood pressure (BP), chest discomfort, palpitations
DERM: Urticaria
EENT: Tinnitus, blurry vision, red eye, altered depth perception
GI: Abdominal discomfort, pain, flatulence, nausea, vomiting
GU: Dysuria, urinary incontinence, urinary tract infections
META: Body temperature increases
MS: Arthralgia, back pain, myalgia, neck pain
NEURO: Headache, mild anterograde amnesia, anxiety, apathy, attention, balance disorder

Interactions

- These agents have an additive effect with benzodiazepines and alcohol.
- These drugs are metabolized by the CYP-3A4 isoenzyme. Thus, drugs that compete for this isoenzyme will decrease the blood levels of these agents and render them less effective. Such agents include cimetadine, rifampin, phenytoin, and carbamazepine.
- Drugs that increase blood levels of these hypnotics are ketoconazole, erythromycin, clarithromycin, and protease inhibitors.

Contraindications

- Hypersensitivities
- Pregnancy

Conscientious Considerations

- Transient sleep problems can often be treated by sleep hygiene programs and should be suggested before prescribing these agents.
- Because many patients diagnose their own insomnia and take OTC sleep aids, a routine health history often does not reveal the patient's complete use of OTC medicines. A careful OTC and herbal drug history is needed to help avoid drug interactions and other problems before prescribing any sleep aids.
- All prescription sleep aids are U.S. Food and Drug Administration (FDA) classified as category C and should not be used during pregnancy.

■ Although no clinical evidence of abuse exists, it is best if these agents are used no longer than 2 weeks (acutely) or 3 months (chronically) without careful evaluation of the treatment.

■ Use with care in patients with alcoholism.

■ Use lower doses in the elderly.

■ Prescription sleep aids are monitored by the federal government as Class IV agents under the Controlled Substances Act.

Patient/Family Education

■ Patients should be told there is little to distinguish between these drugs other than their clinical response. Thus, if one does not work, perhaps another will.

■ Do not use if drinking alcohol, using OTC sleep aids, or taking any other CNS depressant.

■ Patients should take these agents directly before bedtime and only if they will be able to get at least 4 hours of sleep because they work very quickly (usually in about 20 minutes). However, all patients should be told that unless they plan to get 6 to 8 hours of sleep, they shouldn't be using these agents.

■ Until their effects are known, there may be daytime drowsiness, thus avoiding driving and other hazardous activity is recommended.

■ Patients need to know that prescription sleep aids are for short-term use only (no more than 7 to 10 days) because they have habit-forming features.

■ Any use beyond 2 weeks will likely result in withdrawal symptoms (fatigue, nausea, flushing, uncontrolled crying, nausea, vomiting, GI upset, panic attacks, nervousness) and psychological dependence.

DRUGS USED TO TREAT MIGRAINE HEADACHES

Headache is a very common symptom that presents challenges to every clinician. Headaches, including migraines with or without aura, tension headaches, and cluster headaches are diagnosed primarily by clinical features and exclusion of secondary etiologies.

Migraine headaches are considered a complex condition resulting from the interplay of several factors, but there is a genetic/familial component to them and they affect women two to three times more often than they do men (i.e., men = 0.6%, women = 18%) (Lay & Broner, 2009). Women who report migraines often notice an increased incidence about the time of their menstrual cycle or when taking estrogen-containing oral contraceptives. Alcohol, strong lighting, blinking lights, fatigue, certain foods, and strong smells are other migraine triggers.

There are three categories of **migraines**: migraine with aura (classic migraine), migraine without aura (common migraine), and complicated migraine (migraine associated with focal neurological deficits). Complicated migraines occur in 2% of patients with migraines. Although the classification is important for an accurate diagnosis, the pharmacological management remains the same.

Serotonin levels are usually high before a migraine attack, causing constriction of brain blood vessels and a lowering of the pain threshold. During an attack, serotonin levels drop, resulting

in expansion of the brain's blood vessels and throbbing pain, especially behind the eye. The area around the expanding and contracting blood vessels becomes inflamed and triggers the migraine (Goadsby & Spierings, 2009). This is what led clinicians and researchers to treat migraines with medications such as the triptans, because these serotonin agonists have been found to cause vasoconstriction in large intracranial arteries and thus relieve severe migraine headaches.

Medications are used to either abort the migraine attack or prophylactically to prevent further attack. The goal of therapy is to minimize the impact these headaches have on the patient's quality of life and the patient's ability to work. Simple analgesics such as aspirin, acetaminophen, and NSAIDs are often used first, then therapy progresses to either the triptans or ergotamine. A key distinction is that only migraine headaches respond to triptans and ergotamine; tension (muscle contraction) headaches do not respond to these agents. The conscientious clinician starts by taking a thorough medication history to check for secondary causes of migraine headache. Patients should then be given a trial of a medication to test for side effects and efficacy.

Patient education is a key factor in the treatment of migraine headache, and often the clinician will require the patient to keep a diary of potential triggers to search for specific ones. This process will likely take months. The goal of prophylactic therapy is to minimize triggers such as lights and sounds and migraine incidence by at least 50%. Patients may never be migraine free, but with accurate medication usage they may be able to control the frequency of attacks. For example, rather than take a medication to stop migraine, agents such as topiramate (Topamax) are given on a daily basis as a prophylaxis therapy that reduces the frequency of migraine attacks. The FDA has also approved the beta blockers propanolol (Inderal), timolol (Blocadren), the anticonvulsants divalproex (Depakote), and Botox as agents for the prevention of migraine. If patients have had a stroke and are also experiencing migraines, they should not be placed on beta blockers for migraine prevention. Clinicians can expect research to continue in this area and new therapies to arrive.

Serotonin Receptor Agonists for Migraine Headache

Serotonin receptor agonists, or triptans, constitute a group of agents specifically targeted to relieve the pain, sensitivity to light and noise, and nausea and vomiting associated with migraine, especially if the migraine is moderate or severe. They include almotriptan (Axert), naratriptan (Amerge), rizatriptan (Maxalt), and zolmitriptan (Zomig), which bind to 5-HT-1B and -1D receptors; frovotriptan (Frova) and sumatriptan (Imitrex), which bind to 5HT-1D receptors; and eletriptan (Reelpax), which binds to 5-HT-1B, -1D, and -1F receptors. Compared to older agents, their pharmacology is selective and precise. They vary only in their pharmacokinetic properties and in the ways that individuals respond to them.

Mechanism of Action

Serotonin receptor agonists act selectively on serotonin receptors in cranial arteries, causing vasoconstriction, and they also block the release of vasoactive substance that causes sterile inflammation associated with migraine. The cerebral receptors in cranial arteries that mediate 5-HT–induced vasoconstriction has proven difficult to characterize. but what is known today is that all triptans have an "indole" structure similar in chemistry to that of the neurotransmitter 5-HT agents.

Pharmacokinetics

- Absorption: Onset is quick (about 30 minutes).
- Distribution: Protein binding is minimal.
- Metabolism: Primarily hepatic.
- Excretion: Urine, as an indole acetic metabolite.
- Half-life: Sumatriptan tabs, rizatriptan, zolmitriptan: 2.5 hours; naratriptan, 6 hours.

Dosage and Administration

Generic Name	Trade Name	Route	Usual Adult Daily Dose to Abort a Migraine
sumatriptan	Imitrex	PO, SC, nasal spray	PO 25–100 mg initially, repeat every 2 hr for up to 24 hr. 300 mg/day, 4 headaches per month 6 mg SC or 20 mg via nasal spray
zolmitriptan	Zomig	PO, ODT	2.5 mg initially; repeat in 2 hr if headache returns. Max is 10 mg/24 hr
rizatriptan	Maxalt	PO, ODT	5–10 mg at onset; repeat in 2 hr if needed. Max 30 mg/24 hr
almotriptan	Axert	PO	6.25 or 12.5 mg once; may repeat once in 2 hr
eletriptan	Relpax		20 or 40 mg at onset; may repeat once in 2 hr
naratriptan	Amerge	PO	One 1-mg or 2.5-mg tab at onset; repeat in 4 hr if needed
frovotriptan	Frova	PO	2.5 mg with fluids; may repeat in 3 hr
Combination of 500 mg naproxen and 85 mg sumatriptan	Treximet	PO	No more than 2 tablets in 24 hr

Clinical Use

- Relief of migraine, either to abort an attack or to be used prophylactically

Adverse Reactions

CV: Chest pain, hypotension
DERM: Tingling, warm sensation, flushing
EENT: Vision disturbances
GI: Abdominal discomfort, nausea, vomiting, diarrhea
GU: Hematuria
META: Warm/hot sensations, heaviness, fatigue
MS: Neck/joint/throat and jaw pain
MISC: Injection site reactions
NEURO: Vertigo, paresthesia, dizziness
PUL: Throat discomfort, allergic rhinitis

Interactions

- ALL TRIPTANS CAN INTERACT WITH THE SSRIs, POSSIBLY CAUSING SEROTONIN SYNDROME (for a description of serotonin syndrome, see Chapter 15, Drugs Used in Psychiatric Disorders, p. 277)
- Zolmitriptan and naratriptan interact with oral contraceptives and cimetidine, decreasing the effect of both.
- All triptans interact with MAOIs and should not be used within 2 weeks of discontinuing the MAOI, nor should they be used concurrently.

Contraindications

- All triptans are contraindicated in pregnancy and in patients with ischemic heart disease, cerebral vascular syndromes, or uncontrolled hypertension because of their ability to constrict coronary artery vessels.
- No triptan can be used if ergotamine derivatives have been used in the preceding 24-hour period, because vasospastic reactions may be increased.
- All triptans are contraindicated in complicated migraine.

Conscientious Considerations

- Triptans may be used in children with migraine, but it is always best to have a pediatric consultation first.
- Watch for hypersensitivity reactions. It is always best to administer the first dose of a triptan in the clinician's office so that the clinician can monitor the patient for any adverse cardiovascular event as well as observe the patient's ability to self-administer the medication.

Patient/Family Education

- Triptans should be administered at any sign of an impending migraine attack or during an attack. If the symptoms return, a second dose may be given if there has been at least 1 to 2 hours between doses.
- Patients should not use any more than two doses in any 24-hour period because additional doses are not likely to be effective and could cause side effects.
- Alcohol can aggravate the headache during use of these drugs.
- Patients will need instruction on the proper loading, SC injection, and discarding of the auto injectors.
- Patients should be taught that soreness or redness at the injection site usually lasts about 1 hour.
- If using the intranasal form of administration, the patient should be instructed in proper administration and taught that a dosage interval of greater than 2 hours is needed if the first dose does not produce relief.

The Ergotamines

The alkaloids from the ergot plant have been used for decades to treat vascular migraine headaches because of their vasoconstrictive properties. As a fungus growing on fermented rye plants, it has a history of being used in obstetrics, as a hair restorative, and as a hallucinogen because of its relationship to lysergic acid (LSD). Because chemists have isolated about 80 different types of ergot alkaloids, medicinal ergot is made either by isolation from a natural wheat/rye hybrid plant in fields, as a byproduct from fermenting rye in large vats, or by semisynthesis in a laboratory from its known peptides. Today's pharmaceuticals include ergotamine (Ergostat, Ergomar), ergot with caffeine (Cafergot), and dihydroergotamine (DHE 45, Migranol). They are used in aborting about 70% of migraine headaches if taken very early after symptoms first appear. However, due to their unpredictable oral absorption and adverse effects, their use has been severely curtailed since the triptans came on the market.

Mechanism of Action

The ergotamines act as direct-acting vasoconstrictors that stimulate vascular smooth muscle, leading to a decrease in the amplitude of extra cranial artery pulses and a decrease in the hyperperfusion of the basilar artery area.

Pharmacokinetics

■ Absorption: Oral absorption is erratic, but it is enhanced in the presence of caffeine.
■ Distribution: Widely distributed.
■ Metabolism: Extensively in the liver.
■ Excretion: In feces as inactive metabolite.
■ Half-life: 2 hours.

Dosage and Administration

Generic Name	Trade Name	Route	Usual Adult Daily Dose
ergotamine	Ergostat Ergomar	PO	1 tab sublingually at start of attack; may repeat in 30 min. Max 3 tabs per attack
dihydroergotamine	DHE 45	IV/IM	Inject 1 mg/IM/IV; repeat 1 dose/hr for total 3 mg
	Migranol	Intranasal	1 spray at onset in each nostril. Repeat in 15 min.
ergotamine/ caffeine combination	Cafergot	PO	2 tabs at onset, then 1 tab every 30 min up to 6 per attack.

Clinical Uses

■ To abort or prevent vascular-based headaches, such as migraine

Adverse Reactions

EENT: Rhinitis from nasal spray
GI : Nausea, vomiting
META: Hot flashes
NEURO: Dizziness, somnolence

Interactions

■ Any CYP450 drugs will interfere with ergotamines

Contraindications

■ Pregnancy: Because of their ability to constrict uterine muscle, these drugs are FDA pregnancy category X. The risks clearly outweigh the potential benefits. These drugs should not be used in pregnant women.
■ Uncontrolled hypertension, hemiplegic or basilar migraine, peripheral or cerebral vasoconstrictors, and ischemic heart disease.
■ Do not use with strong/potent CYP3A inhibitors, such as azole antifungals and macrolides.
■ Patients with severe renal impairment.
■ All ergotamines are contraindicated in complicated migraine.

Conscientious Considerations

■ Nausea will often limit the dose or lead to nonadherence, so caution must be exercised when first starting patients on these medications.

Patient/Family Education

■ Drinking grapefruit juice may increase blood levels of the drug, leading to increased toxicity.
■ Avoid coffee, tea, and cola, because caffeine may increase absorption and effects.
■ If an initial dose has failed, repeating the dose rarely mitigates the migraine.

DRUGS USED TO TREAT PARKINSON'S DISEASE

Parkinson's disease (PD) is a chronic, progressive disorder of motor function involving the extrapyramidal system of the brain and particularly basal ganglia. It affects approximately one million Americans, with 60,000 diagnosed yearly. Although the incidence of PD increases with age, 4% of those diagnosed with it are under the age of 50 (Parkinson's Disease Foundation, 2011). The cause of Parkinson's disease remains unknown, and most cases are sporadic, idiopathic, and multifactorial, likely involving genetic predisposition, environmental toxins, aging (when there is a progressive loss of dopamine neurons), and drug-induced cases (iatrogenic).

Degeneration of the dopamine-producing neurons produces a dopamine/acetylcholine imbalance ending in loss of dopamine (an inhibitory neurotransmitter) and an increase in acetylcholine (an excitatory neurotransmitter). This imbalance in neurotransmitters results in the motor function disturbance associated with the disorder—namely, its four classical features:

■ Tremor (a pin-rolling movement involving the thumb and forefinger is usually the first noticeable sign)
■ Muscle rigidity
■ Slowness of movement
■ Postural disturbances

Interestingly, the amounts of other neurotransmitters, such as norepinephrine and serotonin, are also decreased in the brains of patients with Parkinson's disease. According to the National Institute of Neurological Disorders and Stroke (NINDS, 2011), although some people become severely disabled, others experience only minor motor disruptions. Tremor is the major symptom for some patients, whereas for others tremor is only a minor complaint and other symptoms are more troublesome. No one can predict which symptoms will affect an individual patient, and the intensity of the symptoms also varies from person to person. Patients with dementia have a worse prognosis because dementia limits the dosage of medications that could be helpful without exacerbating underlying confusion or psychosis.

No cure is known for Parkinson's disease. Treatment is symptomatic, and a long-term, individualized treatment plan is beset with frequent dosage adjustments because of the chronic and progressive nature of this disease. Clinicians will stage the disease into one of six stages to help with assessment of disease progression relative to treatment regimens. When recommending a course of treatment, a clinician will assess how much the symptoms disrupt the patient's life and then tailor therapy to the person's particular condition. Because no two patients will react the same way to a given drug, it may take time and patience to get the dose just right. Even then, symptoms may not be completely alleviated because most patients' responses to medications are complicated by the development of motor fluctuations and dyskinesias so that age-specific incidence rates increase sharply after age 60 and decline after age 90 (Driver, Logoscino, Gaziano, & Kurth, 2009). Parkinson's disease research remains active, and the U.S. government reports that as of January 2011, 783 clinical trials are ongoing in the United States to find help and hope for the many people who suffer from it.

The observation that the neurotransmitter dopamine is markedly reduced in Parkinson's disease led to the development of its stable precursor, L-dopa. First used as a single agent and then later with a decarboxylase inhibitor (carbidopa and benserazide), L-dopa therapy remains key in the treatment of Parkinson's disease symptoms. L-dopa should be thought of as a treatment that allays symptoms and not a cure. One of the issues with L-dopa is that after using it for several years, it typically loses effectiveness, and/or unwanted side effects (dyskinesias, on-off phenomena) develop. Why there is a progressive degeneration of L-dopa's effectiveness remains unclear. However, newer agents have been introduced to be used as either adjuvants or as monotherapy to help keep dopamine levels level.

Thus, today medications typically used to treat Parkinson's patients include at least five classes of agents:

- Anticholinergic agents: benztropine (Cogentin), and trihexyphenidyl (Artane)
- Dopamine replacement drugs (dopamine precursors): Carbidopa-levodopa (Sinemet)
- Dopamine agonists: Bromocriptine (Parlodel), pramipexole (Mirapex), and ropinirole (Requip)
- COMT inhibitors or catechol-O-methyltransferase inhibitors: Entacapone (Comtan) and Tolcapone (Tasmar)
- MAOB inhibitor: Selegiline (Eldepyrl) and rasagiline (Azilect)

The therapeutic goals of these agents, whether used alone or in combination, is to restore the dopamine/acetylcholine balance back to normal by increasing the supply of dopamine being released, preventing its destruction by enzymes, or protecting the neurotransmitter.

Another goal of these agents is to protect current dopamine ratios **(MAOB inhibitors),** and finally to manage the associated symptoms of Parkinson's disease (anticholinergics, dopamine agonists).

Conscientious Prescribing of Agents for Parkinson's Disease

- These agents need to be used with caution in patients with dysrhythmias, psychoses, peptic ulcer disease, hypertension, and liver function impairment.

- The clinician must monitor symptoms and watch for the on-off syndrome when using these drugs (Box 14-1).

Patient/Family Education Regarding Use of Agents for Parkinson's Disease

- Caregivers of Parkinson's patients need as much as or more support as do patients.
- Caregivers and patients need education on the need for taking these medications exactly as prescribed.
- Patients should be instructed that any missed dose should be taken within 2 hours of the missed dose and not to double up doses if one is missed.

Anticholinergics

Anticholinergics cross the blood-brain barrier to exert a direct inhibitory effect on acetylcholine. They are useful in treating many of the symptoms of Parkinson's disease that can be attributed to having excessive cholinergic activity (muscle rigidity and muscle tone). Anticholinergics have been used for decades to treat Parkinson's disease; however, their usefulness is limited because of their side effects and noticeable drop in effectiveness over time. They are also useful for the patient who has some tremor but little rigidity or bradykinesia. Like cholinergics, they are also used to control salivation and drooling. The anticholinergic drugs used today to treat Parkinson's disease are benztropine (Cogentin) and trihexyphenidyl (Artane).

Mechanism of Action

Anticholinergics block the excitability of central neuron pathways of the parasympathetic nervous pathway so that the

---

BOX 14-1 The On-Off Syndrome

On-off syndrome is a complication typically appearing after 2, or as many as 7, years of levodopa therapy. The patient goes from being totally symptom free to presenting with a sudden onset of severe Parkinson's symptoms. The on-off phenomenon may last minutes, hours, or a few short days. It is believed to be caused by any of the following:

- The dopamine receptors momentarily lose their sensitivity.
- There is a fluctuation in the kinetics of levodopa, especially metabolism.
- A decrease occurs in the central delivery of dopamine.
- A combination of all of these occur.

Treatment typically is to give more levodopa or more carbidopa-levodopa combinations or to add another drug such a dopamine agonist. In some cases, the patient is given a drug holiday—a week or so free of levodopa—in the hopes that when levodopa is again introduced, the patient will have regained dopamine receptors that are sensitive to the drug. The symptoms may worsen during any drug-free holiday, and because many patients needed to be institutionalized during this period, the practice has almost disappeared from use.

dopamine/acetylcholine balance in the brain can return to normal. They also have a direct relaxing effect on smooth musculature, both directly and indirectly, through parasympathetic nervous system inhibition.

Pharmacokinetics

- Absorption: Well absorbed and can act in about an hour
- Distribution: Well distributed and crosses brain-barrier
- Metabolism: Liver
- Excretion: In the urine
- Half-life: 3-4 hours

Dosage and Administration

Generic Name	Trade Name	Route	Usual Adult Daily Dose
benztropine	Cogentin	PO	1–3 mg 1–2 times/day
trihexyphenidyl	Artane	PO	1–2 mg/day increased by 1–2 mg every 3–5 days

Clinical Uses

- As antidyskinesics, to treat drug-induced extrapyramidal effects
- As adjunctive treatment of Parkinson's disease

Adverse Reactions

CV: Tachycardia
DERM: Dry skin, rash, photosensitivities
EENT: Blurry vision, mydriasis, increased IOP, dry eyes
GI: Nausea, vomiting, dysphagia, constipation, dry mouth
GU: Urinary hesitancy, pain on urination, urinary retention
NEURO: Confusion, euphoria, drowsiness, headache, hallucinations, delusions, paranoia

Interactions

- **CNS depressants** of any kind will have additive effects when coadministered with anticholinergics.

Contraindications

- Hypersensitivities
- Narrow-angle glaucoma
- Pyloric/duodenal obstruction
- Prostate hypertrophy or bladder neck obstruction

Conscientious Considerations

- Elderly patients require strict dosage monitoring and regulation.
- Clinicians should monitor patients' IOP.
- In addition, clinicians must be aware of the important considerations that apply to *all* antiparkinson's agents (see p. 256, Conscientious Prescribing of Agents for Parkinson's disease).

Patient/Family Education

- Use with caution during hot weather or during exercise.
- In addition, the clinician must be aware of the advisories that apply to patients taking *any* antiparkinson's agent (see p. 256, Patient/Family Education Regarding the Use of Agents for Parkinson's disease).

Dopamine Agonists

By correcting the imbalance of the brain's dopamine to acetylcholine, dopamine agonists are able to minimize or correct the dyskinesia and tremor associated with early onset of Parkinson's disease. Although effective in the early course of the disease, dopamine agonists are most useful in treating middle-aged patients who have tremors but little rigidity and in whom drooling and salivation need to be controlled. Bromocriptine (Parlodel) is an ergot-derived dopamine agonist; pramipexole (Mirapex) and ropinirole (Requip) are non-ergot derivatives.

Mechanism of Action

Bromocriptine activates postsynaptic dopamine receptors stimulating the production of dopamine. Pergolide also stimulates dopamine receptors but in the nigrostriatal area. Unlike bromocriptine, pergolide acts independently of dopamine synthesis or dopamine storage sites. Pramipexole and ropinerole are non-ergot dopamine receptor agonists, but their exact mechanism of action is not well understood.

Pharmacokinetics

- Absorption: Bromocriptine is only 28% absorbed, with 6% reaching the circulation; the others are well absorbed and serum binding is high.
- Distribution: Well distributed.
- Metabolism: All in the liver.
- Excretion: In urine.
- Half-life: Pramipexole: 8 hours; ropinerole: 6 hours; bromocriptine (biphasic half-life): 4 hours and 15 hours.

Dosage and Administration

Generic Name	Trade Name	Route	Usual Adult Daily Dose for Parkinson's Disease
bromocriptine	Parlodel	PO	1.25 mg 2 times/day, increase by 2.5 mg/day in 2- to 4-week intervals
pramipexole	Mirapex	PO	0.375 mg/day in 3 divided doses; increase gradually by 0.125 mg/dose every 5–7 days
ropinirole	Requip	PO	0.25 mg 3 times/day; increase weekly by 0.75 mg 3 times a day and balance against side effects of nausea, dizziness, somnolence, dyskinesia.

Clinical Uses

- Treatment of Parkinson's disease, either alone or as an adjunctive treatment in combination with carbidopa-levodopa.
- Ropinerole and pramipexole are also used in the treatment of restless leg syndrome.

Adverse Reactions

CV: Hypotension
GI: Nausea, distress, constipation, dry mouth, dyspepsia, tooth disease
GU: Urinary frequency
MS: Leg cramps
NEURO: Drowsiness, weakness, headache, confusion, hallucinations, dizziness, sedation, abnormal dreams, compulsive

gambling, compulsive sex, falling asleep, TARDIVE DYSKINESIA (characterized by uncontrolled movements of body, face, tongue, arms, hand, and head) (see Special Case: Extrapyramidal Syndrome, p. 271, in Chapter 15, Practical Pharmacotherapy of Drugs Used to Treat Psychiatric Disorders, for a description of tardive dyskinesia.)

Interactions

- Concurrent use of **alcohol** may result in a disulfiram-like reaction.
- Use of pramipexole and ropinerole results in increased serum levels in presence of **cimetadine.**
- Concurrent use with **drugs excreted renally** may result in decreases of drug excretion.
- Concurrent use with levodopa increases the risk of hallucinations and dyskinesia.

Contraindications

Sensitivities to ergot alkaloids

Conscientious Considerations

- Use with caution in patients with psychoses, hypertension, liver function impairment, and in the elderly, because these people show increased risk of hallucinations.
- In addition, clinicians must be aware of the important considerations that apply to *all* antiparkinson's agents (see p. 256, Conscientious Prescribing of Agents for Parkinson's disease).

Patient/Family Education

- Patients should be advised to avoid use of alcohol.
- Patients should be advised they may experience drowsiness and unexpected episodes of falling asleep.
- Patients should be advised to change positions slowly to minimize any orthostatic hypotension, which usually occurs in the early days of therapy.
- Female patients should be advised to report if they are pregnant or planning pregnancy.
- Patients may experience nausea at the beginning of therapy, but this usually resolves over time. Administering with meals may minimize the nausea.
- In addition, the clinician must be aware of the advisories that apply to patients taking *any* antiparkinson's agent (see p. 256, Patient/Family Education Regarding the Use of Agents for Parkinson's disease).

Dopamine Precursors

Dopamine precursors, such as levodopa (Larodopa, L-Dopa) and its combination with carbidopa-levodopa (Sinemet) have been used since the1960s to restore the dopamine/acetylcholine balance by resupplying the body with dopamine. Levodopa is a stable form of dopamine and is directly converted to it once it passes through the intestinal wall. It may be used alone or with carbidopa, a decarboxylase inhibitor, to help reduce the dosage required to meet therapeutic levels of levodopa. Carbidopa competes for the enzyme decarboxylase, which helps reduce the peripheral metabolism of levodopa. Carbidopa does not cross the blood-brain barrier; thus

more of the levodopa that crosses into the brain is available to be converted into dopamine. About 50 to 100 mg per day of carbidopa is needed to block the peripheral conversion of levodopa to dopamine. Being able to use a smaller dose of levodopa (20% to 25% less) to achieve therapeutic effects also means patients will have a lower incidence of side effects from the levodopa (nausea, vomiting, cardiac dysrhythmias being common). However, the CNS side effects are greater when more levodopa reaches the brain. Elderly patients usually cannot tolerate the side effects of these drugs (anxiety, paranoia, confusion, hallucinations). Administration of the dopamine precursors begins with low doses and builds over several weeks, as tolerance to side effects also builds.

Mechanism of Action

A small percentage of levodopa enters the brain through the blood-brain barrier intact. It is acted upon by an enzyme that decarboxylates it into dopamine. It can then be used as a neurotransmitter to stimulate dopamine receptors and help restore balance to dopamine and acetylcholine levels. Carbidopa is a dopa decarboxylase inhibitor and prevents peripheral destruction of the levodopa, allowing more per dose to enter the brain.

Pharmacokinetics

- Absorption: Levodopa is well absorbed from the GI tract by active transport. Between 30% to 40% of a dose of levodopa reaches the systemic circulation, and about 40% to 70% of a dose of carbidopa is absorbed.
- Distribution: Levodopa and carbidopa are distributed to most body tissues, but because of peripheral metabolism, only 1% of levodopa reaches the brain and no carbidopa reaches the brain.
- Metabolism: The enzyme dopa decarboxylase converts levodopa to dopamine in the stomach, liver, and intestines.
- Excretion: Both by the kidneys.
- Half-life: The half-life of levodopa is about 50 minutes, but in the presence of carbidopa it may be as long as 90 minutes.

Dosage and Administration

Generic Name	Trade Name	Route	Usual Adult Daily Dose
carbidopa-levodopa	Sinemet, Parcopa	PO carbidopa 10 mg/levodopa 100 mg	Immediate-release tablets of carbidopa 25 mg/levodopa 100 mg; use 3 times/day
	Sinemet CR	PO SR carbidopa 25 mg/levodopa 120 mg	Give 2 times/day at intervals of no less than 6 hr
carbidopa-levodopa/ entacapone	Stalevo	Carbidopa 25 mg/ levodopa 100 mg/ entacapone 200 mg	Individualize the dose and titrate slowly

Clinical Use

- Treatment of idiopathic Parkinson's disease

Adverse Reactions

CV: Orthostatic hypotension, irregular heart rate
DERM: Rash, alopecia, malignant melanoma
GI: Nausea, vomiting (can be severe), anorexia, dry mouth
GU: Difficult urination, discolored urine, increased libido

HEM: Hemolytic anemia, leucopenia, plastic anemia

MISC: Darkening sweat

MS: Involuntary movement of body, face, tongue, head, upper body (note eyelid twitching/spasm is an early sign of overdose)

NEURO: Anxiety, confusion, hallucinations, nervousness, nightmares, depression, mood changes, increased aggressiveness, involuntary movements

PUL: Cough, dyspnea

Interactions

■ Antipsychotics, benzodiazepines, haloperidol, phenytoin, and reserpine have been known to reverse the effects of levodopa and decrease its effectiveness.

■ Additive hypotension may result when given concurrently with antihypertensives.

■ Foods containing kava and pyridoxine will reverse the effect of levodopa.

■ Cocaine and MAOIs may induce a hypertensive crisis when used with levodopa alone. The combination of levodopa with carbidopa helps prevent this.

Contraindications

■ Hypersensitivity
■ Narrow-angle glaucoma
■ Undiagnosed skin lesions
■ Safety for children and during pregnancy have not been established

Conscientious Considerations

■ Because of its adverse effects and poor tolerability, administration begins with low doses and builds over several weeks.

■ Watch the patient for mental or mood changes, which are early signs of overdose, especially in the elderly.

■ Do not use in children under 12 years because dosage is not established.

■ Watch for on off syndrome (see Box 14-1).

■ Titrate upward until desired effect or undesired side effects occur (nausea, GI distress, HTN).

■ Watch for the limiting side effect *altered mental status* (visual hallucinations, paranoia). If this side effect persists at dosage levels needed to control motor symptoms, consider adding an SSRI.

■ Eyelid twitching/spasm is an early sign of overdose.

■ More carbidopa-levodopa is absorbed if it does not compete with dietary protein (amino acids).

■ In addition, clinicians must be aware of the important considerations that apply to *all* antiparkinson's agents (see p. 256, Conscientious Prescribing of Agents for Parkinson's disease).

Patient/Family Education

■ Watch for mental or mood changes as early signs of overdose, especially in the elderly, and report them to the clinician.

■ Take medication exactly as instructed.

■ Eating food immediately after administration of a dose may alleviate gastric irritation, but high-protein foods will impair the effects of levodopa.

■ Avoid driving or using machinery until response to the medication is known because drowsiness or dizziness is likely to occur.

■ Frequent oral rinses, good mouth hygiene, and chewing sugarless gum are helpful for dry mouth.

■ Monitor any skin lesions for changes because carbidopa-levodopa may activate malignant melanoma.

■ Large amounts of pyridoxine (vitamin B) supplements may inactivate levodopa.

■ Darkening of urine or sweat is a harmless reaction.

■ In addition, the clinician must be aware of the advisories that apply to patients taking *any* antiparkinson's agent (see p. 256, Patient/Family Education Regarding the Use of Agents for Parkinson's disease).

Catechol-o-Methyltransferase (COMT) Inhibitor

Tolcapone (Tasmar) and entacapone (Comtan) were approved by the FDA in 1998 as a new class of drugs used to treat PD. These drugs are catechol-O-methyltransferase (COMT) inhibitors, which means they metabolize catechol compounds (such as dopamine and levodopa), converting them into inactive compounds. Because COMT is present in the periphery as well as the CNS, inhibition of peripheral COMT results in an increase in the plasma level of levodopa, thereby making more available for transfer into the brain and raising levels of it there.

Mechanism of Action

These agents are reversible, and they are selective inhibitors of catechol-O-methyltransferase (COMT). When they are taken as adjuncts with levodopa, the pharmacokinetics of the levodopa are altered, resulting in higher and more sustained serum levels of levodopa. The resulting sustained levels of levodopa provide increased levels available to cross the blood-brain barrier, thus providing increased levels of dopamine, the active metabolite of the levodopa.

Pharmacokinetics

■ Absorption: Very rapid
■ Distribution: Well distributed; bound to protein
■ Metabolism: Through glucuronidation in the liver
■ Elimination: In the feces
■ Half-life: 0.4 to 0.7 hours

Dosage and Administration

Generic Name	Trade Name	Route	Usual Adult Daily Dose
tolcapone	Tasmar	PO	100 mg 3 times/day; may increase up to 200 mg 3 times/day
entacapone	Comtan	PO	200 mg taken with each dose of carbidopa-levodopa

Clinical Uses

■ Used as an adjunct to carbidopa-levodopa therapy in patients with Parkinson's disease who experience a wearing off of the effects of carbidopa-levodopa (called fluctuating patients) following a long course of therapy

Adverse Reactions

CV: Orthostatic hypotension, syncope
DERM: Alopecia, rash
EENT: Cataracts, tinnitus
GI: Nausea, anorexia, diarrhea, flatulence, tooth disorders, transaminase increases
MS: Rhabdomyolysis, muscle cramps
NEURO: Sleep disorders, excessive dreaming, dizziness, headache, confusion, dyskinesia, dystonia, NEUROLEPTIC MALIGNANT SYNDROME
PUL: Upper respiratory infections

Interactions

■ Effects of these agents on mental status may be additive in the presence of **CNS depressants** and **hypnotics.**
■ Concurrent use with selective MAOIs is not advised because both agents inhibit metabolic pathways of catecholamine.
■ Other drugs that are metabolized by COMT, such as isoproterenol, epinephrine, dopamine, and methyldopa may increase the risk of tachycardia, elevated blood pressure, and arrhythmias.

Contraindications

■ Hypersensitivities.
■ The FDA has issued a **black box warning** that tolcapone (Tasmar) should be used with caution and held in reserve for those with inadequate responses to other antiparkinson's drugs, owing to the potential to develop fatal liver toxicities.
■ Safety in children, pregnancy, and lactation has not been established.

Conscientious Considerations

■ Tolcapone should only be used in patients who do not respond to other therapy because they can cause fatal hepatotoxicities (clinicians need to closely monitor liver enzymes for signs of hepatic change).
■ In addition, clinicians must be aware of the important considerations that apply to *all* antiparkinson's agents (see p. 256, Conscientious Prescribing of Agents for Parkinson's Disease).

Patient/Family Education

■ Patients need to be instructed that liver enzymes, blood pressure, and Parkinson's symptoms must be closely monitored for the first 6 months of therapy.
■ Patients can take these medications without or without food.
■ Educate patients that nausea may occur at initiation of therapy and that urine may change to a brownish-orange.
■ Patients should be advised to avoid alcohol because CNS effects such as drowsiness may increase.
■ **In addition, the clinician must be aware of the advisories that apply to patients taking *any* antiparkinson's agent (see p. 256, Patient/Family Education Regarding the Use of Agents for Parkinson's Disease).**

Selegiline (Eldepryl, Carbex)

Selegiline (Eldepryl, Carbex) is a selective monoamine oxidase B (MAOB) inhibitor that may prevent the progression of Parkinson's disease by serving as a neuroprotectant. Selegiline is also used in conjunction with carbidopa-levodopa in later stage Parkinsonism to reduce levodopa dosage requirements and to minimize or delay the onset of dyskinesias and motor fluctuations that typically accompany long-term use of levodopa.

Mechanism of Action

Because selegiline prevents the breakdown of dopamine (by blocking MAOB enzyme), it makes more dopamine available at the synapse at doses of 10 mg per day or less. It is believed that selegiline slows the progression of PD by reducing the formation of toxic free radicals produced during the metabolism of dopamine.

Pharmacokinetics

■ Absorption: Oral absorption occurs within an hour, but drug has low bioavailability once bound to plasma proteins
■ Distribution: Well distributed, but highly bound to plasma protein
■ Metabolism: Hepatic by CYP 2B6 isoenzymes
■ Excretion: As inactive metabolites in the urine
■ Half-life: 1.5 to 2 hours

Dosage and Administration

Generic Name	Trade Name	Route	Usual Adult Daily Dose
selegiline	Eldepryl, Carbex	Oral tab	Either 5 mg 2 times/day with breakfast or lunch, or 10 mg in the morning
	Zelapar	Oral disintegrating tablet	1.25 mg, place on tongue and let dissolve. Note: Reduce the patient's carbidopa-levodopa dosages several weeks after starting selegiline or rasagiline.

Clinical Use

■ To manage Parkinson's disease as an adjunct to carbidopa-levodopa in those patients who fail to respond to carbidopa-levodopa alone or may be used prior to beginning carbidopa-levodopa therapy.

Adverse Reactions

CNS: Agitation, COMA, confusion, dizziness, delirium, fainting, hallucinations, insomnia, vivid dreams
GI: Nausea, dry mouth, abdominal pain

Interactions

■ Selegiline should not be taken with meperidine (Demerol), dextromethorphan, MAOIs, methadone, propoxyphene, or tramadol because a serious drug interaction occurs, resulting in stupor, muscle rigidity, elevated temperature, agitation, muscle rigidity, or death.
■ Selegiline should not be given with TCAs or SSRIs because of the possibility of developing serotonin syndrome.

Contraindications

■ Hypersensitivity.
■ Concurrent use of opioid or meperidine may lead to fatal reactions.

Conscientious Considerations

■ Clinicians need to consider selegiline as an agent to be used only when patients fail to respond to carbidopa-levodopa therapy alone.
■ Clinicians should consult the medication guides available from the FDA, especially if this drug is to be used in children and adolescents.
■ Doses of greater than 10 mg per day increase the risk of hypertensive reactions should the patient be ingesting foods high in tyramine.
■ **In addition, clinicians must be aware of the important considerations that apply to *all* antiparkinson's agents (see p. 256, Conscientious Prescribing of Agents for Parkinson's Disease).**

Patient/Family Education

■ Patients should be shown how to place the tablet on top of the tongue and let it dissolve and be reminded to not eat or drink 5 minutes before.
■ Patients should be advised that selegiline 5 mg should be taken at breakfast, and if taking 10 mg, then take 5 mg at breakfast and 5 mg at lunch so that optimum blood levels can occur due to selegiline's low oral bioavailability.
■ Patients need to avoid tyramine-containing foods and beverages (e.g., aged cheese, red wine, cured meats, tap beer, sauerkraut, soy).
■ Patients and caregivers need to be informed of the signs and symptoms of selegiline overdose (hypertensive crisis, vomiting, photosensitivity, enlarged pupils).
■ Patients should inform their clinician if they experience new or increased gambling urges, increased sexual urges, or other intense urges while taking selegiline. Clinicians should consider dose reduction or stopping the medication if a patient develops such urges while taking selegiline.
■ In addition, the clinician must be aware of the advisories that apply to patients taking *any* antiparkinson's agent (see p. 256, Patient/Family Education Regarding the Use of Agents for Parkinson's Disease).

DRUGS USED TO TREAT ALZHEIMER'S DISEASE

Named after Aloysius "Alois" Alzheimer who described this disease in 1907, **Alzheimer's disease (AD)** is a gradually progressing dementia affecting both cognition and behavior. It is not a disease of the elderly because persons as young as 40 have suffered from early onset, and today 5.3 million Americans suffer from it (Alzheimer's Association, 2011). It is the sixth leading cause of death in the United States. It affects females twice as often as it does men (Alzheimer's Association, 2011).

The definitive causes of Alzheimer's disease remain unknown, but it is characterized by a buildup of proteins in the brain. These brain proteins can now be measured in the spinal fluid in living patients. Deposits of the protein beta-amyloid accumulate in the spaces between nerve cells as plaques. Neurofibrillary tangles are deposits of Tau protein that accumulate inside nerve cells. What beta-amyloid plaques and tangles do remains theoretical, but many scientists believe they block the ability of nerve cells to communicate with each other, thus making it difficult for the cells to survive. The probability of being diagnosed with Alzheimer's disease nearly doubles every 5 years after age 65. Family history plays a role; the probability of developing AD is two or three times higher if a parent or sibling developed it (NIA, 2010). A genetic test is now available for the ApoE allele to see if a patient has a genetic type of dementia.

Prognosis for survival of Alzheimer's disease is such that patients can live as little as 3 years (average 8 years) to as long as 20 years. For those with longer survival rates, the costs of medical care can be staggering (Health-cares.net, 2005).

The expected rise in prevalence rates of Alzheimer's disease over the next several decades has generated a great deal of attention at all levels of society, including governmental and scientific communities. These concerns have resulted in a vast number of research studies; however, treatment still focuses primarily on the symptomatic relief of the cognitive, neuropsychiatric, and behavioral alterations thought to be part of the underlying pathology of the disease. The American College of Physicians recently published clinical practice guidelines with recommendations for pharmacological treatment in the patient with AD (Qaseem et al., 2008). The document emphasizes an individualized approach to pharmaceutical therapy based on evaluating the benefits and risks of treatment as well as the ease of use, adverse effect profile, patient tolerability, and cost of medication. For patients with mild-to-moderate AD, cholinesterase inhibitors have the strongest evidence of being effective in treating cognitive symptoms. Because a primary pathology of AD is a deficiency in acetylcholine, agents in this category exert their pharmacological effect by inhibiting the enzyme acetyl cholinesterase, reducing the hydrolysis of acetylcholine, and subsequently increasing levels of acetylcholine available in the synaptic space.

Since 1993, few new drugs have been marketed for the treatment of AD, and those that have entered the market are regarded as having only symptomatic rather than disease-modifying effects. For example, tacrine (Cognex) is no longer a drug in favor because of its side effects (hepatotoxicity) and because any benefits seem to disappear after about 30 weeks. Although donepezil (Aricept), rivastigmine (Exelon), and galantamine (Razadyne) have been approved by the FDA, there is no strong clinical evidence that one agent is superior in efficacy to another. The benefits of galantamine and rivastigmine, which are approved for mild-to-moderate AD, last only about 2 years. Memantine is approved for moderate-to-severe AD. The drugs currently used to treat AD demonstrate modest benefits on patient cognitive and functional scales, and this may translate into improvement in the patient's daily life. The medications, especially the combination of one of the cholinesterase inhibitors with memantine, can significantly extend the time before a patient requires care in an institutional setting such as a nursing home.

The Agency for Healthcare Research and Quality guidelines (AHRQ, 2009) ask clinicians to use pharmacological interventions only when nonpharmacological interventions are not working and then to make choices based on the symptoms that are being targeted because adverse effects of drugs may be serious and significant. One nonpharmacological intervention is the preparation caprylidine (Axona), which is a prescription medicinal food made of caprylic triglycerides. Axona is prescribed to combat the well-documented decline in glucose metabolism that occurs in Alzheimer's disease. When taken once a day, caprylidine is converted in the liver to ketone bodies that provide an efficient source of fuel for brain cells suffering from glucose hypometabolism. Patients taking Axona have shown real cognitive improvement (Henderson et al., 2009).

Conscientious Prescribing of Antidementia Agents

■ It is important to remember that the higher the dose, the higher the risk for adverse events and reactions.

■ Treatment must include both pharmacological and non-pharmacological approaches because of the profound effect this disease has on the patient and the family.

■ Patients may also need secondary medications to control depression, psychosis, and agitation.

■ With all agents, the most common adverse event is GI complaints, which can often be alleviated by dosage reductions.

Patient/Family Education Regarding the Use of Antidementia Agents

■ All of the drugs used in AD must be taken exactly as prescribed, and doses should not be skipped or doubled if one is missed.

■ Increasing the dose may not improve symptoms, and may, in fact, only increase side effects, especially dizziness and GI upset.

■ Abrupt discontinuance of any of these drugs is likely to induce a decrease in cognitive functioning as soon as the drug's effect wears off. Lost cognitive function cannot be completely regained by restarting the medication.

■ Safety measures to prevent falls should be taken because the patient may experience dizziness.

■ Administration with food may mitigate GI upset with donepezil and tacrine.

■ Rivastigmine should be given *with* food, whereas memantine and galantamine can be given with or without food.

■ Patients should be advised to notify their clinician if nausea, vomiting, diarrhea, or changes in the color of stool occur or if new symptoms appear.

■ Patients and caregivers need to know their treatment is not a cure but rather a means to control symptoms and improve cognition. They need to understand that slowing the decline in cognitive function is a treatment success, even though the memory continues to worsen.

■ Advise patients to wear a MedicAlert-type bracelet that identifies their disease and the medications they are taking.

■ Beginning with the time of diagnosis, families need to be involved in decisions regarding course of treatment, options of treatment, legal decisions, and quality of life to minimize the stress on every person involved.

■ Caregivers must be prepared to accept and face the changes that will occur in their loved ones. Encourage caregivers to take part in a support group and counseling as soon as possible.

Acetylcholinesterase Inhibitors

Patients with AD show reduction in cerebral choline acetyl transferase. This in turn leads to a decrease in acetylcholine synthesis and impaired cortical cholinergic function. This early discovery of a marked cholinergic deficit in the brains of patients with AD led to research designed to therapeutically augment cholinergic activity. Early studies failed to demonstrate that using acetylcholine precursors would augment cholinergic activity. A second line of research led to agents that could block acetylcholinesterase at the postsynaptic cleft, but these agents had too many side effects to become marketable. Research focused on cholinesterase inhibitors, which increase cholinergic transmission by inhibiting cholinesterase at the synaptic cleft, led to FDA approval of four cholinesterase inhibitors—tacrine, donepezil, rivastigmine, and galantamine—for use in AD.

Mechanism of Action

These agents are reversible, noncompetitive, centrally acting acetylcholinesterase inhibitors, which means they impede the breakdown of what little acetylcholine remains in the brain of an AD patient. By inhibiting this enzyme, the drug permits accumulation of acetylcholine in the brain. Donepezil has the longest-acting profile, permitting it to be used as once-a-day dosing.

Pharmacokinetics

■ Absorption: **Donepezil:** Has complete bioavailability with 96% protein binding. **Tacrine:** Has poor bioavailability, made worse by meals; short half-life requires it a four-times-a-day dosing. **Galantamine:** Absorption is rapid and complete. **Rivastigmine:** Also rapidly absorbed.

■ Distribution: Primarily to albumin; levels in brain are two to three times higher than serum.

■ Metabolism: **Donepezil:** Metabolized in the liver to four metabolites, two of which are active. **Tacrine:** Metabolized in the liver to multiple inactive metabolites. **Galantamine:** Metabolized in the liver to two inactive metabolites. **Rivastigmine:** Undergoes some metabolism in the brain, but mostly hepatic to an inactive metabolite.

■ Excretion: All metabolites excreted primarily by the kidneys into the urine.

■ Half-life: Tacrine: 1 to 4 hours; **donepezil:** 70 hours; **galantamine:** 7 hours; **rivastigmine:** 1.5 hours.

Dosage and Administration

Generic Name	Trade Name	Route	Usual Adult Daily Dose
donepezil	Aricept	PO	5 mg daily at bedtime for 1 week, if tolerated; may take 10 mg/day for mild to moderate to severe Alzheimer's dementia; dose may be increased after 4 months to 23 mg once daily for moderate to severe Alzheimer's dementia
tacrine	Cognex	PO	10 mg 4 times/day between meals for 4–6 weeks, then may titrate upward at 4-week intervals up to a max of 160 mg/day, depending on results of alanine aminotransferase (ALT) testing
galantamine	Razadyne, Reminyl	PO	4 mg daily with meals; increase to 8 mg daily after 4 weeks. If tolerated, increase up to 12 mg daily, thereafter
rivastigmine	Exelon	PO	1.5 mg in a.m. and p.m. with food; increase to 3 mg 2 times/day after 2 weeks if tolerated, then titrate up to 4.5 and 6 mg 2 times/day after 2-week intervals

Clinical Use

■ Symptomatic treatment of mild to moderate dementia of the Alzheimer type

Adverse Reactions

Note: All of these adverse reactions are the result of having too much acetylcholine (ACh) in the CNS.
CV: Bradycardia, hypertension
DERM: Red scaly itching skin, bruising of skin
EENT: Miosis, increased tears
GI: Increased secretions, abdominal cramps, nausea, vomiting, diarrhea, loss of appetite, weight loss, HEPATOTOXICITY with tacrine requiring routine testing of patient's ALT
GU: Frequent urination
MS; Muscle aches/cramps, joint pain
NEURO: Abnormal dreams, dizziness, headache, nervousness, confusion, changes in behavior
PUL: Excessive secretion in lungs, bronchospasm, cough

Interactions

■ These drugs are metabolized by the CYP-450 system, thus drug levels and effects may be altered by other drugs that affect this metabolic pathway, especially theophylline levels, to a risk of toxicity.
■ Alcohol may increase risk of sedation as well as GI irritation.

Contraindications

■ Avoid in people with hypersensitivities
■ Use cautiously in people with a history or risk of GI bleed or are using NSAIDs

Conscientious Considerations

■ Use cautiously in patients with a history of asthma, COPD, convulsions, liver impairment, urinary tract obstructions, cardiac disease, history of ulcers, use of NSAIDs.

■ Overdosage may bring on a *cholinergic crisis* with dangerously high levels of acetylcholine, which can cause symptoms such as slowed heart rate and low blood pressure, leading to fainting and muscle weakness. Also, patients may experience respiratory depression, salivation, sweating, and vomiting.
■ **In addition, clinicians must be aware of the important considerations that apply to *all* antidementia agents (see p. 262, Conscientious Prescribing of Antidementia Agents).**

Patient/Family Education

■ Patients, families, and caregivers should be told:
　■ Drugs used to treat Alzheimer's disease are not a cure, but are treatments only to delay progression.
　■ Any improvement seen with these drugs may be so modest so that family members and patients may not see any benefit at all.
　■ All drugs used to treat Alzheimer's disease are expensive.
　■ There are no serious risks associated with medications for Alzheimer's disease but side effects may be troublesome (nausea, vomiting, diarrhea, indigestion, loss of appetite).
　■ If cholinesterase inhibitors are used there is an increased risk of GI bleed.
　■ Treating Alzheimer's disease symptoms may be a better plan in some cases, but this also brings the risk of side effects, thus it is a choice that should be delayed as long as possible.
　■ If the Alzheimer's disease is moderate to severe, drugs such as nemantine (Nemand) may be used but it will only delay progression for about 1 year.
■ Clinicians must be aware of the advisories that apply to patients taking *any* antidementia agent (see p. 262, Patient/Family Education Regarding the Use of Antidementia Agents).

NMDA Receptor Agonist

Memantine (Namenda) is an N-methyl-D-aspartate receptor (NMDA) antagonist. Memantine has been approved for moderate to severe Alzheimer's disease. It is a noncompetitive inhibitor of NMDA receptors located throughout the brain. Memantine is well tolerated and causes a moderate decrease in the clinical deterioration seen in moderate to severe Alzheimer's disease.

Mechanism of Action

Memantine owes its mechanism of action to the role it plays in the regulation of glutamate receptors found throughout the brain. Glutamate is an excitatory amino acid in the CNS that is involved in information processing, storage, and retrieval. Glutamate plays an essential role in learning and memory by how it triggers NMDA receptors of nerve cells to allow a controlled amount of calcium ions to flow into and out of nerve cells, creating the environment for storage of information. If excessive amounts of glutamate exist, these receptors are overstimulated, and the resulting neurotoxicity allows too much calcium to flow into nerve cells, leading to disruption and cell death. Memantine attaches to the NMDA receptors and protects them from the overstimulation caused by excessive glutamate.

Pharmacokinetics

- Absorption: Completely from the GI tract with 100% bioavailability.
- Distribution: Rapidly passes the blood-brain barrier and CNS in under 30 minutes while being 45% protein bound.
- Metabolism: Metabolized by glucuronidation, hydroxylation, and N-oxidation to inactive metabolites. CYP-450 plays no role.
- Excretion: As a glucuronide in the urine.
- Half-life: 60 to 80 hours.

Dosage and Administration

Generic Name	Trade Name	Route	Usual Adult Daily Dose
memantine (tabs/oral solution)	Namenda, Namenda XR	PO	5 mg once a day, with a target dose of 20 mg/day; titrate initial dose up by 5 mg/week.

Clinical Use

- Treatment of moderate to severe dementia of the Alzheimer type

Adverse Reactions

CV: Hypertension, cardiac failure, AV BLOCK
DERM: Rash, STEVENS JOHNSON SYNDROME
EENT: Cataracts, conjunctivitis
GI: Constipation, vomiting, LIVER FAILURE
GU: Frequent micturition
MISC: Fatigue, pain
MS: Back pain
NEURO: Confusion, somnolence, hallucinations, dizziness, TARDIVE DYSKINESIA
PUL: Coughing, dyspnea

Interactions

- Clearance of memantine is decreased at urinary pH of 8 or higher (alkaline), and at that level it is decreased by as much as 80%. **Drugs that raise urinary pH** (e.g., sodium bicarbonate) therefore should be avoided.

Contraindications

- Known hypersensitivity to memantine HCl or to any of its excipients

Conscientious Considerations

- The combined use of memantine with other NMDA antagonists (amantadine, ketamine, and dextromethorphan) has not been systematically evaluated and such use should be approached with caution.
- It is not known whether memantine is excreted in human breast milk. Because many drugs are excreted in human milk, caution should be exercised when memantine is administered to a nursing mother.
- There are no adequate and well-controlled studies of memantine being used in in pregnant women. Thus, memantine should be used during pregnancy only if the benefits outweigh the risks to the fetus.

- Because the clearance of memantine is reduced by about 80% under alkaline urine conditions at pH 8, alterations of urine pH toward the alkaline condition may lead to an accumulation of the drug with a possible increase in adverse effects. Urine pH is altered by diet, drugs (e.g., carbonic anhydrase inhibitors, sodium bicarbonate), and the clinical state of the patient (e.g., renal tubular acidosis or severe infections of the urinary tract). Memantine should therefore be used with caution under these conditions.
- This drug has not been studied properly in patients who have seizure disorders.
- In patients with renal insufficiency, dosage adjustment is needed for estimated creatinine clearance of 29 mL/min or less.
- Patients and their caregivers particularly require assurances and support throughout the treatment of moderate to severe AD.
- **In addition, clinicians must be aware of the important considerations that apply to *all* antidementia agents (see p. 262, Conscientious Prescribing of Agents for Antidementia drugs).**

Patient/Family Education

- There are no dietary restriction on the use of this drug, and it may or may not be taken with food.
- Patients should be advised dosages will likely go up as therapy continues and to monitor for any side effects.
- **In addition, the clinician must be aware of the advisories that apply to patients taking *any* antidementia agents (see p. 262, Patient/Family Education Regarding the Use of Agents for Antidementia drugs).**

DRUG TREATMENT OF MULTIPLE SCLEROSIS

Multiple sclerosis is the most common cause of chronic neurological disability in young adults, causing about half of them to be unable to walk without assistance about 15 years after onset of the disease. However, no drug treatment can halt its impact on disability despite progress in understanding the disease's underlying pathology. The FDA-approved medications (disease-modifying drugs) are able to generate favorable outcomes on the progression of the disease but are far from being a cure. Many other drugs are used to treat patients for their symptoms and rehabilitation.

An exacerbation of MS (also known as a relapse, attack, or flare-up) causes new symptoms to appear or cause a worsening set of old symptoms. Exacerbations can range from being mild to severe, but usually they interfere with home and work functioning, with no two exacerbations being alike. Exacerbations such as optic neuritis, issues with impaired balance and walking (e.g., footdrop), or severe fatigue may appear individually or as multiple symptoms. To be called a MS exacerbation, the attack must last at least 24 hours and be separated from the previous attack by at least 30 days. Most exacerbations last from a few days to several weeks or even months.

A number of disease-modifying drugs have been shown to slow disease activity and the progression of MS and its exacerbations in relapsing form of MS, including those with secondary progressive diseases, but there is no one drug that works all the time in one person. Treatments include interferon beta-1a (Avonex, Rebif), interferon beta-1b (Betaseron, Extavia), glatiramer acetate (Copaxone), mitoxantrone (Novantrone), natalizumab (Tysabri), and fingolimod (Gilenya) (Table 14-3).

Treatment of multiple sclerosis is complex because there is no known cause for why the myelin sheath on nerves develops plaques and breaks down nerve transmission. The FDA-approved drugs work by suppressing or altering the activity of the body's immune system. Thus, these therapies are based on the theory that MS is, at least in part, a result of an abnormal response.

TREATMENT OF PERIPHERAL NEUROPATHIES

The term *peripheral neuropathy* is used to describe damage to the peripheral nervous system. There are more than 100 types of peripheral neuropathies, each with its own defining set of symptoms, patterns of development, and prognosis. Clinical signs and symptoms depend on the type of nerves that are damaged, that is, motor, sensory, or autonomic. Whereas some patients may experience temporary numbness, tingling, pricking sensations, sensitivity to touch, or muscle weakness, others may experience pain (especially at night), muscle wasting, paralysis, or organ/gland dysfunction.

Peripheral neuropathy may be either inherited or acquired (trauma, tumors, toxins, autoimmune responses, nutritional deficiencies, alcoholism, and vascular and metabolic disorders). Acquired peripheral neuropathies are caused by systemic diseases such as diabetes or autoimmune disorders affecting nerve tissue. Inherited forms of peripheral neuropathy are caused by inborn errors in genetic coding or by new genetic mutation. Many types of medications can be used to relieve the pain of peripheral neuropathy, but there is no cure, especially for inherited neuropathies (NIH, 2011) (Table 14-4). When the patient has a diabetic neuropathy, the first goal of treatment is to get blood glucose under control to prevent further deterioration.

TABLE 14-3 Drug Treatment of Multiple Sclerosis

NAME OF DRUG (GENERIC, TRADE)	WHEN USED	HOW ADMINISTERED	FREQUENCY OF ADMINISTRATION	COMMON SIDE EFFECTS
interferon beta-1a (Avonex, Rebif)	Relapsing-remitting MS, secondary progressive MS	IM, SC	30 mcg IM once/week self-injection 44 mcg SC, 3 times/week self-administered	Mild flu-like symptoms
interferon beta-1b (Betaseron, Betaferon, Extavia)	Relapsing-remitting MS, secondary progressive MS	SC	30 mcg SC injection once every 2 days	Mild flu-like symptoms
glatiramer acetate (Copaxone)	Relapsing-remitting MS	SC	20 mg SC as daily self-injection	Possible reaction at injection site
mitoxantrone (Novantrone)	Rapidly worsening relapsing-remitting MS and for progressive-relapsing MS	IV	12 mg/M² once every 3 months or 4 times/year	Nausea, thinning hair Decreases in WBC counts
natalizumab (Tysabri)	Relapsing forms of MS	IV	300 mg infused over 1 hr every 4 weeks	Headache, lethargy, joint pain
fingolimod (Gilenya)	Relapsing-remitting MS	PO	0.5 mg as a daily pill	Eye toxicity, increased risk of infection

TABLE 14-4 Medications for Peripheral Neuropathies

CATEGORY	ACTION
PAIN RELIEVERS	Mild symptoms of pain may be relieved by over-the-counter pain medications such as acetaminophen or NSAIDs. Severe symptoms require agents as strong as the opioids, with all their inherent adverse effects.
ANTICONVULSANT DRUGS	gabapentin (Gralise, Neurontin), topiramate (Topamax), pregabalin (Lyrica), carbamazepine (Carbatrol, Tegretol), and phenytoin (Dilantin, Phenytek) treat neuropathies. However, there are many adverse effects such as drowsiness and dizziness.
WARMING AGENTS	Derived from hot peppers, capsaicin when formulated as a cream is applied to alleviate foot neuropathies and may cause modest improvements of peripheral neuropathy. Some patients have trouble getting used to its warming sensation.

Continued

TABLE 14-4 Medications for Peripheral Neuropathies—cont'd

CATEGORY	ACTION
TOPICAL ANESTHETICS	Lidocaine in a patch dosage form brings relief to many because of its action as a topical anesthetic. Apply up to 4 patches a day to relieve pain. It has no side effects. However, it may cause a rash at the site to which it is applied.
TRICYCLIC ANTIDEPRESSANTS	amitriptyline (Elavil) and nortriptyline (Aventyl, Pamelor) relieve pain by interfering with serotonin and norepinephrine and diminish the sensation of pain. One popular agent used today is the serotonin and norepinephrine reuptake inhibitor duloxetine (Cymbalta). It is effective when the peripheral neuropathy is caused by diabetes.
TRANSCUTANEOUS ELECTRICAL NERVE STIMULATION (TENS)	Although not a drug therapy, electrical stimulation of nerves for pain control is centuries old. TENS is used to relieve peripheral neuropathy symptoms by placing electrodes onto the skin and delivering a small gentle electric current at varying frequencies onto the skin in an attempt to stimulate nerve transmission. For any effectiveness to be achieved it needs to be done regularly and at frequencies that are either below motor contraction or at a frequency that does produce motor contraction.

IMPLICATIONS FOR SPECIAL POPULATIONS

Pregnancy Implications

When prescribing for the pregnant female, clinicians should carefully consider their choice of drugs. Following is a selected list of drugs used in treating CNS disorders along with their assigned FDA safety category.

FDA PREGNANCY SAFETY CATEGORY	DRUGS
B	memantine (Namenda), bromocriptine (Parlodel), pergolide (Permax), pramipexole (Mirapex), ropinirole (Requip)
C	benzphetamine (Didrex), diethylpropion (Tenuate), mazindol (Mazinor), phendimetrazine (Bontril), phentermine (Adipex), ethosuximide (Zarontin), eszopiclone (Lunesta), zolpidem (Ambien), zalepon (Sonata), almotriptan (Axert), eletriptan (Relpax), frovotriptan (Frova), sumatriptan (Imitrex), naratriptan (Amerge), rizatriptan (Maxalt), zolmitriptan (Zomig), benztropine (Cogentin), trihexyphenidyl (Artane), carbidopa-levodopa (Sinemet), entacapone, tolcapone (Tasmar), selegiline (Eldepyrl), donapezil, galantamine, rivastigmine
D	phenytoin (Dilantin), fosphenytoin (Cerebyx), carbamazepine (Tegretol), oxcarbazepine (Trileptal)
X	ergotamine (Ergostat), ergot with caffeine (Cafergot), dihydroergotamine (DHE 45, Migranol)

LEARNING EXERCISES

Case 1

Mrs. P.T. is a 75-year-old widowed white female brought to your office by her two daughters with the complaint of memory loss over the past 2 years. She had been independent until experiencing a stroke 2 years ago; since then, "it has been a struggle." She has trouble remembering people's names and finding appropriate words. She has had progressive difficulties with organization and planning. Her elder daughter needs to help her grocery shop, pay bills, and balance her checkbook. The patient has lost interest in daily activities, and she is less able to concentrate and see tasks through to completion. She has no residual motor deficits from her ischemic CVA. She takes Prinzide 20/25 twice daily for hypertension, fluoxetine 20 mg daily for depression, Ditropan XL 15 mg daily for overactive bladder, Caltrate D two tablets daily, baby aspirin 81 mg (1 tablet) daily, and Centrum Silver 1 tablet daily. Her husband died 4 years ago, and the elder daughter notes that she is drinking more vodka now, going through a quart every week and a half or so. There is no known family history of AD.

On examination, she is an awake, alert, pleasant, frail-appearing woman in no acute distress. No clinical signs of malnutrition or dehydration are noted. She appears indifferent and confabulates during the interview. She has obvious short-term memory deficits and has difficulty following complex instructions. Mini Mental Status Exam (MMSE) score is 21.

1. What are your clinical impressions of this patient?

2. What are appropriate medical approaches to treat Mrs. P.T.?

3. How would you treat behavioral disturbances in patients with AD?

Case 2

A 32-year-old married woman presents with severe headache, nausea, and vomiting. Her headache started 24 hours ago as a mild tightness behind her eyes and in her neck, then the pain gradually became more intense, throbbing, and localized to the right forehead region. Her pain is exacerbated by loud sounds, bright light, and moving her head. Tylenol and Advil have not helped. She has experienced similar headaches lasting 2 to 3 days on four prior occasions. She reports having tension headaches weekly since age 20. She has never sought medical care for her headaches until today.

Upon entering the examination room, you observe her to be lying in the fetal position on the examination table in a dark room. She appears to be in obvious distress due to her pain. Her face is pale and she is holding an emesis basin.

1. **What are your clinical impressions of this woman?**

2. **How would you treat this woman's headache? Provide a rationale to support your management decisions.**

3. **Identify appropriate options to prevent recurrence of migraine headache. Which agents should be avoided in pregnant women?**

References

Agency for Healthcare Research and Quality (AHRQ). National Guideline Clearinghouse (2009). Guideline for Alzheimer's disease management. Retrieved February 5, 2013, from www.guideline.gov/content.aspx?id=12691

Alzheimer's Association. (2011). Alzheimer's Facts and Figures. Available at www.alz.org/alzheimers_disease_facts_and_figures.asp#key

Driver, J., Logroscino, G., Gaziano, J. M., & Kurth, T. (2009). Incidence and remaining lifetime risk of Parkinson's disease in advanced age. *Neurology, 72*(5), 432–438.

Goadsby, P., & Spierings, E. H. (2009). The vascular theory of migraine—a great story wrecked by the facts. *Brain, 132*(2): 6, 7.

Health-cares.net. (2005). What is the prognosis of Alzheimer's disease? Retrieved February 3, 2013, from http://neurology.health-cares.net/alzheimers-disease-prognosis.php

Henderson S. T., Vogel, J. L., Barr, L. J., Garvin, F., Jones, J. J., & Costantini, L. C. (2009). Study of the ketogenic agent AC-1202 in mild to moderate Alzheimer's disease: A randomized, double-blind, placebo-controlled, multicenter trial. *Nutrition & Metabolism (Lond), 6*: 31.

Lay, C. L., & Broner, S. W. (2009). Migraine in women. *Neurologic Clinics, 27*(2): 503–11.

Lowenstein, D. H., & Alldredge, B. K. (1998). Status epilepticus. *New England Journal of Medicine, 338*(14): 970–976.

National Institute on Aging. (2010). Alzheimer's Disease Education and Referral Center. About Alzheimer's disease: Alzheimer's basics. Retrieved February 2, 2013, from www.nia.nih.gov/Alzheimers/AlzheimersInformation/GeneralInfo

National Institutes of Health (NIH). (2011). National Institute of Neurological Disorders and Stroke. NINDS Peripheral Neuropathy Information Page. Retrieved February 5, 2013, from www.ninds.nih.gov/disorders/peripheralneuropathy/peripheralneuropathy.htm

National Institute of Neurological Disorders and Stroke (NINDS). (2011). Parkinson's disease research web overview. Retrieved February 3, 2013, from www.ninds.nih.gov/research/parkinsonsweb/index.htm

Parkinson's Disease Foundation. (2011). Statistics on Parkinson's. Retrieved February 3, 2013, from www.pdf.org/en/parkinson_statistics

Qaseem, A., Snow, V., Shekelle, P., Casey, D., Cross, J. T., & Owens, D. (2008). Evidence-based interventions to improve the palliative care of pain, dyspnea, and depression at the end of life: A clinical practice guideline from the American College of Physicians. *Annals of Internal Medicine, 148*(2), 141–146.

chapter 15

Practical Pharmacotherapy of Drugs Used to Treat Psychiatric Disorders

William N. Tindall, John M. Boltri, Mona M. Sedrak

Key Terms

Anticholinergic effects

Anxiety disorders

Bipolar disorder

Extrapyramidal Syndrome(EPS)

Extrapyramidal Side Effects (EPSE)

Hypertensive crisis

Mania

Serotonin syndrome

Tardive dyskinesia (TD)

Torsade de pointes

Tyramine

CHAPTER FOCUS

To properly treat patients with a mental illness, clinicians must be knowledgeable about the pathophysiology of mental health disorders, starting with an understanding of how the mind and body work together to affect cognition, emotion, and social behavior. This chapter presents information on agents that affect cognition, emotion, and social behavior through actions that affect the central nervous system. Agents discussed in this chapter include both first-generation and second-generation antipsychotics, antidepressants, mood stabilizers and drugs to alleviate anxiety. Special attention is given to the side effects that patients may experience when taking these medications. Also discussed is the importance of patient counseling when using these agents.

OBJECTIVES

After carefully reading and studying this chapter, the student should be able to:

1. Describe the role pharmaceuticals play in the management of mood disorders, psychoses, and anxiety as well as their important conscientious prescribing elements.
2. Describe the four receptors that antipsychotics block and the effects they produce once each receptor is blocked.
3. Describe the signs, symptoms, and management of extrapyramidal adverse effects reported with antipsychotic agents.
4. Compare and contrast the differences between the first generation antipsychotics (FGA) and the second generation antipsychotics (SGA), giving particular attention to their adverse effects and the need for patient and family teaching.
5. Define *major depressive disorder* and differentiate it from depression and bipolar disorder.
6. Recall the conscientious considerations and patient teaching that should occur when clinicians prescribe antidepressants.
7. Recall the mechanism of action for the monoamine oxidase inhibitors (MAOIs), tricyclics, and SSRIs.
8. Compare and contrast the pharmacology of the four classes of non-TCA antidepressants.
9. Briefly describe the medical management of depression.
10. List the distinguishing features of the three classes of mood elevator medications: lithium, valproate, and carbamazepine.
11. Recall the distinguishing features of the benzodiazepines that make them useful in treating generalized anxiety.

DRUGS USED FOR TREATING PSYCHIATRIC DISORDERS

Antipsychotic Agents
First Generation Antipsychotics (FGA)
- chlorpromazine (Thorazine)
- fluphenazine (Prolixin)
- mesoridazine (Serentil)
- perphenazine (Trilafon)
- prochlorperazine (Compro)
- thioridazine (Mellaril)
- trifluoperazine (Stelazine)
- haloperidol (Haldol)
- loxapine (Loxitane)
- molindone (Moban)
- pimozide (Orap)
- thiothixene (Navane)

Second Generation Antipsychotics (SGA)/Atypicals
- aripiprazole (Abilify)
- asenepine (Saphris)
- clozapine (Clozaril)
- iloperidone (Fanapt)
- lurasidone (Latuda)
- olanzapine (Zyprexa, Zydis)
- olanzapine and fluoxetine combination (Symbyax)
- quetiapine (Seroquel)
- paliperidone (Invega)
- risperidone (Risperdal)
- ziprasidone (Geodon)

Antidepressant Agents
Monoamine Oxidase Inhibitors (MOAI)
- phenelzine (Nardil)
- selegiline (Emsam)
- tranylcypromine (Parnate)

Tricyclic Antidepressants (TCA)
- amitriptyline (Elavil)
- clomipramine (Anafranil)
- doxepin (Sinequan)
- imipramine (Tofranil)
- trimipramine (Surmontil)
- amoxapine (Asendin)
- desipramine (Norpramin)
- nortriptyline (Pamelor)
- protriptyline (Vivactil)

Related Tetracyclic Antidepressants (TeCA)
- amoxapine (Amokisan, Asendin, Asendis, Defanyl, Demolox, Moxadil)
- maprotiline (Deprilept, Ludiomil, Psymion)

Selective Serotonin Reuptake Inhibitors (SSRI)
- citalopram (Celexa)
- escitalopram (Lexapro)
- paroxetine (Paxil)
- fluvoxamine (Luvox)
- fluoxetine (Prozac)
- sertraline (Zoloft)

Serotonin-Norepinephrine Reuptake Inhibitors (SNRIs)
- duloxetine (Cymbalta, Ariclaim, Xeristar, Yentreve, Duzela)
- desvenlafaxine (Pristiq)
- venlafaxine (Effexor)

Norepinephrine and Dopamine Reuptake Inhibitors (NDRIs)
- bupropion (Wellbutrin)

Serotonin Reuptake Inhibitor (SRI)
- trazodone (Desyrel)

Tetracyclic Antidepressant
- mirtazapine (Remeron, Avanza, Zispin)

Antimanic (Mood Stabilizer) Agents
- lithium (Eskalith)
- valproate (Depakote)
- carbamazepine (Tegretol)

Nonclassified Mood Stabilizers
- gabapentin (Neurontin)
- topiramate (Topamax)
- lamotrigine (Lamictal)

Antianxiety Drugs
Benzodiazepines and Others
- alprazolam (Xanax)
- buspirone (Buspar)
- diazepam (Valium)
- chlordiazepoxide (Librium)
- clonazepam (Klonopin)
- clorazepate (Tranxene)
- gabapentin (Fanatrex, Gabarone, Gralise, Neurontin, Nupentin)
- hydroxyzine (Vistaril)
- lorazepam (Ativan)
- oxazepam (Serax)
- pregabalin (Lyrica)
- triazolam (Halcion)

DRUGS USED IN THE TREATMENT OF PSYCHOTIC DISORDERS

Advances in drug treatment over a period of six or seven decades has brought better drugs to the treatment of psychiatric disorders, but not a cure. Newer drugs improve a patients' quality of life (QOL), and they do so because they are better able to control symptoms and reduce adverse effects of their older siblings. The introduction of second-generation antipsychotics (SGAs) has not helped alleviate the burden of mental illness for patients, their families, and society, but it has helped alleviate the prevalence of adverse effects, such as tardive dyskinesia. Because the incidence of extrapyramidal effects has been reduced, although not entirely eliminated, the SGAs have made it possible for more patients to be treated on an outpatient basis than ever before. However, making appropriate drug choices to treat mental health conditions is not an easy task because single mode treatments are usually less effective than a multimode approach.

Additionally, drugs used to treat mental diseases and disorders are very potent, have significant adverse effects, and always present the challenge of long-term patient compliance. Antipsychotic drugs must also be considered in the context of comorbid conditions that increase both the risk of side effects and drug interactions. Finally, clinicians must educate patients to understand that these drugs only help with symptoms and that psychotherapy or counseling will be part of their treatment to learn coping skills.

Psychiatric Disorders and Comorbid Conditions

Psychiatric illness and medical diseases, such as heart disease, stroke, cancer, and diabetes, will often exist together in the same patient. The interrelationship between these concomitant conditions is very real, and failure to recognize this fact often leads to an underdiagnosis of the mental health disorder. There is a need for early identification and long-term integration of treatment for both the mental and medical illnesses. For example, there is an increased prevalence of depression among patients who suffer from type 2 diabetes, stroke, and cancer (Canto et al., 2005). This interplay of a psychiatric and other medical conditions results in the need for a collaborative care plan to improve the patient's quality of life. Additionally, treatment of medical conditions is often hampered by coexisting psychiatric illnesses. For example, it is difficult to achieve recommended glucose targets in patients with both depression and diabetes.

Coexisting psychiatric and medical conditions can lead to unintended consequences. Patients treated with selective serotonin reuptake inhibitors (SSRIs), for instance, often complain of easy bruising and do not know the reason—namely, that SSRIs can cause abnormalities in the clotting cascade, which in turn can result in clot formation. This effect is especially serious in patients who have had a stroke, myocardial infarction (MI), or heart failure (HF). Also, tricyclics are contraindicated in patients with heart disease because they can reduce heart rate to the point of causing serious life-threatening orthostatic hypotension or may induce arrhythmias.

When making treatment choices for patients with psychiatric illness, it is important to consider that there is no drug of choice or prototype drug for psychiatric illnesses. Any selection of a drug is highly individualized when one attempts to balance patient characteristics, clinical improvement, and tolerance of side effects. All clinicians who use mental health drugs must have a therapeutic relationship with the patient as an empathic, supportive, and trusted clinician. If the clinician believes in the efficacy of a medication and shares this belief with the patient, the patient is more likely to believe in the drug and be more compliant when taking it. Most clinicians believe that for many psychotic disorders, first-line treatment is psychotherapy, with medications being only an adjunct. For other mental health disorders, such as depression, treatment may include lifestyle changes, social support, psychotherapy, cognitive therapy, and even alternative treatments.

Antipsychotic agents can be divided into three broad categories: phenothiazines; typical antipsychotics, also called first-generation antipsychotics (FGA); and atypical antipsychotics or second-generation antipsychotics (SGA). Furthermore, these drugs can be classified by their potency: low, intermediate, and high potency. The basis for this classification system is the quantity of the drug needed to produce an equivalent effect when compared with other agents in the same category.

Antipsychotic agents are used to treat a wide variety of psychotic symptoms such as delusions, hallucinations, or paranoid behavior, as well as treating some other nonpsychiatric disorders such as nausea and intractable hiccups. Antipsychotics block various receptors (cholinergic, muscarinic, histamine, and dopamine) throughout the body. Their antipsychotic action comes from their blocking of central nervous system (CNS) dopamine receptors in the mesocortical/mesolimbic dopamine tracts of the brain, which in turn affects irritability, hallucinations, and delusions. However, the blocking of dopamine in other parts of the body leads to the following:

■ Extrapyramidal effects when dopamine receptors are blocked in the nigrostriatal pathways, which can lead to parkinsonian effect, tardive dyskinesia, and akathisia.
■ Hypersecretion of prolactin when dopamine is blocked in the tuberoinfundibular pathway, which includes the pituitary, leading to amenorrhea, infertility, and impotence.

■ Antiemetic action when dopamine receptors are blocked in the medulla.
■ Sedation and weight gain when histamine receptors are blocked by higher doses. Some antipsychotics such as quietiapine and olanzapine block histamine at low doses.
■ Dry mouth, constipation, urinary retention, and cycloplegia when the antipsychotic blocks muscarinic receptors.
■ At higher doses may see confusion, memory loss, delirium, tachycardia, and dry skin.
■ Dilated arterioles, decreased peripheral resistance and orthostatic hypotension when some antipsychotics block alpha-1 adrenergic receptors.

Conscientious Prescribing of Antipsychotic Agents

■ Clinicians should understand that the dosage of antipsychotic agents varies according to the individual, the reason for treatment, comorbid conditions, and the patient's response to the medication.
■ Long-term use of these drugs will increase the odds of an idiosyncratic arrhythmia or neuroleptic syndrome. Other long-term use of these agents can affect weight, cholesterol, and glucose metabolism. However, there is a paucity of information about their long-term use in the elderly. Researchers have found the rapid onset of cardiometabolic risks among teens and young adults using second-generation antipsychotics is alarming (Correll et al., 2009).
■ Some of these drugs can cause or exacerbate metabolic syndrome. Although the manufacturer's literature states that weight gain of 20 pounds can occur, some clinicians have experience with patients gaining as much as 100 pounds or more. In one study young people added 8 to 15% of their total body weight in less than 3 months of using antipsychotics and their waists expand 2 to 3 inches. These are alarming statistics especially since these drugs are often prescribed for off-label use such as for attention deficit hyperactivity disorder (ADHD).
■ Overdoses are quite common, but rarely fatal, thus clinicians should watch for worsening of CNS depression, hypotension, or worsening of extrapyramidal reactions.
■ When antipsychotic agents have been given at high doses and are suddenly stopped, patients may experience nausea, vomiting, dizziness, tremors, and withdrawal dyskinesia.
■ When stopping antipsychotic therapy, gradually reduce the dose over 2 to 3 weeks.
■ High-potency drugs (haloperidol, fluphenazine) produce the greatest extrapyramidal effects. Low potency drugs (thioridazine, chlorpromazine) produce the greatest anticholinergic, antihistamine, and anaphylactic effects.
■ Clinicians need to understand the potential of these drugs to interfere with cognitive and motor skills, to produce drug interactions, and the risk factors for neuroleptic malignant syndrome (see box on page 272 for definition of NMS). Monitor blood pressure (BP), heart rate, and movement regularly.

Patient/Family Education Regarding Use of Antipsychotics

- Patients should be instructed to rise slowly from any reclining position.
- Patients should be instructed to avoid abrupt withdrawal of any antipsychotic medications.
- Patients on phenothiazines (first-generation antipsychotics) should be instructed to use sunscreen anytime they have exposure to the sun.
- Patients should be instructed to use caution or discretion if driving a car or using machinery requiring alertness.
- Patients should be reminded always to communicate with their clinician before discontinuing or adding medications, including over-the-counter medications.
- Patients and caregivers need to be informed of all possible side effects, including tardive dyskinesia and neuroleptic syndrome.

Phenothiazines

The first group of psychotropic agents entered the market during the 1950s. At that time they were called the *phenothiazines* because they have similar chemical structures, being either aliphatic compounds, piperidine compounds, or piperazine compounds. They were hailed as breakthrough medication because patients with psychoses could be treated on an outpatient basis. Today it is more correct to call them first-generation antipsychotics (FGAs).

Mechanism of Action

Although their exact mechanism of action is unknown, it is theorized that FGAs' major therapeutic effects are a result of dopamine blockade in specific areas of the CNS. FGAs also produce an alpha-blocking effect, inhibit or block dopamine at the chemoreceptor trigger zone, and peripherally inhibit the vagus nerve in the gastrointestinal (GI) tract. Furthermore, they produce an antianxiety effect by depressing the brainstem's reticular system.

Pharmacokinetics

- Absorption: Absorbed well orally with an onset of action between .5 and 1 hour. Intramuscular (IM) onset of action is usually within 30 minutes, with the exception of a long-acting parenteral form. Antipsychotic effect is achieved gradually and requires several weeks. The peak therapeutic effect is between 6 weeks and 6 months.
- Distribution: These drugs are widely distributed, being greater than 90% protein bound, and reach high CNS concentrations. They will cross the placental barrier and enter breast milk.
- Metabolism: Highly metabolized by the liver and GI mucosa. Some liver metabolites are active.
- Excretion: Excreted primarily by the kidney.
- Half-life: Usually long; for example, chlorpromazine is 30 hours.

Dosage and Administration

Generic Name	Trade Name	Route	Usual Adult Daily Dose for Treating Psychoses
chlorpromazine	Thorazine	PO, IM	PO: 10–25 mg, 2–4 times/day, may increase every 3–4 days up to 30 or as much as 300 mg taken once/day or 3 times/day IM (for severe psychoses): 25–50 mg initially; repeat in 1 hr, then repeat with up to 400 mg every 3–12 hr, if needed
fluphenazine	Prolixin	PO, IM	PO: 0.5–10 mg, every 6–8 hr. Max dose is 40 mg/day IM: 5 mg, every 6–8 hr
perphenazine	Trilafon	PO, IM	PO: 8–16 mg, 2–4 times/day IM: 5 mg, every 6 hr
prochlorperazine	Compazine	PO, IM, IV	PO: 5–10 mg, 3–4 times/day IM: 10–20 mg, every 2–4 hr IV: 2.5–10 mg/day Rectal (antiemetic) 25 mg, 2 times/day
trifluoperazine	Stelazine	PO, IM	PO:15–20 mg, 2 times/day IM: 1–2 mg, every 2 hr as needed
thioridazine	Mellaril	PO	50–100 mg, 3 times/day

Clinical Uses

- Acute, idiopathic psychotic illnesses marked by agitation
- Manic phase of bipolar disorder
- Schizophrenia

Adverse Reactions

CV: Dizziness, fainting, orthostatic hypotension, tachycardia

DERM: Photosensitivity

EENT: Blurry vision, increased intraocular pressure, mydriasis, retinal pigmentation

ENDO: Hyperglycemia, weight gain, impaired thermoregulation

GI: Dry mouth, constipation, jaundice

GU: Decreased libido, inhibited ejaculation, urinary retention

NEURO: Extrapyramidal syndrome (EPS) (see Special Case: Extrapyramidal Syndrome for description of EPS and its symptoms), impaired memory

SPECIAL CASE: Extrapyramidal Syndrome

Extrapyramidal syndrome (EPS) may occur with both the typical and atypical antipsychotics. The severity of these effects varies with the drug class being administered. In addition, EPS is not related to any particular dosage regimen but rather is a result of accumulated use over several years of exposure. EPS may present as the following:

Akathisia: Inability to sit still, tapping of feet, restlessness

Dystonia: A state of muscle spasms of face, tongue, back, and neck that are dramatic, frightening, and painful and usually occurs in the first 5 to 30 days of use of the medication. However, dystonia can occur with just the FIRST dose of the antipsychotic.

Continued

Parkinson-like symptoms: Mask-like face, tremors, shuffling gait, and hypersalivation, which mimic the four classic signs of Parkinson's disease. These are akinesia/bradykinesia or decreased motor activity, tremor known as pill-rolling, cogwheel rigidity seen as jerky ratchet-like movement, and postural abnormalities, especially stooping.

Tardive dyskinesia (TD): Tardive dyskinesia may occur after 3 months of exposure to an antipsychotic, but it usually occurs after several years of exposure to the offending agent. TD is characterized by rhythmic tongue protrusion, puffing of cheeks, and puckering of mouth. This condition is rare, it may not remit, and it can be irreversible in patients, even when the drug is withdrawn. The development of TD's frequent blinking, brow arching, grimacing, upward deviation of the eyes, and lip-smacking symptoms has often lead to a misdiagnosis of stereotypical schizophrenia.

Neuroleptic malignant syndrome (NMS): NMS is a life-threatening neurological emergency that includes a combination of hyperthermia, rigidity (extrapyramidal effect), and autonomic dysregulation, that occur as an adverse event when using neuroleptics. It is considered a medical emergency because it can be fatal. It affects 0.5% to 1% of patients taking phenothiazines, but its frequency rises if the patient is dehydrated, exhausted, or has mental disorders. The risk of NMS is lower with the use of atypical agents. Onset of the syndrome varies from early on in the treatment to months following use; however, once started, it develops rapidly over 24 to 72 hours. Neuroleptic malignant syndrome is characterized by body temperature exceeding 38°C (100.4°F), and may go as high as 41.7°C (107°F), altered level of consciousness, tachycardia, labile blood pressure, diaphoresis, tachypnea, urinary or fecal incontinence, rigidity, stupor, coma, and acute renal failure. Possible mechanisms for this happening appear to be disruption of the central thermoregulatory process or excess production of heat due to skeletal muscle contractions.

Treatment of NMS: This begins with recognizing it as a medical emergency and stopping the offending drug. Supportive therapy is used to aggressively treat the hypothermia. Circulatory and ventilation support should be provided. Agents such as dantrolene, a direct skeletal muscle relaxant that can block calcium from signaling muscles to contract as well as affect heart rate, respiratory rate, and temperature, or one of the two dopamine agonists, bromocriptine (Parlodel) or amantadine (Symmetrel), can be used to reverse dopamine blockage and free up the rigidity.

Knowing what this syndrome is and initiating rapid discontinuation of the responsible antipsychotic has caused death rates to fall from 20% in the 1980s to less than 4% today.

Interactions

■ Alcohol and CNS depressants: May result in enhanced CNS depression, respiratory depression, and increased hypotensive effects

■ Anticholinergic drugs: May result in increased anticholinergic side effects
■ Amphetamines: Decrease antipsychotic effect of the phenothiazides
■ Dopaminergic antiparkinson drugs (Levodopa): Antagonize the antipsychotic effect of the phenothiazides
■ Insulin/oral hypoglycemics: Weakens control of diabetes
■ Lithium: Decreases the antipsychotic effect of the phenothiazides
■ Beta blockers (propranolol): When coadministered, effect of both or either increased

Contraindications

■ Parkinsonism
■ Blood dyscrasias
■ Severe liver impairment
■ Severe cardiac disease
■ Severe CNS depression
■ Reye's syndrome

Conscientious Considerations

■ It is recommended that titration be slow, starting from a low dose, increasing when necessary to produce a therapeutic effect.
■ Overdoses are quite common, but rarely fatal. Signs of overdose include worsening of CNS depression, hypotension, or worsening of extrapyramidal reactions.
■ Long-term use of these drugs can lead to cardiac arrhythmia, hyperreflexia that is life threatening, hypertension, rigidity, and tardive dyskinesia.
■ The low-potency agents are the most frequent offenders, and the elderly are the most common sufferers of adverse reactions to these medications.
■ In addition, clinicians must be aware of the important considerations that apply to all antipsychotic medications (see p. 270, Conscientious Prescribing of Antipsychotics).

Patient/Family Education

■ The advisories for patients who are taking phenothiazines are the same as for patients taking any other antipsychotic medication (see p. 271, Patient/Family Education Regarding the Use of Antipsychotics).

Second Generation—Atypical Antipsychotics

The introduction of the first second-generation antipsychotic agent, clozapine, in the early 1990s was considered a breakthrough in treating schizophrenia as a chemical imbalance disorder. Use of these drugs has allowed many people with psychoses to return to society and assume relatively normal lives. They are easily administered orally, and patients are easily monitored. As a drug group, they have diverse and differing pharmacodynamic profiles but are considered atypical because of their superior ability to not induce **extrapyramidal side effects (EPSE)** or elevation of prolactin levels. However, the drugs most likely to cause prolactin elevation are risperidone (Risperdal) and paliperidone (Invega), both of which are atypical antipsychotics.

Clozapine (Clozaril) is the only atypical antipsychotic with clear evidence of efficacy in treatment-resistant schizophrenia.

However, all first-generation and second-generation antipsychotics have a U.S Food and Drug Administration (FDA) BLACK BOX WARNING that they may increase mortality among elderly patients with dementia-related **psychosis**. Also, patients who take clozapine (Clozaril) are at increased risk of agranulocytosis, seizures, and myocarditis. As a group, the atypical antidepressants are associated with an unhealthy weight gain profile, which can lead to diabetes or metabolic syndrome.

Mechanism of Action

These agents partially interfere with the binding of serotonin at its receptor sites in the cortex, blocking serotonin, which inhibits the release of dopamine. Their main activity is binding to dopamine receptors in the CNS. Thus, by these two antagonist activities on serotonin and dopamine receptors, they cause more dopamine to be released to the frontal cortex, which reduces the negative symptoms of schizophrenia. These agents also have some anticholinergic and alpha-adrenergic-blocking activity.

Pharmacokinetics

- Absorption: Rapidly and well absorbed through GI tract.
- Distribution: 99% protein bound, mostly to albumin, reaching steady state in 2 weeks.
- Metabolism: All are metabolized by the liver.
- Excretion: Mostly through the renal system.
- Half-life: Usually fairly long, for example, aripiprazole: 75 hours, olanzapine: 21 to 54 hours, quetiapine: 6 hours.

Dosage and Administration for Schizophrenia

Generic Name	Trade Name	Route	Usual Daily Oral Adult Dose and Titration Schedule
aripiprazole	Abilify	PO	10–15 mg once a day; may increase up to 30 mg/day in 2 weeks
asenapine	Saphris	PO	5–10 mg sublingual tablets in black cherry flavor twice a day
clozapine	Clozaril	PO	25 mg 1–2 times/day and titrate up to target dose of 300–450 mg/day over 2 weeks. Max dose is 900 mg/day in divided doses.
iloperidone	Fanapt	PO	1 mg 2 times/day on day 1; titrate up over 7 days to a target dose of 12 mg 2 times/day
lurasidone	Latuda	PO	40 mg 1 time/day, max dose 80 mg/day
olanzapine	Zyprexa	PO	10–15 mg/day; increase to 20/mg day over 2 weeks
olanzapine/ fluoxetine	Symbyax	PO	olanzapine 6 mg/fluoxetine 25 mg combo/ day at bedtime
paliperidone	Invega	PO	6 mg PO every a.m.; may titrate up or down, but do not exceed 12 mg/day
		IM	234 mg in deltoid muscle on day 1, then 156 mg 1 week later, then maintain at 117 mg IM every month
quetiapine	Seroquel	PO	25 mg 2 times/day; increase by 25 mg/day in divided doses up to 300–400 mg/day, not to exceed 800 mg/day
risperidone	Risperdal	PL	1 mg 2 times/day, increase on third day to 3 mg 2 times/day, then use weekly intervals to increase by 1 mg/day, not to exceed 6 mg/day due to risk of extrapyramidal side effects.
ziprasidone	Geodon	PO	20 mg 2 times/day; may increase daily up to 80 mg 2 times/day
		IM	10–20 mg as needed up to 40 mg/day

Clinical Uses

- Psychosis in patients with schizophrenia
- Depression or mania with psychotic features
- Bipolar disorder
- Severe agitation and delusions in patients with dementia

Adverse Reactions

CV: Risperidone can produce a dose-related fall in blood pressure and reflex tachycardia, prolonged QT intervals, orthostatic hypotension. Clozapine can cause orthostatic hypotension, tachycardia, and myocarditis. Quetiapine may cause palpitations and postural hypotension.

GI: Vomiting, nausea.

GU: Sexual dysfunction (risperidone).

HEM: Clozapine can cause agranulocytosis (see Conscientious Prescribing for monitoring).

MISC: Weight gain; hypersalivation (clozapine). Risperidone may change sleep architecture because of its blockage of 5-HT receptors.

NEURO: Headache, insomnia, light-headedness, akinesia, somnolence, extrapyramidal symptoms, and neuroleptic malignant syndrome.

Interactions

- Any drug, including alcohol, that requires liver metabolism, will compete for the drug and require the dosage to be adjusted by as much as half or even doubled.

Contraindications

- Liver impairment

Conscientious Considerations

- Selecting one agent over another must be based on specific patient risk factors, the patient's history of responding to any other agent, and adverse effects experienced by any other agent.
- Any change from one atypical antipsychotic to another must be done by slow titration of one agent to another with either a "wash out" or a "cross-titration." If the appearance of psychotic symptoms makes a wash out unfeasible, then lowest doses and a short time duration of the switch is needed. Most experts cross-titrate rather than wash out because washing out one antipsychotic without another onboard may lead to a worsening of symptoms.
- In addition, clinicians must be aware of the important considerations that apply to all antipsychotic medications (see p. 270, Conscientious Prescribing of Antipsychotics).

Patient/Family Education

- The advisories for patients who are taking atypical antipsychotics are the same as for patients taking any other antipsychotic medication (see p. 271, Patient/Family Education Regarding the Use of Antipsychotics).

Miscellaneous Antipsychotics

As a group, these agents are dopamine receptor antagonists. This means that they block dopamine receptors in the basal ganglia, hypothalamus, limbic system, brainstem, and medulla. By doing so, they reduce the symptoms of schizophrenia. For example, haloperidol is a antipsychotic with effects on dopaminergic D1 and D2 receptors. Molindone is a dihydroindolone antipsychotic whose action closely resembles chlorpromazine, but it has more EPS effects. Thiothixene is a thioxanthene antipsychotic, and loxapine is a dibenzoxapine. These agents are likely to induce extrapyramidal side effects, and they have similar efficacies when used in equivalent potency doses. Lower-potency doses tend to cause sedation, whereas higher-potency doses are more likely to induce EPS.

Because these agents were the first in a new class of agents used to treat psychoses in the late 1940s, they have also been labeled as the typical antipsychotics and may be included in some writings as first-generation antipsychotics (FGA). However, their use is waning. A parenteral version of haloperidol (Haldol) exists for the patient needing rapid control of severe agitation or dangerous psychosis. Typical antipsychotic agents are more effective in treating the more severe psychotic patient. Patients are more likely to continue taking atypical antipsychotics, however, because they are better tolerated. Additionally, the newer atypical agents carry less risk for extrapyramidal side effects, but as mentioned previously, they carry a greater risk for an unhealthy weight gain, which in turn can lead to metabolic syndrome.

Mechanism of Action

These drugs competitively block postsynaptic dopamine receptors, interrupt nerve impulse movement, and increase turnover of dopamine in the basal ganglia, hypothalamus, limbic system, brainstem, and medulla. Thus, they cause strong side effects (suppressed locomotor activity, antiemetic effects, weak **anticholinergic effects**, and some sedating effects). The clinical manifestations of cholinergic blockade, can be seen in a number of systems including CNS, cardiovascular system, salivary glands, gastrointestinal tract, and urinary tract system.

Clinical effectiveness is seen when 60% to 70% of dopamine receptors are blocked.

Pharmacokinetics

- Absorption: Quickly absorbed orally, with onset of action within 1 to 2 hours; IM injection produces results in 10 to 30 minutes.
- Distribution: Stored in fat tissues because they are strongly lipid soluble, which hinders their antipsychotic effects from being seen for several weeks.
- Metabolism: Metabolized by the liver to active metabolites.
- Excretion: In the urine.
- Half-life: 4 hours (loxapine)

Dosage and Administration

Generic Name	Trade Name	Route	Usual Oral Adult Daily Dose
haloperidol	Haldol	PO	0.5–5 mg dose 2 to 3 times/day; usual maximum is 30 mg/day
pimozide	Orap	PO	1–12 mg/day
loxapine	Loxitane	PO	10 mg 2 times/day; increase until symptoms are controlled, usually 100 mg twice/day
molindone	Moban	PO	50–75 mg/day STAT, then titrate up to 225 mg/day every 3–4 days if needed
thiothixene	Navane	PO	2–3 mg/day; increase gradually to 30 mg/day; severe cases 60 mg/day

Clinical Uses

- Treatment of psychotic episodes when a tranquilizing effect is also needed.
- Treatment of Tourette's syndrome (pimozide).
- The clinical use of these agents is essentially identical to the FGAs.

Adverse Reactions

CV: Orthostatic hypotension, peripheral edema
EENT: Blurred vision
GI: Constipation, nausea, vomiting, dry mouth
MISC: Allergic reactions, decreased sexual functioning, breast swelling
NEURO: Drowsiness, lethargy, extrapyramidal syndrome (see Special Case: Extrapyramidal Syndrome for description of EPS and its symptoms), including PSUEDO-PARKINSONISM, TARDIVE DYSKINESIA, torsade de pointes, and neuroleptic malignant syndrome (NMS)

Interactions

- CNS depressants, such as barbiturates, hypnotics, narcotics, alcohol, or antihistamines, taken with a typical antipsychotic further increase CNS depression.
- Anticholinergic drugs, when taken with a typical antipsychotic, can increase risk of hyperthermia.
- Beta blockers cause an increased effect of both drugs results.
- Lithium interacts with typical anti-psychotics and manifests as increased EPS and neurotoxicities.

Contraindications

- Pimozide should not be coadministered with other drugs that prolong the QT interval.
- Haloperidol is contraindicated in patients with Parkinson's disease.

Conscientious Considerations

- Clinicians must monitor closely for any adverse signs. There is a higher incidence of dystonia among young males and EPS effects among elderly females.
- The typical antipsychotics have many adverse effects, making patient adherence a common problem.

■ Instruct patients to take the medication with food or milk.
■ At signs of tardive dyskinesia (TD), its effects can be decreased best by a change in dose or a switch to another agent.
■ Monitor motor function of individuals taking typical antipsychotics by using the Abnormal Involuntary Movement Scale (AIMS). This test rates joint rigidity and patient balance on a numerical scale to help the clinician monitor for early signs of EPS.

■ In addition, clinicians must be aware of the important considerations that apply to all antipsychotic medications (see p. 270, Conscientious Prescribing of Antipsychotics).

Patient/Family Education

■ The advisories for patients who are taking typical antipsychotics are the same as for patients taking any other antipsychotic medication (see p. 271, Patient/Family Education Regarding the Use of Antipsychotics).

SPOTLIGHT ON SCHIZOPHRENIA

Schizophrenia is a thought disorder marked by delusions, hallucinations, disorganized speech and behavior, flat affect, withdrawal from interpersonal relationships, and poor grooming and hygiene. Symptoms usually last for 6 months, with at least 1 month of active symptoms. Variations in daily routines or stressors in the environment may exacerbate or cause symptoms. A diagnosis must include two or more of the following: delusions, hallucinations, disorganized speech, disorganized behavior, and/or catatonic behavior. It appears as an illness characterized by periods of relapse and recovery. It has an equal male/female distribution, affecting about 1% of the population, and it appears in adolescence or early adulthood as a lifelong condition. Patients may be able to function marginally in society, but if not, long-term hospitalization is necessary. A family history of similar mental disorders is a contributing factor for increased morbidity of schizophrenia as is a patient's history of substance abuse, incidence of suicide attempts, and complex partial epilepsy.

Medical Management

It is important for the clinician to understand that there is no cure and that these drugs only decrease acute symptoms, decrease frequency and severity of episodes, and optimize social functioning during episodes. Clinical effectiveness occurs when 60% to 70% of dopamine receptors are blocked; however, too much dopamine blockage leads to symptoms resembling parkinsonism. These effects are usually decreased or eliminated by a decrease in dose or changing to a different antipsychotic.

Most patients benefit from a combination of psychotherapy and antipsychotic drugs, where choice of an agent is dependent upon past responses to the medication class, family history, side effect profile of the agent, and monitoring of the initial response.

Typical antipsychotics are used for both short-term and long-term therapy. In cases of acute psychoses, rapid and effective sedation is usually achieved by combining an antipsychotic with a benzodiazepine (intramuscularly or intravenously). Benzodiazepines are also useful in the acute treatment of akathisia (e.g., motor restlessness secondary to antipsychotics).

Lower-potency agents are more sedating than high-potency agents, but they are more likely to cause orthostatic hypotension. Thus, lower-potency agents are generally used for evening sedation of elderly patients, especially if they suffer from sundowning, disorientation, and psychotic episodes at night. However, the anticholinergic side effects of the low-potency antipsychotics may make them poor choices for use among the elderly.

The atypical antipsychotics offer major benefits over typical agents, such as fewer anticholinergic effects, less dystonia and parkinsonism, lower risk of tardive dyskinesia, and potential minimization of other adverse effects such as orthostatic hypotension. Anticholinergic agents are used in the treatment of acute dystonic reactions and in chronic prophylaxis of dystonia, akathisia, and parkinsonian symptoms (such as EPS) secondary to antipsychotics (especially high-potency agents). Table 15-1 shows the relative potency of select antipsychotics.

Patient Education

Relapse is common with this disorder, and a support structure—a caring and compassionate family—is important. Medication compliance is mandatory to avoid a psychotic relapse. Most families also need support and education on how best to care for the patient.

TABLE 15-1 Relative Potency of Several Antipsychotics				
ANTIPSYCHOTIC AGENT	INCIDENCE OF SEDATION	INCIDENCE OF EXTRAPYRAMIDAL SIDE EFFECTS	INCIDENCE OF ANTICHOLINERGIC SIDE EFFECTS	INCIDENCE OF ORTHOSTATIC HYPOTENSION
aripiprazole (Abilify)	Low	Very low	Very low	Very low
clozapine (Clozaril)	High	Very low	High	High
haloperidol (Haldol)	Low	High	Low	Low
loxapine (Loxitane)	Moderate	Moderate	Low	Low
olanzapine (Zyprexa)	Moderate/high	Low	Moderate	Moderate
quetiapine (Seroquel)	Moderate/high	Very low	Moderate	Moderate
risperidone (Risperdal)	Low/moderate	Low	Very low	Moderate
ziprasidone (Geodon)	Low/moderate	Low	Very low	Low/moderate

DRUGS USED IN THE TREATMENT OF DEPRESSIVE DISORDERS

Affective disorders such as major depressive disorder, dysthymia, bipolar disorder, and cyclothymia often coexist with other mental and somatic disorders. For example, anxiety is a common comorbidity with major depression. Although much is known about the mechanism of action of various antidepressants, much is still unknown about the exact etiology of mood disorders. Following are three broad treatment goals for mood disorders:

■ Treatment should be based on the chronic and recurrent nature of the mood disorders.
■ Treatment should focus on eliminating acute symptoms in manic and depressive episodes.
■ Maintenance therapy is important in preventing relapse and recurrence of symptoms.

Depression is considered an affective disorder characterized primarily by a long-term change in mood; it is not to be confused with "having a bad day," "feeling down," or "feeling blue," which healthy people all do from time to time. When clinical depression does occur, it is associated with an imbalance of neurotransmitters (demodulation), especially serotonin, norepinephrine, and dopamine, which leads to clinical symptoms of depressed mood, fatigue and low energy, low motivation, reduced interest in pleasurable things, feelings of worthlessness and hopelessness, and poor concentration. Depression must be taken seriously because it is associated with significant morbidity and mortality, and it can present with a myriad of somatic symptoms.

The prevalence of major depression in the general population is estimated to be 5% to 9%, and yet among institutionalized patients it is as high as 30% (NIMH, 2008). According to the World Health Organization (WHO, 2001), approximately 450 million people suffer from a mental or behavioral disorder, yet only a small minority of them receives even the most basic treatment. Left untreated, an episode of depression can last 6 to 13 months, but if treated quickly, patients may feel better in 3 months or less. Finally, because the symptoms of depression overlap extensively with that of hypothyroidism, laboratory studies are required to rule it out.

When a person has his or her first episode of depression, reaching full remission may take 6 to 9 months of treatment, even after symptoms have resolved, to avoid relapse. Maintenance therapy may be continued for extended periods in patients with multiple depressive episodes or very severe episodes. For example, when a person has three or more episodes of depression, lifelong maintenance therapy is usually required. The spectrum of what constitutes depressive symptoms varies widely, and thus its treatment must also be varied.

There are many treatment options for individuals with mood disorders. Selection of an antidepressant drug therapy for a patient as well as the rationale for combination therapy is based on the differences in mechanism of action offered by the different classes of drugs. Prior to 1990, tricyclic antidepressants were most commonly used. Because of their many side effects, adverse effects, and issues of noncompliance, they have mostly been replaced with the selective serotonin reuptake inhibitors because of their consistent onset of action, ease of dosing, and side effect profile. The monoamine oxidase inhibitors, however, have limited use. Their drug-drug interactions (DDI), food-drug interactions, and titration and dosing issues have made many clinicians wary of using them.

One study has shown that among patients receiving treatment for depression in primary care settings, only one in five was being adequately treated. Overall, more than half of them received at least one form of depression care, but only about one in five (21.3%) received at least one form of therapy conforming to established treatment guidelines. Psychotherapy was more commonly used than was pharmacotherapy, and individuals undergoing psychotherapy were more likely to receive treatment in alignment with clinical guidelines than were individuals taking medications. Mexican American and African American individuals with depression consistently had lower odds of receiving any type of care or care in agreement with treatment guidelines during the previous year (Gonzales, Vega, & Williams, 2010).

Conscientious Prescribing of Antidepressant Agents

■ Patients will discontinue or fail to adhere to new medication regimens at the same rate as with older medications if they find the newer medications are not effective or have the same adverse effects.
■ For patients who recover from a major depression, continued treatment for at least 6 months decreases the risk of relapse by 70% (Kim, Lee, Paik, & Kim, 2011).

Patient/Family Education for Patients Using Antidepressant Agents

■ Inform patients that therapeutic effects may take 4 to 8 weeks to manifest.
■ Advise patients to avoid alcohol; CNS depressants; cough/cold preparations, especially OTC cough/cold products containing dextromethorphan; decongestants; and diet aids.
■ Advise patients not to discontinue these medications abruptly.
■ Inform patients that blurred vision, drowsiness, and dizziness may occur.
■ Advise patients to use caution when driving or undertaking any activity requiring alertness.
■ Advise patients to avoid rising quickly from either sitting or lying down (especially elderly patients).
■ Instruct patients to wear sunscreen and a hat while taking certain of these drugs to prevent sunburn from photosensitivity.
■ When these medications are used in adolescents, it is imperative that an FDA-approved medication guide be distributed to them and their caregivers because of the possibility of suicide ideation.

Monoamine Oxidase Inhibitors (MAOIs)

These third-line agents, tranylcypromine (Parnate), selegiline (Emsam), and phenylamine (Nardil) are rarely used today. The monoamine oxidase inhibitors were introduced 50 years ago. Today, their use as drugs to treat depression has largely been superseded by the selective serotonin reuptake inhibitors (SSRIs), the serotonin-norepinephrine reuptake inhibitors (SNRIs), and other newer agents.

These drugs irreversibly inhibit monoamine oxidase; thus, before any other drugs are administered for depression, the MAOIs must be stopped for 10 to 14 days or longer, for example, if switching to fluoxetine (Paxil). It is also important to be aware that interactions with certain other drugs can cause **serotonin syndrome,** a potentially life-threatening drug reaction that causes the body to have too much serotonin. **Hypertensive crisis** can be precipitated by ingestion of foods rich in **tyramine,** especially cheese and fermented beverages (such as beer and wine), by sympathomimetic drugs (cough medicines containing ephedrine), or by taking a tricyclic antidepressant (TCA) with a MAOI.

Monoamine oxidase is found in nearly all tissue. It exists in two similar molecular forms, MOA-A and MOA-B. MOA-A has a substrate preference for 5-HT (serotonin) and is the target for the antidepressant drugs. MOA-B has a preference for phenylamine, and both MOA-A and MOA-B enzymes act on noradrenaline and dopamine. The drugs phenelzine (Nardil) and tranylcypromine (Parnate) are nonselective inhibitors of MOA-A and MOA-B and are discussed together.

Mechanism of Action

MAOIs are irreversible, nonselective inhibitors of the enzyme monoamine oxidase in its CNS storage sites. This inhibition of activity leads to increased levels of the four neurotransmitters, epinephrine, norepinephrine, serotonin, and dopamine, making them more available at neuronal receptor sites. By inducing adaptive changes in the synapse physiology by protecting norepinephrine and serotonin degradation over a few weeks of time, these agents relieve symptoms of depression. Whereas the tricyclics and the SSRIs have long half-lives, requiring 3 to 4 weeks before any therapeutic effects are noticed, the MAOIs are able to provide relief of depression symptoms immediately, if not at least within 14 days. Typical onset of effect is 1 week.

Pharmacokinetics

- Absorption: Administered orally, MAOIs are rapidly and thoroughly absorbed from the GI tract.
- Distribution: Highly distributed.
- Metabolism: There is a major first-pass metabolism of these drugs in the liver because they have a cytochrome P450 enzyme as a substrate.
- Excretion: Excreted by the liver and the kidneys.
- Half-life: Is variable within 1 to 3 hours; however, the long duration of action that they exhibit is due to their irreversible binding to protein.

Dosage and Administration

Generic Name	Trade Name	Route	Usual Adult Daily Dose
tranylcypromine	Parnate	PO	15 mg, twice/day
phenelzine	Nardil	PO	15 mg, 3 times/day
isocarboxazid	Marplan	PO	20–60 mg/day, 2–4 times/day
selegiline	Emsam	Transdermal patch	6.0 mg/24 hr to start; may be increased at 2-week intervals in increments of 3 mg to a total of 12 mg/24 hr

Clinical Use

- Refractory unipolar depression

Adverse Reactions

EENT: Dilated pupils
GU: Sexual dysfunction
NEURO: Hypertensive crisis, serotonin syndrome
MISC: Weight gain

Interactions

- The MAOIs have interactions with numerous drugs. Among them are the following:
  - All amphetamine types.
  - Antidiabetic drugs.
  - SSRIs, tricyclic antidepressants, and other drugs with CNS effects, including alcohol, when interacting with MAOIs, can cause SEROTONIN SYNDROME and increased risk of HYPERTENSIVE CRISIS.
  - Foods high in tyramine can cause HYPERTENSIVE CRISIS.
  - Concomitant use of St. John's wort and MAOIs has resulted in SEROTONIN SYNDROME, and some FATALITIES.
  - HYPERTENSIVE CRISIS can also occur with large amounts of caffeine.

Contraindications

- Liver impairment

Conscientious Considerations

- If it is necessary to switch from an MAOI to an SSRI, allow a 2-week wash-out period to occur (this is approximately five half-lives and a good rule to follow for most any drug).
- In a patient taking an MAOI, it takes as little as 10 mg of tyramine from aged wines and cheeses to produce severe headache, increased blood pressure, and occasionally intracranial hemorrhage. This is because tyramine is normally metabolized by monoamine oxidase in the gut wall and liver and thus very little of it reaches the systemic circulation.
- In addition, clinicians must be aware of the important considerations that apply to all antidepressants (see p. 276, Conscientious Prescribing of Antidepressant Agents).

Patient/Family Education

- Discuss the medications used in the treatment of bipolar disorder in acute as well as chronic/maintenance situations.

- Advise patients to avoid any food high in tyramine, such as aged cheese, beer, wine, pickled products, liver, raisins, bananas, figs, avocados, chocolate, yogurt, and meat tenderizer.
- In addition, the clinician must be aware of the advisories that apply to patients taking *any* antidepressant agent (see p. 276, Patient/Family Education Regarding the Use of Antidepressant Agents).

Tricyclic Antidepressants (TCAs)

The tricyclic antidepressants, so-named because of their three-ringed structure ("tri-cyclic"), can be divided into tertiary amines and secondary amines. The first to be used were imipramine (1957) and amitriptyline (1961), which were developed from chlorpromazine when it was discovered they had the ability to elevate mood rather than act as antipsychotics. Since then about 10 drugs have come onto the market. These agents are considered second-line agents today mainly because of their side effect profiles. The tertiary amines cause more sedation and orthostatic hypotension than do the secondary amines, and they work best when taken at nighttime.

Mechanism of Action

In the late 1950s TCAs were found to elevate mood by increasing levels of norepinephrine and serotonin in the synaptic cleft. These drugs have anticholinergic properties as well as blocking H1-histamine, and alpha-adrenergic receptors, and these actions account for a large proportion of their side effects. These drugs *do not* stimulate the CNS system, and their ability to increase mood is not clearly understood. Their clinical effects include elevating mood, increasing physical activity, improving appetite and sleep patterns, and reducing morbid preoccupations. Their clinical effects begin gradually and are spread out over from 2 to 8 weeks. All of the tricyclics are equally efficacious in relieving depression within that time frame.

Pharmacokinetics

- Absorption: All are well absorbed orally, and they easily penetrate into the CNS.
- Distribution: Well distributed with peak plasma concentration in 3 to 4 hours.
- Metabolism: They undergo significant first-pass metabolism in the liver, where they are conjugated with glucuronic acid.
- Excretion: Through the kidneys.
- Half-life: Typically 24 hours, but this varies considerably.

Dosage and Administration

Generic Name	Trade Name	Route	Usual Oral Adult Daily Dose
amitriptyline	Elavil	PO	50–300 mg at night
clomipramine	Anafranil	PO	25–250 mg at night
doxepin	Silenor	PO	25–300 mg at night
imipramine	Tofranil	PO	30–300 mg at night
trimipramine	Surmontil	PO	50–300 mg at night
amoxapine	Asendin	PO	50–600 mg at night
desipramine	Norpramin	PO	25–300 mg daily
nortriptyline	Pamelor	PO	30–100 at night
protriptyline	Vivactil	PO	5–60 mg, 3–4 times/day

Clinical Uses

- Endogenous depression
- Reactive depression
- Depression related to alcohol and cocaine withdrawal, anxiety (clomipramine)
- Neuropathic pain (amitriptyline)
- Enuresis
- Obsessive compulsive disorder
- Panic disorder

Adverse Reactions

Anticholinergic side effects: blurred vision, confusion, dry mouth, hot dry skin, constipation, urinary retention.

CV: Orthostatic hypotension, palpitations, tachycardia, ECG abnormalities, and ventricular arrhythmia (including **torsade de pointes,** an uncommon form of polymorphic ventricular tachycardia (VT) characterized by a gradual change in the amplitude and twisting of the QRS and is associated with a prolonged QT interval, which may be congenital or acquired). In the event of an overdose, fatal arrhythmias and seizures could occur.

DERM: Greater susceptibility to photosensitivity.

GI: GI distress, jaundice, metallic taste when eating, nausea, weight gain.

NEURO: Confusion (especially in patients over 40), sedation, delusions and hallucinations, suicidal thoughts or behavior, aggressiveness, engaging in unusual or dangerous activities, restlessness or inability to sit still, extreme elation or feelings of happiness that may alternate with a depressed or sad mood, anxiety, agitation, panic attacks.

GU: Breast changes, including breast enlargement or breast discharge; swelling of the testicles

Drug Interactions

- Drug-drug interactions include a wide range of medications such as any anticholinergic, any barbiturate, chlorpropamide, cimetidine, clonidine, epinephrine, ethanol, fluoxetine, neuroleptics, norepinephrine, propoxyphene, quinidine, and SSRIs.

Contraindications

- MAOI use.
- Not recommended during the recovery phase of MI.
- Doxepin is contraindicated in patients with glaucoma or urinary retention.

Conscientious Considerations

- Many clinicians believe that tricyclics should be considered as second-line treatments today even though they were introduced first into the market.
- Most effective in patients suffering from severe depression, especially those with greater disturbances and melancholia.
- All TCAs have shown efficacy in depression, panic disorder, enuresis, and chronic neuropathic pain, but due to their serotonergic and noradrenergic effects, they are especially

helpful with anxiety disorders such as obsessive-compulsive disorder.

- Overdoses of more than 2,000 mg (a 10-day supply) of a TCA can be fatal. For this reason, when treating someone with a new diagnosis of unstable depression, limited doses of TCA are given. Overdose can result in fatal arrhythmias and seizures.

- Abrupt discontinuation after long-term use may lead to withdrawal syndrome in 36 to 72 hours, including dizziness, nausea, paresthesias, anxiety/insomnia lasting for 3 to 7 days.

- To avoid withdrawal syndrome, decrease dose by 10% to 25% over 1 to 2 weeks.

- Nortriptyline has a long duration of effect and is the least sedating of the group.

- Because of the sedating effects of tricyclics, they should be taken at night after establishing the drug's effective daily dose, particularly if the patient has insomnia.

- The tertiary amines (amitriptyline, doxepin, and imipramine) are most sedating, whereas the secondary amines (desipramine, nortriptyline) and the dicyclic venlafaxine are less sedating.

- Concurrent use with SSRIs should be avoided, and thus 2 weeks should elapse before stopping one drug and continuing with another; with fluoxetine allow a minimum of 5 weeks for a wash out.

- Therapeutic/beneficial effects may take 2 to 3 weeks.

- Monitor complete blood count (CBC), weight, and mental status, especially suicidal tendencies.

- Determination of tricyclic plasma levels is not routinely recommended, but may be useful in determining toxicity and drug interactions. Noncompliance or adjustments in dosage should be made according to clinical response not plasma concentrations.

- Monitoring of cardiac disturbances (using a baseline electrocardiogram [ECG]) is important.

- For anxious or agitated patients with depression, the more sedating TCAs are preferred (amitriptyline, doxepin), whereas the less-sedating drugs (protriptyline) are found to be better for patients who have psychomotor withdrawal.

- In addition, clinicians must be aware of the important considerations that apply to all antidepressants (see p. 276, Conscientious Prescribing of Antidepressants).

Patient/Family Education

- The advisories for patients who are taking tricyclic antidepressants are the same as for patients taking any other antidepressant medication (see p. 276, Patient/Family Education Regarding the Use of Antidepressant Agents).

Selective Serotonin Reuptake Inhibitors (SSRIs)

Use of tricyclics has been superseded by SSRIs, which are less lethal upon overdose, lack cardiovascular and anticholinergic effects, and offer convenient dosing. However, the SSRIs do have side effects such as sexual dysfunction and GI disturbances. (See Special Case: Treatment of Depression in Children, Adolescents, and Young Adults Using SSRIs.)

SPECIAL CASE: Treatment of Depression in Children, Adolescents, and Young Adults Using SSRIs

The media often focuses on the topic of adolescents, young adults, and children being treated for depression because of concerns about the safety of antidepressants being prescribed for them. Depression is common among this age group and in most cases is goes unrecognized. Depression among 15- to 18-year-olds is estimated at 15%. Depressive episodes in this age group last for 7 to 9 months and may induce suicide, the third leading cause of death among this age group (SAMHSA, 2007).

In 1994, the Pediatric Labeling & Extrapolation Regulation was passed. This regulation permits pediatric indications to be based on adult studies as well as other pharmacokinetic studies. This enabled treatment for children who were not adequately being managed due to lack of FDA-approved pediatric indications for medications. This act stemmed from the ongoing problem that only about 20% of the available drugs on the market had indications for use in children. On September 16, 2004, the FDA supported recommendations made by the Psychopharmacologic Drugs Advisory Committee and the Pediatric Advisory Committee that antidepressants should include warnings about increased risk of suicidal ideation and suicide attempts in children and adolescents taking these medications (FDA, 2004). These recommendations were made following an ongoing review of controlled clinical trials.

Conscientious Prescribing of SSRIs

- To avoid withdrawal syndrome, some SSRIs require a tapering down of the dosages over a 1 to 2 week period, depending on the drug.

- SSRI antidepressants are equally efficacious as the older first-generation and second-generation tricyclics, but they are easier to administer and better adhered to because they are dosed once a day rather than three times day. In addition, the SSRIs demonstrate better side effect profiles.

- SSRIs are safer in an overdose because they do not have the cardiotoxicity of TCAs.

- SSRIs are less likely to cause the orthostatic hypotension caused by TCAs because they do not have the alpha-adrenergic activities of the TCAs.

- Fluvoxamine (Luvox) is indicated only for obsessive-compulsive disorder and produces no anticholinergic side effects.

- Fluoxetine (Prozac), paroxetine (Paxil), and sertraline (Zoloft) are usually taken in the morning because they often induce insomnia.

Patient/Family Education for Patients Taking SSRIs

- The patient should be advised not to take NSAIDs concurrently because any bleeding problem could be aggravated.

■ Patients on SSRIs must be taught not to withdraw the drug suddenly; it must be done slowly over 1 to 2 weeks. The exception is fluoxetine (Prozac) because its half-life is approximately 14 days.

■ In addition, the clinician must be aware of the advisories that apply to patients taking *any* antidepressant agent (see p. 276, Patient/Family Education Regarding the Use of Antidepressant Agents).

Mechanism of Action

The SSRIs selectively inhibit 5-HT neuronal reuptake at selected nerve terminals in the central nervous system and inhibit cytochrome P450. They also have a weak or no effect on norepinephrine reuptake and dopamine. The increased availability of serotonin at the receptors results in mood elevation and reduced anxiety. However, the SSRI drugs may take as long as 6 weeks to relieve depression.

Pharmacokinetics

■ Absorption: All are well absorbed orally and they easily penetrate into the CNS.

■ Distribution: Well distributed by protein binding, with peak plasma concentration in 3-4 hours.

■ Metabolism: They undergo significant first-pass metabolism in the liver where they are conjugated with glucuronic acid.

■ Excretion: Excreted through the kidneys.

■ Half-life: Averages up to 24 hours for most SSRIs, but half-life varies considerably. For example, fluoxetine (Prozac) has a half-life that ranges from 4 to 6 days, but its active metabolite makes its effects last up to 14 days; sertraline (Zoloft) ranges from 24 to 26 hours.

Dosage and Administration

Generic Name	Trade Name	Route	Usual Adult Oral Dose Per Day for Depression
citalopram	Celexa	PO	20 mg/day, increase by 20 mg weekly to max of 60 mg/day
fluoxetine	Prozac	PO	20 mg/day in a.m.; after several weeks, increase by 20 mg/day at weekly intervals not to exceed 80 mg/day
fluvoxamine	Luvox	PO	50 mg at bedtime, adjust in 50 mg intervals every 4–7 days to max of 100–300 mg/day. If over 50 mg/day, divide doses.
paroxetine	Paxil	PO	20 mg as single a.m. dose to start, increase by 10 mg weekly to no more than 50 mg/day.
sertraline	Zoloft	PO	50 mg/day as single a.m. dose for several weeks, then increase up to 200 mg/day depending on response.
escitalopram	Lexapro	PO	10 mg 1 time/day; may be increased to 20 mg 1 time/day after 1 week

Clinical Uses

■ Major depression
■ Depression in patients with concurrent illnesses, such as coronary artery disease, glaucoma, hypertension
■ In elderly patients with depression
■ Panic disorder

Adverse Reactions

GI: Nausea, diarrhea
GU: Anorgasmia in both men and women, and ejaculatory disturbances in men
NEURO: Agitation, headache, insomnia, nervousness, sedation, SEROTONIN SYNDROME, tremor

Interactions

■ Buspirone
■ Diazepam
■ Lithium
■ MAOIs: May cause serious and fatal interactions if do not allow at least 14 days between escitalopram (Lexapro) and MAOIs
■ Neuroleptics
■ Tricyclics

Contraindications

■ MAOI use (within 14 days of use).
■ Female patients should not use these drugs if the risk of pregnancy in imminent, or if they are pregnant or lactating.

Fluoxetine (Prozac)

Prozac is slowly eliminated and has a half-life of 21 hours. Thus, patients with any liver problems must have their doses reduced because fluoxetine (Prozac) is a potent inhibitor of the cytochrome P450 system. Prozac can also elevate drug levels of other drugs, including antiarrhythmics, other antidepressants, phenothiazines, risperidone, theophylline, and antiarrhythmics such as quinidine. Prozac is one of the most stimulating of the SSRIs, thus it is used in patients who present with flat affect and fatigue. A form of Prozac that is dosed once a week is available for use by persons who are already being treated for depression and are stable on daily dosages of Prozac: It is not for use by people with newly diagnosed depression.

Paroxetine (Paxil)

As the most sedating of the SSRIs, paroxetine (Paxil) is used in patients whose depression presents with anxiety and agitation and severe insomnia. Unlike other SSRIs, paroxetine accumulates in breast milk. Paxil is highly bound to plasma proteins, thus it requires special attention when coadministered with drugs that are highly protein bound (e.g., warfarin). Because it may cause more weight gain and side effects than its sister agents, its use may need close monitoring. Paxil has been reported to cause a flu-like syndrome if discontinued abruptly. Cases have occurred in which Paxil has been confused with Taxol because of like-sounding names.

Sertraline (Zoloft)

Sertraline (Zoloft) is a middle-of-the-road SSRI that is less sedating than Paxil but less stimulating than Prozac. It is eliminated after 25 hours and thus can be given once a day. Sertraline produces more GI side effects than fluoxetine; this may be because it is less activating than fluoxetine.

Citalopram (Celexa)

Citalopram (Celexa) is a newer SSRI; it is highly bound to plasma protein (80%). Among this group of drugs, it has the least effect on the cytochrome P450 system and thus presents with the most favorable drug-drug interaction profile. Citalopram is approved for use in obsessive-compulsive disorder (OCD).

Non-TCA Antidepressants

At one time, the nontricyclic antidepressants were a group known as miscellaneous antidepressants, but they are correctly classified into the four following groups: serotonin and norepinephrine reuptake inhibitors (SNRI), norepinephrine and dopamine reuptake inhibitors (NDRI), serotonin reuptake inhibitor (SRI), and tetracyclic antidepressants (TeCA).

Serotonin and Norepinephrine Reuptake Inhibitors (SNRI)

SNRIs such as duloxetine (Cymbalta), desvenlafaxine (Pristiq), and venlafaxine (Effexor) work much like SSRIs in that they block not only the reabsorption of serotonin, but also norepinephrine. Many of the side effects of SNRIs are similar to those of SSRIs. The FDA has approved these agents for treatment of anxiety, panic disorder, obsessive-compulsive disorder (OCD), and bulimia as well as depression. They are also heavily marketed for off-label treatment of insomnia, and chronic pain syndromes such as diabetic neuropathy.

These agents are effective antidepressants, similar in effect and chemical structure (they are dicyclic) to the tricyclics, but they have no affinity for cholinergic receptors. Duloxetine (Cymbalta) is much like venlafaxine (Effexor) in that they both block serotonin and norepinephrine transporters, but duloxetine appears to be more potent and has more ability to block both serotonin and norepinephrine than does venlafaxine. As with all other antidepressants, increased suicidal thinking may occur during the first few weeks of use, which necessitates weekly monitoring and dosage adjustments.

Mechanism of Action

These agents inhibit both serotonin and norepinephrine reuptake in the CNS and, to a much lesser extent, dopamine. Blocking serotonin and norepinephrine transporters inhibits their availability to bind with postsynaptic receptors. At lower doses, less than 200 mg per day, venlafaxine affects serotonin reuptake, which contributes more to its effectiveness as an anxiety-reducing agent than as an antidepressant. These agents are used in treating diabetic peripheral neuropathic pain because their antidepressant and pain inhibition are centrally mediated. Desvenlafaxine (Pristiq) is FDA approved for major depressive episodes.

Pharmacokinetics

■ Absorption: Well absorbed from the GI tract following oral administration.
■ Distribution: Protein binding in the serum is only 25% to 30%.

■ Metabolism: Metabolized in the liver to an active metabolite primarily by CYP450 pathways (CYP2D6, CYP1A2). Metabolite 9 to 13 hours; increased if renal impairment.
■ Excretion: In the urine.
■ Half-life: Venlafaxine: 3 to 7 hours, but its active metabolite will extend that half-life up to 9 to 11 hours; duloxetine: 12 hours; desvenlafaxine: 11 hours.

Dosage and Administration

Generic Name	Trade Name	Route	Usual Adult Daily Dose for Depression
venlafaxine	Effexor, Effexor SR	PO	75 mg/day administered in 2–3 divided doses and taken with food depending on tolerability; may increase to 150 mg/day every 4–5 days, up to 225 mg/day. If needed, the max dose is 375 mg/day in 3 divided doses.
duloxetine	Cymbalta	PO	20–30 mg given 2 times/day
desvenlafaxine	Pristiq	PO	50–400 mg 1 time/day, with or without food.

Clinical Uses

■ Major depressive disorder (MDD), generalized anxiety disorder (GAD), social phobia, panic disorders (ER only), vasomotor symptoms.

Adverse Reactions

CV: Sustained increase in diastolic BP of 10 to 15 mm Hg, diaphoresis
DERM: Increase sweating, pruritus, rash
EENT: Blurred vision, increase in intraocular pressure
GI: Nausea, dry mouth, constipation, anorexia, increase in liver enzymes
GU: Ejaculatory disturbances, erectile dysfunction, decreased libido, urinary hesitation
NEURO: Tremor, seizures fatigue, drowsiness, insomnia, headache

Contraindications

■ MAOI use (within 14 days of use)

Conscientious Considerations

■ Because its total half-life (drug plus active metabolite) is in the range of 9 to 11 hours, twice a day dosing is necessary. However, formulations such as Effexor SR have made once-a-day regimens possible, resulting in better tolerance and compliance.
■ Venlafaxine is associated with frequent early onset side effects, especially nausea, vomiting, and diarrhea, and up to 40% to 50% of patients experience these side effects.
■ Venlafaxine has among the greatest risk of withdrawal reactions (along with paroxetine), and its extended release (ER) capsules are associated with withdrawal reactions.
■ The risk of rhabdomyolysis has been reported after venlafaxine ingestion, but only at high doses of more than 150 mg per dose (Wilson, Howell, & Waring, 2007).

■ In addition, clinicians must be aware of the important considerations that apply to all antidepressants (see p. 276, Conscientious Prescribing).

Norepinephrine and Dopamine Reuptake Inhibitors (NDRIs): Bupropion (Wellbutrin)

Bupropion (Wellbutrin) is an NDRI. Although the precise mechanism of its action is not known, bupropion is believed to block the reuptake of norepinephrine as well as dopamine, hence its effect on mood. Bupropion is used as an antidepressant, for treatment of ADHD, and to relieve nicotine withdrawal symptoms. Like many of the antidepressants it, carries a BLACK BOX WARNING for increased risk of suicide when used in children, adolescents, and young adults with major depression or other psychiatric disorders.

Mechanism of Action

Bupropion, as an antidepressant, has no appreciable effect on blocking the reuptake of serotonin, but it does diminish neuronal uptake of dopamine and norepinephrine at CNS presynaptic membranes by increasing the availability of dopamine and norepinephrine at postsynaptic receptor sites. It also reduces the firing rate of noradrenergic neurons, but how and why it works as an antidepressant remains unknown. Bupropion affects sexual functioning much less than the other antidepressants.

Pharmacokinetics

■ Absorption: Well absorbed orally from GI tract. Bupropion usually requires 1 to 3 weeks of administration before its onset of action is seen, and it may take several weeks in some patients.
■ Distribution: Unknown.
■ Metabolism: Metabolized in the liver on first pass.
■ Excretion: Eliminated in the urine.
■ Half- life: 14 hours.

Dosage and Administration

Generic Name	Trade Name	Route	Usual Adult Daily Dose for Depression
bupropion	Wellbutrin, Zyban	PO	For depression, the usual adult dose is 300 mg/day given as 100 mg, 2 times/day; based on clinical response after 3 days, may adjust upward to 100 mg, 3 times/day, but no more than 450 mg/day

Clinical Uses

■ Depression, especially in patients with seasonal affective disorder (SAD)
■ Smoking cessation programs (as Zyban only) when it is combined with behavior modification therapy
■ Off-label use in treating ADHD in adults (sustained release [SR] form only
■ Short-term (up to 4 weeks) management of anxiety disorders
■ To increase sexual desire in women

Adverse Reactions

CV: Tachycardia.
DERM: Photosensitivity.
ENDO: Hyperglycemia, hypoglycemia.
GI: Anorexia, weight loss, nausea, constipation, and dry mouth.
META: Weight loss.
NEURO: Tremors and seizures may occur if the medication is not taken as directed, or if it is taken at higher doses, or used for a longer time than recommended. Seizures may also occur with the use of alcohol, which should be avoided while taking this medication. Because the risk of seizures is dose-dependent, there is a 10-fold increase in the risk of seizures at doses above 450 mg per day.

Interactions

■ Because of its first-pass metabolism in the liver, bupropion can affect hepatic metabolism of drugs undergoing the same metabolism. This can lead to drug-drug interactions that alter effectiveness of both drugs. Common examples are carbamazepine and phenobarbital.

Contraindications

■ Current or prior history of seizures, anorexia, and bulimia
■ MAOI use (within 14 days)

Conscientious Considerations

■ This medication is equally as effective as the tricyclics, causes fewer anticholinergic effects, and does not cause orthostatic hypotension, cardiac conduction problems, or weight gain. It produces less sedation (preferable in the elderly). The risk of seizures increases after patients take more than 150 mg per dose of the immediate release formulation.
■ Because insomnia is a frequent side effect, it is recommended that patients do not take it after 5 p.m.
■ Because it is a dopamine reuptake inhibition, bupropion can also occasionally cause psychotic side effects (delusions, hallucinations).
■ In addition, clinicians must be aware of the important considerations that apply to all antidepressants (see p. 276, Conscientious Prescribing of Antidepressants).

Patient/Family Education

■ Patients should be told that optimal results may take 2 to 4 weeks of treatment, but some improvement may be seen after 7 to 10 days.
■ The advisories for patients who are taking tricyclic antidepressants are the same as for patients taking any other antidepressant medication (see p. 276, Patient/Family Education Regarding the Use of Antidepressant Agents).

Serotonin Reuptake Inhibitor (SRI): Trazodone (Desyrel)

SRIs inhibit the overall reuptake of serotonin. It has strong sedating effects, thus it is used primarily as a nighttime medication for the person with depression who is also suffering from insomnia. Trazodone has a chemical structure similar to that of alprazolam (Xanax), a benzodiazepine; however, trazodone is more specific with its ability to inhibit serotonin reuptake.

Mechanism of Action

Trazodone alters serotonin reuptake in the CNS, thus it works as an antidepressant after several weeks of use because it causes alterations in the presynaptic 5-HT adrenoreceptors.

Pharmacokinetics

■ Absorption: Well absorbed orally, with two-thirds of patients showing relief of depression after several weeks of use; usually some change is seen at the end of the second week.
■ Distribution: Peak plasma levels occur after 1 hour on an empty stomach or 2 hours on a full stomach.
■ Metabolism: Metabolized in the liver by the cytochrome P-450 enzymes.
■ Excretion: Minimal excretion of unchanged drug in the kidneys.
■ Half-life: 5 to 9 hours.

Dosage and Administration

Generic Name	Trade Name	Route	Usual Adult Daily Dose for Depression
trazodone	Desyrel	PO	Initial dose is 150 mg/day in 3 divided doses. May titrate up by 50 mg/day every 3–4 days until desired response is reached. Do not exceed 400 mg/day in outpatients or 600 mg/day in institutional patients.

Clinical Uses

■ In patients with major depression who also have insomnia, anxiety, and chronic pain syndromes.
■ Off-label use as a sedative-hypnotic at 50 to 100 mg per day.
■ Other off-label uses of trazodone are treatment of panic attacks, agoraphobia, cocaine withdrawal, and aggressive behavior.

Adverse Reactions

CV: Orthostatic hypotension for 4 to 6 hours after taking a dose
GI: Mild nausea, vomiting
GU: Priapism
NEURO: Drowsiness

Interactions

■ Digoxin and warfarin. Trazodone (Desyrel) may increase the free plasma concentration of protein-bound drugs, such as digoxin and warfarin, and thus should be taken in divided doses.

Contraindications

■ Hypersensitivity to the drug

Conscientious Considerations

■ Use cautiously in patients following a myocardial infarction.
■ Use cautiously in any patient who is a suicidal risk.

■ Because it is so sedating, it is often prescribed in low doses to counteract the agitation or insomnia caused by other agents.
■ In addition, clinicians must be aware of the important considerations that apply to *all* antidepressants (see p. 276, Conscientious Prescribing of Antidepressants).

Patient/Family Education

■ Inform patients that trazodone may enhance alcohol, barbiturates, and other CNS depressants.
■ Inform patients that this medication may cause dry mouth and constipation.
■ Inform patients that they should not suddenly stop taking this medication without first speaking to their clinician because it may need to be tapered.
■ Every patient prescribed trazodone (male and female) must be counseled regarding priapism. Failure to recognize this condition and stop the trazodone can lead to permanent erectile dysfunction.

Tetracyclic Antidepressant (TeCA): Mirtazapine (Remeron)

Currently, the only agent on the market in this classification is mirtazapine (Remeron). It is used to treat major depressive disorder and post-traumatic stress disorder (PTSD).

Mechanism of Action

This medication is a tetracyclic compound that directly acts as an antagonist at presynaptic alpha receptors, which in turn increases levels of synaptic norepinephrine and serotonin. By increasing both norepinephrine and serotonin transmission, it relieves depression after several weeks of use, but it causes some sedative effects because it has a potent antihistamine action. As a serotonin blocker it inhibits serotonin 5-HT2 and 5-HT3 receptors, leading to selective 5-HT1 effects.

Pharmacokinetics

■ Absorption: Rapidly and completely absorbed after oral administration. Absorption not affected by food.
■ Distribution: Believed to be 85% by protein binding, but exact nature remains unknown.
■ Metabolism: Rapidly metabolized in the liver by cytochrome enzymes, resulting in 50% bioavailability.
■ Excretion: Excreted in urine and feces.
■ Half-life: 20 to 40 hours; longer in males than females.

Dosage and Administration

Generic Name	Trade Name	Route	Usual Adult Daily Dose
mirtazapine	Remeron	PO	Initially 15 mg at night; may increase by 15 mg/day over 1–2 weeks, but no more than 45 mg/day and half that if elderly

Clinical Use

■ Major depressive disorder

Adverse Reactions

GI: Weight gain, constipation, dry mouth, increased appetite, nausea, vomiting.

MISC: Flu-like symptoms and abnormal dreams.

NEURO: Sedation. Mirtazapine has a lower risk of side effects than other antidepressants; however, it does have a 0.08% risk of inducing a seizure among those with no history. Clinicians use the slow-release dosage form in the belief it may reduce the risk of an induced seizure.

Interactions

■ MAOIs. Taken with MAOIs, this drug may induce hypertension, seizures, and even death (serotonin syndrome), especially if both are used within 14 days of each other.

■ CNS depressants. When taken with other CNS depressants, especially with alcohol and benzodiazepines, this drug may cause increased CNS depression.

■ Any drug affecting cytochrome P450 enzymes may alter the effects of mirtazapine.

Contraindications

■ Hypersensitivity

Conscientious Considerations

■ As is true with all antidepressants, anyone with suicidal tendencies, especially adolescents, may develop suicidal ideation during early treatment or dosage adjustment.

■ One advantage of mirtazapine is its sedation side effect, which can be helpful to depressed patients with insomnia.

■ Another advantage of mirtazapine is its lack of sexual side effects.

■ Weight gain is significant with this drug, but this to can be an advantage if an elderly person is cachectic.

■ An overdose may produce cardiovascular events such as orthostatic hypotension, dizziness, tachycardia, palpations, and arrhythmias.

■ Advise patients to avoid alcohol or other antidepressants during therapy and for at least 3 to 7 days after discontinuing therapy.

■ Patients should also be cautioned that therapy for depression may be prolonged and while on therapy to change positions slowly to avoid orthostatic hypotension.

■ If patients experience an increase in appetite, they may need to monitor their diet to avoid unnecessary weight gain.

■ Abrupt discontinuation after prolonged therapy may produce headache, malaise, nausea, and vomiting.

■ Caution should be taken in patients with impaired renal or hepatic function as well as with the elderly.

■ In addition, clinicians must be aware of the important considerations that apply to *all* antidepressants (see p. 276 Conscientious Prescribing of Antidepressant Agents), such as watching for increased suicide ideation during early treatment or dosage adjustment.

Agents Used in the Treatment of Mania and Bipolar Disorder

Mania is a constellation of symptoms that manifest as speech and motor hyperactivity, flight of ideas, and feeling of grandiosity. When manic symptoms are associated with depressive symptoms, the condition is called **bipolar disorder**. The patient may exhibit euphoria and show little insight into his or her behavior. This behavior can turn into irritability if the patient feels inhibited or confined. According to the American Psychiatric Association's publication, *Diagnostic and Statistical Manual of Mental Disorders*, 4th edition (DSM-IV), a patient who experiences one manic episode can be diagnosed with bipolar disorder. Historically, the drug of choice for bipolar disorder is lithium, but carbamazepine and valproic acid can be used in bipolar patients who cannot tolerate lithium. The role of these two agents is also changing due to the increasing use of second-generation psychotics. The mood stabilizers lithium, carbamazepine (CBZ), and valproate (VPA), have differing pharmacokinetics, structures, mechanisms of action, efficacy spectra, and adverse effects.

Lithium (Carbolith, Eskalith, Duralith)

Lithium is a mood stabilizer that is used for both prophylaxis and treatment of the manic phase of manic-depressive/bipolar disorder. Lithium is a light alkali metal, a monovalent cation that is similar to Na^+ and K^+. The precise mechanism by which it produces its therapeutic effect is poorly understood; however, there is a low margin of safety between lithium's effectiveness as a therapeutic agent and as a toxic agent, making it mandatory to monitor lithium blood levels. Before lithium therapy begins, all patients should have a baseline of data that includes serum urea, electrolytes, thyroid function test, and an ECG. Once stabilized, a test for serum lithium, serum urea, and electrolytes should be done every 3 months because a serum lithium level of 1.5 mmol/L can be fatal.

Mechanism of Action

Lithium's mechanism of action remains unknown, even after decades of its use. Its antimanic and antidepressant effects are theorized to be the result of stimulating exit of Na^+, where Na^+ is elevated (as in depression), by stimulating the Na^+/K^+ pump mechanism. This influences Ca^{++} and Na^+ transfer across cell membranes, including the Ca^{++} release of neurotransmitters, increasing norepinephrine reuptake, and increasing serotonin receptor sensitivity, or interacting with Ca^{++} and Mg^{++}, thereby increasing cell membrane permeability.

Pharmacokinetics

■ Absorption: Given orally, it is quickly and completely absorbed from the gut. It causes no discernible effect for the first 5 to 10 days.

■ Distribution: Peak blood levels occur in 1 to 3 hours. Blood levels are closely linked to sodium levels, thus reduction in salt intake will prolong lithium's half-life to the level at which toxic levels are produced. There is no protein binding of lithium because it is a cation.

■ Metabolism: Lithium is a monovalent cation that is not metabolized and is excreted unchanged by the kidneys.

■ Excretion: Over 95% is excreted in the urine; the rest in other body fluids.

■ Half-life: 18 to 27 hours in patients with normal renal function; this may increase by 50% in the elderly or those with impaired renal function.

Dosage and Administration

Generic Name	Route	Usual Adult Daily Dose
lithium	PO	Precise dosing is based on serum lithium levels using 300-mg lithium carbonate tablets (containing 8–12 mEq lithium) Adults and children over 12 years of age usually start with 300–600 mg lithium 3 times/day, then are maintained on 300 mg 3 times/day as the dosage is adjusted by monitoring serum lithium concentrations Extended-release tablets are available to allow 2 times/day dosing.

Clinical Uses

■ Bipolar disorder (both manic and depressive episodes respond)
■ Adjuvant with other antidepressants to treat major depression
■ Adjuvant with antipsychotics to treat schizophrenia

Adverse Reactions

There are many side effects, which are related to serum levels, but at normal doses will see few side effects.

CV: Edema, hypotension
DERM: Acne, folliculitis, alopecia, pruritus
EENT: Aphasia, blurred vision, tinnitus
ENDO: Hyperglycemia, hypothyroidism, hyponatremia
GI: Nausea, vomiting diarrhea, abdominal pain, anorexia, bloating, metallic taste, weight gain
GU: Polyuria, glycosuria
META: Weight gain
MS: Muscle weakness
NEURO: Seizures, fatigue, impaired memory, confusion, drowsiness, hand tremor, incoordination, muscle twitching, headache, irritability, rigidity

When serum levels rise to 2.0–2.5 mEq/L or greater, the following can be anticipated as serious adverse events and signs of toxicity:

CV: Severe hypotension, ARRHYTHMIAS, ECG changes, circulatory failure
NEURO: Ataxia, blurred vision, giddiness, tinnitus, SIEZURES
CV: Circulatory failure
GU: Oliguria, nephrogenic diabetes insipidus

Interactions

■ The list of drugs that interact with lithium is long. Some examples are as follows:
    ■ Sodium depletion raises lithium's serum levels and may lead to lithium toxicity. Patients should avoid the use of

diuretics including acetazolamide, sodium bicarbonate, aminophylline, caffeine, theophylline, and thiazide, as well as NSAIDs.

■ Drugs that inhibit absorption of lithium from the GI tract such as fluoxetine decrease its effectiveness.

■ Angiotensin-converting enzyme inhibitors raise serum levels of lithium.

Contraindications

■ Significant renal impairment or disease
■ Significant cardiovascular disease
■ Significant thyroid disease
■ Diabetes
■ Severe dehydration
■ Sodium depletion
■ Pregnancy

Conscientious Considerations

■ Serum lithium concentrations should be drawn biweekly until stable, then every 2 to 3 months thereafter.
■ During acute phase treatment, a serum lithium concentration of 1.0–1.4 mEq/L is required. For long-term control, the desired level is 0.5–1.3 mEq/L. Thus, serum drug concentrations must be monitored.
■ 5% of patients who have taken lithium for more than 1 year develop symptoms of hypothyroidism, thus clinicians should follow thyroid status as part of routine care regimen.

Patient/Family Education

■ Advise patients to take lithium with meals to reduce nausea and GI upset.
■ Advise patients to drink 10–12 glasses of fluid per day to reduce thirst and maintain normal fluid balance.
■ Suggest that the patient elevate the feet if ankle edema appears.
■ Advise patients to maintain consistent dietary intake of sodium.
■ Instruct the patient to contact the clinician if the patient experiences vomiting, severe tremor, sedation, muscle weakness, or vertigo.
■ Advise female patients not to become pregnant while taking lithium because this medication is teratogenic.

The Valproates: Valproic Acid (Depakene), Valproate Sodium (Depacon), and Divalproex Sodium (Depakote)

These chemically related agents act as anticonvulsant, antimanic, and antimigraine agents, but their mechanism of action is largely unknown. It is believed they directly increase concentrations of the inhibitory neurotransmitter gamma-aminobutyric acid, or GABA. As an anticonvulsant, they decrease sodium and calcium ion influx in nerves and control the manic phase of bipolar disorder. They also have the potential for serious toxic reactions, which include blood dyscrasias, cardiovascular disturbances, and dermatological effects, especially rash and photosensitivities. Abrupt withdrawal or noncompliance among those with epilepsy may result in an episode of status epilepticus. Clinicians should caution patients with epilepsy to avoid activities that require alertness, such as driving, until cleared by a clinician. Clinicians should also assess location, duration, and seizure characteristics as well as mood, ideation, and behavior on a frequent basis.

The valproates are prescribed as monotherapy and adjunctive therapy for simple and complex seizures, decreasing the frequency of manic episodes associated with bipolar disorder, and for prevention of migraine headache. As a mood stabilizer, an initial dose of 750 mg per day of Depakote (regular release tablets) is usually prescribed in divided doses to reduce manic episodes. It is then titrated rapidly to the desired clinical effect or a dose not to exceed 2.5 gm per day in divided doses, or a trough plasma level of 50–125 mcg/mL, but not exceeding a dose of 60 mg/kg/day. Serious side effects such as severe hepatic and pancreatic toxicity and thrombocytopenia can occur. Lesser side effects are weight gain, transient alopecia, drowsiness, nausea, abdominal pain, agitation, dizziness, headache, rashes, irregular menses, and tremors. Despite the need for conscientious and frequent monitoring of the patient

valproic acid, valproate remains a widely prescribed medication, highly regarded as effective and a first-line agent.

Carbamazepine (Carbatrol, Tegretol)

Carbamazepine (CBZ) is both an anticonvulsant and a mood stabilizer, and like valproic acid it decreases sodium and calcium ion influx into neuronal membranes, thus reducing their potentiation ability. It is used more often in the treatment of seizures, trigeminal neuralgia, and diabetic neuropathy than in the treatment of mania. Some clinicians use it for off-label treatment of alcohol withdrawal, bipolar disorder, and neurogenic pain. Its side effects are frequent and include drowsiness, ataxia, nausea, vomiting, and visual abnormalities. Serious blood dyscrasias may also appear, and its abrupt withdrawal may initiate status epilepticus, but this is not likely unless the patient is epileptic. Because its half-life is 25 to 65 hours and it is metabolized in the liver to an active metabolite, its dosing parameters are a challenge to any clinician owing to the autoinduction of its metabolism, which leads to changes in serum concentration even when the patient is adherent to the dosing regimen. Autoinduction is usually complete after about 3 months. Clinicians who use it must monitor CBCs because aplastic anemia is a risk in these patients, with a prevalence rate of five to eight times more than in the general healthy population. Liver function tests and serum drug levels must also be monitored.

SPOTLIGHT ON BIPOLAR DISORDER

Diagnostic criteria for bipolar depression, or more correctly, manic-depressive disorder (MDD), is put forth by two respected sources, the American Psychiatric Association (APA) in its DSM-IV TR manual and the World Health Organization in its ICD-1 coding. Each has similar definitions for what constitutes a major depressive episode (MDE), what is unipolar depression, and what is bipolar depression. The DSM IV TR is used by mental health professionals in the United States to diagnose mental health conditions and by insurance companies to reimburse mental health professionals for their work.

The two major types of bipolar disorder are bipolar I and bipolar II. Patients with bipolar I have experienced at least one manic episode or one mixed episode. Patients with bipolar II have experienced at least one major depressive episode (MDE) and at least one hypomanic episode, but not a full manic or mixed episode. Bipolar II patients exhibit symptoms that incapacitate them in some way, especially in relationships at home or at work. Both the bipolar I and bipolar II diagnoses include subcategories to further refine them based on the patient's symptoms.

Chronic bipolar disorder (cyclothymic disorder) or bipolar-like illness is a mild form of manic-depressive disorder. Patients with this disorder often cycle through short episodes (usually a matter of days) of mild hypomania and depression. If this cycling occurs over a period of 2 years, especially in children and adolescents, and if symptoms do not resolve for more than 2 months, then the diagnosis can be made. The symptoms of this disorder cause significant stress on the patient and manifest in strained relationships and inability to function at work.

A substantial number of patients who have been diagnosed as unipolar depressive for decades eventually experience a hypomania,

manic, or a "mixed mood" state, causing uncertainty regarding their diagnosis. As many as 60% of patients with bipolar disorder are initially misdiagnosed with unipolar depression (Singh & Rajpit, 2006), indicating the difficulty of making the correct diagnosis. This issue is understandable because bipolar disorder usually starts with an episode of depression in a young person, and its manic episodes usually do not occur until later in life, usually before the age of 50. Most patients find it takes 10 years from the time of their first manic or depressive episode to get an accurate diagnosis (Fink & Gayak, 2005). Left untreated, the manic disorder may last up to 3 months. As the patient's age increases and the disorder progresses, there may be more frequent episodes that last longer periods. Suicides are more common in persons with bipolar disorder than in those with major depressive disorder. If the patient is suicidal, hospitalization is required.

Medical Management

Mood stabilizers, such as lithium carbonate, sodium divalproex, or carbamazepine, have traditionally been the mainstays of treatment for patients with bipolar disorder. Benzodiazepines generally are avoided, but they may be temporarily useful in restoring sleep or in modulating irritability or agitation not caused by psychosis. Between 20% and 40% of manic patients do not respond adequately to lithium, but they will likely respond if tried on valproic acid/valproate sodium/divalproex sodium (Depakote) or carbamazepine (Tegretol, Carbatrol). Many clinicians believe that lithium is the agent of choice, and it is usually continued for 4 to 6 months, with frequent serum levels taken.

Selective serotonin reuptake inhibitors may also be used; however, because of the risk of inducing a manic episode, SSRI doses should be low and titration should be done slowly. The only SSRI

SPOTLIGHT ON BIPOLAR DISORDER—cont'd

that currently has FDA approval for the management of unipolar depression in adolescents is fluoxetine (Prozac). This agent should be used carefully in patients with bipolar disorder because of its long half-life and because of its potential to exacerbate manic symptoms when not coadministered with an antimanic or mood-stabilizing agent. Three mood stabilizers, olanzapine (Zyprexa), quetiapine (Seroquel), and aripiprazole (Abilify), are increasingly being used in bipolar disorder with or without psychotic symptoms. Their usage is warranted because they affect both dopamine and serotonin receptors and have a lower incidence of producing extrapyramidal side effects than do the first-generation antipsychotics. Additionally, quetiapine (Seroquel) is the only drug accepted for treating bipolar depression according to the World Federation of Societies of Biological Psychiatry (WFSBP) Guidelines (Grunz et al., 2010).

The second-generation antipsychotics have become good choices for some clinicians treating bipolar disorder because they can be used as maintenance therapy in patients who have episodes of acute mania and mixed episodes. However, their side effect profiles are a challenge due to metabolic syndrome effects (elevated glucose levels, weight and lipid abnormalities) and extrapyramidal

side effects (CNS effects, headaches, agitation, anxiety, insomnia, and somnolence), which seem to occur more commonly in patients with affective disorders than in patients in whom the same drugs are being used to treat schizophrenia.

Clinicians should supervise prescription compliance carefully during the manic phase. Clinicians must recognize that depressive episodes carry a high risk for suicide by overdosing. Other options for the clinician are electroconvulsive therapy (ECT), which is highly effective in all phases of bipolar disorder. Psychosocial therapy is also warranted, and it should consist of three short-term psychotherapies—cognitive, interpersonal, and behavioral—for the patient as well as the patient's family. Family therapy is advisable for immediate family members affected by the patient's disorder because they have a serious role in how the patient responds to relationships.

Patient Education

This disorder is a lifelong problem, and patients must have continued psychological evaluation and treatment, pharmacotherapy, and psychosocial therapy and support aimed at disengaging the patient from situations that trigger either mania or depressive episodes.

Agents Used in the Treatment of Anxiety Disorder

The National Institutes of Mental Health (NIMH, 2011) describes the existence of several types of **anxiety disorders**, including panic disorders, obsessive compulsive disorder, post-traumatic stress disorder, social phobia, specific phobias, and generalized anxiety disorder. Anxiety disorders are common to the point that during any one year, 18% of people experience an anxiety to the extent that its physical symptoms cause them to visit a clinician. For example, generalized anxiety disorder, a condition in which excessive anxiety about several events or activities is experienced for most days during a 6-month period, is a frequent mental health disorder seen in primary care (Kessler, Chiu, Demler, Mcrikangas, & Walters, 2005). Because GAD patients show impairment in many aspects of their life (20% are at increased risk for suicide), they need special help from their clinicians. Yet, 47% of those diagnosed with GAD receive no treatment (Stein, et al., 2005). Despite the high prevalence of all anxiety disorders, they often are under-recognized and undertreated clinical problems.

Conscientious Prescribing of Anxiolytics

- The management of individual anxiety disorders is dependent on the specific diagnosis.
- SSRIs are considered first-line agents for panic disorder, OCD, PTSD, and social phobias by many clinicians.
- Sometimes low-dose benzodiazepines are used for 1 or 2 weeks as adjunct treatment until the SSRI takes full effect.
- GAD is frequently treated with low-dose diazepam or lorazepam, but their ability to generate physical dependence is

always a concern. Venlafaxine, which does not cause physical dependence, is becoming more popular in treating GAD.

- Dosing in panic disorder must start low and go slow due to risk of side effects in patients with this condition. Patients frequently need high doses to prevent attacks, which is the goal when treating panic disorder.
- Because each disorder is fairly chronic, the SSRIs remain the mainstay. If the patient has a history of alcohol or drug dependence, buspirone (BuSpar) may be used because it is nonaddicting.
- Hydroxyzine is FDA approved for anxiety, and there is substantial data to support the use of pregabalin.

Patient/Family Education Regarding the Use of Anxiolytics

- Advise patients to avoid driving and other activities requiring alertness.
- Advise patients to avoid alcohol or other psychotropic medicines unless supervised carefully because concurrent administration of both has often proven fatal.
- Instruct patients not to discontinue abruptly after long-term use because withdrawal syndrome can occur.
- Remind patients that these drugs only relieve anxiety; they do not relieve the perception of pain.

Benzodiazepines (BZDs)

Benzodiazepines are especially useful in the management of acute situational anxiety disorder and adjustment disorder where the duration of pharmacotherapy is anticipated to be 6 weeks or less. They are also used for the rapid control of panic attacks. Chronic benzodiazepine use, however, may be associated with tolerance, withdrawal, and treatment-emergent anxiety.

Tolerance does not usually develop to the beneficial effects of the anxiolytic; rather, it develops to the sedation and the euphoria experienced by the patient.

The risk of addiction to benzodiazepines is very low and is probably only a problem in patients with a preexisting history of substance abuse. However, most patients taking benzodiazepines on a regular, scheduled daily basis, even at therapeutic doses, for longer than 8 weeks, will demonstrate some physical dependence. The popularity of these drugs is probably owing to their hypnotic and anxiolytic dose-related effects, but they also offer the following advantages:

■ Lower fatality rates with acute overdose
■ More favorable side effects and adverse effects profiles
■ Fewer potentially serious drug interactions
■ Patient acceptance is high. Patients often ask for them and ask to be continued on them

Benzodiazepines are categorized as hypnotics (flunitrazepam, flurazepam, and triazolam), anticonvulsants (clorazepate), and anxiolytics. Their use as anticonvulsants and hypnotics is discussed in Chapter 14.

The use of benzodiazepines as anxiolytics is discussed here.

Mechanism of Action

Benzodiazepines depress all levels of the CNS by enhancing the action of GABA, a major inhibitory neurotransmitter in the brain and CNS. Their anxiolytic effect comes from their ability to increase the action of GABA, which, as an inhibitory neurotransmitter, thereby decreases the effect of any neuronal excitation. The benzodiazepines are categorized by their pharmacokinetic properties.

Pharmacokinetics of BZDs Used as Anxiolytics

Drug	Onset	Peak Effect	Duration	Half-Life
diazepam (Valium)	Fast	0.5–2 hr	Long	20–80 hr
midazolam (Versed)	Fast (5–15 min)	30–60 minutes (IM)	2–6 hr	2–6 hr
clorazepate (Tranxene)	Fast	1–2 hr	long	40–50 hr
alprazolam (Xanax)	Intermediate	1–2 hr	intermediate	8–37 hr
chlordiazepoxide (Librium)	Intermediate	0.5–4 hr	long	5–30 hr
clonazepam (Klonopin)	Intermediate	1–4 hr	long	30–40 hr
lorazepam (Ativan)	Intermediate	2–4 hr	intermediate	10–20 hr
prazepam (Centrax)	Slow	6 hr	long	30–100 hr
oxazepam (Serax)	Slow	2–4 hr	intermediate	8 hr

■ Absorption: Given orally, they are well absorbed from the gut. Given intramuscularly, onset is 5 minutes (midazolam). Given orally, onset is 30 to 60 minutes (diazepam) to 6 hours (prazepam). Peak effects usually occur in 1 to 2 hours, and duration lasts up to 2 to 3 hours. Given intramuscularly, effects can start in 1 to 5 minutes, but lorazepam (Ativan) and midazolam (Versed) are rapidly absorbed and widely distributed after intramuscular injection, making them useful as preanesthetic drugs. Diazepam (Valium) is poorly absorbed from an injection site, and its oral absorption is better than intramuscular, thus the popularity of it in tablet form.

■ Distribution: Peak blood levels occur in 1 to 3 hours because protein binding is 85% to 98%.

■ Metabolism: Depending on the benzodiazepine given, metabolism may increase by 50% in the elderly or in those with impaired hepatic function because the metabolite is an active substance. Oxazepam, lorazepam, and temazepam are not metabolized in the liver and therefore are useful in those with liver disease.

■ Excretion: Over 95% is excreted in the urine.

■ Half-life: See the preceding table for normal half-life. Agents such as lorazepam are metabolized to an oxidated metabolite that is biologically active and extends their effective half-life from 10 to 20 hours to 100 hours. Valium also has a long half-life.

Dosage and Administration of Benzodiazepines Used as Anxiolytics

Generic Name	Trade Name	Route	Usual Oral Adult Daily Dose for Anxiety
alprazolam	Xanax	PO	0.5–3 mg, 2–3 times/day
chlordiazepoxide	Librium	PO, IM, IV	5–100 mg, 3–4 times/day
clonazepam	Klonopin	PO	0.5–2 mg, 1–3 times/day
clorazepate	Tranxene ER	PO	11.25–45 mg daily
diazepam	Valium	PO, IV, IM, PR	2–10 mg, 2–4 times/day
lorazepam	Ativan	PO, IV, IM	1–3 mg, 2–3 times/day
oxazepam	Serax	PO	10–30 mg, 2–4 times/day
triazolam	Halcion	PO	0.125–0.25 mg at night

Clinical Uses

■ Anxiety disorders, anticonvulsants, muscle relaxants, adjuvants in anesthesia, and for treatment of alcohol addiction and drug withdrawal

Adverse Reactions

CV: Orthostatic hypotension
DERM: Rashes
EENT: Blurry vision
GI: Constipation, nausea, vomiting, diarrhea, weight gain (unusual and rare)
MISC: Pain at injection site, swelling, carpal tunnel syndrome, physical dependence, psychological dependence, tolerance
NEURO: Ataxia, dizziness, drowsiness, lethargy, headache, slurred speech, forgetfulness, confusion, fatigue, somnolence. Too rapid withdrawal can lead to hand tremor, cramping, diaphoresis, seizures. Memory dysfunction and anterograde amnesia (which is why midazolam is used preoperatively)
PUL: Respiratory depression

Interactions

■ Enhanced CNS depressant effects can occur when used with alcohol and CNS depressants, opiod analgesics, anesthetics, or TCAs.

Contraindications

■ Triazolam (Halcion) and aprazolam (Xanax) are contraindicated in persons receiving ketoconazole and itraconazole.
■ Cross-sensitivity with other benzodiazepines may exist.
■ Contraindicated in patients who are comotose, in uncontrolled severe pain, or have severe hypotension, angle-closure glaucoma, or sleep apnea.
■ Use cautiously in patients with renal impairment, history of depression, or suicidal ideation.

Conscientious Considerations

■ As a class, the benzodiazepines have widespread CNS effects and affect memory, mood, and motor, sensory and cognitive functioning.
■ These agents are DEA Schedule IV drugs.
■ Diazepam is very lipophilic with a very rapid onset of action, but once in the CNS, it rapidly redistributes out to other tissues. For this reason, its duration of action following intermittent dosing is less than an immediate-acting benzodiazepine, such as lorazepam.
■ Lorazepam, which is less lipophilic than diazepam, has a slower onset of action but a longer duration after a single dose.
■ In addition, clinicians must be aware of the important considerations that apply to all anxiolytic agents (see p. 287, Conscientious Prescribing of Anxiolytics).

Patient/Family Education

See p. 287, Patient/Family Education Regarding the Use of Anxiolytics.

Meprobamate (Equanil, Miltown)

This is a DEA Schedule IV drug that is a carbamate derivative. Its use today is extremely limited because of its adverse effects and abuse over the years. Meprobamate affects the thalamus and limbic systems as well as inhibits multineuronal spinal reflexes. Its major use today is to relieve the pain of muscle spasms or other types of muscle rigidity, including headache and premenstrual tension. Side effects, especially drowsiness and dizziness, are frequent. It is known for causing agranulocytosis, hypotensive crisis, Stevens Johnson syndrome, and bullous dermatitis, as well as enhanced CNS depression in the presence of alcohol. Its use today is almost nonexistent.

Implications for Special Populations
Pregnancy Implications

When prescribing psychotherapeutics for the pregnant female, clinicians should carefully consider their choice of drugs. Following is a selected list of psychotherapeutic drugs along with their assigned FDA Safety Category.

FDA SAFETY CATEGORY	DRUGS
B	bupropion, buspirone, clozapine, fluoxetine, maprotiline, sertraline
C	amitriptyline, amoxapine, clomipramine, desipramine, haloperidol, loxapine, mirtazapine, nefazodone, nortriptyline, olsalazine, pimozide, phenelzine, quetiapine, risperidone, trazodone, trimipramine, venlafaxine
D	alprazolam, lorazepam, lithium, midazolam, valproic acid, carbamazepine
X	temazepam, triazolam
Unclassified	doxepin, imipramine, isocarboxazid, molindone, phenothiazines (not recommended during pregnancy), protriptyline, thiothixene, tranylcypromine

Pediatric Implications
Antidepressants

■ TCAs are not recommended for the treatment of depression in children younger than 12 years of age. Several agents such as amitriptyline and Norpramin have been used in children older than 6 years of age for the treatment of major depression. Some of these drugs have also been used in the treatment of enuresis and ADD. Children are very sensitive to an acute overdose, and adolescents also are sensitive and require a reduced dose.
■ Children taking TCAs have experienced changes on their ECGs, sleep disorders, increased nervousness, and hypertension.
■ Young people taking any drug with an antidepressant effect need to be monitored for suicide ideation, especially during the early treatment phase. It is often wise to limit access to large amounts of these drugs. In addition appetite, nutritional intake, weight, and mental status should be continually assessed. (Review page 279, Special Case: Treatment of Depression in Children, Adolescents, and Young Adults Using SSRIs, as the widespread use of SSRIs among this population has created many problems throughout the USA.)
■ Cases have occurred where Paxil has been confused with Taxol, because of like-sounding names.

Antimanics

■ Lithium should be used with caution and monitored closely in children because it decreases bone density and bone formation.

Anxiolytics

■ Young children are more susceptible to the CNS depressant effects of benzodiazepines. In neonates this is especially true because of the lower rate of drug metabolism by the immature liver.

- Although diazepam may be used in infants 6 months and older, this drug should not be used to treat psychosis of hyperactive children.
- Children with excessive sedation and lethargy should be monitored carefully, and doses should be adjusted.
- Paradoxical reactions have been reported in children with the use of these drugs.

Antipsychotics

- Children are at a greater risk for developing extrapyramidal side effects, especially dystonias. Thus, they should be monitored closely.
- Phenothiazine antiemetic therapy should be avoided in children with chickenpox, CNS infections, measles, dehydration, or other acute illnesses because they may have a greater risk of adverse reactions and possibly Reye's syndrome.

Geriatric Implications

Antidepressants

- TCAs may cause increased anxiety in the geriatric patient. Additionally if the patient has cardiovascular disease, the use of TCAs increases the risk of arrhythmias, tachycardia, stroke, congestive heart failure, and myocardial infarction, and especially in the older adult male, they cause **Benign prostatic hyperplasia** (BPH) and CNS effects.

Antimanics

- Lithium can be more toxic in the geriatric patient. Thus, a lower lithium dosage and close monitoring is advised in this age group. The elderly are more prone to develop CNS toxicity, lithium-induced goiter, and clinical hypothyroidism than is the average adult. Excessive thirst and elimination of large volumes of urine may be early side effects of lithium toxicity. Any decrease in renal function as a result of aging is likely to increase the risk of toxicity from lithium.

Anxiolytics

- The elderly and those with CNS dysfunction may experience paradoxical reactions.
- Medications with short-acting durations are preferred. When longer-acting medications are used, patients may experience sedation, ataxia, and memory deficits. Benzodiazepines that are glucuronidated by avoiding phase I metabolism are safer for use in the older adult whose liver function may be impaired.

Antipsychotics

- The elderly have higher serum levels of antipsychotics and antidepressant drugs because of changes in drug distribution that results from decreased lean body mass, less total body water and albumin, and an increase in body fat. Thus, patients should be given lower drug doses and titrated slowly.

- Elderly patients are more prone to orthostatic hypotension, anticholinergic side effects, extrapyramidal effects, and sedation. Thus, close supervision and prescribing the lowest dose possible is advised.
- Elderly patients should receive half the recommended adult dose. Patients with organic brain syndrome should only receive 33% to 50% of the usual adult dose, with increases in dosage at the 7- to 10-day period.

LEARNING EXERCISES

Case 1

JF is a 20-year-old student at the local community college. She comes in to see you with a concern of feeling very anxious about leaving her room. Her symptoms started 5 months ago after her boyfriend broke up with her. Shortly after this, she experienced lightheadedness and dizziness and was told by the school doctor that symptoms would abate in a few weeks. The symptoms started rather suddenly, and in addition to the lightheadedness and dizziness, also include heart pounding and sweating. Her symptoms have persisted, and now she has frequent "spells." These spells have been occurring a few times a week for the past 6 weeks. She is afraid she is going crazy. Now she also feels faint and at times feels as if she is "out of her body," and becomes sweaty and short of breath. She is afraid to leave her room for fear of having a spell in public. Routine laboratory test results, including thyroid testing, are all normal.

1. Write a prescription for the medication you would recommend for a patient with a diagnosis of panic disorder.
   Rx: _____
   M: _____
   Sig: _____

2. Why did you choose this medication?

3. What patient advisories would you give?

   There are a number of effective treatments for panic disorder, including SSRIs, TCAs, MAOIs, and cognitive behavioral therapy. Benzodiazepines are also effective, but they may cause depression and are associated with adverse symptoms during and after use.

Case 2

HG is a 19-year-old college student who comes into the university clinic complaining that he is tired, has low energy, difficulty focusing on his classes, has low appetite, and has lost 20 pounds over the last 2 months. He states he has lost interest in his one hobby, the college marching band. His major complaint, however, is insomnia. One of his "professors who cares" noticed his declining interest and grades and suggested he come to the clinic to find out if something is wrong. During his workup it is discovered that he is feeling "down," feeling guilty over loss of a scholarship, drinks little alcohol, has no suicidal thoughts, takes no prescription or recreational drugs, and finally that his brother, sister, and mother were all treated successfully for depression. His physical finding shows his blood work is normal, especially thyroid, blood counts, and blood chemistry. You now believe your patient is depressed.

1. Write a prescription for the medication you would recommend.

   Rx: _____

   M: _____

   Sig: _____

2. Why did you choose this medication?

3. What patient advisories would you give?

References

Canto, J. G., Shipek, M. G., Rogers, W. G., Malmgren, J. A., Frederick, P. D., Lambrew, C. T., et al. (2005). Prevalence, clinical characteristics, and mortality among myocardial infarction patients without clinical symptoms. *Journal of the American Medical Association, 283*(24), 3223-3229.

Correll, C. U., Manu, P., Olshanshy, V., Napolitano, B., Kane, J. M., Malhotra, A. K. (2009). Cardiometabolic risk of second-generation antipsychotic medications during first-time use in children and adolescents. *Journal of the American Medical Association, 302*(16):1765-1773.

Fink, C., & Guyak, J. (2005). *Bipolar disorder for dummies* (p. 11). Hoboken, NJ: Wiley Publishing.

Food and Drug Administration. (2004). FDA launches a multi-pronged strategy to strengthen safeguards for children treated with antidepressant medications. Press release. Retrieved February 8, 2013, from www.fda.gov/NewsEvents/Newsroom/PressAnnouncements/2004/ucm108363.htm

Gonzales, H. M., Vega, W. A., & Williams, D. R. (2010). Depression care in the USA: Too little for too few. *Archives of General Psychiatry, 67*(1), 37-46.

Grunz, H., Vieta, E., Goodwin, G. M., Bowden, C., Licht, R. W., Möller, H. J. et al. (2010). The World Federation of Societies of Biological Psychiatry: Guidelines for the biologic treatment of bipolar disorders, 2010 update. *The World Journal of Biological Psychiatry, 11,* 81-109.

Kessler, R. C., Chiu, W. T., Demler, O., Merikangas, K. R., Walters, E. E. (2005). Prevalence, severity, and comorbidity of 12-month DSM-IV disorders in the National Comorbidity Survey Replication. *Archives of General Psychiatry, 62,* 617-627.

Kim, K. H., Lee, S. M., Paik, K. S., & Kim, N. S. (2011). The effects of continuous antidepressant treatment during the first 6 months on relapse or recurrence of depression. *Journal of Affective Disorders, 132*(1), 121-129.

National Institute of Mental Health (NIMI). (2008). Prevalence of serious mental illness among U.S. adults by age, sex, and race in 2008. Table. Retrieved February 6, 2013, from www.nimh.nih.gov/statistics/pdf/NSDUH-SMI-Adults.pdf

Singh, T., & Rajpit, M. (2006). Misdiagnosis of bipolar disorder. *Psychiatry, 3*(10), 57-63. Retrieved February 7, 2013, from www.ncbi.nlm.nih.gov/pmc/articles/PMC2945875

Stein, M. B., Roy-Byrne, P. P., Craske, M. G., Bystritsky, A., Sullivan, G., Pyne, J. M., et al. (2005). Functional impact and health utility of anxiety disorders in primary care outpatients. *Medical Care, 43,* 1164-1170.

Substance Abuse and Mental Health Services Administration (SAMHSA). (2007). Mental health: A report of the U.S. Surgeon General: Depression and Suicide in children and adolescents. Retrieved from www.surgeongeneral.gov/library/mentalhealth/pdfs/c1.pdf

Wilson, A. S., Howell, C. W., & Aring, C. S. (2007). Venlafaxine ingestion is associated with rhabdomyolysis in adults: A case series. *Journal of Toxicological Sciences, 32*(1), 97-101.

World Health Organization. (2001). Cross-national comparisons of the prevalence and correlates of mental disorders. *Bulletin of the World Health Organization, 78*(4), 413-426.

chapter 16

Drugs Used in the Treatment of Skin Disorders

Alice A. House, Mona M. Sedrak, William N. Tindall

Key Terms

Comedone
Eczema
Epidermis
Plaque
Pressure
Psoriasis
Sebum
Seborrhea
Shingles
Sore
Thermoregulation
Urticaria

CHAPTER FOCUS

Dermatological conditions can be treated with both oral and topical medications, which are available in multiple formulations and delivered as creams, gels, ointments, suppositories, sprays, patches, and other forms. Clinicians must understand not only which medications are appropriate for a given condition, but also which formulation is appropriate for that condition and the patient who will use it. The availability of many dermatological treatments over-the-counter (OTC) complicates the work of a clinician because many patients will try multiple OTC products or home remedies before seeking treatment.

The majority of patients who present to clinicians' offices with dermatological conditions have common conditions such as rashes, acne, tumors, and warts, as well as chronic conditions such as eczema and psoriasis. The proper treatment of dermatological complaints is paramount to a patient's general well-being because there is often a social stigma associated with lesions of the skin, especially when associated with the face and hands. This chapter presents a general introduction to dermatological principles to aid the clinician in treating the skin.

OBJECTIVES

After reading and studying this chapter, the student should be able to:

1. Properly use common dermatological preparations, considering cost, convenience, efficacy, and side effects.
2. Discuss the unique challenges in treating pediatric, geriatric, and pregnant patients.
3. Describe the various treatment modalities and the appropriate rationale for the use of oral versus topical treatment of dermatological disorders.
4. Describe the various topical treatment modalities in dermatology and the appropriate use of each one.
5. Discuss the treatment of common skin conditions such as acne, eczema, psoriasis, seborrhea, and dermatitis (allergic and contact).
6. Discuss the treatment of infectious skin disorders, including bacterial, viral, fungal, and parasitic disorders.
7. Discuss the treatment of burns and pressure sores and prevention of sun damage and sunburn.

KEY DRUGS USED TO TREAT SKIN DISORDERS*

Topical Corticosteroids
- betamethasone
- fluocinonide (Lidex)
- triamcinolone
- hydrocortisone

Anti-Acne Agents

Retinoic Acid Derivatives
- isotretinoin (Accutane)
- tretinoin (Retin A)
- tazarotene (Tazorac)
- adapalene (Differin)

Keratolytics
- benzoyl peroxide (Benzac)
- salicylic acid (Aveeno)

Oral Antibiotics
- tetracycline (Sumycin)
- doxycycline (Vibramycin)
- minocycline (Minocin)
- erythromycin (E-Mycin)
- clindamycin (Cleocin)
- dapsone (Aczone)

Sunscreens
- zinc oxide
- titanium oxide
- octocrylene

Anti-itch/Anti-Urticarics
- diphenhydramine (Benadryl)
- loratadine (Claritin)

- fexofenadine (Allegra)
- cetirizine (Zyrtec)
- cyproheptadine (Periactin)
- hydroxyzine (Vistaril)

Topical Antibiotics
- mupirocin (Bactroban)
- neomycin/polymyxin B/bacitracin (Neosporin)

Topical Antifungals
- imidazole
- triazoles

Topical Antivirals
- acyclovir (Zovirax)
- docosanol (Abreva)
- penciclovir (Denavir)
- famciclovir (Famvir)
- valacyclovir (Valtrex)

Cleansing and Disinfecting Agents
- isopropyl alcohol
- chlorhexidine (Hibiclens, Chlorohex)
- cationic surfactants (benzalkonium chloride)
- hydrogen peroxide
- povidone-iodine
- phenol derivatives (hexachlorophene, triclosan, Phisohex)

Agents for Burns
- silver sulfadiazine
- mafenide

Agents for Psoriasis
- cyclosporin A
- methotrexate
- fumaric acid
- hydroxyurea (Droxia, Hydrea)
- thioguanine (Tabloid)
- sulfasalazine (Azulfidine)
- mycophenolate mofetil (CellCept)

Agents for Seborrhea
- pyrithione
- selenium sulfide (Selsun, Selsun Blue)
- ketoconazole (Extina, Nizoral A-D, Xolegel)
- sulfanilamide
- tar shampoo

Agents for Skin and Hair Infestations
- crotamiton (Eurax)
- lindane (Kwell)
- malathion (Ovide)
- permethrin (Elimite, Nix)

Topical Anesthetics
- benzocaine
- lidocaine (Xylocaine)
- lidocaine /prilocaine (Emla)

*When appropriate, trade names are placed in their respective sections within the chapter.

The skin is composed of two principle layers, the **epidermis** and its various structures and the dermis. The epidermis is composed of four or five layers, depending on the region of skin. They include, in descending order: (1) the cornified layer (stratum corneum), (2) the clear/translucent layer (stratum lucidum), (3) the granular cell layer (stratum granulosum), (4) the spinous layer (stratum spinosum), and (5) the basal layer (stratum basale). Thirty days are generally required for a cell to fully transform from a basal layer cell to a keratinized cell in the outer layers of the skin. The chief functions of the skin include protection, **thermoregulation**, water regulation, and some vitamin production. The functions of the appendages (hair and nails) include protection and thermoregulation for the hair and protection for the nails. Hair follicles can extend into the subcutaneous layers and may help in the sensation of touch.

Pharmacological agents used topically are often active ingredients contained in an inactive base, although the moisturizing or drying properties of the vehicle may also aid in healing (Box 16-1). Moisturizing agents aid in the absorption of the active ingredients through the skin. Occlusion with plastic wrap will also aid in absorption by increasing the moisturizing properties and by warming the skin.

Care should be taken when applying topical medications to the face, scrotum, axilla, and scalp because of increased permeability in those areas. Dosages may need to be decreased in these areas. In general, lesions that are weeping, oozing, vesicular, or crusting should be treated with lotions, tinctures, and wet dressings to aid in drying. Lesions with xerosis, lichenification, or scaling should be treated with creams and ointments to aid in moisturizing. Aerosols, lotions, and gels may aid in the application of topical medications to hairy areas and the scalp. Patients may express irritation to the inactive ingredients, emulsifiers, or moisturizers added to topical preparations and care should be taken to avoid known triggers. Finally, it is important to consider the effects of skin disorders such as disfigurement, discomfort (both physical, with pain and itching, and mental, with anxiety or depression), and loss of function on the quality of a patient's life.

TOPICAL CORTICOSTEROIIDS

Topical corticosteroids decrease inflammation, reduce itching, and are often the mainstay of treatment in both acute and chronic dermatitis. Potency of the medication differs due to formulation, vehicle, and site of application. In general, low-potency formulations should be used in chronic conditions such as eczema, irritant dermatitis, seborrhea, and atopic dermatitis whereas the more potent formulations may need to be used for conditions such as psoriasis, lichen planus, and allergic contact dermatitis.

Many vehicle types, including ointments, gels, aerosols, creams and lotions, are available for delivery of the topical corticosteroids. Chronic lesions often require the moisturizing properties of creams and ointments, whereas acute lesions may

---

BOX 16-1 Drug Vehicles

Aerosol—A substance, such as a drug containing therapeutically active ingredients, packaged under pressure with a gaseous propellant for release as a spray of fine particles.

Bath—A medium such as water, vapor, sand, or mud, in which the body is wholly or partially immersed for therapeutic or cleansing purposes.

Colloid—A suspension of finely divided particles in a continuous medium from which the particles do not settle out rapidly and are not readily filtered.

Cream—A pharmaceutical preparation consisting of a semisolid emulsion of either the oil-in-water or the water-in-oil type.

Emollient—An agent that softens or soothes the skin.

Gel—A colloid in which the components combine to produce a semisolid material.

Lotion—A liquid suspension or dispersion for external application to the body.

Ointment—A highly viscous or semisolid preparation usually containing medicinal substances and often in a petroleum base.

Paste—A semisolid preparation containing one or more drug substances.

Powder—A dry mass of pulverized or finely dispersed solid particles.

Skin protectant—Any number of preparations designed to protect the skin from noxious stimuli particularly the sun.

Solution—A liquid preparation of one or more soluble chemical substances usually dissolved in water.

Tincture—A solution of active ingredients with alcohol as the solvent.

Wet dressing—A dressing that is soaked prior to application to aid in débridement and cleansing.

---

only require lighter creams, lotions, or gels. Creams are generally preferred over ointments because of their nonocclusive nature and less greasy feel after application. Ointments are better absorbed but are often messy and unacceptable to the patient. Weeping lesions and lesions on the scalp may require aerosols to aid in delivery of the medication. Lotions are easy to apply but often contain alcohol that may lead to stinging in the already irritated skin. Gels spread easily and may be used on the scalp and hairy areas to facilitate delivery.

When considering a topical corticosteroid, the site and extent of the affected area must be considered. The axilla, groin, face, and neck more readily absorb topical corticosteroids, and a lower dose should be used when they are applied in these areas. Large surface areas that require treatment may also lead to significant side effects due to increased local and systemic absorption. The most common adverse effect of topical corticosteroid absorption use is cutaneous atrophy, which is manifested by thinning of the skin accompanied by telangiectasia. It occurs more often with increasing potency and length of use. Other adverse effects of topical corticosteroid use include striae, acne, hypopigmentation, alopecia, and glaucoma. Adrenal suppression, which could be life threatening, may also occur.

Conscientious Prescribing of Topical Steroids

- The anti-inflammatory effect of topical steroids is nonspecific, thus they act against most cases of inflammation.
- Variable amounts of drug will be systemically absorbed depending on the steroid chosen and the vehicle used to apply it to the skin. Drug absorption is enhanced by increased skin temperature, skin hydration, and application to denuded areas.
- Topical steroids *cannot* be used for extensive periods in women who are or may become pregnant.

- There are too many topical steroids in the marketplace for any practitioner to be familiar with them all, thus familiarity with one or two in each category is all that is needed to be effective in most cases.
- The most commonly used low-potency steroid in topical formulations is 1% hydrocortisone.

Patient/Family Teaching

- Any patient given oral steroids for eczema or other conditions must understand the effects are short term and that these agents *cannot* be used frequently.
- Patients must also be advised that any feeling of euphoria or well-being because they feel that their condition has been cured is a false impression because improvement in any acute exacerbation may be dramatic and symptoms may reappear after the steroids wear off.

Mechanism of Action

Controls the rate of protein synthesis; depresses the migration of polymorphonuclear leukocytes, fibroblasts; reverses capillary permeability and lysosomal stabilization at the cellular level to prevent or control inflammation.

Pharmacokinetics

- Absorption: Topical application assumes no systemic absorption, but these agents can be absorbed through intact skin.
- Distribution: If systemically absorbed, will be about two-thirds protein bound.
- Metabolism: Hepatic metabolism if absorbed.
- Excretion: Urine (less than 5% as unchanged drug).
- Half-life: 6.5 hours.

Dosage and Administration of Topical Corticosteroids

POTENCY	MEDICATION	COMMON TOPICAL APPLICATIONS
I. SUPER HIGH (maximum of 45 gm/week)	betamethasone dipropionate gel and ointment 0.05% (Diprolene)	Apply 1–2 times/day less than or equal to 2 weeks
	clobetasol propionate 0.05% (Temovate)	Apply 2 times/day for 2–4 weeks maximum
	diflorasone diacetate ointment 0.05% (Psorcon)	Apply 1–3 times/day
	halobetasol propionate cream 0.05% (Ultravate)	Apply 1–2 times/day for 2 weeks maximum
II. HIGH POTENCY	amcinonide ointment 0.1% (Cyclocort)	Apply 1–2 times/day for 2 weeks maximum
	betamethasone dipropionate ointment 0.1% (Diprosone)	Apply 1–2 times/day for 2 weeks maximum
	desoximetasone diacetate cream and ointment 0.25%, gel 0.05% (Topicort)	Apply 1–2 times/day for 2 weeks maximum
	diflorasone diacetate cream and ointment 0.05% (Florone)	Apply daily for 2 weeks maximum
	fluocinonide 0.05% (Lidex)	Apply 2–4 times/day
	halcinonide cream 0.1% (Halog)	Apply 1–3 times/day
III. HIGH POTENCY	betamethasone dipropionate lotion 0.05% (Diprosone)	Apply 1–2 times/day for 2 weeks maximum
	betamethasone valerate ointment 0.01% (Valisone)	Apply 2 times/day for 2 weeks maximum
	diflorasone diacetate cream 0.05% (Florone, Maxiflor)	Apply 1 time/day for 2 weeks maximum
		Apply 1 time/day for 2 weeks maximum
	mometasone furoate ointment 0.1% (Elocon)	Apply 1–3 times/day for 2 weeks maximum
	triamcinolone acetonide cream 0.05% (Aristocort)	
IV. MEDIUM POTENCY	desoximetasone cream 0.05% (Topicort)	Apply 1–2 times/day for 2 weeks
	fluocinolone acetonide cream 0.2%, ointment 0.025% (Synalar)	Apply 2–4 times/day
	flurandrenolide ointment 0.05% (Cordran)	Apply 1–4 times/day
	triamcinolone acetonide ointment 0.1% (Aristocort, Kenalog)	Apply 1–3 times/day for 2 weeks maximum
V. MEDIUM POTENCY	betamethasone valerate cream and lotion 0.1% (Valisone)	Apply 2 times/day for 2 weeks maximum
	fluocinolone acetonide cream 0.025% (Synalar®)	Apply 2–4 times/day
	flurandrenolide cream 0.05% (Cordran)	Apply 1–4 times/day
	hydrocortisone butyrate cream 0.1% (Locoid)	Apply 2–3 times/day
	hydrocortisone valerate cream 0.2% (Westcort)	Apply 2–3 times/day
	prednicarbate emollient cream 0.1% (Dermatop)	Apply 2–3 times/day
	triamcinolone acetonide cream and lotion 0.1% (Kenalog)	Apply 3 times/day for 2 weeks maximum
VI. MEDIUM POTENCY	triamcinolone acetonide cream 0.1% (Aristocort)	Apply 1–3 times/day for 2 weeks maximum
	alclometasone dipropionate cream and ointment 0.05% (Aclovate)	Apply 2–3 times/day for 2 weeks
	betamethasone valerate lotion 0.1% (Valisone)	Apply 1–3 times/day
	desonide cream 0.05% (Tridesilon)	Apply 1–3 times/day
	desonide lotion 0.05% (DesOwen)	Apply 2–3 times/day
	fluocinolone acetonide cream and solution 0.01% (Synalar)	Apply 2–4 times/day
VII. LOW POTENCY	hydrocortisone cream, ointment, and lotion 1% and 2.5% (Hytone)	Apply 2–4 times/day

Clinical Uses

■ Inflammatory dermatoses, such as seborrheic or atopic dermatitis
■ Reduce itching
■ Acute and chronic dermatitis: eczema, irritant and allergic dermatitis, seborrhea and atopic dermatitis
■ Psoriasis
■ Lichen planus

Adverse Reactions (Systemic Absorption)

CV: Congestive heart failure
DERM: Ecchymoses, facial erythema, fragile skin, hirsutism, hyperpigmentation/hypopigmentation, striae, wound healing impaired, acneiform eruptions
EENT: Cataracts, glaucoma, intraocular pressure increased
ENDO: Cushing's syndrome, diabetes mellitus, growth suppression, hyperglycemia
GI: Appetite increased
MS: Necrosis (femoral and humeral heads)
NEURO: Dizziness, headache

Interactions

■ None if topical

Contraindications

■ Hypersensitivity to the steroid or any component in the formulation
■ Contraindicated in systemic fungal infections

Conscientious Considerations

■ Choice of vehicle used depends on site and type of lesion. Use ointments for dry scaly lesions, creams for oozing areas or aesthetic reasons. Gels, ointments, and aerosols are useful for hairy areas.
■ Apply ointments, creams, and gels sparingly as a thin film and only to clean skin **Note:** Occlusive dressings can be a problem because the occlusion increases absorption of the medication.
■ Aerosols need to be shaken thoroughly before use. Spray carefully for 2 seconds and cover an area no larger than the size of a hand.
■ Do not inhale aerosols or spray near eyes.

Patient/Family Education

■ Instruct patients regarding proper use (as above).
■ Caution patients on occlusive dressings (unless indicated).
■ Caution patients to avoid use in infants with diapers because the diapers act as an occlusive.
■ Caution women who are pregnant not to use these agents for any length of time.
■ Caution patients to ask for help from a clinician if symptoms worsen because it could be a sign of another underlying condition.

SPOTLIGHT ON DERMATITIS AND ECZEMA

Eczema is characterized by an inflammatory process that leads to weeping vesicles, followed by crusting and lichenification. Dermatitis caused by inflammation due to irritant contact, allergic contact, or atopy display similar lesions. Pruritus is a common feature of all types of dermatitis and should be treated to prevent scratching and possible sequelae such as scarring and secondary infections. A search for causes of irritation should be initiated regardless of the type of dermatitis because even endogenous atopic eczema may have exogenous triggers (stress, allergies, and irritants).

Hand eczema is a special case where eczema begins as a mild dryness and redness. It can progress to the point at which it interferes with an adult's daily work. Emollients are the first line of treatment to halt progression and protect the hands. Topical steroids are the mainstay of treatment.

Medical Management

Treatment consists of pruritic control with antihistamines and lesion control with corticosteroids. The lowest-potency formulation should be used for the shortest period of time possible to avoid systemic effects. Fluorinated corticosteroids should not be used on the face, genital area, or mucosal area to avoid excessive systemic absorption and side effects or a rosacea-like reaction on the face.

Acute eczema is best treated with mild to moderate corticosteroids and wet dressings to decrease weeping. Chronic eczema is treated by decreasing triggers, maintaining moisture to the skin, and the use of corticosteroids. When there is an inadequate response to conventional therapies, or when patients cannot tolerate medium-potency corticosteroids, tacrolimus (Prograf) and pimecrolimus (Elidel), topical formulations of immunosuppressive agents, may be used for short-term or maintenance therapy of intermittent atopic dermatitis.

Protecting the Skin From UV Radiation

Sunscreens are used to prevent or decrease the effects of ultraviolet (UV) radiation on the skin. Two types of UV radiation, UVA and UVB, are chiefly responsible for most sun damage to the skin. UVA radiation penetrates the skin more deeply than does UVB and is responsible for wrinkling, the darker pigmentation of photoaging, and leathering of the skin. UVB radiation is most commonly associated with sunburn, although UVA may also be minimally responsible for sunburns. Both UVA and UVB radiation can lead to several types of skin cancer, and decreased exposure to all UV radiation has been shown to decrease the risk of skin cancer. No sunscreen can prevent all exposure to UV radiation, and UVA radiation is only minimally reduced by some sunscreens.

When evaluating a sunscreen for efficacy, the sun protection factor (SPF) is often used to determine the ability of a given sunscreen to adequately protect from short-term and long-term effects of the sun. The SPF is a measure of a sunscreen's ability to protect against UVB. In general, an SPF of 15 or greater will be needed to offer adequate protection for most people (if it takes someone 10 minutes to burn, use of a product with an SPF of 15 will enable him or her to spend approximately 150 minutes in the sun before burning). Because UVA radiation is responsible

for the long-term effects of the sun, much damage can occur irrespective of the presence or absence of sunburn. Sunscreen should be applied 15 minutes before exposure to the sun and reapplied 30 minutes to 2 hours after exposure to the sun. Frequent reapplication (every 2 hours) is needed if one is swimming or sweating.

Many of the sunscreens available in the United States today combine several active chemical sunscreen ingredients to provide protection against both UVA and UVB radiation. There are two types of sunscreens popular today: physical sunscreens and chemical sunscreens. Physical sunscreens contain zinc oxide or titanium dioxide to protect against UVB and UVA by deflecting UV radiation. Zinc oxide is a preferred ingredient because it blocks more UV radiation than does titanium dioxide. Chemical sunscreens work by absorbing or scattering sun rays. Octocrylene is a chemical sunscreen that has both UVA- and UVB-absorbing properties. Benzophenones (such as avobenzone) absorb both UVA and UVB rays and prevent them from reaching the skin.

DRUGS USED IN THE TREATMENT OF ACNE AND ROSACEA

Acne vulgaris (common acne) is thought to be caused by a disruption in the normal function of the pilosebaceous unit of the skin. Excessive **sebum** production, caused by sebaceous gland hyperplasia under the influence of androgens, and hyperkeratinization of the hair follicle results in obstruction of the follicle and the formation of a small **comedo**. This provides an environment that can become colonized by *Propionibacterium acnes*. The presence of bacteria begins an immune response that includes the production of inflammatory mediators. These inflamed lesions are most commonly seen in areas of the body that have the highest concentration of sebaceous glands (face, chest, back, neck, upper arms). A number of factors are thought to lead to the formation of acne, including androgenic activity, mechanical obstruction, cosmetics, stress, medications, and possibly diet.

Comedones (the plural of comedo) can develop into open (blackhead) lesions or closed (whitehead) lesions. Inflammatory papules or pustules may develop and may progress to larger lesions (nodules). In severe cases, scars and hyperpigmentation may occur. The American Academy of Dermatology notes three levels of severity: mild, moderate, and severe. In mild acne, there are a few to several papules and pustules, but no nodules. In moderate acne, there are several papules and pustules and a few nodules. In severe disease, there are extensive papules and pustules, along with many nodules.

Rosacea, which is often mistaken for acne, is a chronic condition characterized by a redness of the central area of the face that may or may not include comedones. This condition can progress across the cheeks, nose, and forehead. It is considered a harmless condition unless it affects the eyes. It primarily affects Caucasians and is more common in women. Treatment with topical steroids is likely to aggravate the condition.

Drugs Used for Acne: Keratolytics, Antibiotics, Vitamin A Derivatives

Mild keratolytics such as benzoyl peroxide and salicylic acid cause the cells of the epidermis to shed more readily and help prevent pores from clogging. Highly concentrated formulations may lead to hyperpigmentation and an increased risk of skin irritation. Benzoyl peroxide converts to benzoic acid in the skin and releases free-radical oxygen, which oxidizes bacteria proteins and leads to a decrease in the number of anaerobic bacteria in the follicles. All concentrations of benzoyl peroxide seem to work equally; however, the higher strengths seem to lead to more topical irritation. These compounds are absorbed via the skin, with gels showing more penetration than creams. Side effects include irritation, contact dermatitis, dryness, erythema, peeling, and stinging.

Antibiotics can be used to decrease the bacterial load and the inflammation and infection resulting from the presence of bacteria. Treatment may be topical or oral, although oral antibiotics should be reserved for resistant cases. The addition of benzoyl peroxide to topical antibiotic treatment provides better results than either agent alone. Tetracycline, doxycycline, minocycline, erythromycin, and clindamycin are oral antibiotics commonly used in the treatment of acne. Tetracycline and minocycline are bacteriostatic antibiotics that have a long half-life of 24 to 48 hours when given orally. However, when applied topically, the mechanism by which they improve acne remains unknown. Tetracycline itself is active against *P. acnes*. Because resistance is an issue, clinicians prefer other tetracyclines such as doxycycline and minocycline. Clindamycin and metronidazole are sometimes included in a compounded formulation. All tetracyclines become more potent after their expiration date; therefore, their use should be avoided after that date. Side effects include light sensitivity, gastric upset, and diarrhea. Caution should be taken in prescribing these medications to children under the age of 8 years (because their teeth are still forming) and pregnant women to avoid the blue-gray/yellow-brown discoloration or mottling of the teeth and bones of a developing fetus or those in early childhood. Topical antibiotic formulations often include erythromycin and clindamycin alone or in combination with benzoyl peroxide because the peroxide has activity against *P. acnes*, the predominant organism in sebaceous follicles and comedones. Topical antibiotics offer decreased systemic effects; however, clindamycin may still lead to infection with *Clostridium difficile*, and patients should be informed to report unexplained diarrhea to their clinician while taking this medication.

Vitamin A is a fat-soluble vitamin, and derivatives of this vitamin (retinoids) are used in the treatment of many skin disorders, including acne. Retinoids prevent the formation of comedones by normalizing the desquamation of the follicular epithelium. Tretinoin (Retin A) has been in use much longer than have been the other agents, adapalene and tazarotene. All retinoids are known to lead to excessive drying, burning, and inflammation of the skin. This can be decreased by using the medication every other day or by decreasing the dosage. Tretinoin has been rated pregnancy category C and should not be used in pregnant women or in those who may become pregnant. Tazarotene and isotretinoin (Accutane) have been designated pregnancy category X and should never be used in those who might be pregnant. All agents are available in various strengths and vehicles. The choice of vehicle is determined by the patient's skin type and the patient's response to the treatment. Details about drugs used to treat acne are summarized in Table 16-1.

TABLE 16-1 Drugs Used in the Treatment of Acne

	GENERIC NAME	TRADE NAME	ROUTE	DOSAGE
MILD KERATOLYTICS	benzoyl peroxide	Benzac, Brevoxyl, Desquam-X	Topically	Apply 1–3 times/day
	salicylic acid	Aveeno Clear Complexion	Topically	Apply 2 times/day
ANTIMICROBIAL THERAPY	dapsone*	Aczone	Gel	Apply a pea-sized amount to acne lesions 2 times/day for up to 12 weeks
	tetracycline, minocycline	Sumycin, Minocin, Solodyn	PO	Taken orally 2 times/day
	erythromycin	Akne-Mycin	Topically	Applied 2 times/day
	clindamycin	Generic	PO	Taken orally 2 times/day
		Cleocin T, Clindagel	Topically	Topically 2 times/day
RETINOIC ACID DERIVATIVES	adapalene	Differin	Topically	Apply daily in the evening
	tazarotene	Avage, Tazorac	Topically	Apply daily in the evening
	tretinoin	Retin A	Topically	Apply daily in the evening
	isotretinoin	Accutane	PO	2 times/day

*Note: All drugs have side effects, and dapsone is one of them, even though applied topically. Dapsone may lead to hemolytic anemia in those with glucose-6-phosphate dehydrogenase deficiency and should not be used in patients with this deficiency.

DRUGS USED IN THE TREATMENT OF URTICARIA

Urticaria derives from the Latin word for nettle and means "to burn or to itch." It can result from allergic reactions, viral illnesses, autoimmune causes, exercise, cold, sunlight, and idiopathic causes. Histamine release from cells leads to wheals, erythema, and itching and is the common result regardless of the initiating stimulus. Treatment is geared toward decreasing the triggers and combating the effects of the histamine release. Antihistamines act at the histamine receptor to decrease the release of histamine from the mast cells. First-generation antihistamines (diphenhydramine) are effective, but can lead to drowsiness. Diphenhydramine is usually taken orally, but it is also found in many creams, lotions, gels and sprays for topical application; these formulations do not cause drowsiness. Second-generation antihistamines (loratadine, fexofenadine, cetirizine) are effective in relieving itching and cause very little drowsiness when used at the commonly prescribed lower dosages. Details about drugs used to treat urticaria are summarized in Table 16-2.

DRUGS USED FOR SUPERFICIAL BACTERIAL INFECTIONS

Impetigo is a superficial bacterial infection that is caused by *Staphylococcus aureus* and *Streptococcus pyogenes*. It is common in children, but may occur at any age, and it is most commonly contracted due to physical contact (e.g., in sports such as wrestling). It is characterized by lesions with a honey-colored crust and is highly contagious. The best treatment is prevention, with attention to hand washing and hygiene. Prior to antibiotics, treatment consisted of gentian violet, which was moderately effective but left violet stains on the patient and clothing. Topical antibiotics are often sufficient to resolve these infections; however, oral treatment with dicloxacillin, erythromycin, or amoxicillin with clavulanate may be required. One of the topical antibiotics, mupirocin, is effective against gram-positive bacteria, including methicillin-resistant *Staphylococcus aureus*, and acts by inhibiting RNA synthesis in the bacterial cell. Triple antibiotic ointment is a combination of neomycin, bacitracin, and polymyxin B, and it is fairly effective against most superficial infections. Because many people are allergic to the neomycin component, a double antibiotic formulation was fashioned containing only bacitracin and polymyxin B.

Mechanism of Action

Mupirocin binds to bacterial transfer-RNA synthetase, which results in the inhibition of protein synthesis and, ultimately, the protein used for cell wall synthesis. The antibiotic formulations, whether single, double, or triple, affect either gram-positive bacteria, gram-negative bacteria, or are broad spectrum.

Pharmacokinetics

- Absorption: Topical, penetrates outer layers of skin with minimal systemic absorption.
- Metabolism: Skin.
- Excretion: Urine (10% to 40%) within 24 hours.
- Half-life: Systemic absorption is no more than 0.3% of which half-life is 20-40 minutes as it converts to an inactive metabolite. Topical removal is by normal skin desquamation.

Dosage and Administration

GENERIC NAME	TRADE NAME	ROUTE	DOSAGE
mupirocin	Bactroban	Topically	apply 3 times/ day, for 3–5 days
neomycin/ bacitracin/ polymyxin B	Neosporin triple antibiotic ointment	Topically	apply 1–5 times/day for 10 days
bacitracin/ polymyxin B	Polysporin	Topically	apply 1–5 times/day for 10 days

TABLE 16-2	Antihistamine Drugs Used in the Treatment of Urticaria			
CLASS	GENERIC NAME	TRADE NAME	ROUTE	DOSAGE FOR URTICARIA
FIRST-GENERATION ANTIHISTAMINES	diphenhydramine	Benadryl	PO Topically	6–11 years old: 1 tablet (tab) or capsule (cap) every 4–6 hr as needed Younger than 12 years old: 1–2 tabs, caps, or strips every 4–6 hr as needed Apply as needed; max 4 times a day
	cyproheptadine	Periactin	PO	Over 14 years: 4 mg every 8 hr 2–6 years: 2 mg every 8–12 hr 6–14 years: 2–4 mg every 8–12 hr
	hydroxyzine	Atarax Vistaril	PO	25–100 mg 3–4 times/day
SECOND-GENERATION ANTIHISTAMINES	loratadine fexofenadine	Claritin Allegra-12 hr Allegra-24 hr	PO PO PO	Older than 6 years: 1 tab or cap daily, as needed Older than 12 years: 1 tab every 12 hr, as needed Older than 12 years: 1 tab daily
	cetirizine	Zyrtec	PO	Older than 6 years: 1 tab/ or cap daily

Clinical Use

■ Superficial skin infections

Adverse Reactions

DERM: Cellulitis, dermatitis, dry skin, erythema, hives, pruritus, rash
EENT: Blepharitis
GI: Anorexia, nausea, vomiting, diarrhea
MISC: Burning, edema, pain, stinging, tenderness
NEURO: Dizziness, headache

Interactions

■ Nasal mupirocin should not be used concurrently with other nasal products.

Contraindications

■ Hypersensitivities to the agent or any ingredient in its formulation

Conscientious Considerations

■ Wash affected area with soap and water *before* applying. Apply only a small amount and gently rub in.
■ Treated area may be covered with gauze if desired.

Patient/Family Education

■ Instruct patient on correct application.
■ Advise patients to adhere to the recommended dosage and length of use for best results.
■ Teach patients proper techniques to avoid spread of any condition.
■ Instruct patients to inform a school nurse for monitoring, screening, and prevention of transmission.

DRUGS USED FOR SUPERIFICAL FUNGAL INFECTIONS

Fungal infections are common, can affect any part of the body, and they affect millions of people worldwide. They are generally caused by *Trichophyton* or *Microsporum* species and are categorized by the location of the infection, for example, athlete's foot (tinea pedis), vaginal yeast infections (candidiasis), ring worm (tinea corporis or tinea capitis if on the scalp), jock itch (tinea cruris), or nails (onychomycosis or tinea unguium). Intact skin is normally an adequate defense against fungal infections; however, a weakened immune system, antibiotic use, or prolonged exposure to fungi, along with a moist and warm environment, may allow the fungi to penetrate that defense. Treatment for fungal infections can be topical or oral, and they generally clear easily and without further sequelae. These medications may be obtained over the counter and by prescription.

Mechanism of Action

■ Imidazole and triazole agents inhibit the cytochrome P450 system and thereby inhibit the conversion of lanosterol to ergosterol, which is required for fungal cell wall synthesis. These medications can also interfere with steroid synthesis in humans.
■ The triazoles act in a similar fashion but are less toxic and more effective.
■ The allylamines inhibit squalene epoxidase, which is required for ergosterol and fungal wall synthesis; they may also inhibit human steroid synthesis, but do so less than the imidazoles.
■ Griseofulvin binds to fungal microtubules and inhibits fungal mitosis and reproduction.
■ The mechanism of action for the other agents is not fully understood, but it is believed that they inhibit cell wall synthesis in a fashion similar to the allylamines.

Pharmacokinetics

■ See Chapter 18 for pharmacokinetics of oral dosage forms.
■ Most agents are not absorbed; if there is any absorption, it is minimal through intact skin.
■ Distribution if absorbed is unknown; however antifungal action is local.
■ Metabolism and excretion following topical application are unknown.

Clinical Uses

■ Tinea cruris: Topical treatment with any agent is sufficient for most cases unless the infection has spread to the lower thighs or buttocks. In these cases, oral treatment with itraconazole or terbinafine may be needed.
■ Tinea capitis: Although topical itraconazole and terbinafine may be effective, oral griseofulvin is generally used for treatment because topical agents usually do not clear this infection well.
■ Tinea corporis: May be treated topically if only one or two lesions are present, but will require oral therapy with terbinafine or itraconazole; fluconazole may be used once a week for 4 weeks with good results.
■ Tinea pedis: Most cases may be treated with any topical agent; however, highly keratotic lesions may require oral treatment with itraconazole or terbinafine.
■ Onychomycosis (tinea unguium): Requires oral therapy; itraconazole and terbinafine are effective, and griseofulvin is effective to a lesser extent. Pulse therapy (short bursts of large doses of drug, followed by a rest period of a week or more) with itraconazole is effective and offers less concern regarding side effects and better patient compliance.
■ Candidiasis: Often requires only topical treatment, but fluconazole may be used orally and offers much better patient acceptance.

Adverse Reactions

DERM: Burning, itching, stinging for topical agents
GI: Nausea, hepatotoxicity for oral agents

Dosage and Administration

CLASS	GENERIC NAME	TRADE NAME	ROUTE	DOSAGE
IMIDAZOLES	clotrimazole	Lotrimin AF Cream	Topically	Apply 2 times/day for 2–4 weeks depending on site
	Econazole	Spectazole 1% cream	Topically	Apply 1–2 times/day for 2–4 weeks depending on site
	Ketoconazole	Extina 2% foam	Topically	Apply 2 times/day for 4 weeks
		Nizoral A-D	Topically	Apply 3–4 times/day for 8 weeks, then as needed
		generic	PO	200–400 mg PO daily until cleared
	Miconazole	Desenex	Topically	Apply 2 times/day for 2–4 weeks depending on site
	Oxiconazole	Oxistat 1% cream	Topically	Apply 1–2 times/day for 2–4 weeks depending on site
	Sulconazole	Exelderm 1% cream	Topically	Apply 1–2 times/day for 2–4 weeks depending on site
TRIAZOLES	itraconazole	Sporanox	PO	200 mg 1–3 times/day depending on site
ALLYLAMINES	butenafine	Lotrimin Ultra	Topically	1–2 times/day for 1–2 weeks depending on site
	Naftifine	Naftin	Topically	Apply daily for 1–4 weeks depending on site
	Terbinafine	Lamisil	PO	250 mg daily orally for 6–12 weeks depending on site
		Lamisil AT	Topically	Apply daily for 1–2 weeks depending on site
OTHERS	ciclopirox	Loprox 0.77% gel, cream, or suspension	Topically	Cream, topical suspension, or gel, apply 2 times/day for 4 weeks
	griseofulvin*	Grifulvin V	PO	250–500 mg orally as a single dose or 2 doses daily for 4–6 weeks; i.e., 10–20 mg/kg/day
		Gris-PEG	PO	Children: 5–10 mg/kg/day in single or two doses. Adults: 330–375 mg/kg/day in single or divided doses

*Ultramicrosized pellets are in Gris-PEG, and Grifulvin has only microsized pellets of the active drug, griseofulvin. The microsized form of the drug is absorbed variably (25% to 70%); dietary fat will enhance absorption. The ultramicrosize form of the drug may be nearly 100% absorbed. Generally, the ultramicrosize form is absorbed 1.5 times as well as the microsized form for a given patient. Griseofulvin is concentrated in skin, hair, nails, fat, skeletal muscle, and the liver, and can be found in the stratum corneum within 4 hours of dosing.

Interactions

■ None

Contraindications

■ Hypersensitivities

Conscientious Considerations

■ Inspect involved areas of skin and mucous membranes during therapy; they are at risk for compromise of skin integrity or for other infections.
■ Watch for increased skin irritation as a sign to discontinue treatment.
■ Work with other learned and specialty clinicians because there is often a knowledge deficit when it comes to fungal infections, as with most infestations.

Patient/Family Education

■ See above regarding other topical medications, especially choice of vehicle and application.
■ Caution patients that antifungals, especially the imidazoles, usually stain clothing, bedding, etc., including skin and hair.
■ Patients being treated for athlete's foot should wear well-ventilated shoes and change their socks every day.
■ Advise patients to return to their clinician if symptoms worsen.
■ Women should remove any nail polish/lacquer during treatment and for at least a week after their treatment is successful.

AGENTS USED TO TREAT VIRAL INFECTIONS

Herpes simplex and herpes zoster are common viral disorders of the skin. Herpes simplex, caused by the herpes simplex virus 1 (HSV-1) and herpes simplex virus 2 (HSV-2), can infect the face and mouth (cold sores), the genitalia, the eyes, and the brain. It is characterized by episodic vesicular lesions that may be painful or pruritic followed by periods of remission. Although the periods of remission may last for years, the virus is not cleared from the body; once infected, a person remains so for life. Treatment may be topical, depending upon the location and the severity of the lesions, or oral in more severe cases or for prophylaxis.

Herpes zoster is commonly known as **shingles** and results from a recurrence of symptoms from a varicella zoster virus infection (chicken pox). It is characterized by a painful, vesicular rash that is usually localized on one side of the body along a single dermatome. Like herpes simplex, the virus is not cleared from the body after the initial bout of chicken pox, and recurrences of the rash as shingles can occur periodically. Postherpetic neuralgia may occur, with pain lasting for months to years after the rash has cleared. Antiviral medications may reduce the severity and duration of herpes zoster, but they should be started within 72 hours of the onset of lesions. Vaccines are available to prevent both chicken pox and herpes zoster. The vaccine may be given even after the onset of herpes zoster lesions and may lessen the symptoms and help prevent postherpetic neuralgia.

Mechanism of Action

■ Antiviral agents act by inhibiting DNA synthesis and therefore decreasing viral replication.

Pharmacokinetics

■ Absorption and Distribution: See Chapter 18 for pharmacokinetics of antivirals.
■ Metabolism: By the liver.
■ Excretion: Excreted in the urine.
■ Half-life: 8 to 10 hours.

Dosage and Administration

	GENERIC NAME	TRADE NAME	ROUTE	DOSAGE
AGENTS FOR TREATING COLD SORES	acyclovir	Zovirax	topically	Apply 4–6 times per day for 10 days
	docosanol OTC	Abreva	topically	Apply 5 times a day for 10 days
	penciclovir	Denavir	topically	Apply every 2 hr while awake for 4 days
AGENTS FOR TREATING THE FIRST EPISODE OF GENITAL HERPES	acyclovir	Zovirax	PO	400 mg, 3 times/ day for 7–10 days 200 mg 5 times/ day for 7–10 days
	famciclovir	Famvir	PO	250 mg, 3 times/ day for 7–10 days
	valacyclovir	Valtrex	PO	1 g, 2 times/day for 7–10 days
AGENTS FOR TREATING RECURRENT GENITAL HERPES	acyclovir	Zovirax	PO	400 mg, 3 times/ day for 5 days 200 mg 5 times/ day for 5 days 800 mg 2 times/ day for 5 days
	famciclovir	Famvir	PO	125 mg 2 times/ day for 5 days
	valacyclovir	Valtrex	PO	500 mg 2 times/ day for 3–5 days 1 gm 2 times/day for 5 days 2 gm 2 times/day for 1 day
AGENTS FOR SUPPRESSIVE TREATMENT OF GENITAL HERPES	acyclovir		PO	400 mg 2 times/day
	famciclovir	Famvir	PO	250 mg 2 times/day
	valacyclovir	Valtrex	PO	500 mg–1 gm daily (depends on number of outbreaks per year)
AGENTS FOR THE TREATMENT OF HERPES ZOSTER	acyclovir	Zovirax	PO	800 mg, 5 times/ day for 7–10 days
	famciclovir	Famvir	PO	500 mg 3 times/ day for 7 days
	valacyclovir	Valtrex	PO	1 gm 3 times/day for 7 days

Clinical Uses

■ HSV-1
■ HSV-2
■ Shingles

Adverse Reactions

DERM: Urticaria
GI: Nausea, abdominal pain, elevated liver enzymes
NEURO: Disorientation, hallucinations, headache

Interactions

■ Concurrent use of other nephrotoxic drugs will increase the risk of renal effects.
■ Probenecid will increase drug levels of these agents.
■ There is a risk of toxicity when given with theophylline, thus dosage adjustments are necessary.

Contraindications

■ There is often a hypersensitivity to acyclovir and valacyclovir.

Conscientious Considerations

■ Treatment should begin as soon as symptoms appear.

Patient/Family Education

■ Advise patient to take medication exactly as directed and for the full course of treatment.
■ Advise patient that use of ancillary OTC creams may delay healing and cause spread of lesions.
■ If therapy does not bring relief within 7 days, it is usually a sign the medication is not working and the patient needs to return to the clinician.
■ Instruct women to be sure they have a yearly Pap test, if being treated for genital herpes, because they are at risk for cervical cancer.
■ Inform patients that these drugs may just control symptoms rather than cure the condition, because viruses may lie dormant and reappear later under times of stress or other cause of immunocompromise

DRUGS USED FOR CLEANING AND DISINFECTING THE SKIN

Cleaning and disinfecting the skin is done to decrease bacterial load and the likelihood of infection (Box 16-2). In general this should be done to intact skin because many of the agents used are toxic to the deeper tissues. Normal saline is usually sufficient for irrigation and cleansing of open wounds, although copious amounts will be needed. Chlorhexidine is used as an active ingredient in skin cleansers and mouthwashes and is bactericidal to both gram-negative and gram-positive organisms. It is more effective than povidone-iodine at killing bacteria and may have residual effects for up to 6 hours after application. Povidone-iodine is less toxic than iodine disinfectant and demonstrates good antibacterial activity. Free iodine is slowly liberated from the povidone-iodine complex and interrupts the cell membranes of bacterial, fungal, protozoal, and viral cells.

The phenol derivatives, such as hexachlorophene, are disinfectants that are found in soaps and toothpaste. It was available

---

BOX 16-2 Agents Used for Cleansing and Disinfecting the Skin

Isopropyl alcohol

Chlorhexidine (Hibiclens, Chlorohex) used diluted 1:100

Cationic surfactants (benzalkonium chloride)

Hydrogen peroxide

Povidone iodine

Phenol derivatives (hexachlorophene, triclosan, Phisohex) found in Dial and Lever 2000 soap

---

over the counter until the 1970s when concerns over carcinogenesis led to its availability only as a prescription. It is useful in the treatment of acne.

Hydrogen peroxide is useful as a disinfectant and antiseptic, but it is mildly caustic to tissues in open wounds. Patients should be cautioned not to use hydrogen peroxide after the initial cleansing of an open wound to avoid delay in wound healing.

Cationic surfactants act by disrupting the cell membrane lipid bilayer and are found in skin cleansers, hygienic towelettes, and as a preservative in eye and nasal drops. Used as an antiseptic, it does not burn when applied to the skin, but in long-term use (eye drop users), allergic reactions have been reported. Isopropyl alcohol also works by disrupting the cell membrane lipid bilayer, but burns when applied to open skin; it is most useful for cleansing the skin prior to injections or procedures.

DRUGS USED IN THE TREAMENT OF BURNS

The treatment of burns depends on the burn's severity. Burns are categorized as first degree, second degree, or third degree. First-degree burns exhibit erythema and pain only, second-degree burns exhibit blisters and pain, and third-degree burns are full-thickness burns that are insensate and usually require more than outpatient treatment. First-degree burns do not usually require any treatment but may be treated with a topical antibiotic such as silver sulfadiazine and covered with gauze, especially if sloughing occurs. Second-degree burns should be treated with silver sulfadiazine and covered with gauze; the dressing should be changed twice a day until the burn is healed. Ruptured blisters or dead tissue may be debrided, and special care should be given to circumferential burns because these may compromise blood flow. Silver sulfadiazine acts on the cell wall and is bactericidal for many gram negative and gram positive bacteria. Mafenide interferes with bacterial folate synthesis and DNA synthesis and is effective on many gram positive and gram negative bacteria.

Dosage and Administration of Agents Used to Treat Burns

GENERIC NAME	TRADE NAME	ROUTE	DOSAGE
silver sulfadiazine	Silvadene	Topically	1% cream applied 1-2 times/day
mafenide	Sulfamylon	Topically	Apply 1-2 times/day with a sterile gloved hand

DRUGS USED TO TREAT PRESSURE SORES

Pressure sores (decubitus ulcers) are caused by ischemic injury resulting from prolonged pressure on the skin over a bony prominence complicated by the presence of shear force and friction. They are most common in those who are limited in their mobility and who do not have the ability to adjust their posture (often seen in the elderly). Prolonged immobility, decreased vascularity, neurological disorders, and malnutrition also play a role in the development of pressure sores. Lesions progress from areas of erythema to full-thickness lesions that expose the bone. There four stages of pressure sores: Stage I exhibits blanchable erythema, stage II exhibits extension through the dermis, stage III exhibits full thickness involvement, and stage IV exhibits full-thickness loss with extension into the muscle or bone. The lesions can be colonized by bacteria and may require antibiotics for full recovery. The mainstay of treatment is removal of the pressure; cleansing; correction of malnutrition; débridement; and less commonly, surgical reconstruction to cover the exposed area (Box 16-3).

BOX 16-3 Agents Used in the Treatment of Pressure Sores

Stage I/II

Polyurethane film (OpSite, Tegaderm): Helps protect from friction and provides a moist wound bed; aids in autolytic débridement.

Hydrocolloid dressing (DuoDERM, Restore): Provides a moist environment and aids in autolytic débridement.

Stage III/IV (treatment is additive to medications for stage I/II lesions)

Absorptive dressing (calcium alginate, Sorbsan, Aquacel): Absorbs exudates in highly exudative lesions, should be changed when saturated.

Autolytic débridement: The use of moist dressings with some level of occlusion to allow for the body's intrinsic proteases to complete the débridement process. This is a very slow process and requires a great measure of patience.

Enzymatic débridement: Can be papain-urea based or collagenase based and works by breaking down proteins in the wound bed to aid in débridement. *Papain-urea* (Accuzyme) is purified from the carica papaya fruit and acts by breaking down proteins containing cysteine residues. This is a nonselective process and breaks down necrotic tissue as well as healing tissue. Collagen does not contain cysteine residues and is unaffected by papain. There can be pain and inflammation associated with the use of papain, and some formulations have added chlorophyllin (Panafil) to decrease inflammation. These preparations have the added benefit of increased fibrin deposition and control of odors. Collagenase preparations (Santyl) are water-soluble proteinases that break down collagen into gelatin and are most effective in a narrow pH of 6 to 8. Collagenase has been noted to be gentle on viable cells, which further aids in wound healing.

DRUGS USED IN THE TREATMENT OF PSORIASIS

Psoriasis is an inflammatory disorder associated with erythematous plaques and adherent silvery scales. It is a chronic disorder with periods of exacerbations and remissions that begins between 15 and 40 years of age. Genetic disposition and environmental triggers have been implicated as a causative factor, although the exact cause is not fully known. Regardless of the cause, two factors predominate in a **psoriatic plaque**: hyperproliferation of keratinocytes and inflammation (neutrophils and T cells). Plaques are often located on the elbows, knees, back, and scalp, although they may be generalized as in guttate psoriasis. The nails, palms, soles, and joints can be affected, and infants may present with napkin psoriasis in the diaper area. The treatment of psoriasis depends upon the patient's desire to control the disorder and the severity of the lesions.

Treatments include topical corticosteroids, vitamin D analogues, retinoids, emollients, and keratolytics (Tables 16-3, 16-4, and 16-5).

Treatment of Seborrhea

Seborrhea is an inflammatory disorder of the skin that is most common in infancy and adolescence due to increased activity of the sebaceous glands. Less severe lesions can persist into adulthood. Although increased activity of the sebaceous glands is associated with an increase in severity of disease, the cause of seborrhea is not fully known. *Pityrosporum ovale* has been implicated in many studies but has not been proven to be the causative agent. Lesions can be localized or generalized and typically are

TABLE 16-3   Topical Agents Used in the Treatment of Psoriasis

DRUG CLASS	MECHANISM OF ACTION	DOSAGE
corticosteroids	Inhibit the transcription of genes to decrease inflammation	Apply 2–4 times/day for 2–4 weeks, then intermittently to achieve control while minimizing exposure
vitamin D analogues	Bind to vitamin D receptors and promote the differentiation of keratinocytes	Apply Calcipotriene 0.005%, 2 times/day
tazarotene	Metabolites bind to retinoic acid receptors and normalize epidermal differentiation	Available in 0.05% and 0.1% cream and gel. Applied daily at bedtime
calcineurin inhibitors	Inhibit transcription of cytokines including interleukin-2	Apply 2 times/day to affected area

TABLE 16-4   Oral Agents Used in the Treatment of Psoriasis*

DRUG	MECHANISM OF ACTION	DOSAGE	OTHER IMPORTANT INFORMATION
cyclosporin A (Neoral)	Inhibits interleukin-2 and other cytokines	2.5–5 mg daily to max of 5 mg/day, then taper when ready to discontinue	Requires periodic laboratory evaluation to ensure safety. Is contraindicated with uncontrolled hypertension, abnormal renal function and history of malignancy.
methotrexate	Blocks dihydrofolate and therefore DNA synthesis	Start at 2.5 mg test dose, and titrate up to a dose of 10–15 mg/week	Requires periodic laboratory evaluation to ensure safety. Contraindicated in pregnancy and lactation and caution should be used in patients with hepatic dysfunction.
acitretin	Binds to retinoic acid receptors and normalizes keratinization	Start at 25–50 mg/day, and titrate until desired response is achieved	Requires periodic laboratory evaluation to ensure safety. Contraindicated in pregnancy and lactation. Pregnancy should be avoided for 3 years after this medication is discontinued.
fumaric acid esters	Interferes with T-cell response	Initiate at low dose, and titrate up to a maximum dose of 1.2 gm/day	Requires periodic laboratory evaluation to ensure safety. Contraindicated in patients with renal or GI tract disease, in pregnancy or lactation, and with a history of malignancy.

Continued

TABLE 16-4 Oral Agents Used in the Treatment of Psoriasis—cont'd

DRUG	MECHANISM OF ACTION	DOSAGE	OTHER IMPORTANT INFORMATION
hydroxyurea	Inhibits DNA synthesis	Initiate with 500 mg/day, and titrate to 1–1.5 gm/day based on response and patient's tolerance	Requires periodic laboratory evaluation to ensure safety. Contraindicated in those with a history of bone marrow depression, in pregnancy or lactation.
thioguanine	Arrests cell cycle and leads to cellular apoptosis	Start at 80 mg 2 times/week; titrate by 20 mg every 2–4 weeks, with a max dose of 160 mg 3 times/week	Requires periodic laboratory evaluation to ensure safety. Contraindicated in those with liver disease and in pregnancy.
sulfasalazine	Inhibits 5-lipoxygenase and inflammation	Initiate therapy at 500 mg 2 times/day. Increase slowly, based on tolerance to a max of 1 gm 4 times/day	Requires periodic laboratory evaluation to ensure safety. Use with caution in those with hypersensitivity to sulfa medications and in those with G6PD deficiency.
mycophenolate mofetil	Selectively cytotoxic for cells that rely on purine synthesis	Initiate treatment at 500–750 mg 2 times/day, and increase to 1–1.5 gm 2 times/day	Requires periodic laboratory evaluation to ensure safety. Contraindicated in those with severe infections or malignancy.

Note: A number of agents are applied in psoriasis treatment; however, they should only be used when patients using FDA-approved medications for the indication of psoriasis are not responding to them positively. Thus, use of such agents are considered an "experiment of one" when they are being used for "off-label" indications. Such agents may include fumaric acid, hydroxyurea, thioguanine, sulfasalazine and mycophenolate mofetil.

G6PD, glucose-6-phosphate dehydrogenase.

TABLE 16-5 Injectable/Intravenous Agents Used in the Treatment of Psoriasis

DRUG	MECHANISM OF ACTION	DOSAGE	OTHER IMPORTANT INFORMATION
alefacept	Binds to CD-2 on the T cell, interferes with T-cell activation, and leads to T-cell apoptosis.	Given IM at 50 mg biweekly for 3 months	Should check CD4 T-cell counts every 2 weeks
etanercept	Binds TNF-α and neutralizes its activity.	Given subcutaneously at 25–50 mg 2 times/week	Check purified protein derivative (PPD) at onset of therapy
infliximab	Binds to TNF-α and neutralizes its activity.	Given intravenously over 2 hr at 5–10 mg/kg at 0 weeks, 2 weeks, and 6 weeks	Check PPD at onset of therapy
adalimumab	Binds TNF-α and neutralizes its activity	Given 40 mg SC for 2 weeks, then 40 mg SC for 1 week, then 40 mg SC every other week	Check PPD at onset of therapy
ustekinumab (Stelara)	A human monoclonal antibody directed against interleukin-12	Give 45 mg SC to start and again in 4 weeks; then give 45 mg SC every 12 weeks	Side effects tend to be a nasopharyngitis and upper respiratory infections
salicylic acid	Is FDA approved as a keratolytic	Is used topically 2–4 times/day to decrease hyperkeratosis and scaling	Side effects include headache, tinnitus, and drowsiness
phototherapy UVB-nm 311	UV light at a wavelength of 311 nm has been shown to be the most effective in the treatment of psoriasis while limiting adverse effects. UV light penetrates the	Present in natural sunlight. UVB light may worsen psoriasis before it starts to heal. Treatment usually begins in a clinic and then patients may use home equipment	It can be used in pregnancy, making it preferred over previously used UVA therapy

Continued

TABLE 16-5	Injectable/Intravenous Agents Used in the Treatment of Psoriasis—cont'd		
DRUG	MECHANISM OF ACTION	DOSAGE	OTHER IMPORTANT INFORMATION
	dermis and depletes T cells, and therefore decreases the symptoms of psoriasis and does not require a photosensitizer	with daily exposure times increased over several weeks	
tar preparations	The phenols in these compounds give them antipruritic properties but can irritate acute lesions and lead to irritant folliculitis. They may aid in decreasing hyperkeratotic buildup	Scalp psoriasis: use tar oil bath or coal tar solution sparingly to the lesions 3–12 hr before shampooing Body psoriasis: use at bedtime. If thick scales are noted, then may use tar product with salicylic acid and apply many times per day	Phototoxicity and allergic contact dermatitis have been seen with these preparations and should be avoided in those with a history of sensitivity

macular lesions with yellowish-brown scaling associated with inflammation. In susceptible persons, the lesions may begin in the first month of life but usually will be evident within the first year of life. The lesions will often be generalized in infancy and localize to the scalp (dandruff), axillae, and face (areas with high concentrations of sebaceous glands) as the person ages. In the elderly, blepharitis is common and may be incorrectly treated with antibiotics because it can be confused with an infectious etiology. In infants, cradle cap is commonly seen as scaling and crusting of the scalp, which can be quite thick. These scales may be difficult to remove and should be pretreated with mineral oil to soften the lesions, followed by gentle débridement with a toothbrush or washcloth and shampooing with baby shampoo. No other treatment for cradle cap is generally needed. Treatment of seborrhea consists of mild-strength topical corticosteroids due to the need for prolonged treatment over a large surface area. Shampoos containing selenium are useful in the treatment of scalp lesions as are antifungal creams and shampoos (Table 16-6).

TABLE 16-6	Drugs Used in the Treatment of Seborrhea		
DRUG	MECHANISM OF ACTION	DOSAGE	OTHER IMPORTANT INFORMATION
selenium sulfide (Selsun, Selsun Blue, Head and Shoulders Intensive)	Thought to slow the growth of epithelial tissue	Apply 10 mL to scalp and leave in place for 2–4 min for scalp lesions. May apply foam into affected areas of the body 2 times/day.	May cause burning or irritation to open skin lesions and can damage jewelry, which should be removed prior to application.
pyrithione zinc (Head and Shoulders, Tegrin)	Zinc has some antibacterial properties and is found in many dandruff shampoos	Shampoo 2–3 times/week	It is useful in conjunction with pretreatment with salicylic acid to help remove crusts and scales. Zinc can cause some skin irritation and is toxic when ingested.
ketoconazole (Nizoral)	Alters the formation of the cell wall by blocking fungal cytochrome P450	Is available in many formulations, including cream, foam, gel, and shampoo. Creams and foams are applied to the affected area 2 times/day for 4 weeks, gels are applied daily for 2 weeks, and shampoos are applied 2 times/week for 4 weeks, with a minimum of 3 days between shampoos.	Adverse reactions include irritation, allergic reaction, hair loss, and dryness.
sulfacetamide lotion (Sebizon)	Interferes with bacterial growth by the inhibition of folate synthesis	Apply at bedtime and allow to remain overnight for 8–10 applications. May use to prevent recurrence by applying once a week.	May cause burning or irritation and infrequently Stevens-Johnson syndrome. May lead to kernicterus in the newborn.

Continued

TABLE 16-6	Drugs Used in the Treatment of Seborrhea—cont'd		
DRUG	MECHANISM OF ACTION	DOSAGE	OTHER IMPORTANT INFORMATION
tar shampoos (Zetar, Tegrin, Denorex, Neutogena T-Rex)	May aid in decreasing hyperkeratotic buildup	Tar preparations may be applied to skin lesions 1–4 times/day with a decrease in frequency as control is reached	May use a tar-containing soap in place of normal soap to help control symptoms. May use as an additive to the bathwater with a soak of 10–20 minutes. Shampoos containing tar are used by rubbing onto wet hair and leaving on for 5 minutes. May be used 2 times/week for 2 weeks, then 1 time/week. Phototoxicity and allergic contact dermatitis have been seen with these preparations; they should be avoided in those with a history of sensitivity.

Treatment of Skin and Hair Infestations

Lice and scabies have infested humans since the beginning of recorded history. Both of these disorders lead to intense itching; the word *scabies* is actually derived from the Latin word for "scratch." Lice are insects that live their entire life cycle on their hosts feeding on skin and debris, although some species feed on sebaceous oils and blood. They attach tenaciously to the hair with claws and are difficult to remove. Scabies is caused by a mite that burrows under the skin and lays eggs. The host responds with an allergic reaction to the mite and their waste with an intense itching reaction. The mite cannot live apart from the host for more than 14 days. Eggs laid in the burrows will hatch within 3 to 10 days, and the adult can survive for 3 to 4 weeks in the host. Agents available to treat scabies and lice include over-the-counter medications and prescription medications. Most treatments are topical, however ivermectin may be used orally to treat scabies (Table 16-7).

TOPICAL ANESTHETICS

Pain is experienced as a result of disease as well as during procedures to diagnose and treat dermatological disorders. Pain control can be systemic, local, or topical. Medications used to treat pain on a local level all act by blocking the voltage-gated sodium channels and slowing impulse conduction along nerve fibers. Slowing continues until conduction is temporarily halted and pain control is achieved. The half-life of these preparations is short, making them ideal for procedures with quick recovery times. Epinephrine may be used in conjunction with topical anesthetics to hinder systemic absorption, decreasing the clearance of these medications and prolonging their effects.

TABLE 16-7	Drugs Used as Scabicides (scabies) and Pediculicides (lice)		
DRUG	MECHANISM OF ACTION	DOSAGE	OTHER IMPORTANT INFORMATION
crotamiton (Eurax) for scabies	The mechanism of action is known to be toxic to the scabies mite, but the exact mechanism is not known	It is applied to the whole body and left on for 48 hr. It may be repeated 2–3 times before the desired effect is reached.	The most common side effect is skin drying and irritation.
lindane (generic) for lice and scabies	Is FDA approved for the treatment of both scabies and lice	Apply 1 oz of shampoo to dry hair and leave on for no longer than 4 minutes. Add enough water to make a good lather and rinse immediately. After application, lindane should be washed off with warm, not hot, water to avoid increased absorption.	Should not be used as first line of defense but rather in those patients for whom permethrin has failed or is contraindicated. Serious neurotoxicity has been reported and even deaths after multiple applications for recurrent mite infestations. Lindane shampoo 1% should not be used in those with a seizure disorder, pregnant women, low-weight infants, children, elderly, or premature infants to avoid neurotoxicity.

TABLE 16-7 Drugs Used as Scabicides (scabies) and Pediculicides (lice)—cont'd			
DRUG	**MECHANISM OF ACTION**	**DOSAGE**	**OTHER IMPORTANT INFORMATION**
malathion 0.5% lotion (Ovide) for lice	Is an organophosphate and is pediculicidal (kills living lice) with some ovicidal activity (kills some lice eggs)	Apply and leave in place for 24 hr. May require second treatment in 7–10 days if lice are still present. This is recommended for children over the age of 6 years.	Some irritation to the scalp and eyes has been noted. The lotion is flammable and care should be taken around heat and flames.
pyrethrins (RID, Pronto, A-200) for lice	Are extracts from the chrysanthemum flower and are safe and effective	These agents kill lice but not eggs (nits), and a second treatment is recommended in 7–10 days to kill any recently hatched eggs.	Should be avoided by those allergic to the flower or to ragweed.
permethrin (Elimite, NIX) for lice and scabies	Is a neurotoxin effective against scabies and lice	It is applied to the skin at bedtime, left in place for 8–16 hr, and then showered off. It must be applied from the top of the head to the bottom of the feet to be effective, but care should be taken to avoid the eyes and mucous membranes. Permethrin is available in a 1% and 5% preparation.	The FDA has approved the 1% solution for the treatment of head lice. It is safe and effective against live lice but is not very effective against unhatched eggs. A second treatment in 7–10 days will kill the newly hatched eggs before they are able to reproduce. It is not approved in children younger than 2 years of age. The chief adverse reaction is irritation and dryness.
sulfur ointment in petroleum jelly for scabies	Has been shown to be somewhat effective in the treatment of scabies	A 10% ointment is applied daily for several weeks.	Is safe in children and pregnant women.
ivermectin (Stromectol)	An antihelminthic used against many nematodes worldwide	An oral dose of 150–200 mcg/kg as a single dose. Follow-up stool exam is needed, and retreatment may be needed every 3–12 months until the parasite dies.	Can be used in children.

Care should be taken to avoid epinephrine in areas where compromised blood flow would be detrimental (ears, nose, fingers, toes, and penis).

Mechanism of Action

Blockage of voltage-gated sodium channels with slowed conduction along nerves and disruption of the action potential

Pharmacokinetics

■ Absorption: Topical anesthetics are not absorbed.
■ Distribution: Not a factor in topical application.
■ Metabolism: Esters are converted in the plasma, and amides are converted in the liver.
■ Excretion: Both esters and amides are excreted in the urine after conversion.
■ Half-life: Benzocaine: less than 10 minutes; lidocaine: 10 minutes; prilocaine: 5 minutes.

Available Formulations

■ Benzocaine: Topical: 5%, 6% creams; 15%, 20% gels; 5%, 20% ointments; 0.8% lotion; 20% liquid; 20% spray

■ Lidocaine (Xylocaine):
   ■ Local: 0.5%, 1%, 1.5%, 2%, 4% for injection; 0.5%, 1%, 1.5%, 2% with 1:200,000 epinephrine; 1%, 2% with 1:100,000 epinephrine, 2% with 1:50,000 epinephrine
   ■ Topical: 2.5%, 5% ointments; 0.5%, 4% cream; 0.5%, 2.5% gel; 2%, 2.5%, 4% solutions; 23mg and 46 mg per 2 cm^2 patch
   ■ **Note:** Clinicians should avoid using more than 4.5 mg/kg of plain lidocaine or more than 7 mg/kg in lidocaine with epinephrine, because it can become toxic.
   ■ Prilocaine (Citanest): Local: 4% with epinephrine

Clinical Uses

■ Topical anesthetics
■ IV doses are used as antiarrhythmics

Adverse Reactions

All adverse reactions are signs of systemic absorption.

CV: Depresses cardiac pacemaker activity
HEM: Conversion of hemoglobin to methemoglobin and cyanosis

MISC: ALLERGIC REACTIONS: converted to *p*-aminobenzoic acid derivatives, which leads to allergic reactions in some patients

NEURO: Sleepiness, lightheadedness, visual and auditory disturbances, restlessness, nystagmus, muscular twitching, tonic-clonic convulsions

Interactions

■ None, but skin, scalp, and hair products may increase systemic absorption.

Contraindications

■ Hypersensitivities

Conscientious Considerations

■ Assess application site for open wounds; apply only to intact skin.

Patient/Family Education

■ Explain the use and purpose to patients and that all sensation to the treated skin may be blocked.

■ Caution patients to avoid any scratching or trauma to the area until all sensation has returned.

Implications for Special Populations

Pregnancy Implications

When prescribing for the pregnant female, clinicians should carefully consider their choice of drugs. A selected list of dermatological drugs along with their assigned FDA Safety Category follows.

CATEGORY	DRUGS
B	sulfasalazine, alefacept, etanercept, infliximab, adalimumab
C	corticosteroids, vitamin D analogues, calcineurin inhibitors, cyclosporin, fumaric acid esters, mycophenolate mofetil, efalizumab, salicylic acid, selenium, ketoconazole, sulfacetamide, tar shampoos
D	hydroxyurea, thioguanine
X	tazarotene, methotrexate, acitretin
Unclassified	

Pediatric Implications

Corticosteroids

May affect growth velocity; growth should be routinely monitored in pediatric patients. Topical use in patients 12 years of age or younger is not recommended, but if necessary then use in lowest dose and amount.

Drugs for Acne

Care should be taken in children under the age of 10 years or in prolonged use of the tetracyclines to avoid graying of the teeth.

Oral Antihistamines

Oral antihistamines should be avoided or used with caution in pediatric patients because of concerns about increased morbidity and mortality.

Anesthetics

Care should be taken to avoid toxic levels of anesthetics in this age group.

Geriatric Implications

Corticosteroids

Systemic corticosteroids should be used cautiously in the elderly in the smallest possible effective dose for the shortest duration to avoid systemic effects, which are more common in the elderly.

Oral Antihistamines

Anticholinergic effects may worsen dementia and can lead to increased falls. They should be avoided or used with caution in this age group.

LEARNING EXERCISES

Case 1

You are a physician's assistant on your first family medicine clerkship. You are making rounds at the local nursing home that is reported to have had an outbreak of scabies. You are examining a patient in her room and have been told that her roommate has recently been diagnosed with scabies. You examine your patient and find the characteristic burrows of scabies between her fingers and she complains of having intense itching.

1. What is the best treatment for this patient? What are the considerations for the elderly in the treatment of scabies?

2. What steps should you take to avoid spreading this infestation or contracting it yourself?

Case 2

A 6-year-old girl complains of itching, especially at the elbows and the ankles. You suspect eczema and instruct her mother on proper hydration of the skin. You arrange to see the child again in 4 weeks. At that time her rash and itching are no better, and you elect to start a corticosteroid.

1. What is the best corticosteroid for this patient, and what vehicle would be most appropriate?

2. Would an occlusive dressing be appropriate for her?

chapter 17

Modern Approaches to Managing Bacterial Infections

W. P. Roche III, William N. Tindall, Mona M. Sedrak

CHAPTER FOCUS

This chapter focuses on drugs used to treat bacterial infections. When bacterial infections occur, clinicians must be knowledgeable about the physiology and pathophysiology of the organ systems affected by the infection and the cellular biology of the invading microbe. Understanding both is necessary to make appropriate drug choices. Clinicians must also be aware that drugs used to treat bacterial infections are categorized by their effect on an organism. They must also understand that, although a bacterial infection can wreak havoc on its host, the medications used to eradicate that infection can likewise be deleterious to the patient.

OBJECTIVES

After carefully reading and studying this chapter, the student should be able to:

1. Compare and contrast the pharmacokinetics, mechanism of action, adverse effects, interactions, and contraindications of antimicrobial drugs used for the treatment of bacterial infections.
2. Describe how antibiotic resistance develops and what can be done about it.
3. Explain how empirical prescribing has developed and how it can best be used.
4. Differentiate between natural, beta-lactamase-resistant, and expanded-spectrum penicillins.
5. Restate and explain the patient advisories that every clinician should ensure patients on antibiotics understand.
6. Differentiate between antibiotics that are bacteriostatic and bacteriocidal, and give examples of each.
7. Explain the significance of methicillin-resistant *Staphylococcus aureus* (MRSA) and what antibiotics can be used to treat it.
8. Explain the significance of folic acid synthesis on bacterial metabolism.

Key Terms

- 30S ribosomal subunit
- 50S ribosomal subunit
- Antibiotic resistance
- Bacteriocidal antibiotic
- Bacteriostatic antibiotic
- Beta-lactamase
- *Clostridium difficile* (C. diff)
- Disulfiram-like reaction
- Empirical prescribing
- Folic acid synthesis
- Gram-negative
- Gram-positive
- Penicillin-binding protein (PBP)

KEY DRUGS IN THIS CHAPTER

Penicillins
Penicillins (Penicillinase Sensitive)
  penicillin G potassium (Pfizerpen, Wycillin)
  penicillin V potassium (Veetids, Pen-VeeK, V-Cillin K)
  penicillin G procaine
  penicillin G benzathine (Bicillin LA)
  penicillin G benzathine/penicillin G procaine (Bicillin CR)
Penicillins (Beta-Lactamase Inhibitors)
  amoxicillin (Amoxil, Trimox)
  amoxicillin/clavulanate (Augmentin)

ampicillin sodium (Polycillin, Principen)
ampicillin sublactam (Unasym)
carbenicillin indanyl sodium (Geocillin)
cloxacillin (Tegopen, Cloxapen)
dicloxacillin (Dynapen)
methicillin (Staphcillin)
oxacillin (Prostaphilin, Bactocill)
nafcillin IM (Unipen)
piperacillin (Pipracil)
piperacillin/tazobactam (Zosyn)
piperacillin/clavulanate (Timentin)
ticarcillin (Ticar)

Cephalosporins (Expanded Spectrum Penicillins)
First Generation
  cefadroxil (Duracef)
  cephalexin (Keflex)
  cefazolin (Ancef, Kefzol)
  cephapirin (Cefadyl)
  cephradine (Velosef)
Second Generation
  cefaclor (Ceclor)
  cefamandole (Mandol)
  cefonicid (Monocid)

continued

cefuroxime axetil (Ceftin)
cefuroxime (Zinacef)
cefprozil (Cefzil)
cefotetan (Cefotan)
loracarbef (Lorabid)
Third Generation
cefdinir (Omnicef)
ceftibuten (Cedax)
cefoperazone (Cefobid)
cefotaxime (Claforan)
cefixime (Suprax)
ceftazidime (Ceptaz, Fortaz, Tanicef)
ceftizoxime (Cefizox)
ceftriaxone (Rocephin)
Fourth Generation
cefepime (Maxipime)
Penicillin-Like Monobactam
aztreonam (Azactam)
Penicillin-Like Carbepenems
imipenem-cilastatin (Primaxin)
meropenem (Merrem)
Aminoglycosides
amikacin (Amikin)
gentamicin (Garamycin)
kanamycin (Kantrex)

netilmicin (Netromycin)
neomycin (generic)
streptomycin (generic)
tobramycin (Nebcin)
Tetracyclines
demeclocycline (Declomycin)
doxycycline (Vibramycin)
methacycline (Rondomycin)
minocycline (Minocin)
oxytetracycline (Terramycin)
tetracycline HCL (Achromycin V, Sumycin, Doxycin)
Macrolides
azithromycin (Zithromax, Z-Pak)
clarithromycin (Biaxin)
clindamycin (Cleocin)
erythromycin (E-Mycin)
dirithromycin (Dynabac)
troleandomycin (Tao)
Lincosamides
lincomycin (Lincocin)
Quinolones and Fluoroquinolones
cinoxacin (Cinoxacin)
ciprofloxacin (Cipro)

enoxacin (Penetrex)
gatifloxacin (Tequin)
levofloxacin (Levaquin)
lomefloxacin (Maxaquin)
moxifloxacin (Avelox)
norfloxacin (Noroxin)
ofloxacin (Floxin)
sparfloxacin (Zagam)
trovafloxacin (Trovan)
Sulfonamides
sulfamethoxazole (SMX, Gantanol)
sulfamethoxazole/trimethoprim (Bactrim, Spectra, Cofatrim, Primsol)
Special Use
Streptogramins for Vancomycin-Resistant Enterococci (VRE) and Methicillin-Resistant *Staphylococcus aureus* (MRSA)
quinupristin/dalfopristin (Synercid)
Glycopeptides
vancomycin (Vancocin, Lyphocin)
linezolid (Zyvox)

Antimicrobial agents may be synthetic, semisynthetic, or made by a fermentation process of natural substances. Antimicrobial agents or *antibacterials* (*anti* means "against," *bios* means "life") are unique for their ability to negatively affect the biological processes of invading bacteria (benefit) while not harming a host to whom they are given (risk). However, antimicrobial agents can and do cause many adverse or unwanted effects in a person, especially to the gastrointestinal (GI) system. To affect invading pathogens, an antimicrobial agent must be able to reach its site of action; thus, clinicians need a good understanding of agents' pharmacokinetic properties to successfully use them.

Because bacteria, viruses, protozoa, and other pathogens are a huge part of the natural world, our bodies are constantly in contact with microbes that are potentially harmful. Many bacteria are helpful, such as those that colonize the gastrointestinal tract and help with digestion of food or those that act on the skin and keep bacterial flora in balance. These bacteria are part of human normal flora. When the body, or a part of it, is invaded by either normal flora (an internal microbe) or pathogenic flora (external microbe), it is called an *infection*.

Organisms capable of causing infections typically do so because some of the body's natural barriers to them have failed. Some of these natural barriers are as follows:

▪ Skin and mucous membranes
▪ Lactic acid in sweat and long-chain fatty acids in sebum
▪ Lysozymes found in conjunctiva, respiratory, genital, and intestinal mucosa.

▪ The reticuloendothelial system of phagocytic macrophages found in the lining of the gastrointestinal tract, as well as in the spleen, liver, lymph nodes, bone marrow, and connective tissue.

A person's ability to resist invading microorganisms depends on more than natural barriers; it is also a function of the host's overall health, age, nutritional state, and the presence of other diseases, especially those of metabolic origin, such as diabetes. Other considerations include the function of the blood supply near the location of an infection, and the presence of natural and acquired antibodies.

All organisms and pathogens are identified by how they fit into a simple classification system that is based on the following:

▪ Morphology (cocci, bacilli, spirochetes, coccobacilli)
▪ Growth characteristics (anaerobes, aerobes)
▪ Physical characteristics (gram-positive organisms vs. gram-negative organisms). Gram staining is a means of identifying two broad classes of bacteria by their ability to uptake crystal violet to stain cell walls, using iodine as a mordant and sapphrine as a counterstain.

Antibiotics are also classified by their ability to match against microbes placed in this system. For example, an antibiotic that affects **gram-positive** cocci aerobes will likely not affect **gram-negative** bacilli anaerobes. Although there are several classification schemes for antibiotics based on bacterial spectrum (broad vs. narrow), route of administration (injectable versus oral versus topical), or type of activity (bactericidal or bacteriostatic), the most useful is that based on chemical structure. Antibiotics within a structural class will generally have similar patterns of effectiveness, toxicity, and allergic potential. The most commonly used classes of antibiotics are the penicillins, fluoroquinolones, cephalosporins, macrolides, and tetracyclines. Although each class contains a number of agents, each drug has its own unique properties as well.

THE RELATIONSHIP BETWEEN MICROORGANISMS AND ANTIBIOTICS

Bacteria are distinct living organisms that are encased by both a cell membrane and a cell wall (Fig. 17-1). The cell wall is the outside layer of bacteria and is essential to the survival of the organism. The cytoplasm inside the cell membrane is hypotonic, and without a rigid cell wall, bacteria cannot survive. If the cell wall were not rigid, the cell membrane would bulge through the nonrigid/damaged cell wall and rupture, spilling the contents of the bacterium into the surrounding area. When a cell wall is formed, its strength comes from the cross-linking of peptides (peptidoglycan synthesis).

In the human body, the skin and much of the gastrointestinal tract is teaming with bacteria known as normal flora, which compete for space and which will promptly reestablish itself once disturbed (e.g., by an oral antibiotic). These internal microbes are generally helpful to the host organism and cause no harm, especially because they are effectively excluded from sterile spaces by the barriers mentioned previously. There is also transient flora that

may colonize the host for hours or weeks after it invades the body, but it does not permanently establish itself in the host. However, both resident and transient floras have the potential to cause sickness should the host's defense mechanisms become disrupted. One example of this is the bacteria *Haemophilus influenzae*. This organism often colonizes the bronchial tree in patients with chronic obstructive pulmonary disease (COPD). When the microbe becomes virulent (disease producing), it does so by doing the following:

■ Producing certain toxins or enzymes that may destroy tissue and damage blood vessels causing hemorrhage or edema
■ Blocking lymphatic drainage by clot formation
■ Dissolving blood clots and allowing the infection to spread

Thus, to combat any invading or colonizing bacteria that have become virulent, antimicrobial drugs are used to take advantage of the biochemical differences between microorganisms and humans. It is again worth pointing out that even though these agents are harmful to the microorganism, but they may also be toxic to humans.

Antibiotics work by bactericidal or bacteriostatic activity. **Bacteriocidal antibiotics** have the ability to kill the susceptible organism once it has been exposed to a high enough concentration of the antibiotic for a specific period of time. **Bacteriostatic antibiotics** have the ability to stop growth of a microorganism, which then enables the host to overcome the pathogen using its native immune system and bodily defenses. Most antibiotics are bactericidal at high serum concentrations but may be bacteriostatic at lower concentrations. These drugs are able to achieve an

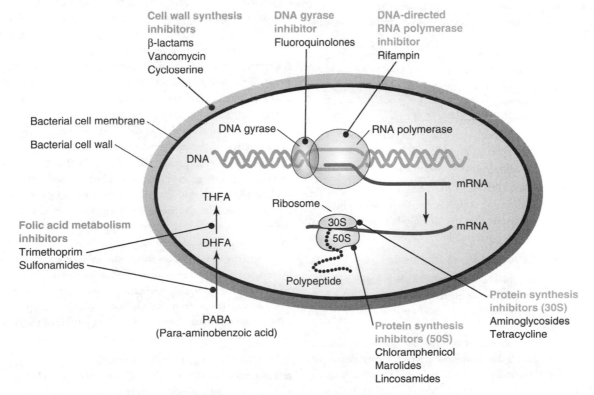

FIGURE 17-1 Sites of action for antibiotics.

antimicrobial effect by one of five mechanisms that are specific to the life cycle of the microbe:

1. Inhibition of cell wall synthesis and repair (e.g., penicillin, cephalosporin)
2. Inhibition of protein synthesis (e.g., aminoglycosides, macrolides, tetracycline)
3. Disruption of the permeability of cell membranes (e.g., amphotericin)
4. Inhibition of nucleic acid synthesis (e.g., antivirals, fluoroquinolones, quinolones)
5. Inhibition of specific biochemical pathways (e.g., sulfonamides)

INHIBITION OF CELL WALL SYNTHESIS For bacteria to maintain their size and integrity, they must depend on a well-functioning bacterial cell wall. Several antibiotics (penicillins, cephalosporins) prevent synthesis and repair of cell walls and thus, expose the bacteria to a hypotonic environment in the host, leading to eventual lysis of its cell contents. For example, gram-positive bacteria have a simpler cell wall structure and appear to be easier to damage than do their gram-negative counterparts. This explains, in part, their susceptibility to narrow-spectrum antibiotics such as the penicillins and cephalosporins.

INHIBITION OF PROTEIN SYNTHESIS Antibiotics can inhibit or interfere with protein synthesis. Therefore, a microbe's ability to grow and thrive is halted. Drugs such as the aminoglycosides cause production of bacterial proteins that have incorrect sequencing of amino acids, which are lethal to bacterial cells.

DISRUPTION OF THE PERMEABILITY OF CELL MEMBRANES Cell membranes in some bacteria and fungi are disrupted by drugs such as amphotericin B, nystatin, and polymyxins, leading to the death of a cell.

A bacteria's cell membrane is made of two layers of many lipids and proteins. Water and gases can flow freely back and forth through the cell membrane, but any nutrients must be actively transported through it by specific proteins in the membrane; thus, the energy-driving system of bacteria lies within its cell membrane. Consequently, any disruption of this process, such as by attached molecules of an antibiotic to the bacterial cell membrane, disrupts this transport system and kills the bacteria.

INHIBITION OF NUCLEIC ACID SYNTHESIS Antiviral agents inhibit synthesis of a virus's DNA or RNA, thus inhibiting replication. Some agents that use this mode of action against viruses include acyclovir, amantadine, zidovudine, and ribavirin.

Conscientious Prescribing of Antibiotics

The ideal antimicrobial agent is one with a high degree of selectivity—able to target the microorganism but not the host. However, every medicine has a potential for host toxicity. When any drug enters the body, it is affected by the body's defense systems for absorption, distribution, metabolism, and excretion. In practice, there is a therapeutic index or window in which there is differential activity between the action on the microbe and the effect (toxicity) on the host. However, every clinician should be aware of the toxicity of the agent to the host if the therapeutic efficacy is exceeded.

Frequent prescribing of antibiotics is associated with multidrug resistance to pathogens. In cases in which the etiology is known, the antibiotic that is most cost effective, least toxic, and most narrow in spectrum is recommended. In reality, however, the conscientious clinician always considers whether or not antibiotic therapy is even necessary by weighing the benefits (clinical efficacy, rapid recovery, patient comfort) against the risks (**antibiotic resistance**, allergic responses, adverse effects, pharmacokinetics) and costs of treatment. Clinicians should also keep in mind that many infections are self-limiting and that many patients just need supportive therapy to deal with the symptoms. Selection of an antibiotic is typically done in one of two ways: by definitive means, using definitive tests to identify the organism, or by empirical means, using previous experience with cases of similar nature.

Antimicrobial drug resistance is one of the world's most pressing health problems (CDC, 2011a), and since 1995, the Centers for Disease Control and Prevention (CDC) has campaigned nationally to stop the overuse of antibiotics by asking patients to implement smarter and more appropriate approaches to their use of antibiotics. The CDC encourages patients to do the following:

■ Ask their clinicians about antibiotic resistance and whether taking one is absolutely necessary.
■ Take antibiotics exactly as prescribed, finishing the entire prescription.
■ Not take antibiotics for viral infections such as the common cold or flu.
■ Never take antibiotics prescribed for someone else (CDC, 2011b).

Selection of an appropriate antimicrobial and its regimen should be based on appropriate dosing guidelines, as well as the patient's age and weight. Age is an important factor because many antibiotics are renally eliminated. The elderly and neonates are at greater risk of drug toxicity when taking these medications. For patients of heavier weight, there is a larger volume of distribution of medications or an increased storage of drug in fat tissues. This leads to reduced drug efficacy and need for dosage adjustment. Clinicians should also carefully consider the pharmacokinetics of the medication they are prescribing. For instance, highly plasma protein- bound drugs such as sulfonamides and penicillinase-resistant drugs should be avoided in late pregnancy and in neonates. Other important considerations when prescribing include the site of infection, any barriers to antimicrobial access, such as the cerebral spinal fluid (CSF), and the route of drug elimination and organ function.

Clinicians should follow their patients' responses to therapy by reviewing laboratory evidence indicating whether there was an infection and inquiring whether or not the patient experiences adverse effects from the antimicrobial. For example, every clinician who initiates, continues, or discontinues an antibiotic should consider the following questions:

■ Has the causative agent been identified?
■ Have adequate doses of the antibiotic been provided?
■ Have resistant pathogens evolved?
■ Has the patient's symptoms persisted?

Additionally, clinicians should work together with patients to ensure safe antibiotic use. For instance, clinicians should remind their patients of the following:

■ Not to share medications with anyone.
■ To use sunscreens and protective clothing to prevent photosensitivity reactions if patient is taking macrolides, sulfonamides, or tetracycline antibiotics.
■ To discard any unused medication.
■ To be careful when using some antibiotics, such as minocycline, because they may experience dizziness.
■ To take medications as prescribed because absorption of certain medications may be decreased due to certain foods or other medications. For instance, quinolones should be taken at least 2 hours before or 6 hours after ingesting any agent that could chelate them, such as foods or drugs rich in multivitamins with zinc, food or drugs with iron, or antacids with Ca, Mg, or Al salts, because the chelation will prevent absorption from the GI tract.

Empirical Prescribing of Antibiotics

When the pathogen is not known, but is suspected, and the illness requires treatment with antimicrobials before a microbiology laboratory can assist by identifying the pathogen, treatments become empirical. **Empirical prescribing** is based on the clinician's working knowledge or experience of what is most likely to be the pathogen causing the patient's condition. Certain organisms can present in a predictable manner, and over time the experienced clinician can identify which pathogen is causing the illness. Certain elements of the presenting illness (such as the site of infection, age, environment, immunosuppression, and prior antibiotic usage) help the clinician to predict the most likely organism. Ideally, selection of the most appropriate antimicrobial agent should wait until the results of culture and sensitivity tests are available. However, in many cases treatment is initiated immediately before results are known in an effort to expedite a cure or avert a catastrophic outcome resulting from an overwhelming infectious disease.

Because all organisms are classified according to morphology (cocci, bacilli), growth characteristics (anaerobic, aerobic), and other qualities (gram-positive or gram-negative), a better way to prescribe antibiotics comes from knowing these characteristics and then matching the therapy to the evidence. As antimicrobial resistance increases, many institutions have infectious control committees that review local, regional, national, and even global trends of microorganism susceptibility so that they may make recommendations for empirical prescribing. The clinician also needs an accurate patient history, especially any history of pregnancy, lactation, or allergies. Many antibiotics should not be given to pregnant or nursing women, and some may interact with other medications the patient is taking. Furthermore, as noted earlier, some antibiotics are contraindicated in patients with renal or hepatic insufficiency.

Recommendations for the empirical selection of an antibiotic are broadly and variably accepted and used. Some recommendations are published by specific societies or organizations, such as the American Thoracic Society, whereas others are based on a set of commonly accepted criteria (Arnold, 2009), such as the following:

■ Evaluation of evidence supporting infection (fever, leukocytosis, erythema)
■ Severity of illness (hemodynamic, neurological, respiratory, cellular changes)
■ Pathogen probabilities at site of infection
■ Resistance patterns; especially in *Streptococcus pneumoniae*, to specific antimicrobials
■ Comorbid conditions in the patient that compromise therapy

Drug Interactions Between Antibiotics and Other Medications

Antibiotics are commonly prescribed to patients who are also taking other medications. Many pharmacology textbooks contain long lists of potential interactions between antibiotics and other drugs, but only a few of these interactions have serious clinical consequences. Quinolones and macrolides are the groups of antibiotics most commonly associated with clinically significant drug interactions. Warfarin interacts with many antibiotics, although the incidence of this interaction can range from predictable to rare. The association between most antibiotics and oral contraceptive failure is weak, with only sporadic case reports in the literature. However, it is still common practice to advise patients using oral contraceptives as a form of birth control to use another, nonhormonal method of contraception while taking penicillin V and to wait until the next menstrual period to restart oral contraceptives. Some antibiotics, such as erythromycin and sulfonamides, inhibit the metabolism of other drugs via enzyme inhibition. Such changes in drug metabolism result in drug interactions, clinically significant changes in drug dosages, and adverse effects.

SPOTLIGHT ON MANAGING METHICILLIN-RESISTANT *STAPHYLOCOCCUS AUREUS* (MRSA)

Staphylococcus aureus is a constantly evolving versatile pathogen. It can cause a variety of infections, and it can adapt to a variety of environments with the propensity to acquire resistance to most antibiotics. In 1959 methicillin was first introduced into clinical practice, and the first cases of methicillin-resistant *S. aureus* (MRSA) were reported in the United Kingdom 2 years later (Jevons, 1961). Seven years later, after this resistant strain of *S. aureus* had spread to Japan, Europe, and Australia, the first case of MRSA was discovered in the United States (Barrett, McGehee, & Finland, 1968). By 1969 MRSA was considered a nosocomial infection tied to hospitals (hospital-acquired MRSA, or HA-MRSA), but currently community-acquired MRSA (CA-MRSA) has a higher prevalence than does HA-MRSA. CA-MRSA causes 14% of all infections and is resistant to methicillin, amoxicillin, penicillin, and other antibiotics (Levine, 2010). Every segment of society is at risk for acquiring this type of infection, especially children and the elderly who seem more prone to soft tissue and skin infections.

This organism's virulence is due to the fact that it has 2,500 genes acquired by transfer from other organisms; thus, 60% to 70% of them are resistant to typical antibiotics (VacZine Analytics, 2008). Two strains (USA 300 and USA 400) are widely found in community settings and are rapidly able to spread into institutions, such as

Continued

SPOTLIGHT ON MANAGING METHICILLIN-RESISTANT *STAPHYLOCOCCUS AUREUS* (MRSA)—cont'd

hospitals. The USA 300 strain carries a sequence of genes that helps increase its resistance to antibiotics. The bottom line is that *S. aureus* infections are much harder to treat today than when this bacterium was initially isolated 70 years ago. Routine methicillin use has been discontinued in the United States, and most of the penicillinase-resistant penicillins have limited utility against *S. aureus* in the developed world. However, methicillin resistance remains a term by which a laboratory can alert a clinician about the sensitivity of one isolate of *Staphylococcus* to one of the drugs listed in Table 17-1.

Interestingly, the only method that seems to work to prevent the spread of MRSA, both in the community and in the hospital, is hand washing (CDC, n.d.). That technique, although simple, has not been fully embraced by many clinicians. Consequently, clinicians and patients have to cope with many adverse effects resulting from using powerful antibiotics to treat MRSA. Such effects include cytopenia, elevated liver enzymes, clotting abnormalities, drug-drug interactions, and diarrhea, especially Clostridium difficile.

Several antibiotics are used today to treat MRSA (Table 17-1), but the gold standard remains parenteral vancomycin (1 gm every 12 hours). However, even at the recommended dosage of 1 gm every 12 hours, vancomycin use brings a risk of underdosing when the infection is very virulent. Thus, clinicians confronting MRSA have some serious questions to ponder:

■ Should treatment be started before or after conducting a culture and sensitivity test?
■ Should treatment be done at home or in a hospital?
■ Because science and professional literature differ, which drug is the most appropriate to prescribe?

TABLE 17-1	Empirical Prescribing of Oral and Parenteral Antibiotics for the Treatment of CA-MRSA, HA-MRSA, and Other Infections*		
GENERIC NAME	**TRADE NAME**	**INDICATION**	**DOSE**
clindamycin	Cleocin	Bronchitis (not *H. influenzae*) Bronchitis with *H. Influenzae* MRSA	250 mg every 12 hr 500 mg 2 times/day for 10 days 300–400 mg every 6–8 hr
sulfamethoxazole/ trimethoprim	Bactrim, Septra	General infections Urinary infections MRSA	2 gm initially, then 1 or 2 double-strength tabs every 12 hr for 10 days 1 or 2 double-strength tablets every 8–12 hr
doxycycline	Vibramycin	Most infections Gonorrhea MRSA	100 mg 2 times/day on first day then 100–200 mg 1 time/day 300 mg at once, then another 300 mg 1 hr later 100 mg every 12 hr
minocycline	Minocin	Acne MRSA	50 mg 1–3 times/day 100 mg every 12 hr
linezolid	Zyvox	Uncomplicated skin infections MRSA	400 mg every 12 hr for 10–14 days Linezolid is not recommended for MRSA, especially for outpatients. An infections specialist should be consulted for institutional use.
rifampin	Rifadin	Tuberculosis	600 mg daily
Parenteral Antibiotics for Institutional Use			
vancomycin	Vancocin	MRSA	1 gm every 12 hr
clindamycin	Cleocin	MRSA	600–900 mg every 6–8 hr
daptomycin	Cubicin	MRSA	4–6 mg/kg every 24 hr
tigecycline	Tygacil	MRSA	100 mg loading, followed with 50 mg 2 times/day
linezolid	Zyvox	MRSA	600 mg every 12 hr but data are inconclusive in support of its indication
quinupristin/ dalfopristin	Synercid†	MRSA	7.5 mg/kg every 8–12 hr

*Every clinician who prescribes drugs should consult the manufacturer's literature and an authoritative drug reference because recommended dosages change in relation to patients (children, adults, elderly), comorbidities, general health, and other factors, and in relation to the pathogen(s) involved.

†Synercid, a combination of two drugs (quinupristin and dalfopristin) was introduced in 2001 and is the first in a distinct class of antibiotics known as the streptogramins. Synercid has activity against a range of gram-positive bacteria that are usually resistant to other agents, including VREF, nosocomial infections, and infections related to the use of intravenous catheters. Synercid can be dosed at 8- to 12-hour intervals. There is no demonstrable ototoxicity, nephrotoxicity, bone marrow suppression, or cardiovascular adverse effects; however, reversible arthralgias, myalgias, and peripheral venous irritation are the major side effects of Synercid. Some clinicians use this product only through a central line because of venous irritation.

BACTERIOCIDAL ANTIBIOTICS THAT AFFECT CELL WALL SYNTHESIS

Bacteriocidal antibiotics that affect cell wall synthesis are known as the penicillins and cephalosporins. All the drugs in these two groupings have a shared chemical moiety called a *beta-lactam ring* (Fig. 17-2). It is this ring structure that gives these drugs their bacteriocidal activity. The problem with using these agents is that some microbes produce an enzyme called **beta-lactamase**, which will lyse the beta-lactam ring on the antibiotic and render it ineffective. Thus, the microbe is resistant to the medications sent to fight it.

When first introduced during World War II, penicillin came in only one form, penicillin G, which was produced in fermentation tanks. Since then, significant limitations to this antibiotic led to modifications that gave it expanded coverage, or the capacity to kill more organisms. To understand the need for the various groups of penicillins, one must first understand the limitations of penicillins V and G. The penicillins are grouped into narrow-spectrum penicillins, penicillinase-resistant penicillins, and expanded-spectrum penicillins.

There are several disadvantages of penicillin, both because it is a narrow-spectrum antibiotic and because its chemical moiety, the beta-lactam ring, is unique. Modifications to the penicillin molecule have been made over the last five decades in hopes of overcoming this limitation and its narrow-spectrum of activity:

Disadvantage: Penicillin is a narrow spectrum antibiotic and is ineffective against gram-negative organisms.

Solution: Ampicillin is a synthetic penicillin designed to overcome penicillin's limited ability to affect gram-negative organisms. Ampicillin is *not* penicillinase resistant.

Disadvantage: Penicillin is destroyed by gastric acid; thus, its GI absorption is erratic.

Solution: A more stable salt form of penicillin G has been created, penicillin V; it is more reliably absorbed when given by mouth.

Disadvantage: Penicillin is rapidly excreted; to maintain high blood levels, it must be given often.

Solution: Benzathine penicillin (Bicillin) was created to develop and sustain high tissue levels. This intramuscular formulation will maintain therapeutic levels for up to a week.

Disadvantage: Penicillins are all hydrolyzed by beta-lactamase or penicillinase produced by many bacteria, especially *staphylococci*.

Solution: Penicillins have been synthesized with structures that prevent the splitting of the beta-lactam ring of the penicillin moiety, for example, cloxacillin, dicloxacillin, nafcillin, and oxacillin.

Disadvantage: Penicillin causes hypersensitivities and toxicities; there are skin rashes in 2% to 4% of patients and anaphylaxis in 0.05% of patients.

Solution: A new category of drugs was created to avoid these reactions because penicillin can be so dangerous. This new category of drugs is called the *cephalosporins*.

Natural Penicillins

There are four groups of penicillins: the natural penicillins, penicillin G, penicillin V, and the aminopenicillins (amoxicillin and ampicillin). Penicillin G was the first antibiotic; it was discovered in 1876 by the Irish physician John Tyndall, who described a battle between bacteria and mold. However, it was Dr. Alexander Fleming in London, England, who in 1928 found that penicillium fungus on moldy bread secreted a substance that exhibited antibacterial properties. Penicillin (PCN) did not come into widespread use until World War II, when through a fermentation process large batches could be produced. It thus became possible to save the lives of many soldiers suffering battle-induced infections. The discovery of penicillin could be considered to be the most famous of all medical advances; however, shortly after its introduction, cases of resistance prompted scientists to develop new and different antibiotics. Therefore, today's penicillins differ considerably in their spectrum of activity. Penicillins still remain the drug of choice for syphilis, group A streptococci, *Listeria monocytogenes*, *Pasteurella multocida*, actinomycetes, some enterococci, and anaerobic infections.

Conscientious Prescribing of Penicillins

■ Clinicians should watch for abdominal cramps; fever; and severe, watery diarrhea, which may indicate a superinfection.

■ Hypersensitivity reactions include angioedema, serum sickness, anaphylaxis, and a severe local inflammatory reaction at the site of injections (Arthus reaction) may occur.

■ Any patient with renal impairment may require dosage adjustments.

■ Penicillin can cause a false-positive direct Coombs' test.

■ Aqueous penicillin G potassium or sodium, when given intravenously and when given in high doses, should be administered slowly because of the possible side effect of electrolyte imbalance caused by the K salt or Na salt.

Patient/Family Education Regarding Penicillins

■ In general, penicillins should be taken on an empty stomach.

■ Patients should be instructed to take oral penicillin 1 or 2 hours after meals to increase absorption of the drug.

■ If taking a reconstituted oral product, patients should take all medication within 14 days. Patients should shake the

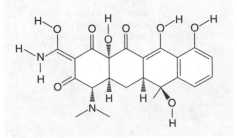

FIGURE 17-2 Tetracycline structure showing its four cyclic rings.

bottle each time a dosage is withdrawn and use a calibrated measuring device, *not* a teaspoon.

■ Advise women patients taking oral contraceptives to use another, nonhormonal method of contraception while taking penicillin V and to wait until the next menstrual period to restart oral contraceptives.

■ Patients should take this medication around the clock (that is, the time between dosages should be divided equally) and finish the medication, even if they are feeling better.

■ Patients should notify the clinician if fever and diarrhea develop, especially if there is any blood, pus, or mucus in the stool.

Mechanism of Action

Penicillins exert both a bacteriocidal and bacteriostatic effect on susceptible bacteria by interfering with the final stages of cell wall synthesis (see Fig. 17-1). All bacteria have protective cell walls made of cross-linked peptides. Because penicillins and cephalosporins are structurally similar to these peptides, they can compete for and bind to the bacterial enzyme (peptidoglycan) in the bacterial cell wall that catalyzes the peptides that build the cell wall and give a cell wall its strength. As the cell wall of a bacterium incorporates the penicillin (or cephalosporin), it gradually deteriorates, becoming too weak to support its underlying cell membrane. When the cell wall ruptures, bacterial cytoplasm oozes out due to the hypertonic osmolarity of the surrounding tissue, and thus the microorganism dies. Despite their relative low toxicity for the host, these agents are active against many bacteria, especially gram-positive pathogens, streptococci, staphylococci, clostridia; certain gram-negative forms; certain spirochetes (*Treponema pallidum* and *Treponema pertenue*); and certain fungi. Certain strains of some target species, for example *Staphylococcus* bacteria, secrete the enzyme penicillinase, which inactivates penicillin and confers resistance to the antibiotic. Some of the newer penicillins, for example methicillin, are more effective against penicillinase-producing organisms. An additional class of extended-spectrum penicillins has been approved for use; it includes piperacillin and mezlocillin.

Penicillins contain a thiazolidine ring connected to a beta-lactam ring, which is then connected to a side chain (see Fig. 17-2). The beta-lactam ring is responsible for penicillin's antibacterial properties; it is structurally similar to the polypeptides in the bacteria cell wall and disrupts the peptides. However, the beta-lactam ring is quite fragile, which makes it easy for bacteria to neutralize penicillin. The thiazolidine side chain determines many of penicillin's other distinguishing characteristics.

Pharmacokinetics

■ Absorption: Rate and degree of absorption from GI tract varies 33% to 76%. Generally, these medications are well absorbed from the GI tract.

■ Distribution: Widely distributed and will cross placenta and mother's milk; distribution into CSF is minimal, but sufficient with meningeal inflammation. Protein binding is about 20%.

■ Metabolism: Partial metabolism occurs in the liver yet most is eliminated unchanged.

■ Excretion: Primarily occurs in the urine.

■ Half-life: 30 to 60 minutes.

Clinical Use

■ Pneumococcal pneumonia, streptococcal pharyngitis, sexually transmitted diseases such as certain gonorrheal strains and syphilis, rheumatic fever (when used in combination with an aminoglycoside), Lyme disease.

■ Treats infections caused by gram-positive cocci and susceptible gram-negative cocci (e.g., gonorrhea); used prophylactically before surgical procedures in patients with a history of rheumatic fever, rheumatic heart disease, congenital heart disease.

Dosage and Route of Administration

Generic Name	Trade Name	Route	Adult Dose	Indications
penicillin V potassium	Veetids, Pen-VK, V-Cillin K	PO	Adults and children 12 years old: 125–500 mg every 6–8 hr	*Streptococcus*, pharyngitis, erysipelas, gingivitis, Lyme disease
penicillin G benzathine/ penicillin G procaine	Bicillin CR	IM	Group A strep: 2.4 million units as a single dose. Syphilis: For primary, secondary, or late (<1 year), 2.4 million units as one single dose. For indeterminate-duration latent syphilis, without CNS involvement, 2.4 million units IM once a week for 3 doses. Penicillin G (3–4 million units IV every 4 hr) for 10–14 days is recommended for neurosyphilis	Moderately severe infections: respiratory, skin, soft tissue, otitis media
penicillin G procaine	Pfizerpen, Wycillin	IM	Adults: 600,000 to 1.2 million IU/day Syphilis: 2.4 million IU 4 times/day for 10–14 days	Syphilis, diphtheria, antibacterial
penicillin G benzathine	Bicillin LA	For deep IM use only in large muscle mass*	Pharyngitis: 1.2 million IU as a single dose Syphilis: 2.4 million IU weekly for 3 weeks (adults)	Prophylaxis for streptococcal infections in patients with history of rheumatic fever Group A streptococcal pharyngitis, acute glomerulonephritis, and rheumatic fever.

*An injection given IV has caused embolisms, toxic reactions, and death.

Adverse Reactions

DERM: Rash, urticaria

GI: Mild diarrhea, nausea, vomiting

NEURO: Headache, seizures

MISC: Oral or vaginal candidiasis owing to suppression of normal flora. HYPERSENSITIVITY CAN BE SEVERE AND CAN INCLUDE ANAPHYLAXIS AND INTERSTITIAL NEPHRITIS. SUPERINFECTIONS: THE ALTERING OF A BODY'S NORMAL BACTERIAL BALANCE WITH BACTERIOCIDAL AGENTS LIKE PENICILLIN CAN RESULT IN POTENTIALLY FATAL SUPERINFECTIONS AND ANTIBIOTIC-ASSOCIATED COLITIS.

RENAL: Renal failure

Drug Interactions

- Inhibited antibacterial activity of penicillin can occur with coadministered chloramphenicol, macrolide antibiotics, methotrexate, and tetracycline.
- Advise patients taking oral contraceptives to use another form of contraception because penicillins occasionally hamper the efficacy of oral contraceptives.
- Probenecid potentiates the activity of penicillin and cephalosporins by raising their blood levels. It does this by competing with the penicillin for excretion at the organic ionic transport system in the kidney.

Contraindications

- Cross-sensitivity with cephalosporins is about 10%.
- Hypersensitivity to any penicillin is a possibility.
- A person with infectious mononucleosis should not be on penicillins, as they have propensity to cause extensive rash in these patients.

Expanded-Spectrum Penicillins: The Cephalosporins

The cephalosporins are widely used semisynthetic agents. These drugs are not the first drug of choice for most infections, even though they are highly effective in a variety of mild to severe infections caused by both gram-positive and gram-negative bacteria. They are structurally similar and chemically related to penicillins but are produced synthetically. However, because of their large spectrum of activity over gram-negative organisms, they have achieved widespread use in cases in which there is uncertainty about the cause of an infection or while culture results are still pending.

Cephalosporins are also frequently used when there has been intolerance to other antimicrobials. There is, however, a cross sensitivity to penicillin that precludes their use in patients with a history of immunoglobulin E–mediated allergic reactions to a penicillin (i.e., anaphylaxis, angioneurotic edema, immediate urticaria). In addition to the classic anaphylactic response, toxicity issues with cephalosporins are the same as for penicillins, but toxicity is likely to be less severe.

The cephalosporins are grouped in four generations (first, second, third, and fourth) based on their antimicrobial properties.

As a general rule, the first generation cephalosporins have the best activity against gram-positive organisms, with relatively modest activity against gram-negative bacteria. As the designation increases from first to third generation, there is increased activity against gram-negative organisms and anaerobes (and less against gram-positive), along with increased ability to withstand destruction by beta-lactamase. Thus, the first-generation cephalosporins are active against gram-positive cocci, including *S. aureus* and *Staphylococcus epidermitis*. They are not active against MRSA and have a limited effect against anaerobes, such as *Escherichia coli*. They do not enter the CSF.

The second-generation cephalosporins are active against the same organisms as the first, but have improved gram-negative coverage (*Klebsiella, Proteus,* and *E. coli*). In addition, they have some activity against beta-lactamase-producing strains of *H. influenzae* and *Moraxella catarrhalis*. The third- and fourth-generation cephalosporins are active against the same organisms as the first two generations, but they have a wider spectrum of activity against gram-negative organisms, especially some of the more uncommon bacteria such as the *Enterobacter*.

Clinicians should keep in mind the usefulness of cephalosporins comes from their low toxicity and their broad spectrum of activity. However, none of them have reliable activity against MRSA, penicillin-resistant *S. pneumoniae* or enterococcal infections, all of which are common pathogens of the integument, respiratory, and gastrointestinal tracts. This again reinforces the need for culture and sensitivity testing before prescribing.

Most often, clinicians learn to separate those cephalosporins that treat infections above the diaphragm from those that treat infections below the diaphragm. Typically, clinicians have problems with the fact that so many of the names of these drugs all sound so similar. However, each generation contains a few more popularly used agents that are usually prescribed by trade name, and as clinicians gain experience, they place them in their personal formulary. However, most managed care plans usually have a limited number of these drugs listed in their formularies. Therefore, clinicians may need to allow substitutions within a class to save patients money.

Conscientious Prescribing of Cephalosporins

- Use cautiously in those sensitive to penicillins. PCN-allergic patients have 5% to 10% incidence of cross-allergy. ANY PATIENT WITH A HYPERSENSITIVITY OR HISTORY OF ALLERGIES TO PENICILLIN IS AT RISK FOR A SEVERE HYPERSENSITIVITY REACTION. Most people who give a history of allergy to penicillin should be treated with a different antibiotic.
- Use cautiously in patients with renal impairment.

Patient/Family Education Regarding Cephalosporins

- Instruct patient to take medications around the clock at evenly spaced times and to finish the medication, even if feeling completely better.
- Missed doses should be taken as soon as possible, unless it is time for the next dose. Instruct patients to not double the doses.

Dosage and Administration

Generic Name	Trade Name	Route	Adult Dose	Indications
FIRST GENERATION				
cefadroxil	Duricef	PO	500 mg–1 gm daily as 2 divided doses	Urinary tract infections (UTIs), skin and skin structure,* tonsillitis/pharyngitis, impetigo
cephalexin	Keflex	PO	250–500 mg every 6 hr for strep pharyngitis, skin and skin structures	Otitis Media (OM), skin and skin structure,* bone, genitourinary, respiratory
cefazolin	Ancef	IV or IM	1–1.5 gm every 6 hr	skin and skin structure,* bone, genitourinary, respiratory
cephradine	Velosef	PO	250–500 mg every 6 hr	skin and skin structure,* genitourinary, respiratory
SECOND GENERATION				
cefuroxime axetil	Ceftin	PO	Adults (>13 years): Mild to moderate bronchitis, sinusitis, uncomplicated skin and skin structures, 250–500 mg 2 times/day for 7–10 days Uncomplicated gonorrhea: 1 gm single dose Pharyngitis/tonsillitis: 250 mg 2 times/day for 10 days Children: 20–30 mg/kg/day divided 2 times/day for pharyngitis, OM	Mild to moderate bronchitis, sinusitis, uncomplicated skin and skin structures, UTIs, gonorrhea, OM, pharyngitis/tonsillitis
cefprozil	Cefzil	PO	Adults (>13 years): bronchitis 500 mg every 12 hr; sinusitis 250–500 mg every 12 hr, uncomplicated skin and skin structures 250–500 mg every 12 hr; pharyngitis/tonsillitis 500 mg daily. All administered for 10 days.	Mild to moderate acute and chronic bronchitis, sinusitis, uncomplicated skin and skin structures, OM, pharyngitis/tonsillitis
loracarbef	Lorabid	PO	200–400 mg every 12 hr for 7–10 days	Mild to moderate acute and chronic bronchitis, sinusitis, uncomplicated skin and skin structures, OM, pharyngitis/tonsillitis
cefotetan	Cefotan	IV or IM	1–2 gm every 12 hr for UTI and gynecological infections	Lower respiratory, UTI, skin and skin structure, gynecological, intra-abdominal surgical prophylaxis
cefuroxime	Zinacef	IV and IM	750 mg–1.5 gm every 8 hr	Lower respiratory, UTI, skin and skin structure, surgical prophylaxis
cefaclor	Ceclor, Raniclor	PO	250–500 mg 3 times/day	Bronchitis, sinusitis, otitis media, UTIs, soft tissue infection, cellulitis
THIRD AND FOURTH GENERATION				
ceftibuten	Cedax	PO	400 mg daily 10 days	Mild to moderate acute bacterial exacerbations of chronic bronchitis, OM, pharyngitis/tonsillitis
ceftriaxone	Rocephin	IM or IV	1–2 gm daily or in 2 divided doses. Gonorrhea:125–250 mg IM once	Septicemia, lower respiratory, OM, skin and skin structures, genitourinary, pelvic inflammatory disease (PID), intra-abdominal, meningitis, surgical prophylaxis (orthopedic, hip)
cefotaxime	Claforan	IV and IM	1–2 gm every 6–12 hr	Bacteremia, septicemia, lower respiratory, skin and skin structures, genitourinary, gynecological, intra-abdominal, meningitis, surgical prophylaxis
cefixime	Suprax	PO	400 mg/day as a single dose or 2 divided doses for otitis media, acute bronchitis, uncomplicated UTI. Single dose therapy (400 mg) for uncomplicated gonococcal infection of genitourinary tract	OM, pharyngitis/tonsillitis, sinusitis, mild to moderate acute bacterial exacerbations of chronic bronchitis, UTI, gonorrhea
FOURTH GENERATION				
cefdinir	Omnicef	PO	300 mg every 12 hr or 600 mg every 24 hr for 10 days for community-acquired pneumonia	Mild to moderate acute bacterial exacerbations of chronic bronchitis, OM, pharyngitis/tonsillitis, sinusitis, community-acquired pneumonia, skin and skin structure
cefepime	Maxipime	IV or IM	1–2 gm every 8–12 hr	Treating febrile neutropenic patients and antibiotic-resistant gram-negative bacteria.

*It should be noted that with increasing prevalence of MRSA, most cephalosporins are no longer used to treat skin and soft tissue infections unless culture has been performed to direct therapy.

- Advise patients not to share the medication.
- Advise patients to report signs of superinfection (black furry tongue, vaginal itching, loose foul smelling stool, or allergies).
- Caution patient not to treat diarrhea without consulting a clinician, especially if diarrhea and fever develop together.

Mechanism of Action

Cephalosporins have a mechanism of action identical to that of the penicillins. However, the basic chemical structure of the penicillins and cephalosporins differ in other respects, resulting in some difference in the spectrum of antibacterial activity. Like the penicillins, cephalosporins have a beta-lactam ring structure that interferes with synthesis of the bacterial cell wall and thus they are bactericidal. Cephalosporins are derived from cephalosporin C, which is produced from *Cephalosporium acremonium*, a microbe found in soil. However, being semisynthetic agents, another structure is fused to their beta-lactam ring, making them more resistant to degradation by beta-lactamase-producing bacteria.

Pharmacokinetics

- Absorption: All are well absorbed following either intramuscular or oral administration.
- Distribution: All are widely distributed, but CSF penetration is poor; all enter breast milk; all cross placenta barrier.
- Metabolism: 85% excreted unchanged in urine.
- Excretion: Primarily excreted unchanged by the kidneys.
- Half-life: About 2 hours, but increased in renal impairment (ceftriaxone is a notable exception, with half-life of 8 hours).

Clinical Use

- Respiratory tract infections, pneumonia
- Otitis media
- Skin and skin structure infections not caused by MRSA or methicillin resistant *Staphylococcus epidermidis* (MRSE)
- Bone and joint infections (not cefmetazole, cefprozil, or loracarbef)
- Urinary tract infections (not cefprozil)
- Septicemia (not cefmetazole, cefprozil, loracarbef)
- Sexually transmitted diseases and most gonorrheal infections

Adverse Reactions

GI: Nausea, mild diarrhea, mild abdominal cramping, antibiotic associated colitis
GYN: Vaginal candidiasis
HEM: Anemia and leukopenia
MISC: Anaphylaxis, oral candidiasis, serum sickness (usually after second course of therapy and it resolves when drug is discontinued). ANY PATIENT WITH A HYPERSENSITIVITY OR HISTORY OF ALLERGIES TO PENICILLIN IS AT RISK FOR A SEVERE HYPERSENSITIVITY REACTION THAT CAN MANIFEST AS SEVERE PRURITUS, ANGIOEDEMA, BRONCHOSPASM, ANAPHYLACTIC SHOCK, AND DEATH.
RENAL: Nephrotoxicity, interstitial nephritis

Interactions

- Aminoglycosides can add to the nephrotoxicity.
- Loop diuretics can increase nephrotoxicity.
- Oral anticoagulants can create hypoprothrombinemia.

Contraindications

- Hypersensitivity to any cephalosporin. Patients who are hypersensitive to one cephalosporin will likely be hypersensitive to them all.

Beta-Lactamase-Resistant (Penicillinase-Resistant) Penicillins

Resistance to penicillins is largely due to the production of beta-lactamase (penicillinase) by the invading microbe, which, in turn, hydrolyzes the beta-lactam ring of the antibiotic, rendering it ineffective. The most notorious bacteria that does this is *S. aureus*. The genetic information for making beta-lactamase is encoded in the microbe, and it is easily transferred to other bacteria, making them also resistant to the penicillins. Thus, penicillinase resistant penicillins, with expanded coverage against *S. aureus*, were developed 50 years ago to address this continuing and growing worldwide problem. Today, these make up a large group of antibiotics that include carbenicillin (Geocillin), cloxacillin, dicloxacillin, methicillin, and many others.

Mechanism of Action

Resist the action of penicillinase and bind to the cell wall, leading to cell death (bactericidal).

Pharmacokinetics

- Absorption: Rate of absorption and degree of absorption from GI tract varies (33% to 76%).
- Distribution: Widely distributed; will cross placenta and into breast milk; distribution into CSF is minimal, but sufficient if meninges are inflamed.
- Metabolism: Partial metabolism occurs in the liver.
- Excretion: Partially unchanged excretion occurs in liver.
- Half-life: 0.5 to 1 hour

Clinical Uses

Used to treat the following infections when penicillinase producing staphylococci are present or suspected:

- Infections of soft tissues and bone
- Respiratory tract infections
- Sinusitis
- Urinary tract infections
- Endocarditis
- Septicemia
- Meningitis

Dosage and Administration

Generic Name	Trade Name	Route	Adult Dose	Indications
carbenicillin	Geocillin	PO	382 mg every 6 hr	Serious UTIs, prostatitis caused by gram-negative aerobic bacilli
cloxacillin	Tegopen Cloxapen	PO	200–250 mg every 6 hr	Mild to moderate infections produced by penicillin-resistant *S. aureus*
dicloxacillin	Dynapen Pathocil	PO	125–1,000 mg every 6 hr	Pneumonia, septicemia, skin/ soft tissues, osteomyelitis
oxacillin	Prostaphilin Bactocill	IM or IV	1–2 gm every 4–6 hr	Osteomyelitis, septicemia, endocarditis, CNS infections
piperacillin*	Pipracil	IM or IV	200–300 mg/kg/day divided every 6 hr	*Pseudomonas, Proteus,* uncomplicated UTI
ticarcillin and clavulanate potassium†	Timentin	IV	75–300 mg ticarcillin every 4–6 hr if <60 kg	Infections of lower respiratory tract, UTI, skin, skin structure, bone and joints, septicemia
piperacillin and tazobactam‡	Zosyn	IM or IV	IM for moderate infection, 2.25 gm IV every 4–6 hr	Bone and joint infections, septicemia, intra-abdominal infections (appendicitis)
ticarcillin*	Ticar	IM or IV	1–4 gm every 4–6 hr	Septicemia, acute/ chronic respiratory infections, skin/soft tissue infections, UTIs

*Piperacillin and ticarcillin are sometimes classified as extended-spectrum penicillins because their spectrum covers many other species. They are usually administered with an aminoglycoside antibiotic (e.g., gentamycin, tobramycin, amikacin, or netilmicin). The inhibition of cell wall synthesis by piperacillin and ticarcillin permits better cell wall penetration by one of the aminoglycosides and subsequently better inhibition of protein synthesis.

†The combination of the broad-spectrum penicillin, ticarcillin, and clavulanate produces an antibiotic (Timentin) that is able to resist beta-lactamase. Its spectrum of activity is like all penicillins, but is now extended to include several gram-negative aerobic pathogens, especially pseudomonas. The drug is usually reserved for hospital use and is given intravenously.

‡Piperacillin is combined with a beta-lactamase inhibitor, tazobactam, to extend its spectrum of activity. It is often coadministered with an aminoglycoside. This drug is well absorbed from intramuscular sites and will enter the CSF when meninges are inflamed.

Adverse Reactions

DERM: Urticaria, rashes
GI: Pseudomembranous colitis, nausea, vomiting, diarrhea
GU: Interstitial nephritis
HEM: Blood dyscrasias
MISC: Pain at IM site, phlebitis at IV sites
NEURO: Seizures

Interactions

■ Gastric acids and acidic juices decrease absorption.
■ Other interactions: See p. 318 regarding penicillins.

Conscientious Considerations

■ Side effects are frequent, and mild hypersensitivity reactions such as fever, rash, pruritus, and GI effects such as nausea, vomiting, and diarrhea may occur.
■ If given orally, these drugs should be given on an empty stomach (1 hour before or 2 hours after meals).
■ In addition, clinicians must be aware of the same important considerations that apply to all penicillins (see p. 316).

Extended Spectrum Penicillins

Because penicillins are narrow-spectrum antibiotics, they are ineffective against gram-negative bacteria. Extended spectrum penicillins such as amoxicillin and ampicillin, however, pass through the pores in the outer membrane and can reach **penicillin-binding proteins (PBPs)** on the inner cell's cytoplasmic membranes. Although ampicillin and amoxicillin are not resistant to penicillinase secreted by *S. aureus*, they do have increased effectiveness against certain gram-negative bacteria (*E. coli, H. influenzae, Proteus mirabilis, Salmonella,* and *Shigella*), and this is their major advantage over penicillin G or V. Amoxicillin is preferred over ampicillin because it is more completely absorbed and has a lower incidence of diarrhea. Scientists have found that combining some agents with antimicrobials provide increased effectiveness of the antibiotic. For example, the addition of clavulanate to the penicillin amoxicillin creates Augmentin. Clavulanate inhibits bacterial released beta-lactamase and protects the penicillin against enzymatic degradation.

Amoxicillin/Clavulanate (Augmentin)

This combination agent is formed by adding clavulanate to amoxicillin creating a wider spectrum of activity than amoxicillin used alone. It allows penicillin a broader killing power against common pathogens, such as *H. influenzae, E. coli, P. mirabilis, Neisseria meningitidis, Shigella, Salmonella,* and *M. catarrhalis.* This fixed-dose combination is only available for oral dosing, but it has recently been marketed in an extended-release formulation.

Ampicillin/Sulbactam (Unasyn)

The addition of sulbactam sodium to ampicillin increases the resistance of ampicillin to beta-lactamase enzymes, which may inactivate it. Patients may be sensitive to both ampicillin and the sulbactam. This drug should be restricted to infections in which there is known to be beta-lactamase-producing strains. It is not indicated for pseudomonal infections. It is sold only for parenteral use.

SPOTLIGHT ON *STREPTOCOCCUS PNEUMONIAE*

Streptococcus pneumoniae is a gram-positive, aerobic, spherical-celled bacterium that is a common cause of community-acquired pneumonia, especially in children, the elderly, and those with compromised host defenses. It is the leading cause of respiratory tract infections (sinusitis, bronchitis, pneumonia, and emphysema), otitis media, and a host of other syndromes, including pericarditis, endocarditis, osteomyelitis, septic arthritis, epidural abscess, brain abscess, and skin and soft tissue infections. Pneumococci are transmitted person to person by close contact; thus, transmission among children in day-care centers and among the elderly in nursing homes is a common problem. The incidence of infection by *S. pneumoniae* varies drastically by age, being highest among children under 2 years and adults over 65 years, and in the immunocompromised. However, acute lower respiratory infections continue to be the leading cause of acute illnesses worldwide and remain the most important cause of infant and young children mortality, accounting for about two million deaths each year and ranking first among causes of disability-adjusted life-years lost in developing countries (Madhi, 2006). In the United States, in 2007, *S. pneumoniae* was responsible for about 5.6 million cases of bacterial community-acquired pneumonia (CAP), resulting in 4.5 million visits to physician offices and as many as 1.1 million hospitalizations. The highest rates occurred in children under 5 years of age with treatment being macrolides (34%), cephalosporins (22%), and penicillins (14%) (Kronman et al., 2011).

The spleen is the principal organ that cleanses the blood stream of pneumococci; thus, serious infection will likely result in those who are absent their spleen or have a compromised splenic function. In this setting, an individual may be at up to a 100-fold risk of developing serious pneumococcal infection. Clinicians should be aware that higher case-fatality rates from *S. pneumoniae* occur among those with the following:

■ HIV infections
■ Diabetes
■ Sickle cell disease
■ Chronic obstructive pulmonary disease (COPD)
■ Coronary heart disease/congestive heart failure
■ Renal failure, especially those needing dialysis
■ Reduced or defective polymorphonuclear cells, as in chemotherapy-induced leucopenia and in those on corticosteroids
■ History of cigarette smoking

Medical Management

S. pneumoniae was first isolated and grown by Louis Pasteur in 1881, and, as we enter the 21st century, it is still a challenge to treat it successfully because of its growing resistance to penicillins, cephalosporins, macrolides, and (recently) quinolones. The prevalence of resistance varies, but overall it is near 10%. Historically, streptococci organisms were susceptible to any of the penicillin class of agents or beta-lactam agents, and typically at low dosages. But since the late 1960s, there has been increasing report of the organism resisting the bactericidal effect of penicillin and placing a greater burden on society such that now CAP is the sixth leading cause of death in the United States and the leading cause of death (5% in outpatients and 12% in hospitalized inpatients) around the world.

Among the resistant strains there are moderately resistant (or intermediately sensitive) and highly resistant strains. Moderately resistant strains will respond to high-dose penicillin, ampicillin, a cephalosporin, or a macrolide; highly resistant strains will not respond to any of the penicillins or macrolide antibiotics and occasionally resist third-generation cephalosporins. Choice of therapeutic agents to treat pneumococcal infections should be based on the following:

■ The site of infection
■ The results of antimicrobial sensitivity tests
■ The severity of the infection
■ Host factors such as age, allergies, drug interaction possibilities, renal and hepatic function, and pregnancy status

Susceptible strains should be treated with either penicillin (penicillin G), amoxicillin, or a first- or second-generation cephalosporin. Patients allergic to penicillin or cephalosporins should receive a macrolide if the infection is not serious. If the infection is life-threatening, patients should be treated with vancomycin. All drugs should be dose-adjusted for the patient's renal function, hepatic function, weight, and manufacturer's instruction for administration. For patients with a serious infection that is penicillin resistant, cephalosporin resistant, and vancomycin resistant, fluoroquinolones (levofloxacin, moxifloxacin) or doxycycline should be administered.

ANTIBIOTICS THAT INHIBIT PROTEIN SYNTHESIS: MACROLIDES

This is a unique class of antibiotics that inhibit protein synthesis at the level of the 50S ribosome unit. Thus, these agents may be bacteriostatic against susceptible organisms, or they may be bactericidal, depending on their dosage, infection site, and susceptibility of the bacteria. Many susceptible organisms to this class are aerobic gram positive as well as gram negative. Macrolides do not bind to mammalian or human 50S ribosomes, and this partly accounts for their selective toxicity. They include erythromycin, clarithromycin, and azithromycin. Clindamycin, which binds to the 50S subunit of bacterial ribosomes at a different location, can be considered with the macrolides, although it technically can be effective when there is macrolide resistance. However, because the macrolides and clindamycin act at sites in close proximity, binding of one of these antibiotics to the ribosome can inhibit the interaction of the others. Therefore, they are not complementary to each other.

Conscientious Considerations for Macrolides

■ Patients need to be properly assessed for a treatable infection.
■ Obtain cultures for sensitivity testing; may give first dose while waiting for results.
■ Observe for signs and symptoms of ANAPHYLAXIS.
■ Watch for signs of nonadherence.

Patient/Family Education for Macrolides

■ May be taken without regard to food or antacids (some references say concomitant use of food and antacids hinders absorption).

■ Use sunscreen and protective clothing to prevent photosensitivity reaction.

■ May cause drowsiness and dizziness, so be careful driving or operating machinery.

■ Report to clinician any signs of superinfection, especially black, hairy tongue.

■ Instruct patient to take medication around the clock and to finish drug as directed.

■ If a dose is missed, take next dose, but do not double up.

■ If abdominal cramps, diarrhea, fever, bloody stool develop, get professional help.

■ When administered intravenously, inform patient that a bitter taste in the mouth is *not* clinically significant.

■ When used vaginally, insert high into vagina at bedtime, remain lying down for 30 minutes after application, and use sanitary napkin to prevent staining of clothing and bedding. Refrain from sexual intercourse during therapy.

■ For topical use, avoid smoking or open flame, because topical clindamycin is flammable. Notify clinician if skin gets excessively dry when using topical formulation. Wait 30 minutes after washing or shaving before applying clindamycin cream.

Azithromycin (Zithromax, Z-Pak, Zmax)

Azithromycin is in the family of antibiotics known as the macrolides. It is a subclass of these agents because it is a derivative of erythromycin. Because it is so effective against so many gram-positive bacteria, and some gram-negative bacteria (broad spectrum), it has become one of the best-selling antibiotics in the United States for treating respiratory infections, skin infections, and sexually transmitted diseases. As an altered molecule, this macrolide's most distinguishing feature is its long half-life; thus, a once-a-day tablet taken for a short time provides active serum levels for several days beyond. By contrast, erythromycin has such a short half-life it must be dosed four times a day, and this leads to compliance and adherence issues over a course of therapy.

Mechanism of Action

This macrolide is different from the older macrolides (erythromycin and clarithromycin) in that it inhibits more gram-negative organisms.

Pharmacokinetics

■ Absorption: Rapidly absorbed when given orally, but the absolute bioavailability is about 40% because of protein binding in plasma

■ Distribution: Widely distributed in body tissues and fluids except CSF; has high concentration within cells, resulting in much greater concentration in tissues than in serum

■ Metabolism: Some hepatic metabolism to inactive metabolites

■ Excretion: Mostly excreted unchanged in bile

■ Half-life: 11 to 14 hours after one dose; 2 to 3 days after several doses

Dosage and Administration

Generic Name	Trade Name	Route	Adult Dose	Indications
azithromycin	Z-Pak Tabs	PO	500 mg/day for 3 days	Bacterial sinusitis
azithromycin	Zithromycin	IV	500 mg as a single dose for 1–2 days; follow with oral route of 250 mg daily to complete 7 days of therapy	PID
azithromycin	Zmax	PO	10 mg/kg on day 1, followed by 5 mg/kg/day 1 time/day on days 2–5	Community-acquired pneumonia

Clinical Uses

■ As an alternative to treat mild to moderate pharyngitis/tonsillitis caused by streptococcal species.

■ Mild to moderate bacterial exacerbations of chronic bronchitis, sinusitis, otitis media, and soft tissue infections.

■ Community-acquired pneumonia believed to be caused by penicillin-sensitive *S. pneumoniae* or *H. influenzae* or any atypical pathogen (*Mycoplasm, Legionella*, or *Chlamydia* species).

■ Nongonococcal urethritis and cervicitis such as PID.

■ Bacterial exacerbations in COPD.

Adverse Reactions

CV: Chest pain, palpitations
DERM: Photosensitivity
ENDO: Hyperglycemia
GI: Pseudomembranous colitis, diarrhea, nausea, vomiting, abdominal pain
GU: Nephritis, vaginitis
MISC: Angioedema, local pain or inflammation at injection site
NEURO: Dizziness, drowsiness, fatigue headache

Interactions

■ Aluminum- and magnesium-containing antacids decrease peak serum levels.

■ Digoxin, theophylline, and phenytoin triazolam increase serum levels.

Contraindications

■ Known sensitivities
■ Pregnancy or breastfeeding
■ Liver impairment

Erythromycin (E-Mycin), Clarithromycin (Biaxin, Biaxin XL)

Erythromycin has a long history of being the alternative drug to tetracycline, especially when an antibiotic is needed to treat chlamydial infections. However, the drug is far from ideal because its absorption in oral doses is somewhat erratic, and its ability to cause GI upset is frequent and is often the source of noncompliance. Unlike tetracycline, erythromycin does not discolor teeth or bind to bone, a factor favoring its use in young people in whom it is commonly used to treat acne.

Mechanism of Action

Macrolide antibiotics may be bacteriostatic or bactericidal depending on the concentration of the drug, target organism and its susceptibility, growth rate, and size of the inoculum. Macrolides do not bind to the 50S mammalian ribosome, but do so in bacteria, and interfere with the elongation of a peptide chain.

Pharmacokinetics

■ Absorption: Well absorbed orally and intramuscularly; minimal absorption topically and vaginally
■ Distribution: Wide distribution does cross placenta and breast milk as 90% protein bound
■ Metabolism: In the liver
■ Excretion: Mostly in feces by bile
■ Half-life: 1.4 to 2 hours

Dosage and Administration

Generic Name	Trade Name	Route	Adult Dose	Indications
erythromycin	Erythrocin, E-Mycin, Ilosone	PO	250 mg every 6 hr or 500 mg every 12 hr	Upper and lower respiratory infections, skin infections, acne, PID, syphilis,* Legionnaire's disease (use when penicillin is appropriate, but hypersensitivity reactions prohibit use of penicillin)
clarithromycin	Biaxin	PO	250–500 mg 2 times/day for 10 days	As above, but has use in cocktail regimen for gastric ulcer or Helobacter pylori. Bronchitis, pneumonia, endocarditis, streptococcal pharyngitis

*Data to support the use of penicillin alternatives in the treatment of early syphilis are limited. However, several therapies might be effective in nonpregnant, penicillin-allergic patients who have primary or secondary syphilis. For example, doxycycline 100 mg PO twice daily for 14 days and tetracycline (500 mg PO four times a day) are regimens that have been used for many years. Because tetracycline causes many patients to experience GI upset, patient compliance with doxycycline is usually better. Other alternatives to PCN are ceftriaxone (1 gm daily IM or IV for 14 days), which is also effective for treating early syphilis. Another choice for early syphilis is azithromycin (a single 2-gm oral dose); however, treatment failures are being documented, and thus it should only be used if treatment with PCN or doxycycline has failed (CDC, 2010). Additionally, erythromycin, azithromycin, or any other nonpenicillin treatment during pregnancy is unlikely to reliably cure an infection in the fetus (Pickering et al., 2006).

Clinical Uses

■ Legionnaire's disease
■ Diphtheria
■ Management of late and early syphilis

■ Atypical pneumonias, such as legionella, mycoplasma, and chlamydia pneumonia
■ Topical dosage forms: Acne vulgaris

Adverse Reactions

■ EENT: Hearing loss (reversible)
■ GI: Disabling nausea, vomiting, diarrhea, and abdominal pain

Interactions

■ Ethanol reduces plasma erythromycin concentrations.
■ If coadministered with penicillin, the activity of penicillin is diminished.
■ The list of drug interactions between erythromycin and a number of drugs is long and requires a thorough review of all patient medications.

Contraindications

■ Any patient having a history of hepatic disease or a history of sensitivity to macrolides

Conscientious Considerations

■ Often used as an alternative for penicillin in patients allergic to it.
■ Topical dosage forms are used to treat acne vulgaris because it can eradicate *Propionibacterium acnes*, the anaerobic bacteria in pilosebaceous glands that secrete a variety of enzymes capable of disrupting follicular epithelium and causing inflammation.

Clindamycin (Cleocin, Cleocin T, Clinda-Derm, Clindets)

Clindamycin is of the class of antibiotics known as lincosamides, even though it is considered a member of the macrolide family. It is used to treat serious infections, especially anaerobes and some protozoa. Its popular use today is based on the fact it can be used to treat conditions ranging from acne to MRSA. Its most serious side effect is the ability to cause *Clostridium difficile* (*C. difficile*) diarrhea, a precursor to pseudomembranous colitis.

Mechanism of Action

Clindamycin is an anti-infective that can be either bacteriostatic or bactericidal, depending on susceptibility and concentration, thus its spectrum is similar to erythromycin. It inhibits protein synthesis in susceptible bacteria at the level of the 50S ribosome.

Pharmacokinetics

■ Absorption: Well absorbed following oral/intramuscular administration; minimal absorption through topical/vaginal use
■ Distribution: Widely distributed; does *not* cross blood-brain barrier, but does cross placenta and enters breast milk; 90% protein bound
■ Metabolism: Mostly metabolized by the liver to active metabolites
■ Excretion: Primarily in the urine
■ Half-life: 2 to 3 hours; increased in patients with impaired renal function and infants

Dosage and Administration

Generic Name	Trade Name	Route	Adult Dose	Indications
clindamycin	Clinda-Derm Cleocin T	IM, IV, vaginal or topical	1 applicator full of 2% gel at bedtime for 3–7 days, or use 100-mg suppositories, 300–600 mg every 6 hr	Topical creams and solutions: severe acne and bacterial vaginosis IV/IM: Septicemia, intra-abdominal infections, gynecological infections, osteomyelitis, endocarditis prophylaxis, empyema of lung, and skin and skin structure infections, especially MRSA.
clindamycin	Clindets	PO	150–300 mg every 6 hr 1,200–1,800 mg/day	Oral tablets: Treatment of most infections, including *Pneumocystis jiroveci* (previously called *Pneumocystis carinii*

Clinical Use

■ Used to treat most infections with gram-positive *Staphylococcus* and *S. pneumoniae*

Adverse Reactions

GI: Nausea, vomiting, abdominal pain; disabling diarrhea, and pseudomembranous colitis.
HEM: Cytopenia
MISC: Skin rashes, urticaria, angioedema

Interactions

■ Kaolin/pectin preparations decrease absorption of clindamycin.

Contraindications

■ Hypersensitivities
■ Previous pseudomembranous colitis
■ Severe liver impairment
■ Diarrhea
■ Known alcohol intolerance
■ Pregnancy or lactation

Conscientious Considerations

■ Because of its high incidence of diarrhea and its potential to cause pseudomembranous colitis, clindamycin use should be limited to infections in which it is clearly superior to other agents.
■ There is strong unlabeled support for using clindamycin to treat *P. jiroveci* pneumonia when trimethoprim/sulfamethoxazole is contraindicated.
■ These agents have major drug interactions caused by inhibition of the cytochrome P450 system.

Lincomycin (Lincocin)

Lincomycin (Lincocin) is an antibiotic that is rarely used today because of its adverse effects and toxicity. Thus, it is largely reserved for the patient who is allergic to penicillin or for the patient in whom bacterial resistance has developed. Although similar in structure, spectrum, and mechanism of action to the macrolides, lincomycin is effective against *Actinomycetes, Mycoplasma,* and *Plasmodium* bacteria. It is administered by intramuscular injection or intravenous infusion over 2 hours, where it has a biological half-life of 5 to 6 hours but yields therapeutic levels for up to 14 hours per dose. Adults with serious infections typically receive 600 mg (2 mL) intramuscularly every 24 hours, and if the infection is more severe, the same dose is given every 12 hours. When an infection is severe or life threatening, clinicians have given intramuscular injections of up to as much as 8,000 mg/day.

SPOTLIGHT ON LOWER RESPIRATORY TRACT INFECTIONS (LRTI)

Lower respiratory infections are infections in the respiratory tract below the level of the vocal cords or voice box. Many of the LRTIs involve the lower alveolar sacs, and when they do, the resultant disease is called pneumonia. There are several other lower respiratory infections involving the air conduits such as trachelitis, bronchitis, and bronchiolitis. In children, lower respiratory tract infections are usually caused by viruses, but in others they can be caused by bacteria such as *Mycoplasma pneumoniae, Chlamydophilia pneumoniae, and Bordetella pertussis.* Sputum cultures are notoriously unreliable, and sputum smears examined by Gram stain often show multiple organisms. Thus, noninvasive diagnostic tests are not helpful in establishing the etiology of LRTIs. The incidence of LRTIs is increasing largely because of the high numbers of immunocompromised people living in the United States, because of the expanding numbers of mutating pathogens, and possibly because of poorer air quality, all leading to higher and higher numbers of multidrug-resistant strains invading people with lower and lower resistance to fight them off. Acute bronchitis is the most common of the LRTIs and is usually diagnosed clinically (a cough that lasts 1 to 3 weeks with or without sputum production).

Pneumonia is one of the most life-threatening conditions in the immunocompromised host, and treatment requires identifying the pathogen quickly so that the right antimicrobial agent can be used. In treating the immunocompromised patient with pneumonia, it is helpful to know the common pathogens in the local area, any episodes of pneumonia treated before in that patient, and which type of immune compromise exists. These and other elements of the patient history can make the work of the infectious disease specialist less daunting.

Continued

SPOTLIGHT ON LOWER RESPIRATORY TRACT INFECTIONS (LRTI)—cont'd

Medical Management

An important factor in treating LRTI is to decide whether or not an antibiotic is needed because many LRTIs are caused by viruses. If an antibiotic is to be used, the usual indications for it are presence of purulent sputum, the age of the patient, the severity of the illness, underlying comorbidities, drugs that are already being used, history of drug reactions, and likelihood of patient adherence to the selected regimen.

In acute bronchitis, treatment is directed at controlling the cough, and routine antimicrobial use is not recommended (because the usual cause is viral). However, when the patient has underlying lung disease (such as COPD), antibiotics are used to treat common gram-positive pathogens. If influenza is suspected, antivirals may also be useful. In cases of chronic bronchitis or pneumonia in which sputum volume is increased and purulent, and when dyspnea is reported, antibiotics are appropriately warranted. Most pathogens seem to respond well to doxycycline or amoxicillin, although amoxicillin has a high failure rate against bacteria that produce beta-lactamase. Thus, many clinicians like to start with amoxicillin/potassium clavulanate, cefaclor, erythromycin (500 to1000 mg four times a day for 14 days), or azithromycin (500-mg single dose followed by 250 mg daily for 3 days).

TETRACYLINES

Tetracyclines are derived from a species of *Streptomyces* bacteria and today are synthesized and not produced by fermentation means, as is penicillin. Tetracycline antibiotics are broad-spectrum bacteriostatic agents that inhibit bacterial protein synthesis. Tetracyclines may be effective against a wide variety of microorganisms, including rickettsia and amebic parasites.

Mechanism of Action

These agents bind to the **30S ribosome unit** (Note: A ribosomal subunit carries out the process of translating genetic information encoded in messenger RNA and does so one amino acid at a time allowing for the formation of new synthesized polypeptide chains. Thus ribosomal are protein factories found in every cell of every organism of the planet. There are two ribosomes disrupted by antibiotics, the 30S unit by tetracyclines and the 50S unit disrupted by aminoglycosides) in mammalian cells, thus they are bacteriostatic to susceptible organisms. Tetracyclines have the same basic shared chemical structure (think of *tetra* and *cycle* as meaning "four rings"; thus, as in Fig. 17-2, tetracyclines have four fused six-member rings.) Because tetracyclines have a similar chemical structure, they all exhibit the same bacteriostatic mechanism of action. Once ingested, tetracyclines become concentrated in sensitive gram-negative and gram-positive bacterial cells by an energy-dependent process that occurs in bacteria but not in mammalian cells. Once inside the bacteria, these drugs depress protein synthesis blocking the attachment of aminoacyl transfer RNA to a receptor site on a messenger RNA ribosome complex. This binding of a tetracycline occurs primarily at the bacterial 30S ribosomal subunit, and this accounts for the tetracycline's ability to stunt growth of the bacteria rather than kill it.

Pharmacokinetics

- Absorption: 60% to 80% is well absorbed following oral administration.
- Distribution: Distribution varies widely, but the drugs are widely distributed. Some CSF penetration, crosses placenta, and enters breast milk.
- Metabolism: Doxycycline: some activation in intestine and by bile; minocycline: most metabolism by the liver; tetracycline: concentrated by the liver and excreted as active drug into the bile.
- Excretion: Doxycycline: 20% to 40% excreted unchanged in urine; minocycline: some unchanged in bile and liver; tetracycline: 60% excreted unchanged by kidneys and the rest unchanged in feces and in a highly active form. Because renal clearance is by glomerular filtration, the state of renal function is critical to elimination.
- Half-life: 6 to 12 hours for tetracycline; 15 to 22 hours for doxycycline and minocycline.

Dosage and Administration

Generic Name	Trade Name	Route	Adult Dose
doxycycline	Vibramycin	PO	100 mg 2 times/day
tetracycline	Achromycin V	PO	250–500 mg 4 times/day
minocycline	Minocin, Dynacin	PO	250–500 mg 4 times/day
oxytetracycline	Terramycin	PO	500 mg every 6 hr for 6 weeks concurrent with streptomycin

Clinical Uses

- Chlamydia and chancroid.
- Syphilis in penicillin-allergic patients.
- Lyme disease (doxycycline).
- Anthrax (doxycycline only).
- Inflammatory acne with papules and pustules.
- Many zoonoses (Rocky Mountain spotted fever, typhus, Q fever, and others).
- Treatment and prevention of malaria and leptospirosis (doxycycline only).
- To control oral mucosal ulcers in conjunction with steroids, both given topically.
- Tetracycline is adjunctive to proton pump inhibitor, metronidazole, and bismuth subsalicylate in treating *Helicobacter pylori* gastritis or ulcers induced by *H. pylori.*
- Treatment of infections caused by susceptible strains of gram-positive and gram-negative bacteria; treatment of *Mycoplasma pneumoniae.*
- Adjunctive treatment of acute intestinal amebiasis.
- Treatment of nongonococcal urethritis.
- Preferred monotherapy for community-acquired pneumonia includes doxycycline or a respiratory quinolone, although some prefer doxycycline and a penicillin combination.

Adverse Reactions

DERM: Photosensitivities, seen as abnormal sunburn reactions.
GI: Nausea, vomiting, GI distress, esophagitis; when given orally, hepatotoxic.
MISC: By suppressing the normal natural flora of the body, they can produce superinfections, especially in the oral, anogenital (i.e., allow *Candida* to proliferate), and intestinal areas.

Interactions

■ May increase the effect of warfarin
■ May decrease the effect of sucralfate and barbiturates

Contraindications

■ Contraindicated in children younger than 8 years of age and pregnant women (especially after 4 months gestation) because it binds to calcium and consequently stains teeth and has an effect on long bone development.

Conscientious Considerations

■ Several species of bacteria are becoming increasingly resistant to these drugs because of their overuse. Many strains of staphylococci, streptococci, and pneumococci are no longer susceptible. Ironically, MRSA does show some susceptibility, and minocycline and doxycycline are currently listed as preferred treatments for CA-MRSA. Emergence of resistant *N. gonorrhea* strains is common around the world.

■ Regular doses are used to control a variety of unusual organisms because of the broader spectrum, but they only control growth of some gram-positives and some gram-negative bacteria.
■ Calcium, magnesium, and iron products block absorption by forming insoluble compounds (chelates). As tetracyclines bind to calcium, they are retained by bones and teeth for long periods. They can damage developing teeth (softening and giving them a yellow-brown color) and delay development of long bones. Because of their effect on tooth staining and long bone development, these drugs are contraindicated in children under 8 years of age, pregnant women (especially after 4 months gestation), and breast-feeding women.

Patient/Family Education

■ Instruct patient to take medication around the clock and finish the medication.
■ Advise patient to avoid milk and other dairy products, antacids, sodium bicarbonate, or iron supplements within 1 to 3 hours of taking tetracycline.
■ If the patient is female, instruct her to use nonhormonal contraceptives.
■ Advise patient to contact clinician if signs of superinfection occur.
■ Advise patient to tell clinician of any drugs being used before surgery or before the addition of tetracyclines.

SPOTLIGHT ON COMMUNITY-ACQUIRED PNEUMONIA (CAP)

According to *The Merck Manual of Geriatrics*, community-acquired pneumonia (CAP) is the most common cause of death in the United States among the elderly, and it is the fourth leading cause of death overall (Merck Manual, 2010). CAP costs the U.S. health system about $23 billion annually, despite improved diagnostic measures and improved antibiotics to treat it. Two of the biggest clinical challenges are identifying the etiology (causative organism) and selecting appropriate treatment. Cultures of sputum are notoriously unreliable, and sputum gram stain and blood culture will yield the organism in less than half the cases.

Without knowledge of bacterial etiology, pneumonias can be categorized as community acquired versus hospital acquired (and sometimes nursing home acquired), or by mechanism of onset—aspiration pneumonia. They are also sometimes categorized according to the pattern of lung infiltration on x-rays. The treatment varies according to the age and condition of the patient, as well as the type of pneumonia, all of which signal the clinician to the most likely offending microbe. Oral flora, normally occurring bacteria found in the gingival crevices, are the pathogens usually associated with pneumonia, which is felt to be almost always due to micro- or macroaspirations. Whereas *S. pneumoniae* is the most common organism among community-acquired pneumonias, gram-negative bacilli and anaerobes are frequent pathogens seen in nosocomial (hospital or nursing home) aspiration

pneumonias. Older patients tend to have poorer oral hygiene with higher rates of gram-negative colonization; these organisms end up in the lung after aspirating oral contents, sometimes causing abscess formation.

In the elderly, pneumonia is often fatal. Aspiration pneumonia (considered macroaspiration as compared to the aerosolization of *S. pneumoniae* from the nasopharynx) is usually a consequence of any condition that impairs consciousness or interferes with swallowing, although (micro) aspiration of saliva and its flora occurs in normal individuals during sleep and is not usually associated with development of pneumonia. The aspiration of gastrointestinal secretions or contents may cause chemical damage to the alveoli or surrounding tissue (pneumonitis, as opposed to pneumonia), and many episodes of aspiration do not cause infection nor mandate antibiotics. Only when there are bacteria in the material aspirated that cannot be killed by the defense systems that normally protect hosts do individuals develop infections known as aspiration pneumonia. This commonly occurs in patients with strokes, dementias, and other neurological diseases (epilepsy, Parkinson's disease, amyotrophic lateral sclerosis), but can also occur with intoxication, during or after intubation for surgeries, and in a variety of other settings.

The conscientious clinician should realize the classic signs and symptoms of pneumonia (cough, fever, production of sputum). However, these classic signs and symptoms are often not present in

SPOTLIGHT ON COMMUNITY-ACQUIRED PNEUMONIA (CAP)—cont'd

the elderly or in those who are immunocompromised. In these cases, the presenting signs are more likely as follows:

■ Tachypnea
■ Tachycardia
■ Fever (30% to 60% with high fever)
■ Cough (foul-smelling sputum and productive cough in 60% of patients)
■ Weight loss
■ Anemia

Medical Management

Empiric antibiotics should be broad-spectrum antibiotics effective against the likely pathogen. Clinicians should take special care to counsel their patients and caregivers about compliance with and duration of therapy to help prevent relapse. Specific guidelines for the management of community-acquired pneumococcal pneumonia in outpatients come from well-respected authorities such as the Infectious Disease Society of America (IDSA), the American Thoracic Society (ATS), and the Centers for Disease Control and Prevention (CDC). Yet no matter the thoughtfulness and care that goes into creating them, the various prescribing guidelines are not always 100% in sync. For example, according to the IDSA, antibiotic choices for CAP include a macrolide or doxycycline *or* fluoroquinolone antibiotic.

As alternatives, amoxicillin and clavulanate potassium combination, cefuroxime, axetil or cefpodoxime or cefprozil can be used (Mandell et al., 2007). According to these guidelines, patients with low-risk, nonhospitalized CAP, with no cardiopulmonary disease and no modifying factors, should be treated with a macrolide (such as azithromycin or clarithromycin), with doxycycline as a second choice. The ATS believes that broader-spectrum coverage with a new antipneumococcal fluoroquinolone antibiotic such as levofloxacin, moxifloxacin, or gatifloxacin would be effective but unnecessary and could lead to the overuse of this valuable class of antibiotics, thereby contributing to the growing problem of antibiotic resistance.

According to the CDC, the antibiotic of choice for CAP is doxycycline, a macrolide, an oral beta-lactam (amoxicillin, amoxicillin/clavulanate), or a fluoroquinolone. A fourth guideline developed by the Therapeutic Working Group of the CDC, however, recommends using fluoroquinolones sparingly because of resistance concerns (Heffelfinger, 2000). The bottom line is that, when it comes to treatment of CAP on an outpatient basis, the consensus among the CDC and others is that empirical oral antibiotics with a macrolide, doxycycline, or an oral beta-lactam (amoxicillin, cefuroxime [Ceftin], or amoxicillin/clavulanate) are the choices to start with and that clinicians should be conservative with the newer antibiotics in case resistance develops.

AMINOGLYCOSIDES

The aminoglycosides (gentamicin, netilmicin, streptomycin, tobramycin, and amikacin) are all similar in their properties, but their differences allow them to be used in differing clinical situations. Aminoglycosides are a group of bactericidal drugs that are structurally related. Their name comes from the fact they contain at least one sugar—that is, a glycoside attached to one or more amino groups. These drugs are used mostly to treat gram-negative aerobic bacteria.

Mechanism of Action

By binding *irreversibly* to both the ribosomal 30S and 50S subunit of susceptible streptococci and other bacteria, they cause a misreading of the messenger RNA genetic codes in the translation that creates protein out of amino acids. Hence, they inhibit bacterial protein synthesis, resulting in a defective cell membrane that cannot sustain the bacteria.

Pharmacokinetics

■ Absorption: These drugs are very polar, that is, they are very water soluble, and thus cannot pass through the gastrointestinal membrane (less than 1% of an oral dose is absorbed). However, they are rapidly absorbed when given intramuscularly, with peak concentrations occurring in about an hour.
■ Distribution: Widely distributed throughout extracellular fluid; poor penetration into meninges.
■ Metabolism: None; 90% is excreted as unchanged drug.
■ Excretion: Aminoglycosides are eliminated by renal excretion, and if a neonate or adult has any renal impairment, dosages must be adjusted downward.
■ Half-life: 2 to 4 hours, which increases with renal impairment.

Clinical Uses

■ To treat infections caused by sensitive strains of Enterobacteriaceae (*E. coli, Klebsiella, Proteus*), and *Pseudomonas* (see p. 318, Conscientious Considerations); serious bacteremia, respiratory and urinary tract infections, infected wounds, infected bones and soft tissue, peritonitis, and burns complicated by sepsis. Serious infections with *Pseudomonas aeruginosa* may require combined therapy with ticarcillin, carbenicillin, piperacillin, or ceftazidime.

Adverse Reactions

EENT: Most unwanted effects of these drugs are dose related and many are reversible; however, watch for irreversible ototoxicity. Prolonged treatment at high doses can lead to accumulation of an aminoglycoside in the inner ear, resulting in both vestibular and cochlear disturbances that affect hearing and balance. Note this ototoxicity is enhanced when the patient is taking loop diuretics. Although becoming deaf is not life threatening, this adverse event is serious because it is *not* reversible.

GU: Nephrotoxicity can occur when these drugs accumulate in the renal tubules of the kidney, and it can develop even with recommended and conventional doses, especially if the patient is dehydrated. However, generally, the renal damage is reversible.

MISC: Hypersensitivity reactions.

MS: In hospitals, when an aminoglycoside is administered along with an anesthetic, acute neuromuscular blockade can occur, resulting in muscle paralysis, usually the result of high doses.

Dosage and Administration

Generic Name	Trade Name	Route	Dose	Indications
amikacin	Amikin	IV only	7.5 mg/kg every 12 hr or 15 mg/kg 1 time/day in a patient with normal renal function, until doses can be based on peak and trough levels. **Note:** Use ideal body weight for dosing rather than actual body weight. Individualization of dosing is critical because of low therapeutic index.	Serious gram-negative infections as *Proteus* and *Pseudomonas*
gentamicin	Gentamicin Garamycin	IM or IV Sterile eye-drops	2 mg/kg as loading dose, then 1.7 mg/kg of lean body weight every 8 hr 1 or 2 drops in affected eye(s) every 4 hr*	Bacterial infections especially *S. aureus* and *S. pneumoniae* Ophthalmic solutions for eye infections
netilmicin	Netromycin	IV	4 mg/kg as 1 time/day	Reserved for serious sepsis infections in neonates and infants
streptomycin		IM	IM administration *only* children 29–40 mg/kg/day; adults 15–30 mg/kg/day	Reserved for combination therapy in treating tuberculosis, endocarditis, plague, tularemia†
tobramycin	Tobrex	IM or IV	2 mg/kg as loading dose, then 1.7 mg/kg of lean body weight every 8 hr	Meningitis, cystic fibrosis, diverticulitis, endocarditis, PID, plague, hospital-acquired pneumonia, tularemia, UTI

*CAUTION: Rare allergic reactions have occurred, as well as bacterial and fungal ulcerations of the cornea.

†Streptomycin has a high toxicity index causing neurotoxicity, nephrotoxicity, neuromuscular blockade, and respiratory paralysis.

Interactions

■ A long list of drug interactions can occur with these drugs, most of which result in additive nephrotoxicity or ototoxicity. Thus, clinicians should take a thorough drug history. For example, these drugs exhibit an increased risk of nephrotoxicity when used with cephalosporins and loop diuretics (furosemide).

Contraindications

■ Cross-sensitivity exists among the whole family of aminoglycosides.

Conscientious Considerations

■ Aminoglycosides are poorly absorbed by mouth and are given either IM or IV. They can be given on a once-daily schedule or by multiple daily doses (every 8 to 12 hours).

■ Dose adjustments are necessary for renal impairment. Dosing is adjusted based on peak and trough serum levels, which should be monitored to avoid toxicity. Alternatively, a single daily dose of 5.1 mg/kg is appropriate if the renal function is normal (creatinine clearance greater than 80).

■ Therapy lasting 5 to 7 days can cause dose-dependent damage in proximal tubular epithelium. Because the drug also accumulates in the inner ear's cochlear and vestibular sensory cells, the patient may experience tinnitus, hearing loss, and dizziness, usually with some degree of permanence.

■ Although tobramycin and netilmicin are less nephrotoxic than gentamicin, concomitant therapy with furosemide, ethacrynic acid, or cephalosporins will increase the risk of nephrotoxicity with any of the aminoglycosides.

■ Bacterial resistance varies widely, and these drugs can be inactivated by many methods. The prevalence of inactivating enzymes varies widely by hospital, county, district, and even wards of a hospital. Therefore, it is critical that sensitivity tests be done before using these drugs, especially with gentamicin because it is the most widely used in this class.

Patient/Family Education

■ Clinicians should warn patients of serious adverse effects and then should monitor for nephrotoxicity and neurotoxicity (muscle twitching, visual issues, seizures, tingling).

■ Instruct patients to watch for signs of hypersensitivity, especially tinnitus, rash, and difficulty urinating.

■ For topical use, patients should wash area and gently pat dry before applying. Instruct the patient to apply a thin film to not apply an occlusive dressing unless the clinician so directs. The moist wound healing technique, where an occlusive gauze dressing is applied over the antibiotic, is done in cases of burns or where dehydration of the skin is to be prevented and collagen synthesis and angiogenesis are to be stimulated.

BACTERIOSTATIC ANTIBIOTICS AFFECTING FOLIC ACID METABOLISM

The Sulfonamides

Sulfamethoxazole (SMX) is a sulfonamide drug that slowly kills bacteria by inhibiting bacterial **folic acid synthesis**. Humans absorb folic acid from food, but bacteria must synthesize it. Para-aminobenzoic acid (PABA) is an essential component of folic acid, and sulfonamides are structurally similar to PABA. Thus, sulfonamides compete with PABA, preventing folic acid formation and inducing bacteriostasis.

Trimethoprim (TMP) is a competitive inhibitor of an enzyme responsible for a converting step in the last step in the production of folic acid, taking it from its inactive form to its active form.

Trimethoprim/sulfamethoxazole is a combination of these two drugs in a ratio of 1:5; that is, 1 unit trimethoprim to 5 units of sulfamethoxazole. Taken together, they are more effective in reducing folic acid formation and folic acid activation than when either is given alone. Thus, they are used to treat a variety of systemic infections caused by both gram-positive and gram-negative organisms, including upper and lower respiratory, urinary, gastrointestinal, and uncomplicated genitourinary tract infections, as well as superficial infections of the skin and soft tissues. They are also used in *P. jiroveci* (previously called *P. carinii*) infections and serious septicemias, such as meningitis. And they have found use against CA-MRSA infection.

Mechanism of Action

Unlike humans, bacteria cannot use external folic acid, a nutrient essential for cell growth. Folic acid is used to manufacture purines for incorporation into bacterial DNA. Bacteria must synthesize their folic acid from PABA, and because sulfonamides are structurally similar to PABA, they compete for a critical enzyme in the pathway of synthesizing folic acid. Should the bacteria find high concentrations of PABA, it can overcome the effectiveness of sulfonamides against it. Thus, sulfonamides have a bacteriostatic action.

Pharmacokinetics

■ Absorption: Both SMX and TMP are rapidly and well absorbed from the small intestine.
■ Distribution: Distributes well throughout the body, including the CSF. In the blood it can be found in one of three forms: unbound, protein bound (85%), or conjugated; the free (unbound) form is considered to be therapeutically active.
■ Metabolism: Mainly in the liver.
■ Excretion: Most of TMP is excreted unchanged in the urine, and 85% of the SMX is inactivated prior to renal secretion.
■ Half-life: Each is about 10 hours.

Dosage and Administration

Generic	Trade Name	Route	Adult Dose	Indications
sulfamethoxazole	Gantanol	PO	Tablets, suspension: 2–4 gm initially, then 1 gm every 8–12 hr	Treatment of acute UTI Toxoplasmosis, malaria
sulfamethoxazole/ trimethoprim	Bactrim, Septra	PO	160 mg TMP/ 800 mg SMX, 2 tabs to start, then 1 tab 4 times/day	Most adult infections
sulfamethoxazole/ trimethoprim double strength	Bactrim DS Septra DS	PO	Double strength offers good bioavailability and 2 times/ day dosing	Most adult infections
				P. jiroveci pneumonia

Clinical Uses

■ Their bacteriostatic action gives them a spectrum of activity over a wide range of gram-positive and gram-negative organisms.
■ Used in the treatment of infection with toxoplasma, *Pneumocystis jiroveci* pneumonia, Shigella enteritis, and urinary tract infections; prophylaxis of pneumocystis in HIV and immunocompromised patients.

Adverse Reactions

GI: Nausea, vomiting, and anorexia in 5% to 10% of patients.
HEM: Acute or chronic hemolytic anemias can develop within 2 to 7 days of starting therapy. Agranulocytosis and thrombocytopenia can also occur.
MISC: STEVENS-JOHNSON SYNDROME, which can cause death (see p. 331, Conscientious Considerations).

Interactions

■ Warfarin: Trimethoprim/sulfamethoxazole can increase the hypoprothrombinemia response to warfarin by inhibition of metabolism.

Contraindications

■ Patients with a known hypersensitivity to sulfonamides

Conscientious Considerations

■ STEVENS-JOHNSON SYNDROME, also known as anaphylaxis erythema multiforme, is an adverse effect that may grow into a manifestation known as toxic epidermal necrosis, which is serious. Stevens-Johnson syndrome is life-threatening; 5% to 15% of cases result in death because a person's skin literally falls off. This is an immune complex hypersensitivity that presents first as a rash and moves to serious skin peeling in which the epidermis separates from the dermis. Because it is a hypersensitivity, early withdrawal of the offending agent and supportive/symptomatic treatment are all that can be done. In the United States, about 300 cases per year are reported.
■ Be cautious in patients who may be folate deficient, for example, the elderly, alcoholics, or malnourished individuals, and those with malabsorptive syndromes.
■ Beware of use in those with glucose-6-phosphate dehydrogenase (G-6-PD) deficiency. G-6-PD deficiency is a common genetic condition in which abnormal X chromosomes in genes cause red blood cells to prematurely die at a rate faster than the body can replace them. This results in hemolytic anemia and is triggered by bacteria or viruses. It most commonly affects people of African American, Asian, and Mediterranean heritage. Treatment is usually discontinuing the offending drug and/or blood transfusions.
■ Hypersensitivity reactions can occur 10 to 12 days *after* initiation of therapy or within hours, if previously exposed. Thus, assess patient for sulfonamide sensitivity.

Patient/Family Education

■ Advise the patient to notify his/her clinician if skin rash, sore throat, fever, unusual bleeding, or mouth sores occur.

■ Until patients know how they will respond to this medication, they should avoid driving.

■ Advise patients to stick to the prescribed regimen and to take the tablets until finished.

■ Instruct patients to drink fluids liberally to help prevent crystalluria as a result of the sulfamethoxazole in Bactrim.

SPOTLIGHT ON GRAM-NEGATIVE BACTERIAL INFECTIONS

Infections caused by gram-negative bacilli (*Salmonella, Shigella, Escherichia, Klebsiella, Enterobacter, Proteus,* and others) often result in watery or bloody diarrhea, pus-filled abscesses, and/or other signs of bacteremia. A common pathogen is *E. coli.* It is an opportunistic microbe causing disease in patients with compromised host defenses, likely due to other comorbidities (cancer, diabetes, cirrhosis) or treatment with corticosteroids, radiation, antineoplastics, or antibiotics.

Medical Management

Gram-negative bacterial treatment may be started empirically, but it should always be modified by the results of antibiotic culture and sensitivity testing. An acute, uncomplicated infection of the lower urinary tract (cystitis or urethritis) in females can be treated with the trimethoprim/sulfamethoxazole (TMP/SMX) combinations (Bactrim, Spectra). Three days of therapy is quite successful without having to collect cultures, even though 15% to 20% of *E. coli* is now resistant to the TMP/SMX (Litwin & Saigal, 2007).

Among U.S. women, about 11% experience one UTI per year (Foster, 2008). In men with urinary tract infection, or in either sex with an upper urinary tract infection (or pyelonephritis), empirical therapy frequently calls for a fluoroquinolone until cultures and sensitivities are reported, after which antibiotics can be adjusted against specific organisms. In upper urinary tract infections, antibiotics are usually given for 10 to 14 days, because shorter courses are associated with frequent relapses.

Beta-lactams are less effective on cases of gram-negative infections as they are associated with frequent resistance and show higher recurrence rates. First- and second-generation cephalosporins are fairly effective against *E. coli, P. mirabilis,* and *K. pneumoniae,* but have less activity against other gram-negative nosocomial infections. These are often infections for which the third-generation antibiotics can help. If the organism is resistant to a cephalosporin, it will likely respond to one of the aminoglycosides (gentamicin, tobramycin, amikacin).

If the gram-negative organism is *P. aeruginosa,* it will likely respond to ticarcillin, ceftazidime, aztreonam, and piperacillin. Gram-negative aerobic bacteria cause most UTIs, 95% of which are the result of bacteria ascending from a colonized vagina or urethra. Eighty percent of the bacteria in a UTI are *E. coli.* Many strains are susceptible to ampicillin and tetracyclines, but there is increasing use of ticarcillin, piperacillin, cephalosporin, and fluoroquinolone (National Guidelines, 2008). In fact the federal government has specific guidelines for the medical management of UTIs and distinguishes between upper UTI, lower UTI, and UTI in women who are pregnant. These comprehensive guidelines also recommend the use of cranberry products as a means of preventing recurrent UTIs.

FLUROQUINOLONES AND QUINOLONES

Drugs such as ciprofloxacin (Cipro), norfloxacin (Noroxin), and levofloxacin (Levaquin) were introduced as broad-spectrum antibiotics to be active against a wide variety of both gram-positive and gram-negative organisms in cases in which resistance to penicillins, cephalosporins, and aminoglycosides is evident. However, over time, fluoroquinolone-resistant strains are appearing. These agents are synthetically produced broad-spectrum antibiotics with a chemical structure similar to nalidixic acid. A "fluorine" chemical moiety and a piperazine group added to the structure of nalidixic acid resulted in a greatly enhanced antibiotic with greater potency and broader spectrum.

Mechanism of Action

Fluoroquinolones inhibit DNA synthesis by specific action on the enzyme responsible for the unwinding and supercoiling of bacterial DNA before its replication. They are synthetic antibiotics and are not derived from bacteria. The older quinolones are not well absorbed and are used to treat mostly urinary tract infections. The newer fluoroquinolones are broad-spectrum bacteriocidal drugs that are chemically unrelated to the penicillins or the cephalosporins. Because of their excellent absorption, fluoroquinolones can be administered not only intravenously, but orally as well.

Pharmacokinetics

■ Absorption: All are rapidly, but variably, absorbed following oral administration.

■ Distribution: All appear to distribute widely in body and body fluids, such as blister fluid, pus, saliva, lung, liver, and kidney.

■ Metabolism: Variable among the quinolones, 5% to 15% have changed to active metabolites found in the urine.

■ Excretion: Mostly unchanged and by the kidney (all can be recovered in the urine), and dosages must be adjusted for renal failure. The exception is moxifloxacin (Avelox), which is metabolized predominantly in the liver and should not be used in liver failure.

Clinical Uses

■ Fluoroquinolones are effective against most aerobic gram-positive bacteria such as *H. influenzae, Haemophilus ducreyi,* and some gram-negative cocci such as *N. meningitidis, Neisseria gonorrhoeae,* and *M. catarrhal.*

■ Gemifloxacin, levofloxacin, and moxifloxacin are considered respiratory quinolones; they all have good activity against penicillin-resistant strains of strep pneumonia and are useful in treating severe pneumonia, especially if the patient has been on other antibiotics in the previous 3 months. Levofloxacin and moxifloxacin are also frequently used as alternatives to ciprofloxacin for infections below the diaphragm.

■ Ciprofloxacin is used widely to treat patients with enteric infections (bacterial enteritis and diverticulitis), urinary tract infections (including prostatitis), and bone and joint infections.

Dosage and Administration

Generic	Trade Name	Route	Dosage	Indications
ciprofloxacin	Cipro	PO and IV	500 mg every 12 hr for 60 days 250 mg 2 times/day for 3 days 500–700 mg every 12 hr 250-mg single dose	Inhalation anthrax Uncompli-cated UTI Most infections Gonorrhea
gatifloxacin	Tequin	Ophthalmic drops	1 drop in affected eye every 2 hr while awake for 2 days, then 1 drop 4 times/day for next 5 days	0.3% ophthalmic solution for bacterial conjunctivi-tis
		PO, IV	400 mg daily for 7–14 days PO or IV: 400 mg every 24 for 7–10 days	community-acquired pneumonia (CAP)
gemifloxacin	Factive	PO	320 mg once a day for 7 days	CAP caused by multi-drug-resistant strains of *S. pneumonia*
levofloxacin	Levaquin	PO and IV	500 mg every 24 hr for 7 days 500 mg ever 24 hr for 28 days	Chronic bronchitis, diverticuli-tis, prostatitis
moxifloxacin	Avelox	PO and IV	400 mg every 24 hr for 10 days	Sinusitis, bronchitis, skin infections, abdominal infections
ofloxacin	Floxin Ocuflox	Ophthalmic drops Otic drops	Instill 5 drops in affected ear/eye 2 times/day for 10 days	Acute otitis media in <12 with tubes
		PO	400 mg every 12 hr for 10 days	Sinusitis, pro-statitis, PID, cervical gonorrhea, bronchitis

■ Oxyfloxacin, norfloxacin, gatifloxacin, and ciprofloxacin have U.S. Food and Drug (FDA) approval for treatment of uncomplicated gonorrhea; resistant strains are now present worldwide, and a minimum of 7 days of therapy is recommended by the CDC.

Adverse Reactions

CV: QT interval may be prolonged with any fluoroquinolone, and major risk is use of fluoroquinolones with concomitant drugs that prolong QT.

DERM: Photosensitivities (rare).

GI: Nausea, vomiting, abdominal pain, dyspepsia, flatulence, diarrhea, stomatitis.

MS: Pain and inflammation in tendons, with Achilles tendon rupture increased in frequency in those over age 60.

NEURO: Effects may include drowsiness, weakness, insomnia, agitation, confusion.

Interactions

■ The plasma concentrations of theophylline, warfarin, and cyclosporine are all increased by ciprofloxacin and norfloxacin through inhibition of hepatic metabolism.

■ Avoid concomitant drugs with a potential to prolong QT, because mixture could potentially trigger lethal arrhythmia.

Contraindications

■ Hypersensitivity to any drug in this class

Conscientious Considerations

■ Ciprofloxacin (Cipro) gained attention for treating urinary tract infections in nursing home patients, and clinicians should reserve its use for complicated UTI or until pathogen is confirmed.

■ Most recently used as the drug of choice for bioterrorism anthrax.

■ The incidence of unwanted side effects is low, adding to their popularity. However, no fluoroquinolone is approved for use in children younger than 16 years of age based on studies showing joint cartilage injury in immature animals.

Patient/Family Education

■ Patients should be instructed to drink fluids liberally to help prevent crystalluria.

■ Patient should understand the significance of being adherent to the regimen of these drugs.

■ Quinolones may be taken with or without meals, but they should be taken at least 2 to 6 hours before or after taking any agent that is able to chelate them, such as iron salts, multivitamins with zinc, antacids with Mg, CA, Al salts, or sucralfate, because the chelation would prevent their absorption from the GI tract.

■ Patients should discontinue treatment and inform clinician if pain, inflammation, or tendonitis occur.

SPECIAL USE ANTIBIOTICS

Many consider *antibiotics* to mean the same as *antibacterial*, but such is not the case because the human body is often invaded with anaerobes, protozoa, and other organisms. Thus, a host of drugs cross classes. These drugs are effective in both parasitic and bacterial diseases.

Metronidazole (Flagyl, Metro21, Trikacide)

Metronidazole is a special antibiotic that crosses classes. It is used as a systemic and topical antibiotic (effective in some skin disorders and as an intravaginal drug for bacterial vaginosis), and it is also useful because of its activity against anaerobic bacteria (bactericide) as well as having direct trichomonacidal and amebicidal, activity. It provides good effectiveness against intestinal protozoa (*Trichomonas, Amoeba, Giardia*). Two agents similar to metronidazole have been introduced in the past 10 years: nitazoxanide (Alinia) and tinidazole (Tindamax). Both are used for the treatment of the same conditions as metronidazole.

Mechanism of Action

■ Metronidazole (as well as nitazoxanide and tinidazole) is ta nitroimidazole chemical that interferes with the pyruvate ferredoxin reductase, an enzyme in the bacteria's electron transfer system, which is essential for its production of energy. Thus, the susceptible organism accumulates metabolites that disrupt its DNA and protein synthesis.

Pharmacokinetics

■ Absorption: 80% absorbed after oral administration. Minimal absorption after cream or gel is used on skin or vagina.
■ Distribution: Widely distributed in most tissues, including CSF. Crosses the placenta and enters fetus; will appear in breast milk in the same concentration as plasma serum levels.
■ Metabolism: Partially metabolized in the liver.
■ Excretion: Partially excreted unchanged in urine; metabolites excreted in feces.
■ Half-life: For adults, 6 to 12 hours for metronidazole.

Dosage and Administration

Generic Name	Trade Name	Route	Adult Dose	Indications
metronidazole	Flagyl	PO or IV	250–750 mg every 8–12 hr for 5–10 days*	Anaerobic infections
metronidazole	Flagyl creams and gels Metro-Cream, MetroGel	Vaginal	One applicator full (0.75%) 2 times/day for 5 days	Bacterial vaginosis

Patients with decompensated liver disease need dosage reductions.

Clinical Uses

■ Metronidazole is most notable for its action against anaerobic bacteria and some protozoa.
■ Used for treatment of infections such as intra-abdominal infections, gynecological infections, lower respiratory infections, bone and joint infections, septicemia, endocarditis.
■ Used as a prophylactic agent in colorectal surgery, especially because of its excellent tissue penetration into abscesses, cavities, bones, and CNS.
■ Intestinal parasite Giardia.
■ Vaginitis caused by *Trichomonas* or bacterial vaginosis.
■ Management of amebic dysentery, trichomoniasis; used as a component of the treatment of peptic ulcer disease caused by *H. pylori*.

■ Treatment of intra-abdominal abscesses (in combination with another antibiotic).
■ Treatment of pseudomembranous colitis (*C. Difficile colitis*).
■ Topical cream is used for treatment of acne rosacea and bacterial vaginosis.
■ Metronidazole is also useful for treating pseudomembranous colitis caused by *C. difficile* when it is an overgrowth because normal GI flora are suppressed by another drug and it is not prudent to stop the offending drug.

Adverse Reactions

EENT: Tearing.
DERM: Rashes urticaria.
GI: Nausea, abdominal pain diarrhea, dry mouth, furry tongue, unpleasant metallic taste in the mouth.
GU: Dysuria, cystitis, and a sense of pelvic pressure sometimes reported.
HEM: Leukopenia.
MISC: Superinfections, disulfiram-like reaction. Disulfiram is an alcohol antagonist drug that blocks the oxidation of alcohol during its metabolism stage. By doing so it allows aldehyde to build up in the blood stream which causes unpleasant reactions such as headache, dizziness, flushing, nausea, sweating, hyperventilation, and disorientation. Severe reactions are respiratory distress, irregular heartbeat, congestive heart failure, and death. The drug is used as part of an alcohol treatment plan so that when the patient drinks alcohol they experience the unpleasant side effects called the "disulfiram-alcohol" reaction. Because several drugs, especially metronidazole, can also induce these same side effects, they are said to cause a "disulfiram-like reaction", so patients using these drugs should stay away from alcohol use.
NEURO: Peripheral neuropathy, seizures, dizziness, headache.

Interactions

■ Cimetidine may reduce the metabolism of metronidazole.
■ Phenobarbital can increase the metabolism of metronidazole.
■ Disulfiram-like reactions occur with alcohol ingestion.

Contraindications

■ Hypersensitivities
■ First trimester of pregnancy

Conscientious Considerations

■ Patients with decompensated liver disease need dosage reductions.
■ Metronidazole should be used cautiously in patients with CNS disease because of its potential for neurotoxicity.
■ Patients should be warned about the severe alcohol intolerance reaction that can ensue if they combine metronidazole and alcohol (disulfiram-like reaction). This reaction manifests as changes in taste, flushing, throbbing headache, breathing difficulties, nausea, copious sweating and vomiting, chest pain, tachycardia, syncope, weakness, blurry vision. It varies in severity and can be fatal.

- Advise patients of a possible furry tongue and possible unpleasant metallic taste.
- Advise patients that good oral hygiene, rinsing the mouth after each oral tablet, and using sugarless gum, may help against dry mouth.
- Advise patients that dizziness and lightheadedness are common and to use caution around machinery or driving.
- Advise patients their urine may turn dark color.
- Advise patients of proper use of vaginal gel applicator and to refrain from intercourse while on this medication.
- Advise patients that the drug may be taken with food to minimize GI upset. Also tablets may be crushed if there is difficulty swallowing.

The Special Case of *Clostridium Difficile* or *"C. Diff."*

C. Difficile is a bacterium found in soil, air, water, and the large intestine (feces) and increasingly has been found in hospitals and long term care facilities (LTCF). It typically flares after use of antibiotics have suppressed normal GI flora. Recently it has become more common and more severe as resistant strains are developing. Its incidence among the elderly and hospitalized has resulted in tens of thousands of deaths per year resulting from its inflammation and perforation of the bowels, dehydration, or kidney failure. Treatment for mild cases is to stop all antibiotics, and in moderate to severe cases, to start another kind (metronidazole [Flagyl] or vancomycin). Thus clinicians should advise patients to report watery stools of as much as 10 times a day, cramping, fever, pus or blood in stool, nausea, or dehydration, or it could lead to inflamed colon (pseudomembranous colitis). Note that 1 in every 4 patients that experience C. Diff will get it again either because the original episode was not cleared sufficiently or another strain has been introduced.

Daptomycin (Cubicin)

The first in a new class of antibacterial agents, this is a cyclic lipopeptide that exhibits rapid bacteriocidal activity against a wide variety of gram-positive bacteria as well as many of the bacteria that have become resistant to vancomycin and methicillin. Its special niche as an intravenous-only drug is to treat complicated infections of the skin and skin structures, especially those that are *Staphylococcus* types, including methicillin-resistant strains.

Mechanism of Action

Daptomycin is bacteriocidal because it binds to bacterial cell membranes and causes rapid depolarization of the membrane potential, resulting in death of the bacteria.

Pharmacokinetics

- Absorption: Poorly absorbed by oral route, this product is only available for parenteral use, and direct toxicity precludes intramuscular injection.
- Distribution: Reversibly bound to albumin, 92% protein bound

- Metabolism: Not known
- Excretion: By the kidneys
- Half-life: 8 hours

Dosage and Administration

Generic Name	Trade Name	Route	Adult Dosage	Indications
daptomycin	Cubicin, 500 mg powder for reconstitution	IV	Infuse over 30 min 4 mg/kg 1 time/day for 7–14 days*	Skin and soft tissue infections

*Dosing adjustments are recommended for those with creatinine clearance less than 30 mL/min

Clinical Uses

- Treatment of complicated skin and skin structure infections
- *S. aureus* bacteremia
- Right-sided endocarditis

Adverse Reactions

GI: Pseudomembranous colitis (diarrhea, cramping, fever, bloody stools), elevated liver function tests
MISC: Injection site reactions, paresthesias
MS: Skeletal muscle effects (weakness, pain) and elevations of creatine phosphokinase may occur.

Interactions

- No clinically relevant drug interactions have been reported.
- Manufacturer recommends against statin drugs when daptomycin is being used because of the risk of myopathy.

Contraindications

- Hypersensitivities

Conscientious Considerations

- The clinician should assess for signs of possible pseudomembranous colitis as well as for signs of further infection and/or abatement during therapy.
- Because resistance to this drug can develop, the clinician should always be sure to drain any abscesses to help minimize the risk.

Patient/Family Education

- Patients should be informed of the risk of pain and/or phlebitis at the injection site.

Tigecycline (Tygacil)

This is the first member in a new class of antibiotics called the glyclines. As its name implies, it is similar to the tetracyclines in that it, too, has a four-ring structure. Bearing a very similar resemblance to the minocycline molecule, tigecycline is bacteriostatic in nature, but its molecular structure offers a wider spectrum of activity over minocycline as well as more protections against resistant bacteria.

Mechanism of Action

Categorically, this is another of the agents that inhibits bacterial protein synthesis by binding to the 30S ribosomal subunit of susceptible bacteria. However, as a new agent it is only available for intravenous infusion. It is of a chemical class called glycylcycline, so technically it is not a tetracycline. However, its glycyl side chain gives it an expanded spectrum of activity over bacteria normally susceptible to tetracycline and minocycline.

Pharmacokinetics

- Absorption: Intravenous administration gives it 100% bioavailability
- Distribution: Good penetration into gallbladder, colon, lung
- Metabolism: Very minimal metabolism
- Secretion: Primary biliary/fecal route as unchanged drug
- Half-life: 27.1 hours after one dose, 42.1 hours after multiple doses

Dosage and Administration

Generic Name	Trade Name	Route	Adult Dose	Indications
tigecycline	Tygacil	IV	Infuse through dedicated line over 30–60 min; 100 mg STAT, then 50 mg every 12 hr for 5–14 days	Complicated skin and skin structure infections, and complicated intra-abdominal infections including those caused by vancomycin-resistant enterococci (VRE) and MRSA

Clinical Uses

- Tigecycline has a broad spectrum of activity against gram-positive, gram-negative, and anaerobic bacteria, and it is bacteriostatic.
- Currently, the FDA has cleared it only for use in severe skin and soft tissue infections and complicated intra-abdominal infections having resistant pathogens, such as vancomycin-resistant enterococci (VRE) and MRSA.

Adverse Reactions

CV: Changes in heart rate, hypotension, phlebitis
DERM: pruritus, rash
GI: Nausea and vomiting, altered taste, potential for pseudomembranous colitis
NEURO: Somnolence, fever, headache, dizziness
PUL: Increased coughing

Interactions

- May decrease the effectiveness of hormonal contraceptives

Contraindications

- Age younger than 18 years.
- Pregnancy and breastfeeding.
- Because its structure is similar to tetracycline, it is contraindicated in children less than 8 years of age and pregnant women (especially after 4 months gestation) because of its binding to calcium and consequent possible tooth staining and effect on long bone development.

Conscientious Considerations

- Its use should be reserved for resistant pathogens, such as VRE, and until more experience and data are available, it is not a first-line antibiotic.

Patient/Family Education

- Giving food concomitant to intravenous administration is said to lessen nausea and vomiting.

Linezolid (Zyvox)

The first FDA drug approved in a new class of antibiotics called the oxazolidinones is linezolid (Zyvox). This agent is noted for its ability to treat nearly all gram-positive resistant bacteria, thus it is kept as the drug of choice and in reserve for treating MRSA and VRE. Reversible thrombocytopenia is its major drawback, and this may occur when treatment is given for more that 10 to 14 days.

Mechanism of Action

Linezolid binds to the 50S subunit of the ribosome and blocks the bacteria's ability to assemble transfer RNA-ribosomal complex and thus protein synthesis. It is bacteriostatic against enterococci and staphylococci and bacteriocidal against most streptococci.

Pharmacokinetics

- Absorption: Rapid and complete following oral administration
- Distribution: Readily distributes to well-perfused tissue
- Metabolism: About two-thirds is metabolized by liver
- Excretion: About 30% excreted unchanged in the kidneys
- Half-life: 4 to 6 hours

Dosage and Administration

Generic Name	Trade Name	Route	Adult Dose	Indications
linezolid	Zyvox	PO	400 mg every 12 hr for 10–14 days	Uncomplicated skin infections
			600 mg every 12 hr for 10–14 days	Nosocomial pneumonia and CAP caused by MRSA and VRE
linezolid	Zyvox IV infusion 200 mg/100 mL bag	IV	600 mg every 12 hr for 14–28 days	VRE

Clinical Use

- The intravenous and oral formulations are bacteriocidal against gram-positive bacteria such as streptococci but bacteriostatic against resistant enterococci and staphylococci.

Adverse Reactions

GI: Pseudomembranous colitis, taste alteration, vomiting, diarrhea
HEM: Thrombocytopenia, anemia, and neutropenia reported, generally reversible
MS: Lactic acidosis
NEURO: Headache, insomnia, optic and peripheral neuropathy

Interactions

■ Because linezolid is a mild monoamine oxidase inhibitor, use of dopaminergic agents, vasopressors, sympathomimetics should have doses reduced because of the inhibiting properties of linezolid.

■ Coadministration of linezolid with over-the-counter (OTC) cold remedies that contain pseudoephedrine or phenylpropanolamine should be avoided, because blood pressure (BP) can be elevated by the combination.

Contraindications

■ Hypersensitivities.

■ No safety profiles exist on use in pregnancy, lactation, or use in children.

■ Use cautiously if there is concurrent use of antiplatelet drugs.

Conscientious Considerations

■ When using this drug, the clinician should be prepared to monitor bowel status during therapy, monitor visual function if the therapy is longer than 3 months, and monitor complete blood and platelet counts.

■ Against MRSA, linezolid is as effective as vancomycin, but it should be considered as an alternate to vancomycin or in patients sensitive to vancomycin or as oral MRSA therapy when intravenous access is unavailable. Resistance to this antibiotic is also possible.

■ Use cautiously in anyone with bleeding or coagulation issues.

Patient/Family Education

■ Patients taking the oral medicine should be advised against ingesting foods high in tyramine because elevated BP may occur.

■ Patients should also be advised to talk to their clinician about any use of OTC decongestants, cold remedies, antidepressant medications, history of hypertension, or other OTC or prescribed herbal medicines being taken.

Quinupristin/Dalfopristin (Synercid)

Quinupristin and dalfopristin are the first in a new class of agents that act to form complexes with bacterial ribosomes to inhibit protein synthesis. Quinupristin and dalfopristin are two semisynthetic streptogramins that have been lyophilized into a sterile powder and placed in a vial to be reconstituted for injection. The streptogramin molecules are produced by certain strains of streptomyces and then altered in a laboratory and made into an injectable antibiotic to be used when there are life-threatening skin infections caused by VRE and MRSA and no other antibiotics have worked.

Mechanism of Action

Quinupristin inhibits the late phase of protein synthesis and dalfopristin inhibits the early phase of protein synthesis, making them both bacteriostatic. However, in many bacterial species, synergistic binding of these two molecules to the ribosome results in bactericidal activity.

Pharmacokinetics

■ Absorption: Because it is administered intravenously, it is 100% bioavailable.

■ Distribution: Unknown

■ Metabolism: Both agents are conjugated in the liver and converted to active metabolites.

■ Excretion: Parent drugs and metabolites are mostly excreted through bile and into feces.

■ Half-life: Quinupristin: 0.85 hour; dalfopristin: 0.7 hour.

Dosage and Administration

Generic Name	Trade Name	Route	Adult Dose	Indication
quinupristin/ dalfopristin	Synercid	IV	7.5 mg/KG every 8 hr for 7 days *	Vancomycin-resistant *Enterococcus faecium*

*Patients with hepatic impairment may require a dosage adjustment, in which case the dosing frequency should be reduced from 8 to 12 hours.

Clinical Use

■ Treatment of infection with antibiotic-resistant gram-positive organisms, especially VRE, MRSA, and vancomycin-resistant *Enterococcus faecium* (VREF).

Adverse Reactions

MISC: Intravenous infusion site pain and thrombophlebitis are common.

MS: Arthralgias and myalgias can cause discontinuation of therapy.

Interactions

■ The drug interaction list is long and includes delavirdine, indinavir, ritonavir, vinca alkaloids, docetaxel, paclitaxel, verapamil, diltiazem, methylprednisolone, quinidine, lidocaine, and disopyramide. Interactions usually result in an increased risk of toxicity because multiple drugs compete for the cytochrome enzyme (CYP450-3A4) system because quinupristin-dalfopristin (Synercid) significantly inhibits the cytochrome P450-3A4 enzyme system.

Contraindications

■ Hypersensitivity

Conscientious Considerations

■ Consider this new product when vancomycin cannot be tolerated.

■ Use these agents cautiously in any patient using drugs metabolized by the cytochrome P450 system, including some antihistamines, macrolide antibiotics, some fluoroquinolones, and some antimalarials.

■ Use cautiously if severe hepatic impairment is present because dosage may need reduction.

■ Use cautiously in any signs of GI disease.

■ Pregnancy, lactation, and pediatric safety have not been established.

Patient/Family Education

- Patient needs to watch for changes in stool as well as symptoms of muscle and joint aches or any anaphylaxis/hypersensitivity reaction.
- Patients need to watch for pain or discomfort at the injection/infusion site.

Implications for Special Populations

Pregnancy Implications

When prescribing for the pregnant female, clinicians should carefully consider their choice of drugs. A selected list of drugs used to treat bacterial infections along with their assigned FDA Safety Category follows.

FDA PREGNANCY SAFETY CATEGORY	DRUGS
B	penicillins, cephalosporins, clindamycin, erythromycin, sulfonamides, quinupristin /dalfopristin, daptomycin, metronidazole
C	quinolones: ciprofloxacin, gatifloxacin, levofloxacin, moxifloxacin, norfloxacin, ofloxacin, linezolid, macrolides: clarithromycin, azithromycin
D	aminoglycosides: gentamicin, etc.; tetracyclines, tigecycline

Pediatric Implications

Pediatric antibiotics are usually reconstituted suspensions and have expiration dates of 10 to 14 days.

Many children do not take the full course of treatment even though it is the parent's role to supervise the regimen. Discontinuation of oral antibiotics occurs in the pediatric population occurs because the parent or guardian judges the infection to be cured; the child refuses to take the drug; and the side effects appear, especially diarrhea.

Geriatric Implications

Because of declining renal function in the elderly, antibiotic dosing should be based on lean body weight and calculated creatinine clearance. Note that estimates of renal function are less accurate as patients age.

Total absorption of antibiotics is not affected by aging unless it has been blunted by atrophy of the GI mucosa and decreases in blood supply.

The elderly will always consider their cost to acquire an antibiotic, any discomfort, side effects, potential treatment success (life sustaining vs. life prolongation), and their health beliefs because these affect their decision to be adherent or not.

LEARNING EXERCISES

Case 1

MG is a 29-year-old female who calls her clinician to complain she has had painful urination over the past few days that comes with great urgency to void. Although her history indicates that in the past 2 years she has had a urinary tract infection on four occasions, this one seems the worst of them. MG is otherwise healthy. She exercises regularly, is sexually active with a new boyfriend, and uses oral contraceptives. She reports she does not feel that she has an infection because she has no fever, sweats or chills, discharge from the vagina, nor does she have a headache or flank pain.

1. How would you approach this case?

2. What would be a good antibiotic for MG?

Case 2

JD brings her six-year-old son to your Family Medicine Clinic. She tells you her child has a runny nose. She thinks he is running a temperature, and he is refusing to eat. She adds further, "His runny nose is something he just picked up from his older brother, and what he needs is an antibiotic." Upon examination you note: Temperature is 102.2°F, clear lungs, copious nasal discharge, eardrums red but mobile, no retractions in the chest, no appearance of dehydration. Although you tell the mother you believe the child has a virus, and a virus needs to clear up on its own, the mother then replies, "I believe an antibiotic would be best for my child, and I insist on it."

1. How would you handle this situation?

References

Arnold, F. W., LaJoie, A. S., Brock, G. N., Peyrani, P., Rello, J. Menéndez, R. et. al. (2009). Improving outcomes in elderly patients with community-acquired pneumonia by adhering to national guidelines: Community-acquired pneumonia organization international cohort study results. *Archives of Internal Medicine, 169*(16), 1515–1524.

Barrett, F. F., McGehee, F. F., & Finland, M. (1968). Methicillin-Resistant *Staphylococcus aureus* at Boston City Hospital. Bacteriologic and epidemiologic observations. *New England Journal of Medicine, 279*, 441–448.

Centers for Disease Control and Prevention. (n.d.). Prevention of MRSA infections. Retrieved February 12, 2013, from www.cdc.gov/mrsa/prevent/index.html

Centers for Disease Control and Prevention. (2011a). Antibiotic/antimicrobial resistance. Updated May 5, 2011. Retrieved February 12, 2013, from www.cdc.gov/drugresistance/index.html

Centers for Disease Control and Prevention. (2011b). Get smart: know when antibiotics work. Updated April 4, 2011. Retrieved February 12, 2013, from www.cdc.gov/getsmart/index.html

Centers for Disease Control and Prevention. (2010). Sexually transmitted diseases: treatment guidelines. *Morbidity and Mortality Weekly*

Report, 59, no. RR5912. Retrieved February 13, 2013, from www.cdc.gov/std/treatment/2010/STD-Treatment-2010-RR5912.pdf

Foster, R. T. (2008). Uncomplicated urinary tract infections in women. *Obstetrics and Gynecology Clinics of North America, 35*(2), 235–248.

Heffelfinger, J. D., Dowell, S. F., Jorgensen, J. H., Klugman, K. P., Mabry, L. R., Musher, D. M., et al. (2000). Management of community-acquired pneumonia in the era of pneumococcal resistance: a report from the Drug-Resistant *Streptococcus pneumoniae* Working Group. *Archives of Internal Medicine, 160*, 1399–1408.

Jevons, M. (1961). "Celbenin"-resistant staphylococci. *British Medical Journal, 1*, 124–125.

Kronman, M. P., Hersh, A. L., Feng, R., Huang, Y. S., Lee, G. E., & Shah, S. S. (2011). Ambulatory visit rates and antibiotic prescribing for children with pneumonia: 1994–2007. *Pediatrics, 3*(127), 411–418.

Levine, M. (2010). Understanding MRSA infections: the basics. Retrieved February 14, 2013, from www.webmd.com/skin-problems-and-treatments/understanding-mrsa-methicillin-resistant-staphylococcus-aureus

Litwin, M. S., Saigal, C. S., editors. (2007). *Urologic diseases in America*. U.S. Department of Health and Human Services, Public Health Service, National Institutes of Health, National Institute of Diabetes and Digestive and Kidney Diseases. Washington, DC: US Government Printing Office, NIH Publication No. 07-5512.

Madhi, S. A., Klugman, K. P. (2006). Acute Respiratory Infections: National Library of Medicine Bookshelf, Chapter 11. Available at www.ncbi.nlm.nih.gov/books/NBK2283

Mandell, L. A., Wunderink, R. G., Anzueto, A., Bartlett, J. G., Campbell, G. D., Dean, N. C., et al. (2007). Infectious Diseases Society of America/American Thoracic Society consensus guidelines on the management of community-acquired pneumonia in adults. *Clinical Infectious Diseases, 44*(suppl), S27–S72.

Merck Manuals Online Medical Library, a publication of Merck, Sharpe, & Dohme. (2010). Retrieved from www.merckmanuals.com/professional/sec23.html?WT.z_section=Geriatrics

National Guideline Clearing House of the Agency for Healthcare Research and Quality (AHRQ). (2008). Management of suspected bacterial urinary tract infections in adults: a national clinical guideline. Retrieved February 25, 2013, from www.guideline.gov/content.aspx?id=34098&search=bacterial+urinary+tract+infections+adults

Pickering, L. K., Baker, C. J., Long S. S., et al. (2006). *Red book: report of the Committee on Infectious Diseases* (27th ed., pp. 640–641). Elk Grove Village, IL: American Academy of Pediatrics.

VacZine Analytics. (2008). Disease Info Pak, Community Acquired MRSA: May 2008. Retrieved February 13, 2013, from www.vaczine-analytics.com/VADIP003_TOC.pdf

chapter 18

Drugs Used in the Treatment of Nonbacterial Infections

W.P. Roche III, William N. Tindall, Mona M. Sedrak

Key Terms

Acquired immunodeficiency syndrome (AIDS)

Ergosterol

Genome

Nucleoside reverse transcriptase inhibitors

Nonnucleoside reverse transcriptase inhibitors

Helminths

Human immunodeficiency syndrome (HIV)

Highly active antiretroviral therapy (HAART)

Opportunistic infections

Protease inhibitors

Retrovirus

Stevens-Johnson syndrome

CHAPTER FOCUS

This chapter focuses on drugs used to treat infections caused by viruses, fungi, and other nonbacterial microbes. It introduces the student to anti-infective medications that are different from those considered typical antibiotics, although many of the same basic principles of using typical antibiotics apply to antiviral, antifungal, and antiparasitic therapies. This chapter discusses how appropriate drug choices can be made by weighing the risks and the benefits of these drugs to a hosting individual and how to provide these individuals with special education about their medicines. This chapter spotlights drugs for some of the simplest of viral infections, such as influenza and herpes, to drugs for the most devastating viral infection, human immunodeficiency virus (HIV) and its sequel, acquired immunodeficiency syndrome (AIDS). In addition, drugs used for fungal infections and against other microbes such as protozoa and helminths are discussed.

OBJECTIVES

After reading and studying this chapter, the student should be able to:

1. Recognize and understand the different types of targets for chemotherapeutic drugs for nonbacterial infections and how their mechanisms of action relate to selective toxicity.

2. Recall the pharmacokinetics and mechanisms of action of the nonbacterial therapeutic drugs.

3. Describe what highly activated antiretroviral therapy (HAART) is and recall the pharmacology of the antiretroviral drugs that make up its regimens.

4. Describe the pharmacology of the drugs used to treat herpes.

5. Compare and contrast the antifungal medications, whether sold by prescription or over the counter.

6. List the clinical uses and adverse effects associated with metronidazole.

7. Describe the pharmacology of drugs used in the United States to fight intestinal and extra-intestinal parasites such as the helminths, known as ascaris, pinworm, hookworm, and tapeworm.

KEY DRUGS IN THIS CHAPTER

Antivirals for Treating HIV-AIDS

Nucleoside Reverse Transcriptase Inhibitors (NRTIs)
abacavir (Ziagen)
didanosine (Videx, formerly ddI)
emtricitabine (Emtriva)
lamivudine (Epivir, formerly 3TC)

stavudine (Zerit, formerly d4T)
zalcitabine (Hivid, formerly ddC)
zidovudine (Retrovir, formerly AZT)
zidovudine + lamivudine (Combivir)
zidovudine + lamivudine + abacavir (Trizivir)

Protease Inhibitors (PI)
amprenavir (Agenerase)

atazaniavir (Reyataz)
fosamprenavir (Lexiva)
indinavir (Crixivan)
nelfinavir (Viracept)
ritonavir (Norvir)
saquinavir (Fortavase, Invirase)

continued

338

KEY DRUGS IN THIS CHAPTER—cont'd

Nonnucleoside Reverse Transcriptase Inhibitors (NNRTIs)
delavirdine (Rescriptor)
efavirenz (Sustiva)
nevirapine (Viramune)

Antivirals for Treating Viral Herpes
valacyclovir (Valtrex)
acyclovir (Zovirax; ACV)
famciclovir (Famvir)
ganciclovir (Cytovene)
ribavirin (Virazole)
trifluridine (Viroptic)

Antivirals for Treating Viral Influenza
amantadine (Symmetrel)
rimantadine (Flumadine)
zanamivir (Relenza)
oseltamivir (Tamiflu)

Antifungals
amphotericin B (Fungizone)
nystatin (Mycostatin, Nilstat)
miconazole (Monistat, Micatin)
fluconazole (Diflucan)
econazole (Spectazole)
ketoconazole (Nizoral)
clotrimazole (Gyne-Lotrimin, Mycelex)
flucytosine (Ancobon)
griseofulvin (Fulvicin, Grifulvin)
terbinafine (Lamisil)
tolnaftate (Aftate, Dr. Scholl's Athlete's Foot Cream, Quinsana, Tinactin)

Antiprotozoals
metronidazole (Flagyl, Protostat)

Antimalarials
chloroquine (Aralen)
mefloquine (Lariam)

primaquine (generic and Malirid)
pyrimethamine with sulfadoxine (Fansidar)

Antimycobacterials
isoniazid (Nydrazid, Laniazid)
ethambutol (Myambutol)
rifampin (Rifamate)
cycloserine (CycloSERINE, Seromycin)
ethionamide (Trecator)
capreomycin (Caprocin)

Antihelminthics
Treatment of Intestinal Nematodes
mebendazole (Vermox)
albendazole (Zentel)
thiabendazole (Mintezol)
pyrantel pamoate (Antiminth)
Treatment of Systemic Nematodes
ivermectin (Eqvalan, Ivomec)

The extensive and worldwide use of antibiotics for the treatment of bacterial infections has led to the emergence of many superinfections of viral and fungal etiology, especially in patients who are immunocompromised, have HIV-AIDS, or who are in need of transplant or neoplastic therapy. The number of antiviral and antifungal medications available today is the result of much research by scientists into the genetic and molecular functioning of small organisms. By better understanding the structure of viruses, fungi, yeasts, and other nonbacterial infestations (i.e., protozoa, helminthes, etc.), researchers have been able to find much more effective and specific medications during a time when the world added pressure to those doing research because of the human immunodeficiency virus (HIV) that resulted in the worldwide AIDS pandemic. For example, designing any safe and effective antiviral was difficult because of the rapid mutations that led to drug resistance. However, most antivirals today are able to deal with HIV viruses, herpes viruses, hepatitis B and C viruses, and influenza A and B viruses. Additionally, the increase in global travel has led to people acquiring parasitic diseases more readily than ever before. Thus, clinicians are likely to encounter varying infections and infestations that require a very specific drug to eradicate them, yet they remain challenged to use drugs that do no harm to the patient.

Viruses are among the simplest of living organisms, but only recently has their full genetic sequence been known in detail so that the mystery of how they reproduce could be unraveled. Viruses are composed of a **genome** (one or more strands of either DNA or RNA) and a few enzymes, which may be stored in a capsule made of protein (capsid). The protein capsule is sometimes covered with a light layer of lipid material (called an envelope). However, a mature virus differs from a bacteria in that it has no definitive cell wall to help it survive and so it must penetrate through the cell wall of a host to survive and replicate. A virus can remain outside of its host cell for a long time and still retain its infective properties; however, to reproduce, it must enter a host cell and take over that cell's protein and nucleic acid synthesis and thwart it so that it can direct the host cell to make new viral particles or copies of itself. In essence, viruses are intracellular parasites living off the host cell's biochemical mechanisms, and as parasites, they have a life cycle that allows researchers to target drugs to stop one or more of the following steps in the replication process:

1. Attachment of the virus to the host cell
2. Release of the virus's genes into the host cell
3. Replication and assembly of new viral components
4. Release of viral components into a new host cell

To the clinician, it becomes important to find a drug that inhibits virus replication but does not harm the host. Because current antiviral agents only affect viral replication, this also implies that in cases of viral infections, the host's immune response system must be working in order to cure the infection. Similarly, this approach to therapeutics is also true when certain human infections are caused by fungi. Because these infections can be caused by any one of 50 known but different simple fungi, agents such as griseofulvin, the azoles, and terbinafine exert their activity by disrupting the mitotic spindle structure of the fungal cell, effectively halting metaphase cell division.

UNDERSTANDING HUMAN IMMUNODEFICIENCY VIRUS AND ACQUIRED IMMUNODEFICIENCY VIRUS

Acquired immune deficiency syndrome or **acquired immunodeficiency syndrome (AIDS)** is a disease of the immune system caused by the **human immunodeficiency virus (HIV)**. HIV/AIDS is one of the most significant diseases of the 20th century, killing thousands worldwide every year and repeatedly defying all the best epidemiological modeling by the best minds available. In 2007 the

United Nations reported between 30 and 36 million people were living with HIV, 2.3 to 3.2 million became infected with the virus, and 1.2 to 3.2 million people died that year from HIV-related causes. The first cases of HIV were reported in 1981, and the first therapy to treat HIV was made available in 1987. However, after 25 years of HIV drug treatments being available, the number of people who acquire HIV every year continues to outstrip the number of people who need treatment by a ratio of 2.5 to 1. Thus, much of the world, especially people living in developing countries or those who cannot afford expensive drugs are left to suffer on their own (Walensky, 2006).

AIDS is a clinical syndrome caused by a **retrovirus**, human immunodeficiency virus (HIV). Once acquired (e.g., through blood, sexual contact, passed from mother to child), HIV leads to a progressive compromised immune system, which in turn results in **opportunistic infections** (e.g., *Pneumocystis jiroveci*, toxoplasmosis, Mycobacteria, hepatitis), cancer, or both. Immediately following infection with HIV, there is dissemination of the virus to lymphatic systems and organs, allowing the virus to be easily detected in blood and sexual secretions. However, at about 6 months postinfection, there is a set point at which the virus can remain stable for a period of months or years before it progresses to AIDS, with the average time course being 10 to 11 years in the absence of antiretroviral therapy. During this time, the patient may be asymptomatic or may only show signs of enlarged lymph glands. A warning sign, however, is that common infections (recurrent herpes zoster, thrush) become more severe and persistent. Figure 18-1 shows the life cycle of a virus.

HIV is a member of a family of retroviruses, and in order for it to replicate, it must first reverse transcribe its RNA genome into DNA. This means it is able to create DNA copies of its RNA genome, thus reversing or retro-enacting the usual flow of genetic information (RNA transcribed to DNA rather than DNA transcribed to RNA). Once transcribed into DNA, this viral genome is incorporated into the host cell genome, allowing it to take full advantage of the transcription/translation system for the purpose of replication. In other words, the pathology of HIV is a result of damage done to the lymphocytes (HIV virus has an affinity to the CD4+ T lymphocytes) and, subsequently, a loss of these T lymphocytes, which are needed to maintain cell-mediated immune function. This loss of immune function provides opportunities for other viruses, bacteria, and fungi to overtake the host, and over time, it leads to the downward spiral into full-blown AIDS.

Drugs used to treat AIDS are part of a regimen known as **highly active antiretroviral therapy (HAART)**. These drugs attack the virus itself and achieve suppression of HIV replication so that further immune damage does not occur and host immune function is restored so that it can fight opportunistic infections. Also, these drugs treat infections that arise as a result of the host's reduced immune response system (supportive therapy) so that survival is lengthened.

The clinical management of HIV is not an easy task. It has become very complex, especially as new drug combinations are constantly being evaluated and as adherence to a heavy multidose and expensive regimen remains a problem. The bottom line,

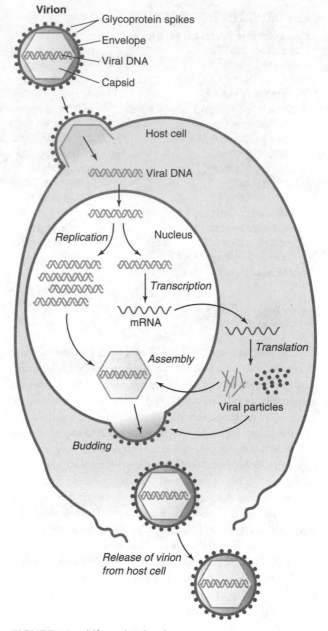

FIGURE 18-1 Life cycle of a virus.

however, is that persons with acute primary HIV infections should be treated with combination HAART to suppress viral replication to undetectable plasma HIV RNA levels and then should be counseled to avoid risky behaviors associated with transmission of the HIV; they should remember to consider themselves infectious. Long-term survival is not an unusual event because of the HAART protocol and because treatment decisions are individualized.

One major issue for the clinician treating HIV-AIDS patients is their high degree of nonadherence to the drug regimen. Factors that influence adherence to the treatment regimen include the treatment needs to be continued for years; the medications can cause adverse effects that impact the quality of life; the drugs are expensive, costing as much as $2,000 per month; and patients may become frustrated at constantly changing regimens when resistant strains develop.

There is also controversy regarding when to start therapy. Some clinicians argue that if therapy is started too soon or not managed well, then future options become compromised. Here again, patient wishes and preferences need to be balanced against costs, adherence potential, and immune system decline. Once a decision has been made to start therapy, the clinician must decide which drugs should be used. Generally, three agents are superior to two in suppressing viral replication. The decision of which drug combination to use is based on potency of the drugs, expected duration of therapy, adverse drug reactions expected and their impact on quality of life, potential interactions with each other and other medications being taken, cost, and ease of administration. Drug choice is also based on what other therapy might be needed in case of virologic failure and the probability of cross-resistance within drug classes.

Because the intensive antiretroviral regimens such as HAART are imperative in the treatment of HIV disease, the complexity of the regimens make it imperative the patient be a full partner. The clinician must educate patients regarding the following:

■ How to take the medication
■ What adverse events they can expect
■ How to fit the regimen into their daily lifestyle for a long period of time
■ How to manage the costs
■ How to adjust their life to include safe sex practices, which minimize transmission of the virus
■ How to avoid opportunistic infections
■ How to live with a chronic infectious (potentially lethal) disease

All clinicians can benefit from developing a working knowledge of the therapeutics and pharmacology of HAART medications and of the various classes of approved drugs because they will probably be asked about them at some point.

Because of the development of new and more accurate diagnostic tests for HIV-associated opportunistic infections during the past 5 years and because of the more effective treatments for these infections, the National Institutes of Health and the Centers for Disease Control and Prevention (CDC) in cooperation with the HIV Medicine Association of the Infectious Diseases Society of America (IDSA) have worked together to create a consensus for new guidelines, called Guidelines for Prevention and Treatment of Opportunistic Infections in HIV-Infected Adults and Adolescents.

Additionally, the U.S. Department of Health and Human Services has convened a panel of experts that have given their consensus on how best to treat HIV with antiretroviral drugs. Their work was released in January 2011 (DHHS, 2011).

Antiretrovirals Used in the Treatment of HIV/AIDs Infections

Patients with acute primary HIV infections should be treated with combinations of drugs that will suppress viral replication to undetectable plasma HIV RNA levels because this will prevent further immune system damage as well as any possibility of emerging resistant strains. The most effective means of accomplishing this is to use highly active antiretroviral therapy. The U.S. Department of Health and Human Services publishes recommendations for antiretroviral therapy for adults and adolescents (AIDSinfo, 2011). These guidelines state that initial treatment should include combinations taken from the six classes of antiretroviral drugs, i.e.:

a) Nucleoside reverse transcriptase inhibitors (NRTI)
b) Non-nucleoside reverse transcriptase inhibitors(NNRTI)
c) Protease inhibitors (PI)
d) CCR5 Antagonists (CCR5)
e) Fusion Inhibitors (FI) and
f) Integrase Inhibitors (INTEGRASE)

It appears the most common combinations are two nucleoside analogues, **nucleoside reverse transcriptase inhibitors (NRTI)** in combination with one **protease inhibitor (PI)**, or one **nonnucleoside reverse transcriptase inhibitor (NNRTI)**. An initial antiretroviral (ARV) regimen generally consists of two NRTIs (e.g., tenofir, zidovudine) in combination with anNNRTI, (e.g., efavirenz) a Protease Inhibitor (PI) (e.g., atanzavir, but preferably boosted with ritonavir [RTV]), an Integrase Inhibitor (e.g., raltegravir [RAL]), or a CCR5 antagonist (e.g., maraviroc [MVC]). In clinical trials, NNRTI, PI, INTEGRASE, or CCR5 antagonist-based regimens have all resulted in HIV RNA decreases and CD4 cell increases in a large majority of patients (DHHS, 2011).

If patients can comply and tolerate the drugs, dramatic reductions in viral loads are seen. The disadvantage to this regimen is that if treatment is started with drugs from more than one class and therapy fails, then cross-resistance to one or more of the remaining drugs in these classes of drugs is likely. If the clinician believes there may be a chance of resistance to an antiviral cocktail, initial therapy can be started with one NRTI and one PI and the more potent NNRTI classes can be reserved until later.

Despite the continuing introduction of potent ARV drugs, HIV resistance to all categories of existing ARV drugs continues, and it limits the successful treatment of many patients with HIV infection to the point that they do not enjoy long-lasting remission of symptoms. Clinicians will suspect resistance when the patient does not respond well to treatment and exhibits symptoms such as tiredness, development of opportunistic infections, high plasma viremia, and virus detection in sexual organs and secretions. But not all of this treatment failure is the result of drug resistance: Most is the result of poor adherence to complex therapy, adverse effects from the drugs, use of suboptimal or inappropriate dosing and therapies, and the inevitable ability of HIV to mutate under the selective pressure of ARV agents. From a public health perspective, though, wider access to ARV therapy and an increasing number of patients who fail combination therapy has led to transmission of drug-resistant HIV-1 to the next generation of patients, both from treatment-experienced and treatment-inexperienced individuals.

Conscientious Prescribing of Antiretroviral Therapy

■ Treatment decisions need to be individualized, weighing the risks to benefits in a rapidly changing dynamic.

■ The extent of HIV-induced immune system damage is measured by the level of CD4+ T-cell counts. Thus, CD4+T levels and plasma HIV RNA counts must be measured regularly to initiate or modify antiviral therapy in adults, children, pregnant women, or anyone else. Therapy is likely to be initiated if a person has symptomatic disease, decreasing CD4 T-cell counts, high viral load, and primary HIV infection.

■ HIV care is highly complex, rapidly evolving, and without concrete guidelines. Specific regimens must always be individualized and never fixed; they must be seen as only a starting point.

■ Because of the rapid emergence of resistance and toxicities of any individual agent, combinations of agents remain the mainstay of treatment, and these combinations commonly include up to four agents.

Patient/Family Education for Antiretroviral Therapy

■ Patients must be taught to take the medications exactly as prescribed; this will likely be around the clock and interrupt their sleep.

■ Missed doses should be taken as soon as they are remembered, unless it is time for another dose, in which case it is not recommended to double the dose.

■ Patients need to know they can still infect others; unprotected sex, sharing needles, and giving blood spread the AIDS virus.

■ Patients need to realize the importance of frequent follow-ups with their treating clinician.

Nucleoside Reverse Transcriptase Inhibitors (NRTIs)

Seven NRTIs are approved for use in the United States: zidovudine, didanosine, zalcitabine, stavudine, lamivudine, lamivudine/zidovudine combination (Combivir), abacavir, and emtricitabine. The NRTIs are synthetic agents able to mimic natural nucleotides, the molecules that are the building blocks of DNA and RNA.

Mechanism of Action

NRTIs compete with natural nucleotides in the HIV virus that would otherwise be incorporated by HIV's reverse transcriptase enzyme into newly synthesized viral DNA chains. By inhibiting a natural substrate in the enzymatic reaction (i.e., the HIV's reverse transcriptase), NRTIs prevent its incorporation into the process that would create new viral DNA chains, thereby slowing the progression of HIV infection. Figure 18-2 shows the mechanism of action of ARV drugs.

Pharmacokinetics

■ Absorption: Rapidly and extensively absorbed after oral administration

■ Distribution: About 50% protein bound, widely distributed in cerebrospinal fluid (CSF) and erythrocytes

■ Metabolism: In liver to inactive metabolites or minimal; however, zalcitabine is phosphorylated intracellularly to an active metabolite

■ Excretion: In the urine

■ Half-life: Lamivudine: 2 to 11 hours (adults); all others: approximately 1.5 hours

Dosage and Administration of Antiretrovirals

Generic Name	Trade Name	Route	Typical Adult Dose*
abacavir	Ziagen	PO	300 mg 2 times/day; take without regard to meals
didanosine	Videx	PO	200 mg 2 times/day; take 30 min before or 1 hr after meals
emtricitabine	Emtriva	PO	200 mg once a day; if results of creatinine clearance test (Ccr) is acceptable, take medication without regard to meals. If Ccr indicates kidney malfunction, adjust dosage.
lamivudine	Epivir	PO	150 mg 2 times/day; take without regard to meals
zidovudine	Retrovir	PO, IV	600 mg/day in divided doses; take without regard to meals. Patient should receive IV infusion only until oral therapy can be initiated
zalcitabine	Hivid	PO	0.75 mg every 8 hr; if over 60 kg, take without regard to meals
stavudine	Zerit	PO	20 mg 2 times/day; if over 60 kg, take without regard to meals

*When in combination with other retrovirals.

Clinical Uses

■ Treatment of HIV infection in combination with other antiretrovirals.

Adverse Reactions

Each of the NRTI agents has unique adverse effects; however, the following are common to all of them.

DERM: Rash

GI: Abdominal pain, diarrhea, nausea, anorexia, hepatitis, dyspepsia, vomiting

HEM: Thrombocytosis

META: Fatigue and LACTIC ACIDOSIS, presumed to be the result of mitochondrial toxicity

MS: Back pain, myopathy

NEURO: Tremor, headache, weakness, anxiety, confusion, decreased mental acuity, dizziness, depression, restlessness, syncope

Adverse effects unique to individual agents

zidovudine: ANEMIA, LEUKOPENIA
lamivudine: ANEMIA, NEUTROPENIA, ANAPHYLAXIS
didanosine: PANCREATITIS, retinal and visual changes
zalcitabine: HEPATOMEGALY
abacavir: HEPATOMEGALY, HYPOTENSION

Interactions

■ Zidovudine and stavudine can compete with each other and antagonize any therapeutic effect, so concomitant use of these two drugs in any HAART or cocktail is not recommended.

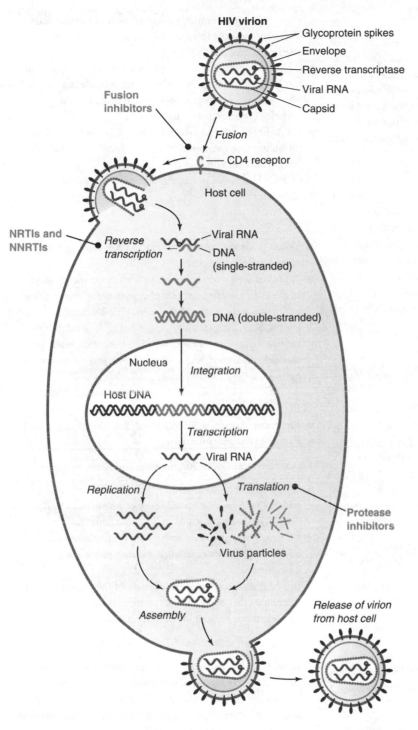

FIGURE 18-2 Mechanism of action of antiretroviral (ARV) drugs: i.e., cellular targets.

■ Zidovudine has an additive effect with any drug that works to suppress bone marrow.

Contraindications

■ Suspected hypersensitivity

Conscientious Considerations

■ These drugs require special monitoring of complete blood counts (CBC), metabolic panel, CD4 lymphocytes, and HIV RNA levels.

■ It is recommended that all patients be tested for chronic hepatitis B virus before initiating therapy.

■ Severe hepatomegaly and lactic acidosis, including some fatal cases, have been reported with NRTIs, with the majority being in obese women or those having prolonged exposure.

■ Patients on abacavir must be monitored for signs of hypersensitivity (abdominal pain, cough, diarrhea, dyspnea, fatigue, fever, nausea, rash, vomiting) and elevated liver function.

Protease Inhibitors (PI)

HAART involves the use of one protease inhibitor combined with one or two NRTIs. The resultant management of HIV-AIDS with this combination has been remarkable. The most common adverse effect of these agents is gastrointestinal intolerance. Because of their metabolism by the cytochrome P450 isoenzymes, they have a great number of potential drug interactions, requiring careful monitoring of concomitant medications.

Mechanism of Action

Protease inhibitors target a later stage in the viral replication cycle than do the NRTIs. The protease inhibitors bind to an active site used by viral protease enzymes, thus they cannot process viral precursors critical to the maturation of an HIV virus. Since the development of structural elements is hampered, the HIV virus is immature, noninfectious, and unable to replicate and proliferate. However, resistant mutations can occur if the protease inhibitor is unable to suppress the viral load in the patient.

Pharmacokinetics

■ Absorption: Rapidly absorbed after oral administration.
■ Distribution: Protein binding is high.
■ Metabolism: In the liver by Cyp-450 system.
■ Excretion: In the feces.
■ Half-life: 7 to 10 hours.

Dosage and Administration of Protease Inhibitors

Generic Name	Trade Name	Route	Typical Adult Dose*
amprenavir	Agenerase	PO	1,200 mg 2 times/day; not affected by food, but dosing requires 16 caps a day
atazaniavir	ATV, Reyataz	PO	300 mg atazaniavir with 100 mg ritonavir as a single daily dose with food
fosamprenavir	Lexiva, Telzir	PO	1,400 mg daily or 700 mg 2 times/day without regard to food
indinavir	Crixivan	PO	800 mg orally every 8 hr; take before or after a low-fat meal
ritonavir	Norvir	PO	600 mg orally every 12 hr; take with food, if possible
saquinavir	Fortovase	PO	500 mg 2 times/day; no food effect
nelfinavir	Viracept	PO	1,250 mg 2 times/day; take with meals or snack

Clinical Use

■ Treatment of HIV-1 infections in combination with other antiretrovirals

Adverse Reactions

DERM: Amprenavir has severe hypersensitivity reactions and can cause STEVENS-JOHNSON SYNDROME (also known as toxic epidermal necrosis [TEN], a disorder of the immune system triggered by infections, herpes simplex virus, influenza, mumps, cat-scratches, and Epstein Barr Virus; its leading causes are sulfa drugs and antibiotics as severe allergic reactions).

GI: Diarrhea, vomiting, acid regurgitation, anorexia, metallic taste, elevated transaminase levels, hyperlipidemia.

HEM: Thrombocytopenia, possible increased bleeding episodes in patients with hemophilia.

META: Exacerbation of diabetes, loss of fat from face and limbs, increased abdominal girth (paunch), and pads of fat behind neck and on back.

NEURO: Headache, insomnia, dizziness, somnolence, mood disorders.

Interactions

■ When given with other drugs in its class, mild increases in plasma levels may occur.
■ A host of drug interactions occur with drugs metabolized in the liver, causing increased clearance of the non-PI drug and creating the potential for serious life-threatening adverse events. Such drugs include nonsedating antihistamines, sedative hypnotics, astemizole, triazolam, midazolam, ergot alkaloid preparation, and antiarrhythmics such as amiodarone, quinidine.

Contraindications

■ Hypersensitivities, especially to sulfonamides
■ Patients taking vitamin E

Conscientious Considerations

■ Caution must be considered when using these drugs in patients with hepatic insufficiency or impairment as these drugs have been known to induce viral hepatitis.
■ GI toxicities, especially diarrhea, are the first adverse effects that patients experience and may play a role in nonadherence.
■ In addition, clinicians must be aware of the important considerations that apply to all antiretroviral agents (see p. 343, Conscientious Prescribing of Antiretroviral Therapy).

Patient/Family Education

■ Patients need to be aware that GI intolerance is likely to occur.
■ Because the agents have been associated with metabolic abnormalities such as body fat redistribution, glucose intolerance, and increases in triglycerides and cholesterol, patients must be educated about these effects.

Nonnucleoside Reverse Transcriptase Inhibitors (NNRTIs)

Currently, three NNRTIs are approved for use in the United States: delavirdine (Rescriptor), efavirenz (Sustiva), and nevirapine (Viramune). Although the NNRTIs are structurally different from the NRTIs, they do bind near the catalytic site of HIV reverse transcriptase and are quite specific as noncompetitive inhibitors of this enzyme. They are typically used for their additive or synergistic effect with other antiretrovirals, but their large number of potential drug interactions requires dosage adjustments when used with protease inhibitors.

Mechanism of Action

The three NNRTIs differ structurally, but they all have the same mechanism of action. They bind to the active site of HIV reverse transcriptase, and their antiviral activity is additive or synergistic with most other antiretrovirals.

Pharmacokinetics

- Absorption: Rapidly absorbed after oral administration.
- Distribution: Protein binding is high in plasma.
- Metabolism: Metabolized in the liver.
- Excretion: In feces and urine.
- Half-life: Delavirdine: 2 to 11 hours; efavirenz: 55 hours; nevirapine: 45 hours (single dose).

Dosage and Administration of NNRTIs

Generic Name	Trade Name	Route	Typical Adult Dose
delavirdine	Rescriptor	PO	400 mg 3 times/day (12 tabs per day); take with or without food
efavirenz	Sustiva	PO	600 mg once a day; avoid high-fat meal
nevirapine	Viramune	PO	200 mg daily for 14 days; take with or without food, then 200 mg 2 times/day

Clinical Uses

- Treatment of HIV infection in combination with other appropriate antiretroviral agents

Adverse Reactions

DERM: Skin rash, itching (rash may progress to TOXIC EPIDERMAL NECROSIS), increased sweating, pruritus

GI: Nausea, vomiting, diarrhea, increased liver enzymes

GU: Hematuria, renal calculi

MISC: Fever, anorexia

NEURO: Hypoesthesia; with efavirenz: headache, fatigue, and psychiatric symptoms such as abnormal dreams, depression, impaired concentration, nervousness

Interactions

- BECAUSE OF POSSIBLE EFFECTS OF THESE DRUGS ON HEPATIC METABOLISM, ADMINISTRATION WITH NONSEDATING ANTIHISTAMINES, SEDATIVE HYPNOTICS, ANTIARRHYTHMICS, CALCIUM CHANNEL BLOCKERS, ERGOT ALKALOID PREPARATIONS, AND AMPHETAMINES CAN RESULT IN SERIOUS LIFE-THREATENING EVENTS.

Contraindications

- Use of nonsedating antihistamines, sedative hypnotics, antiarrhythmics, calcium channel blockers, ergot alkaloid preparations, and amphetamines

Conscientious Considerations

- The skin rash associated with these drugs usually occurs within the first 28 days of treatment. As a class, they must be monitored for mild to moderate skin rashes that can rarely fulminate into Stevens-Johnson syndrome.
- Efavirenz should be taken at bedtime to improve the tolerability of the central nervous system (CNS) and psychiatric effects.
- Because rapid emergence of resistance is a problem, these agents should be given in combination with other antiretrovirals.
- Dosage adjustments must be made if they are given with protease inhibitors.
- Patients taking Stavudine must be monitored for any signs of peripheral neuropathy (tingling, burning, numbness, pain in hands and feet).
- In addition, clinicians must be aware of the important considerations that apply to all antiretroviral agents (see p. 343, Conscientious Prescribing of Antiretroviral Therapy).

Patient/Family Education

- Patients need to learn to stay well hydrated to ward off renal failure.

Antiviral Drugs for Herpes Infections

Herpes is a family of double-stranded DNA viruses that includes herpes simplex 1 and 2, varicella-zoster, cytomegalovirus, Epstein-Barr virus, and human herpes virus (HHV) 6, 7, and 8. These common pathogens cause a variety of infections (Table 18-1). HHV 8 appears to cause Kaposi's sarcoma. HHV 7 is a ubiquitous virus, not currently recognized to cause any human disease. Genital herpes is caused by two serotypes (HSV-1 and HSV-2); it is incurable and recurrent. Fifty million people in the United States have either serotype, and according to a bulletin of the World Health Organization, 536 million people have it worldwide (Looker, 2008). Unfortunately, medications are only 75% effective at suppressing symptoms. A healthy immune system, exercise, nutrition and diet, and rest play a significant role in healing. Because most people are asymptomatic and shed the virus in the genital tract, additional spread occurs frequently.

After an initial (primary) infection, herpes viruses can develop a latent state and live in the human host without causing illness, and they can become reactivated later in life. An example is the varicella virus, which causes chickenpox in a primary infection, generally in the nonimmunized toddler. Later, the virus becomes latent and lives in a sensory nerve ganglion. Following a stressed state or a period of depressed cellular immunity, the latent virus begins to replicate and migrate to the skin of that nerve root, creating the rash of zoster, commonly termed *shingles*.

Medical management is typically through suppressive therapy when symptoms manifest six or more times per year. After

TABLE 18-1   The Treatment of Herpes Viruses with Antivirals

HERPES VIRUS	TRANSMISSION	CLINICAL DISEASES	NUCLEOSIDE ANALOGUE USED FOR TREATMENT
Herpes simplex 1 (HSV-1)	Direct contact to mucous membranes and sexual transmission	Cold sores, corneal infections, encephalitis, genital herpes (occasional), neonatal infection	acyclovir, valacyclovir, famciclovir, trifluridine eyedrops, for corneal infection
Herpes simplex 2 (HSV-2)	Direct contact to mucous membranes and sexual transmission	Similar to HSV-1, but more often seen in genital infections and less often seen in oral, ocular, or CNS infections	acyclovir, valacyclovir, famciclovir
Varicella zoster	Aerosolized respiratory secretions, contact with vesicle (pox) fluid, nasal, and oral secretions	Chicken pox, sometimes with pneumonia and encephalitis. Shingles/zoster, occasionally affecting the ophthalmic area and potentially leading to blindness.	vaccine, zoster immune globulin, acyclovir, valacyclovir, and famciclovir
Cytomegalovirus (CMV)	Breast milk, saliva, urine, tears, and sexual contact	Congenital infections, mononucleosis-like illness, reactivation in the immunocompromised (pneumonia, retinitis, esophagitis, disseminated infection).	ganciclovir, foscarnet, cidofovir, valganciclovir
Epstein-Barr virus (EBV)	Saliva (intimate contact like kissing)	EBV is a common human virus that causes infectious mononucleosis and plays a role in the emergence of two rare forms of cancer: Burkitt's lymphoma and nasopharyngeal carcinoma.	Numerous drugs inhibit EBV replication in vitro. These include acyclovir,* ganciclovir, interferon-arabinoside, and phosphonoacetic acid.
Human herpes 6 (HHV-6)	Saliva	Roseola (exanthum subitum) in toddlers and occasional seizures and encephalitis. May have role in multiple sclerosis.	No specific treatment beyond rest and plenty of fluids. AVOID giving aspirin to toddlers because it can cause Reye's syndrome; use acetaminophen instead.
Human herpes 8 (HHV-8)	Sexual, especially in homosexual men	Primary infection: Fever and rash of 2–10 days duration. Reactivation during immunosuppression. Associated with Kaposi's sarcoma.	penciclovir, acyclovir

*Acyclovir, which inhibits viral shedding from the oropharynx, is the only antiviral drug used to treat infectious mononucleosis in placebo-controlled clinical trials. However, the clinical course is not significantly affected in patients with uncomplicated EBV, and typically treatment is by steroids and supportive therapy.

a year of this therapy, most people experience fewer outbreaks, but this does not eliminate subclinical shedding of the virus to other partners. Episodic therapy is effective in shortening the duration of an outbreak if started within 24 hours of lesions appearing or as soon as the patient feels some itching, tingling, or burning sensations. For this reason, clinicians typically give the patient a prescription so they can self-medicate as the need arises.

Mechanism of Action

These agents are all nucleic acid analogues. As synthetic molecules, they are able to convert to active compounds (i.e., acyclovir triphosphate) in the presence of host enzymes, becoming part of the DNA chain where they interfere with DNA synthesis and viral replication through their inhibition of viral RNA. Valacyclovir (Valtrex) is an ester form of acyclovir (Zovirax), but this drug is rapidly converted to acyclovir when administered orally. Thus, its mechanism of action is the same as acyclovir; however, serum levels are three to five times greater than the parent acyclovir and are nearly that of acyclovir when administered intravenously.

Pharmacokinetics

■ Absorption: Absorption following oral administration varies by drug. Acyclovir is poorly absorbed (15% to 20%), but therapeutic levels are still achieved. Famciclovir is absorbed in the intestine for conversion to its active form. Penciclovir is a topical drug only. Valacyclovir is a prodrug that is converted to acyclovir, and absorption is then 54%.

■ Distribution: Acyclovir, famciclovir, and valacyclovir are widely distributed, with CSF concentrations being about 50% of serum concentrations. All cross the placenta and enter breast milk.

■ Metabolism: Acyclovir is not metabolized, but is excreted in the urine as unchanged drug; all the others are metabolized in the liver.

■ Excretion: In the urine.

■ Half-life: About 2 to 3 hours.

Dosage and Administration

Generic Name	Trade Name	Route	Dose	Indication
acyclovir	Zovirax	PO & IV	PO: 200 mg 5 times/ day while awake for 7–10 days, or IV: 5 mg/kg every 8 hr for 5 days PO: 20 mg/kg 4 times/ day for 5 days	Treatment of initial herpes zoster (genital herpes, less active vs. cytomegalovirus [CMV]), Epstein-Barr virus (EBV) chickenpox in adults
cidofovir	Vistide	IV	IV 5 mg/kg 1 time/week for 2 weeks, then 5 mg/kg every 2 weeks; administer with robenecid	CMV retinitis in persons with HIV
ganci-clovir	Cytovene	IV & PO	5 mg/kg every 12 hr for 14–21 days, then 5 mg/kg/day 5 days/ week for prevention	Inhibitory viruses, best reserved for CMV for all herpes
famci-clovir	Famvir	PO	500 mg every 8 hr for 7 days	Treatment of herpes zoster, herpes simplex, and genital herpes
penci-clovir	Denavir	Topical use as a 1% cream	Apply 1% cream every 2 hr for 4 days	Treatment of herpes labialis (cold sores), topical formulation only
foscarnet	Foscavir	IV as 6,000 mg/250 mL	60 mg/kg every 8 hr for 2–3 weeks. Dosage reduction for any renal impairment	For acyclovir-resistant herpes infections and ganciclovir-resistant CMV infections, including retinitis
trifluri-dine	Viroptic	Eye-drops	Instill 1 drop on cornea every 2 hr (up to 9 drops/day) until cornea has reepithe-lialized, then 1 drop/ eye every 4 hr for another 7 days	For herpes simplex viral infection of the eye
valacy-clovir	Valtrex	PO	2 gm 2 times/day for 1 day 1 gm 3 times/day for 7 days 1 gm 2 times/day for 10 days	Herpes simplex (cold sores) Herpes zoster Genital herpes
valganci-clovir	Valcyte	PO, each tablet with 450 mg	900 mg 2 times/day for 21 days 900 mg daily for 100 days posttransplant	CMV retinitis and prevention of CMV after transplant

Clinical Use

■ Treatment of various herpes virus diseases (see Table 18-1)

Adverse Reactions

Side effects vary by drug, but typically they are few when these drugs are given orally. When the drugs are used short term, occasionally (3%) patients may develop the following:

DERM: Skin rash
GI: Nausea, diarrhea
NEURO: Headache

Interactions

■ Drug interactions are minimal and are not a real issue for the nucleoside analogues; however, bioavailability may be affected if acyclovir and famciclovir are administered with antihistamines.

Contraindications

■ Hypersensitivity

Conscientious Considerations

■ Cautious use of these agents is indicated for those with renal impairment. The most important variable in selecting the dosage of these drugs and the dosing interval is renal function.

■ Use cautiously in patients with preexisting neurological, hematological, hepatic, or fluid and electrolyte abnormalities.

■ Therapy with these drugs needs to be started within 3 days of any outbreak of a herpes zoster rash.

■ Valacyclovir has a higher incidence of SERIOUS REACTIONS (THROMBOCYTOPENIA, HEMOLYTIC UREMIC SYNDROME) IN PATIENTS WHO ARE IMMUNOCOMPROMISED.

■ Valacyclovir is made by Glaxo Smith Kline, and they maintain a registry for monitoring use of the drug in pregnant patients. Clinicians are urged to register their pregnant patients so that maternal-fetal outcomes can be monitored, especially because acyclovir and valacyclovir pass readily into breast milk and could expose an infant to fairly high doses from the nursing mother.

Patient/Family Education

■ Inform patients that these agents are *not* a cure. Although they improve the rate of healing, they do not prevent recurrence (usually 6 to 10 times a year is common). Development of drug resistance is likely to increase as recurrence increases.

■ Inform patients that application of creams, lotions, or any occlusive dressing may delay healing and may cause spread of lesions.

■ Instruct women with herpes to get yearly Pap smears.

■ If using ointment, apply every 3 hours at least 6 times a day using a gloved finger, and wear loose clothing.

Antiviral Drugs for Respiratory Infections

Amantadine and rimantadine are used for the prevention and treatment of respiratory infections caused by influenza A virus strains. Their greatest value may be prophylaxis of the at-risk elderly in nursing homes. They do not interfere with immunization against influenza, and patients often receive it while waiting for the influenza vaccine to take effect. Clinical studies seem to indicate that these agents shorten the duration of influenza by only 1 or 2 days, when the virus is not resistant. Oseltamivir and zanamivir are used in the prevention and treatment of either influenza A or B.

Mechanism of Action

Amantadine (Symmetrel) is a dopaminergic agonist with the ability to block the uncoating of influenza A virus, preventing its penetration into the host and inhibiting the assembly of proteins in any progeny, because has the ability to block reuptake of dopamine into presynaptic neurons. It is also used as an antiparkinsonian agent. Rimantadine (Flumadine) is a tricyclic amine that, as a potent inhibitor of virus surface enzymes, affects the release of newly replicated virus strands from host cells, possibly by inhibiting uncoating of the virus. Oseltamivir (Tamiflu) is an analogue of sialic acid and is a potent selective inhibitor of influenza A and B virus neuraminidases. Zanamivir (Relenza) also prevents viral replication by inhibiting the enzyme neuraminidase, which is essential for viral replication.

Pharmacokinetics

- Absorption: Amantadine, rimantadine, and oseltamivir are well absorbed after oral administration. Only 4% to 15% of the inhaled dose of zanamivir is absorbed.
- Distribution: Amantadine is protein bound and widely distributed including saliva and nasal secretion; distribution for the other three is not known.
- Metabolism: Amantadine, zanamivir, and oseltamivir and its active form are excreted unchanged with no detectable metabolites. Rimantadine is metabolized in the liver.
- Excretion: All in the urine.
- Half-life: Amantadine: 24 hours; rimantadine: 25.5 hours, prolonged in elderly; zanamivir: 2.5 to 5.1 hours; oseltamivir: 6 to 10 hours.

Dosage and Administration

Generic Name	Trade Name	Route	Dosage
amantadine	Symmetrel	PO	100 mg daily for 5–8 days
oseltamivir	Tamiflu	PO	75 mg 2 times/day for 5 days for treatment, 75 mg daily for prophylaxis
rimantadine	Flumadine	PO	Treatment of adults 100 mg 2 times/day for 5–8 days Prophylaxis of elderly in nursing homes: 100 mg/day
zanamivir	Relenza	Powder for inhalation	Inhale dry powder (10 mg) 2 times/day for 5 days; not for children under 5

Clinical Uses

- Amantadine and rimantadine: Prevention and treatment of respiratory infections caused by influenza A virus.

- Oseltamivir and zanamivir: Prevention and treatment of either influenza A or B. Amantadine and rimantadine are used for the prevention and treatment of respiratory infections caused by influenza A virus strains. According to the CDC, through November 2009, about 99% of typical influenza viruses were H1N1, with the vast majority of H1N1 viruses tested for drug resistance being susceptible to oseltamivir and zanamivir but resistant to the adamantanes (amantadine, rimantadine) (CDC, 2009a).

Adverse Reactions

CV: Hypotension heart failure (HF) (amantadine, rimantadine)
DERM: Urticaria
EENT: Blurred vision, dry mouth
GI: Throat/tonsil irritation, nausea, vomiting, constipation
HEM: Leukopenia, neutropenia (amantadine)
MISC: ANAPHYLACTIC REACTIONS, STEVENS-JOHNSON SYNDROME, TOXIC EPIDERMAL NECROSIS (with oseltamivir and tamivir).
MS: Muscle pain
NEURO: Headache, dizziness, depression, fever, fatigue, CNS excitation, insomnia, vertigo
PUL: Cough/bronchospasm (Zanamivir)

Interactions

- May cause dry mouth, blurry vision, and constipation if administered with antihistamines or antidepressants.
- Amantadine and rimantadine: When used with triamterine, increased amantadine/rimantadine toxicity may result.

Contraindications

- Amantadine and rimantadine should not be used in pregnancy.

Conscientious Considerations

- Clinical studies seem to indicate that these agents shorten the duration of influenza by only 1 or 2 days when the virus is not resistant; this effect was reported by the Advisory Committee on Immunization Practices (ACIP) of the CDC in 1994 and remains true today (CDC, 1994).
- Half-life may be increased in the elderly or those with renal impairment.

Patient/Family Education

- Take at least 4 hours before bedtime to reduce chance of insomnia.
- If patient is using powder for inhalation (i.e. oseltamivir [Tamiflu] 75mg twice a day for 5 days, at a cost of $115 for 10 doses or using zanamivir [Relenza] 5mg twice a day for 5 days at a cost of about $70), tell the patient to take exactly as directed and to finish the entire 5-day course even if feeling better before the five days are up. Also instruct patient on use of disk haler.
- Alcohol should be avoided because it can compound any dizziness and hypotension.

SPOTLIGHT ON INFLUENZA

Influenza is a seasonal illness caused by the influenza virus, a negatively stranded RNA virus that has a very high attack rate and spreads through tiny respiratory droplets from person to person. It causes a variety of symptoms, typically fever, muscle aches, headache, and cough; symptoms typically last 3 to 5 days. Approximately 20% of the world's population gets infected with the "flu" every year, generally during the "flu season," which the CDC indicates starts the 40th week of the year (about September) and peaks in January (CDC, 2013). This upper respiratory illness can spread rapidly and can lead to hospitalization and death for many persons who develop secondary bacterial infections, generally the elderly or those with underlying chronic illness. Death is rare in previously healthy children and adults, but occasionally, when new strains of the virus surface, the mortality trends afflict different age groups, as occurred with the H1N1 flu in 2009.

The structure of the virus is important in our understanding of its virulence, as well as how it is prevented (with immunization) and treated (by antivirals). The virus has a nucleocapsid, or helical, RNA protein at its center and is surrounded by a membrane. On the outer surface of the surrounding membrane, there are two distinct types of glycoproteins: hemagglutinin (HA) protein spikes create the points of attachment for sialic acid receptors on host cells, such as red blood cells or respiratory epithelial cells. Neuraminidase (NA), the second type of glycoprotein on the virus, cleaves neuraminic acid, which is an important part of mucin, a component of the gelatinous matter that generally covers the respiratory epithelium and prevents attachment of the virus.

There are three types of influenza: A, B, and C. These types have many antigenic strains separated by antigenic differences in HA and NA. Because flu is an annual phenomenon, and many people are exposed to the circulating strain on a yearly basis, the general population develops herd immunity for the most recent strains. Hence, based on a host's immune "memory," these pathogens are partially attacked by the immune system, and the result is a mild disease.

In some years, the influenza virus undergoes a more massive change, and the HA and NA glycoproteins are almost completely changed, giving the virus a makeover and leading to an unrecognizable virus, even in mature (older) hosts. This complete change of the antigens on the surface of the virus is called *antigenic shift*. Because the virus now wears a new "jacket," the entire population is susceptible, and devastating pandemics can occur because there is no antigenic overlap or partial immunity in the host population. Hence, during years in which there is an antigenic shift, the attack rate and virulence of the influenza virus are higher and the mortality greater. Although epidemiologists attempt to predict the antigenic strains that will be present from year to year, vaccination programs occasionally fail when the virus shifts the glycoprotein composition. This can lead to devastating respiratory infections, and compels clinicians to have knowledge of antiviral therapy for influenza.

Medical Management

Amantadine (Symmetrel) and rimantadine (Flumadine) are approved by the Federal Drug Administration (FDA) for influenza A virus infections, and zanamivir (Relenza) and oseltamivir (Tamiflu) are approved for acute influenza A in adults and children older than 7 years of age. According to the FDA, "Tamiflu (oseltamivir phosphate) is an oral antiviral drug approved for the treatment of uncomplicated influenza in patients 1 year and older, whose flu symptoms have not lasted more than 2 days. This product is approved to treat type A and B influenza. However, the majority of patients included in the studies were infected with type A, the most common in the United States. Efficacy of Tamiflu in the treatment of influenza in subjects with chronic cardiac disease and/or respiratory disease has not been established. Tamiflu is also approved for the prevention of influenza in adults and children aged 1 year and older. Efficacy of Tamiflu for the prevention of influenza has not been established in immunocompromised patients, patients at high risk for influenza infection, patients in whom vaccination is contraindicated, and protection of patients waiting for immunity to develop following vaccination" (FDA, 2011). These drugs should never be considered substitutes for vaccination.

THE ANTIFUNGALS

In the 1950s, amphotericin B was released to help fight fungal infections in humans. Since then only a few more agents have been added to the armamentarium used to treat fungal disease because amphotericin B is still available and effective. Newer agents offer expanded spectrums over amphotericin B, but they have brought additional adverse reactions and drug interactions. Understanding the pharmacokinetics and pharmacodynamics of fungal agents is important so that each clinician is able to effectively manage fungal infections in patients. Amphotericin B emerged as the preferred polyene over the more toxic agent in its class, nystatin. Today nystatin is used only topically. Although an expanded list of agents is available for fighting fungal infections, none of them is 100% effective at fungal infection eradication.

Conscientious Prescribing of Antifungals

■ Patients and their clinicians need to work together to prevent the overuse of antibiotics, which in many cases has led to the growth of fungal superinfections and bacterial resistance.

■ Because of the differences in the pharmacokinetic properties of antifungals, clinicians need to be well educated regarding their use or they will be ineffective.

Patient/Family Education for Antifungals

■ Patients should be advised that therapy with antifungal agents, especially those applied topically, is usually a long process. This is especially true of fungus infections under nails of the hands and feet.

■ Patients taking an oral fungal medicine in solution need to swish it around in their mouth for as long as they can and then spit it out.

■ Advise patients that topically applied antifungals can and will stain clothing and bedding. It is best to use creams and lotions that can be washed with soap and water.

■ Intravenously administered antifungals often cause some discomfort at the injection site.

Polyene Macrolides: (Amphotericin B and Nystatin)

Amphotericin B was the drug of choice for deep-seated or invasive fungal infections, such as aspergillus, candida, *Cryptococcus*, and coccidiomycosis, but it is now reserved principally for cryptococcal meningitis or invasive and rapidly progressing fungal infections failing other treatments. Nystatin (Mycostatin) is the drug of choice for topical fungal infections.

Mechanism of Action

Amphotericin and nystatin bind to sterols in the fungal cell membrane (**ergosterol**), altering the membrane's permeability to K^+, Mg^{2+}, and other components of the cell. They do this by creating pores or channels in the cell membrane, which causes leakage of these ions and other cellular components, leading to the death of the fungal cell.

Pharmacokinetics

- Absorption: Both amphotericin B and nystatin are poorly absorbed from the GI tract thus they are not given orally. Amphotericin is given intravenously when high plasma levels are needed or intrathecally when there is meningitis due to fungus, but specific dosages and length of therapy depend on the nature of the infection being treated. Because it is not absorbed from intact skin, it is formulated as various salts, that is, amphotericin B deoxycholate (Fungizone) or amphotericin B cholesteryl sulfate (Amphotec).
- Distribution: When given intravenously and absorbed, these agents are bound to plasma protein but with poor penetration into the CSF. The "cholesteryl" salt is taken up by the liver, spleen, and bone marrow, then slowly released.
- Metabolism: Mostly metabolized in the liver over a long period. Amphotericin is detectable in the urine up to 7 weeks after treatment stops.
- Excretion: Nystatin, taken orally, is eliminated unchanged in the feces; the metabolic fate of amphotericin is unknown.
- Half-life: Amphotericin B deoxycholate: 380 hours; amphotericin B lipid complex: 174 hours; amphotericin B cholesteryl: 28 hours; amphotericin B liposome: 100 to 150 hours.

Dosage and Administration

Generic Name*	Trade Name	Route	Dosage	Comments
amphotericin B deoxycholate	Fungizone	IV	0.25 mg/kg/day	Deoxycholate is a bile salt that forms a dispersion with amphotericin so it can be given in IV infusion
amphotericin B cholesteryl sulfate	Amphotec	IV	IV 3–4 mg/kg per 24 hr	Use if intolerant or refractory to Fungizone
amphotericin B lipid complex	Abelcet	IV	IV 5 mg/kg every 24 hr	Use if intolerant or refractory to Fungizone
amphotericin B liposome	AmBisome	IV	3 mg/kg every 24 hr	Use if intolerant or refractory to Fungizone
nystatin	Mycostatin, Nilstat, Nystex	PO	Oral suspension (100,000 units/ 5 mL) 500,000 units/ tablet 100,000 units/ 30 gm	For candida infections: 400,000–600,000 units 4 times/day (oral suspension)
		Vaginally, tablets		Insert 1 tablet daily.
		Topical creams		Apply 2–3 times a day to mucocutaneous lesions. If very moist, use Mycostatin powder.

*To date, amphotericin B remains the broadest-spectrum antifungal agent available, with activity against many clinically relevant yeasts and molds. During the 1990s, newer lipid preparations of amphotericin B, including amphotericin B lipid complex (Abelcet), liposomal amphotericin B (Am-Bisome), and amphotericin B colloidal dispersion (Amphotec), were developed to alleviate amphotericin adverse reactions and drug toxicity. These agents possess the same spectrum of activity as amphotericin B deoxycholate, but with less incidence of nephrotoxicity than the parent amphotericin B deoxycholate.

Clinical Uses

- Amphotericin B: Treatment of cryptococcal meningitis in HIV patients; invasive and rapidly progressing, potentially fatal fungal infections; and treatment of visceral leishmaniasis.
- Nystatin (Mycostatin): Treatment of topical fungal infections such as oral candidiasis, vaginal infections, GI and cutaneous candidal infections.

Adverse Reactions

For nystatin, there are no serious effects from oral administration, but occasionally a skin or vaginal irritation can occur upon topical application. Large doses can lead to GI upset, nausea, vomiting, and diarrhea.

Amphotericin B has several serious side effects that have continued to limit its usage since its development 60 years ago.

CV: HYPOTENSION (in patients with preexisting cardiac or pulmonary disease) arrhythmias
GU: NEPHROTOXICITY, hematuria
HEM: Prolonged treatment with amphotericin B usually results in anemia or blood dyscrasia.
MISC: Infusion reaction, chills, fever, hypersensitivity
NEURO: peripheral neuropathy
PUL: HYPOXIA (in patients with preexisting cardiac or pulmonary disease)

Interactions

- Synergistic nephrotoxicity occurs when used with aminoglycosides or cyclosporine.

Contraindications

- Hypersensitivities to sulfites, otherwise any compound in the formulation

Conscientious Considerations

- Amphotericin and nystatin are fungistatic, but amphotericin B can be given in higher doses, where it becomes fungicidal. Amphotericin does not readily pass the blood-brain barrier. If a patient has a fungal infection in the CNS, it can be treated with intrathecal administration. It has serious side effects and is therefore rarely used when other options are available.
- It is available in combination with a corticosteroid (nystatin + triamcinolone acetonide [Mycolog II]), which may decrease inflammation and itching associated with topical fungal infections.
- Infusion reaction when giving any amphotericin B formulation is common. Watch for fever, chills, nausea, headache, vomiting, and hypotension 1 to 3 hours after administration.
- Clinicians need to monitor CBC, renal function, electrolytes, and liver function tests, as well as total dosage (generally recommended not to go beyond 3 or 4 gm).
- Nephrotoxicity is a limiting factor in the use of amphotericin B; this is less likely with lipid formulations, and generally reverses upon stopping the medication.

Patient/Family Education

- Inform patients that long-term therapy may be needed to clear infections (a few weeks to 3 months).

The Azoles: Imidazoles and Triazoles

The only orally available imidazole, ketoconazole, has been associated with hepatic toxicity. It has been largely replaced by itraconazole for the treatment of all mycoses except when the lower cost of ketoconazole outweighs the advantage of itraconazole. Topical imidazoles are safer and are still widely used for many superficial fungal infections, that is, those confined to the skin or cornea. They do not work well in nail or hair infections. Many topical imidazoles are available without prescriptions. Aside from ketoconazole, commonly prescribed agents are itraconazole, fluconazole, and triazole derivatives.

Mechanism of Action

Imidazoles and triazoles impair the synthesis of ergosterol, which is necessary in fungal cell membranes, by inhibiting the fungal demethylase, a cytochrome P450–dependent enzyme present in fungi. The azoles thus affect synthesis of the fungal cell wall and cause leakage of the cell's contents. In general the azoles are fungistatic in low doses and fungicidal in higher doses.

Pharmacokinetics

These drugs vary widely in their pharmacokinetic characteristics. The following are the pharmacokinetic features of the *systemic* antifungals:

- Absorption: Well absorbed from GI tract
- Distribution: Widely distributed, including CSF; only partially bound to protein
- Metabolism: Itraconazole: metabolized in the liver into active metabolites; ketoconazole: metabolized in the liver to inactive metabolites; fluconazole: metabolized partially in the liver, but essentially excreted unchanged
- Excretion: Fluconazole: cleared by renal excretion as unchanged drug in urine; itraconazole: 40% in urine as inactive metabolite; ketoconazole: 90% in bile and feces
- Half-life: Fluconazole: 30 hours; itraconazole: 21 to 64 hours; ketoconazole: 8 hours.

Dosage and Administration of Oral Azoles

Generic	Trade Name	Dosage	Route	Indication
fluconazole	Diflucan	PO	150 mg as a single dose	Vaginal candidiasis
ketoconazole	Nizoral	PO	200–400 mg 1 time/day for 5 days	Vaginal candidiasis
itraconazole	Sporanox	PO	200 mg 1 time/day with meals for 12 weeks	Vaginal candidiasis Onychomycosis

Clinical Uses

- Oral antifungals are used for treatment of superficial (mucocutaneous) infections by yeasts (vulvovaginal candidiasis) and dermatophytes (tinea corporis, tinea capitus), and invasive systemic mycoses (aspergillosis, blastomycosis, candidiasis, histoplasmosis, and paracoccidiomycosis).
- Topical forms such as miconazole (Monistat) and clotrimazole (Gyne-Lotrimin) are used for treatment of tinea infections and superficial yeast infections.

Adverse Reactions

DERM: Rash (with higher doses), photosensitivity, alopecia, STEVENS-JOHNSON SYNDROME
GI: GI upset, nausea, vomiting, diarrhea, (with higher doses), HEPATOTOXICITY
HEM: Thrombocytopenia
NEURO: Confusion, drowsiness, dizziness

Interactions

- There are many drug interactions, which either increase the plasma concentration of the azole or the competing agent. Always consult a drug reference when prescribing these drugs if other drugs are being used concurrently.

Contraindications

- Hypersensitivity to any drugs in this class.
- Concommitant use of medications that may lead to prolonged QT interval and arrhythmias are contraindicated.
- All of the imidazoles and triazoles are metabolized by the cytochrome P450 enzyme system.
- Heart failure is potentially aggravated by itraconazole; it should not be used when there is a history of HF.

Conscientious Considerations

- Try to avoid any coadministration of antibiotics because it can lead to fungal resistance and fungal superinfection.
- Conduct liver function testing before prescribing. Use cautiously in any patient with liver disease.
- Any patient who develops a rash while on these agents needs careful monitoring because exfoliative conditions can occur.
- Topical imidazoles do not work well in nail or hair infections (tinea capitus).
- Although oral azole antifungal drugs are often used to treat superficial (mucocutaneous) infections by yeasts (*Candida*) and dermatophytes (tinea corporis, tinea capitus), most tinea infections and superficial yeast infections can (and should) be treated with topical agents alone, which are well tolerated and efficacious when used twice daily over 2 weeks.

Patient/Family Education

- Itraconazole: Take with food to enhance absorption, and avoid any use of antacids within 2 hours of ingestion.
- Because all oral antifungals can cause hepatotoxicity, any use of alcohol should be discouraged, and patients should watch for signs of liver damage (anorexia, nausea, pale stools, dark urine, tiredness, and jaundice).
- Because of photosensitivities associated with ketoconazole, exposure to sunlight should be minimal.
- Caution patients that all topical products may stain clothing and fabrics (underwear, bedding, towels), as well as skin and hair. Products stained by creams can usually be washed with soap and warm water; Those stained by ointments need standard cleaning fluids.

Terbinafine (Lamisil)

Terbinafine is a synthetic allylamine, structurally similar to the topical agent naftifine. It is available in both oral and over-the-counter

(OTC) topical formulation. It is well absorbed when given orally, and the drug accumulates in the skin, nails, and fat, making it useful in the treatment of onychomycosis. Oral terbinafine is at least as effective as itraconazole for the treatment of nail infections. It is also used as a pulse therapy, given once or twice daily for the first week of each month for up to 6 months.

Mechanism of Action

Terbinafine inhibits squalene 2, 3-epoxidase, an enzyme needed for ergosterol synthesis in the cell wall, making terbinafine fungicidal to a wide range of dermatophytes. It is fungistatic against *Candida albicans.*

Pharmacokinetics

■ Absorption: Minimal, if any, absorption through skin.
■ Distribution: Action is topical. When used orally, it is extensively distributed to dermis and epidermis, concentrating in the stratum corneum of the hair, scalp, and nails.
■ Metabolism and excretion: If any is absorbed through the skin, it is metabolized in the liver by first-pass effects to about 15 nonactive metabolites; the rest is eliminated in the feces. Kinetic properties remain unknown when used as a topical agent.
■ Half-life: With systemic use, 22 days.

Dosage and Administration of Terbinafine

Generic Name	Trade Name	Route	Dosage and Indication
terbinafine	Lamisil	PO	250 mg 1 time/day for 6 weeks for onychomycosis
terbinafine	Lamisil AT	Topical	Apply 2 times/day for tinea pedis, tinea cruris, tinea corporis for 1–4 weeks

Clinical Uses

■ Treatment of superficial fungal infections of hair, nails, and skin, such as tinea pedis (athlete's foot), tinea cruris (jock itch), or tinea corporis (ringworm).

Adverse Reactions

Adverse effects with systemic use include the following:

CV: CHF
DERM: Toxic epidermal necrosis, STEVENS-JOHNSON SYNDROME, itching, rash
GI: Anorexia, diarrhea, altered taste
GU: Hepatotoxicity
HEM: Neutropenia
NEURO: Headache
PUL: Cough

Interactions

■ Alcohol consumption is likely to increase the risk of hepatotoxicity.
■ Any drug that inhibits hepatic drug metabolism enzymes (e.g., cimetidine, rifampin) may decrease the effectiveness of terbinafine.
■ Side effects may increase with any caffeine or caffeine-containing herbs.

Conscientious Considerations

■ There is a high risk for noncompliance and superinfections.

Patient/Family Education

■ Instruct patient to take the medication exactly as indicated and for the full course of therapy. Doses should be taken at the same time every day.
■ If a dark urine, rash, or pale stool should appear, the clinician should be notified as soon as possible and the drug discontinued.
■ Patients should discuss OTC and herbal medications with a clinician before using them.

Griseofulvin (Fulvicin)

Griseofulvin is an older, cheaper alternative to the oral antifungals in the azole class. It is fungistatic, and indicated for fungal infections of the skin, hair, and nails. It is *not* effective for subcutaneous or deep fungal infections, nor will it work against candidiasis or tinea versicolor. Griseofulvin is produced by certain species of *Penicillium.*

Mechanism of Action

Griseofulvin binds to microtubules comprising the spindles and inhibits fungal mitosis. It incorporates into affected keratin where it is fungistatic to dermatophytes only.

Pharmacokinetics

■ Absorption: Ultramicrosize granules are formulated into tablets to allow for systemic absorption (which ranges between 25% and 70% of an oral dose) but which is enhanced by ingestion of a fatty meal.
■ Distribution: Widely through the body, especially skin, hair, and nails where it links to keratin.
■ Metabolism: Hepatic conjugation.
■ Excretion: About half in urine, the rest in feces.
■ Half-life: 9 to 22 hours.

Dosage and Administration

Generic Name	Trade Name	Route	Dose
griseofulvin	Ultramicrosize	PO	330–375 mg/day in single or divided tinea corporis (2–4 weeks), tinea capitis (4–6 weeks and perhaps up to 12 weeks), tinea pedis (4–8 weeks), and tinea unguium (3–6 months or longer doses where the duration of therapy is dependent upon the site)

Clinical Uses

■ Treatment of superficial fungal infections of hair, nails, and skin

Adverse Reactions

DERM: Rash, urticaria, photosensitivity
GI: Nausea, vomiting, diarrhea, GI bleed, excessive thirst, flatulence
GU: Menstrual irregularities
HEM: Leukopenia, granulocytopenia
MISC: Oral thrush, a rare drug-induced lupus-like syndrome
MS: Paresthesia

NEURO: Headache, fatigue, dizziness, insomnia, mental confusion

RENAL: Hepatotoxicity, proteinuria, nephrosis

Interactions

■ When taken with aspirin, griseofulvin reduces plasma salicylate levels.

■ Griseofulvin taken with oral contraceptives increases the chance of menstrual irregularities and possible pregnancy.

■ Griseofulvin taken with warfarin reduces the anticoagulant response of the warfarin.

■ Griseofulvin can increase the effects of alcohol, causing the patient to experience tachycardia, diaphoresis, and flushing.

Contraindications

■ Any hypersensitivity to the medication or its components

■ Any person with severe liver disease

■ Any person who is an active alcoholic

Conscientious Considerations

■ Prior to initiating antifungal therapy, the type of fungus responsible should be identified.

■ Several weeks to months of therapy are needed, especially when nail beds are affected.

■ Avoid use in pregnant women because it is Pregnancy Category C drug and has caused spontaneous abortions and congenital abnormalities.

Patient/Family Education

■ Avoid prolonged exposure to sunlight or sunlamps.

■ Be sure to report the appearance of its most common adverse reaction: skin eruptions and rash, and sore throat.

■ Avoid use of alcohol.

■ Oral suspensions should be stored away from direct sunlight and at room temperature.

SPOTLIGHT ON FUNGAL INFECTIONS

Unlike viruses, fungi are free living, that is, independent and highly organized cells. They have a nucleus bound by a nuclear membrane and enclosed by a rigid cell wall. They occur naturally in water, dirt, and air, often residing on plants, where they also go through a dormant "spore" stage. While there are a few fungi that can cause serious disease in healthy subjects (so called endemic mycoses), most fungi are innocuous inhabitants of the everyday world and rarely cause consequential problems for healthy individuals. Most fungal infections are superficial—involving the mucocutaneous tissues—and they are easily treated. If fungi create deeper infections, it is usually when the immune system of the host is weakened. In this environment, a fungus may multiply and spread to form an opportunistic mycotic infection. Opportunistic mycoses are increasingly common because of the huge increases in antibiotic usage and the widespread use of drugs that are associated with suppressed immune systems. When the immunological response of the host becomes ineffective, opportunistic fungi will transition from harmless commensals to invasive pathogens. An example is Candida, which causes yeast infections in the mouths of some neonates or in the skin covered by their diapers. Candida is a common resident of the human GI tract, skin, and female genitalia; in healthy individuals, it is kept in check by the other normal bacterial flora. However, in the severely ill hospitalized patient, it is now being isolated quite commonly from blood cultures. In fact, candidemia is the fourth most common nosocomial bloodstream infection, with up to 30% mortality.

Medical Management

Because fungi are resistant to conventional antibiotics, they require specific antifungal drugs to treat them. However, human cells and fungal cells share many functional and anatomical characteristics, and therefore the use of antifungal drugs becomes problematic because it is difficult to harm a fungal cell without harming a human cell of the host. Over time, most fungi have become resistant to conventional antibiotics, thus new classes of medicines have been developed to treat them. The azoles and terbinafine have been associated with hepatotoxicity and with rare hepatitis. These are usually reversible once the drugs are stopped.

Selection of antifungals is like selection of other antibacterials: It is based on susceptibility, pharmacokinetics, and adverse effects, especially the need to monitor liver response on a monthly basis if therapy extends 3 to 4 months.

ANTIPROTOZOALS

Protozoa are free-living, single-celled organisms with a nucleus. They can reproduce sexually and asexually, and they cause a variety of human diseases. In the United States, Trichomonal vaginitis (a common sexually transmitted disease) and intestinal giardiasis (a waterborne intestinal parasite) are frequent pathogens. Amebiasis is a cause of dysentery (bloody diarrhea). All three pathogens are treated with metronidazole or tinidazole. Giardia can also be treated with nitazoxanide. In asymptomatic amebiasis, patients carry cysts in the intestine. Protozoal cysts can evade metronidazole or tinidazole; therefore, these individuals warrant treatment with paromomycin or iodoquinol, the so-called luminal agents because the primary site of their action is on the lumen of the gut.

Conscientious Prescribing of Antiprotozoals

■ If prescribing for trichomoniasis, include sexual partner in treatments.

■ Be careful of a disulfiram-like reaction caused by the alcohol base in other intravenous preparations.

■ The efficacy of these medicines in immunocompromised patients remains unclear.

■ If retreatment is necessary, conduct a CBC with white blood cell differential.

Patient/Family Education for Antiprotozoals

■ Because drug may cause GI upset, be sure to take it with food.

■ Avoid use of alcoholic beverages for at least 24 hours after last dose.

- Drug may cause darkening of urine (reddish-brown color).
- Patients should expect a metallic taste.

Metronidazole (Flagyl), Nitazoxanide (Alinia), Tinidazole (Tindamax)

These three agents, metronidazole, nitazoxanide, and tinidazole, cross classes; they are all used to treat both parasitic and bacterial diseases.

Mechanism of Action

Metronidazole (Flagyl) is an anaerobic bactericide and a trichomonacide as well as an amebicide. It works by disrupting DNA and protein synthesis after diffusing into a susceptible organism. Metronidazole is a prodrug; its mechanism of action is not completely understood, but its metabolic by-product is a ferredoxin, which appears to cause a loss of helical DNA strand structure, resulting in cell death through inhibition of protein synthesis in anaerobes and protozoa.

Nitazoxanide (Alinia), a recent addition to this drug class, also interferes with the pyruvate ferrodoxin enzyme pathway, which is essential for energy metabolism in anaerobic bacteria.

Tinidazole (Tindamax) has a mechanism of action similar to metronidazole, but it is converted to an active metabolite by cell extracts of the pathogen, which then causes DNA damage to the pathogen.

Pharmacokinetics

- Absorption: Well absorbed (80%) after oral administration.
- Distribution: Well distributed, even into CSF, breast milk, and fetus, because of limited protein binding.
- Metabolism: Partially in liver.
- Excretion: In urine and feces.
- Half-life: Metronidazole: 6 to 8 hours; nitazoxanide: unknown; tinidazole: 12 to 14 hours

Dosage and Administration

Generic Name	Trade Name	Route	Dose	Comments
metronidazole	Flagyl	PO 500 mg tabs / 0.75% cream	For anaerobes: oral 500 mg every 6–8 hr / For acne rosacea: apply cream once a day.	Avoid all ethanol use.
		0.75% gel	Vaginosis: Apply one applicator full 2 times/day for 5 days	For vaginosis, recommend sex partner be treated as well.
tinidazole	Tindamax	PO tabs and suspension	Antiprotozoal: Children 4–11 years: 200 mg every 12 hr for 3 days / Adults: 500 mg every 12 hr for 3 days	Shake suspension before dosing. Suspension contains sucrose. Administer with food.
nitazoxanide	Alinia	100 mg/5 mL powder for oral suspension / 500-mg tablets	For infectious diarrhea, especially caused by Giardia and Cryptosporidium.	Take 1 tablet every 12 hr for 3 days. Do not use tablets in children younger than 11 years of age; use suspension instead.

Clinical Uses

- Metronidazole: oral therapy for anaerobic infections, amebiasis, giardiasis, trichomoniasis, and colitis due to *Clostridium difficile* (overgrowth colonic infection).
- It is often used with a cephalosporin or as a perioperative prophylactic agent in colorectal surgery.
- Used in combination therapy to treat peptic ulcer disease caused by *Helicobacter pylori*.
- Used topically for acne rosacea and for bacterial vaginosis.
- Nitazoxanide: Treatment of diarrhea associated with *Giardia lamblia* and *Cryptosporidium parvum*, especially in children.
- Tinidazole: Treatment of intestinal amebiasis, giardiasis, and trichomoniasis.

Adverse Reactions

CV: Flattening of the T-wave, flushing
GI: Nausea, diarrhea, furry tongue, unpleasant taste, abdominal pain, anorexia
GU: Reddish-brown or darkened urine, diminished libido, dysmenorrhea
HEM: Neutropenia, leukopenia
MISC: Phlebitis at injection site, SERIOUS ANTABUSE-TYPE REACTIONS CAN OCCUR WITH ANY ALCOHOL USE, teratogenicity
NEURO: Headache, dizziness, fatigue, malaise, peripheral neuropathy, SEIZURES
PUL: Nasal congestion, rhinitis, flu-like syndrome

Interactions

- Warfarin used with metronidazole may induce bleeding as prothrombin times increase.
- Cimetidine may decrease the metabolism of metronidazole.
- Disulfiram-like reactions may occur with alcohol ingestion, resulting in acute psychoses and confusion.
- CYP-34A substrates are inhibited, so watch for many drug interactions.

Contraindications

- First trimester of pregnancy
- Unsafe in lactating women

Conscientious Considerations

- Watch for signs of leukopenia.
- For most conditions, resolution of symptoms indicates a cure, but with giardiasis, symptoms may persist for weeks or even months after the organism is eradicated because of the lactose intolerance brought on by the infection.
- Tinidazole is more expensive than metronidazole. Therefore, metronidazole, which is equally efficacious, remains the drug of choice.
- Forty percent of patients will suffer a disulfiram-like reaction (Antabuse reaction) if they ingest alcohol.

Patient/Family Education

- Patients should refrain from intercourse if they are being treated for trichomoniasis. Partners should be treated because they may be asymptomatic but a source of reinfection.

- Patients may experience an unpleasant metallic taste. Chewing sugarless gum or sucking hard candy or ice can help overcome the dry mouth and metallic taste associated with metronidazole.
- Suggest good oral hygiene and mouthwash to minimize dry mouth.
- Report signs of superinfection or if there is no improvement in 2 to 4 days.
- The common headache associated with these drugs can be treated with acetaminophen.
- The darkening of urine is harmless.

THE ANTIHELMINTHICS

The antihelminthics are used to treat parasitic infections caused by **helminths**, or parasites, such as roundworms (nematodes), tapeworms (cestodes), and flukes (trematodes). Helminths are a class of arthropods that can cause serious infections in many parts of the world, not just in underdeveloped areas. These multicellular parasites are usually controlled in developed countries, but they can still be passed through the skin by contaminated food, insect vectors, and fecal matter in contaminated soils. Hookworm and onchocerciasis (river blindness) are still issues throughout the world.

Drugs for use against soil-transmitted helminths (STHs) are albendazole (Albenza), mebendazole (Vermox), thiabendazole (Mintezol) and pyrantel. However, reinfection is high unless the environment that spawned them is cleaned of fecal matter that allows the helminth to reenter the GI tract or other tissue. The antihelminthic drugs used today are quite specific, and therefore the infecting parasite must be identified before starting treatment.

Conscientious Prescribing of Antihelminthics

- Either mebendazole 100 mg twice a day for 3 days or albendazole 400 mg once a day is appropriate for all helminthic infestations except pinworms.
- The most pressing concern of fighting a nematode infestation is seeing resistance develop; thus the clinician needs to monitor patients very closely.
- Patients should be monitored when taking a benzimidazole because of the propensity of benzimidazoles to cause bone marrow depression, aplastic anemia, or agranulocytosis.
- Antihelminthics were originally developed to fight infestations in farm animals; thus clinical pharmacology in humans is incomplete, and their use in widespread infections in areas of poor resources remains a challenge for clinicians.
- Patients should be asked about all the medications, including both prescription and OTC, they are taking before starting these drugs.

Patient/Family Education for Antihelminthics

- Patients should be advised to avoid herbal and folk remedies such as tobacco, pumpkin seed, garlic, and wormwood because when given in sufficient volume to kill the worms,

they are equally poisonous to humans, and there is no scientific evidence that these remedies are effective.
- Patients should be advised to avoid people with the flu, colds or other infections.
- If a dose is missed, the next dose should be taken at its regular time; doses should not be doubled up.

Benzimidazoles

The benzimidazoles include mebendazole (Vermox), thiabendazole (Mintezol), and albendazole (Albenza).

Mechanism of Action

Although each of the drugs in this class acts in different ways, they all act directly on a parasite to relieve systemic infections. For example, mebendazole inhibits formation of the protozoa's microtubules, which irreversibly blocks uptake of glucose so that the infesting worm starves to death. Thiabendazole suppresses production of eggs and larva. Albendazole also inhibits tubulin polymerization, which results in loss of microtubule cytoplasm, decreased ATP production, and depleted energy.

Pharmacokinetics

- Absorption: Thiabendazole is well absorbed from the GI tract, but the others are poorly absorbed from the GI tract; with fatty food, their absorption is increased by approximately twofold to fivefold.
- Distribution: Widely distributed, including cyst fluid (in flatworm infections) and CSF.
- Metabolism: Extensively in the liver. Albendazole is converted to an active metabolite.
- Excretion: Primarily in feces and bile, some urine.
- Half-life: Albendazole: 8 to 12 hours; mebendazole: 2.5 to 9 hours; thiabendazole: 1.2 hours

Dosage and Administration

Dosage varies depending on the parasite treated and the site of the infection. A few important indications deserve comment.

Generic Name	Trade Name	Indication	Route	Dosage
albendazole	Albenza	Parenchymal neurocysticercosis	PO	400 mg 2 times/day for 8–30 days
		Pinworms (enterobiasis)	PO	400 mg as a single dose, repeat in 2 weeks
		Tapeworm	PO	400 mg 2 times/day for up to 6 months
mebendazole	Vermox	Pinworms, roundworms, hookworms	PO	One 100-mg tablet, then repeat in 2 weeks One 100-mg tab 2 times/day for 3 days; check in 3 weeks to see if a second course is indicated
thiabendazole topical cream		Use to treat cutaneous larvae	15% topical lotion	Apply 2–3 times/day for 5 days
		Trichinosis	PO	25 mg/kg 2 times/day, for up to 5 days

Clinical Uses

- Mebendazole: Treatment of ascariasis, trichuriasis, hookworm and pinworm infection.
- Thiabendazole: used as an alternative drug to ivermectin for treatment of strongyloidiasis (threadworm).
- Albendazole: Treatment of ascariasis enterobiasis (pinworm), hookworm, and after surgical removal or aspiration of hydatid cysts.

Adverse Reactions

CV: Angioedema
DERM: Rash, itching, alopecia
GI: Abdominal pain, nausea, vomiting, diarrhea
HEM: Neutropenia (see warning signs of sore throat, unusual fatigue). Unusually high doses or overdosing with mebendazole may induce myelosuppression.
NEURO: Unusual weakness, dizziness, headache, seizure

Interactions

- Cimetidine and anticonvulsants, such as phenytoin, inhibit the metabolism of mebendazole.
- Thiabendazole competes for metabolism with xanthene derivatives (e.g., theophylline) and can result in toxic levels of these drugs if given concomitantly without dosage adjustment.

Contraindications

- Pregnancy
- Renal disease
- Cirrhosis
- Hypersensitivities

Conscientious Considerations

- Because these drugs are specific to parasites, precautions and contraindications are minimal.
- Drugs extensively metabolized by the liver require cautious administration in patients with liver impairment.
- There have not been any well-controlled studies in pregnant women so each of these drugs is a Pregnancy Category C drug.
- Mebendazole and albendazole are not recommended in children younger than 2 years old.

Patient/Family Education

- Tablets should be chewed before swallowing.
- Stool should be retested to check for residual ova because worms may still be present 3 days after treatment.
- Strict hygiene at home is required to prevent reinfection.

Pyrantel Pamoate (Pin-Rid Antiminth, Combantrin, Pin-X)

Pyrantel pamoate is effective only within the GI lumen because it is poorly absorbed. Pyrantel is therefore not effective against migratory stages in tissues or against ova. It is highly effective for treatment of pinworm and roundworm infections and moderately effective against hookworm. It is not effective against trichuriasis or strongyloidiasis.

Mechanism of Action

Pyrantel pamoate is an antihelminthic that acts as a neuromuscular blocking agent in susceptible mature and immature helminths within the GI tract. It causes release of acetylcholine (Ach) and inhibition of cholinesterase, resulting in a spastic paralysis of the worm. This allows expulsion of the worm from the host's intestinal tract.

Pharmacokinetics

- Absorption: Poorly absorbed from the GI tract. Over half of the drug is recovered unchanged in the feces.
- Distribution: Unknown.
- Metabolism: Partial metabolism in the liver.
- Excretion: Primarily unchanged in the feces.
- Half-life: Unknown.

Dosage and Administration

Generic Name	Trade Name	Route	Dose
pyrantel pamoate	OTC as Pamix, Pin-X, Combantrin, and others.	PO	The patient is instructed to take 11 mg/kg of body weight as a SINGLE dose. (Maximum dose is 1 gm). **Note:** If treating pinworm infections, a second dose is suggested after 2 weeks, as well as treatment of all family members.

Clinical Uses

- Treatment of pinworm, roundworm, and hookworm infections.

Adverse Reactions

DERM: Rash
GI: Abdominal cramps, anorexia, cramps, nausea, vomiting, liver enzymes increase
NEURO: Dizziness, drowsiness, insomnia, headache

Interactions

- Pyrantel and piperazine mutually antagonize each other.

Contraindications

- Pyrantel is contraindicated in those sensitive to it or any part of its formulation.

Conscientious Considerations

- Use with caution in patients with liver dysfunction (aminotransferase elevations have been noted in a small number of patients).
- *All* family members in close contact with the patient should be treated.

Patient/Family Education

- Taking with food or milk may help relieve any mild GI upset.
- Using a laxative to help with expulsion of worms is not necessary.
- Strict hygiene at home, including sterilizing underclothing and bed cloths, is essential to prevent reinfection.

Ivermectin (Stromectol)

Ivermectin is an antiparasitic drug that is related to the macrolide antibiotics.

Mechanism of Action

Ivermectin selectively binds to chloride ion channels in the invertebrate's nerve and muscle cells, increasing their permeability to chloride ions and effectively causing paralysis and death of the parasite.

Pharmacokinetics

- Absorption: Well absorbed, and plasma concentrations rise and fall as dosage levels rise and fall. Its bioavailability is increased 2.5 times following a high-fat meal. However, its peak effect takes place 3 to 6 months after first ingestion.
- Distribution: Ivermectin is well distributed, but it does not cross the blood-brain barrier.
- Metabolism: In the liver.
- Excretion: In the feces over a period of 12 days.
- Half-life: 16 to 35 hours.

Dosage and Administration

Generic Name	Trade Name	Route	Dose
ivermectin	Stromectol	PO	Onchocerciasis (river blindness): either 150 mcg/kg or 200 mcg/kg as a single dose. Treatment may be required every 3–12 months until the worm dies.

Clinical Uses

- Treatment of infection with organisms susceptible to ivermectin, generally with a single dose.
- *Strongyloides stercoralis* (intestinal) and *Onchocera volvulus* (which causes river blindness in Africa); control of head lice and scabies.

Adverse Reactions

DERM: Skin rash (when ivermectin is used for skin infestation), STEVENS-JOHNSON SYNDROME

EENT: Blurry vision, mild conjunctivitis
GI: Nausea, fever, vomiting, diarrhea or constipation
MISC: Ivermectin can cause Mazzotti reaction (a syndrome consisting of arthralgia, edema, fever, lymphadenopathy, ocular damage, pruritus, rash, and synovitis).
MS: Myalgia, tremor, weakness
NEURO: Lightheadedness, headache
PUL: Asthma exacerbation

Interactions

- Ivermectin can affect liver function tests.
- Avoid use with barbiturates and benzodiazepines to avoid increased sedation.

Contraindications

- Hypersensitivity
- Pregnancy
- Women who are lactating

Conscientious Considerations

- Monitor stool for parasites and blood for microfiliaria and eosinophils.
- Monitor skin and eye, especially for ophthalmological reaction.
- A follow-up stool examination is required to be sure the adult worms are dead.

Patient/Family Education

- Warn patient that rapid killing of parasites may induce a systemic or ocular response known as Mazzotti reaction.
- Tablets should be taken with a full glass of water, on an empty stomach, 1 hour before breakfast.
- Advise patients that treatment may be lengthy and repeated.

SPOTLIGHT ON LARGER PARASITIC INFECTIONS

Helminths are disease-producing multicellular parasites that feed on host tissue. Colloquially known as *worms*, they infect over 2 billion people worldwide where adequate water and sanitation is lacking, usually sub-Saharan Africa, Eastern Asia, China, India, and South America (Brooker and Clements, 2006). They are also a significant public health issue in the United States, contributing to malnutrition, iron deficiency anemia, and deficient physical and mental growth of children in parts of the country. The CDC offers advice on how to recognize and treat helminths (CDC, 2012).

There are three major classes of worms that affect humans: roundworms (nematodes), flukes (trematodes), and tapeworms (cestodes). Although roundworms are not uncommon in the developed world, flukes and tapeworms are rare owing to public health measures aimed at eradicating them. A useful resource for identifying treatments for flukes and tapeworms is the Drug Service section of the Centers for Disease Control and Prevention available at http://www.cdc.gov/parasites/taeniasis/.

Intestinal roundworms present in the United States include *Ascaris lumbricoides* (ascariasis), *Necator americanus* (hookworm),

Trichuris trichuria (whipworm), *Enterobius vermicularis* (pinworm), and *S. stercoralis* (threadworm). *Enterobius* infections are the most common helminth infections, with over 400 million people infected worldwide (Kucik, Martin, & Sortor, 2004), but all of the roundworms cause disease. For example, a larva form of the dog hookworm (*Ancyclostoma braziliense*) can cause an itching skin rash called cutaneous larva migrans (creeping eruption), and it does so especially in parts of the southeastern United States.

Tapeworms have no digestive tract and depend on nutrients they find in the host, causing the host to suffer malnutrition as more and more nutrients feed the tapeworm.

Trematodes (flukes) are found in water contaminated by human feces; these flat parasites can be ingested in contaminated fish or water. They attach to the host with suckers, and grow into worms that cause ulceration and necrosis of surrounding tissue. If the liver and spleen become infected, death usually results.

Nematodes (roundworms) are nonsegmented worms that look like tiny cylinders, but they have a mouth, anus, and digestive tract. They reside in the upper GI tract and feed on undigested food. Their

Continued

SPOTLIGHT ON LARGER PARASITIC INFECTIONS—cont'd

fertilized eggs are eliminated in the feces and can contaminate ground soil for a long time. In less than sanitary conditions, a person may become reinfected, resulting in the egg hatching in the host and beginning a new cycle.

A type of roundworm called the pinworm is prevalent in the United States in areas where children may go barefoot. Contamination may also occur when children scratch their anus and touch bedding, clothing, furniture, and rugs, because the female lays her eggs in the perianal region.

Medical Management

The antihelminthic drugs used today are quite specific, which is why the invading creatures must be identified before starting treatment. This is usually done by finding eggs or larvae in feces, urine, blood, sputum, or tissue. Once identified, they can be treated with the benzimidazole derivatives (mebendazole, thiabendazole, or albendazole) or pyrantel pamoate.

Drugs Used in the Treatment of Malaria

Malaria is a mosquito-borne disease that leads to the death of 1 to 3 million persons annually, especially in subtropical areas of the Americas, Asia, and Africa (CDC, 2010). Malaria has been eliminated from the United States and Canada, as well as Europe, and it is considered a disease of the tropics. However, because the number of people traveling outside the United States to vacation or work has increased, every clinician should know something about the prevention and treatment of the illness.

Malaria is a febrile disease caused by four different protozoa, all in the *Plasmodium* family. The parasite is carried by the anopheles mosquito. Malaria infects the human host after a mosquito bite from a carrying mosquito. Once injected into the human bloodstream, the parasitic organisms travel to the liver, where they reproduce and then spread to the human red blood cells.

The different species of *Plasmodium* grow at different rates, expand, and then burst the red blood cells at different time intervals. Upon the rupture of the red blood cells by the malaria protozoa, high fevers and chills occur in the host. Diagnosis is typically made by identifying the protozoan inside the red blood cell on a smear of the peripheral blood.

Severe malaria is almost always associated with the *falciparum* species, which can cause profound anemia, renal failure, pulmonary edema, jaundice, impaired consciousness, and seizures. Cerebral malaria is a serious complication of the infection, and frequently causes seizures and sometimes coma and death among those affected. Children younger than 5 years seem especially at risk for death from malaria.

Treatment is based on the organism's susceptibility, because increasingly there are chloroquine-resistant strains discovered in Africa and South America. Two subtypes (ovale and vivax) are associated with having dormant larvae in liver cells of the host, and therefore relapses are known to occur unless liver protozoa are also killed when types ovale and vivax are diagnosed. Treatment with primaquine will kill dormant protozoa in the liver.

Chloroquine is the most widely used drug for patients with malaria. It is useful for both prophylaxis of the disease, often used by travelers, and for treatment (but with different dosing schedules for these uses). Quinidine gluconate and quinidine sulfate, two drugs used for prophylactic treatment of cardioversion of atrial fibrillation/flutter to maintain normal sinus, also have activity against *Plasmodium falciparum* malaria. Adults who need

treatment for malaria are usually given a test dose to identify any idiosyncrasies. This is followed by a treatment dose of 324 to 972 mg by mouth every 8 hours, or if given intravenously, 200 to 400 mg/dose where it is diluted and given at a rate of 10 mg/minute.

Quinine sulfate is not to be confused with quinidine sulfate. Quinine is the cornerstone of malarial treatment, especially when there is uncomplicated chloroquine-resistant *Plasmodium falciparum* malaria. Quinine is extracted from the cinchona tree bark and is a cinchona alkaloid. As an antimalarial, it decreases oxygen uptake, decreases carbohydrate metabolism, and elevates pH in intracellular organelles of the malarial parasite. The adverse effects of taking quinine, including nausea, headache, tinnitus, and slight visual disturbances (mild cinchonism), are frequent and have limited its use in favor of primaquine and mefloquine. Also, quinine overdose can lead to severe cinchonism, which manifests as severe headache, intestinal cramps, apprehension, severe cardiac conduction problems, decreased hearing, confusion, seizures, blindness, and respiratory depression.

Primaquine and mefloquine are also antiprotozoals used for malarial prophylaxis and treatment in areas where there is known resistance to chloroquine. They may be used in pediatric and obstetric patients. Primaquine is used for postexposure prevention for "relapsing" malaria or eradication of malaria when there is liver involvement. Primaquine is mainly used to treat the *P. vivax* or *P. ovale* malaria. Once the parasite has been eliminated from the bloodstream, the remaining hypnozoites must be removed from the liver; this is done by administering a 14-day course of primaquine (called radical cure). If primaquine is not administered to patients with proven *Plasmodium vivax* or *Plasmodium ovale* infection, there is a very high likelihood of relapse within weeks or months (sometimes years). When attempting a radical cure, primaquine requires the presence of quinine or chloroquine to work. If primaquine is given alone, the cure rate is only 21%.

Mechanism of Action

The mechanism of action of chloroquine is not well understood. Chloroquine is a synthetic molecule that has been shown to inhibit the parasitic enzyme heme polymerase, resulting in the accumulation of toxic heme within the parasite, which affects the biosynthesis of nucleic acids. In other words, it interferes with parasite protein synthesis and inhibits its growth. However, chloroquine kills only the erythrocyte form of the malarial parasite; it does not kill liver forms. With species that have a sleeping or dormant liver form, primaquine is necessary to supplement chloroquine.

Primaquine and mefloquine act by destroying the asexual blood forms of malarial pathogens (e.g., *P. falciparum*). They also disrupt mitochondria and bind to DNA, effectively inhibiting parasite growth. Pyrimethamine with sulfadoxine (FANSIDAR) is a combination drug that has been found to inhibit tetrahydrofolic acid synthesis in *Plasmodium* and *Toxoplasma gondi* organisms.

Pharmacokinetics

- Absorption: All are well absorbed.
- Distribution: All are well distributed, including in the CSF.
- Metabolism: All in the liver; primaquine and chloroquine to an active metabolite.
- Excretion: Primarily in the urine.
- Half-life: Mefloquine: 21 to 22 days; primaquine: 4 to 6 hours; chloroquine: 3 to 5 days.

Dosage and Administration

Generic Name	Trade Name	Route	Indication	Average Adult Dose
chloroquine	Aralen	PO	Malaria treatment	1 gm on day 1 to start, then 500 mg 6 hr later, then 500 mg/day on days 2 and 3
chloroquine	Aralen	PO	Malaria prophylaxis	500 mg once weekly on same day for 2 weeks before travel, then throughout travel, and continue for 4–6 weeks after returning from the endemic area
mefloquine	Lariam	PO	Malaria treatment	5 tablets (1250 mg) as 1 dose
mefloquine	Lariam	PO	Malaria prophylaxis	1 tablet (250 mg) 1 week before travel, then 250 mg throughout travel, and continue for 4 weeks thereafter
primaquine	Primaquine generic	PO	Malaria treatment (radical cure)	*P. vivax*: 30 mg 1 time/day for 14 days *P. ovale*: 15 mg 1 time/day for 14 days
primaquine	Primaquine generic	PO	Malaria prophylaxis	30 mg 1 time/day starting 1 day before travel and continuing 7 days after returning

Clinical Uses

- Chloroquine: Prophylaxis and treatment of malaria; also used as a disease-modifying therapy in treating rheumatoid arthritis and for treatment of discoid and systemic lupus erythematosus.
- Primaquine: Prophylaxis and treatment of malaria in areas where there is known resistance to chloroquine and in pediatric and obstetric patients; postexposure prevention for "relapsing" malaria or eradication of malaria when there is liver involvement; also used in treatment (usually combined with clindamycin) of *Pneumocystis pneumonia*.

- Mefloquine: Prophylaxis and treatment of malaria in areas where there is known resistance to chloroquine and in pediatric and obstetric patients.

Adverse Reactions

CV: Arrhythmias
DERM: Pruritus
EENT: Tinnitus, blurry vision (as drug interferes with visual accommodation)
GI: Abdominal pain, nausea, vomiting
HEM: LEUKOPENIA, AGRANULOCYTOSIS, HEMOLYTIC ANEMIA (in patients with a deficiency of glucose-6-phosphate dehydrogenase)
MS: Myalgia, muscle weakness
NEURO: Headache

Interactions

- Drug interactions with drugs that alter cardiac conduction (beta blockers, calcium channel blockers, quinidine) can increase the toxicity of these agents, leading to dysrhythmias, cardiac arrest, and seizures. If concurrent administration cannot be avoided, the patient should try to space the dosing of the beta blocker or calcium channel blockers at least 12 hours after the antimalarial drug.

Contraindications

- People with a history of seizures, psychiatric disorders, cardiac abnormalities, or hypersensitivities.
- Pregnancy.

Conscientious Considerations

- Periodically monitor CBC if the patient is on long-term therapy.
- If liver function tests, hemoglobin concentration, or leukocyte counts drop, discontinue the drug.
- Patients with glucose-6-phosphate dehydrogenase deficiency may experience hemolytic anemia or leukopenia when taking chloroquine or primaquine.

Patient/Family Education

- Taking mefloquine or primaquine with food decreases gastric irritation.
- Take medication with a full glass of water.
- Urine may turn brown when taking primaquine.

Special Case: Atovaquone/Proguanil (Malarone)

Atovaquone 250 mg/proguanil 100 mg is a combination product sold as Malarone. It can be used as a self-initiated treatment for emergency situations where medical care is not available, for example, if someone is traveling in a malaria-infested area and develops an acute case of malaria. In these cases the usual emergency dose is four adult tablets orally every day for 3 days. Malarone's more popular use is for the prophylaxis of malaria for which a person takes one tablet daily for 2 days prior to leaving, one tablet every day while

Continued

in the malaria-infested area, and one tablet a day for 7 days after leaving the malaria-ridden area.

Malarone contains atovaquone, an agent that selectively inhibits malaria mitochondria, and proguanil is an agent that inhibits dihydrofolate reductase; together they inhibit the ability of the parasite to mature. Malarone is hard on the renal system and so is contraindicated in renal insufficiency and used cautiously in the elderly. It must be taken with food or milk products because its main side effects are abdominal pain, nausea, and vomiting. Its oral dosing makes it easily transportable in a traveler's emergency medicine kit.

Implications for Special Populations

Pregnancy Implications

■ When prescribing antiprotozoal, antifungal, antiviral, and other such antibiologics for the pregnant female, clinicians should carefully consider their choice of drugs. Below is a selected list of drugs along with their assigned FDA Safety Category. Because most antibiotics have a specific effect on a limited range of microbes, the prescriber must formulate a specific diagnosis *before* prescribing an antimicrobial.

FDA CATEGORY	DRUGS
B	metronidazole, nitazoxanide, valacyclovir (Valtrex), acyclovir (Zovirax, ACV), famciclovir (Famvir), ganciclovir (Cytovene), ribavirin (Virazole), trifluridine (Viroptic), amphotericin B (Fungizone), nystatin (Mycostatin, Nilstat), miconazole (Monistat, Micatin), fluconazole (Diflucan), econazole (Spectazole), ketoconazole (Nizoral), clotrimazole (Gyne-Lotrimin, Mycelex), flucytosine (Ancobon), griseofulvin (Fulvicin, Grifulvin), ethambutol (Myambutol), rifampin (Rifamate), cycloserine (CycloSERINE, Seromycin), ethionamide (Trecator), capreomycin (Caprocin)
C	tinidazole, abacavir (Ziagen), didanosine (Videx), emtricitabine (Emtriva), lamivudine (Epivir), stavudine (Zerit, d4T), zalcitabine (Hivid), zidovudine (Retrovir), amprenavir (Agenerase), atazanavir (Reyataz), fosamprenavir (Lexiva), indinavir (Crixivan), nelfinavir (Viracept), ritonavir (Norvir), saquinavir (Fortavase, Invirase), delavirdine (Rescriptor), efavirenz (Sustiva), nevirapine (Viramune), amantadine (Symmetrel), isoniazid (Nydrazid, Laniazid), rimantadine (Flumadine), zanamivir (Relenza), oseltamivir (Tamiflu), chloroquine (Aralen), mefloquine (Lariam), primaquine (generic and Malirid), pyrimethamine with sulfadoxine (Fansidar), ivermectin
D	
X	
Unclassified	

Pediatric Implications

■ Pyrantel and mebendazole are not recommended for children under 2 years of age.
■ Ivermectin and thiabendazole are not recommended for children under 15 kg.
■ Tablets of nitazoxanide contain more than the recommended dose for children 11 years or younger; use oral suspension and reduce dose.
■ Fungal infections are growing as a larger incidence of infections among pediatric patients who are immunocompromised, HIV positive, premature infants, or on cytotoxic regimens. Newer antifungals are available in oral dosage form to help fight these infections, but thorough knowledge of them and their dosing and administration is essential. Of all the pediatric fungal infections, *Candida* is the most common, especially among those with indwelling catheters.
■ Pediatric dry powder antimalarial medications have been found to not be consistent in preservative or stated amounts; thus, although they may be convenient for travel, they should be avoided.
■ Pediatric helminth control is better aimed at cleaning up the environment because it has been shown that children tend to harbor more than one species of helminth at a time, making eradication a difficult and burdensome task. The same dosage is applied to adults, children, and elders, and the tablets may be chewed, swallowed, or crushed and mixed with food.

Geriatric Implications

■ Antiretrovirals: In addition to HIV-AIDS, many older patients have higher incidences of mental illnesses, substance abuse, and other comorbidities. In the early days of HIV transmission, the elderly mostly obtained their infections through transfusion, but today they have the same risk factors as do younger cohorts (risky sexual habits, IV drug use, and contact with drug users). The major comorbidity associated with HIV-AIDS in the older population is psychiatric issues, especially depression, making care of the elderly with HIV a special challenge.
■ Antihelminthics: The same dosage is applied to adults, children, and the elderly, and the tablets may be chewed, swallowed, or crushed and mixed with food.
■ Antifungals: The elderly are at greater risk for oral lesions from candidal infection and reactivation of varicella-zoster infection because of the decreased salivary gland function and use of dental prostheses. Treatment is typically with topical antifungal drugs such as nystatin oral suspension (100,000 units/mL; 5 mL, four times a day, swished for 5 minutes and swallowed) or clotrimazole troches (10 mg, four times a day). Both agents are used for 10 to 14 days. Therapy with antifungal agents is usually a long process of several months; this is especially true of fungus infections under nails of hands and feet. Thus with the elderly, adherence to the regimen is likely to be a problem, which ends up in delaying cure or worsening the infection.

LEARNING EXERCISES

Case 1

A 55-year-old male who frequents sushi bars comes to you with abdominal pain, weakness, tingling, dizziness, and irritability. His neurological exam produces no abnormal findings. A stool study finds that he has a tapeworm infestation.

1. What would you prescribe for him?

Case 2

A 32-year-old woman has been coming to you for treatment of HIV-AIDS. After several months of treatment, when she was beginning to be symptom free, she has started showing signs of symptoms again.

1. Is it possible that the HIV-AIDS virus is developing resistance to the HAART therapy?

2. What might be the cause of the returning symptoms?

References

AIDSinfo. (2013). A service of the U.S. Department of Health and Human Services. Adult and Adolescent Guidelines, January 2011. Retrieved February 15, 2013, from http://aidsinfo.nih.gov/guidelines/html/1/adult-and-adolescent-arv-guidelines/0

Brooker, S., Clements, A. C. A., Bundy, D. (2006). Global epidemiology, ecology and control of soil transmitted helminth infections, *Advances in Parasitology*, *62*, 221-261. Retrieved February 17, 2013, from www.ncbi.nlm.nih.gov/pmc/articles/PMC1976253/?tool=pubmed

Centers for Disease Control and Prevention (CDC). (1994). Prevention and control of influenza: Part II, Antiviral agents recommendations of the Advisory Committee on Immunization Practices (ACIP). *Morbidity and Mortality Weekly Report*, *439*,(RR150), 1-10. Retrieved February 16, 2013, from www.cdc.gov/mmwr/preview/mmwrhtml/00035666.htm

Centers for Disease Control and Prevention. (2009a). 2009 HiNi flu. Updated August 11, 2010. Retrieved February 16, 2013, from www.cdc.gov/h1n1flu

Centers for Disease Control and Prevention (CDC). (2009b). Updated interim recommendations for the use of antiviral medications in the treatment and prevention of influenza for the 2009–2010 season. December 07, 2009. Available from www.cdc.gov/h1n1flu/recommendations.htm

Centers for Disease Control and Prevention. (2010). Malaria Facts. Updated December 9, 2010. Retrieved February 15, 2013, from www.cdc.gov/malaria

Centers for Disease Control and Prevention. (2012). Other infectious diseases related to travel, 2012. In *Travelers health—Yellow book* (Chapter 5). Retrieved February 15, 2013, from wwwnc.cdc.gov/travel/yellowbook/2012/table-of-contents.htm

Centers for Disease Control and Prevention. (2013). Key facts about influenza (flu) and influenza vaccine. Retrieved February 17, 2013, from www.cdc.gov/flu/keyfacts.htm

Kucik, C. J., Martin, G. L., & Sortor, B. V. (2004). Common intestinal parasites. *American Family Physician*, *69*, 1161-1168.

Looker, J. K., Garnet, G. P., & Schmidt, G. P. (2008). An estimate of the global prevalence and incidence of herpes simplex type 2 virus infection. *Bulletin of the World Health Organization*, *86*(10), 737-818. Retrieved February 17, 2013, from www.who.int/bulletin/volumes/86/10/07-046128-ab/en/index.html

United Nations. 2008 Report of the Global Aids Epidemic (Chapter 2). Retrieved from www.unaids.org/en/dataanalysis/knowyourepidemic/epidemiologypublications/2008reportontheglobalaidsepidemic/

U. S. Department of Health and Human Services (DHHS). (2011). *Panel on Antiretroviral Guidelines for Adults and Adolescents. Guidelines for the use of antiretroviral agents in HIV-1-infected adults and adolescents.* January 10, 2013. Retrieved from http://aidsinfo.nih.gov/contentfiles/AdultandAdolescentGL.pdf

U. S. Food and Drug Administration (FDA). (2011). Drugs: Tamiflu (oseltamivir phosphate) information. Retrieved February 17, 2013 from www.fda.gov/Drugs/DrugSafety/PostmarketDrugSafetyInformationforPatientsandProviders/ucm107838.htm

Walensky, R. P., Paltiel, A. D., Losina, E., Mercincavage, L. M., Schackman, B. R., Sax, P. E., Weinstein, M. C., et al. (2006). The survival benefits of AIDS treatment in the United States. *Journal of Infectious Diseases*, *194*, 11-19.

Conscientious Prescribing for Special Populations

Drugs Used in the Treatment of Neoplasms

chapter 19

Hugh S. McLaurin, William N. Tindall, Mona M. Sedrak

CHAPTER FOCUS

This chapter focuses on general knowledge about neoplasms (new growth) and the application of agents used to combat them. This is done first by describing the pathogenesis of cancer and then through a general discussion of the classes of drugs used to treat them. The emphasis of the drug discussion is on how these agents are classified to impact the cell cycle. The adverse effects of chemotherapeutic (cytotoxic) agents is presented as a group because the importance of these adverse effects presents significant problems no matter what class of agent is being used. In addition, these drugs are presented in a general and comprehensive manner because their specificity and efficacy against growing tumors is rapidly changing because of new scientific discoveries. This chapter's focus and design emphasizes that cancer cells and normal cells are so similar in many respects that it is difficult to find exploitable biochemical differences between them, and thus the research into cancer treatments must go on.

OBJECTIVES

After reading and studying this chapter, the student should be able to:

1. Summarize the steps in the cell cycle and its relationship to the pathobiology of disease.
2. Understand and explain the cell kill theory.
3. Recall and describe the basics of chemotherapy as it relates to treating cancer.
4. Recall the four characteristics of cancer cells not found in normal cells.
5. Compare and contrast the eight classes of chemotherapeutic agents and describe their mechanism of action.
6. Recall what biological response modifiers (BRMs) are, how they are used, and how they work, and give examples of each.
7. State the role monoclonal antibodies play in cancer chemotherapy.
8. Illustrate how vascular access devices (VADs) are used in the intravenous administration of chemotherapy.
9. State the significance of a drug's nadir.
10. List six management strategies for the treatment of anemia induced by chemotherapy.
11. Recall the relationship between cancer chemotherapy, neutropenia, and infections.
12. Describe the management of thrombocytopenia.

Key Terms

Adjuvant therapy

Biological response modifier (BRM)

Blood-brain barrier

Chemotherapy

Cell cycle

Cell cycle time

Cell kill theory

Chemoprotective agents

Combination chemotherapy

Consolidation therapy

Extravasation

Grade

Growth fraction

Irritant

Leukemogenic

Metastasize

Nadir

Stage

Tumor-associated antigens

Tumor burden

Vesicant

KEY DRUGS AND CLASSES IN THIS CHAPTER

Alkylating Agents

Nitrogen Mustards
- mechlorethamine (Mustargen)
- cyclophosphamide (Cytoxan, Neosar)
- ifosfamide (Ifex)
- phenylalanine mustard, melphalan (Alkeran)
- chlorambucil (Leukeran)
- uracil mustard (Uramustine)
- estramustine (Emcyt)
- bendamustine (Treanda)

Ethyleneamines
- thiotepa (Thioplex)

Alkyl Sulfonates
- busulfan (Myleran)

Nitrosoureas
- lomustine (CeeNU)
- carmustine (BiCNU, BCNU)
- semustine (methyl-CCNU)
- streptozocin (Zanosar)

Triazenes
- dacarbazine (DTIC-Dome)
- procarbazine (Matulane)

Platinum Coordination Complexes
- cis-platinum, cisplatin (Platinol, Platinol AQ)
- carboplatin (Paraplatin)
- oxalaplatin (Eloxatin)

Antimetabolites

Folic Acid Analogues
- methotrexate (MTX), (Amethopterin, Folex, Mexate, Rheumatrex)
- pemetrexed (Alimta)

Pyrimidine Analogues
- 5-fluorouracil (5-FU) (Adrucil, Efudex, Fluoroplex)
- floxuridine (FUDR)
- capecitabine (Xeloda)
- cytosine arabinoside (Cytarabine, Cytosar, Ara C)

Purine Analogues
- 6-Mercaptopurine (6-MP) (Purinethol)
- 6-Thioguanine (6-TG) (Thioguanine)
- cladribine (Leustatin)
- gemcitabine (Gemzar)
- fludarabine (Fludara)
- deoxycoformycin pentostatin (Nipent)
- hydroxyurea (Hydrea, Droxiua, Mylocel)

Antitumor Antibiotics
- bleomycin (Blenoxane)
- dactinomycin (Actinomycin-D, Cosmegen)
- mitomycin-C (Mutamycin)
- mithramycin (Mithracin)
- daunorubicin (Daunomycin, Cerubidine)
- doxorubicin (Adriamycin)

Vinca Alkaloids
- vinblastine sulfate (Velbane, Velsar)
- vincristine (Oncovin, Vincasar PFS, Vincrex)
- vinorelbine (Navelbine)

Taxanes
- paclitaxel (Taxol), and albumin bound paclitaxel
- docetaxel (Taxotere)

Hormonal Agents

Estrogens
- diethylstilbestrol (Stilbestrol, Stilphostrol)
- estradiol, estrogen (many brands)
- esterified estrogens (Estratab, Menest)
- estramustine (Emcyt)

Antiestrogens
- tamoxifen (Nolvadex)
- toremifene (Fareston)

Aromatase Inhibitors
- anastrozole (Arimidex)
- letrozole (Femara)

Progestins
- 17-OH progesterone (many brands)
- medroxyprogesterone (many brands)
- megestrol acetate (Megace)

Gonadotropin-Releasing Hormone (GnRH) Agonists
- goserelin (Zoladex)
- leuprolide (Leupron)

Androgens
- testosterone (many brands)
- methyltestosterone (many brands)
- fluoxymesterone (Android-f, Halotestin)

Antiandrogens
- flutamide (Eulexin)
- bicalutamide (Casodex)
- nilutamide (Nilandron)

Biological Response Modifiers (Monoclonal Antibodies)
- rituximab (Rituxan)
- alemtuzumab (Campath)
- cetuximab (Erbitux)
- denileukin (Ontak, Diftitox)
- levamisole (Ergamisol)
- trastuzumab (Herceptin)
- bacillus Calmette-Guerin, BCG (TheraCys, TICE BCG)
- interferon alpha-2a, alpha-2b (Roferon-A, Intron A)
- interleukin-2, aldesleukin (ProLeukin)

Cytoprotective Therapy
- dexrazoxane (Zinecard)
- amifostine (Ethyol)

Antinauseants
- dolasetron (Anzemet)
- granisetron (Kytril)
- ondansetron (Zofran)
- tropisetron (Navoban)

Cancer affects people of all ages and does not differentiate who, when, or where it will strike. Cancer is a leading cause of death worldwide, and it was responsible for 7.9 million deaths in 2007 (Centers for Disease Control and Prevention [CDC], National Cancer Institute [NCI], and North American Association of Central Cancer Registries [NAACCR]). This chapter aims to introduce the building blocks of a good working vocabulary and a basic understanding about cancer chemotherapy, how chemotherapy agents work, their limitations, why early detection and aggressive treatment are essential to successful treatment so that this knowledge can help with a basic dialogue with patients and other professionals.

CANCER TERMS AND CONCEPTS

Even with all our advances in science and technology it is still difficult to answer the question of what causes cancers.

Although its causes may not be clear, researchers are clear about risk factors that increase an individual's chances of developing cancer. These risk factors include increasing age; tobacco use; excessive exposure to sunlight; exposure to ionizing radiation; exposure to certain chemicals; exposure to bacteria, viruses, and hormones; family history of cancer; excessive use of alcohol; a poor diet; lack of physical exercise; and being overweight.

The term *neoplasm* comes from the Latin *neo*, which means "new" and *plasma*, which means "life." Neoplasm refers to a group of cells that undergo cell division and replication at rates that distinguish them from normal cells. Thus, there are distinguishing characteristics of cancer cells that separate them from normal cells:

- Uncontrolled differentiation
- Decreased cell differentiation from normal cells, ending in loss of function

■ Invasiveness
■ Metastasis

Once uncontrolled differentiation begins, abnormal cells can either invade surrounding cells within an organ or tissue or they can **metastasize**, or spread, to other cells, organs, or tissues via entry into lymph and blood systems. The risk factors are well-known: It is believed that 95% of cancer cases result from risk factors (tobacco use: 25% to 30%), unhealthy diet and obesity (30% to 35%), and infections (15% to 20%). Tobacco use is the single most important risk factor for cancer because tobacco smoke contains about 300 chemicals known to be toxic to cells. If 95% of cancers are induced by risk factors, then only 5% of cancers have genetic origins, that is, lung, stomach, liver, colon, and breast cancer, the causes of most cancer deaths. However, the most frequent types of cancer have different prevalence rates between men and women (CDC, NCI, & NAACCR, n.d.), especially cancers of the prostate, ovarian, and breast. Prognosis of any cancer treatment depends upon the type of cancer, the staging of the cancer at the time of diagnosis, the presence of histological markers, and early detection.

Histological Markers

By definition, a cancer malignancy means that there is evidence of uncontrolled growth of tissue. There is a correlation between this uncontrolled growth and the ability to diagnose late-stage tumors, but histological appearances of malignancy are difficult to detect during the early stages of malignancy. This is because the boundary between premalignant and malignant states blur upon histological examination because dysplasia and early growth neoplasm share many common histological features. Dysplasia is not always a precursor to a malignancy, and some lesions may disappear or remain unchanged over the years or decrease in size and then develop malignancy. Regardless of the histological characteristics a lesion may exhibit, if it is not growing, it is not malignant, and therefore may not need treatment. Diagnostic tools such as ultrasound and biopsies have increased the ability to distinguish between benign and malignant lesions and to identify lesions earlier and with greater precision. Early detection followed by early treatment has proven to the best way to ensure a curative outcome.

Malignancies

The terms *malignancy* and *cancer* can be used interchangeably. Both terms refer to the situation in which abnormal cells divide uncontrollably and have the ability to spread to nearby tissues. Malignant cells may spread throughout the body using blood and lymph systems, but they can also do so through tissue-tissue contact. There are several types of malignancies:

■ *Carcinoma*: A malignancy that begins in the skin or in tissues that line or cover internal organs.
■ *Sarcoma*: A malignancy that begins in bone, cartilage, fat, muscle, blood vessels, or other connective or supportive tissue.
■ *Leukemia*: A malignancy that starts in blood-forming tissue, such as the bone marrow, and causes large numbers of abnormal blood cells to be produced and enter the blood.

■ *Lymphoma and multiple myeloma*: Malignancies that begin in the cells of the immune system.

Common Cancers

The most common cancer in the United States is skin cancer; more than 3.5 million skin cancers are diagnosed per year (Skin Cancer Foundation, n.d.). The most common types of skin cancer are nonmelanoma skin cancers (NMSCs) that usually start either in the basal cells of skin as basal cell carcinoma (BCC) or in the squamous cells of the skin as squamous cell carcinoma (SCC), typically on skin that has been exposed to the sun. Skin cancers can be either local or invasive, and 2% of them do metastasize into highly dangerous and sometimes fatal malignant melanomas. Since the 1970s, the incidence of malignant melanoma in the United States has increased significantly, on average by 4% every year.

Because 65% to 90% of skin melanomas are caused by exposure to ultraviolet (UV) light, preventive measures are well studied and well advertised to the public. However, even with many public service campaigns educating the public on the harm that results from excessive sun exposure, one in every five Americans will develop skin cancer during their lifetime (Stern, 2010).

For U.S. men, the cancers that most commonly result in death are lung, prostate, and colorectal cancer. For women, they are lung, breast, and colorectal cancer. Again, the incidence and death rate for all causes of cancer are declining in the United States due to early detection, aggressive treatment, and newer agents.

Lung cancer is the most common cause of death among both males and females in the United States, but it is the cancer most easily prevented given its low prevalence in those who do not smoke. Lung cancers are classified as being either small cell lung cancer or non-small cell lung cancer. There are major treatment and prognostic differences between the two categories. Non-small cell lung cancers are mainly composed of squamous cell, adenocarcinoma, and large cell lung cancer.

Colorectal cancer arises from adenomatous polyps (abnormal growths from the wall of the colon), which is why colonoscopy exams are so important for its early detection. Risk factors for developing colon cancer are advancing age, presence of polyps, history of ulcerative colitis or Crohn's disease, a diet high in fat and low in fiber, a positive family history of colorectal cancer, and lifestyle issues such as alcohol and smoking use.

Breast cancer arises from malignant transformation of the epithelial cells lining the ducts and lobules of the breast. Risk factors relative to the development of breast cancer include early age of menarche, late age of first pregnancy and late age of menopause, estrogen exposure, and genetic predisposition resulting from inheriting abnormal tumor suppressor genes, including the *BRCA-1* and *BRCA-2* gene mutations. *BRCA-1* and *BRCA-2* stand for *Br*east *Ca*ncer Susceptibility Gene-1 and *Br*east *Ca*ncer Susceptibility Gene-2, respectively. Not everyone with an altered *BRCA-1* or *BRCA-2* gene will develop breast cancer because these mutations only increase the risk from 13% to between 36% and 85% over a woman's lifetime. *BRCA-1* and *BRCA-2* are tumor suppressor genes that help assure the stability of normal genetic material in a cell, but once a mutation occurs, the risk of breast, ovarian, cervical, colon, uterine, pancreatic, stomach, gallbladder, and bile duct cancers rise. Men can also develop mutations in their *BRCA-1* and *BRCA-2* genes and have an increased risk of developing breast, testicular, pancreatic, and early onset prostate cancer.

Prostate cancer tends to develop in men over 50 years of age. It is mostly a slow-growing tumor that is often asymptomatic because it affects the prostate, the walnut-sized muscular gland between the bladder and rectum. The prostate gland functions to mix sperm-containing fluid created in the testicles with a prostate secretion containing citric acid, enzymes, and calcium. This fluid secretion is added to the semen before ejaculation. It also contains the enzyme prostate-specific antigen (PSA), which aids in liquefying the semen after ejaculation. This mix of fluid makes the semen alkaline, which protects sperm from the acidic environment encountered in the vagina during intercourse. The addition of this prostate secretion to the semen aids sperm mobility and survival, ultimately increasing the chances of fertility. The PSA enzyme is the basis of a test that is highly recommended by the American Urological Association (2009) for men over the age of 40 to follow their risk for developing prostate cancer. Other risk factors are increasing age, race (occurs more often in African-American men), lifestyle factors such as smoking and high dietary fat, genetics, and *BRCA-2* mutations. Treatment includes surgery (radical prostatectomy), chemotherapy, radiation, immunotherapy, and vaccine therapy.

Oncology Is a Team Effort

Oncology is the branch of medicine focused on treatments of cancer. Clinicians who work as oncologists may come from a variety of specialties:

- Surgical oncologists who perform and manage the surgical treatment of cancer.
- Radiation oncologists who treat tumors with X-ray radiation.
- Medical oncologists who prescribe cytotoxic agents to treat cancer. Medical oncologists are also trained in hematology.

Surgical, medical, and radiation oncologists mostly treat cancers as part of an interprofessional team. It is not uncommon for cancer patients to receive surgical resection of their tumors followed by local radiation treatment and systemic chemotherapy. Other members of the interprofessional team treating cancer patients may include specialty oncology nurses, pharmacists, nutritionists/dieticians, physical therapists, occupational therapists, dentists, social workers, primary care physicians (PCP), physician assistants (PA-C), and many other trained clinicians. Supportive systems such as hospice also provide comfort and care and are very much a part of the team and community efforts.

Chemotherapy

In the most general sense **chemotherapy** is the use of chemicals to treat disease. More specifically, the term refers to the use of medications to kill or inhibit the growth and spread of disease. Being even more specific, chemotherapy can refer to both the use of antimicrobials to treat infectious disease and the use of antineoplastics, drugs that harm or destroy malignant cells, and cytotoxics, agents that are cell-toxic or can harm or kill living cells, whether targeted or not. These agents treat cancer because both attempt to eradicate or influence the life cycle of a living cell. The term *chemo-* refers to the use of chemical agents that are destructive to malignant cells or tissues.

The general principle guiding both the use of medications to fight infectious and those to fight malignant cells are similar, in that both are being used to exploit the differences between foreign cells and normal cells of the host. Viruses, bacteria, and most parasites have cells that are significantly different from mammalian cells, and this allows use of medications that are extremely toxic to the invading organism but relatively harmless to the human host (see Chapter 18). However, two major problems arise in the use of chemotherapeutic drugs whether or not they are used to treat infections or cancers and these are the emergence of resistant organisms and cells and the adverse effects they can cause to the host.

Because cancer cells arise from a host's own cell lines, the ability to exploit differences between normal cells and cancer cells is more challenging than if treating invading bacteria, viruses, and fungi, and it is these challenges that give rise to how some chemotherapists conscientiously select a cancer-fighting medication. For example, some cancer cells have antigens attached to surface membranes. The antigens are not found on normal cells, so it makes sense to use cytotoxic medications that target those antigens because they will attack the cancer cells while leaving normal cells alone. Another common difference between normal cells and cancer cells is that cancer cells undergo unregulated and rapid cell division. Thus, normal cells most susceptible to the adverse effects of cytotoxic medications are the human cells that naturally divide and multiply rapidly, such as hair, skin, blood, and stomach lining cells. It is not surprising that common side effects of cancer chemotherapy involve the hematological, gastrointestinal, and integumentary systems because this is where the body's most rapidly dividing and multiplying cells reside.

Cancer cells, like invading bacteria, also have the ability to develop resistance to chemotherapeutic medications. Although most cytotoxic medications target rapidly dividing cells, there are different treatment modalities to minimize the adverse effects this can cause. For example, many cancer cells will respond to a single agent, but more commonly a combination of these medications is used in smaller doses to stop the rapid cell turnover in the cancer cells and minimize their toxicity in the human host. By using combinations of medications (cocktails), oncologists are also attempting to lower the possibility of inducing drug resistance.

Cytotoxic Medication Protocols

Cytotoxic medications are often prescribed according to protocols that have been shown over time to be effective for a particular type of cancer. These protocols typically involve the following:

- Dosing by body surface area
- Dosing in cycles

- Grouping similar cytotoxic agents together in categories
- Understanding of the cell kill theory to determine treatment length

Chemotherapeutic protocols typically require medications to be dosed by the body surface area (BSA) of the patient. BSA is less affected by adipose mass than weight and is therefore a better indicator of the patient's metabolic mass. Surface area is calculated by one of several formulas that consider the patient's height and weight together. There are no less than five commonly used formulas for BSA calculations, but at best they are only an estimate of the true surface area of the body. For example, the Mosteller formula is easily applied; it is often found as an application on a calculator, smartphone, or Internet site.

$$\text{BSA (M}^2) = (\{\text{Height (cm)} \times \text{Weight (kg)}\}/3600)^{1/2}$$

For example, a common dose of an agent such as carboplatin used alone for treating ovarian cancer is 360 mg/M^2 given intravenously once every 4 weeks, likely for six cycles.

Using body surface area to calculate doses has led to much underdosing and overdosing. BSA dosing overlooks the fact that there is a fourfold to tenfold variation in cytotoxic drug clearance among individuals because of differences in genetics, drug elimination processes, and environmental factors. It has been shown, for example, that underdosing women with breast cancer has led to an almost 20% relative reduction in breast cancer survival. For this reason, some oncologists ask a patient to collect urine over a 24-hour period and submit it so that it can be tested for renal clearance.

Cytotoxic medications are administered in cycles, with rest periods between these cycles. Some medications are infused over a short period of time, whereas others may take several hours. An administration cycle may take one or more days. Cycles are often given every 1, 2, 3, or 4 weeks. A course of chemotherapy often consists of multiple cycles set by protocols chosen by knowing the type of cancer being treated, its **stage**, and its **grade**.

Cytotoxic medications cause cell death in a variety of ways, and there are over 100 available for use. Many cytotoxic medications have similar chemical structures or modes of action, which allow them to be grouped into categories. There are several ways of placing drugs in these categories, but no one way is perfect. Some drugs overlap categories, and some do not fit well into any category. Drugs placed into a category may not effectively treat a certain cancer as well as other drugs in the same category. Knowing the value of creating artificial divisions, while being mindful of their limitations, allows groupings of chemotherapeutic medications into the eight categories (including some subcategories) used in this chapter.

Cell Kill Theory

Cell Kill Theory proposes that a set percentage of cells are killed with each dose of chemotherapy. The percentage of cells killed depends on the specific drugs used. For example, if a tumor has 1,000,000 cells and is exposed to a drug that has an 80% cell kill rate, the first chemotherapy dose will kill 80% or 800,000 of the targeted cancer cells. The second dose will kill another 80% of the remaining cancer cells. However, because only a percentage of cells die with each exposure to a cytotoxic agent, additional doses of chemotherapy must be repeated to reduce the cancer cells to just a few remaining cells. When only a few cancer cells remain, it is hoped that the body's immune response system will take over and kill, or eradicate, the final few cells.

Cell Division and Replication

Cell-Division Cycle

One helpful way to categorize cytotoxic medications is to consider their effect on a particular phase of the cell division cycle or whether they are toxic to cells regardless of what phase of cell division they are in. Agents that exert their cytotoxic activity during a particular phase of the cell division cycle are referred to as cell-cycle specific (CCS) agents. Those that have cytotoxic activity unrelated to the cell cycle are referred to as cell cycle nonspecific (CCNS) agents.

In eukaryotic cells (cells that have a distinct membrane surrounding a nucleus), cell replication is divided into interphase and mitosis cycles. Cells that are not actively dividing or are preparing to divide are in a resting phase referred to as G-0. CCS agents are not active against cells in the resting phase. During mitosis (M), the cell splits itself into two identical cells, often called daughter cells. During interphase, the cell grows, accumulates nutrients needed for mitosis, and duplicates its DNA. Interphase is subdivided into a postmitotic phase (G-1), a synthesis phase (S), and a premitotic phase (G-2).

The body has a sophisticated system for maintaining normal cell repair and growth. It is thought that the body responds to a feedback system that signals a cell to enter the G-1 phase of the cell life cycle in response to cell death. In persons who have cancer, this feedback system doesn't work normally, and cancer cells enter the cell cycle independently of the body's feedback system. The failure of cells to respond to the normal mechanisms that control normal cell birth and death results in cancer (neoplasm).

Five Phases of Cell Cycle Replication

The **cell cycle**, or cell replication cycle, refers to the series of events that take place in a cell that complete the cell's division and replication (duplication). In a typical cell cycle, a cell doubles it size, mass, and volume of chromosomes so that when it divides, the offspring, or daughter cells, are genetically identical. This phenomenon of life occurs in from approximately 8 minutes in a human embryo to between 10 to 24 hours for most human cells, except liver cells, which take about a year to divide. The cell replication occurs as a distinctive process involving a network of protein kinases. These protein kinases regulate DNA synthesis, mitotic entry, and mitotic exit.

In humans and animals, not all cells replicate on a set continuous cycle; however, deregulation of cell-cycle control proteins plays a key role in the development of cancer. This is through either overactivation of proteins, especially cyclins that favor cell cycle progression, or inactivation of proteins that impede cell progression because, in human tumors, genes encode the proteins to cause transition from one cell phase to the next. There is much evidence to suggest that cyclins can act as oncogenes to induce cells to become cancerous.

Phases of the Cell Cycle

Refer to Figure 19-1, which illustrates the phases of the cell cycle.

Phase 1—Resting Phase (G-O): In this phase, cells are not dividing and are temporarily out of the cell cycle. Depending on the type of cell, this phase can last for a few hours to several years. When the cell is signaled to reproduce, it moves into the G1 phase.

Phase 2—Postmitotic phase (G-1): This is the first gap (G) phase. In this phase, the cell starts making more proteins in preparation for cell division. Enzymes needed for DNA and RNA synthesis are produced. DNA is an essential nucleic acid composed of deoxyribose, a phosphate, and four nitrogenous bases: adenine, guanine, cytosine, and thymine. Adenine and guanine are purine derivatives. Cytosine and thymine are pyrimidine derivatives. Chemical reactions occur between the bases, leading to the formation of the double-stranded DNA helix, which serves as the genetic template for cell division. The duration of the G-1 phase can last from hours to days.

Phase 3—Synthesis (S): In this phase, the proteins containing the genetic code (DNA) are copied so that both of the new cells formed will have the right amount of DNA. The S phase lasts approximately 10 to 20 hours and is where chromosome replication takes place.

Phase 4—Premitotic phase (G-2): This is the second gap phase, which occurs just before the cell starts splitting into two cells. Additional protein and RNA synthesis occurs as well as organelle development. The G-2 phase lasts from 1 to 3 hours in most cells.

Phase 5—Mitosis (M): Cellular division occurs in this phase under five distinct steps that cause the chromosomes to separate and form two distinct nuclei: These steps are prophase; (where replicated chromosomes condense); prometaphase (where the nuclear membrane dissolves and spindle fibers form as chromosomes attach to spindle fibers, which pull them apart); metaphase (where replicated chromosomes form at the center); anaphase (where daughter chromosomes move to the poles); and the telophase (where nuclear membranes form and spindle fibers disappear). The spindle fibers are composed of microtubules and proteins and are necessary for moving chromosomes within the dividing nucleus. Once mitosis has occurred, the cell then divides, creating two identical cells (called cytokinesis). The M phase lasts about 1 hour.

Cell Cycle Time

Cell cycle time refers to the amount of time required for a cell to move from one mitotic phase or cell division to another. The length of the total cell cycle varies with the specific type of cell. The length of the cell cycle is important because it determines how quickly an organism can multiply. For single-celled organisms, like an amoeba, this rate determines how quickly the organism can reproduce new, independent organisms. For higher-order species, like animals and humans, the length of the cell cycle determines how long it takes to replace damaged cells. Thus, duration of the cell cycle varies from organism to organism and from cell to cell. For example, certain fly embryos have cells that cycle every 8 minutes per cycle, and some mammals have cells, such as certain liver cells, that can take as much as a year to cycle. Generally, however, for fast-dividing human cells, the length of the cycle is approximately 24 hours.

The **growth fraction** of a tumor refers to the percentage of cells actively dividing at a given point in time. A higher growth fraction causes more cancer cells to be killed when they are exposed to cell cycle-specific drugs. Tumors with a greater fraction of cells in G-0 are more sensitive to cell cycle-nonspecific agents.

Tumor burden refers to the number of cancer cells present in the tumor. Cancers with a small tumor burden are usually more sensitive to cytotoxic therapy, because they have a high number of cells reproducing. As the tumor burden increases, the growth rate slows, and the numbers of cells actively dividing slow down.

Understanding the stages of cell cycles is important because many chemotherapy drugs work only on actively reproducing cells. Knowing how specific drugs kill cancer cells helps oncologists predict which drugs are likely to work well when administered together. Cell cycle–specific drugs exert their major killing effect on cells that are actively dividing at specific phases during the cell cycle. Cell destruction occurs when cancer cells attempt to divide. Cell cycle–specific agents are not active against cells in the resting state (G-0).

CLASSIFICATION OF CHEMOTHERAPEUTIC AGENTS

Besides being classified as cell cycle–specific or –nonspecific agents, cytotoxic drugs are also classified on the basis of their biochemical structure and mechanism of action. There are several classes of cytotoxic drugs; they include the following and may include others as they are discovered: alkylating agents,

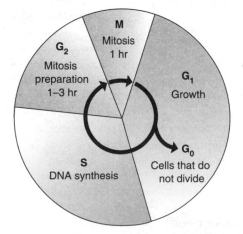

FIGURE 19-1 The Phases and Timing of a Cell's Replication Cycle.

antimetabolites, antitumor antibiotics, vinca alkaloids, taxanes, biological response modifiers (BRM), gene therapy, and chemoprotective agents.

Alkylating Agents

Alkylating agents were the first chemotherapeutic drugs used. It was noted during World War II that soldiers exposed to mustard gas developed low white blood cell (WBC) counts. This observation led to early attempts at treating leukemia with intravenous nitrogen mustard. Alkylating agents interfere with DNA replication to prevent cells from reproducing, and most are cell cycle nonspecific. Alkylating agents can produce major toxicities affecting the hematopoietic system (the blood-producing system of the bone marrow) and the gastrointestinal and reproductive systems. In addition to causing acute bone marrow suppression, alkylating agents are **leukemogenic** (causing leukemia).

These drugs are active against chronic leukemia, non-Hodgkin's lymphoma, Hodgkin's lymphoma, multiple myeloma, and some cancers of the lung, breast, and ovary. Certain alkylating agents, like cyclophosphamide (Cytoxan), help empty bone marrow prior to bone marrow transplant to allow new cells to engraft. When used as a single agent, resistance to alkylating agents develops quickly.

There are a number of cytotoxic drugs commercially available that are classified as alkylating agents (Table 19-1).

TABLE 19-1 Cytotoxic Alkylating Agents

CLASS	DRUGS
NITROGEN MUSTARDS	mechlorethamine (Mustargen)
	cyclophosphamide (Cytoxan, Neosar)
	ifosfamide (Ifex)
	phenylalanine mustard, melphalan (Alkeran)
	chlorambucil (Leukeran)
	uracil mustard (Uramustine)
	estramustine (Emcyt)
	bendamustine (Treanda)
ETHYLAMINES	thiotepa (Thioplex)
ALKYL SULFONATES	busulfan (Myleran)
NITROSOUREAS	lomustine (CeeNU)
	carmustine (BiCNU, BCNU)
	semustine (Methyl-CCNU)
	streptozocin (Zanosar)
TRIAZENES	dacarbazine (DTIC-Dome)
	procarbazine (Matulane)
PLATINUM COORDINATION COMPLEXES	cis-platinum, cisplatin (Platinol, Platinol AQ)
	carboplatin (Paraplatin)
	oxaliplatin (Eloxatin)
OTHERS	altretamine (Hexalen)

Antimetabolites

Antimetabolites interfere with DNA and RNA formation. They are chemicals that inhibit the normal use of a metabolite by cells. Metabolites are chemicals that are needed for normal cell development. Most antimetabolites are structurally very similar to the metabolite they mimic. The similarities of their chemical structure cause the cell to incorporate antimetabolites into normal metabolic processes necessary for cell growth and division, but the small differences in chemical structure cause inhibition of growth and cell division, thus initiating cell death. Antimetabolites are used to treat chronic leukemias as well as tumors of the breast, ovary, and the gastrointestinal tract. Most antimetabolites are cell cycle specific and act in the S phase of the cell cycle. Major toxicities occur in the hematopoietic and gastrointestinal systems. Table 19-2 lists antimetabolites by their parent chemical analogue.

Antitumor Antibiotics

Antitumor antibiotics interfere with DNA by stopping enzymes needed for cell division or by altering the membranes that surround cells (Box 19-1). These agents are cell cycle nonspecific. Major toxicities occur in the hematopoietic, gastrointestinal, reproductive, and cardiovascular systems. The anthracycline antibiotics are toxic to the heart, leading to cardiomyopathy.

Vinca Alkaloids (Mitotic Inhibitors)

Vinca alkaloids are also referred to as plant alkaloids because they were originally derived from the periwinkle plant Vinca rosea. They are inhibitors of tubulin, which forms the microtubules of the spindle apparatus. The spindle apparatus is necessary for

TABLE 19-2 Antimetabolites Classed by Analogue of a Parent Chemical

SUBCLASS	DRUG
FOLIC ACID ANALOGUES	methotrexate (MTX), (Amethopterin, Folex, Mexate, Rheumatrox)
	pemetrexed (Alimta)
PYRIMIDINE ANALOGUES	5-fluorouracil (5-FU) (Adrucil, Efudex, Fluoroplex)
	floxuridine (FUDR)
	capecitabine (Xeloda)
	cytosine arabinoside (Cytarabine, Cytosar, ARA-C)
PURINE ANALOGUES	6-Mecaptapurin (6-MP) (Purinethol) 6-Thioguanine (6-TG) (Thioguanine)
	cladribine (Leustatin)
	gemcitabine (Gemzar)
	fludarabine (Fludara)
	deoxycoformycin/pentostatin (Nipent)
	hydroxyurea

BOX 19-1 Antitumor Antibiotics That Are Derivatives

Generic Name (Trade Name)

bleomycin (Blenoxane)

dactinomycin (Actinomycin D, Cosmegen)

mitomycin-C (Mutamycin)

mithramycin (Mithracin)

daunorubicin (Daunomycin, Cerubidine)

doxorubicin (Adriamycin)

idarubicin (Idamycin)

mitoxantrone (Novantrone)

procarbazine (Matulane)

valrubicin (Valstar)

TABLE 19-3 Examples of Monoclonal Antibodies Used in Cancer Therapy

GENERIC NAME	TRADE NAME	CANCER
rituximab	Rituxan	Non-Hodgkin's lymphoma, chronic lymphocytic leukemia, rheumatoid arthritis
alemtuzumab	Campath	Chronic lymphocytic leukemia
cetuximab	Erbitux	Metastatic colon cancer, head and neck cancer
denileukin	Ontak, Diftitox	Recurrent T-cell lymphoma
levamisole	Ergamisol	Stage III colon cancer
trastuzumab	Herceptin	Metastatic breast cancer
interferon alpha-2a, alpha-2b	Roferon-A, Intron A	chronic hepatitis C, hairy cell leukemia, and AIDS-related Kaposi's sarcoma
interleukin-2 aldesleukin	Proleukin	Metastatic melanoma and renal cell cancer

mitosis. Most plant alkaloids are cell cycle specific, acting in the M phase. Cells unable to complete metaphase die. Major toxicities occur in the hematopoietic, integumentary, neurological, and reproductive systems. Frequently used plant alkaloids include vinblastine sulfate (Velbane, Velsar, VLB); vincristine (Oncovin, Vincasar, PFS, Vincrex); vinorelbine (Navelbine); and taxanes (mitotic inhibitors).

Taxanes

Taxanes also affect the spindle apparatus. In normal cell growth, microtubules are formed when a cell starts dividing. Once the cell stops dividing, the microtubules are broken down or destroyed. Taxanes stop the microtubules from breaking down, and cancer cells become so clogged with microtubules that they cannot grow and divide. Paclitaxel is an example of the taxanes; it is used for advanced ovarian cancer and as an initial treatment for ovarian cancer in combination with cisplatin. The U.S. Food and Drug Administration (FDA) has also approved paclitaxel for the treatment of breast cancer that recurs within 6 months after chemotherapy or that has spread to nearby lymph nodes or other parts of the body. Paclitaxel is also used for other cancers, such as AIDS-related Kaposi's sarcoma and lung cancer. Taxanes include paclitaxel (Taxol), albumin-bound paclitaxel, and docetaxel (Taxotere).

Biological Response Modifiers

Biological response modifiers (BRMs) are naturally occurring substances that stimulate and enhance the body's response to disease, infection, and cancer. Several have been synthesized in pharmaceutical laboratories and are available commercially. BRMs stimulate the patient's immune system to protect the body from foreign substances such as tumor cells. BRMs include substances such as monoclonal antibodies and cytokines, including tumor necrosis factor (TNF).

Tumor necrosis factor (TNF) is a natural substance produced by many cells in response to the presence of tumor cells and infectious agents. It is a key mediator of inflammation. TNF exerts a direct cytotoxic effect on tumor cells.

Monoclonal antibodies are agents that are able to target specific antigens (Table 19-3). Certain tumor cells have unique antigens on the cell surface that lend themselves to this type of therapy. Once the antibody has attached to the tumor cell, the immune system is stimulated to destroy the cell. The first monoclonal antibodies came from mouse (murine) cells. They are designated by the suffix *-omab*. Because they came from mouse cells, they tended to be immunogenic in humans. This led to the development of chimeric (suffix *-ximab*) and humanized (suffix *-zumab*) antibodies, which are modifications of the murine antibodies. Human monoclonal antibodies (suffix *-mumab*) are fully human antibodies.

Cytokines are naturally occurring substances secreted by immune system cells. They act as signals between cells. Cytokines can strengthen the activities of the immune system, altering the growth and metastatic ability of tumor cells. Cytokines include interferons, interleukins, colony-stimulating factors (CSF), and erythropoietin.

Interferons are proteins produced by the body in response to biological agents such as viruses and tumor cells. Interferons inhibit the growth and division of cancer cells. They also stimulate **tumor-associated antigens** on tumor cell surfaces, making the tumor cell more apparent to the immune system. Interferon-alpha is useful in treating lymphomas and renal tumors.

Interleukins are regulatory substances produced by lymphocytes and monocytes. Interleukins demonstrate a wide range of biological effects that enhance the immune system response. *Colony-stimulating factors* are naturally occurring proteins that regulate the growth and development of blood cells. CSFs bind to the surface of hematopoietic stem cells, stimulating them to proliferate and differentiate. For example, G-CSF or GCSF (granulocyte colony-stimulating factor) increases the number of granulocytes or neutrophils, white blood cells that are vital to fighting infection. As a result, patients can better tolerate standard treatment protocols and may be able to tolerate higher doses of chemotherapeutic agents, which may improve outcomes.

Erythropoietin is another substance that is naturally produced by the kidneys in response to decreased red cell production or hypoxia. Erythropoietin stimulates the bone marrow to produce more red blood cells and to speed up red blood cell maturation. Laboratory-manufactured erythropoietin can be given to patients experiencing anemia as a result of chemotherapy.

Additional biological agents and approaches such as *vaccine therapy* are based on the idea that there are tumor-associated antigens on the cell surface of tumors not found on normal cells. Potentially, the body's immune system can be taught, through immunization, to recognize these tumor-specific antigens, and to activate the immune system to prevent the recurrence of cancer.

Gene therapy is a technique in which new genetic material is inserted into a patient's cell to correct an inborn genetic error or to introduce a new biological function to the cell. In the future, gene therapy may be useful in cancer treatment if it can be proven to improve patient immune response.

Hormone Therapy

Hormone therapy is most often used in breast and prostate cancer therapy because these tissues are dependent on hormone stimulation for growth and development. Hormone therapy includes antiestrogen therapy, luteinizing hormone–releasing hormone (LHRH) agonists, glucocorticoids, and some progestins.

Tamoxifen is the most widely used *antiestrogen therapy*. It binds to the estrogen receptor and exerts either estrogenic or antiestrogenic effects, depending on the specific organ. Tamoxifen is the most widely studied antiestrogenic treatment in breast cancer. It competes for binding at the estrogen receptor in breast tissue, causing an antiestrogenic effect. It is prescribed as **adjuvant therapy** (additional treatment) of early-stage breast cancer, for therapy of advanced breast cancer, and for the prevention of breast cancer in high-risk patients.

Luteinizing hormone–releasing hormone agonists cause tonic stimulation of the LHRH receptor that results in decreased output of luteinizing hormone (LH) by the anterior pituitary. Decreased LH production results in decreased elaboration of testosterone by the testicle, resulting in decreased tumor growth. Examples are leuprolide (Leupron) and goserelin (Zoladex).

Commonly used *glucocorticoids,* including prednisone and dexamethasone, suppress mitosis in lymphocytes. Glucocorticoid therapy can be used to treat acute leukemia in children as well as lymphoma in both adults and children. They can also be used to limit edema related to tumors, especially those of the brain and spinal cord. Prolonged use of glucocorticoids requires tapering the dose because abrupt discontinuation can precipitate adrenal crises.

Progestins have been used in breast and endometrial cancer. They are also used to stimulate appetite in cachectic patients. Examples of these medications include hydroxyprogesterone, medroxyprogesterone, and megestrol (Table 19-4).

Chemoprotective Agents

Chemoprotective agents are a class of drugs that are designed to protect the body against specific toxic effects of chemotherapy. For example, dexrazoxane (Zinecard) is a cardioprotective agent used in combination with the antitumor antibiotic drug

TABLE 19-4	Commonly Used Hormones in Cancer Treatments
HORMONE	**DRUGS**
ESTROGENS	diethylstilbestrol (Stilbestrol, Stilphostrol)
	estradiol, estrogen (many brands)
	esterified estrogens (Estratab, Menest)
	estramustine (Emcyt)
ANTIESTROGENS	tamoxifen (Nolvadex)
	toremifene (Fareston)
AROMATASE INHIBITORS	anastrozole (Arimidex)
	letrozole (Femara)
PROGESTINS	17-OH-progesterone (many brands)
	medroxyprogesterone (many brands)
	megestrol acetate (Megace)
GNRH AGONISTS	goserelin (Zoladex)
	leuprolide (Lupron)
ANDROGENS	testosterone (many brands)
	methyltestosterone (many brands)
	fluoxymesterone (Android-F, Halotestin)
ANTIANDROGENS	flutamide (Eulexin)
	bicalutamide (Casodex)
	nilutamide (Nilandron)

doxorubicin to help prevent cardiotoxicity. Another example of chemoprotection is amifostine (Ethyol), a cytoprotective agent used to reduce potential renal toxicity associated with cumulative doses of platinum-containing agents (e.g., cisplatin). It can also be used to reduce the incidence of neutropenia-related fever and infection induced by DNA-binding chemotherapeutic agents, including alkylating agents (e.g., cyclophosphamide; see formulary list at the beginning of the chapter for others).

PROTOCOLS FOR ADMINISTERING CYTOTOXIC AGENTS

Cancer chemotherapy dosing is more an art than an exact science because the majority of cytotoxic agents being administered are being done so at a recommended fixed dosage that is finalized based either body surface area (BSA), weight, Creatinine Clearance (CRCl) or other adjustments made for each patient. Because these compounds have a narrow therapeutic index and lack a simple means by which to monitor treatment effects, they are ideal candidates for therapeutic drug monitoring programs. There are too many patient, drug, and treatment variables, making it difficult to identify only one correct standardized protocol. There are many cytotoxic drug protocols, but the following are the most common themes in their approaches.

Combination Chemotherapy

Combination chemotherapy involves using two or more drugs simultaneously. The development of this strategy has accounted for major advances in cancer treatment. Combining drugs that act in different phases of the cell cycle increases the number of cells exposed to cytotoxic effects. Tumors in their early stages have a high growth fraction, allowing for rapid growth. Over a period of time the number of cancer cells grows and the tumor burden increases. This results in a decreased supply of nutrients, causing the tumor's growth fraction to decrease.

Combinations of drugs are often effective in patients with large tumors containing a small number of cells that are reproducing. Cell cycle specific (CCS) and cell cycle–non-specific drugs (CCNS) are given in combination, because the CCS drugs reduce the tumor growth factor and CCNS drugs help to reduce the tumor burden. By killing a high proportion of tumor cells, the CCNS drug stimulates the remaining tumor cells to enter the cell reproduction cycle, making them vulnerable to CCS agents. Combining drugs allows for the use of lower doses of each component. This often decreases the incidence and severity of side effects of therapy. Combining agents also decreases the development of drug resistance. An example of an agent in this class is filgrastim, also known as a granulocyte-colony stimulating factor (GCSF). It is indicated in adult and pediatric patients receiving mylosuppressive therapy and in whom filgrastim can be used to decrease neutropenia and fever during acute myelocytic leukemia induction or in patients receiving **consolidation therapy** (treatment given after the initial therapy to kill any remaining cancer cells).

The number of chemotherapy courses or cycles varies, depending on the type of cancer, the cytotoxic drugs used, and the patient's response to therapy. Combination-therapy protocols are usually described by abbreviations that use the first letter of each drug in the protocol. For example, CAF (cyclophosphamide + adriamycin + fluorouracil) is a combination protocol used to treat breast cancer.

Administering Chemotherapy

Cytotoxic agents can be administered in a variety of ways (Table 19-5). The term *parenteral* is used to describe drugs given intravenously, intramuscularly, or subcutaneously. The intravenous route is most often used. Intramuscular and subcutaneous injections are used less often, because many drugs can be very irritating or even destroy skin or muscle tissues. Giving cytotoxic drugs via an IV route distributes the drugs quickly throughout the body.

There are several types of *vascular access devices* (VADs). The choice of which device to use is often based on determining the length of time it will be needed. Peripheral devices can be used for several weeks. Surgically implanted devices are nearly permanent. *Midline catheter* is a VAD that is not inserted as far as a peripherally inserted central catheter (PICC). It may be used for intermediate length therapy when a regular peripheral IV is not advisable or available. PICC lines provide continuous access to a peripheral vein in the arm for several weeks or longer.

TABLE 19-5	Routes of Administration
Oral	By mouth
Topical	On the surface of the skin as a cream or lotion
Intravenous	Into a vein or IV
Intramuscularly	Into a muscle or IM
Subcutaneous	Under the skin or SQ
Intra-arterial	Into an artery
Intrathecal	Into the central nervous system via the cerebrospinal fluid
Intrapleural	Into the chest cavity
Intraperitoneal	Into the abdominal cavity
Intravesical	Into the bladder
Intralesional	Into the tumor

Tunneled central venous catheter is a type of VAD with multiple lumens, surgically placed in a large central vein, with a catheter tunneled under the skin. Implantable devices include a port of plastic, stainless steel, or titanium with a silicone septum attached to a catheter surgically placed under the skin of the chest or arm in a large or central vein. The port can be accessed with a needle when cytotoxic drugs need to be given.

Intravesical chemotherapy is especially effective for early stage bladder cancer. Each treatment involves the placement of a urinary catheter to give the drug into the bladder. The drug is retained in the bladder for several hours and then drained.

Intrapleural and intraperitoneal routes of administering chemotherapy are useful for some people with mesothelioma (cancer that involves the lining of the lung), ovarian cancer that has spread to the peritoneum, and lung or breast cancers that have spread to the pleura.

Intraperitoneal chemotherapy is given through a catheter that is specially designed to remove or add large amounts of fluid from or into the peritoneum through an implanted port. *Intrathecal chemotherapy* is given directly into the cerebrospinal fluid to reach cancer cells in the central nervous system. Most chemotherapy drugs that are given intravenously are unable to cross the **blood-brain barrier**—a special characteristic of the capillary walls of the brain that prevents potentially harmful substances from moving from the bloodstream to the brain and cerebrospinal fluid. Intrathecal chemotherapy may be done via a lumbar puncture or through a special reservoir called an Ommaya shunt or Ommaya reservoir that is designed to deliver chemotherapy medication directly into the cerebrospinal fluid. It is placed into the skull with access to the ventricles (spaces inside the brain filled with cerebrospinal fluid).

Many cytotoxic agents can cause severe tissue damage if an intravenous needle or catheter delivers the drug into tissues rather than into the bloodstream. **Extravasation** is a term used when a drug infiltrates into local tissues. In some instances, locally applied antidotes may help minimize the effects of infiltration. **Irritants** are drugs that can cause a short-lived and localized/limited cellular damage to a vein. **Vesicants** are drugs that cause severe redness, blistering, and severe tissue damage (chemical cellulites) at an injection site, and it be may severe enough to require skin grafting (Table 19-6). Symptoms of damage due to vesicants may start to appear 6 to 12 hours after administration. To avoid infiltration with vesicant drugs, the larger veins of the arm are used for intravenous administration.

Exposure to cytotoxic drugs poses a potential health risk to personnel who handle, administer, and dispose of these drugs. Potential routes of exposure include both direct and indirect contact. Examples of direct contact include skin and mucous membrane contact and absorption, inhalation, or ingestion. Indirect contact can occur through handling body fluids and excreta of clients who have received cytotoxic drugs. Clinicians involved with preparing, administering, or caring for patients who are receiving cytotoxic drugs take special precautions to decrease their risk of exposure.

Adverse Reactions of Cytotoxic Drugs

Although chemotherapy is given to kill cancer cells, it also can damage normal cells. The cells most likely to be damaged are normal cells that are rapidly dividing, such as bone marrow cells, hair follicle cells, and cells in the reproductive and gastrointestinal tracts. Damage ranges from mild to severe. The toxicity of the medications is dependent on the dosage and route given. Most of the symptoms such as nausea and hair loss are reversible. Some cytotoxic medications have cumulative toxicity limiting lifetime dosage. Side effects are different for each chemotherapy drug. Patients have differing abilities to tolerate certain side effects.

Adverse Effects on Hematological System

The hematological or hematopoietic system is responsible for producing new blood cells. The bone marrow in all the bones of the body contains stem cells, the precursors to the main blood components. Stem cells are able to reproduce and differentiate into red blood cells, white blood cells, and platelets, depending on the body's need for cell replacement. Because the cells of the bone marrow are almost always in some phase of cell division, many cytotoxic drugs damage bone marrow stem cells. Depressed bone marrow function is called myelosuppression. It is one of the most common side effects of chemotherapy. The main effects of myelosuppression are anemia (less than normal number of red blood cells), leukopenia (less than normal number of white blood cells), and thrombocytopenia (less than normal number of platelets).

As blood cells wear out, they are constantly being replaced by the bone marrow stem cells. Following chemotherapy, worn-out blood cells are no longer being replaced. The drugs temporarily prevent formation of new blood cells by the bone marrow stem cells. Because the drugs do not destroy the cells in circulation, decreases in blood cell counts do not occur immediately after chemotherapy. Normally, white blood cells have an approximate 6-hour life span, platelets live for about 10 days, and red blood cells have a life span of 120 days.

The lowest count that blood cell levels fall to is called the **nadir**. The nadir for each blood cell type will occur at different times, but usually WBCs and platelets reach their nadir within 7 to 14 days. At this point, patients are most susceptible to infection and bleeding. Red blood cells (RBCs) live longer and will not reach a nadir for several weeks after a cycle of medication. Another blood test, the absolute neutrophil count (ANC), refers to the percentage of neutrophils plus the number of cells that will become neutrophils multiplied by the white blood cell count. If the ANC is below 2,000, the patient is considered neutropenic. If the ANC is between 1,000 and 15,000, there is a slight risk (low-risk) of infection. If the ANC is between 500 and 1,000, there is a moderate risk of infection. Finally, if the ANC is below 500 there is a high risk of infection.

Anemia

Red blood cells, or erythrocytes, carry oxygen from the lungs to the tissues and transport carbon dioxide back to the lungs. There are normally between 4 and 6 million red blood cells per milliliter of blood. The hematocrit is a measurement of the percentage of total blood volume occupied by red blood cells. A normal hematocrit ranges between 36% and 42%. Hemoglobin is the red pigment in RBCs; its function is to carry oxygen. Normal hemoglobin is between 12 to 16 grams per deciliter. Anemia caused by chemotherapy is temporary. Patients with anemia will most often complain of fatigue and dyspnea on exertion. A CBC will show a reduction in red blood cell count and decreased hemoglobin and hematocrit levels. Profound anemia can result in hypotension and shock.

Transfusions of packed red blood cells may be needed when a patient's hematocrit and hemoglobin fall too low. Transfusion therapy may be required until the bone marrow has recovered its normal ability to produce more blood cells. Because blood transfusions have some risks, this procedure is used only if there are serious symptoms. An option for treating anemia caused by chemotherapy is giving erythropoietin. Erythropoietin, a therapy

TABLE 19-6	Vesicants and Irritants That Can Lead to Extravasation*	
VESICANTS	**IRRITANTS**
5-FU	bleomycin
dactinomycin	carboplatin
doxorubicin	carmustin
idarubicin	cisplatin
mechlorethamine	dacarbazine
mitomycin-c	daunorubicin
mitoxantrone	doxorubicin
paclitaxel	liposome
streptozocin	etoposide
teniposide	ifosfamide
vinblastine	streptozocin
vincristine	teniposide
vindesine	thiotepa
vinorelbine	vinorelbine

Some agents cause both.

usually reserved for patients with long-standing anemia, can stimulate RBC production by bone marrow stem cells, thus relieving symptoms and reducing the need for blood transfusions. Patients with anemia should be encouraged to eat foods that are rich in iron, vitamins, and minerals. They should modify and pace activities to get sufficient sleep and rest.

Leukopenia

White blood cells help the body resist infection. Bacteria can invade many areas of the body, including the skin, respiratory tract, oral cavity, sinuses, and perianal area. A normal WBC count ranges between 4,000 and 10,000 per milliliter of blood. An overall decrease in the total white blood cell count is known as leukopenia.

Leukocytes are divided into two main categories, granulocytes and agranulocytes, depending on the presence or absences of granules in the cell's cytoplasm. Neutrophils, eosinophils, and basophils are granulocytes. Agranulocytes include lymphocytes and monocytes.

Granulocytes, especially neutrophils, provide an important defense against infections and are the most numerous type of WBC. The normal range of neutrophils is between 2,500 and 6,000 cells per milliliter. A lower than normal number of neutrophils is referred to as neutropenia. Neutropenia is the most common factor that puts people with cancer at risk of potentially life-threatening infection. A patient with an absolute neutrophil count of 1,000 or less is considered to be neutropenic. Patients with a neutrophil count of 500 or less are severely neutropenic and at high risk of infection.

The myelosuppressive effects of a cycle of cytotoxic drugs can be predicted by knowing the type of agents used, the dose, and the mode of administration. Neutropenia is most severe with the use of cell cycle–specific drugs, particularly those that are active in the S and M phases. However, cell cycle–nonspecific drugs can have a delayed and prolonged effect on the bone marrow. The use of high-dose or combination regimens can cause persistent nadirs because of intense damage to the stem cell population. If WBC counts are very low, the patient may be given antibiotics as a preventative measure. Cancer patients with neutropenia (ANC less than 500 or expected to be so within 24 hours) and a fever (defined as being greater than 38.5°C or greater than 101.5°F) is usually treated with broad-spectrum antibiotics and colony-stimulating factors in a hospital until neutrophils begin to recover and they are infection free.

Growth factors, granulocyte-macrophage colony-stimulating factor, and granulocyte colony-stimulating factor are used to stimulate production of granulocytes and macrophages. These drugs may be given the day after chemotherapy. In some situations, clinicians may prescribe growth factors to prevent the white count from falling too low, allowing chemotherapy to be given on schedule.

Thrombocytopenia

Thrombocytes are critical for maintaining homeostasis and are vital to the formation of blood clots. The normal range for platelet counts is between 150,000 and 450,000 per milliliter of blood.

The term for a low platelet count is *thrombocytopenia*. Symptoms of thrombocytopenia include easy bruising and abnormal bleeding. Patients may also develop small (1 to 2 mm) red or purple spots called petechiae. Sites of bleeding can include the skin, mucous membranes, gastrointestinal system, genitourinary system, respiratory system, and the brain. Chemotherapy can depress the platelet count and drugs containing acetylsalicylic acid (aspirin) or NSAIDS can worsen the potential for thrombocytopenia while increasing the risk of gastrointestinal bleeding.

Although thrombocytopenia resulting from chemotherapy is temporary, it can result in serious and potentially life-threatening blood loss. If platelet counts are very low (below 10,000), or if a person with moderately low counts has greater than normal bleeding, platelet transfusions may be given. Transfused platelets last only a few days, and some people who have received multiple platelet transfusions can develop an immune reaction that destroys donor platelets. A platelet growth factor may be given to people with severe thrombocytopenia to decrease the need for platelet transfusions.

Patients with thrombocytopenia should postpone any invasive medical or surgical procedures if possible and should avoid the use of razors, nail clippers, and scissors. These patients should be encouraged to use stool softeners to avoid straining, which can cause rectal tearing and bleeding. They should be encouraged to eat a high-fiber diet and drink plenty of fluids to avoid constipation.

Adverse Effects on Integumentary System

The integumentary system comprises the skin and its appendages, including hair and nails. It is the organ system that protects the body from external damage, including infection and sun injury (i.e., severe sunburn). The integumentary system is composed of rapidly dividing cells that are sensitive to cytotoxic medications. One of the most psychologically devastating side effects of chemotherapy is the development of hair loss, or alopecia. Chemotherapy affects the rapidly growing hair follicle cells. The hair may become brittle and break off at the surface of the scalp, or it may simply fall out from the hair follicle. Alopecia is individual. Some people may lose all their hair, whereas others may experience hair thinning. Loss of eyebrows, eyelashes, pubic hair, and body hair is usually less severe, because the growth is less active in these hair follicles than in the scalp.

The extent of hair loss depends on which drugs are given, drug doses, and the length of treatment. Hair loss is almost always temporary. Unlike some other side effects of chemotherapy, hair loss is not life threatening. However, it is often extremely distressing to cancer patients because hair loss is often a visible, constant reminder of cancer and has a severe negative impact on body image. Hair loss usually begins within 2 weeks after chemotherapy begins. After chemotherapy is completed, hair regrowth may take 3 to 5 months. When hair grows back, the color or texture may be different.

Radiation Recall Reactions

The synergistic effects of both radiation and chemotherapy on some body tissues, such as the skin, lung, heart, and gastrointestinal tract, can cause radiation enhancement and recall. Symptoms may include skin reddening, blistering, hyperpigmentation, edema, exfoliation, and ulceration. Enhancement reactions may occur if chemotherapy is given within a week of radiation therapy. Radiation recall reactions or radiation recall dermatitis is an inflammatory reaction that occurs in a previously irradiated area precipitated by certain drugs. These reactions may happen within weeks to months to years following radiation exposure. Recall reactions encompass a wide range of clinical presentations from mild erythema to necrosis and ulceration. In addition to the cutaneous findings, recall reactions have been reported in the oral or genital mucosa, larynx, lungs, gastrointestinal tract, and also the central nervous, lymphatic, and musculoskeletal systems. The onset of recall reactions vary considerably as well, with intravenous medications causing recall dermatitis in a few minutes to 14 days (median onset being 3 days) and oral medications causing them typically within 2 days to 2 months (median onset being 8 days). The vast majority of cases have been associated with the administration of chemotherapy medications that contain actinomycin D, bleomycin, cytarabine, doxorubicin, daunorubicin, idarubicin, hydroxyurea, lomustine, methotrexate, paclitaxel, and vinblastine.

Acral Erythema

Acral erythema, also known as hand-foot syndrome, can occur with high doses of drugs such as cytarabine, methotrexate, 5-fluorouracil, hydroxyurea, capecitabine, and etoposide. Symptoms include burning, swelling, tingling, and a rash (erythema) on the palms and fingers of the hands and the soles of the feet. The initial rash can progress to painful blistering of the affected areas. Patients should be advised to keep their feet elevated and receive proper instruction on foot hygiene.

Adverse Effects on the Gastrointestinal System

The cells of the gastrointestinal tract are metabolically very active and are, therefore, quite susceptible to the damaging effects of cytotoxic drugs. Toxic effects to the gastrointestinal system can cause life-threatening infection, malnutrition, and fluid and electrolyte disturbances. Commonly occurring chemotherapy-induced toxicities affecting the gastrointestinal system include anorexia, stomatitis, nausea and vomiting, constipation, and diarrhea.

Anorexia

Most chemotherapy drugs cause some degree of anorexia. Anorexia can be mild, or it may lead to cachexia, a severe form of malnutrition. Cancer treatments and the cancer itself can alter the way some food tastes. Taste changes may include a dislike for or an increased desire for meat and sweet foods, a dislike of foods with bitter tastes, tomatoes and tomato products, and a metallic or medicinal taste in the mouth. These changes occur because chemotherapy drugs can alter the taste receptor cells in the mouth that are responsible for flavor sensations. Decreased appetite is generally temporary and returns when chemotherapy is finished. Medications can be prescribed to help improve appetite.

Stomatitis (Mucositis)

Stomatitis, also called *mucositis*, refers to the development of inflammation and sores in the mouth occurring in approximately 40% of cancer patients. Similar changes in the throat or the esophagus are called *pharyngitis* and *esophagitis*. Stomatitis, pharyngitis, and esophagitis can lead to bleeding, painful ulcerations, and potentially life-threatening infections. The first signs of mouth sores occur when the lining of the mouth appears pale and dry. Later, the mouth, gums, and throat feel sore and become red and inflamed. The tongue may be coated and swollen, leading to difficulty swallowing, eating, and talking. Mouth, throat, and esophageal sores are temporary and usually develop 5 to 14 days after receiving chemotherapy.

Other alterations in the oral mucosa include dryness of the mouth (xerostomia), unusual taste perceptions, and decreased taste perception. Stomatitis can lead to life-threatening problems such as sepsis and malnutrition. Factors that increase the incidence of stomatitis include the type of cancer, the patient's age and oral health, and the types of drugs used. Drugs most commonly associated with stomatitis include antimetabolites, such as 5-fluorouracil and methotrexate, and the antitumor antibiotics, such as doxorubicin and actinomycin. Patients should have instruction in good oral hygiene. If mild stomatitis occurs, mouth care should be done every 4 hours around the clock. Mouth care should be done every 2 hours, day and night, if the patient develops severe stomatitis/mucositis. It is important to note that stomatitis is not just limited to the mouth area; its sores, or ulcers, can occur anywhere along the gastrointestinal tract.

Nausea and Vomiting

Nausea and vomiting are extremely distressing side effects of cancer chemotherapy treatment. Approximately 70% to 80% of patients receiving cytotoxic drugs have some degree of nausea and vomiting. Chemotherapy drugs cause nausea and vomiting because they both irritate the lining of the stomach and duodenum and stimulate nerves that lead to the vomiting center in the brain. Vomiting can be acute, occurring within minutes to hours after chemotherapy, or delayed, developing or continuing for 24 hours after chemotherapy and sometimes lasting for days.

Anticipatory emesis is a conditioned or learned aversion to chemotherapy experienced by approximately 10% to 44% of cancer patients. A patient with anticipatory emesis may start vomiting before chemotherapy. Acute emesis usually begins shortly after treatment. Delayed emesis persists for 1 to 4 days after chemotherapy. Delayed emesis is usually associated with high doses of cisplatin and some combination chemotherapy regimens. Protracted nausea and vomiting can severely affect the patient's food intake and nutritional status.

Although it is not possible to predict the onset, severity, or duration of nausea and vomiting for individual patients, the following drugs are notable for being emetogenic (inducting nausea): cisplatin, carmustine, dacarbazine, daunorubicin, actinomycin-D, doxorubicin, mechlorethamine, epirubicin, streptozocin, idarubicin, carboplatin, cytarabine, cyclophosphamide, ifosfamide, and lomustine.

Some patient characteristics increase the potential for nausea and vomiting. Younger patients tend to have more nausea and vomiting than older patients. Females, especially those who had nausea and vomiting with their pregnancies, are at higher risk than males. Patients who are prone to motion sickness or have had symptoms with previous rounds of chemotherapy tend to have worse symptoms than others.

The most effective intervention for nausea and vomiting is prevention, including using both drugs and behavioral interventions. Behavioral approaches include guided imagery, relaxation, hypnosis, and distraction. Recent advances in antiemetic (antivomiting) therapy include drugs that can decrease the incidence and distress associated with nausea and vomiting. Serotonin receptor antagonists are an important class of antiemetic drugs that provide effective emetic control with minimal side effects. These drugs, given before chemotherapy, include dolasetron (Anzemet), granisetron (Kytril), ondansetron (Zofran), and tropisetron (Navoban). Many other drugs are used alone or in combination to prevent or decrease nausea and vomiting.

Constipation

Constipation affects half of people with cancer and almost all of those with advanced disease. Constipation can be caused by the cancer itself, changes in food and fluid intake, decreases in activity, and by some cytotoxic drugs and other drugs used to treat cancer symptoms. Agents that commonly produce constipation are the vinca alkaloid drugs, vincristine and vinblastine, opioids given for pain relief, and antiemetics, particularly the serotonin receptor antagonists.

Diarrhea

Diarrhea is more common than constipation and can cause potentially serious side effects, including dehydration, electrolyte imbalances, and malnutrition. Diarrhea occurs in 75% of people who receive chemotherapy due to damage to the rapidly dividing cells of the gastrointestinal tract. Cytotoxic drugs often associated with causing diarrhea are 5-fluorouracil, methotrexate, docetaxel, and actinomycin-D. Factors affecting diarrhea include the drugs given, the drug dose, and the length of treatment. Patients who have a stomach tumor, are lactose intolerant, or are receiving radiation therapy in conjunction with chemotherapy have an increased incidence of diarrhea. Diarrhea is managed by pharmacological interventions with anticholinergic drugs and opioids.

Adverse Effects on the Cardiovascular System

Certain chemotherapy drugs can cause heart damage or cardiotoxicity. Young children and adults over age 50 are at an increased risk for cardiotoxicity. Signs and symptoms of cardiotoxicity may range from subtle changes on an electrocardiogram (ECG) to life-threatening problems such as cardiac arrhythmias, congestive heart failure, and ischemia. Patients may complain of increasing fatigue or shortness of breath with mild exertion. They may also report a dry cough and an inability to lay flat without becoming short of breath. On physical exam they may demonstrate signs of fluid overload, including peripheral edema and jugular venous distention (JVD). Their pulse may be fast and irregular. A chest x-ray may show an enlarged heart (cardiomegaly).

Cytotoxic drugs associated with causing cardiotoxicity include dactinomycin, Dapacin, doxorubicin, cyclophosphamide, 5-fluororuracil, and paclitaxel. The prescribing information for cytotoxic drugs lists the maximum dose that should be given to avoid such adverse effects as cardiotoxicity. Because of its cardiotoxicity, the maximum lifetime dose of doxorubicin is 550 mg per meter squared. Doses above this limit significantly increase the risk of cardiotoxicity. The new cardioprotectant drug, dexrazoxane (Zinecard), may be given to help decrease the effects of cardiac toxicity. The maximum cumulative dose is reduced if the patient has received or is currently receiving radiation therapy to the mediastinum or is also receiving cyclophosphamide therapy. Patients who have had past radiation to the midchest area, have existing heart problems, uncontrolled high blood pressure, or who smoke, will be at increased risk of heart damage.

Prior to prescribing cardiotoxic chemotherapeutic agents, patients should be asked specifically about their cardiac history. A history of chest pain, dyspnea upon exertion, and the presence of fatigue should be noted. A physical examination should focus on the circulatory system, including heat sounds, blood pressure, and peripheral pulses. The presence or absence of JVD and peripheral edema should be documented. The presence of any abnormal breath sound such as rales may indicate cardiac dysfunction.

A baseline ECG should be obtained prior to therapy. The ECG should be repeated at intervals throughout the course of therapy. For patients at high risk for pulmonary complications, a baseline assessment of pulmonary function (including chest x-ray, pulmonary function tests, and arterial blood gas analysis) should be obtained. These patients should undergo periodic assessment looking for signs of pulmonary toxicity, including a dry persistent cough, dyspnea, tachypnea, cyanosis, or rales.

Adverse Effects on the Neurological System

The nervous system regulates and maintains body function through stimuli reception and response. The brain and spinal cord compose the central nervous system. The peripheral nervous system (PNS) includes the motor and sensory nerves leading to and from the spinal cord, the cranial nerves, and the nerves of the autonomic nervous system. The cranial nerves, part of the peripheral nervous system, are connected directly to the brain and are important for movement and touch sensations of the head, face, and neck. Cranial nerves are also important for special senses of vision, hearing, taste, and smell.

Some cytotoxic drugs can cause changes in the central nervous system (CNS) and the PNS. Central nervous system toxicity can produce symptoms such as confusion, dizziness, and an unsteady gait. Toxicity to the PNS, which comprises the sensory and motor nerves, causes abnormal sensations known as paresthesias, including numbness and tingling of the hands and feet. Patients at high risk for neurotoxicity include patients who have received localized treatment to the central nervous system, including radiation to the brain and intrathecal administration of cytotoxic drugs. The use of vinca alkaloids is associated with neurological dysfunction. Patients with chronic kidney disease or who are also taking nephrotoxic medications such as aminoglycosides are at risk for neurotoxicity.

Adverse Effects on the Respiratory System

Some anticancer drugs are associated with causing significant damage to the respiratory system. Alveolitis, interstitial pneumonitis, and pulmonary fibrosis can occur, all of which can be precursors to life-threatening respiratory failure. The two cytotoxic agents that commonly cause pulmonary damage are bleomycin and busulfan. The pulmonary damage caused by bleomycin is dose-related. Patients who receive a cumulative dose of greater than 450 units have an increased risk of pulmonary toxicity. Other factors that increase the risk of pulmonary toxicity include having preexisting lung disease, age older than 60, renal dysfunction, smoking or smoking history, high-dose oxygen therapy, and radiation to the chest area. Primary signs and symptoms of chemotherapy-induced pulmonary toxicity include shortness of breath, difficulty breathing (dyspnea), and cough. Patients may develop tachypnea (increased respiratory rate) and abnormal breath sounds.

Adverse Effects on the Reproductive System

Because of the growth in numbers of cancer survivors, the effect of chemotherapy on male and female sexual function has become increasingly important. In addition, because many cytotoxic medications affect DNA, chemotherapy can be teratogenic, causing abnormal fetal structural development and leading to genetic mutations. Many agents can cause gonadal dysfunction leading to infertility. In males, chemotherapy-associated infertility results from the destruction of sperm-producing cells. Males over 13 years of age, who may wish to have children later in life, should be given the option of banking sperm. Depending on the drug used and the duration of treatment, some recovery of spermatogenesis after completion of therapy is believed to be possible. Most men on chemotherapy still have normal erections. Erections and sexual desire often decrease after a course of chemotherapy, but recur within several weeks. Some cytotoxic drugs, such as cis-platinum or vincristine, can permanently damage parts of the nervous system. These drugs may interfere with the nerves that control erection. Chemotherapy can sometimes affect sexual desire and erections by slowing down the amount of testosterone produced.

As a consequence of receiving chemotherapy, women may experience various degrees of gonadal dysfunction, including premature menopause. Patients may complain of vaginal irritation, dryness, and itching. They may experience pain with intercourse (dyspareunia) as a result of vaginal dryness and atrophy. These medications can cause amenorrhea, hot flushes, and sterility. Many chemotherapy drugs can either temporarily or permanently cause ovarian damage, reducing hormonal output affecting fertility and libido. Chemotherapy-associated infertility occurs from direct injury to the ova. Some women regain ovarian function after treatment, some do so with time, and some never do. Vaginal infections are common during chemotherapy, particularly in women taking steroids or the powerful antibiotics used to prevent bacterial infections. Flare-ups of genital herpes or genital warts may also occur during chemotherapy. Women over 30 years of age are less likely to regain ovarian function after chemotherapy. Although it is possible to conceive during chemotherapy, the toxicity of some drugs may cause birth defects.

Adverse Effects on the Urological System

Many of the breakdown products of chemotherapy drugs are excreted through the kidneys. These drug by-products can damage the kidneys, ureters, and bladder. Some of the cytotoxic agents known for their potential nephrotoxic effects are ifosfamide, cyclophosphamide, cisplatin, methotrexate, streptozocin, carmustine, and lomustine.

Symptoms of urinary tract dysfunction include dysuria, oliguria, and flank pain. Patients may develop hemorrhagic cystitis and complain about hematuria. Direct kidney damage resulting in renal dysfunctions will often present with an increased creatinine level. It is important to assess whether the patient is on other drugs that may also be nephrotoxic, such as aminoglycoside antibiotics. Alkalinizing the urine to a pH of more than 7 can minimize adverse effects of high-dose methotrexate. This helps prevent precipitate formation. Amifostine is a cytoprotective agent used to reduce potential renal toxicity associated with cumulative doses of platinum-containing medications such as cisplatin.

Prior to starting chemotherapy, patients should have baseline renal function tests. The dosing of many drugs is affected by creatinine clearance. Renal function tests should be closely monitored throughout the treatment process. Medication or dose adjustment may be required in the event of any signs of toxicity. Patients should be well hydrated either intravenously or by oral intake of fluids prior to receiving cytotoxic mediations. It is important to stay well hydrated and to maintain diuresis after receiving the medications. This can be complicated when patients are having nausea and vomiting.

Patients should be encouraged to report signs and symptoms of urinary toxicity, including dysuria, hematuria, urinary urgency, and flank pain. Providers should be reminded that common symptoms associated with chemotherapy such as fatigue, weakness, nausea, and vomiting are also symptoms of renal toxicity. Hemorrhagic cystitis may arise in those who undergo chemotherapy or radiation of the pelvic area or immune suppression as part of cancer therapy. This diffuse inflammation of the bladder, if temporary, can usually be resolved with antibiotics. Cyclophosphamide (Cytoxan) and ifosfamide (Ifex) are two of the Mustargen class agents known for causing hemorrhagic cystitis.

Adverse Hypersensitive Reactions to Cytotoxic Agents

Hypersensitivity reactions are common in patients receiving chemotherapy. Hypersensitivity reactions range from a mild localized skin reaction to severe anaphylaxis. Clinicians giving cytotoxic drugs that are associated with hypersensitivity reactions should know the symptoms of a reaction so they can anticipate symptoms and manage them quickly. When a patient develops a hypersensitivity reaction to a chemotherapeutic agent, the drug is usually stopped. The decision to use the drug again depends on the severity of the reaction, the treatment plan, and the availability of alternative drugs.

Long-Term Adverse Effects

Long-term side effects of chemotherapy depend on the specific drugs received and whether the patient has received other treatments, such as radiation therapy. Permanent damage to some organs and systems, such as the reproductive system, may not be apparent until after chemotherapy is finished. When young children receive chemotherapy for cancer treatment, it may affect their growth and development, including their ability to learn. The impact on a child's development varies, depending on the child's age, the specific drugs that are given, the dosage and length of treatment, and whether or not chemotherapy is used along with other types of treatment such as radiation.

Future Trends

Those who specialize in oncology realize that nearly all anticancer therapies are going to target cell proliferation and most will do so as nonspecific cell inhibitors. Thus, somewhere during the treatment regimen multidrug resistance is likely. Total elimination of malignant cells is not entirely possible with many tumors and cancers using recommended therapeutic doses, and thus the patient's immune response system must adequately deal with remaining cancer cells; in many cases it will not.

New approaches in the treatment of neoplasms will be developed as advances in the pathobiology of cancer are revealed so that better targeting of anticancer compounds can occur. Other research will likely bring solutions to the need for reversing anticancer drug resistance and for boosting or augmenting the body's immune system.

Patient and Family Education

- Hematological effects: Patients need to be taught about signs of infection such as fever, sore throat, new cough or shortness of breath, nasal congestion, burning during urination, shaking chills, redness, swelling, and warmth at the site of an injury. They should be advised to avoid people who have colds or any communicable diseases. Patients known to be neutropenic should be advised to avoid eating raw fruits and vegetables, handling fresh flowers or plants, or handling pet excrement due to the possibility of acquiring a fungal or bacterial infection. Additionally, hand hygiene and aseptic and isolation techniques are especially important for patients (due to their compromised immune systems) as well as caregivers and any professionals who have physical contact with patients. For example, neutropenic precautions are created and enforced by most institutions or care service organizations.

- Thrombocytopenia: Patients with thrombocytopenia should postpone any invasive medical or surgical procedures if possible. This would include surgery, dental extractions, and procedures requiring multiple venipunctures, or injections. These patients should be encouraged to use stool softeners and to avoid straining, which can cause rectal tearing and bleeding. They should be encouraged to eat a high-fiber diet and drink plenty of fluids to avoid constipation. Additionally, they should avoid things that can puncture the skin, such as scissors, nail clippers, razors, and hobby knives, and they should use a soft toothbrush.

- Hair and skin: Patients should be taught proper hair-care techniques, including using a mild shampoo, avoiding chemical hair treatments such as permanents or coloring, and avoiding using heated rollers and vigorous brushing. Wigs can be helpful in helping patients maintain self-esteem. Some cytotoxic drugs increase the risk of a painful photosensitivity reaction. Photosensitivity is a skin reaction characterized by exaggerated sunburn, accompanied by itching and stinging. Patients should be encouraged to avoid direct sunlight and use sunscreen (SPF 30 or greater). Patients should be instructed to wash the skin with mild soap using a soft cloth, to avoid vigorous rubbing of the skin, to use an electric razor for shaving, to apply sunscreen as appropriate. Mild detergents should be used to launder clothing.

- Gastrointestinal upset and stomatitis: Patients should be urged to eat high-protein, high-calorie foods. They may tolerate small, frequent meals better than large ones. Food supplements should be encouraged in the face of protein caloric malnutrition. To help with stomatitis there are mouthwashes that, if used two times a day, can help reduce risk. Brushing teeth frequently is also advised.

- Nausea: Patients should avoid eating for 2 hours prior to chemotherapy. They should avoid hot spicy foods because bland foods served cold or at room temperature are better tolerated. Small, light meals served frequently during the day not only help decrease nausea, but also help patients avoid malnutrition. Patients should also be reminded to ask for medicine when they believe they need it because not all nausea happens according to a dosage schedule.

- Constipation: Patients should be encouraged to increase intake of foods rich in fiber and bulk and to drink 8 to 10 glasses of water daily. They should establish a daily bowel program and remain as physically active as possible.

- Diarrhea: Patients with diarrhea should be instructed to eat a low-residue, high-protein, high-calorie diet, increase fluids, and avoid foods and substances such as spicy foods, beans, milk, caffeine, alcohol, and tobacco. They should rest and decrease activity during periods of diarrhea. Their fluid and electrolyte intake must compensate for losses. Intravenous replacement may be necessary.

- Cardiotoxicities: Patients should be advised to avoid alcohol and tobacco due to their stimulant effect on the heart muscle. They should be made aware of the symptoms of cardiac toxicities and adverse effects and the importance of reporting those symptoms as soon as they occur.

- Fatigue: Patients should be advised to get rest and sleep during the day as needed. Good nutrition and a realistic exercise program should be encouraged.

- Respiratory system: Patients should avoid smoking and exposure to respiratory irritants such as noxious gases and aerosol sprays.

■ Genitourinary system: All patients, both men and women, should take precautions and use some type of birth control if they are sexually active. They should be advised that reproduction after chemotherapy remains controversial because some cytotoxic drugs, in a laboratory setting, have been shown to cause birth defects and genetic mutations. Patients should void frequently when using some chemotherapy agents to prevent bladder toxicities such as hemorrhagic cystitis.

Implications for Special Populations

Pregnancy Implications

When prescribing for the pregnant female, clinicians should carefully consider their choice of drugs. Following is a selected list of drugs along with the assigned FDA Safety Category.

FDA PREGNANCY CATEGORY	DRUGS
B	None
C	None
D	**Alkylating Agents:** busulfan, ifosfamide, carboplatin, mechlorethamine hydrochloride, chlorambucil, melphalan, cisplatin, procarbazine, cyclophosphamide, thiotepa, dacarbazine, uracil
	Nitrosoureas: carmustine, lomustine, streptozocin
	Antimetabolites: 5-fluorouracil injection, 6 mercaptopurine, capecitabine, cytosine arabinoside, floxuridine, and fludarabine
	Antitumor antibiotics: dactinomycin, daunorubicin, doxorubicin, idarubicin, mitomycin-C, and mitoxantrone
	Plant Alkaloids: vinblastine, vincristine, and vinorelbine
	Taxanes: paclitaxel
	Hormones: tamoxifen

Pediatric Implications

The most common cancers in children are acute leukemias. However, because all cells in a child, including cancerous cells, are growing rapidly, children and adolescents usually respond quite well to chemotherapy (yet there are many cancers that do not) and also seem to tolerate the adverse effects better than do adults.

Geriatric Implications

The elderly typically have other diseases, such as diabetes, hypertension, blood disorders, and/or Parkinson's disease that are being treated concurrently with their treatments for cancer. Those diseases all play a role in the ability of the elderly to withstand the good as well as the adverse effects of chemotherapy. Among the geriatric population, it is not always feasible to reduce dosages to help ward off adverse effects. The clinician must choose agents and doses appropriate for the individual and not based only on the patient's age.

LEARNING EXERCISES

Case 1

Mrs. H is a moderately obese Latino woman who is being treated with lisinopril and hydrochlorothiazide for hypertension and Paxil for depression. She presents at your clinic complaining of "pain in my right breast and pain under my arm." A full work up and a mammogram reveal a mass, suggestive of malignancy, in the right quadrant of her breast. She has no history of having had a mammogram done before, and states there is no family history of breast cancer. She does have a history of tobacco use but quit smoking 8 years ago at age 40. A needle biopsy confirms the diagnosis of stage II breast cancer.

1. What adverse events will Mrs. H likely experience if she is given drug therapy?

2. What important information should Mrs. H be given regarding the use of chemotherapy for breast cancer?

Case 2

During a routine physical exam, Mr. G, a 40-year-old Caucasian obese male with a history of smoking, tells you about his father who was diagnosed with prostate cancer and recently died from it. He asks, "What are my chances of getting cancer, and what can I do about it?"

1. What would you say to him?

2. Where would you send Mr. G for unbiased help that he could understand in laypersons' language?

References

American Urological Association. (2009). Prostate-Specific Antigen Best Practice Statement: 2009 Update. Retrieved May 4, 2011, from www.auanet.org/content/guidelines-and-quality-care/clinical-guidelines.cfm

Centers for Disease Control and Prevention, National Cancer Institute, & North American Association of Central Cancer Registries. (n.d.). United States Cancer Statistics. 1999-2007 cancer incidence and mortality data. Retrieved May 4, 2011, from http://apps.nccd.cdc.gov/uscs

Skin Cancer Foundation. (n.d.). Skin Cancer Facts. Retrieved May 4, 2011, from www.skincancer.org/Skin-Cancer-Facts

Stern, R. S. (2010). Prevalence of a history of skin cancer in 2007: Results of an incidence-based model. *Archives of Dermatology, 146*(3), 279-282.

chapter 20

Drugs Used to Affect Women's Health

Monique Davis-Smith, Roberta Weintraut, Mona M. Sedrak

Key Terms

Abnormal uterine bleeding (AUB)

Amenorrhea

Combined oral contraceptives

Intravaginal ring

Iron deficiency anemia

Menorrhagia

Metrorrhagia

Monophasic oral contraceptives

Oligomenorrhea

Osteoporosis

Premenstrual dysphoric disorder

Premenstrual syndrome

Transdermal contraception

Triphasic oral contraceptives

CHAPTER FOCUS

This chapter discusses some of the most commonly encountered medications specific to women's health needs in primary care settings. This chapter also addresses how a woman's nutritional status, exercise habits, and tobacco and alcohol use are important assessments that are necessary when prescribing many drugs. Although it is impossible for this chapter to cover the full spectrum of pharmaceutical therapies for all medical conditions that are unique to women, it does provide an overview of certain pharmaceuticals commonly used by women and their special needs relative to uterine bleeding, contraception, anemia, osteoporosis, and menopause.

OBJECTIVES

After reading and studying this chapter, the student should be able to:

1. State the pharmacological interventions for menstrual disorders.
2. Discuss therapy for iron deficiency anemia.
3. List contraceptive options and modalities.
4. Understand the use of pharmacological therapies for menopausal symptoms.
5. Describe treatment modalities for the prevention of osteoporosis.
6. Differentiate between the various treatment options for osteoporosis.
7. Review medication use during pregnancy and lactation.

KEY DRUGS AND CLASSES OF DRUGS MENTIONED IN THIS CHAPTER

All drugs mentioned in this chapter are discussed fully in other chapters; however some of the pharmacology of the following drugs is mentioned in this chapter because of their unique application to women.

Drugs for Premenstrual Syndrome (PMS) and Premenstrual Dysphoric Disorder (PMDD)
Supplements and herbals
selective serotonin reuptake inhibitors (SSRIs) e.g., citalopram (Celexa), fluoxetine (Prozac), fluvoxamine (Luvox), paroxetine (Paxil), sertraline (Zoloft)
NSAIDS e.g. aspirin, ibuprofen

Drugs for Abnormal Uterine Bleeding (AUB) and Dysfunctional Uterine Bleeding (DUB)
oral estrogens
oral progestins

Drugs for Iron Deficiency Anemia
ferrous sulfate, ferrous fumarate, ferrous carbonate

Drugs for Reversible Contraception
low-dose monophasic contraceptives
multiphasic contraceptives
combination oral contraceptives (COC)
transdermal contraceptives
injectable contraceptives
implantable contraceptive devices

intravaginal rings
contraception prevention using barriers and spermicides
spermicides, diaphragms, caps, sponge, condom

Drugs for Emergency Contraception
high-dose estrogen
high-dose progestin

Drugs Used for the Treatment of Osteoporosis and Osteopenia
calcium and vitamin D
bisphosphonates
selective estrogen receptor modulators (SERMS)
calcitonin

continued

Gender differences affect all phases of pharmacokinetics and pharmacodynamics. Clinicians must consider the following before prescribing medications for women, especially during the childbearing years.

- A fetus could be harmed through teratogenicity.
- Inadequate prenatal care could harm a fetus.
- Breastfeeding could pass medicines onto an infant.
- Teenage pregnancy can give rise to smaller infants and preterm infants.
- Cultural beliefs may influence how a women considers and accepts health counseling from a clinician.

GENDER DIFFERENCES AFFECTING PHARMACODYNAMICS AND PHARMACOKINETICS

Drug Absorption

Women have longer gastric emptying times and thus the bioavailability and absorption of many oral drugs is different when compared to men. Drug absorption is also one area mainly affected by estrogen levels as well as enzyme levels. For example, gastric levels of alcohol dehydrogenase, the enzyme in the gastrointestinal (GI) tract that oxidizes alcohol, are lower in women than men, which causes higher levels of alcohol to appear in the plasma/bloodstream of women compared with men when women and men drink equal amounts of alcohol.

Drug Distribution

Women generally have lower body weights and body mass indexes (BMIs) than do men. They also have a higher proportion of body fat, which results in lipophilic drugs being more readily absorbed in women. Women have lower levels of lipophilic drugs circulating in plasma. One example of this is when estrogens are free analogues or are exogenous as they initiate an increase in several serum-binding globulins that in turn can bind them to other circulating agents and cause fewer estrogens to be free and bioavailable. This is borne out by the evidence that shows one estrogen being more active than another in a specific tissue or organ, such as breast, uterus, or bone. The most striking example of this is the synthetic estrogen analogue tamoxifen, which blocks estrogen actions in breast tissue but has estrogen-like activity on bone. These new findings have stimulated extensive research into new pharmaceuticals that could have selective actions on specific tissues and thus might provide beneficial hormone replacement therapy without some of the undesirable side effects and as well as research into how estrogens could be useful in the treatment of cancer or other conditions.

Drug Metabolism

There is inconsistent evidence in the literature regarding whether or not there are gender differences among all the CYP450 isomers, but women seem to have more of the CYP450 3A4 substrate than do men and are thus a better able to metabolize drugs that are affected by the cytochrome P450 system.

Drug Excretion

Excretion of drugs by the kidneys is a function of weight, body surface area, age, gender, and glomerular filtration rate (GFR). Thus, any drug excretion differences between men and women are likely the result of weight differences.

Drug Pharmacodynamics

Research supports that pharmacodynamic differences exist when comparing men to women. One exception, however, is when women use cardiovascular drugs. It has been shown that because women between the ages of 15 and 50 have longer QT intervals than do men, they are more susceptible to cardiac arrhythmias (Kligfield, Lax, & Okin, 1996). A second example would be the opiate analgesics, which have been shown to produce greater analgesia in women as well as increased nausea and vomiting. This is postulated to be due to women having a greater drug receptor affinity and receptor density for the opiates than men. However, the differences seen by opioid administration in patients indicates that gender alone cannot be used as a basis for altering opioid dosages. Thus, clinicians need to titrate their opioid doses for each patient, whether male or female (Fillingham, King, Ribeiro-Dasilva, Rahim-Williams, & Riley, 2009).

Although research on drug-related differences between men and women continues, it has yet to have any significant effect on how drugs are dosed. This is because most drugs have a fairly wide therapeutic index (margin of safety). Thus, minor differences in drug response and pharmacokinetic differences between men and women are not clinically significant. However, a number of factors do influence how drugs are used and dosed in women; these are related to the extraordinary physiological changes that occur during puberty, pregnancy, breastfeeding, menopause, and advancing age. It is the clinician's responsibility to understand women's need when it comes to premenstrual syndrome (PMS), premenstrual dysphoric disorder (PMDD), endometriosis, vaginitis, osteoporosis, infertility, and conditions that can affect women quite variably.

DRUG THERAPY FOR PREMENSTRUAL SYNDROME AND PREMENSTRUAL DYSPHORIC DISORDER

Premenstrual syndrome (PMS) is the recurrence of physical and behavioral symptoms 7 to 14 days prior to a menstrual cycle.

It occurs in almost 40% of menstruating women. **Premenstrual dysphoric disorder (PMDD)** is less common, occurring in about 2% to 5% of women and by definition is a more severe variant of PMS (Halbreich, Borenstein, Pearlstein, & Kahn, 2003). Specifically, the depression, irritability, and tension in PMDD are more severe than what is seen in PMS. The cause of PMS and PMDD is unclear, with several proposed etiologies ranging from hormonal to social factors. Over 150 symptoms have been associated with PMS and PMDD, including acne, irritability, water retention, mood swings, and sugar cravings. It is important to rule out anemia, thyroid disorders, depression, or other mood disorders when considering the diagnosis of PMS or PMDD. Treatment options for PMS and PMDD include conventional medications, exercise, dietary changes, such as caffeine reduction, supplements, mind-body approaches, and counseling (Table 20-1). Regular aerobic exercise has shown to have a positive effect on the symptoms (Pearlstein & Steiner, 2008). It has also been shown that it is the frequency of exercise, not the intensity that resolves the negative mood and physical symptoms associated with these disorders (Mass General, 2010). Similarly, a fiber-rich diet with less than 20% of total calories from fat helps to lower estrogen levels.

TABLE 20-1 Therapeutic Alternatives for PMS and PMDD		
MEDICATION	DOSAGE	COMMENTS AND CAUTIONS
Rx Drugs		
alprazolam (Xanax)	6.25 mg–12.5 mg to start, not to exceed 2 doses/ 24 hr period	• Antianxiety agent • Highly habit forming (Schedule IV-CSA), watch for dizziness, drowsiness, lethargy
danazol (Cyclomen)	200–400 mg daily	• For moderate endometriosis • A synthetic androgen but its use is waning due to androgenic side effects hirsutism, deepening voice, acne, weight gain)
ibuprofen (Advil, Motrin, Nuprin)	400–600 mg every 8 hr	• For dysmenorrhea • Watch for gastrointestinal irritation (bleeding, vomiting, dyspepsia, nausea) as well as hepatitis and heme issues
SSRIs (such as citalopram (Celexa), fluoxetine (Prozac) paroxetine (Paxil) fluvoxamine (Luvox), and sertraline (Zoloft)	Varies per drug: e.g., citalopram and fluoxetine (20 mg/day)	• Very effective for improving behavioral and physical symptoms associated with PMDD • Monitor for suicidal ideation plus CNS and GI adverse events
Herbal Agents, Vitamins, and Dietary Supplements		
evening primrose oil many OTC suppliers available such as Nature's Bounty	1.5 gm 2 times/ day, usually dose is 2–8 gm/day	• Rich source of prostaglandins and gamma-linoleic acid, which can soften the cervix • No studies are able to confirm its effectiveness as a PMS treatment beyond use of a placebo.
chaste tree berry (vitex, Abraham's balm, monk's pepper)	250–1,000 mg/day	• Used for numerous PMS complaints (irritability, anger, headache, breast fullness), and especially cyclical breast pain and polycystic ovary syndrome. • Ancients, Greeks, Romans, and monks started its use as an antilibido medicine. • It has no proven effectiveness, but its fruit, leaves, and flowers do contain some steroidal hormone precursors and many other agents. • Although its mode of action is not clear, the effects mimic the effect when the corpus luteum stimulates the production of luteinizing hormone, thereby increasing progesterone production, hence chaste tree berry's hormonal effects.
calcium salts oral (carbonate, citrate, gluconate, lactate etc.) sold as Chloromag, Citroma, Milk of Magnesia, Magtrate, etc.	1,200 mg/day	• Improves mood and somatic symptoms as it acts as an activator in transmission of smooth, cardiac, and skeletal muscle. • Should not be taken with iron, tetracycline(TCN), phenytoin, calcium channel blockers (CCBs), thyroid hormones, or corticosteroids as PO ingestion of calcium decreases absorption of other agents.
magnesium salts oral (chloride citrate, gluconate, hydroxide)	200–400 mg/day in 3–4 divided doses	• Used for dysmenorrhea, fatigue, insomnia, but watch for side effects of diarrhea, flushing, sweating • Use with caution in presence of any renal disease as excretion can be impaired.

continued

TABLE 20-1 Therapeutic Alternatives for PMS and PMDD—cont'd

MEDICATION	DOSAGE	COMMENTS AND CAUTIONS
alpha-tocopherol (vitamin E)	400 mg/day	• A few studies indicate vitamin E can reduce most symptoms of PMS
pyridoxine (vitamin B$_6$) sold in many vitamin B complex formulations but alternatives are a diet with foods that contain it (e.g., cereals).	50–100 mg/day	• Is required for the synthesis of serotonin norepinephrine, and myelin formation, hence its use to treat depression and other emotional symptoms of PMS • Doses above 100 mg/day may lead to peripheral neuropathy. • May combine vitamin B^6 with chaste tree berry extract for PMS.

DRUG THERAPY FOR ABNORMAL UTERINE BLEEDING AND DYSFUNCTIONAL UTERINE BLEEDING

Normal uterine bleeding is a 21 to 35 day cycle, with the duration of bleeding ranging from 1 to 7 days. The volume of blood should require less than one sanitary napkin or tampon per 3-hour period. **Abnormal uterine bleeding (AUB)** is any bleeding that differs in regularity, frequency, duration or volume from the usual menstrual flow. AUB affects up to one-third of women of reproductive age. A wide range of disorders including anovulation, pregnancy-related conditions, trauma, anatomic abnormalities of the genital tract, infection, endocrinological disorders, malignancies and systemic illness may cause AUB. Dysfunctional uterine bleeding (DUB) is the diagnosis given when no clear systemic, anatomical, or infectious etiology is present. DUB can be anovulatory, which is characterized by irregular, unpredictable bleeding, or ovulatory, which is characterized by heavy regular periods. Anovulatory DUB accounts for 90% of cases of DUB, resulting from unopposed estrogen stimulation in the endometrium. This is most prevalent in women during their perimenarchal or perimenopausal years (Merck Manual, 2012). The mechanisms of ovulatory DUB are not well understood. Table 20-2 defines various abnormal uterine bleeding patterns.

Some abnormal vaginal bleeding may be caused by drugs and herbal products that induce the cytochrome P450 pathway to increase the catabolism of estrogen, leading to breakthrough bleeding (BTB). Oral contraceptive pills (OCPs) may also cause BTB, especially the lower-dose estrogen pills. Although they are associated with fewer serious side effects, such as stroke, pulmonary embolism, and myocardial infarction, as the estrogen dose decreases, the rate of BTB increases. Some of the drugs known to induce abnormal uterine bleeding are listed in Table 20-3.

Medical Management of DUB

Once the diagnosis of DUB is established, the primary goals of management are to stabilize the bleeding and prevent endometrial hyperplasia or cancer. The secondary goals are to prevent future unpredictable bleeding, treat the underlying endometrial and hormonal abnormalities and treat concomitant anemia. The treatment will vary depending on the severity and type of bleeding, fertility status of the patient, contraception needs, patient preference, and side effects.

Severe DUB

When treating a patient with DUB, the clinician should focus first on correcting the patient's volume status and then the uterine bleeding. The rapid onset of intravenous (IV) conjugate equine estrogen therapy is effective in the management of severe, acute bleeding. It can be administered intravenously 25 mg up to six times for 24 hours. Oral estrogen can also be administered, 2.5 mg every 6 hours until bleeding stops (Behara, 2010). Side effects from using high doses of estrogen include nausea, and caution should be taken with women who have a history of liver disease, are older than 35 years, and/or smoke. If a woman has a history of a thromboembolic event or an estrogen-dependent tumor, an alternative treatment should be considered.

Other medical options for the treatment of severe DUB include combination oral contraceptives (COC) and oral progestins.

TABLE 20-2 Terms Used to Describe Abnormal Uterine Bleeding Patterns

TERMS	DEFINITIONS
Menorrhagia	Prolonged (>7 days) or excessive (>80 mL) bleeding occurring at regular intervals
Metrorrhagia	Bleeding occurring at irregular intervals or between periods
Menometrorrhagia	Bleeding occurring at irregular intervals with heavy or prolonged menstrual flow
Polymenorrhea	Bleeding occurring at regular intervals of <21 days
Oligomenorrhea	Infrequent, scanty bleeding occurring at intervals of >35 days
Amenorrhea	Primary: No onset of menarche by age 16 years; Secondary: Absence of bleeding for more than 6 months in a nonmenopausal woman
Postmenopausal	Bleeding >1 year after cessation of menses or at an unanticipated time for women taking cyclic hormone therapy

TABLE 20-3	Drugs and Herbal Products That Induce Abnormal Uterine Bleeding (AUB)
DRUGS KNOWN TO CAUSE AUB	**HERBAL PRODUCTS KNOWN TO CAUSE AUB**
Anticoagulants	Garlic
Antidepressants (more common with tricyclics)	Ginkgo biloba
	Ginseng
Antipsychotics	Soy
Oral contraceptive pills	St. John's wort
Oral corticosteroids	Arnica
Phenytoin	Aspen
Tamoxifen	Bladderwrack
Tranquilizers	Capsicum
	Dong quai
	Omega-3 fatty acids
	Parsley

List compiled from data in the Natural Medicine Comprehensive Database, www.naturaldatabase.com/.

However, COC used for DUB are considered an "off label" use. A monophasic COC, 35 mcg ethinyl estradiol/1 mg norethindrone, can be given three times a day for 7 days followed by once-daily dosing for 3 weeks. The average time to stop bleeding is 3 days. The progestins norethindrone 5 to 15 mg/day and medroxyprogesterone acetate up to 80 mg/day have been used for women with a contraindication to estrogen therapy. Common side effects of progestin therapy include headaches and breast tenderness.

If the patient's condition is not responsive to medical therapy, surgical intervention may be necessary.

Heavy Bleeding

The outpatient management of the hemodynamically stable female will depend on the patient's tolerance to ongoing blood loss, wishes regarding future fertility, willingness and ability to take daily drugs vs. taking drugs only during menses, side effects, and contraindications to various treatments. The levonorgestrel-releasing intrauterine device (IUD) (Mirena) is the medical treatment with the strongest evidence to support its use for **menorrhagia** (heavy menstrual bleeding), and the U.S. Food and Drug Administration (FDA) approved the Mirena IUD in 2009 for such use (Waynine, 2011). It can only be used in a woman whose uterus measure 6 to 9 cm without gross malformations seen on examination. Additionally, the woman should be at low risk for sexually transmitted infections. Estrogen-containing contraceptives such as the pill, patch, or ring are options for daily, weekly, monthly, or extended use. Bleeding may be reduced by 50% with long-term use. Various dosing of progestins can be used during a 14- to 21-day cycle in which blood loss may be reduced by as much as 90% (Lethaby, Irvine, & Cameron, 2008). NSAIDs reduce uterine bleeding by vasoconstriction of the vasculature and decrease levels of prostaglandins by improvement in platelet aggregation. Women with gastritis, peptic ulcer disease, or renal disease should use this option with caution.

Anovulatory Bleeding in Women Younger Than 35 Years of Age

The off-label use of COCs or cyclic progestin therapy is commonly prescribed for the medical management of anovulatory bleeding in women younger than 35 years (Casablanca, 2008). Generally, a low-dose COC is used for 3 months. If the bleeding continues, a higher dose estrogen pill is used. Persistent bleeding will require further evaluation. Polycystic ovary syndrome (PCOS) should be suspected when there are two of the three following symptoms: oligomenorrhea and/or anovulation, clinical and/or biochemical signs of hyperandrogenism, and evidence of polycystic ovaries. Also known as Stein-Leventhal syndrome, PCOS is a hormonal deficiency usually affecting women of childbearing age. It can affect any woman, but typically it is seen in women as obesity (weight gain), acne (skin discoloration), anovulation (irregular menses), excessive amounts of masculinizing hormones (unusual hair growth, dandruff), and diabetes (insulin resistance). Women who have PCOS may have a sister or mother who also has it, but this is not an absolute.

Anovulatory Bleeding in Women Older Than 35 Years of Age

The risk of endometrial atypia or cancer is increased in women older than 35 years of age if they are experiencing anovulatory bleeding. Thus, assessment of their endometrium should be done. Once an evaluation of anovulatory bleeding has been made, the bleeding can be controlled with the off-label use of COC, an IUD, or cyclic progestins.

Postmenopausal Bleeding

Most postmenopausal bleeding is benign; however, the diagnostic evaluation is designed to detect endometrial cancer along with other abnormalities that may cause bleeding after 1 year of no bleeding. If endometrial hyperplasia without atypia is noted, it can be treated with the off-label use of cyclic or continuous progestins. If the atypia persists, other interventional management should be explored.

DRUG TREATMENT OF IRON DEFICIENCY ANEMIA

According to the National Library of Medicine (NLM) menstrual blood loss and increased iron requirements of pregnancy are the most common causes of **iron deficiency anemia** in the developed world (NIH, 2010). The patient may present with the concerns of heavy blood loss, fatigue, or pica (the consumption of substances such as clay, ice, or starch). A peripheral smear will show hypochromic, microcytic red blood cells. Also, the patient will have low serum ferritin and iron levels with an increased total iron-binding capacity. The first treatment option should be to increase the iron consumed in the diet. If that is not sufficient, then an oral supplement of ferrous sulfate, 325 mg, three times a day is recommended. This dose should be taken between meals to enhance absorption.

The use of acid-neutralizing medications can impair the response to oral iron. Iron stores should be replenished over approximately 6 months. Common side effects of iron products include the gastrointestinal symptoms of constipation and nausea. Ferrous gluconate and fumarate may be better tolerated. Noncompliance is a common reason for oral therapy failure.

DRUGS USED TO INFLUENCE CONTRACEPTION

A wide range of contraceptive options are available for use by women of childbearing age. The efficacy, risks and benefits of each differ. Clinicians choosing a contraceptive option must keep in mind the patient's needs by asking a series of questions such as the following:

■ What are the goals of the patient?
■ Is this to be long-term or only temporary use?
■ How quickly does she desire fertility to return?
■ Is she interested in reducing the frequency of bleeding?
■ Is her interest primarily in controlling her cycle predictably?
■ Is she breastfeeding?
■ Does she have a regular routine?
■ How dangerous is conception for her overall health?
■ Is there a family history of ovarian cancer?

Because each mode of contraception carries specific risks and benefits, their use must be tailored to each woman.

Selecting the Right Oral Contraceptive

Selecting an oral contraceptive requires care in selecting the formulation with the lowest dose of estrogen that can be tolerated by the woman who will be taking it. Generally, there is no indication for routine use of high-dose (50 mcg) estrogen pills (oral contraceptives), but they may be used temporarily to manage menorrhagia. The higher dose estrogens in contraceptive pills carry a markedly increased risk of cardiovascular events. Thus, the 20- and 30-mcg estrogen pills offer effective protection from pregnancy at far lower risk to the patient. However, lower dose estrogen pills carry a higher risk of breakthrough endometrial bleeding should one or more doses be missed or if the pill is taken with food or drugs that bind them in GI transit.

The choice of oral contraceptive progesterone should also be tailored to meet a patient's needs. For example, older progesterones (norethindrone and levonorgestrel) are cheaper but quite androgenic, and thus worsen acne and lipid profiles in sensitive patients. Less androgenic pills containing norgestimate and desogestrel are less prone to cause acne. Drospirenone (Yasmin) is a fairly new progestational agent that is related chemically to spironolactone, making it antiandrogenic as well as a mild diuretic. Although Yasmin may cause potassium retention in patients with renal disease, it is generally well tolerated and is an excellent choice for patients with severe acne.

Once a decision to use oral contraceptives is made, the clinician then has to decide on a dosing schedule and a pill formulation that will assure compliance by the patient. Pill formulations are packaged as progesterone only pills (Micronor), extended-cycle contraceptives, or combined COC (low-dose monophasic oral contraceptives and multiphasic oral contraceptives).

Most oral contraceptives are formulated using a regimen that includes taking active-ingredient pills for 21 days, then inactive pills for 7 days. This is done to "regulate" the woman into having a 28-day cycle during which there is a "withdrawal bleed," hence the appearance of a regular menses every month. The low-dose **monophasic oral contraceptives** are used in a continuous or extended daily dosing pattern lasting 2 to 3 months. This allows for continuous use of the contraceptive's active ingredients before stopping them to allow withdrawal bleeding to occur, but it allows a woman to have her menses four times a year. These "extended cycles" induced by monophasic pills offer improved suppression of ovulation and less risk of pregnancy, but they may result in occasional breakthrough bleeding.

Multiphasic pills may only be used for regular monthly cycles and are not suitable for extended cycling. Although claiming to provide a more natural variation of hormone levels, these pills are essentially supraphysiological in dose, and the variation in hormone levels they offer is more likely to produce breakthrough bleeding when doses are missed. Because multiphasic pills are formulated to minimize estrogen deprivation, they are best used for treating women with menstrual migraines. This is also true for the continuous dosing provided by monophasic low-dose pills because in both cases the patient's migraines were induced by estrogen withdrawal.

Combined oral contraceptives are widely used contraceptive choices because they combine both estrogen and progestin agents. Combined agents suppress the pituitary-ovarian axis and generally prevent ovulation. These agents regulate the endometrial cycle by inducing a resting endometrial state that is generally progesterone dominant and by allowing bleeding to occur during the 7-day drug holiday. When used in a regular cyclic pattern (21 days on, 7 days off), they provide effective birth control and monthly withdrawal bleeding cycles that are generally predictable and with less blood loss than a nonmedicated cycle. The lower dose agents may also be used in a continuous cycle pattern, with 2 to 3 months of continuous active pill, followed by a prescribed week off (drug holiday) to allow withdrawal bleeding to occur. When these agents are used continuously, the term *bicycling* refers to the use of the active pill for 2 months, and *tricycling* refers to the use of the active pill for 3 months. Several **triphasic oral contraceptives** are marketed today specifically to provide 3 months of continuous coverage in single packaging, although any of the low dose pills may be used in this fashion (Table 20-4).

Progesterone-only pills are always used in continuous-dose fashion with no withdrawal breaks. These pills are effective only when taken in regular 24-hour intervals, so they require strict schedule adherence. They do not suppress the pituitary-ovarian axis; thus, they allow breastfeeding without inhibition of milk production. For women with a family history of ovarian cancer, use of combined OCPs offers reduced risk of ovarian cancer.

TABLE 20-4	Common Oral Contraceptive Formulations Available in the United States
A: Monophasics 20–30 mcg Estrogen	
20/1 EE/norethindrone acetate/iron	Loestrin FE 1/20
20/0.1 EE/levonorgestrel	Aviane
20/1 EE/norethindrone acetate	Loestrin 1/20
30/1.5 EE/norethindrone acetate/iron	Loestrin FE 1.5/30
30/0.3 EE/norgestrel	Low-Ogestrel
30/3 EE/drospirenone	Yasmin, YAZ
30/0.15 EE/levonorgestrel	Levora
30/1.5 EE/norethindrone acetate	Loestrin 1.5/30
30/0.15 EE/desogestrel	Ortho-Cept
B: Monophasics With 35 mcg estrogen	
35/1 EE/ethynodiol diacetate	Zovia 1/35
35/0.25 EE/norgestimate	Ortho-Cyclen
35/1 EE/norethindrone	Ortho-Novum 1/35
35/0.5 EE/norethindrone	Modicon
C: Monophasics with 50 mcg estrogen	
50/1 EE/ethynodiol diacetate	Zovia 1/50
50/1 ME/norethindrone	Ortho-Novum 1/50
D: Multiphasics	
desogestrel/EE	Mircette
norethindrone/EE	Ortho-Novum 10/11
norethindrone acetate/EE/iron	Estrostep FE
levonorgestrel/EE	Trivora
desogestrel/EE	Cyclessa, Velivet
norethindrone/EE	Tri-Norinyl
norgestimate/EE	Ortho Tri-Cyclen
norgestimate/EE	Ortho Tri-Cyclen LO
norethindrone/EE	Ortho-Novum 7/7/7
E: Progestin Only OC for Breastfeeding Women	
norethindrone 350 micrograms	Ortho Micronor
F: Extended Cycle Formulations	
0.15 mg levonorgestrel and 0.03 mg EE pill-pak has 91 tabs: 84 are active, 7 are placebo	Seasonale
0.15 mg levonorgestrel and 0.03 mg EE. Pill Pak has 91 tabs: 84 active and 7 with low-dose estrogen (0.01 EE) EE, ethinyl estradiol	Seasonique

Conscientious Prescribing for Patients Taking Oral Contraceptive Pills

■ The decision to use a pill that contains estrogen must be made cautiously, keeping in mind the known risks of estrogen, including increased coagulability, liver dysfunction, and enhancement of estrogen-sensitive tissue growth.

■ Patients with a history of cerebrovascular accident CVA, complicated migraines, heart or liver disease, clotting disorders, estrogen-sensitive cancers, undiagnosed vaginal bleeding, or possible pregnancy should not be prescribed oral contraceptives.

■ Women over 35 years old with hypertension or who smoke are frequently prescribed low-dose COCs, with closely supervision and counseling to stop smoking. All women with a personal or family history of deep venous thrombosis (DVT) or gactor V Leiden, protein C or S deficiency, should avoid use of combined oral contraceptives.

■ Patients who have difficulty keeping regular schedules or following daily pill regimens should not use OCPs if pregnancy would be life threatening, because they are at high risk of OCP failure.

■ OCPs should not be used for contraception purposes in women with undiagnosed uterine bleeding or at high risk of breast cancer. Estrogen inhibits milk production by triggering receptors on galactocele membranes (not via pituitary effect).

Patient/Family Education for Patients Taking Oral Contraceptives

■ Instruct patient to use a backup method of contraception when using the first package of OCP.

■ Instruct patient regarding when to begin taking the OCP (day 1 or Sunday start).

■ Patient education for OCP use should include the necessity of regular daily dosing and need for avoidance of other medications that could impair absorption.

■ Patients should be educated not to smoke, and to maintain a normal body mass for their age and height.

■ Patients should be taught to identify possible warning signs of adverse effects that they should bring to their clinician's attention. Symptoms of unilateral numbness, tingling, weakness, slurring of speech, or vision loss could suggest stroke and need to be brought to the clinician's attention.

■ Oral contraceptives have a perfect use failure rate of less than 1% per year; however it can be as high as nearly 9% per year due to missed pills, use of interfering medications, and irregular timing. If pills are missed, patients should be taught appropriate catch-up strategies, and should be warned to use backup methods of contraception for the remainder of their cycle (Women's Health About.com, 2013).

■ OCPs protect against pregnancy, but not against sexually transmitted diseases (STDs) and HIV. Encourage all users to follow safe sex practices such as maintaining mutually monogamous relationships, using condoms, and limiting sexual partners.

■ Prescribe a 3-month supply of OCP and schedule a return visit at 3 months to evaluate the patient.

■ Patients should be cautioned that OCPs do not reduce the risk of cervical cancer.

■ Patients should be told to expect an experience of breakthrough bleeding during at least the first 3 months of using OCPs.

■ Patients should also be told that during their first month of using OCPs they need to use some other form of backup contraception.

■ Patients should be advised that it is a good idea to take their OCP at the same time every day.

Combination Oral Contraceptives

Combination oral contraceptives (COCs), of which there are many (see Table 20-4), all inhibit ovulation through a negative feedback mechanism on the hypothalamus. Combined oral contraceptives in the United States are highly effective when used properly because they contain either a combination of a synthetic estrogen with a synthetic progestin or a progestin alone. As estrogen suppresses follicle-stimulating hormone (FSH), the estrogen in a COC prevents the development of a dominant follicle. Estrogens also potentiate the action of progestin, which in turn suppresses luteinizing hormone (LH). Thus a number of these combinations has various levels of estrogen or none at all because it is the progestin that halts follicle growth. The varying amounts of estrogen serve to stabilize the endometrial lining and hence control bleeding. Due to the side effects of these agents, women may try one pill over another until they find a product that causes minimal side effects. If they must avoid estrogen use, they can use the progestin-only pills.

Mechanism of Action

Interruption of the ovarian cycle through a feedback mechanism that alters the normal pattern of gonadotropin secretion of FSH and LH hormone by the pituitary occurs. This alteration then affects the mid-cycle surge of the ova, rendering the egg immature. Oral contraceptives also produce changes in cervical mucus, making it inhospitable to sperm even if ovulation should occur. They may also alter ova transport through the fallopian tubes. The addition of progestin agents reduces the risk of endometrial hyperplasia and the risk of endometrial cancer in women with an intact uterus.

Pharmacokinetics

■ Absorption: Combinations of estrogen and progestin are rapidly absorbed across the intestine, but undergoes significant metabolism in both the small intestine and liver via cytochrome P450 enzyme systems.

■ Distribution: Once absorbed, the drug readily diffuses across lipid bilayers and across the blood-brain barrier.

■ Metabolism: It is metabolized in the liver, undergoing conversion into 2-hydroxy and 16-hydroxy estrogen metabolites.

■ Excretion: It is excreted enterically.

■ Half-life: 12 to 30 hours

Dosage and Administration

Ortho-Cyclen is provided in a dose-unit packaging format that allows 21 days of active pills containing 35 mcg of ethinyl estradiol and 0.25 mg of norgestimate, with 7 days of inert pills each month to provide a withdrawal bleed.

Clinical Uses

■ Ortho-Cyclen is used for cycle regulation, contraception, and acne relief.

Adverse Reactions

CV: Hypercoagulability, Deep vein thrombosis (DVT) and pulmonary embolism (PE), and CVA risks.
GI: Liver abnormalities, cholelithiasis
MISC: May stimulate estrogen-sensitive cancer cells.

Interactions

■ Interference with antiestrogenic agents used for cancer treatment such as tamoxifen.

■ The older enzyme-inducing anticonvulsants may interact with estrogens causing enhanced metabolism of the estrogen in any contraceptive and rendering the contraceptive unreliable. Other contraceptive means (condom, diaphragm, IUD, spermicide) should be used if the patient must be on one of the older anticonvulsants.

■ Concern regarding the use of oral antibiotics and induced inefficacy of the pills has been raised. In general, however, some literature (Blumenthal & Edelman, 2008; Dickinson, Altman, Nielsen, & Sterling, 2001; Archer & Archer, 2002; Lomaestro, 2009) indicates a low risk of this interaction with the exception of rifampin and griseofulvin. Yet the debate continues, with strong arguments both for and against antibiotics interacting with oral contraceptives. Although occasional case reports of OCP failure occur, they can generally be explained as being part of the normal failure rate of the oral contraceptive itself.

■ Table 20-5 lists common drug interactions with oral contraceptive pills.

TABLE 20-5	Common Drug Interactions with Oral Contraceptive Pills (OCPs)
MEDICATION	CLINICAL EFFECT
Anticonvulsants	Older anticonvulsants such as phenytoin, phenobarbital, carbamazepine, and oxcarbazepine (*except* valproate) induce CYP450 3A4, reducing OCP efficacy.
Benzodiazepines	Estrogen increases benzodiazepine effect (reduces hepatic oxidation).
Corticosteroids	OCPs prolong steroid effect (via increase steroid binding globulin).
Penicillin	Minor effect, reduced efficacy.
Protease inhibitors	Protease inhibitors increase OCP hormone levels (via CYP450 3A4 inhibition).
Rifampin	Rifampin decreases OCP efficacy (via CYP450 3A4 induction).
Griseofulvin	Griseofulvin decreases OCP efficacy (via CYP459 3A4 induction).
St. John's wort	St. John's wort decreases OCP efficacy (via CYP459 3A4 induction).
Topiramate	Topiramate decreases OCP efficacy (via CYP459 3A4 induction).

Contraindications

- Hypertension
- Cigarette smoking (patient over 35 years)
- Liver disease
- Heart disease, thromboembolic disease
- Breast cancer
- Undiagnosed vaginal bleeding
- Pregnancy
- Major surgery with prolonged immobilization
- Complicated migraine
- Diabetic nephropathy
- Breastfeeding

Transdermal Contraception

Transdermal contraception, often called "birth-control patches" or "weekly patches," contains both estrogen and progesterone (Ortho Evra). They are growing in popularity in urban centers where there is greater demand for easy-to-use methods of birth control. These patches are approximately 1 inch square and are placed on the woman's upper torso, upper arm, abdomen, or buttocks. Single hormone progesterone-based subdermal agents (IMPLANON and Norplant) are also available. Chief advantages of transdermal agents include lack of first-pass metabolism through the liver, and the ability to avoid daily dose requirement.

Conscientious Prescribing for Patients Using Transdermal Contraception

- Transdermal combination patches provide a higher steady state of estrogen, although the peak concentration of the agent is much lower than that used in oral pills.
- Though risk of clotting and liver disorders is reduced, patients should be cautioned regarding this side effect. They generally confer the same risks and benefits as OCPs with less risk of noncompliance. They should not be used in patients who would not be candidates for OCPs for any reason.
- Patches should not be placed over the breast or over broken skin.

Patient/Family Education for Patients Using Transdermal Contraception

- Transdermal contraception needs to be replaced once weekly. To achieve a monthly cycle, they may be used for 3 consecutive weeks and then a withdrawal bleed is allowed (patch free week).
- For extended cycling, patches may be used for 6 to 8 weeks and then discontinued for 1 week to allow a withdrawal bleed.
- Transdermal patches may not achieve reliable hormone levels to suppress ovulation in patients weighing over 200 lbs. Such patients should choose a backup method of contraception.
- Patients should know that hyperpigmentation may occur due to the adhesive.
- Breakthrough bleeding is slightly more common with this method.

- Patients who develop sensitivity to adhesive should be encouraged to choose an alternative means of contraception because hyperpigmentation may become severe. The patch works only if completely adhered to the skin. Patients should check daily to ensure that edges are completely adherent.

Mechanism of Action

The transdermal patch is a matrix system consisting of three layers in about a 20 cm^2 area. The first or outer layer is a water-resistant film that protects the patch from the environment, the middle layer is medicated and adhesive, and the third or inner layer is a clear release layer that is removed just before application. Transdermal patches suppress ovulation and cause thickening of cervical mucus. The menstrual periods of women wearing the patch appear to be better regulated because the patch is worn on a planned regimen (i.e., patch-free and patch-on weeks). This assures the patch wearer of a more trouble-free menstrual period. Secondly, because the patch maintains a fairly long period of hormonal control, there is no need for secondary precautions before or after having intercourse. There is still the possibility of an increased risk of venous thromboembolism among women who wear the patch.

Pharmacokinetics

- Absorption: Transdermal patches are slowly absorbed over 1 week. They do not undergo first-pass metabolism in the enterocyte or hepatocyte and will therefore be less affected by use of antibiotics, antacids, and other drugs. Additionally, therapeutic effects are achieved at lower doses because first-pass hepatic metabolism and gastric enzyme degradation do not occur.
- Distribution: Plasma hormone remains level because peaks and troughs do not occur as with pills.
- Metabolism: Same as oral contraceptives.
- Excretion: Same as oral contraceptives.
- Half-life: Due to prolonged absorption, half-life when the patch is removed is approximately 24 hours.

Dosage and Administration

Generic Name	Trade Name	Usual Adult Daily Dose
norelgestromin (NGMN)/20 mcg ethinyl estradiol (EE) 150-mcg transdermal patch	Ortho Evra	Apply one patch to non-hair-bearing skin weekly. Patch-free weeks should occur at regular intervals after 3 weeks to allow withdrawal bleeding unless continuous use is planned.

Clinical Use

Transdermal patches are an excellent option for patients who may be good candidates for hormonal contraception but who are unable to reliably take a daily OCP on schedule. This may include teenagers, shift workers, college students, and other women with hectic schedules.

Adverse Reactions

DERM: Contact dermatitis, adhesive intolerance, or skin hyperpigmentation (darkening of skin).

Interactions

■ Because absorption and metabolism is transdermal and not affected by the cytochrome P450 system, few drug interactions are noted.

Contraindications

■ Patients who are not candidates for OCPs should not use transdermal patches.

Patient/Family Education

■ The effectiveness of the patch remains the same whether it is worn on the arm, upper torso (not breasts), buttocks, or abdomen.
■ The use failure rate for any form of contraceptive is approximately 5%; compliance with the regimen is the best way of ensuring effectiveness.
■ Patients using the patch should be counseled on the risk of thromboembolism because it may be higher than with the use of OCPs.

Injectable Contraceptives

Injectable contraception provides women with a safe and highly effective method of contraception. Injectable contraceptives are formulated either as a progestin-only product that is effective for 2 to 3 months or a combined formulation that contains both a progestin and an estrogen and is effective for 1 month. The progestin-only products consist of depo medroxyprogesterone acetate sold as Depo-Provera (injection) and as Provera (oral tabs) and norethisterone enanthate (Net-En). Depo-Provera is injected every 3 months, whereas Net-En is injected every 2 months. One combined estrogen-progestin (norethisterone and estradiol) formulation is sold under the trade names Mesigyna, others are Cyclofem and Lunelle (medroxyprogesterone and estradiol) and Norigynon; containing the progesterone norethisterone and 5 mg estradiol and is administered intramuscularlydeep into the muscle of the arm or buttock for a 30-day effect. The deep IM injection allows for slow absorption into the bloodstream and sustained levels of effective contraception for the 1, 2, or 3 months between injections, depending on the formulation chosen.

Conscientious Prescribing for Patients Taking Injectable Contraception

■ Users of medroxyprogesterone acetate enjoy 3 months of continuous contraceptive protection without the risks of estrogen. No daily dosing or weekly changing is needed.
■ Disadvantages of injectables include pain of injection, weight gain, and irregular menses. With prolonged use, amenorrhea and decreased bone density are noted.
■ Progestin-only injectables offer a suitable method of contraception for women who are at risk if they take estrogens, especially such risks as thromboembolism.
■ One noncontraceptive health benefit of the progestin-only contraceptives is that they can increase hemoglobin concentration, largely because of reduced menstrual flow, and thus offer an advantage to anemic women.

■ The use of the progestin-only contraceptives possible protects against pelvic inflammatory disease, seizures in women with epilepsy, uterine myoma, and endometriosis.
■ These agents should not be used in women under 16 years.
■ It is advisable to stop these agents about 4 weeks before elective surgery and to restart at least 2 weeks thereafter.

Patient/Family Education for Patients Taking Injectable Contraception

■ Depo-Provera users must remember to obtain their doses on regular 3-month intervals or risk loss of contraceptive protection.
■ Although Depo-Provera offers an excellent safety profile because it contains no estrogen, patients may experience irregular cycles in the first few months of use. This is usually followed by amenorrhea if the injection is used consistently. Other issues may be prolonged menses, spotting between menses, and heavy bleeding. After about 5 years of use, it is fairly common for women to report amenorrhea.

Mechanism of Action

The primary mode of action in progestin-only injectables is to thicken cervical mucus, which occurs within a few hours of the dose, as well as impair ovulation. Reports of failure rates with progestin-only injectables are very low (under 0.1%). The combined injectable contraceptives mainly exert their effect through suppression of ovulation whereas the progestin in the formulations thickens cervical mucus.

Pharmacokinetics

■ Absorption: Intramuscular injection is absorbed slowly over approximately 12 to 14 weeks; subcutaneous injection (104 mg) is similarly slowly absorbed.
■ Distribution: Wide area of distribution; lipophilic; it will cross blood-brain barrier.
■ Metabolism: Hepatocytic metabolism via CYP450 system.
■ Half-life: 50 days.

Dosage and Administration

Generic Name	Trade Name	Dose/Application
medroxyprogesterone acetate in aqueous microcrystalline suspension 150 mg/mL	Depo-Provera	IM injection into thigh, buttocks, or deltoid muscle every 4 months; provides pregnancy protection 1 week after injection. Provided as 150 mg/mL aqueous injection. It is also available as 104 mg/mL SC injection.
200 mg norethisterone enanthate	Noristerat, Norigest, Doryxas, and others	200 mg given IM; the first dose is given within 5 days of the start of any cycle.
50 mg norethisterone enanthate and 5 mg estradiol valerate	Mesigyna, Norigynon	The first injection should be given within 5–7 days of any cycle to avoid chance of pregnancy in first cycle.

Adverse Reactions

CV: Results of a WHO study suggest there is little to no increased risk of cardiovascular events with the use of progestin-only injectables, but there remains the possibility of increased stroke risk among women with high blood pressure.

DERM: Acne.

GI: Liver toxicity and an abnormal lipid profile.

META: Decreased libido, osteoporosis, glucocorticoid activity.

MS: changes in calcium uptake in bone and decreases in urinary calcium excretion have been documented but there is no proof of a long-term relationship between use of the progestin injectable contraceptives and low bone density.

Interactions

Drugs that induce liver enzymes may lessen the efficacy of the injectable hormones. Examples are aminoglutethimide (Cytadren), an agent used to treat breast cancer; rifampin (Rifadin); griseofulvin; phenytoin; carbamazepine; and barbiturates.

Contraindications

■ Not for IV usage; use IM only

■ Contraindicated in women who are pregnant or are suspected of being pregnant

■ Contraindicated in women with any vaginal bleeding, urinary tract bleeding, undiagnosed breast pathology, thrombophlebitis, liver dysfunction, or any known hypersensitivity

Subdermal Implantable Contraceptive Devices

An implantable form of contraception based on a progesterone formulation encased in permeable capsules and implanted under the skin is marketed as Implanon (etonogestrel). Introduced in 2006 as a single-rod implantable system, Implanon is about the size of matchstick, and it inhibits ovulation effectively for 3 years. The Implanon casing is not biodegradable, but remains inert if not removed after all the hormone has eluted. Side effects include irregular bleeding, weight gain, and acne because the progesterone used is androgenic. Benefits include excellent efficacy and rapid reversibility (94% ovulation within 3 to 6 weeks of removal). Implant insertion risks include bleeding and infection, but these risks are rare. Insertion is done in the clinician's office and is a quick outpatient procedure. Implanon is a safe and reliable choice for women who are not candidates for estrogen, including women with heart or liver disease, breastfeeding mothers, women with clotting disorders, and smokers over 35 years of age.

Intravaginal Rings

The **intravaginal ring** offers combined contraceptive hormone therapy with low systemic dose levels. The ring is made of a soft ethylene polymer, which elutes 15 mcg of ethinyl estradiol (EE) daily and 120 mcg of etonogestrel (desogestrel) daily. This results in ovarian suppression locally, but minimizes systemic side effects, because circulating hormone levels remain lower than even low-dose OCP levels. Like the transdermal patch, the intravaginal hormones do not undergo first-pass metabolism. Fewer drug interactions are noted due to the combined effect of lower serum levels and lack of cytochrome P450 passage. The intravaginal ring is available as NuvaRing, which provides 35 days of active use. The preferred method of use is 3 weeks on (in) and 1 week off (out) to allow for withdrawal bleed, but the ring may be worn continuously. Because the ring does contain estrogen, it should not be used in patients with a contraindication to estrogen. but it offers a reliable combined hormone choice for women with irregular daily schedules, nonsmokers over 35 years, and women who are nauseated by OCPs. The ring should be left in place during intercourse, but should not be used with spermicide, due to possible degradation of the ethylene carrier vehicle. Because it is a low-dose product, compliance with it is quite high compared with OCP usage.

Contraception Prevention Using Barriers and Spermicides

Other contraceptive options include barriers and toxins, which prevent effective transport of sperm to the fallopian tube. Barrier contraceptives such as external barriers, like male and female condoms, and internal barriers, like diaphragms, cervical caps, or sponges, are often combined with spermicides.

■ *Diaphragms and cervical caps:* Diaphragms and cervical caps provide internal latex barriers to sperm passage, must be fitted by a clinician for each individual user, and must be obtained by prescription. These devices are used with spermicidal foam or gel and must be inserted prior to each act of intercourse. The failure (pregnancy) rate per year is 11% for the diaphragm and approaches 30% for the cervical cap if it is not fitted correctly. Cap users should be encouraged to use condoms or to maintain a supply of emergency contraception pills because the cap failure rate is so high.

■ *Spermicides:* Chemical spermicides are available as vaginal gels, foams, creams, and coating on condoms. They generally include nonoxynol-9 in the United States, although multiple other chemical compounds are used worldwide. Nonoxynol-9 is an irritant to mucous membranes and may increase transmission of STDs, including HIV. Women and their partners who are at risk of HIV exposure should *not* use nonoxynol-9.

■ *Condoms:* Both male and female condoms are moderately effective barriers to conception. Usually made of latex, these are available over the counter. These products will degrade with age, heat, and lipid-based lubricants, so they should not be carried in wallets for prolonged periods, used with petroleum jelly–type lubricants, or if the risk of tearing is high. Failure rates range from 10% to 20% per year. These should be used with spermicide to improve efficacy, and should not be relied on if pregnancy would be medically contraindicated.

■ *Sponge:* The sponge is a nonprescription, unfitted vaginal insert containing a specified quantity of spermicide, suitable for multiple acts of intercourse over a 24-hour period, but it must remain in place for at least 6 hours after the last intercourse. Failure rates are approximately 9% to 11% when used correctly and 13% to 16% when not used correctly.

EMERGENCY CONTRACEPTION

Emergency contraception (ECP) is intended for use by women who have an unexpected failure of protection from other contraceptive methods (ruptured condom, dislodged diaphragm, etc.), or by women who experience an unanticipated act of intercourse or a rape. The first dose of ECP must be administered within 72 hours of intercourse, with a second dose administered 12 hours later if estrogen-containing pills are used. Two basic strategies are used in emergency contraception.

High-Dose Estrogen Medication Administration

Administration of high-dose estrogen for emergency contraception consists of using 100 mcg of ethinyl estradiol per dose in two doses 12 hours apart. This may be done using two 50-mcg tablets per dose, or multiple tablets of the lower dose pills may be used per dose if the woman wishes to use her regular OCPs so that she may rapidly and conveniently take her first dose as early as possible. This may necessitate using three 35-mcg tablets or four 30-mcg tablets. Use of the 20 mcg would require five tablets. Such a high dose of estrogen (100 mcg/dose) is nauseating to most women, and thus most women will need an antiemetic to tolerate this regimen. Over-the-counter (OTC) Dramamine works quite well for this purpose and should be used 20 minutes prior to each estrogen dose. This strategy involves a brief exposure to very high doses of estrogen and may transiently increase the risk of blood clots. This strategy is generally recommended only if the woman wishes to use pills she already has readily available.

High-Dose Progesterone Administration

Administration of high-dose progesterone consists of using 1.50 mg of levonorgestrel in a single dose within 72 hours of intercourse, or as a divided dose, half within 72 hours of intercourse and the second half 12 hours later. This regimen is commercially available as Plan B, and is a nonprescription drug for patients over 16 years of age. Because Plan B does not use estrogen at all, it is not nauseating, carries no clotting risk, and it can be done as a single dose. When Plan B is unavailable, the prescription drug Ovrette may be used, but it requires 20 pills per dose.

Conscientious Prescribing of Emergency Contraception

Plan B should be the preferred ECP because it carries no estrogen risk, is free of nausea, and may be used as a single dose. *Plan B is safe and effective for over-the-counter use*. However, if a woman requests a prescription, it should be made available routinely without an office visit required. Patients should be reassured that ECPs work by halting the motility in the fallopian tubes and by thickening the mucus in those tubes so that sperm is rendered immobile. Patients also should be counseled that Plan B is not an abortifacient and thus will not interfere with an already implanted pregnancy. Clinicians should ask the following questions if patients inquire about ECP use:

1. First, and most important, are you safe? Was this episode the result of an attack? If a woman has had unprotected sex, she may have been raped and may be fearful to ask for the ECP. In addition to Plan B, she should be offered information about rape crisis support.
2. What is your regular method of birth control and how did it fail? A woman may need to choose a more reliable regular method such as Depo-Provera or NuvaRing.
3. How long has it been since the intercourse, and how long since your last menstrual cycle? Although ECPs can be used up to 5 days after intercourse, effectiveness is dramatically reduced after 3 days. If the woman is already pregnant, ECPs will not cause an abortion, and are not harmful to the embryo.

DRUGS FOR THE TREATMENT OF OSTEOPOROSIS AND OSTEOPENIA

Osteoporosis is a significant public health problem characterized by structural deterioration of bone microarchitecture (bone mass) and a corresponding increase in the propensity for bone fractures. While often considered a disease of postmenopausal women, it also affects men and younger women. Overall, women are five times more likely to develop osteoporosis than are men, but men are very much at risk, especially for hip fractures. A woman with osteoporosis who suffers a hip fracture is 10% to 15% more likely to die within 1 year than other women in her age cohort; for men the risk is 25% for death within 1 year. Osteoporosis is also responsible for half a million vertebral fractures per year and 200,000 wrist fractures per year in the United States.

Osteoporosis is confirmed when there is hip or spinal bone mineral density (BMD) score of 2.5 standard deviations (SD) or more below the mean for healthy young women as measured by dual energy x-ray absorptiometry (DEXA). A spinal or hip BMD score between −1 and −2.5 SD below the mean defines osteopenia.

While its symptoms help define osteoporosis and osteopenia, the exact mechanism by which bone architecture shifts is clearly multifactorial. It seems some of the predisposition toward bone loss are polygenic as structural genes and regulatory genes are becoming known. For example, in a variety of population groups polymorphism has been found in the vitamin D receptor gene. Additionally, because estrogen plays a role in pre- and postmenopausal women, there is speculation there is a genetic mutation of estrogen receptor genes. There is also some suggestion that there is a mutation in a gene that affects bone collagen, a key bone protein. As with many medical conditions, genetic and nongenetic factors are interacting to either exacerbate or ameliorate the condition. What is evident, however, is that with today's modern lifestyles and better health care, many women will live more than a third of their lives in a postmenopausal state, making osteoporosis and osteopenia more visible than ever and making prevention more important than treatment.

Osteoporosis prevention begins in childhood with an adequate consumption of calcium and vitamin D. Maintaining healthy bone through adulthood can be accomplished with continued adequate calcium and vitamin D intake along with weight-bearing exercise, moderate use of alcohol, and avoidance of tobacco. There are no clear follow-up recommendations in place to guide the clinician once the diagnosis of osteoporosis or osteopenia is made and treatment initiated, thus the clinician is left to assess successful treatment based on either lack of fractures or increases in BMD scores. A decrease in BMD may suggest noncompliance, inadequate calcium and vitamin D, treatment failure, or an unidentified secondary cause of bone loss. Morbidity is higher among men who experience hip fractures than it is in women, making osteoporosis not just a disease affecting women (Aharonoff, Zuckerman, Egol, & Koval, 2005). A number of medical conditions and medications known to increase the incidence of osteoporosis and osteopenia are listed in Table 20-6.

Medications for treating osteoporosis are many and varied, but they all have the same goals: to achieve optimal peak bone mass, to minimize further bone loss, and to decrease the risk of fracture if a fall occurs. Non-drug approaches such as diet with adequate calcium and vitamin D, exercise, and smoking cessation are proven means of affecting bone mass density (Tang, Eslick, Nowson, Smith, & Bensoussan, 2007). However, the clinician

must still choose the best drug interventions for an individual patient relative to the use of the following classes of drugs:

■ Calcium and vitamin D
■ Bisphosphonates
■ Monoclonal antibody
■ Zoledronic acid
■ Selective estrogen receptor modulators (SERMS)
■ Calcitonin
■ Recombinant parathyroid hormone

Consequently, several guidelines exist for the treatment of osteopenia and osteoporosis. However, the guidelines offered by the Women's Health Initiative seem to be gaining ground due to their definitive answers about hormone replacement therapy and estrogen replacement therapy, and their comprehensive recommendations about low-fat diets, calcium plus vitamin D, and counseling programs on related cardiovascular disease, fracture risk, and lifestyle changes such as weight-bearing exercise (heavy walking, stair-climbing) (NHLBI Women's Health Initiative, 2010).

Calcium and Vitamin D

Calcium, the most abundant mineral found in the human body, is required for vascular contraction and vasodilation, muscle function, nerve transmission, intracellular signaling, and hormonal secretion. Less than 1% of body calcium is used to support these metabolic functions; the remaining 99% is stored in bones and teeth where it supports continuous remodeling and metabolism. The balance between bone resorption and deposition changes with age. The structure of bones requires both osteoclasts and osteoblasts to be involved in a complex signaling pathway if there is to be adequate growth and differentiation.

Involved with this process is having adequate amounts of calcium, parathyroid hormone (PTH), growth hormone, calcitonin, as well as several cytokines. Calcium and vitamin D levels are related to this process because when there is calcium deficiency, PTH levels rise and the vitamin D axis promotes bone resorption to regain calcium homeostasis. Normally, the body only absorbs about 10% of the calcium it ingests; thus, to prevent secondary hyperparathyroidism and bone loss, adequate calcium must be obtained either as a supplement or in the diet. This knowledge has led to the Office of Dietary Supplements of the NIH recommendation that a daily intake of at least 1,000 to 1,200 mg of calcium is necessary for those under 70 years of age and 1,200 mg for those who are over 71 to maintain adequate bone health and calcium retention (NIH, 2011b).

The Institute of Medicine (IOM) recommends a calcium intake of 1,000 mg/day for males between 51 and 70 years of age and 1,200 mg/day for females between 51 and 70 years of age. Women under 70 years of age have a recommended upper limit of 2,500 mg/day if the larger calcium dose is tolerable to the patient. The IOM recommends daily intake of vitamin D at 600 IU for females between 51 and 70 and 800 IU for females over 71 years of age (IOM, 2010). Actual dosing depends on the

TABLE 20-6	Medical Conditions and Medications Having an Increased Risk Associated with Osteoporosis and Osteopenia	
MEDICAL CONDITIONS	**MEDICATIONS**
Alcoholism	Anticonvulsants (phenytoin, phenobarbital)
Chronic renal disease	Aromatase inhibitors (letrozole, anastrazole)
Cushing's syndrome	Cytotoxic drug (methotrexate, cisplatin)
Cystic fibrosis	Ethanol
Glucocorticoids	Tobacco
Diabetes mellitus	Heparin
Eating disorders	Immunosuppressants
Gastrointestinal disorders (malabsorption syndrome)	Lithium
	Thyroid supplements
Hematological disorders	Gonadotropin-releasing hormone (GnRH) agonist (Lupron)
Hyperthyroidism	Heavy consumption o iodine containing drugs such as some OTC cough and cold remedies
	Amiodarone, propylthiouracil, interferon
Hyperparathyroidism	Lithium, thiazide diuretics
Hypergonadism	Prolonged use of opioids
Hyperprolactinism	Antidepressants, Antipsychotics, Antihypertensives
Drug Induced Neuropathies	Cancer Drug Treatments

individual's age, the reasons for taking calcium and vitamin D, the type of calcium being taken, how much calcium the person gets in his or her daily diet, and the person's medical history and current comorbid conditions.

In addition to calcium, there is increasing interest in the health benefits of vitamin D. It has been called the miracle vitamin because lay literature and scattered reports suggest that the importance of vitamin D extends beyond bone health and that it may reduce the risk for cancer, heart disease, stroke, diabetes, and autoimmune diseases. As the only vitamin that the body is able to manufacture itself, vitamin D's major biological function is to help regulate normal blood levels of calcium and phosphorus and assist in calcium absorption into bone. It does this by promoting calcium absorption from the gut, maintaining serum calcium levels, and aiding in bone remodeling of osteoblasts and osteoclasts.

Vitamin D deficiency can lead to osteomalacia (muscle and bone weakness) as well as rickets (deformed bones). Those at greatest risk for vitamin D deficiency are the elderly, obese, and breast-fed infants with little or no sun exposure, and those with Crohn's disease. Over the past 20 years, mean serum concentrations of vitamin D in the United States have slightly declined among males but not females, likely due to male increases in body weight, reduced milk intake, and women's greater use of sun protection when outside (NIH, 2011a).

Most people meet at least some of their vitamin D needs through exposure to sunlight where ultraviolet (UV) B radiation penetrates uncovered skin and converts cutaneous 7-dehydrocholesterol to previtamin D_3, which in turn becomes vitamin D_3. This is influenced by season, time of day, length of exposure, cloud cover, air quality (smog), skin melanin, and use of sunscreen. However, opportunities exist to form vitamin D and store it in the liver and fat from the sunlight exposure obtained throughout the year. Cloud cover reduces UV energy by 50%. In the shade, UV energy is reduced by 60%, and UV radiation does not penetrate glass, thus exposure to sunshine indoors through a window does not produce vitamin D. As for sunscreens, those with an SPF of 8 or more block vitamin D–producing UV rays, but people generally do not apply sufficient amounts or cover all sun-exposed skin, nor do they reapply it with enough regularity to make a difference. Thus, the skin synthesizes some vitamin D even when it is protected by sunscreen, and the average person will still receive approximately 5 to 30 minutes of sun exposure between 10 a.m. and 3 p.m. at least twice a week to the face, arms, legs, or back, which is sufficient to induce vitamin D synthesis.

Two forms of vitamin D are important for humans, ergocalciferol (vitamin D_2) and cholecalciferol (vitamin D_3). Ergocalciferol is obtained from plants. Cholecalciferol is synthesized first as an inactive form in the skin of humans when exposed to sunlight and then converted to its active form by the liver. Only about 10 to 15 minutes a day of non-peak sunlight exposure two to three times a week is necessary to produce an adequate amount of vitamin D. A daily dose of 400 IU is the recommended dose for supplementing vitamin D.

Conscientious Prescribing of Calcium and Vitamin D

■ Elemental calcium binds to numerous medications such as levothyroxine, fluoroquinolones, tetracycline, phenytoin, angiotensin-converting enzyme inhibitors, iron, and bisphosphonates, which can cause these agents to be significantly decreased when given with calcium. This has led to the recommendation that these medications be given several hours before or after calcium dosing.

■ Calcium carbonate is the salt of choice because it contains the highest concentration of elemental calcium and it is inexpensive. It should be given at mealtimes so that increased acid secretion will enhance absorption.

Patient/Family Education for Patients Taking Calcium and Vitamin D

■ The lighter a person's skin, the more vitamin D a person will make. Thus, skin color can affect dosing of vitamin D as well as the use of high (greater than 8) SPF sunscreens. Patient education is needed about sun exposure and risk of skin cancer.

■ Some people have a genetic predisposition that prevents adequate absorption of vitamin D from sunlight, which may affect dosing of vitamin D.

■ People who live in northern areas may not get adequate sunlight during winter months; encourage sun exposure to help develop "natural vitamin D."

■ To maintain good bone health and prevent osteoporosis, patients need to be taught to eat a balanced diet that includes calcium-rich foods (Table 20-7), especially calcium-rich nondairy foods.

■ Patients must be counseled that calcium potentiates the effects of exercise on bone mineral density. The value of exercise as well as smoking cessation and decreased alcohol use (maximum one drink per day for women or two drinks per day for men) cannot be overemphasized.

■ Patients should be able to distinguish between osteoporosis and osteopenia so that if they have the low bone density of osteopenia, but not osteoporosis, they may wish to use a recommended medication to reduce the risk of developing osteoporosis and fracture.

■ Patients should be directed to the over-the-counter formulations that provide elemental calcium and/or calcium and vitamin D (Table 20-8).

Interactions

Vitamin D is known to interact with at least 141 drugs, but only three drug interactions with it and three of its analogues, calcitrol (Rocaltrol), paricaltrol (Zemplar) and doxercalciferol (Hectoral), are significant. In the presence of vitamin D, these three drugs induce an additive effect, producing symptoms of acute hypercalcemia (headache, nausea, dizziness, vomiting, and loss of appetite). Another drug interaction results from coadministration of both calcium and vitamin D and hydrochlorothiazide. The combination of high doses of calcium and Vitamin D along with hydrochlorthiazide (HCTZ) results in the HCTZ

TABLE 20-7 Calcium Rich Foods (nondairy)

FOOD	SERVING SIZE	CALCIUM (MG)
Soy beverage, calcium fortified	1 cup	368
Collard greens, cooked	1 cup	357
Sardines in oil	3 oz	325
Tofu, firm	½ cup	253
Spinach, cooked	1 cup	245
Turnip greens, cooked	1 cup	197
Pink salmon, canned w/bone	3 oz	181
Okra, cooked	1 cup	176
Molasses, blackstrap	1 tbsp	172
Beet greens, cooked	1 cup	164
Bok-choi, cooked	1 cup	158
Soybean greens, cooked	½ cup	130
Ocean perch, cooked	3 oz	116
White beans, canned	½ cup	96
Kale, cooked	1 cup	93.6
Clams, canned	3 oz	78
Nuts, almonds, oil roasted	1 oz	74.5
Rainbow trout, cooked	3 oz	73

TABLE 20-8 Elemental Calcium and Vitamin D in Common OTC Formulations

PRODUCT (1% ELEMENTAL CALCIUM)	ELEMENTAL CALCIUM PER TABLET (MG)	VITAMIN D PER TABLET (IU)
Calcium carbonate (40%)	200	—
Tums 500 mg	300	—
Tums EX 750 mg	400	—
TUMS ultra 1,000 mg	500	—
Os-Cal 500	500	200
Os-Cal 500+ D.	600	200
Rolaids 550 mg	220	—
Caltrate 600	600	200
Viactiv	500	100
Calcium citrate (40% available calcium)	250–500	Vitamin D3-400
Citracal	200	—
Citracal plus D	315	200
Calcium phosphate (39%–40% available calcium)	500	200–400
Posture-D	600	—
Calcium lactate (13%)	85	—
Calcium gluconate (9%)	60	—

inhibiting the renal secretion of calcium, which in turn leads to hypercalcemia. Finally, steroids, dilantin and phenobarbitol all have their metabolism affected by Vitamin D. While not a true drug interaction, agents such as orlistat (Zenical, Alli) interfere with Vitamin D absorption.

Contraindications

■ Vitamin D is relatively safe except that it is contraindicated in patients with parathyroidism.
■ Contraindications to calcium supplementation include people with a history of ventricular fibrillation, hypercalciuria, hyperphosphatemia and renal stones. It should be used cautiously in people taking digitalis for heart failure.

Bisphosphonates

Bisphosphonates are first-line drugs for treating postmenopausal women with osteoporosis because they have been shown to reduce vertebral fractures by 40% to 70% and reduce the amount of nonvertebral fractures by about 50% (North American Menopause Society, 2010). They also appear to reduce the risk of fracture in men with osteoporosis and in persons who take glucocorticoid medications such as prednisone.

Alendronate (Fosamax), risedronate (Actonel), and ibandronate (Boniva) are administered orally; zoledronic acid (Zometa) and pamidronate (Aredia) are given by intravenous infusion once a year. Alendronate (Fosamax) and risedronate (Actonel) are known for reducing the risk of hip and vertebral fractures, whereas ibandronate (Boniva) has been shown to decrease the risk of vertebral fractures only (Paxianas, Cooper, Ebatino, & Russell, 2010).

The challenges surrounding bisphosphonates include the need for careful administration to avoid serious gastrointestinal upset, including nausea, pain, and dyspepsia. Also, these drugs are poorly absorbed (1% to 5%), and thus have low bioavailability.

Conscientious Prescribing for Patients Taking Bisphosphonates

■ Use cautiously in patients with renal impairment.
■ Bisphosphonate therapy has been associated with osteonecrosis of the jaw.
■ Patients on these drugs may show abnormal diagnostic imaging results in bone scans because of reactions with the diagnostic imaging agent.
■ Monitor patients by periodically testing serum calcium, phosphorous, and alkaline phosphatase.

Patient/Family Education for Patients Taking Bisphosphonates

■ Warn patients about incidences of bone, joint, and muscle pain. These symptoms may be debilitating and severe, last a day or months, but will dissipate when bisphosphonates are discontinued.
■ Oral bisphosphonates must be taken with a full glass of water. Patients are encouraged to remain upright for 30 to 60 minutes before reclining or consuming other medications, beverages, or food to lower the risk of upper gastrointestinal adverse effects such as erosive esophagitis.

■ The intravenous forms of these drugs can be administered once annually, except for ibandronate, which is administered every 3 months.

Mechanism of Action

The bisphosphonates have been known since the middle of the 19th century when it was discovered that they could be used to prevent calcium carbonate scaling in industrial applications. Research into the bisphosphonates has led to compounds that inhibit calcification when given in high doses and inhibit bone resorption, all without being destroyed by enzymes. Bisphosphonates adhere tightly to bone surfaces, and by inhibiting osteoclastic activity, they inhibit both normal and abnormal bone resorption. Because the cycle of bone remodeling takes longer to complete and slows with age, especially in postmenopausal women, bisphosphonates are able to slow and often reverse this process, and thus halt and even reverse loss of bone.

Pharmacokinetics

■ Absorption: Oral formulations are poorly absorbed.
■ Distribution: Transiently distributes to soft tissue, then onto bone.
■ Metabolism: There is no metabolism of this drug.
■ Excretion: Excreted in the urine.
■ Half-life: About 10 years before drug is released from skeletal bone.

Dosage and Administration

Generic Name	Trade Name	Route	Usual Adult Daily Dose For Postmenopausal Osteoporosis
alendronate	Fosamax	PO	5 mg daily or 35 mg once a week for osteopenia
			10 mg daily or 70 mg once a week for osteoporosis
ibandronate	Boniva	PO, IV	2.5 mg/day or 150 mg once a month or 3 mg IV every 3 months
risedronate	Actonel	PO	5 mg daily or 35 mg once a week
raloxifene	Evista	PO	60 mg/day
etidronate	Didronel	PO	400 mg/day for 2 weeks, then no dose for 13 weeks, then repeat cycle
pamidronate	Aredia	IV infusion over 2 hr	12–13.5 mg/dL (60–90 mg) per single dose for hypercalcemia or Paget's disease
zoledronic acid	Zometa	IV infusion	Treatment of hypercalcemia and bone metastasis Provide an IV infusion of 5 mg once a year

Clinical Uses

■ Treatment and prevention of osteoporosis in premenopausal women.
■ Treatment of osteoporosis in males.
■ Treatment of Paget's disease in patients who are symptomatic.
■ Treatment of glucocorticoid-induced osteoporosis in both men and women who have low bone mineral density and are taking steroids.

Adverse Reactions

CV: Atrial fibrillation.
DERM: Erythema, photosensitivity, rash.
GI: Abdominal distention, abdominal cramps, abdominal pain, constipation, GI reflux, dyspepsia, flatulence, GI ulcer, change in taste.
MS: Osteonecrosis of the jaw. This rare complication is seen most often with frequent infusion of intravenous bisphosphonates. 94% of cases occur in patients treated with IV bisphosphonates and 85% of those cases were in patients also being treated for cancer, but this uncommon adverse event is severe and can be associated with oral therapy as well.
NEURO: Headache.

Interactions

■ This medication should not be taken with antacids and calcium supplements because their ions decrease absorption of the bisphosphonate.
■ Medication should not be taken with aspirin or NSAIDS because of the increased risk of GI side effects.
■ Food significantly decreases bisphosphonate absorption.
■ Caffeine, mineral water, and orange juice considerably decrease absorption.

Contraindications

■ Bisphosphonates are contraindicated in patients with decreased creatinine clearance.
■ Contraindicated in patients with hypocalcemia, any history of gastrointestinal disease, and patients with invasive dental procedures due to risk of osteonecrosis.

Conscientious Considerations

■ Intravenous dosing offers an alternative way of taking bisphosphonates for people who are unable to tolerate the oral therapy or who are not compliant with the oral therapy.
■ Oral bisphosphonates should be given along with calcium and vitamin D.

Patient/Family Education

■ Patients must be instructed on the importance of taking oral bisphosphonates at the same time each morning, 30 minutes *before* other medications or food.
■ If a dose is missed, skip the daily dose and resume the following morning.
■ When taking a dose, patients should be instructed to remain upright for 30 minutes to facilitate passage of the drug into the stomach and reduce the risk of esophageal irritation.
■ Patients should be counseled on the need for a balanced diet, supplemental calcium and vitamin D, and regular weight-bearing exercise.
■ To reduce the risk of osteoporosis, patients should be counseled to stop smoking and cut back on alcohol consumption.
■ Patients should also be counseled on the use of sunscreens and use of protective coverings to reduce the risk of photosensitivity, notwithstanding the moderate amount of sun exposure needed to assure adequate vitamin D production.

Selective Estrogen Receptor Modulators

Selective estrogen receptor modulators (SERMs) mimic estrogen agonists in some tissues and antiestrogen in others, and ideally, they provide the bone resorption inhibition of estrogen without its unwanted side effects. SERMs were initially called "antiestrogens," but it was subsequently recognized that this inadequately described their spectrum of activities. The widely used SERMs, tamoxifen (Nolvadex) and toremifene (Fareston), demonstrate estrogen antagonist activity in breast tissue. Tamoxifen (Nolvadex) is used for the treatment of both breast cancer and osteoporosis in postmenopausal women. Raloxifene (Evista) is a popular SERM marketed for its ability to allay the undesirable estrogen agonist actions of other SERMs.

Raloxifene (Evista)

The Multiple Outcomes Raloxifene Evaluation (MORE) study, an international study to determine the effects of raloxifene on bone mineral density and vertebral fractures in 7,705 postmenopausal women with osteoporosis, showed the incidence of new spinal fractures to be reduced by 30% to 50% whether or not there were vertebral fractures at baseline (Conner, 2002). Raloxifene also showed significant no-skeletal effects: It significantly decreased the risk of invasive breast cancer in postmenopausal women, an effect that is sustained over 8 years.

In other research, the National Surgical Adjuvant Breast and Bowel Project conducted the Study of Tamoxifen and Raloxifene on postmenopausal women at high risk of breast cancer. The women were given either raloxifene or tamoxifen. Although results showed similar efficacy of both drugs at reducing the risk of breast cancer, there was a lower risk of adverse events and a better tolerance for raloxifene (Vogel, 2009).

Mechanism of Action

This drug has estrogen agonist activity on the bones and lipids and an estrogen antagonist effect on the breast and uterus.

Pharmacokinetics

- Absorption: About 60% from GI system.
- Distribution: 95% is bound to plasma protein.
- Metabolism: Hepatic, with extensive first-pass metabolism to glucuronide conjugates resulting in only 2% being bioavailable.
- Excretion: Primarily in feces.
- Half-life: 27 to 32 hours.

Dosage and Administration

Generic Name	Trade Name	Route	Dose
raloxifene	Evista	PO	60 mg/day

Clinical Uses

- Prevention and treatment of osteoporosis in postmenopausal women
- Decreases the risk of invasive breast cancer in postmenopausal women with osteoporosis

Adverse Reactions

CV: Increased vasomotor symptoms, increased risk of venous thromboembolism

MS: Leg cramps
MISC: Hot flashes
NEURO: Drowsiness

Interactions

- May alter the effects of warfarin and other highly protein-bound drugs

Contraindications

- Hypersensitivity
- History of thromboembolic events
- Women of childbearing potential and during pregnancy and lactation

Conscientious Considerations

This medication must be used only in postmenopausal women with osteoporosis who have no vasomotor symptoms, no history of venous thromboembolism, are unable to tolerate bisphosphonates, and have a high breast cancer risk score.

Patient/Family Education

- Instruct patients to take their medication for the full course of therapy and as directed.
- If a dose is missed, it should be taken at the time it is remembered, but not if it is almost time for the next dose. Doubling doses is not recommended.
- Advise the patient that raloxifene will not reduce hot flashes or flushing associated with estrogen deficiency and may in fact cause these symptoms.
- Advise the patient that weight bearing exercise is an important part of therapy.
- Advise the patient of the importance of adequate calcium and vitamin D supplements as well as the need to stop smoking and reduce alcohol consumption.
- Because of the risk of leg cramps turning into venous thrombosis, patients should be advised to avoid prolonged travel if it involves long periods of sitting and to discontinue the medication for at least 72 hours before any surgery where long periods of immobilization may result.

Calcitonin

Calcitonin-salmon is a manufactured version of the 32-amino acid polypeptide hormone produced in the thyroid glands of humans. The commercial calcitonins (Miacalcin, Fortical, and Calcimar) are prepared synthetically and are modeled after the calcitonin found in salmon.

Mechanism of Action

Calcitonin acts primarily on bone, but the exact mechanism of its action is not well understood. Old bone is removed by cells called osteoclasts, and new bone is laid down by cells called osteoblasts. Calcitonin inhibits bone removal by osteoclasts and promotes bone formation by osteoblasts. Calcitonin is found in many animal species, but calcitonin-salmon is the one most widely used.

Pharmacokinetics

- Absorption: Nasal as a spray or injected intramuscularly or subcutaneously
- Distribution: Local

■ Metabolism: Is not metabolized
■ Excretion: In the urine
■ Half-life: Subcutaneously: 1.5 hours; intranasally: 143 minutes

Dosage and Administration

Generic Name	Trade Name	Route	Dose
calcitonin	Miacalcin Fortical	Nasal spray 200 IU per spray	200 IU in alternating nostrils each day but *only* for women who are at least 5 years postmenopausal
	Calcimar Miacalcin	Injection 200 IU/mL	Inject SC or IM 100 IU per day for Paget's disease

Clinical Uses

■ Calcitonin is used for treating postmenopausal osteoporosis, Paget's disease of bone, and hypercalcemia.
■ It is indicated for treatment of postmenopausal osteoporosis in women at least 5 years postmenopausal with low bone mass relative to healthy mass.
■ When used as a nasal spray, it protects against spine fractures and is sometimes used to help treat the pain of an acute spine fracture.

Adverse Reactions

EENT: Rhinitis, other nasal symptoms, epistaxis, runny nose.
MISC: Because calcitonin-salmon is a protein, the possibility of systemic allergic reaction exists.
MS: Back pain, arthralgia, bone pain.
NEURO: Headache.

Contraindications

■ Side effects are uncommon, but anyone with a known allergy should not use it.
■ Its use in pregnancy, children, or nursing mothers has not been studied.

Interactions

Concomitant use of calcitonin and lithium may lead to a reduction in lithium concentrations.

Conscientious Considerations

■ Calcitonin has been shown to decrease the occurrence of vertebral fractures. It also has a modest analgesic property in the setting of acute and chronic vertebral compression fractures.
■ It is not considered a first-line treatment for osteoporosis because more effective medications are available.
■ Periodic nasal examinations are recommended; if nasal ulceration occurs, discontinue treatment until healed.

Patient/Family Education

■ Patients should take the medication exactly as indicated. If a dose is missed they should try to take it within 2 hours of the scheduled time, if scheduled daily. If taken every other day, then take missed dose on the next day.
■ Advise patients about signs of hypercalcemic relapse (bone pain, flank pain, anorexia, nausea, thirst, lethargy, vomiting).

■ If patient is using subcutaneous or intramuscular dosage forms, advise that flushing and warmth following injection are transient and usually last about an hour. Nausea following injection will decrease with continued therapy.
■ Patients should follow a low-calcium diet if indicated, but postmenopausal women with osteoporosis should adhere to a diet rich in vitamin D and calcium.
■ Patients will need instruction on the use of an intranasal pump if that is being prescribed: Activate pump by holding upright and depress white side arms six times, then place nozzle in nose with head in an upright position and depress pump toward its bottle.

Recombinant Human Parathyroid Hormone (Parathyroid Hormone Therapy)

Parathyroid hormone causes bone density to increase by its ability to maintain calcium and phosphorus levels as new bone is formed. A synthetic form of naturally occurring parathyroid hormone is approved as therapy for the treatment of postmenopausal women with severe bone loss, men with osteoporosis who have a high risk of fractures, and persons who have not improved on bisphosphonate therapy.

Teriparatide (Forteo)

Once-daily administration of teriparatide stimulates the growth of new bone formation on trabecular and cortical bone surfaces by preferential stimulation of osteoblastic activity over osteoclastic activity.

Mechanism of Action

Forteo, also called rhPTH, contains recombinant human parathyroid hormone and has an identical sequence to the 34 *N*-terminal amino acids (the biologically active region) of the 84-amino acid human parathyroid hormone. Teriparatide is manufactured using a strain of *Escherichia coli* modified by recombinant DNA technology.

Pharmacokinetics

■ Absorption: Absorbed after subcutaneous injection, with about 95% becoming rapidly available. Peak serum concentrations are reached in about 30 minutes and decline to undetectable levels within a few hours.
■ Distribution: Systemic bound to protein.
■ Metabolism and excretion: No studies have been performed because it is believed enzymatic mechanisms occur in the liver followed by excretion by the kidneys into the urine.
■ Half-life: 1 hour when given subcutaneously.

Dosage and Administration

Generic Name	Trade Name	Route	Dose
teriparatide	Forteo	Subcutaneously	20 mcg/day for 2 years

Clinical Use

■ Treatment of postmenopausal women with osteoporosis at high risk for fracture, defined as a history of osteoporotic fracture, multiple risk factors for fracture, or patients who have failed or are intolerant to other available osteoporosis therapy

Adverse Reactions

CV: Orthostatic hypotension

GI: Nausea

META: Increases serum calcium and decreases serum phosphorus, transient hypercalcemia

MS: Arthralgia, leg cramps

Interactions

■ No studies have been able to confirm any drug interactions.

Contraindications

■ Contraindicated in patients with risk of osteosarcoma, such as patients with Paget's disease, previous skeletal radiation, or unexplained elevation of their alkaline phosphatase level.

Conscientious Considerations

■ Patients should also be screened for hyperparathyroidism prior to initiating therapy. If there are high levels of calcium or alkaline phosphatase in the patient's blood, this medication should not be prescribed.

■ Patients with a history of kidney stones should use this medication with caution.

■ Patients should also be screened for use of drugs that increase the risk of osteoporosis or osteopenia (see Table 20-6).

Patient/Family Education

■ Because teriparatide has been shown to increase the rate of bone tumors in animal studies, the risk of its use in humans should be discussed with the patient.

■ Patients should be queried as to whether or not they are taking digoxin (Lanoxin) because dosage adjustments may be needed, and the digitalis could reach toxic levels. Caution is advised if the two are given concomitantly.

■ Because this medication can increase calcium levels in the blood, the patient should be advised to tell any other clinician that they are taking this drug before blood tests are taken or if they suffer any renal insufficiency.

HORMONE REPLACEMENT THERAPY FOLLOWING MENOPAUSE

Menopause is the permanent cessation of menstruation secondary to the loss of ovarian and follicular activity. It may occur naturally or be induced. Vasomotor symptoms (hot flashes and night sweats) and vaginal dryness are the most often reported complaints with menopause. The most effective treatment for the management of these symptoms is estrogen replacement therapy. When estrogen is contraindicated, nonestrogen options may be considered. Many women go through menopause with few or no symptoms. The median age for menopause in the United States is 52 years, which means that a woman with a life expectancy of about 80, will live one-third of her life postmenopausal. Health concerns for this population include bone health, cardiovascular health, breast health, colorectal cancer screening, physical activity, no tobacco, alcohol in moderation, responsible sexual activity, and oral health.

The use of hormone treatment by menopausal women has declined since the results of the Women's Health Initiative, a major 15-year study by the National Institutes of Health (NIH),

were published. This study found hormone replacement therapy (HRT) among women taking a combination of estrogen 0.625 mg plus 2.5 mg of progestin per day was associated with a higher risk of having a myocardial infarction or a venous thromboembolism after one year of HRT, a stroke after 3 years of HRT, and breast cancer after 4 years of HRT, with the risk increasing each year beyond. This study did find a lowering of the prevalence of fractures and colon cancer among women who used HRT, but as more of the data have been analyzed, risks of blood clots, ovarian cancer, and dementia have been identified. The North American Menopause Society recommends extended use of estrogen or estrogen-progestogen agents in women if they are aware of the risks and benefits and are under medical supervision, believe the benefits of symptom relief outweigh the risks, have moderate to severe symptoms and are at high risk of osteoporosis fractures, and have reduced bone mass and want to prevent further bone loss when alternate therapies are inappropriate (North American Menopause Society, 2010).

Conscientious Prescribing of Hormone Replacement Therapy (HRT)

■ Hormone treatment should be prescribed at the lowest effective dose for the shortest duration necessary to control menopausal symptoms.

■ Because of the impact the Women's Health Initiative Trial has had on society and clinicians, estrogen-only replacement therapy (ERT) is used solely for patients without a uterus; otherwise, estrogen and progestin combination HRT may be used in women with a uterus.

■ The U.S. Preventative Services Task Force recommends against the routine use of combined estrogen and progestin for the prevention of chronic conditions such as cardiovascular disease, osteoporosis, and dementia in postmenopausal women.

■ Nonhormonal therapeutic options such as black cohosh, tai chi exercise, soy, and selective serotonin reuptake inhibitors should also be considered.

Patient/Family Education for Patients Taking Hormone Replacement Therapy

■ Patients considering hormone treatment should talk with their clinicians to see if they are good candidates for this treatment option. The process should start with a low dosage, and the treatment should be used for the least amount of time necessary to manage the symptoms.

■ Frequent follow-up with the clinician will be important to discuss the symptoms, side effects, and the dosage of the medication.

Estrogen Replacement Therapy

These medications are synthetic female hormones are used to do the following:

■ Prevent conception for women during childbearing age

■ Reduce menopause symptoms of hot flashes and vaginal dryness

■ Prevent bone loss and osteoporosis in people at high risk

■ Treat certain cancers in men and women

All of the signs, symptoms, and adverse effects of menopause result from declining 17 beta-estradiol production by the ovarian follicles. Exogenous estrogen administration to the perimenopausal and postmenopausal woman obviates most of these changes. The objective of estrogen-replacement therapy should be to diminish the signs and symptoms of ovarian failure and restore estrogen levels. There are several estrogen preparations available through various routes. The conjugated estrogens are unconjugated in the gastrointestinal tract and delivered to the target tissues as estrone. When taken orally, 17 beta-estradiol is oxidized to estrone. However, if administered transdermally or intravaginally, it remains unaltered. The administration of continuous unopposed estrogens can result in endometrial hyperplasia and an increased risk of endometrial adenocarcinoma. Hence, it is essential to administer a progestin in conjunction with estrogens in women who have not undergone a hysterectomy.

Continuous estrogen replacement therapy with cyclic progestin administration results in resolution of symptoms and cyclic endometrial withdrawal bleeding from the endometrium. One of the challenges of this approach is that many postmenopausal women do not want cyclic bleeding and would rather continue on a regimen of daily administration of both an estrogen and a low-dose progestin. The other use of ERT is the use of conjugated estrogen during menopause to reduce moderate to severe hot flashes; treat moderate to severe dryness, itching, and burning in and around the vagina; and to help prevent and treat osteoporosis.

Estrogen replacement therapy is available in many formulations. The mainstay for 50 years has been the conjugated equine estrogen (Premarin), which is extracted and purified from the urine of pregnant mares. Newer formulations contain agents that have been synthesized in a laboratory (Table 20-9) or are taken from plant sources.

Conjugated Estrogen (Premarin)

Conjugated estrogen is used after menopause to reduce moderate to severe hot flashes; to treat moderate to severe dryness,

TABLE 20-9 Common Formulations and Dosages of Estrogens Used in Women's Health

	GENERIC NAME	TRADE NAME	USUAL ADULT DAILY DOSE AND INDICATION
Oral Estrogens	conjugated equine estrogens	Premarin	0.3, 0.45, 0.625 mg/day cyclically, such as 25 days on and 5 days off (osteoporosis)
	synthetic conjugated estrogens	Cenestin	0.3–0.625 mg/day cyclically, such as 25 days on and 5 days off (osteoporosis)
	esterified estrogens	Estratab	10 mg 3 times/day for 3 months (breast cancer)
	estradiol	Estrace	0.5 mg/day cyclically (3 weeks on, 1 week off) (osteoporosis prophylaxis)
	estropipate	Ogen, Ortho-Est	0.625 mg/day for 25 days of a 31-day cycle (osteoporosis prevention)
Transdermal Estrogen	estradiol patch	Alora, Climara, Esclim, Estraderm, FemPatch, Vivelle	0.025 mg/weekly patch (vasomotor symptoms of menopause)
	estradiol	Menostar	1 mg weekly (osteoporosis prophylaxis)
	estradiol	EstroGel	1.25 gm/day (vasomotor symptoms of menopause)
Topical Estrogens			
Vaginal Creams	conjugated equine estrogens	Premarin	0.2–0.4 GM of cream applied daily. Each gram contains 0.625 mg of estrogen. (Treat moderate to severe dyspareunia).
	estradiol	Estrace	Each gram contains 0.1 mg of estradiol. The usual dosage range is 2–4 gm (marked on the applicator) daily for 1 or 2 weeks, then gradually reduced to one-half initial dosage for a similar period. A maintenance dosage of 1 gm, 1–3 times/week, may be used after restoration of the vaginal mucosa has been achieved.
	estropipate	Ortho-Est	2–4 gm/day (atrophic vaginitis)
Vaginal Rings	estradiol	Estring, Femring	2 mg (vaginal atrophy)
Vaginal Table	estradiol	Vagifem	1 tab/day for 14 days (atrophic vaginitis)
Emulsions	estradiol	Estrasorb	3.84 gm once a day in a.m. (for vasomotor symptoms of menopause)

itching, and burning in and around the vagina; and to help prevent and treat osteoporosis. Conjugated estrogen is a blend of estrogen hormones that in fact are not exactly the same as human natural estrogen whether taken from horses, plants, or laboratory flasks, but all have FDA approval for use in treating menopausal symptoms.

Mechanism of Action

Conjugated estrogens contain a mixture of estrone sulfate, equilin sulfate, 17 alpha-hydroequilin, 17 alpha-estradiol, and 17 beta-dihydroequilenin. Because estrogens are responsible for the development and maintenance of the female reproductive system and secondary sexual characteristics following menopause, these conjugated estrogens help modulate the pituitary secretion of gonadotropins, luteinizing hormone (LH), and follicle-stimulating hormone (FSH) through feedback mechanisms. In essence, these hormones reduce elevated levels of gonadotropins, LH, and FSH in postmenopausal women.

Pharmacokinetics

■ Absorption: Are well-absorbed orally
■ Distribution: Circulate protein bound
■ Metabolism: Liver CYP450 converted to active estrogen metabolites
■ Excretion: Urine
■ Half-life: 1 to 2 hours

Dosage and Administration

Generic Name	Trade Name	Route	Form	Dose
Conjugated/equine estrogen	Premarin	PO, IV	Tablets: 0.3 mg, 0.045 mg, 0.625 mg, 0.9 mg, 1.25 mg, 2.5 mg Also IM, IV, and vaginal cream, 0.3 mg, 0.45 mg, 0.625 mg, 0.09 mg, 1.25 mg	For vasomotor symptoms associated with menopause/prevention of osteoporosis: 0.3 mg/day; adjust according to bone mineral density levels and response.
Plant-sourced conjugated estrogen (estrogen derivative)	Enjuvia	PO	Combinations as 0.3 mg estrogen + 1.5 mg medroxyprogesterone, 0.45 mg estrogen + 1.5 mg medroxyprogesterone, 0.625 mg estrogen + 2.5 mg medroxyprogesterone, 0.625 mg estrogen + 5 mg medroxyprogesterone	For vasomotor symptoms associated with menopause, start with 0.3 mg/day and titrate up to 1.25 mg/day
Conjugated estrogen plus medroxyprogesterone	Prempro	PO		For vasomotor symptoms of menopause, start with lower dose formulation and titrate up
Synthetic estrogen (not the same as conjugated estrogen from equine sources; contains only 9 elements)	Cenestin	PO	0.3 mg, 0.45 mg, 0.625 mg, 0.9 mg, 1.25 mg	For vasomotor symptoms of menopause, start with 0.45 mg/day For atrophic vaginitis use 0.3 mg/day.

Clinical Uses

■ Treatment of the symptoms of menopause
■ Prevention of osteoporosis in those at risk

Adverse Reactions

CV: Thromboembolism, retinal thrombosis, myocardial infarction, edema, stroke, hypertension
DERM: Acne, oily skin, increase pigmentation, urticaria
ENDO: Gynecomastia (men), hyperglycemia
GI: Nausea, weight changes, anorexia, jaundice, vomiting
META: hypercalcemia, water retention
MS: Leg cramps
NEURO: Headache, dizziness, lethargy, depression
OB/GYN: Ovarian, breast, and endometrial cancer, endometrial hyperplasia, uterine fibroid enlargement, and hypercalcemia, amenorrhea, breakthrough bleeding, breast tenderness

Interactions

■ Grapefruit juice may increase estrogen levels.
■ Will alter requirements for warfarin, oral hypoglycemic agents, and insulin.
■ Smoking will increase risk of adverse cardiovascular events.

Contraindications

■ Pregnancy
■ Undiagnosed vaginal bleeding
■ Breast cancer
■ Recent or current thromboembolism
■ Estrogen-dependent cancer

Conscientious Considerations

■ Caution should be used with smokers and patients with hypertriglyceridemia.
■ Any unusual vaginal bleeding while taking estrogen should be evaluated by a clinician. Vaginal bleeding after menopause may be a sign of endometrial cancer and should be evaluated with an ultrasound and/or endometrial biopsy.
■ Using estrogens, with or without progestins, may increase the risk of myocardial infarction, stroke, breast cancer, and thromboembolism. Using estrogens, with or without progestins, has been suspected to increase the risk of dementia, but this association remains controversial.
■ The drug should be used at the lowest dose to control the symptoms for the shortest time period required. The risks and benefits as well as alternative therapies should be discussed with the patient.

Patient/Family Education

■ Explain the importance of the medication regimen, that patients should not double dose if they miss a dose, and if they take a week off the drug, withdrawal bleeding will occur.
■ If nausea is a problem, advise patients to take this medication with food.
■ If water retention is noticed, patients should be counseled to return for evaluation.

■ Patients should be instructed to stop the medication if pregnancy is suspected.

■ Patients over 35 years of age should be warned that the risk of adverse events increases dramatically in those who continue to smoke while on this medication.

■ Because increased pigmentation is a risk with these agents, patients need counseling on the use of sunscreens and protective clothing.

■ Remind patients on oral ERT of the importance of routine wellness exams, including a Papanicolaou smear and mammogram. Additionally, all women who are pregnant should undergo cervical cytology screening at the time of their initial prenatal visit.

Progestins

With the advent of menarche the ovaries begin producing steroids, estrogen, and progestin. Progestin causes the following:

■ Thickening of the endometrium in preparation for pregnancy
■ Production of a sticky mucus to plug the cervical os
■ Thinning of the vaginal mucosa
■ Relaxation of smooth muscle along the fallopian tubes and uterus.

Outside the reproductive system, progestin stimulates lipoprotein activity, increases basal insulin levels and responses to glucose, promotes glycogen storage in the liver, increases body temperature, and competes with aldosterone in the renal tubules to decrease sodium reabsorption.

Several progestin preparations are available to alleviate the decline of ovarian hormone function during menopause. Medroxyprogesterone (Provera) and norethindrone (Aygestin) are oral formulations, and micronized progesterone (Prometrium) is available in oral form and as a vaginal gel marketed as Prochieve and Crinone.

Medroxyprogesterone (Provera)

Medroxyprogesterone (MPA), the primary exogenous progestin, has been synthesized and branded as Provera and Cycrin (in 2.5-mg, 5-mg, 10-mg tablet); Depo-Provera (as 150 mg/mL injection and 400 mg/mL injection); and Amen (as 10-mg tablet). All are used in the treatment of secondary amenorrhea and abnormal uterine bleeding caused by hormone imbalance as well as prevention or decrease of endometrial hyperplasia.

Mechanism of Action

Progestin inhibits pituitary gonadotropin release, preventing follicular maturation (contraceptive effect), transforms proliferative endometrium into secretary endometrium, and maintains pregnancy by inhibiting spontaneous uterine contractions. It also produces an antineoplastic effect in cases of endometrial and renal carcinoma.

Pharmacokinetics

■ Absorption: Following oral administration, between 0.6% and 10% is absorbed.
■ Distribution: Well distributed and enters breast milk.
■ Metabolism: Metabolized in the liver.

■ Excretion: In the urine.
■ Half-life: 14 to 16 hours.

Dosage and Administration

	Generic Name	Trade Name	Usual Adult Daily Dose For
ORAL PROGESTINS	Medroxyprog-esterone acetate	Provera	Amenorrhea: 5–10 mg/day for 10 days
TRANSDERMAL PROGESTINS	Levonorgestrel	Mirena, Plan B	Emergency contraception: One 0.75-mg tablet STAT within 72 hr of unprotected sex; take a second tablet 12 hr after the first.

Clinical Uses

■ To decrease endometrial hyperplasia in postmenopausal women receiving concurrent estrogen therapy
■ Treatment of secondary amenorrhea and abnormal uterine bleeding (AUB) caused by hormonal imbalance
■ As an emergency contraceptive

Adverse Reactions

CV: Fluid retention, PULMONARY EMBOLISM
DERM: Alopecia, acne, melasma, chloasma, rashes
EENT: Retinal thrombosis
ENDO: Amenorrhea, breakthrough bleeding, breast tenderness, changes in menstrual flow, spotting, hyperglycemia, edema
GI: Weight changes, nausea, GI-induced hepatitis, gingival bleeding
GYN: Menstrual irregularities, breast tenderness, cervical erosions
MISC: Allergic reactions, including anaphylaxis and angioedema, weight gain or loss
NEURO: Depression

Interactions

■ Use as a contraceptive may be rendered ineffective in the presence of phenobarbital, phenytoin, rifampin.
■ This drug should be given 1 hour before or at least 4 hours after using bile acid binding.
■ Resins (e.g., cholestyramine, colestipol) which will bind to the hormone, reducing bioavailability.

Contraindications

■ Contraindicated in cases of hypersensitivity, pregnancy, thromboembolic or cardiovascular disease, liver disease, cancer, seizure disorders, mental depression, renal disease, and lactation.

Conscientious Considerations

Those who prescribe this medication need to be familiar with its various packaging and dosing parameters. For example, only the 150-mg/mL vial should be used for contraception. If giving the intramuscular dose, the vial should be shaken vigorously before giving dose, which should be injected very deeply into muscle.

Patient/Family Education

■ When used for menstrual dysfunction, patients should be taught that withdrawal bleeding will occur between 3 and 7 days after stopping the medication.

■ Patients should review and understand the list of side effects and be committed to contacting their health professional should any of them occur.

■ Patients should be taught how to do a monthly breast exam and to watch for any increase in breast tenderness.

■ Good oral hygiene should be emphasized with patients because gingival bleeding may occur.

■ If a period is missed or pregnancy is suspected, patients should be instructed on the importance of contacting their clinician.

■ Medroxyprogesterone may cause melasma (brown patches on face) in some patients with exposure to sunlight. Thus, patients need counseling on the use of sunscreens and protective clothing.

■ Patients on these agents need to understand the importance of a yearly routine wellness examinations that include a general physical, blood pressure, pelvic and breast examinations, and a Papanicolaou smear.

Combination Estrogen/Progestin Products

Preparations combining estrogen and progesterone are available in tablets or transdermal patches and with different dosing schedules. Some single tablets have options for various dosages to be taken daily, others use a phase technique with estrogen tablets being taken for 14 days and combined estrogen and progesterone for the next 14 days. Another method (Prefest) uses a pulsed therapy, which has intermittent 3-day bursts of norgestimate in combination with daily low-dose estrogen. The bursts of pulse therapy are thought to reduce the incidence of bleeding by not producing as much endometrial atrophy as the combined therapy. Whether estrogen is used alone or in combination with a progestin, the lowest effective dose possible should be used for the shortest duration of therapy possible, with periodic evaluations to determine if treatment is still necessary.

Dosage and Administration

	Generic Name	Trade Name	Starting Dose Schedule
ORAL	conjugated estrogens (CE)	Prempro	Prempro therapy consists of a single tablet taken orally 1 time/day
	medroxyprogesterone acetate (MPA)	Premphase	Premphase is a 2-tablet regimen, 1 tablet taken daily on days 1–14 (contains 0.625 mg of CE) and 1 tablet taken on days 15–28 (contains 0.625 mg CE and 5 mg of MPA)
	estradiol + norethindrone	Activella	On 1st Sunday after menstruation, take 1st tablet daily for 21 days, then rest 7 days
	ethinyl estradiol + norethindrone	Femhrt	On 1st Sunday after menstruation, take 1st tablet daily for 21 days, then rest 7 days
	estradiol + norgestimate	Ortho-Prefest, Ortho-Cyclen	On 1st Sunday after menstruation, take 1st tablet daily for 21 days, then rest 7 days
	estradiol + norethindrone	Loestrin, Ortho-Novum	Day 1–7: 1 blue tab Day 8–16: 1 yellow-green tab Day 17–21: 1 blue tab Day 22–29: 1 orange inactive tab
	estradiol + levonorgestrel	Climara Pro, Tri-Levlen, Seasonale, Triphasil	On 1st Sunday after cycle, start 1st dose, then 1 tab daily for either 21 days or 28 days, depending on packaging

Implications for Special Populations

Pregnancy Implications

When prescribing for the pregnant or lactating female, clinicians should carefully consider their choice of drugs and their effects on a fetus. The FDA categories of the medications discussed in this chapter follow.

FDA CATEGORY	DESCRIPTION OF RISK
A	Vitamin D compounds
	Calcium
C	All calcium salts
	Bisphosphonates
	Calcitonin-salmon
	Recombinant parathyroid hormone
X	Estrogens and progestins (medroxyprogesterone)
	All contraceptives
	Selective estrogen receptor modulators (SERMS)
	Conjugated estrogens

Most clinicians would prefer *not* to prescribe anything for a pregnant woman because there is always the concern of fetal abnormalities (teratogenicity) occurring. Many women are unaware that their prescription medications can cause teratogenicity. Every clinician must be aware of medication with known teratogenic effects (Table 20-10).

Breastfeeding

Breast milk is known to possess nutritional and immunological properties superior to those found in infant formulas. The long- and short-term effects and safety of maternal drugs on suckling infants is meager. It is important that patients and health professionals consider the risk and benefits of the transport of drugs into breast milk and the possible effects this could have on the infant and milk production. The medications in Table 20-11 are contraindicated in lactating women.

TABLE 20-10	Medications With Known Teratogenic Effects
Alcohol	HMG-CoA reductase inhibitors
Androgens	Iodides
ACE-inhibitors/ARBS	Isotretinoin
Anticonvulsants	Lithium
(valproic acid, phenytoin	Tetracyclines
and carbamazepine)	Thalidomide and DES
Chemotherapeutic agents	Warfarin

ACE, angiotensin-converting enzyme; ARBs, angiotensin II-receptor blockers; DES, diethylstilbestrol

TABLE 20-11	Medications Contraindicated in Lactating Women
ACE inhibitor/ARBs	Isotretinoin
Benzodiazepines	Lithium
Carbamazepine	Methotrexate
Diclofenac	Misoprostol
Ergotamines	Nicotine
Estrogen/combination OCP	Phenobarbital
Flurazepam	Valproate
HMG-CoA reductase inhibitor	Warfarin

ARBs, angiotensin II-receptor blockers; OCP, oral contraceptive pill; ACE, angiotensin-converting enzyme

LEARNING EXERCISES

Case 1

RT is a 62-year-old Native American female radiology technician with a Colles wrist fracture she sustained during a fall. Her 80-year-old mother has osteoporosis. RT is 60 inches tall and weighs 115 lbs. She swims most days and plays softball on the weekends. Her DEXA scan shows she has osteoporosis. RT experienced natural menopause at 54 and does not use hormone treatment. She does not have complaints of vasomotor symptoms of menopause. Her diet is not rich in calcium, and she is not taking a calcium or vitamin D supplement. She smokes and drinks about 5 to 7 alcoholic beverages weekly. She has no history of gastrointestinal disease or esophagitis.

1. What medication, if any, would you recommend? Why would you choose this medication?

2. What patient advisories would you recommend for this patient?

Case 2

MJ is a 27-year-old flight attendant. She travels the world and has a boyfriend who she sees every other weekend. She uses a combination oral contraceptive (COC) to make sure she does not become pregnant when she is at home; she is 100% compliant to its regimen. Upon returning home from a long trip, she feels unwell, and because her medical benefits are good, decides to have her annual check-up. Her physician discovers she has tuberculosis and she is given a 4-month course of antibiotic therapy, which includes the drug rifampin (Rifadin), an antitubercular agent. After 3 months of therapy, MJ believes she may have a urinary tract infection and returns to her physician. At this visit she tests positive for pregnancy. She looks terrified and surprised and shouts, "How did that happen? I have been taking my pills, and haven't missed one, and I've only been with my boyfriend once."

1. How is MJ pregnant?

References

Aharonoff, G. B., Zuckerman, J. D., Egol, K. A., & Koval, K. J. (2005). Gender differences in patients with hip fracture: A greater risk of morbidity and mortality in men. *Journal of Orthopedic Trauma, 19*(1), 29-35.

Archer, J. S., & Archer, D. F. (2002). Oral contraceptive efficacy and antibiotic interaction: A myth debunked. *Journal of the American Academy of Dermatology, 46*, 917-923.

Behara, M. (September, 2010). Dysfunctional uterine bleeding: Treatment and medication. Retrieved February 23, 2013, from http://emedicine.medscape.com/article/257007-treatment

Blumenthal, P. D., & Edelman, A. (2008). Hormonal contraception. *Obstetrics & Gynecology, 112*, 670-684.

Casablanca, Y. (2008). Management of dysfunctional uterine bleeding. *Obstetrics and Gynecology Clinics of North America, 35*, 219-234.

Conner, E. B., Grady D., Sashegi A., Anderson P. W., Cox, D. A., Hoszowski, K., et al. Raloxifene and Cardiovascular Events in Osteoporotic Postmenopausal Women, JAMA 2002; 287(7): 847-857. Accessed February 27, 2013, from http://jama.jamanetwork.com/article.aspx?articleid=194654

Cornforth, T. The Why Behind Contraceptive Failure, April 27, 2009. Women's Health About.com. Accessed February 27, 2013, from http://womenshealth.about.com/od/birthcontrol/a/contraceptive_failure.htm

Dickinson, B. D., Altman, R. D., Nielsen, N. H., & Sterling, M. L. (2001). Drug interactions between oral contraceptives and antibiotics. *Obstetrics & Gynecology, 98*, 853-860.

Fillingim, R. B., King, C. D., Ribeiro-Dasilva, M. C., Rahim-Williams, B., & Riley III, J. L. (2009). Sex, gender, and pain. A review of recent clinical and experimental findings. *Journal of Pain, 10*(5), 447-485.

Halbreich, U., Borenstein, J., Pearlstein, T., & Kahn, L. S. (2003). The prevalence, impairment, impact, and burden of premenstrual dysphoric disorder (PMS/PMDD). *Psychoneuroendocrinology, 28*(Suppl. 3), 1-23.

Institute of Medicine. (2010). Committee to Review Dietary Reference Intakes for Vitamin D and Calcium, Food and Nutrition Board. *Dietary reference intakes for calcium and vitamin D*. Washington, DC: National Academy Press. Available at http://iom.edu/Reports/2010/Dictary-Reference-Intakes-for-Calcium-and-Vitamin-D/DRI-Values.aspx

Kligfield, P., Lax, K. G., & Okin, P. M. (1996). QT interval-heart rate relation during exercise in normal men and women: Definition by linear regression analysis. *Journal of the American College of Cardiology, 28*, 1547-1555.

Lethaby, A., Irvine, G., & Cameron, I. (2008). Cyclical progestogens for heavy menstrual bleeding. Cochrane Database System Review, (3). DOI: 10.1002/14651858.CD001016.pub2

Lomaestro, B. M. (2009). Do antibiotics reduce the efficacy of combined oral contraceptives? Medscape Business of Medicine. Retrieved March 22, 2013 from www.medscape.com/viewarticle/707926

Massachusetts General Hospital (MGH) Center for Women's Mental Health. When PMS Symptoms Interfere with Functioning and Quality of Life: PMS and PMDD. Accessed February 27, 2013, from www.womensmentalhealth.org/specialty-clinics/pms-and-pmdd

Merck Manual for Health Professionals. (2012). Retrieved February 24, 2013, from www.merckmanuals.com/professional/sec18/ch244/ch244c.html

(NHLBI)National Heart Lung Blood Institute, Women's Health Initiative, updated 9/21/2010. Accessed February 27, 2013 from www.nhlbi.nih.gov/whi

National Institutes of Health (NIH). Medline Plus. (2010). Iron deficiency anemia. Available at www.nlm.nih.gov/medlineplus/ency/article/000584.htm

National Institutes of Health (NIH). Office of Dietary Supplements. (2011a). Dietary supplement fact sheet: Vitamin D. Retrieved February 24, 2013, from http://ods.od.nih.gov/factsheets/VitaminD

National Institutes of Health (NIH). Office of Dietary Supplements, (2011b). Dietary supplement fact sheet: Calcium. Retrieved February 24, 2013, from http://ods.od.nih.gov/factsheets/calcium

Natural Medicine Comprehensive Database. Retrieved February 24, 2013, from http://www.naturaldatabase.com

North American Menopause Society. (2010). Management of osteoporosis in postmenopausal women. *Menopause, 17,* 1, 25-54.

Pearlstein, T., & Steiner, M. (2008). Premenstrual dysphoric disorder: Burden of illness and treatment update. *Journal of Psychiatry & Neuroscience, 33*(4), 291-301.

Tang, B. M., Eslick, G. D., Nowson, C., Smith, C., & Bensoussan, A. (2007). Use of calcium or calcium in combination with vitamin D supplementation to prevent fractures and bone loss in people aged 50 years and older: A meta-analysis. *Lancet, 370*(9588), 657–666.

Vogel, V.G. (January, 2009). The NSABP study of tamoxifen and raloxifene (STAR). *Expert Review of Anticancer Therapy, 9*(1), 51-60. Retrieved February 24, 2013, from www.ncbi.nlm.nih.gov/pubmed/19105706

Waynine, Y. (2011). Levonorgesterol IUD approved for women with heavy menstrual bleeding, Medscape Medical News. Available at www.medscape.com/viewarticle/709854

Drugs Used to Affect Men's Health

chapter 21

Fred S. Girton, William N. Tindall

CHAPTER FOCUS

This chapter presents an overview of the pharmacology associated with four health concerns unique to men: erectile dysfunction, benign prostatic hypertrophy (BPH), testosterone insufficiency, and male pattern baldness. Other male concerns such as prostate, testicular, and penile cancer and various urogenital infections are only briefly discussed here because their pharmacology was detailed in Chapter 19, Drugs Used in the Treatment of Neoplasms, and Chapter 17, Modern Approaches to Managing Bacterial Infections.

OBJECTIVES

After reading and studying this chapter, the student should be able to:

1. Describe the role that pharmaceuticals play in men's health, particularly in the treatment of erectile dysfunction, benign prostatic hypertrophy, testosterone insufficiency, and male pattern baldness.

2. Describe the three phosphodiesterase type 5 inhibitors for the treatment of erectile dysfunction, including their mechanism of action and adverse effects.

3. Discuss the two main types of pharmaceuticals (5 alpha-reductase inhibitors and alpha-adrenoceptor blockers) for the treatment of benign prostatic hypertrophy, including the drugs' differences and adverse effects.

4. Explain the main benefits of testosterone treatment for androgen deficiency.

5. Provide recommendations for the treatment of male pattern baldness and discuss the effectiveness of available treatments.

6. Recognize the importance of male self-image and hesitancy to seek care for treatment of their health issues.

Key Terms

Alpha blockers

5-Alpha reductase inhibitors

Andropause

Benign prostatic hypertrophy (BPM)

Erectile dysfunction

Hypogonadism

Male pattern baldness

Penile tumescence

KEY DRUGS IN THIS CHAPTER

Orally Active Phosphodiesterase Type 5 Inhibitors
- sildenafil (Viagra)
- tadalafil (Cialis)
- vardenafil (Levitra)

Prostaglandin E
- alprostadil (Caverject, MUSE)

5-Alpha Reductase Inhibitors (Androgen Inhibitor)
- finasteride (Propecia, Proscar)
- dutasteride (Avodart)

Alpha-1 Adrenoceptor Antagonists (Alpha Blocker)
- prazosin (Minipress)
- doxazosin (Cardura)
- alfuzosin (Uroxatral)
- tamsulosin (Flomax)
- terazosin (Hytrin)
- topical minoxidil (Rogaine)

Testosterone
- oral methyltestosterone (Android)
- oral fluoxymesterone (Halotestin)

- buccal testosterone (Striant)
- testosterone patch (Androderm)
- testosterone transdermal (Testoderm)
- IM testosterone cypionate (Depo-Testosterone)
- IM testosterone enanthate (Delatestryl)
- topical testosterone 1% gel (AndroGel)
- subcutaneous testosterone pellets (Testopel)

According to the U.S. Census Bureau, the average life expectancy for a male born in 2010 is 75.7 years. For men, this is an increase of 3.3 years since 1980. Life expectancies have increased for both genders during the last century, but women have traditionally had a longer life expectancy than do men. In recent years, however, the gender gap in life expectancy has narrowed (U.S. Census Bureau, 2011).

Men generally take more health risks and make fewer visits to their clinicians than do women. Health concerns such as erectile dysfunction, benign prostatic hypertrophy, testosterone insufficiency, and male pattern baldness that are unique to men may evoke significant emotions and affect a man's self-confidence and self-image. Clinicians must be aware of the sensitive nature of these problems.

DRUGS USED TO TREAT ERECTILE DYSFUNCTION

Interest in and treatment of men's health issues has increased tremendously over the last 10 to 15 years. Leading the way was the discovery of phosphodiesterase type 5 (PDE5) inhibitors to treat erectile dysfunction (ED). **Erectile dysfunction** (previously called impotence) is defined by the 1992 National Institutes of Health Consensus Development Panel on Impotence as "the inability of the male to achieve or maintain an erection sufficient for sexual intercourse" (U. S. Department of Health and Human Services, 1992).

The Massachusetts Male Aging Study (MMAS) showed that 52% of 1,290 men aged 40 to 70 had some degree of erectile dysfunction, and almost 10% had total absence of erectile function (O'Donel, Araujo, & McKinley, 2004). Risk for ED rises sharply with age, with a 3.6-fold greater prevalence in men aged 50 to 59 compared with men aged 18 to 29. An estimated 600,000 new cases of ED occur annually in the United States in white males aged 40 to 69 years. ED is associated with comorbidities such as cardiovascular disease and hypertension, diabetes mellitus, lower urinary tract symptoms, prostate cancer, and depression (Rosen, Wing, Schneider, & Gendrano, 2005).

To understand the pharmacological treatment of ED, it is necessary to understand the cascade of events that leads to **penile tumescence** (erection) (Fig. 21-1). Upon sexual stimulation, a neuronal response is sent through the spinal nerves, which results in neurotransmitters being released at the cavernous nerve terminals. As a result, vasoactive relaxing factors are released from the endothelial cells of the penile blood vessels. The smooth muscles of the arterial supply to the cavernosa relax, causing arterial dilatation and a significant increase in blood flow. At the same time nonvascular trabecular smooth muscles of the corpora cavernosa within the sinusoids are also relaxed, allowing the increased blood to flow into the cavernosa to cause an erection. This increase in pressure in the sinusoids results in venous compression and occlusion of venous outflow, thus maintaining the erection.

The neuronal response initiating erection is primarily a parasympathetic response, but there is an important nonadrenergic-noncholinergic neuronal response as well; both appear to result

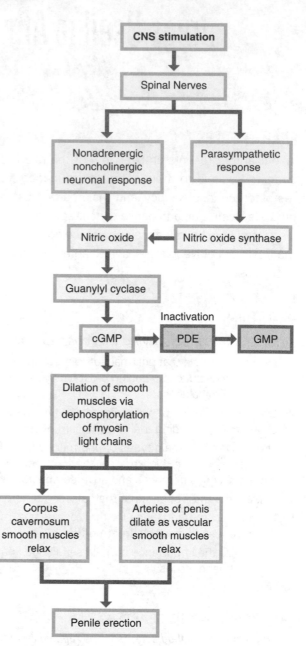

FIGURE 21-1 The physiology/cascade of erection.

in the release of the neurotransmitter nitric oxide, which activates guanylyl cyclase, leading to an increase in production of cyclic guanosine monophosphate (cGMP). cGMP activates a specific protein kinase, which ultimately results in a dephosphorylation of myosin light chains and relaxation of the smooth muscle. Certain other smooth muscle relaxants such as prostaglandin 1 analogues, intestinal polypeptide, neuropeptide Y, substance P, and serotonin are supportive of an erection and, if present in sufficient quantity, can cause penile erection by themselves. A successful erection requires an intact parasympathetic nerve system as well as the release of adequate nitric oxide. The role of testosterone in penile erection is debated, and although libido is definitely affected by low testosterone levels, no relationship has been found between testosterone levels and ED; however, testosterone may be needed to maintain proper function of the nitric oxide pathway.

Etiology of Erectile Dysfunction

The causes of ED are generally classified into six main categories:

1. Vasculogenic (arterial or cavernosal) (e.g., atherosclerosis, hypertension). A significant correlation between hypertension and ED is seen in epidemiological studies; evidence suggests that underlying vascular disease causing hypertension contributes more to ED than the side effects from certain antihypertensive medications. With vasculogenic cases, ED is due to inadequate blood flow to initiate or maintain penile tumescence.
2. Psychogenic (e.g., depression, relationship problems). Loss of libido is associated with the ED.
3. Hormonal (e.g., hypothyroidism, hyperthyroidism, hyperprolactinemia). The ED is associated with impaired nitric oxide release and loss of libido.
4. Neurogenic (e.g., diabetes, spinal cord injury). The ED is caused by failure to initiate neuronal response to activate release of smooth muscle relaxants. More than half of all men with ED have diabetes, a growing epidemic in the United States today.
5. Drug use (e.g., alcohol, tobacco, antihypertensive medications, antidepressants, antipsychotics). The ED may be caused by multiple mechanisms, including neuropathy, loss of libido, and vascular insufficiency. Men treated with two or more drugs have a significantly higher prevalence of ED than do untreated men.
6. Other (e.g., anatomic anomaly, mechanical abnormalities, surgical complications, and the natural result of chronic disease and old age may affect neural, vascular, psychological, and metabolic mechanisms of penile tumescence). Even otherwise healthy aging men often experience a decline in sexual function, including ED.

Although there are many etiologies associated with ED, the newer treatments for ED work at the end of the cascade. Obviously many of the etiologies for ED involve comorbidities or risks that may be of greater concern to the health of the patient than his ED. Although it is not the purpose of this chapter to discuss in detail the differential diagnosis of ED, it is important to know that significant comorbidities may exist that require evaluation and treatment. ED may be the presenting symptom of an unidentified disease or condition such as alcoholism, diabetes, hypertension, or coronary artery disease that requires more acute attention than the presenting ED. It is estimated that 25% of ED is a result of medication side effects (Viera, Clenney, Shenberger, & Green 1999). Therefore, a *complete* medication and nonprescription drug list, including over-the-counter (OTC), herbal, alcohol, tobacco, and illicit drug use, should be determined. Except in the case of alcohol, tobacco, and illegal drugs, many of these medications are needed, and the clinician must weigh the danger of discontinuation versus the side effect of ED.

Vasculogenic erectile dysfunction is one of the most common etiologies. Anything that interferes with the normal flow of blood into and out of the corpus cavernosa of the penis will have an effect on penile tumescence. Although gross arterial and venous anomalies are of concern, by far the most common cause of vasculogenic ED is at the level of the endothelium, where atherosclerosis, diabetes, hypertension, and other factors may alter the normal functioning, resulting in a decrement in endothelial-dependent relaxation of the smooth muscles.

Conditions that cause endothelial dysfunction are risk factors for ED. Chronic cigarette smoking is a major risk factor for ED because of the effects of cigarette smoke on the vascular epithelium and peripheral nerves, a risk that increases as men age. Men with hypercholesterolemia may suffer impairment of endothelium-dependent relaxation in various vascular beds that may be reversible with lipid-lowering drugs. Multivariate analysis shows that ED is positively associated with depression, prostate diseases, diabetes, and use of diuretics.

Treatments for other diseases, such as testosterone for hypogonadism, antidepressants for depression, and anxiolytics for anxiety may also be beneficial in improving ED, but what is really being managed in these cases is a side effect of a primary disease. Some alternative medications (e.g., glyceryl nitrate, saw palmetto, and ginseng) have been found to be of some benefit in treating ED, but they have not been truly studied with great scrutiny.

Depending on the etiology, there are several pharmacological as well as nonpharmacological options for treating ED. The non-pharmacological options include mechanical devices such as vacuum erection devices, which can be purchased over the counter; penile prostheses (implants), which require urologic referral; and penile revascularization, which also requires surgical referral. The pharmacological options include the popular phosphodiesterase type 5 (PDE5) inhibitors such as sildenafil (Viagra), tadalafil (Cialis), vardenafil (Levitra), and the injectable prostaglandins. Like all medications, these come with serious risks and adverse reactions, and patients and their families must be adequately advised before therapy is started.

Conscientious Prescribing of Drugs Used to Treat ED

■ PDE5 inhibitors are expensive, and many insurance companies limit or refuse to pay for them. Many patients request and are usually prescribed 4 to 10 tablets per month.
■ Priapism is rare in PDE5 inhibitors but are more common with alprostadil. This complication can be treated with corpora aspiration, followed by intracavernosal injection with alpha-adrenergic agonists such as phenylephrine (Neo-Synephrine).
■ When patients do not respond to PDE5 inhibitors due to cord injury, alprostadil can be used because it is not dependent on nitric oxide to create an erection.

Family and Patient Education Regarding Drugs for ED

■ Men on nitrates should not take PDE5 inhibitors.
■ None of the treatments for ED are protective against sexually transmitted diseases, including HIV. Patients must be

told that they need to use other methods to prevent pregnancy and STDs.

■ Men using ED medications who experience prolonged erections should seek medical attention immediately.

■ Men using transurethral alprostadil should not have sexual intercourse with a pregnant woman.

Oral Phosphodiesterase Type 5 Inhibitors

The serendipitous discovery of phosphodiesterase type 5 inhibitors in the late 1990s revolutionized the treatment of erectile dysfunction. While searching for a new antihypertensive medication, PDE5 inhibitors were found to have the desirable side effect of enhancing penile erections in those who previously were having difficulty achieving one. It is this PDE5 selectivity that produces the smooth muscle relaxation of arteries in the corpus cavernosum. However, because they are not 100% selective, these agents have many drug interactions, and concomitant administration with any nitrates is absolutely contraindicated because of a possible potentiation of a blood pressure-lowering effect, possibly as much as 80 mm Hg.

Mechanism of Action

Phosphodiesterases are found throughout the body (Fig. 21-2) and perform a myriad of functions by helping to convert various compounds from one form to another. Inhibitors of phosphodiesterases incapacitate their ability to perform these functions.

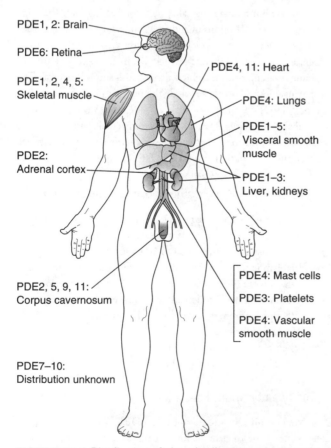

PDE1, 2: Brain
PDE6: Retina
PDE1, 2, 4, 5: Skeletal muscle
PDE2: Adrenal cortex
PDE4, 11: Heart
PDE4: Lungs
PDE1–5: Visceral smooth muscle
PDE1–3: Liver, kidneys
PDE2, 5, 9, 11: Corpus cavernosum
PDE4: Mast cells
PDE3: Platelets
PDE4: Vascular smooth muscle
PDE7–10: Distribution unknown

FIGURE 21-2 Distribution of phosphodiesterase enzymes in tissues throughout the body.

In the corpus cavernosum, PDE5 is the main catalyst responsible for the conversion of cGMP to guanosine monophosphate (GMP). GMP is the inactivated form of cGMP. cGMP acts in the development of an erection by dephosphorylating myosin light chains, which relaxes smooth muscles of the penile arteries and corpus cavernosum, resulting in an erection (see Fig. 21-1). With the inhibition of the PDE5 enzyme by PDE5 inhibitors, cGMP is not converted (broken down) to the inactive form GMP as rapidly, and it can persist in performing its function of creating and maintaining an erection. Because of their locally acting mechanism low in the erectile cascade, PDE5 inhibitors are effective in treating erectile dysfunction owing to multiple and mixed etiologies.

Sildenafil (Viagra) has a 10-fold selectivity for PDE5, tadalafil (Cialis) has a 10,000-fold selectivity, and vardenafil (Levitra) has a 15-fold selectivity; however, there is no drug effect without some type of sexual stimulation because these drugs do not cause penile erections, only the ability of the penis to respond to sexual stimulation.

Pharmacokinetics

■ Absorption: All three drugs are well absorbed orally; however, absorption of sildenafil (Viagra) is inhibited in the presence of food. With sildenafil (Viagra) and vardenafil (Levitra), the onset of action is 30 to 120 minutes, and the duration of effect is approximately 4 hours. Tadalafil (Cialis) has a duration of effect of 36 hours, and its onset of action is approximately 16 minutes.

■ Distribution: Extensive tissue binding.

■ Metabolism: Sildenafil, tadalafil, and vardenafil are metabolized by hepatic (CYP 450) metabolism; with sildenafil, it is metabolized to an active metabolite.

■ Excretion: For sildenafil and vardenafil, 80% is excreted in the feces; for tadalafil, approximately two-thirds is eliminated in feces. The remainder is in urine.

■ Half-life: Sildenafil and vardenafil: about 4 to 5 hours; tadalafil: 17.5 hours.

Dosage and Administration

Generic Name	Trade Name	Route	Usual Oral Adult Daily Dose
sildenafil	Viagra	PO	25–100 mg
vardenafil	Levitra	PO	10–20 mg
tadalafil	Cialis	PO	2.5–5 mg daily or as needed

Clinical Use

■ Treatment of erectile dysfunction

Adverse Reactions

In general, there are few side effects with the use of PDE5 inhibitors.

CV: Flushing.
EENT: Rhinitis, sinusitis.
GI: Dyspepsia, nausea.
GU: Priapism (painful erection lasting over 6 hours) and prolonged erections (lasting over 4 hours) are RARE.

MISC: Flu-like symptoms.

NEURO: Headache.

Interactions

■ **Nitrates.** The most important drug interaction of PDE5 inhibitor medications is their interaction with nitrates (in any form) and sodium nitroprusside. Individuals taking nitrates can have an exaggerated fall in blood pressure (BP) when taking PDE5 inhibitors, which can lead to cardiac arrest and death.

■ **Antihypertensives.** Small additive drops in BP occur when PDE5 inhibitors are given to patients already taking beta blockers, calcium channel blockers, angiotensin-converting enzyme inhibitors, angiotensin receptor blockers, and diuretics. An exception to these findings can be the **alpha blockers**, which in some patients may be associated with an increase in orthostatic hypotension when administered with PDE5 inhibitors. Alpha blockers may be used for treating hypertension.

■ **Other drugs.** Medications that may interact with these medications include macrolides, antifungals, cimetidine, rifampin, non-specific beta blockers, and diuretics because dosage adjustments will need to be made.

Contraindications

■ Contraindicated in patients who are concurrently taking organic nitrate therapy (nitroglycerine, isosorbide mononitrate, or isosorbide dinitrate).

■ Contraindicated in patients with conditions associated with priapism, such as sickle cell disease, myeloma, and leukemia.

■ Contraindicated in patients with retinitis pigmentosa.

■ Use cautiously in patients who are elderly or have any renal impairment.

Conscientious Considerations

■ Because nitrates can cause a significant drop in blood pressure, it is important to determine if PDE5 inhibitors have been ingested within the previous 48 hours prior to administering nitroglycerin.

■ Use caution when prescribing to any person taking antihypertensive medications.

■ Use caution when prescribing to any person taking alpha blockers such as doxazosin (Cardura), tamsulosin (Flomax), and others for benign prostatic hypertrophy.

■ Except in the case of the lower daily dose of tadalafil, it is recommended that these medications only be taken 30 to 60 minutes prior to intercourse and no more often than once a day.

Injectable Prostaglandins Used for Erectile Dysfunction

There are very few vasoactive drugs available for injection therapy, but they include prostaglandin E1 (PGE-1, Caverject, Edex) and papaverine (Regitine), and vasoactive intestinal polypeptides (VIP). Combinations are sometimes used. The drugs are injected using a small-gauge needle into the base of the penis and directly into the corpus cavernosum. Pain sensation is minimal at this point, especially if the drug is injected into the 2 o'clock or 10 o'clock position. The drugs are active in 5 to 10 minutes and their effects last anywhere from 1 to 2 hours. They are very effective and work in 95% of patients. For men who have trouble giving themselves an injection, an auto injector (Ompulse) is available. Papaverine was first available to be used by injection, but its use has fallen because of its high incidence of priapism and liver effects. Vasoactive intestinal polypeptides are available in Europe but not yet in the United States; they are expensive and cause some penile discomfort.

Mechanism of Action

Prostaglandin E1 (Caverject) acts on the arterial smooth muscle cells, causing them to relax by stimulating an increase in levels of intracellular cyclic nucleotides, which in turn causes relaxation of the arterial and trabecular smooth muscles. This results in an increase in arterial blood flow into the corpus cavernosum, allowing the cavernosum to fill with blood and produce an erection. Because prostaglandins bypass many steps in the erectile cascade, they are quite effective at producing an erection even when PDE5 inhibitors cannot. Prostaglandins do not require an intact cord or intact innervations to produce nitric oxide to create an erection. The main impediment to prostaglandin use is that they must be administered by intracavernosal or transurethral injection.

Pharmacokinetics

■ Absorption: Within 10 minutes when injected locally, with an effect that lasts about 1 hour.

■ Distribution: Insignificant.

■ Metabolism: 75% is metabolized through one-pass mechanism in the lungs.

■ Excretion: 90% of metabolites are excreted within 24 hours in the urine.

■ Half-life: alprostadil: about 5 to 10 minutes.

Dosage and Administration

Generic Name	Trade Name	Route	Usual Oral Adult Daily Dose
alprostadil	Caverject	Intracavernosal	2.5–60 mcg given no more than 1 dose/day or 3 times/week as needed
alprostadil	Muse	Intraurethral	125–1,000 mcg given no more than 2 times/24 hr as needed

Clinical Uses

■ Treatment of erectile dysfunction of vascular, psychogenic, or neurogenic etiology

Adverse Reactions

GU: Penile pain (most common adverse reaction, occurring in up to 37% of patients); urethral discomfort; pain in testicles; priapism

Interactions

■ None

Contraindications

■ Penile deformity (e.g., Peyronie's disease)

■ Penile implant

■ Hypersensitivity to alprostadil

■ Patients with conditions predisposing to priapism: sickle cell disease or trait, leukemia, multiple myeloma, polycythemia, thrombocythemia

Conscientious Considerations

■ The first dose should be done under professional supervision to see if it produces an erection lasting under 1 hour.

■ The dose is given using a 0.5 inch 27- or 30-gauge needle along the dorsal aspect of the proximal third of the penis.

Patient/Family Education

■ Patients must be taught to adhere to using the lowest dose that produces a response lasting less than an hour.

■ Patients should also be taught the effects of overdosing (apnea, flushing of face and arms, and bradycardia).

DRUGS USED TO TREAT BENIGN PROSTATIC HYPERTROPHY/HYPERPLASIA (BPH)

Benign prostatic hypertrophy (BPH), the nonmalignant enlargement of the prostate, is a common condition in older men that has become increasingly well known due to the relative aging of the population. According to the National Institutes of Health (NIH), BPH affects more than 50% of men over 60 and as many as 90% of men over the age of 70 (Wei, 2011). Symptoms include weak urinary stream, urinary hesitancy, urinary frequency, frequent nocturnal urination, straining to void, and sensation of incomplete voiding.

A urinary symptom scoring system has been developed by the American Urological Association (AUA) and the Agency for Healthcare Research and Quality (Barry et al., 1998). This scoring system asks patients seven questions about their urinary symptoms and asks them to rate the severity of the symptoms from 0 to 5. Clinicians can use the results to determine the severity of patients' BPH. Once the determination is made that the patient is having symptoms suspicious of BPH, he should be evaluated by careful history, physical examination, and selected laboratory tests for possible other etiology and contributing causes.

The clinical manifestation of BPH is mainly the mechanical compression of the prostatic urethra leading to impaired ability to void. This compression of the urethra may be caused by an enlarged prostate gland and/or increased smooth muscle tone in the bladder neck, prostatic capsule, and prostatic urethra. Prolonged and untreated symptoms of BPH can result in bladder distention and instability of detrusor muscles. Fortunately, benign prostatic hyperplasia condition is such a slow progressive condition it rarely reaches a state of acute urinary retention that may require catheterization due to effective medical management with either pharmaceuticals or the application of minimally invasive therapies.

Etiology

As the name implies, BPH is benign; however, several conditions that are not benign can mimic the symptoms of BPH. The possible causes of BPH-like symptoms besides an enlarged prostate can be neurogenic, infectious, drug induced, and malignant. Particular drugs that may worsen BPH symptoms are first-generation antihistamines, decongestants, narcotics, diuretics, tricyclic antidepressants, and other anticholinergic medications. Medical conditions that may aggravate BPH include diabetes, urinary tract infection, and neurogenic bladder.

Concern for prostate or bladder cancer, especially in this age group, is a primary reason for a thorough evaluation of the BPH symptom etiology. A complete history should be taken, followed by an examination of the genitalia, a digital rectal exam, a urinalysis, and prostate serum antigen (PSA) test. It should be noted that the size of the prostate on physical examination may or may not be helpful in determining the proper diagnosis, but it is necessary to ensure that signs of prostate cancer are not missed. An enlarged prostate may cause increased PSA levels, but these elevated levels should not automatically be assumed to be BPH until cancer has been ruled out.

Pharmacological treatment of BPH is based primarily on the severity of symptoms. For this reason, the patient should be informed fully of the options available to him. The AUA symptom scoring index can help determine the severity of the symptoms. In most cases, when symptoms are mild (usually under 7 on the AUA index scale), the most prudent course to follow is that of watchful waiting.

Since 1992, the FDA has approved the following six drugs to relieve the symptoms commonly associated with an enlarged prostate: the 5-alpha reductase inhibitors finasteride (Proscar) and dutasteride (Avodart) and the alpha blockers terazosin (Hytrin), doxazosin (Cardura), tamsulosin (Flomax), and alfuzosin (Uroxatral).

Alpha blockers relax smooth muscles in the prostate gland. These smooth muscles respond to alpha-adrenergic receptor stimulation and constrict the prostatic urethra. Thus, blockage of these receptors results in relaxation and decreased obstruction of urine flow. Treatment with alpha blockers should result in relatively rapid (1 month) response, but the response does not persist when treatment is stopped.

The **5-alpha reductase inhibitors** are enzymes that inhibit the conversion of testosterone to its more potent form, dihydrotestosterone (DHT), thus suppressing prostate growth, which is stimulated by this androgen. Because they retard prostate growth, the 5-alpha reductase inhibitors may take 2 to 6 months for symptom response, but usually the response is sustained after therapy. The two agents finasteride and dutasteride are not only used for BPH, but find some use in treating prostate cancer, male pattern baldness, and hormone replacement therapy for transgender therapy (male to female).

Alternative therapies, including saw palmetto plant (*Serenoa repens*), rye grass pollen extract (Cernilton), and pygeum, have been used for many years in the treatment of BPH symptoms. In a 2009 Cochrane review, saw palmetto produced mild to moderate improvement, but overall had little or no efficacy over treating with placebo. More needs to be learned about its long-term safety and efficacy (National Center for Complementary and Alternative Medicine [NCCAM], 2009). Studies on rye grass pollen and pygeum have been inconclusive, and presently there are no recommendations for their use.

Conscientious Prescribing of Drugs to Treat BPH

■ The Medical Therapy of Prostatic Symptoms (MTOPS) Trial, supported by the National Institute of Diabetes and Digestive and Kidney Diseases (NIDDK), was the longest running medical trial to see if finasteride and doxazosin used alone or together could stop precancerous prostate growth. This trial found that using finasteride and doxazosin together is more effective than using either drug alone to relieve symptoms and prevent BPH progression (NIDDK, 2010). The two-drug regimen reduced the risk of BPH progression by 67%, compared with 39% for doxazosin alone and 34% for finasteride alone.

■ The antihypertensive effect of alpha blockers requires that attention be paid to other medications that a patient may be taking.

■ Unlike alpha blockers, which are relatively rapid in onset but show no effect on clinical course, the 5-alpha reductase inhibitors are slow to show effect, requiring up to 6 months to reach maximum benefit, but they do show benefit in affecting the clinical course and outcome of BPH.

Family and Patient Education Regarding Drugs for BPH

■ It is important for patients to understand that prior to institution of BPH medication therapy, all prescription medications, over-the-counter medications, and alternative medications need to be evaluated for possible interactions.

■ Men who are on dutasteride and finasteride should avoid donating blood during treatment and for at least 6 months after discontinuing their use.

■ Patients need to understand that treatment will not result in a cure of BPH and that relief of symptoms is the best that can be hoped for.

Alpha-1 Blockers

Medications that block alpha-adrenergic stimulation are called alpha blockers. Alpha adrenergic receptors are located throughout the body, particularly on vascular smooth muscles where they are important in regulating blood pressure through dilation of its vasculature. For that reason, several of these agents, including doxazosin (Cardura), prazosin (Minipress), and terazosin (Hytrin), are also used as antihypertensive medications, though they are not considered first-line treatment for hypertension *because of their ability to produce orthostatic hypotension* as a side effect. This hypotensive side effect in treating BPH with these medications may at times be helpful, but when the decrease in blood pressure is significant, it can be a serious problem resulting in orthostatic hypotension dizziness and even syncope. More selective alpha blockers were therefore developed to target prostatic and bladder smooth muscles only; these newer medications are tamsulosin (Flomax) and alfuzosin (Uroxatral).

Selective and nonselective alpha-1 blocker agents relieve symptoms almost immediately because of their effect on relaxing prostatic smooth muscles. This effect reaches its maximum level within several days to a couple of weeks and is reversible soon after discontinuation of medication.

Pharmacokinetics

■ Absorption: All drugs are well absorbed after oral administration, although tamsulosin is slowly absorbed.
■ Distribution: All are widely distributed throughout the body.
■ Metabolism: All are extensively metabolized in the liver.
■ Excretion: All are excreted both in feces and urine.
■ Half-life: Tamsulosin: 9 to 15 hours; alfuzosin: 10 hours; doxazosin: 22 hours; prazosin: 2 to 3 hours; terazosin: 9 to 12 hours.

Dosage and Administration

Generic Name	Trade Name	Route	Usual Adult Daily Dose
NONSELECTIVE ALPHA BLOCKERS			
doxazosin	Cardura	PO	1–8 mg daily
prazosin	Minipress	PO	0.5–1 mg twice daily
terazosin	Hytrin	PO	1–20 mg at night
SELECTIVE ALPHA BLOCKERS			
alfuzosin	Uroxatral	PO	10 mg daily
tamsulosin	Flomax	PO	0.4 mg daily

All except alfuzosin (Uroxatral) should be started at lowest dose and titrated upward to an effective dose.

Clinical Use

■ Treatment of benign prostatic hypertrophy, hypertension.

Adverse Reactions

CV: Orthostatic hypotension
EENT: Rhinitis
ENDO: Decreased libido
GI: Diarrhea, nausea, stomach discomfort, bitter taste
MS: Muscle pain, back pain
NEURO: Headache, dizziness

Interactions

■ When prescribing alpha blockers, the clinician must consider any medication that may decrease blood pressure, including occasional-use medications such as PDE5 inhibitors (vardenafil, tadalafil, sildenafil) used to treat erectile dysfunction and all antihypertensive medications.

Contraindications

■ Hypersensitivity to medication
■ Concurrent use with any PDE5 inhibitors

Conscientious Considerations

■ First-dose adverse reactions are a possibility. The first dose should be given in the clinic or at bedtime. The first-dose reaction of orthostatic hypotension can be minimized by starting with a low dose and increasing the dose at 2-week intervals.

Patient/Family Education

■ When starting an alpha-1 blocker medication the patient should be cautioned about orthostatic hypotension, especially if he gets out of bed during the night. The patient should be advised to sit up first before standing.

■ Adverse effects often disappear with continued use, but if therapy is interrupted, then started again, side effects may return.

5-Alpha Reductase Inhibitors

Androgenic hormones, particularly dihydrotestosterone (DHT), are responsible for stimulating prostate growth. The 5-alpha reductase inhibitors competitively and specifically inhibit this type 2 isoenzyme that metabolizes testosterone into DHT in the prostate gland. Daily treatment with these inhibitors will cause significant reductions in serum DHT with resultant suppression of prostate growth, decrease in prostate volume (up to 30%), and increase in urine flow rates. With the decrease in prostate volume, the use of 5-alpha reductase inhibitors will result in a significant decrease in PSA levels as well. This is cause for concern because the PSA level is used to screen for prostate cancer. The Prostate Cancer Prevention Trial (PCPT) showed that although finasteride resulted in lower prostate cancers over a 7-year period, the incidence of high-grade cancers was slightly increased, and thus the government stopped the trial. Additionally, because PSA levels were decreased by finasteride, the PCPT trial recommended that when using PSA levels to screen for prostate cancer, the resultant PSA level be doubled to correct for any reduction caused by presence of the 5-alpha reductase inhibitor (National Cancer Institute, 2003).

Pharmacokinetics

■ Absorption: Well absorbed.
■ Distribution: Widely distributed because 90% is protein bound.
■ Metabolism: Metabolized mainly in the liver (40%–50%) to active metabolites.
■ Excretion: More than half is secreted in feces, the rest in urine.
■ Half-life: finasteride: 8 hours in elderly, 6 hours in male adults; dutasteride: approximately 4 weeks. The onset of any clinical effect for both medications is about 3 to 6 months of continued therapy.

Dosage and Administration

Generic Name	Trade Name	Route	Usual Adult Daily Dose
dutasteride	Avodart	Oral	0.5 mg
finasteride	Proscar	Oral	5.0 mg for a minimum of 6 months

Clinical Uses

■ Treatment of benign prostatic hypertrophy (BPH).
■ Finasteride is also used in male pattern baldness and is sold as Propecia.

Adverse Reactions

CV: Postural hypotension
EENT: Rhinitis
ENDO: Impotence, decreased libido, gynecomastia (2%)
GU: Finasteride causes a decrease in prostate specific antigen levels, even in the presence of prostate cancer.
MS: Weakness
NEURO: Dizziness, somnolence
PUL: Dyspnea

Interactions

■ A great many drugs interact with dutasteride and finasteride, including Cimetidine, ciprofloxacin, diltiazem, ketoconazole, ritonavir, verapamil, and St. John's wort, which will result in deactivation of either medication, thus a full drug history of both prescription and OTC drugs is imperative.

Contraindications

■ Hypersensitivity to medication
■ Serious skin reactions to other 5-alpha reductase inhibitors
■ Pediatric patients
■ Pregnancy (or intended pregnancy; see Conscientious Considerations)

Conscientious Considerations

■ Finasteride has been given a pregnancy X category rating because it has been implicated in producing abnormalities in genitalia of male offspring. It should not be handled by a pregnant woman or one who may become pregnant, and men who are on these drugs should avoid donating blood for at least 6 months after taking the drug to avoid exposing women to the drug.

■ Combined therapy with an alpha blocker is becoming more common. Dutasteride 0.5 mg and Tamsulosin 0.4 mg once daily has been approved as an accepted treatment, as has the treatment consisting of 5 mg of Proscar with an appropriate dose of doxazosin. Studies have shown that combination therapy is probably better than monotherapy in reducing clinical progression of BPH (Roehrborn et al., 2008). Side effects are slightly increased in combination therapy, as would be expected.

Patient/Family Education

■ Dutasteride and Finasteride may inhibit development of the genitalia of a male fetus and should not be handled by a pregnant woman or one who may become pregnant.
■ It is important for patients to realize that 3 to 6 months of ongoing therapy may be needed in order to realize significant relief of symptoms.

DRUGS USED TO TREAT TESTOSTERONE DEFICIENCY

Testosterone deficiency is an endocrine deficiency state in which men have a decreased level of testosterone. Signs and symptoms of testosterone deficiency are normal in older men. Although testosterone supplementation is effective in treating testosterone deficiency, testosterone supplementation will not enhance a non-deficient person's vitality, particularly in sexual activities. Despite the benefit of treating those who are truly testosterone deficient, the safety, efficacy, and indications for treatment with testosterone have not yet been clearly defined.

The term **hypogonadism,** often used interchangeably with *testosterone deficiency,* is defined as low serum levels of testosterone associated with certain signs and symptoms. These signs and symptoms include depressed mood, diminished energy, decreased muscle strength and bulk, increased fat mass, impaired cognition, anemia, diminished bone density, fatigue, increased insulin resistance, and multiple sexual dysfunctions, including decreased libido and erectile dysfunction. One can easily see how "normal aging" can easily be misinterpreted as "low testosterone (hypogonadism)" or vice versa.

The causes of hypogonadism in men are many, with aging being the primary cause. Other causes are genetic (Klinefelter syndrome, Kallmann syndrome); androgen receptor defects; 5-alpha reductase deficiency; myotonic dystrophy; cryptorchidism; infectious (mumps, orchitis, HIV, AIDS); pituitary disorders (psychological stress, tumors); medications (glucocorticoids, OTC, illicit drugs); injury/surgical; psychological stress; morbid obesity; and other chronic or serious illnesses. Although these etiologies are multiple, the common finding in all is low levels of testosterone. For that reason, testosterone levels are crucial in making the diagnosis regardless of the signs and symptoms. If the testosterone level is adequate, other causes for the symptoms should be considered. In men it is normal to have a progressive decrease in testosterone levels after the age of 30; this decrease may average 1% to 2% per year. This physiological decrease has been well documented and should be expected (Seidman & Walsh, 1999). This natural decrease is often referred to as "male menopause" or **andropause.** Declining testosterone has been demonstrated to show that about 25% of men develop mild to moderate hypogonadism in mid- to late life (Yassin & Saad, 2008). There is no consistent range of total testosterone that defines hypogonadism, but in general the normal range of total testosterone is considered to be 300 to 1,000 ng/dL (10.4 to 34.7 nmol/L) and hypogonadism is generally considered to be under 200 ng/dL (6.9 nmol/L).

Measurement of total testosterone includes free testosterone and bound testosterone, which differs from bioavailable testosterone (presently bioavailable testosterone is not standardized). The diagnosis of testosterone deficiency is only half of the picture. Next it is necessary to determine if the deficiency is gonadal/testicle failure (primary) or hypothalamic-pituitary complex failure (secondary). Diagnosis therefore requires not only a complete history and physical examination to determine signs and symptoms, but also laboratory tests to include total testosterone, free testosterone, steroid hormone-binding testosterone, luteinizing hormone, and follicle-stimulating hormone levels. Low or normal luteinizing and follicle-stimulating hormone levels in the presence of low testosterone levels may suggest problems with the hypothalamic-pituitary axis and require further investigation, perhaps with magnetic resonance imaging

(MRI) of the head to evaluate the pituitary gland. Because testosterone deficiency can also result in anemia and increased insulin resistance, a complete blood count and fasting blood sugar levels should be obtained as well.

There are no specific nonpharmacological treatments for testosterone deficiency, although numerous nonpharmacological treatments exist for the many vague symptoms associated with this condition, particularly depressed libido. Treatment of testosterone deficiency is accomplished by supplying exogenous testosterone. Secondary causes of testosterone deficiency are also usually treated in this manner unless the secondary condition can be identified and specifically managed.

Exogenous Testosterone

Testosterone is available in multiple forms and can be administered in multiple ways. Testosterone medication is available by oral tablets, buccal systems, intramuscular injection, transdermal patches, transdermal topical gels, and subcutaneous pellets. In general, testosterone deficiency treatment for men is usually done by intramuscular injection. Transdermal patches and gels require greater patient attention because they need to be placed daily. Oral forms of testosterone are not recommended for men owing to the first-pass metabolism and the hepatotoxicity associated with higher doses in men. Pellets and transbuccal troches are relatively new.

Pharmacokinetics

Pharmacokinetics vary according to the ester type of testosterone used and the route of administration.

- Absorption: Absorption is complete when the drug is given intramuscularly.
- Distribution: Testosterone protein binding is about 98% to a sex hormone-binding globulin.
- Metabolism: First-pass metabolism is undergone in the liver, with active metabolites formed.
- Excretion: 90% in urine, the rest in feces.
- Half-life: Varies from 10 to 100 minutes.

Dosage and Administration

Generic Name	Trade Name	Route*	Usual Adult Dose
methyltestosterone	Android	PO	10–50 mg daily
fluoxymesterone	Halotestin	PO	5–20 mg daily
testosterone buccal	Striant	Buccal	30 mg 2 times/day
testosterone patch	Androderm	Applied to nonscrotal skin	2.5–5 mg/24 hr daily
testosterone cypionate	Depo-testosterone	IM	50–400 mg every 2–4 weeks
testosterone enanthate	Delatestryl	IM	50–400 mg every 2–4 weeks
testosterone 1% gel	AndroGel	Applied to nonscrotal skin	5 gm daily
testosterone pellets	Testopel	SC	150–450 mg 3–6 months

*The multiple forms of testosterone give patient and clinician a variety of options to provide the most convenient and cost-effective treatment.

Clinical Uses

- Androgen replacement therapy in the treatment of delayed male puberty
- Male hypogonadism
- Replacement therapy in cases of deficiency of endogenous hormone
- Inoperable female breast cancer

Adverse Reactions

There do not appear to be any major adverse reactions to taking testosterone. However, because both prostate cancer and benign prostatic hypertrophy are thought to be stimulated by testosterone, there is great concern that testosterone supplementation will either cause or have an adverse effect on these two conditions. Nevertheless, to date no convincing data to that effect have been found.

CV: Edema, flushing, hypertension, vasodilation
DERM: Acne, alopecia, dry skin, erythema, hirsutism
ENDO: Breast soreness, gynecomastia, hypercalcemia, hypoglycemia, menstrual issues
GI: Nausea, vomiting, bitter taste, hepatitis, hepatic dysfunction
GU: Bladder irritability, impotence, priapism, testicular atrophy, urination impaired
HEM: Leucopenia, suppression of clotting factors
MISC: Pain and inflammation at injection site.
MS: Weakness
NEURO: Aggressive behavior, amnesia, headache, anxiety, depression, nervousness, sleeplessness, paraesthesia

Interactions

- Oral anticoagulants such as warfarin increase the hypoprothrombinemic response.

Contraindications

- Hypersensitivity to medication or any component of product
- Breast cancer
- Prostate cancer
- Pregnancy (or intended pregnancy)

Conscientious Considerations

- All forms of testosterone treatment require monitoring for side effects and clinical improvement. Such evaluation should be performed by history and physical examination every 3 to 4 months for a year, and then annually.
- If poor or no response has been seen in 3 to 4 months, treatment should be increased, or discontinued if maximum has been reached.
- Testosterone treatment also requires monitoring of lipids, prostate-specific antigen, hematocrit, and digital rectal examination.
- For men taking intramuscular injections of testosterone, levels should be drawn just before the next intramuscular dose to monitor levels until stable.
- For those taking oral preparations of testosterone, liver function tests should be taken every 3 to 6 months.

- Testosterone is a suspected stimulant in certain cancers (breast and prostate). Men starting on testosterone should be made aware of the need to maintain screening for these cancers.
- Men who are smokers, have vascular disease, or have a history of polycythemia should be evaluated and monitored for possible effects of erythropoiesis when taking testosterone. If significant elevations in hematocrit occur, these patients should be taken off the medication.

Patient/Family Education

- Patients should be informed that many of the signs and symptoms of testosterone deficiency are not amenable to treatment, and often a man's age and physical condition may limit the results of treatment with testosterone.
- Pregnant women or women of childbearing age should use caution when handling testosterone-containing medications or when coming in contact with gels or patches containing testosterone because there may be untoward fetal effects should particles be absorbed.
- Men with benign prostatic hypertrophy and abnormal lipid profiles should be told that testosterone treatment may adversely affect these conditions and require close monitoring.

DRUGS USED TO TREAT MALE PATTERN BALDNESS

Although it is not truly a disease, hair loss can impact a man's relations, self-image, and self-assurance. Two-thirds of men will experience hair loss as they age, a natural phenomenon that has resulted in a billion dollar a year industry. Despite this great interest in treatment and obvious willingness to pay, only two pharmacological treatments have been shown to be somewhat effective in maintaining and sometimes regrowing hair (MedlinePlus, 2013).

Male pattern baldness is also referred to as androgenic alopecia due to its close relationship to dihydrotestosterone (DTH). DTH is a metabolite of testosterone as a result of a conversion controlled by a type 2 isoenzyme, 5-alpha reductase. Hair is created in the hair follicles. The hair follicles of humans are completely asynchronous; the individual human hair follicles initiate, grow, mature, and lose hair in a continuous and completely independent manner. For this reason hair is constantly falling out as new hair is regrown. The hair in the area of the scalp where baldness occurs shows shorter, finer, and less pigmented hairs than appears elsewhere. It was found that an increased presence of DHT was associated with this change in hair type and baldness. Once this was determined, treatments to decrease the level of DHT were considered for the treatment of male pattern baldness.

The diagnosis of male baldness would seem to be quite easy and not require a great deal of medical skill or knowledge. In general this is true; however, there are many causes of baldness, and prior to treatment at least a cursory evaluation should be made to rule out other etiology. History is probably the most important element in the diagnosis—family history; medications, illnesses, psychological stresses; and the history of the hair loss itself are almost diagnostic. A family history with the classic gradual progression of hair loss in the characteristic "M" pattern with development of vertex baldness requires little more than a quick examination of the scalp. The scalp examination should reveal no scarring, signs of inflammation, or abnormal growths or defects. Patchy hair loss or abrupt hair loss may indicate etiology other than androgen alopecia and should prompt further investigation.

Two medications are available for the treatment of male pattern baldness: finasteride (Propecia) and minoxidil (Rogaine). The effectiveness of both medications is somewhat variable. Younger men and those with vertex baldness are more successful than older men or those who have hair loss in the temporal and hairline areas. It is difficult to draw conclusions from studies because many report results that are quite subjective. In general, however, most studies show slight to significant satisfaction in the use of either medication because both finasteride (Propecia) and minoxidil (Rogaine) work on the crown and hairline, though mostly the crown area (Leyden & Dunlap, 2000). Minoxidil use is limited to application of 1 mL twice per day according to FDA-approved guidelines. Finasteride is given orally in a dosage of 1 mg daily for male baldness, much lower than the dosage for BPH, which is 5 mg per day.

Mechanism of Action

Finasteride is a 5-alpha reductase inhibitor, its mechanism of action was discussed in the section regarding treatments for BPH. Minoxidil was first developed for its ability to dilate peripheral blood vessels and treat hypertension, but when it was found to be effective in treating baldness, a better market was found. Minoxidil's mechanism of action is less well-defined, but it appears to have a direct effect on hair follicles by stimulating resting hair follicles into active growth. Because minoxidil is also used orally as a third-line antihypertensive medication because of its profound effect in dilating arterioles, it is believed this may be the mechanism for its stimulating hair follicles as well. Minoxidil applied topically does not require a prescription.

Pharmacokinetics of Topical Minoxidil

- Absorption. Does not appear to be systemically absorbed.
- Distribution: Not distributed because it is a topical agent.
- Metabolism: Not an issue because it is not used systemically.
- Excretion: Not an issue because the drug is not absorbed through the scalp.

Dosage and Administration

Generic Name	Trade Name	Route*	Usual Adult Dose
minoxidil	Rogaine 2%	Topical	1 mL 2 times/day
minoxidil extra strength	Rogaine 5%	Topical	1 mL 2 times/day
finasteride	Propecia	PO	1 mg daily

Clinical Uses

- Treatment of male pattern baldness, but patients must be made aware of the fact that results may take 3 to 6 months of daily usage to reach maximum effects and that any hair

regrowth will likely disappear within 4 to 6 months if therapy is discontinued.
- Both medications are about equally effective, but results vary from person to person. Younger men tend to have better results than do older men.

Adverse Reactions

- Minoxidil (Rogaine), when used as directed (limiting amount to 2 mL per day), results in little if any systemic absorption and therefore has almost no adverse reactions other than local skin effects (i.e., allergy) to medication or its constituents.
- Finasteride (Propecia) is given in a much lower dosage for male baldness than for BPH; for this reason, many of its adverse reactions are much less.

Interactions with Minoxidil

As an aerosol applied as a topical foam, there are no drug interactions.

Contraindications

- Hypersensitivity to medication (both)
- Serious skin reactions to other 5-alpha reductase inhibitors (finasteride)
- Pediatric patients (finasteride)
- Women of childbearing potential or who are pregnant because of fetal harm (finasteride)

Conscientious Considerations

- Finasteride has also been given a pregnancy X category rating because it has been implicated in producing abnormalities in genitalia of male offspring.
- Finasteride should not be handled by a pregnant woman or one who may become pregnant.
- The stronger dose of minoxidil 5% (Rogaine Extra Strength) was found to be more effective than the lesser 2% dose.
- Although in treatment of male pattern baldness relatively small doses of the 5-alpha reductase inhibitor finasteride are used, it still must be remembered that there is a possibility of falsely lowered PSA levels. Therefore, when screening men on finasteride for prostate cancer, the clinician should double the patient's PSA levels to account for this decrease.

Patient/Family Education

- Male pattern baldness medication is much less effective in frontal and temporal hair loss than in those who have vertex hair loss.
- New hair is lost within 4 to 6 months when treatment is discontinued.
- Patients must be made aware that results are not immediate and that it may take 2 to 3 months before significant improvement may be seen and 3 to 6 months to reach maximum effect.
- Men who take this drug should avoid donating blood for at least six months after discontinuing it as the blood may transfer a teratogenic agent to a pregnant woman.

DRUGS USED TO TREAT INFECTION/INFLAMMATION OF THE GENITOURINARY TRACT

Other conditions that are of specific concern to men include inflammation and infections of the genitourinary GU tract. Although some of these conditions are unique to the anatomy of the male, the infectious organisms that cause them may affect women as well as men. The specific antibacterial agents mentioned here are discussed in detail in Chapter 17, Modern Approaches to Managing Bacterial Infections.

The usual causes of epididymitis, orchitis, and prostatitis are usually infections of bacterial origin, but certainly viral and even fungal infection can be responsible. In fact, the suffix *-itis* actually refers to inflammation of the various organs, thus in some cases a noninfectious agent can cause the inflammation. Treatment therefore rests on determining the cause of the inflammation. Culture and sensitivity, usually of the urine, gives us our answer in the majority of cases. Unfortunately, this often takes time, and treatment is often required or at least desired before cultures are ready. Empirical treatment is therefore usually provided for most of these conditions.

Epididymitis and Orchitis

Epididymitis and orchitis are closely related because orchitis is usually a result of the spread of infection from the epididymis. The usual cause of this inflammation is bacterial, and the type of bacteria varies with the patient's age. Men 14 to 35 years of age who develop epididymitis often are found to have a sexually transmitted disease such as *Neisseria gonorrhoeae* or *Chlamydia trachomatis*. Those older or younger than this age range are usually found to have a common urinary pathogen such as *Escherichia coli* as the offending agent.

Diagnosis of inflammation is made by physical examination; gentle palpation of the epididymis and testicle will often provide the proper diagnosis. A word of caution should be made to remind clinicians that a patient with acute testicular or scrotal pain and swelling must be considered for testicular torsion; if it is suspected, the patient should be referred for immediate urological evaluation. Usually, the pain of epididymitis is more gradual and occurs in the area of the epididymis, posterior to the testicle. Orchitis may follow epididymitis, but it can also be present concurrently, especially viral orchitis with abrupt and painful swelling. Commonly occurring after mumps infection, orchitis can occur 4 to 7 days after the parotitis.

Medical Management of Male Urinary Tract Infections

In all cases, urine culture and sensitivity should be obtained. Meanwhile, immediate treatment with ceftriaxone (Rocephin), a single 250-mg dose intramuscularly, and doxycycline (Vibramycin), 100 mg orally, twice daily for 10 days, or azithromycin (Zithromax), a single 1-gm dose orally, may be given if the epididymitis is thought to be caused by gonococcal or chlamydial infection. If enteric organisms (coliform bacteria) are suspected, then the treatment should include ofloxacin, 300 mg orally, twice daily, for 10 days, or levofloxacin (Levaquin), 500 mg orally, once daily, for 10 days.

Medical Management of Prostatitis

Prostatitis is one of the most common urological conditions seen by practitioners. Like epididymitis and orchitis, it is usually caused by bacteria, but viral, fungal, and irritative agents can cause inflammation as well. Digital rectal exam usually identifies a boggy, tender prostate as the source of the problem, and again, urinary culture and sensitivity will often provide the etiologic agent. Empiric treatment prior to the culture result is the norm because prostatitis in older men can result in sepsis. Often prostatitis will become chronic, which requires a different treatment strategy, thus empiric treatment is often based on the patient's history of prior infections and duration of symptoms.

Acute prostatitis is usually thought to be caused by gram-positive cocci, and treatment is provided with amoxicillin 500 mg, three times daily for 30 days, or if the patient is allergic to penicillin, trimethoprim-sulfamethoxazole (Septra-DS), twice daily for 30 days. The long treatment is required to ensure adequate antibiotic absorption by prostatic tissue. If chronic prostatitis is diagnosed, then the treatment should consist of a fluoroquinolone such as ofloxacin 300 mg twice daily or ciprofloxacin 500 mg twice daily for 4 to 12 weeks. Treatment of associated fever, pain, and difficulty urinating must accompany the management of epididymitis, orchitis, and prostatitis.

Implications for Special Populations

Pediatric and Female Implications

Many of the agents mentioned in this chapter are not approved for pediatric use and some are contraindicated in women.

Geriatric Implications

A small number of cases in which geriatric patients have used phosphodiesterases inhibitors has prompted the FDA to ask their manufacturers to more clearly display the risk of these events in their labeling. Since being introduced, market research continues for other uses of the phosphodiesterases inhibitors because of their vasodilation effects; thus the scientific literature continues to report on their potential use as an antiplatelet medication in claudication and vascular dementia.

The pharmacokinetics of drugs such as finasteride indicate no dosage adjustments are needed in the elderly or for those with renal insufficiency, although persons over the age of 70 do show decreased elimination rates.

LEARNING EXERCISES

Case 1

You have just completed a comprehensive and completely nonsignificant physical examination with routine laboratory test results on JC, a 55-year-old white male. He has been diagnosed with mild hypertension, but is well controlled on 25 mg of hydrochlorothiazide daily. He notes that he is soon to go on a cruise with his wife and "wants to be in great shape." He stops in the doorway and says, "Oh, by the way, could I have a prescription for Viagra?" After a thorough history and physical you determine that Viagra is appropriate.

1. Write a prescription for the medication you would recommend.

   Rx: _____

   #: _____

   Sig: _____

2. Why did you choose this medication and what patient advisories would you give?

3. What follow-up recommendations would you make?

Case 2

Mr. HH, a patient you seldom see, is upset that his daughter teased him about starting to look like her grandfather, his bald father. He states that he has been losing hair for years, has tried all the over-the-counter creams, lotions, and even some rather expensive electronic scalp stimulators, and nothing has helped. Last week he saw an ad for Rogaine and says that he would like to try it, in the hope of having his hair "look the way it used to when he was young." Your examination reveals a healthy-appearing 60-year-old male with balding of the vertex in a typical androgenic alopecia pattern.

1. Write a prescription for the medication you would recommend.

   Rx: _____

   #: _____

   Sig: _____

2. Why did you choose this medication?

3. What recommendations would you make for follow-up?

References

Barry, M. J., Fowler, F. J., Jr., O'Leary, M. P., Bruskewitz, R. C., Holtgrewe, H. L., Mebust, W. K., et al. (1992). The American Urological Association symptom index for benign prostatic hyperplasia. The Measurement Committee of the American Urological Association. *Journal of Urology, 148,* 1549–1557.

Leyden, J., et al. (2000). Finasteride in the treatment of men with frontal male pattern hair loss. *Journal of the American Academy of Dermatology, 42*(5, Pt 1), 848-849.

Lin, C. S., Xin, Z. C., Lin, G., & Lue, T. F. (2003). Phosphodiesterases as therapeutic targets. *Urology, 61,* 685–691.

MedlinePlus. (2013). Minoxidil Topical. Retrieved March 1, 2013, from www.nlm.nih.gov/medlineplus/druginfo/meds/a689003.html

National Cancer Institute (NIH). (June, 2003). The prostate Cancer Prevention Trial. Retrieved February 28, 2013, from www.cancer.gov/clinicaltrials/noteworthy-trials/pcpt

National Center for Complementary and Alternative Medicine (NCCAM). (2011) Urinary Tract Conditions, Saw Palmetto Extract No More Effective than Placebo for Urinary Symptoms. Retrieved March 4, 2013, from http://nccam.nih.gov/research/results/spotlight/092711.htm

National Institute of Diabetes and Digestive and Kidney Diseases (NIDDK). (January 12, 2010). Medical Therapy of Prostatic Symptoms (MTOPS). Retrieved May 17, 2011, from http://clinicaltrials.gov/ct2/show/NCT00021814

O'Donel, A. B., Araujo, A. B., & McKinley, J. B. (July, 2004). The health of normally aging men: The Massachusetts Male Aging Study. *Experimental Gerontology, 39*(7), 975-984. Retrieved February 28, 2013, from www.ncbi.nlm.nih.gov/pubmed/15236757

Roehrborn, C. G., Siami, P., Barkin, J., Damilao, R., Major-Walker, K., Morrill, B., et al. (2008). The effects of dutasteride, tamsulosin, and combination therapy on lower urinary tract symptoms in men with benign prostatic hyperplasia and prostatic enlargement. *Journal of Urology, 179*(2), 616.

Rosen, R. C., Wing, R., Schneider, S., & Gendrano, N. (2005). Epidemiology of erectile dysfunction: The role of medical comorbidities and lifestyle factors. *Urology Clinics of North America, 32*(4), 403-417.

Seidman, S. N., & Walsh, B. T. (1999). Testosterone and depression in aging men. *American Journal of Geriatric Psychiatry, 7,* 18-33.

U. S. Census Bureau. (2011). The 2011 Statistical Abstract. *The National Data Book,* section 3: Health and Nutrition, 97-140. Retrieved March 1, 2013, from www.census.gov/compendia/statab/2011/2011edition.html

U. S. Department of Health and Human Services, NIH Consensus Development Program. (December 7-9, 1992). Impotence, *10*(4), 1-31. Retrieved March 1, 2013, from http://consensus.nih.gov/1992/1992Impotence091html.htm

Viera, A. J., Clenney, T. L., Shenberger, T. L., & Green, G. F. (1999). Newer pharmacological alternatives for erectile dysfunction. *American Family Physician, 60*(4): 1159-1166. Retrieved March 1, 2013, from www.aafp.org/afp/990915ap/1159.html

Wei, J. T., Calhoun E., Jacobson S. J., Urological Diseases In America: Chapter 2 Benign Prostatic Hyperplasia. Retrieved March 4, 2013, from http://kidney.niddk.nih.gov/statistics/uda/Benign_Prostatic_Hyperplasia-Chapter02.pdf

Yassin, A. A., & Saad, F. (November-December, 2008). Testosterone and erectile dysfunction. *Journal of Andrology, 29*(6), 593-604.

chapter 22

Prescribing for the Geriatric Patient

Florence T. Baralatei, Richard J. Ackerman

Key Terms

Alzheimer's Disease

Anticholinergic effects

Creatinine clearance

Hypertension

Older adults

Polypharmacy

Urinary incontinence

CHAPTER FOCUS

This chapter provides a working knowledge of how pharmacodynamics and pharmacokinetics are altered in older adults. It also introduces medications commonly seen in primary care/family medicine used to treat hypertension, Alzheimer's Disease, and urinary incontinence. Drugs with high rates of adverse events are reviewed, and a general strategy for optimal prescribing for this vulnerable population is provided. Mastery over this chapter's content is presented as an essential first step for clinicians who monitor medications and/or prescribe for older adults.

OBJECTIVES

After reading and studying this chapter, the student should be able to:

1. Recall how pharmacodynamic changes in the aging adult make them more sensitive to many medications as organ function declines.
2. Describe how orally administered drugs may have their absorption, distribution, metabolism, and excretion impaired due to aging.
3. Use the Cockcroft-Gault equation to calculate renal function.
4. Choose and monitor effective and safe medications to treat hypertension in older adults.
5. Describe the pharmacology of the cholinesterase inhibitors and the *N*-methyl-D-aspartate antagonist, memantine, in the treatment of Alzheimer's Disease.
6. Manage medications in the treatment of older adults with urinary incontinence.
7. Describe age-related concerns for the prescribing of digoxin, anticoagulants, antiparkinsonian drugs, antipsychotics, corticosteroids, opiates, NSAIDS, sedative/hypnotics, and drugs with anticholinergic effects.
8. List ways a clinician can prevent polypharmacy and manage drug-related problems in the older adult.

KEY DRUGS IN THIS CHAPTER

Medications for Hypertension
  alpha blockers angiotensin receptor blockers
  angiotensin-converting enzyme inhibitors
  beta blockers
  calcium channel blockers
  diuretics

Medications for Alzheimer's Disease
Cholinesterase Inhibitors
  donepezil (Aricept)
  rivastigmine (Exelon)
  galantamine (Razadyne)
N-methyl-D-Aspartate Antagonist
  memantine (Namenda)

Antimuscarinic Drugs for Overactive Bladder/Urge Incontinence/Urinary Tract Antispasmodics
  darifenacin (Enablex)
  fesoterodine (Toviaz)
  oxybutynin (Ditropan)
  solifenacin (Vesicare)
  tolterodine (Detrol)
  trospium (Sanctura)

Other Medication Classes with Age-Related Concerns
  antiarrhythmic drugs
  antidepressants
  anticholinergics

anticoagulants
antihistamines
antiparkinsonism drugs
antipsychotic drugs
anxiolytic drugs
corticosteroids
digoxin
NSAIDs
opioid analgesics
tricyclic antidepressants

INTRODUCTION TO DRUG USE BY THE OLDER ADULT

Clinicians are seeing and treating an increasingly older population. By the year 2030 one in five American residents will be over the age of 65 (U.S. Census Bureau, 2010). While advances in medicine and pharmaceuticals have greatly prolonged and improved the quality of life for **older adults,** they have also increased the risks for adverse drug reactions (ADRs), concomitant drug-drug interactions (DDI), polypharmacy, and poly-prescribers. ADRs, although mostly preventable, are considered the fourth-to sixth-leading cause of death among the elderly in the United States (Lazarou, Pomeranz, & Corey 1998; WHO, 2010). Note that the boundary between young, middle age, and older adults can NOT be specifically defined as when asked, most people do not categorize themselves as being older because aging has so many physical, functional, psychological, and social parameters (Carr, 2013), however some authors replace being over the age of 65 as being an older adult. In the United States, 12% to 13% of the population is over the age of 65, yet these individuals use about one-third of all prescribed medications. Among the 65 to 74 age group, 51% use two or more prescription drugs, and 12% are using five or more prescription drugs (CDC, 2011). Eighty-one percent of those over 65 are using at least one prescription medication, one over-the-counter (OTC) medication, and one dietary supplement. Twenty-nine percent are concurrently taking five prescription drugs and at least one OTC drug, putting 4% of them at risk for a potentially fatal drug interaction (Qato et al., 2008). Older adult women use more drugs than their male counterparts. Medication use also varies by clinical setting. For example, the average "at home" or "community-dwelling" older adult is using three to four prescription medications, whereas an institutionalized older adult is using an average of seven or eight medications (Slone Epidemiology Center, 2006).

The most common classes of medications used in community-dwelling older adults are analgesics, diuretics, cardiovascular drugs, and sedative hypnotics. Why so many analgesics? Pain is a common symptom in older adults. Half of community-dwelling older adults state that pain interferes with their ability to function (Sawyer, Bodner, Richie, & Allman, 2006). By contrast, some of the most intensive use of medications occurs in nursing homes and among institutionalized elderly, putting them at risk for polypharmacy. Although the mechanisms of the aging process remain unresolved, it is known that aging results in changes in pharmacokinetics and pharmacodynamics (Aymanns et al., 2010; Howland, 2009).

AGE-RELATED CHANGES IN THE OLDER ADULT AFFECTING DRUG DYNAMICS AND KINETICS

Aging, as a process, is characterized by progressive loss of functional capacity among most, if not all, body organs; a reduction in homeostatic mechanisms; a response to receptor stimulation; and a loss of body water along with an increase in body fat. Therefore, understanding the influence of age-dependent changes in composition and function of the body on the pharmacokinetics and pharmacodynamics of drugs is important to clinicians. These age-related changes may lead to drug toxicities and adverse drug reactions, as well as an increased risk of adverse side effects. One theory of aging is that aging events occur because of damage to macromolecules by background radiation, free radicals, environmental toxins, or other environmental factors over time. A second theory purports that aging occurs as a genetically predetermined event. When it comes to specific diseases, however, one study implies that the older adult undergoes a decline in blood-brain barrier function, and this allows circulating beta-amyloid peptides to enter the brain and induce the symptoms of Alzheimer's Disease (Lotrich & Pollock, 2005). Because age-related changes in the older adult affect a drug's pharmacokinetics or pharmacodynamics they can also affect use of other medications (Table 22-1).

TABLE 22-1	Age-Related Physiological Changes that Result in Altered Pharmacokinetics	
	PHYSIOLOGICAL CHANGES DUE TO AGING	**AGING EFFECTS ON PHARMACOKINETICS**
ABSORPTION	• Blood flow to the gastrointestinal tract is decreased but has little effect on drug absorption. • Intestinal motility is decreased. • Gastric acidity is generally unchanged. • Reduced surface area.	• Delays peak effect of drug, especially if drug requires active transport. • Delays symptoms of toxicities. • Drug-drug interactions may delay absorption.
DISTRIBUTION	• Body fluid volume diminished. • Percent of body fat increases. • Reduction in plasma proteins. • Decreased lean body mass.	• Increases serum concentration of water-soluble drugs. • Increases half-life of fat-soluble drugs. • Increases amount of drug availability (concentration).
METABOLISM	• Blood flow and liver function decreases.	• Decreases rate of drug clearance and may lead to increased drug accumulation and toxicity.
EXCRETION	• Kidney function and creatinine clearance (CrCl) decreases.	• Increases body concentration of drugs normally excreted by kidneys.

Pharmacokinetics in the Older Adult

Pharmacokinetics refers to the factors that influence the delivery of an administered drug to the desired site of drug action. These factors include absorption, distribution, metabolism, and excretion of drugs. As people age, they experience decreased ratio of lean mass to body fat, decreased levels of serum albumin, decreased liver function, and decreased renal function, all of which affect how the body responds to a drug. Also, as people age the target organ for a drug may exhibit increased sensitivity to a drug or a decrease in the drug's desirable effects, leading to increases in adverse effects. Additionally, the aging body may exhibit a decrease in its capacity to respond to physiological challenges and adverse drug reactions (i.e., orthostatic hypotension).

Absorption

Changes in the older adult that influence absorption of orally administered drugs include reduced gastrointestinal blood flow and motility, reduced gastric acidity, and reduced absorptive surface from microvilli atrophy. Most drugs, however, are weak organic bases (cocaine, morphine) or acids (acetaminophen) existing in un-ionized or ionized aqueous forms and diffuse readily and passively across cell membranes. Water-soluble vitamins A, D, E, and K are good examples of this.

The absorption of some drugs (e.g., levodopa, propylthiouracil), whose chemical structures are similar to endogenous substances such as sugars, amino acids, peptides, and iron salts, requires active transport. Absorption of these drugs in the elderly will be reduced, resulting in lower bioavailability. The reduction of hepatic first-pass effect may lead to increased bioavailability and significant differences in physiological effect when comparing oral administration to IV administration, for example, oral morphine verses IV morphine, lidocaine, or propranolol. Drugs absorbed from the gastrointestinal (GI) tract normally pass through the portal venous system, then through the liver, and finally into the systemic circulation where they interact with receptors in target tissues. Extensive hepatic metabolism/extraction results in minimal drug delivery to the systemic circulation for certain agents.

There are limited data available on the absorption of drugs delivered via the intramuscular, transdermal, transbronchial, rectal, or transbuccal routes in older adults. For the most part, absorption from these sites is presumed to be no different from the younger population.

Distribution

Total body water and extracellular fluid volume decrease with age, as do cardiac output and brain and cardiac blood flow. Conversely, the percentage of total body fat rises steadily with age, more prominently in women than men, and this leads to a decrease in lean body mass.

Because of these changes, water-soluble drugs have a reduced volume of distribution, leading to increased plasma concentrations of hydrophilic (water-soluble) drugs such as lithium. Because body fat increases with age, lipophilic (lipid-soluble) drugs will have an increased half-life from increased storage in fatty tissue. This can lead to prolonged drug action, exacerbated drug effect, and increased toxic effects. For lipid-soluble drugs, loading doses of medications are often altered to prevent toxic plasma concentrations especially when an elderly person has a lot of body fat because there is more body fat for the drug to disperse into. This prolongs the drug's activity as it slowly returns to the bloodstream.

Many drugs are transported in the body bound to serum proteins, most commonly albumin. However, the active component of the drug is the unbound fraction. In the presence of hypoalbuminemia, the free or unbound fraction increases, thereby increasing the drug's effect and toxicity despite a "normal" or therapeutic serum drug level, which measures both free and bound fractions. A good example of this is phenytoin, which is highly albumin bound. With hypoalbuminemia, the therapeutic range for phenytoin becomes substantially lower. This effect is exacerbated in drugs with narrow therapeutic windows. When possible, measuring the "free" drug level is more helpful in a clinical situation than reviewing total serum concentration or levels.

Normal or therapeutic levels reported in literature were generally derived from younger populations and may not be accurate for older adults. An example is digoxin, with a therapeutic range of 0.8 to 1.2 ng/mL. In older adults, serum levels of 0.6 to 0.8 ng/mL better achieve the therapeutic advantages of the drug, while minimizing side effects. Levels above 0.8 to 1 ng/mL can increase adverse drug events without providing increased effectiveness. Another example is the anticoagulant warfarin, which is very highly protein bound and has a very narrow therapeutic window, thus requiring careful dosage monitoring among the elderly.

Metabolism

For most drugs, the liver is the principal site of metabolism. There is a gradual decline in liver blood flow and its mass over time so that it is reduced to almost at 50% by age 70. Drug metabolism by the liver is usually one of two types: phase I and phase II. Phase I metabolism comprises the oxidation reactions mediated by the cytochrome P450 enzymes, and these are markedly reduced with age. Age-related changes result in reduced clearance and, therefore, increased half-life of medications such as morphine, diazepam, and verapamil. In addition, reduced hepatic blood flow results in reduced first-pass effect, further prolonging availability of drugs such as labetalol and verapamil. Furthermore, the liver is the target of other diseases, medications, and substances such as alcohol and environmental toxins/pollutants, so that in certain individuals, liver reserve may even be smaller than one would expect from the age of the patient.

Excretion

Age-related changes in drug excretion are more important than changes in drug absorption, distribution, or metabolism. Most drugs are excreted through the kidneys, either as the parent drug or its metabolites. For certain drugs, the liver/biliary system, skin, and respiratory system also play roles. Aging is also associated with several anatomical and physiological changes in the kidney. There is reduction in renal mass/number and size of nephrons, blood flow, glomerular filtration rate (GFR), and tubular secretion. The age-associated decline in kidney function is highly variable, but about 30% of those over 70 have a GFR of a little less than one-half that of a normal healthy adult, and that decline has been roughly correlated with a sedentary life style, obesity, and cardiovascular disease (Robinson-Cohen et al., 2009).

The traditional crude markers of renal function in routine medical practice are the serum blood urea nitrogen (BUN) and creatinine (Cr). These markers are often unreliable indicators of kidney function because they can rise if the patient has had recent muscle trauma, such as a car accident or a fall. BUN is made by the liver from ingested protein; thus, inadequate protein intake or marked impairment in liver function will lead to misleading low serum BUN levels. Creatinine comes from the metabolism of muscle creatine. Because older adults have reduced muscle mass, the serum Cr may be falsely low as an indicator of GFR. The most commonly used formula for **creatinine clearance** (CrCl) is the Cockcroft-Gault equation:

$$CrCl = \frac{(140 - age) \times (total\ body\ weight\ in\ kg)}{(72) \times (serum\ creatinine\ in\ mg/dL)}$$

For women, this result is multiplied by 0.85 to account for their lower muscle mass. Another major issue is that because elderly patients have less muscle mass and falsely low serum creatinine (SCr), the end result is an overestimation of the CrCl, making the denominator in the CrCl formula falsely small. Thus if the SCr is less than 1, many clinicians round it up to 1 as a minimum.

Consider the following examples:

1. Estimate the creatinine clearance of a 65-year-old man with a weight of 72 kg and a serum creatinine of 1.5.

$$\frac{(140 - 65) \times 72}{72 \times 1.5} = 50\ mL/min$$

2. If an 85-year-old male has similar weight and serum creatinine values, his CrCl will be

$$(140 - 85)(72)/(72)(1.5) = 37\ mL/min$$

3. If the patient is an 85-year-old woman with characteristics similar to patient no. 2, her CrCl will be

$$(140 - 85)(72)(0.85)/(72)(1.5) = 31\ mL/min$$

Be particularly vigilant when prescribing renally excreted drugs with narrow therapeutic windows, such as digoxin. Antibiotics such as vancomycin, and especially the aminoglycosides, which have direct toxic effects on the kidneys, should be dosed with caution in this age group. Consider consulting a pharmacist for help in choosing a dose or dosing interval for these high-risk drugs.

Pharmacodynamics

Pharmacodynamics refers to different effects of a drug on the patient, despite identical serum concentrations. This happens either by altered sensitivity at the receptor site, a postreceptor effect, or by impairment of physiological and homeostatic mechanisms, with resulting exacerbation of effects and side effects.

Examples of altered receptor sensitivity in older adults include increased central nervous system (CNS) sedation with benzodiazepines, opioids, and neuroleptics. Older adults have a reduced maximal diuretic response to furosemide and decreased responsiveness to both beta blockers and agonists. Older adults often have additive bradycardic responses to combinations of beta blockers and calcium channel blockers (e.g., verapamil, diltiazem).

Examples of impaired physiological reserve include more urinary retention and constipation, more blurry vision, and increased risk to patients with glaucoma from anticholinergic drugs, as well as increased risk of falls from sedative hypnotics. For example, an older patient may develop urinary retention from the use of an ipratropium inhaler to control COPD symptoms. This is particularly a problem with older adults who take multiple medications with **anticholinergic effects**. Anticholinergic effects (blurry vision, constipation, sedation, dry mouth, trouble concentrating, urinary retention) occur when certain medications, e.g., antihistamines such as diphenhydramine (Benadryl), promethazine (Phenergan), or ipratropium (Atrovent), block cholinergic receptors on various types of cells in the body and thus block the action of the neurotransmitter acatylcholine.

DRUG TREATMENT OF HYPERTENSION IN OLDER ADULTS

The prevalence of **hypertension** in older adults increases their risk of myocardial infarction, congestive heart failure, cerebrovascular disease, and peripheral arterial disease. Systolic hypertension has also been well established as a risk factor for dementia.

Systolic blood pressure (SBP) is the primary target for the diagnosis and treatment of hypertension in older adults. As adults age, the systolic pressure continues to rise, whereas the diastolic pressure rises until about 70 years of age, plateaus and then begins to fall. Aging also induces thickening of the left ventricular wall and stiffness of peripheral arteries. Weight loss and reduction of dietary sodium intake can be helpful nonpharmacological approaches to treating hypertension in older adults. Changing from a high sodium diet (4,000 mg/day) to a low-sodium diet (2,000 mg/day) over several years can lower SBP by as much as 10 mm Hg. However, older adults may find reducing sodium intake challenging because their sense of taste is altered due to aging. Reducing body weight by as little as 10% through a moderate exercise and diet program (i.e., moderate physical activity 30 minutes per day at least five times a week) can also decrease SBP by 5 to 15 mm Hg.

Orthostatic hypotension is a major complication of blood pressure treatment in the older adult and may lead to falls and associated complications. Orthostatic hypotension is defined as a drop in SBP of 20 mm Hg or more or a drop of diastolic blood pressure of 10 mm Hg or more.

The following drug classes are discussed in detail in Chapter 6 (Drugs Used to Treat Cardiovascular Conditions) and Chapter 7 (Drugs Used to Regulate Blood Pressure). Discussed here are special considerations that clinicians should know when prescribing these drugs to older adults.

Diuretics

In the largest antihypertensive therapy trial published to date, the Antihypertensive and Lipid Lowering Treatment to Prevent

Heart Attack Trial (ALLHAT, 2006), investigators set out to determine whether treatment with an angiotensin-converting enzyme (ACE) inhibitor, calcium channel blocker, alpha blocker, or diuretic was most effective in reducing the incidence of vascular events in hypertensive patients. ALLHAT showed that a thiazide diuretic was superior in preventing these outcomes. A meta-analysis that incorporated ALLHAT along with many other trials to assess major cardiovascular disease (CVD) end points concluded that low-dose diuretics are the most effective first-line treatment for treating hypertension in older adults.

Diuretics, although very useful in older adults, can contribute to dehydration and electrolyte abnormalities. Impaired thirst sensation and cognitive impairment may also exacerbate these effects. Many clinicians, when dosing the elderly, start with a low dose (e.g., hydrochlorothiazide 12.5 mg/day) and move up to a maximum dose of 25 mg/day should the need arise. If a two-drug regimen is needed to treat hypertension in an older adult, one of the drugs should be a diuretic. It should also be noted that if the patient has significantly impaired renal function (CrCl less than 30 mL/min), some diuretics (especially hydrochlorothiazide) are not very effective in treating hypertension in the elderly. However, as with all diuretics, patients should be monitored for hyponatremia, hypokalemia, and metabolic alkalosis.

Beta Blockers

A seminal study done in 2003 demonstrated the relationship of using diuretics and beta blockers as first-line drug therapy in hypertension. Using data from multiple trials, including the Swedish Trial in Old Patients with Hypertension (STOP) (Dahlof, 1991) and the Systolic Hypertension in the Elderly Program (SHEP) (Furberg et al., 1987), which evaluated the response rate of beta blockers as first-line hypertension therapy in older adults, Messerli and colleagues (2003) found that although beta-blocker monotherapy controls hypertension in many older adults, diuretic therapy is superior in preventing vascular events, especially stroke. The sensitivity of the elderly to sodium and to diuretics enhances rather than reduces the value of a thiazide diuretic as the first-line choice in mainstream treatment. The second option for the conscientious clinician is either to use an ACE inhibitor/angiotensin II-receptor blocker (ARB) or a calcium channel antagonist/blocker (CCB), depending upon the clinical setting, and to use a Step-Care approach (Glynn, Murphy, Smith, Schroeder, & Fahey, 2010).

In contrast to diuretics, beta blockers should not be considered first-line therapy of uncomplicated hypertension for most older adults. However, beta blockers may be an excellent choice as adjunctive hypertensive therapy in patients with heart failure, prior myocardial infarction, or symptomatic coronary disease (Stokes, 2009).

Calcium Channel Blockers

Calcium channel blockers are reasonable second- or third-line drugs in treating hypertension in older adults. The major side effect of this drug class is peripheral edema, which occurs in up to 15% to 20% of patients. This is a type of vasogenic or cerebral edema that occurs when the blood-brain barrier falters and edema builds up in the brain. It usually is the result of trauma, infections, or stroke. It does not respond to diuretics, although it does resolve with discontinuation of the offending drug or by placing the patient on amlodipine.

Angiotensin-Converting Enzyme (ACE) Inhibitors

In the Second Australian National Blood Pressure (ANBP2) trial, 6,083 hypertensive patients above the age of 65 were randomized to receive enalapril or hydrochlorothiazide. The study's purpose was to achieve a goal blood pressure based on the SHEP goal of less than 140 mm Hg. Overall, the study showed little difference between the two treatment groups. These findings suggest that ACE inhibitors should be first- or second-line therapy for hypertension and heart failure (HF) in older adults and for those also who are diabetic and have hypertension. Elderly patients taking ACE inhibitors should be monitored for chronic cough, which occurs in up to 20% of patients. ACE inhibitors also cause dysgeusia, and they should be avoided with use of potassium supplements or other drugs that raise potassium. See Chapter 6, Drugs Used in the Treatment of Cardiovascular Disorders, for more information on ACE inhibitors.

Angiotensin Receptor Blockers (ARBs)

In an open-label, double-blind study, the safety and tolerability of candesartan was tested in 5,464 patients. That study concluded candesartan was equally tolerated by patients above and below the age of 65. Candesartan is a prodrug converted to its active metabolite during its absorption and thus like other ARBs is generally well tolerated by older adults (Ripley, Chonlahan, & Germany, 2006). As with ACE inhibitors, clinicians should monitor patients taking ARBs for hyperkalemia and use them cautiously in patients with chronic kidney disease. Also of note is that ARBs are generally more expensive than generic ACE inhibitors.

Alpha Blockers

The ALLHAT trial had also studied the alpha blocker doxazosin, but this portion of the trial was stopped early because of an increase in cardiovascular events, unlike with diuretics. Alpha blockers should be avoided as first- or even second-line agents in treating hypertension in older adults. Previously, older men who had both hypertension and benign prostate hyperplasia received these drugs. But because of the ALLHAT trial and the existence of safer and more effective alternatives for benign prostatic hypertrophy, nonselective alpha blockers should not be used for either indication.

Other Medications for Hypertension

Clonidine (Catapres) is inexpensive, but it commonly causes significant bradycardia and should be avoided in underlying heart block.

Summary

The clinician should individualize prescribing for hypertension in older adults, generally starting with a low-dose diuretic or an ACE inhibitor. Clinicians should start with a low dose, monitor for side effects, and titrate slowly until blood pressure control is achieved.

DRUG TREATMENT OF DEMENTIA IN THE OLDER ADULT

The diagnosis of dementia is based on its definition, which is that patients experience losses in multiple cognitive domains, such as attention, judgment, language, and spatial skills, not just loss of memory and motor skills. The most common cause of dementia is Alzheimer's Disease (AD). It can be difficult to distinguish between normal aging, dementia, and even depression. Use of standardized neuropsychological tests helps many clinicians find answers to questions about a patient's dementia, whereas challenging cases can be referred to a neurologist or geriatrician (see Special Case: Delirium in Older Adults).

SPECIAL CASE: Delirium in Older Adults

Delirium, or an acute state of confusion, is a transient disorder of cognition that is not a disease but rather a reversible syndrome with many symptoms. Mainly, it is a waxing and waning type of confusion. Unfortunately, it is too often misdiagnosed as dementia or the signs and symptoms of Alzheimer's Disease even though it has been described as far back as Hippocrates's days; its Latin root means "off the track." Once diagnosed, its cause should be sought, but often it is induced by multiple drug regimens.

Treatment is typically a host of supportive therapy including fluid and nutrition as well as environmental supports (i.e., correcting sensory deficits) plus judicious use of some pharmaceuticals: neuroleptics, short acting sedatives, and vitamins. The most common neuroleptics used are haloperidol (Haldol), risperidone (Risperdal), and quetiapine (Seroquel). In the elderly, doses smaller than usual are used. Benzodiazepines once were common but today are reserved for use when the delirium is the result of alcohol or sedative hypnotic withdrawal.

The sedative lorazepam (Ativan) has wide acceptance because it is short acting and can be used intramuscularly or intravenously for patients who need to be sedated for longer than 24 hours. Vitamins are indicated when patients with alcohol or malnutrition, who are prone to delirium induced by vitamin B_{12} and thiamine deficiency, require replacement by use of thiamine (Thiamilate) and cyanocobalamin (Crystamine).

Although care of the elderly patient with delirium will include assessment of daily care needs, daily assessment of mental status, potential for injury, underlying medical conditions, and family interventions, it must also be noted that about one-third of delirium results from drug-drug interactions or as an adverse drug event. Thus, a thorough drug regimen review is always prudent and part of any team effort to act with conscientious consideration.

Alzheimer's Disease is characterized by pathological findings of plaques and neurofibrillary tangles. Plaques are composed of an amyloid peptide called Aβ, and the tangle is made of aggregated tau proteins. Drugs to target these abnormalities are not yet available. Alzheimer's Disease is also associated with a deficiency of the neurotransmitter acetylcholine. Thus, drugs that can increase the effects of acetylcholine are the mainstay of treatment. Initial treatments with precursors of acetylcholine or cholinergic agonists were ineffective or led to intolerable side effects. The current emphasis is on using drugs that inhibit the metabolism of the acetylcholine in the synaptic cleft—the cholinesterase inhibitors (ChEs), for example, donepezil (Aricept), galantamine (Razadyne), rivastigmine (Exelon), and tacrine (Cognex). Cognex is rarely used today because of its side effect profile, especially liver damage and the availability of NMDA (N-methyl D-aspartate) receptor antagonists such as memantine (Namenda). Although two drug classes are approved to treat Alzheimer's Disease—ChEs and the NMDA blocker memantine—clinical trials have not demonstrated that any of the available herbal or alternative agents such as gingko biloba are effective.

Treatment of patients with Alzheimer's Disease does include consideration of medications, but there are other more important aspects of care. For example, patients will need a thorough evaluation for potentially reversible causes of cognitive decline, with particular consideration given to depression and the side effects of medications. Side effects of medications are a major concern because any medication can worsen dementia symptoms. Provide education and support to caregivers, and consider the safety of the patient's living situation. Address advance directives and caregiver stress.

Cholinesterase Inhibitors (ChEs)

Three ChEs—donepezil (Aricept), rivastigmine (Exelon), and galantamine (Razadyne)—are widely used, with no clear advantages of one over the other. These drugs are indicated only for the treatment of Alzheimer's Disease, and their significant effect is delaying the progression of functional decline.

Mechanism of Action

All of these drugs inhibit the enzyme acetylcholinesterase, which increases the concentration of the neurotransmitter acetylcholine in the synaptic cleft. Rivastigmine also inhibits butyrylcholinesterase, whereas galantamine has nicotinic receptor effects, but whether this translates into any differences in clinical effect is unclear.

Clinical Uses

■ These drugs are approved by the U.S. Food and Drug Administration (FDA) only for the treatment of Alzheimer's Disease, thus clinicians should avoid using a ChE for nonspecific memory complaints or even for mild cognitive impairment or dementia believed to be a precursor to Alzheimer's Disease.

■ Older adults with vascular dementia and other dementias, such as Lewy body dementia or the dementia associated with Parkinson's Disease, may benefit from ChE therapy, but the data on this is inconclusive.

■ Rivastigmine and galantamine are FDA approved for the treatment of both the mild and moderate stages of Alzheimer's Disease. Patients with mild AD may be independent in activities of daily living (ADLs), such as walking, transfer, continence, eating, and dressing. Patients with moderate dementia may need help with ADLs.

■ Donepezil is approved for all three stages of Alzheimer's Disease—mild, moderate, and severe—and is the only drug FDA approved for all these stages. These drugs are palliative but do not reverse or cure the dementia. At best, they slow the rate of cognitive decline in a subset of patients, but the magnitude of benefit is small. All patients will eventually progress to end-stage dementia. It is unusual for a patient to "get better" on these drugs. Prescribers may consider discontinuing these drugs in the late stages of dementia when the burdens of taking an extra medication outweigh any benefit.

■ In some patients, behavioral complications of dementia are less common on these drugs, whereas in others these drugs may actually cause or exacerbate agitation and other behavioral symptoms. Sometimes a trial off the drugs may be useful. Clinicians should discuss all risks and benefits with the patient's family and caregivers before making any changes to the plan of care because in most cases any time a drug is stopped the state of dementia declines rather quickly.

Pharmacokinetics

■ Half-life 70 hours, allowing once daily dosage, and the shorter half-lives of rivastigmine (1.5 hours) and galantamine (6 to 8 hours) lead to twice-a-day drug dosing.

■ Absorption: Donepezil is 100% absorbed, without regard to time of day or administration with food. Steady state is reached in about 2 weeks. The drug is both excreted in the urine intact and also extensively metabolized by CYP liver enzymes (by glucuronidation), thus dose reductions are not necessary if the patient has renal impairment.

■ About 40% of an oral dose of rivastigmine is absorbed. However, if the drug is administered with food, it delays its absorption further, making dose administration to an older adult in a regimented institution an issue if drug administration and mealtime coincide.

■ Galantamine is 90% absorbed orally, and food has minimal effects on its absorption. Thus, it is a better agent for the elderly person whose mealtimes are erratic.

■ Dosages of these drugs are not altered by age, gender, or race. Galantamine should not be prescribed in patients with severe hepatic or renal disease, but the other two ChEs are probably safe in these conditions. However, elderly patients with severe liver or kidney failure may not be good candidates for any of these drugs because treating the organ failure is likely to be more clinically important and beneficial than treating any underlying dementia.

Dosage and Administration

Generic Name	Trade Name	Route	Usual Oral Adult Daily Dose
donepezil	Aricept	PO	5 mg once a day in a.m.; if well tolerated, titrate up to target dose of 10 mg once a day, giving each trial 30 days to respond
rivastigmine	Exelon	PO	1.5 mg 2 times/day for 2 weeks, then increase to 3 mg 2 times/day, then 4.5 mg for 2 weeks, then target dose of 6 mg, 2 times/day
		Patch	4.6 mg used once a day
galantamine	Razadyne	PO	4 mg 2 times a day, then titrate to 16 mg/day, then 24 mg/day at 4-week intervals. Option is oral solution of 4 mg/mL.

Adverse reactions

■ The major side effects of all three ChEs are gastrointestinal: nausea, vomiting, diarrhea, and abdominal pain.

■ Titrate slowly. Some patients may not be able to tolerate the target dose but will not have GI side effects at a lower dose.

■ Persons with dementia may not be able to self-report anorexia; therefore, careful observation of oral intake and weight is necessary after starting a ChE. Suspect ChE-induced anorexia if weight loss is not otherwise explained.

■ No routine biochemical monitoring, such as liver function tests, is required unless GI symptoms are severe or persist. However, baseline weight is monitored and reevaluated in 6 weeks.

■ Other side effects of cholinesterase inhibitors include dizziness, fatigue, bradycardia, A-V block, bladder outlet obstruction, seizures, and bronchospasm.

Drug Interactions

■ Because these drugs increase the level of synaptic acetylcholine, clinicians should avoid drugs with anticholinergic side effects, such as antihistamines or antimuscarinic drugs used for urinary incontinence, for example, oxybutynin (Ditropan) or tolterodine (Detrol). The mechanism of action of these drugs is so similar that when used together, each cancels the effect of the other.

■ Because rivastigmine is not metabolized by the liver's CYP system, drug-drug interactions that interfere with or enhance its metabolism are unlikely. Donepezil and galantamine do undergo CYP system metabolism, but there is no clear evidence that these drugs interfere with the metabolism of other drugs or that other drugs alter their metabolism.

Contraindications

■ Although not truly contraindicated, use of these drugs is cautioned in patients with a history of respiratory problems (asthma, chronic obstructive pulmonary disease [COPD]) because their use could induce bronchoconstriction.

■ Caution should also be used in patients with a history of GI problems (ulcers and bleeding) because these drugs could cause spasms that lead to a GI bleed.

■ Further caution should be used in patients with cardiac disorders such as sick sinus syndrome or other conduction disorders; patients can develop bradycardia, especially if they are taking digoxin or a calcium channel blocker, because conduction through the AV node will be slowed.

■ Caution should be taken in patients with problems urinating, such as patients with enlarged prostrate.

Conscientious Considerations

■ These medications can be very expensive and are not necessary for all patients with Alzheimer's Disease. In patients with advanced dementia or significant comorbidities, the risk of these medications may outweigh any potential benefits. Consider discontinuing the ChE if side effects occur, if there are behavioral complications due to medications, or when the goals of care change.

■ When ChE medications are discontinued, rapid deterioration of cognitive impairment may occur. This loss of function may not recover if the drug is restarted. When restarting a ChE, start at a low dose and titrate instead of resuming at the prior dose to reduce the risk of side effects.

Patient/Family Education

■ These drugs must be taken on a regularly scheduled basis and not as needed. Medication treatment is only a small part of caring for patients and families with dementia. It can be very helpful to provide information on the natural course of dementia and how to manage common symptoms and behaviors, as well as advance care planning. Provide referrals to support groups such as the Alzheimer's Association (www. alz.org) and use expert help available in your community, such as geriatricians, neurologists, or clinical pharmacists.

NMDA Inhibitors: Memantine (Namenda)

Mechanism of Action

Memantine (Namenda) is the first drug in a class of agents that inhibits, or blocks, N-methyl-D-aspartate channels. Glutamate is the primary excitatory amino acid in the CNS and may contribute to Alzheimer's Disease by overstimulating NMDA receptors leading to excitotoxicity and neuronal cell death on NMDA receptors located throughout the brain. By binding to the channel pore, memantine prevents magnesium from reentering, and thus the neuroexcitatory effect of the glutamate molecule is reduced. It is thought that this is how memantine improves the symptoms of Alzheimer's Disease without impacting the cholinesterase system or affecting normal neurotransmission.

Clinical Uses

■ Memantine is FDA approved for patients with moderate and severe Alzheimer's Disease, not the mild stage. However, many clinicians prescribe the drug for all stages.
■ Like the ChEs, memantine is FDA approved only for Alzheimer's Disease, although clinicians sometimes use the drug off-label for other dementias.
■ It should not be used to prevent dementia, and there is also no evidence that treating patients with mild cognitive impairment will prevent the development of dementia.
■ Like ChEs, memantine may delay the progression of Alzheimer's Disease in a subset of patients, but the effect is not robust.

Pharmacokinetics

■ Absorption: Memantine is well absorbed after oral administration and can be taken with or without food because its presence does not alter absorption.
■ Distribution: 45% protein bound
■ Metabolism and excretion: Memantine is excreted predominantly unchanged in the urine; however, excretion of the drug is increased in alkaline urine, causing patients with alkaline urine to have lower blood levels. There is some hepatic glucuronidation, but the liver CYP system is uninvolved in its metabolism. No dose reduction is necessary in patients with liver or renal disease, but the drug should be avoided in patients with end-stage liver or renal disease.
■ Half-life: 60 to 80 hours.

Dosage

■ Memantine is available in 5-mg and 10-mg tablets. Dosing usually begins with 5 mg in the morning, and after 2 weeks is increased to 5 mg twice a day. After another week it is increased to 10 mg in the morning and 5 mg at night, and after an additional week it is increased to the target dose of 10 mg twice a day.
■ Limited evidence (Atri et al., 2009) suggests that combining one ChE with memantine may have additive effects in preventing functional cognitive decline in patients suffering from Alzheimer's Disease, but this combination is very expensive.

Adverse reactions

Memantine is usually well tolerated. The most commonly reported side effects (all less than 5%) include dizziness, headache, confusion, coughing, somnolence, pain, vomiting, and hallucinations. Because of this favorable side effect profile in patients where monitoring is more difficult (many of these patients cannot reliably report side effects), many clinicians start with memantine rather than one of the three ChEs.

Drug Interactions

■ No significant drug-drug interactions have been reported with memantine.

Contraindications

■ Avoid use in patients who are hypersensitive.

Conscientious Considerations

■ Clinicians should be alert to discontinue a drug when the patient reaches the end-stage of dementia, or when comorbidities interfere with quality of life issues making the goal of delaying dementia progression less important than the goal of good care for the affected person.
■ Avoid use in those with severely impaired renal function unless dosage adjustments are made. Renal clearance is severely impaired in alkaline urine.

Patient/Family Education

■ Explain to patients and families that this drug is palliative and may only slightly slow progression of the disease. They need to understand that patients generally do not see reversal of their dementia and that all patients eventually progress to end-stage disease.

DRUG TREATMENT OF URINARY INCONTINENCE

Urinary incontinence (UI) is the involuntary loss of urine, which may be severe enough to cause social or health problems. Incontinence is not a normal part of aging, but age-associated changes such as uninhibited bladder contractions, nocturnal excretion during recumbence, diminished bladder capacity, prostate growth, and lower urinary flow rate (in men) do contribute to it. However, older adults with UI should undergo an evaluation by a clinician because in most cases, the problems of UI can be treated even if bladder control problems are found to be associated with many other issues, such as diabetes, infection, obesity, depression, and a sedentary lifestyle.

The bladder fills through relaxation of the detrusor muscle, which is innervated by the muscarinic, parasympathetic nervous system, and at the same time, the bladder sphincters contract. The major neurotransmitter of the muscarinic system is acetylcholine. The urinary sphincter is made up of two parts, the internal sphincter, which contracts under the influence of the sympathetic (α) system, and the external sphincter, which is much less important. When the bladder is filling, the sympathetic system is on and the parasympathetic system is off; this coordination is accomplished by a brainstem center called the pontine micturition center. When the bladder gets full enough, it switches to emptying mode, and the exact opposite occurs: The sympathetic system turns off, relaxing the internal sphincter, and the muscarinic system turns on, causing bladder contraction.

The brainstem can manage this without control by the cortex. For most individuals, however, this would be inappropriate (urinating at an inopportune time), so the frontal lobes, through both conscious and unconscious mechanisms, tonically inhibit this brainstem center until a proper time for voiding. This explains why some patients with dementia are incontinent; they have lost frontal lobe inhibition and simply rely on their brainstem to switch from filling to voiding mode.

There are three major types of incontinence: urge (detrusor too strong), stress (outlet too weak), and obstructive (outlet too strong). In urge incontinence, the patient describes an urge to urinate and can often maintain continence by running to the bathroom. In stress incontinence, any action that raises abdominal pressure, such as sneezing or standing, causes immediate leakage. In urinary obstruction, the patient often has symptoms such as hesitancy, straining, and dribbling. Functional incontinence, the inability to physically get to or onto a toilet, is also seen in patients. The most common cause of UI for both older men and women is urge incontinence. Only the drugs available to treat urge incontinence are discussed in this chapter.

Many older adults, especially women, have a syndrome called overactive bladder, where detrusor overactivity leads to bladder spasms, with symptoms of urinary frequency, urgency, and nocturia. In many of these patients, there is no incontinence because the patient can get to the bathroom in time. This condition is treated in the same way as urge incontinence.

Treatment Options for Urinary Incontinence

In all cases, clinicians should try to correct the underlying problems, such as urinary tract infection, delirium, atrophic vaginitis, depression, restricted mobility, or stool impaction. Bladder training can be useful in most cases of UI, unless the patient is a person with dementia. Ask the patient to void every 30 to 60 minutes, progressively increasing the duration between voids to every 3 to 4 hours during daytime hours. For both urge and stress UI, Kegel exercises can be useful in both men and women. Either show the patient how to do this or refer the patient to an occupational therapist with training in biofeedback-assisted pelvic muscle exercises. Avoidance of caffeine and alcohol, which increase urine production, as well as artificial sweeteners such as sucralose (Splenda), saccharin

(Sweet and Low), and aspartame (Equal, Nutrasweet), which irritate the bladder and cause it to spasm, may help improve symptoms of urinary incontinence. In patients with dementia who have urge UI, prompted voiding can help.

The drugs used to treat urge UI are not very effective; in clinical trials, they have reduced the number of incontinent episodes by about one per day (Burgio et al., 2010). Do not automatically use these drugs in older adults, particularly in patients with cognitive impairment because of the increased risk of confusion. Because all of these drugs work by blocking acetylcholine, if the patient has an underlying disease, such as Alzheimer's Disease, that is associated with loss of acetylcholine, these drugs can make confusion much worse.

Pharmacology of Drugs Used to Treat Urinary Incontinence
Muscarinic Antagonists

There are six medications in the category of muscarinic antagonists that are used to treat incontinence. These include: oxybutynin (Ditropan, Oxytrol patch), tolterodine (Detrol), trospium (Sanctura), darifenacin (Enablex), solifenacin (VESIcare), and fesoterodine (Toviaz).

Mechanism of Action

All six of these drugs are reversible acetylcholine receptor blockers that block the muscarinic or parasympathetic nerve endings on the detrusor muscle of the bladder. They also block muscarinic receptors throughout the body, which helps explain their diffuse anticholinergic side effects. All six drugs have direct spasmolytic action on smooth muscle, including the smooth muscle lining of the GI tract, without affecting vascular smooth muscle. Whether this translates into better clinical efficacy for patients in the form of decreased urge incontinence and decreased number of urinary accidents associated with overactive bladder is still not clear.

Clinical Uses

- These drugs are indicated for urge incontinence in cognitively intact patients. They are not indicated for nonspecific incontinence or other types of UI such as stress or obstructive UI. In fact, using a muscarinic blocker in a patient with obstructive UI could be dangerous, inducing urinary retention.
- Other drugs with anticholinergic side effects such as imipramine (Tofranil), dicyclomine (Bentyl), flavoxate (Urispas), and propantheline (Pro-Banthine) should not be used to treat urge UI. These drugs have doubtful efficacy, and the side effect profile is high in older adults.

Pharmacokinetics

- Absorption: All agents except for trospium and darifenacin are well absorbed, including excellent absorption from the transdermal form of oxybutynin.
- Distribution: Well distributed in serum by being bound to plasma protein.
- Metabolism: All drugs reduce smooth muscle (bladder) tone except for trospium. These drugs have extensive liver metabolism, forming both active and inactive metabolites, whereas trospium is metabolized only by esterase hydrolysis, making it more vulnerable for drug interactions.

■ Excretion: These agents undergo recirculation through the liver and hepatic circulatory system where one metabolite from the liver is active and the others are excreted in the urine.

■ Duration of action: Oxybutynin and tolterodine each have a duration of action of approximately 6 to 8 hours and thus require multiple daily dosing, unless the extended release forms are used. Trospium, darifenacin, and solifenacin have longer durations, allowing once-daily dosing. The newest drug, fesoterodine, has a shorter duration, but it is packaged only in an extended-release format for once-daily use.

Dosage and Administration

For all six of the bladder relaxants, start with low doses, and titrate up slowly, carefully monitoring for efficacy and side effects.

Generic Name	Trade Name	Route	Usual Adult Daily Dose
oxybutynin	Ditropan	PO	5 mg 2–3 times/day
		SR	10–15 mg 1 time/day
		Patch	Change patch every 3 days
tolterodine	Detrol	PO	1–2 mg 1–2 times/day
trospium	Sanctura	PO	20 mg 2 times/day
darifenacin	Enablex	PO	7.5–15 mg/day in a single dose
solifenacin	VESIcare	PO	5- and 10-mg tablets, typically dosed 5–10 mg/day in a single dose
fesoterodine	Toviaz	PO	Extended release 4- and 8-mg tablets dosed 4–8 mg/day in a single dose

Adverse Reactions

NEURO: The common side effects are due to the very mechanism of these drugs, being anticholinergic. Patients may experience dry mouth, blurred vision, constipation, inability to empty the bladder, and tachycardia. Anticholinergic side effects are most worrisome and vary from mild confusion to frank psychosis and agitation. There may be fewer side effects when a patient uses a transdermal patch, because the release of a dosage is even. It is likely this route is clinically effective with a smaller bolus of circulating drug.

REN: Urinary retention may be verified by bladder catheterization, or easier and safer, by bladder ultrasound, if that test is available. Urinary retention is the inability to empty the bladder completely as measured by a postvoid residual volume (PVR) of 100 mcg (in the elderly, a PVR under 200 mL is acceptable).

MISC: Dizziness, headache, and dyspepsia. With the Oxytrol patch, some patients may experience rash or itching.

Interactions

■ Do not combine cholinesterase inhibitors (such as donepezil) with these drugs because they have opposing mechanisms of action.

■ Avoid combining a bladder relaxant with other anticholinergic drugs, such as antihistamines, because excessive drowsiness may occur.

■ Oxybutynin, tolterodine, darifenacin, solifenacin, and fesoterodine may interact with drugs that affect the CYP3A4 system, and tolterodine, darifenacin, and fesoterodine also interact with the 2D6 system. For this reason, be careful in

using any other drugs, for example, antifungals, which interact with these metabolic pathways. Trospium does not have this issue, but it does compete with many more commonly used drugs such as digoxin, metformin, triamterene, and trimethoprim for a common renal tubular transport system.

Contraindications

■ Avoid these drugs in patients with Alzheimer's Disease and other forms of dementia because they are anticholinergic.

■ Ant-muscarinic drugs are contraindicated in patients with bowel or bladder obstruction, myasthenia gravis, and in untreated angle closure glaucoma. Antimuscarinic drugs may worsen the symptoms of gastroesophageal reflux.

■ Information is limited on the use of these drugs in patients with renal or hepatic impairment, thus its best to err on the side of caution even with mild to moderate degrees of either renal or hepatic impairment. For example, consider reducing the typical dose of tolterodine (Detrol) in an elderly patient with a urinary tract infection and a reduced CrCL of less than 30 mL/min to half of the regular dose.

Conscientious Considerations

■ These drugs are modestly more effective than a placebo. Use them only if you and your patients are convinced that the number of incontinent episodes is decreased on the drug.

■ If you have any question about efficacy, try stopping the drug and see what effect that has on urination and possible side effects.

■ Make a firm diagnosis of urge incontinence before using an antimuscarinic drug, and prescribe these drugs in conjunction with behavioral interventions.

■ These drugs, except for generic oxybutynin, are expensive. For many patients, the marginal benefit of the medication may not justify the cost involved.

■ Avoid these drugs in patients with cognitive impairment.

■ If one drug is ineffective, it is reasonable to try another one.

■ Be careful in using these drugs in older men, who may have bladder outlet obstruction.

■ Ensure that the bladder volume is normal, and consider using an alpha blocker or a 5-alpha-reductase inhibitor first.

Patient/Family Education

■ Accept that absolute dryness may not be a realistic goal, but a reduction in the number and severity of UI episodes is usually possible. Reducing the number of episodes can have a substantial impact on both the patient and caregivers.

■ Ask your patients/families to monitor for the anticholinergic side effects, particularly any evidence of cognitive impairment.

■ The drugs are best taken on an empty stomach. Extended-release tablets cannot be crushed or chewed.

DRUGS REQUIRING SPECIAL CONSIDERATION IN OLDER ADULTS

Using caution when prescribing any medications to older adults is always appropriate. However, certain drug classes require extra caution because certain medication use in the older adult comes with increased risks of toxicity or an adverse event. Clinicians should always be wary of extrapolating clinical data from studies where the participants were young and healthy and then applying the same data to frail and older adults. Additionally, because patients in clinical drug trials tend to receive better care than those in a standard-care setting, clinicians should be cautious about generalizing or transferring randomized clinical trial findings to their own patients. Thus, for many clinical trials their evidence is just not good enough to apply its findings to the older adult.

Antiarrhythmics

Specific antiarrhythmic drugs (amiodarone, sotalol, etc.) should only be used for rhythm disorders that are both symptomatic and potentially life-threatening, not for minor problems such as premature ventricular contractions or even asymptomatic runs of ventricular tachycardia. Because of the serious toxicity of these drugs, including inducing arrhythmias themselves, they should almost always be initiated and monitored by a cardiologist or electrophysiologist.

Amiodarone has multiple adverse effects in older adults, including cough and progressive dyspnea, hypothyroidism and hyperthyroidism, liver toxicity, GI effects, corneal microdeposits, confusion, slurred speech, and photosensitivity. It also has a very long half-life (about 2 months), so side effects may take a very long time to resolve when the drug is stopped. Amiodarone also has serious drug interactions with digoxin and warfarin. Use the lowest possible maintenance dose, preferably less than 200 mg/day.

Anticoagulants

This drug class includes aspirin, clopidogrel (Plavix), dipyridamole (usually prescribed with aspirin as Aggrenox), and warfarin (Coumadin). Older adults often have need for these drugs, but for the elderly any increased benefit comes with an increased risk of bleeding because older patients are more sensitive to the effects of anticoagulants, especially because they may have a deficiency in vitamin K clotting factors. All patients with established vascular disease—those with coronary artery disease, carotid disease (including after endarterectomy), and those with peripheral vascular disease—should take aspirin unless there is a contraindication. The dose for all of these patients is 81 mg/day; higher doses are not more effective, but they do lead to more bleeding. Clopidogrel is particularly effective in maintaining the patency of stented coronary arteries. Older adults who have had coronary angioplasty, with either bare metal or drug-eluting stents, and those after acute coronary syndrome should be prescribed clopidogrel (along with aspirin) if at all possible for at least a year. After a year, it is reasonable to consider stopping the clopidogrel. If there are questions, clinicians should consult with a cardiologist. For other types of vascular disease, such as stable coronary artery disease, carotid disease, or patients with multiple cardiac risk factors, prescribe aspirin alone. Clopidogrel can cause serious, life-threatening bleeding, including intracranial hemorrhage.

Aggrenox is a combination of 25 mg aspirin and 200 mg of extended-release dipyridamole. It is dosed twice a day and approved by the FDA to prevent a stroke in patients who have had a previous transient ischemic attack, or nondisabling stroke, but in both cases have had blood clots or the risk of blood clots. Although Aggrenox is expensive, generic aspirin and dipyridamole should not be prescribed to save money because it is unclear if the extended-release formulation of dipyridamole is essential for the clinical effect. A recent clinical trial compared clopidogrel and Aggrenox in patients who had previously had a stroke and found both drugs equally effective, but the Aggrenox produced more bleeding events. Thus, it must be considered as having a very limited role in the older adult, especially to prevent a second stroke (Sacco et al., 2008).

The most common indication for warfarin (Coumadin) in older adults is chronic nonvalvular atrial fibrillation. Although the evidence is not all consistent, most experts recommend that the large majority of elders with this condition be on carefully monitored warfarin, mainly to reduce the risk of stroke. Of course, the major problem is bleeding. At least 2% to 3% of older adults taking chronic warfarin will have a serious or life-threatening hemorrhage every year.

Clinicians should consider a patient's health situation before prescribing anticoagulants, including risk of bleeding, compliance, complexity of the medical regimen, potential drug interactions, comorbidities, and the risk of falling. Also, for patients who are profoundly impaired or near the end of life, for example, a patient with advanced Alzheimer's Disease, prevention of stroke may no longer be a reasonable goal. All older adults on warfarin need very careful monitoring of their international normalized ratio (INR), at least monthly, and often more frequently. There are many, many drugs that interact with warfarin. Consider comanaging these patients with a Coumadin clinic. These programs, usually led by a pharmacist, have been shown to reduce complications.

Antihistamines

Generally avoid antihistamine drugs in the older adult, both the older drugs and the newer less-sedating drugs. The major problem with these drugs is that they are anticholinergics, causing side effects such as blurred vision, dry mouth, constipation, and urinary retention. The most important anticholinergic side effect is confusion. Avoid use of these drugs in older adults with dementia or with any degree of cognitive impairment. Especially harmful to older adults is diphenhydramine (Benadryl), commonly found in over-the-counter products. As an antihistamine that causes drowsiness, it has caused many elderly people to fall. Thus, clinicians again need to ask older adults if they use this drug to help them sleep, and if they do, recommend against it. If an antihistamine is needed, it should be for a short term and be a newer, second-generation agent. For example, chlorpheniramine may be helpful for the older adult who has chronic allergies, and sometimes the newer over-the counter drugs such as loratadine (Claritin) or cetirizine (Zyrtec) are acceptable to older adults.

Antiparkinsonism Agents

Given the great similarity in symptoms, especially tremors at rest, Parkinson's Disease (PD) may on occasion be misdiagnosed in older adults as essential tremor (Villarini-Guell et al., 2010). Parkinsonism can also be caused by antihistamine/antinauseants such as promethazine (Phenergan), prochlorperazine (Compazine), and metoclopramide (Reglan) and antipsychotic drugs, both the older typical drugs (such as haloperidol and chlorpromazine) as and the newer atypical drugs (such as risperidone, olanzapine, and quetiapine). If you suspect drug-induced parkinsonism, taper the patient off the offending drug and reevaluate.

The directly anticholinergic drugs benztropine (Cogentin) and trihexyphenidyl (Artane) should be avoided in older adults. They are minimally effective for tremor, but their strong anticholinergic effects are limiting. Older adults on these medications are at risk for falls and confusion.

The standard treatment of Parkinson's Disease includes dopamine agonists, like pramipexole (Mirapex) or ropinirole (Requip) or the combination drug carbidopa-levodopa (Sinemet). These drugs attempt to replace dopamine, which has been lost as part of the disease. Unfortunately, too much dopamine can cause serious problems. Usually this manifests as either uncontrolled movements, such as grimacing and twisting, or seriously worsened confusion, often with vivid visual hallucinations, even overt psychosis.

Antipsychotics

Antipsychotic drugs are divided into the older, or typical, antipsychotics (such as haloperidol and chlorpromazine) and the newer, or atypical drugs (such as risperidone, olanzapine, quetiapine, ziprasidone, and aripiprazole) (see Chapter 10, Drugs Used in the Treatment of Pulmonary Diseases and Disorders, for detailed information). The newer drugs may have a lower rate of extrapyramidal side effects, but they are markedly more expensive. These agents prolong the QT interval, an electrocardiographic measurement of the interval between depolarization and repolarization within the heart. The length of the QT interval decreases as the heart rate increases, and the QTc is a measurement used to assess conduction status within the heart. As antispsychotic medications, particularly haloperidol, lengthen the QTC interval, they give rise to torsades de pointes.

Antipsychotic medications are most commonly used in geriatrics to treat the behavioral complications of dementia in spite of recent trials showing these drugs have very limited efficacy and serious toxicity in this setting. Unfortunately, their use in nursing homes is increasing once again, despite regulations aimed at slowing their use. Most nursing homes now require that residents be prescribed atypical antipsychotics rather than older conventional agents (Briesacher et al., 2005). In fact, federal and state agencies are enforcing nursing home practices that require monthly drug regimen reviews of all residents and that mandatory dose reductions be implemented as necessary. These reviews are to be done by a consultant pharmacist or nurse who acts independently of the pharmacy from which the nursing home gets its medications. General side effects of the atypical drugs include sedation, orthostatic hypotension, weight gain, hyperlipidemia, even the development of diabetes. The FDA now requires all atypical antipsychotics to carry a black box warning stating that use of these drugs in older adults increases the rate of myocardial infarction, stroke, and vascular mortality. Clinicians who decide to use these drugs should review this mortality risk with either the patient or a caregiver. Clinicians should also routinely check the patient's blood pressure and periodically check glucose and lipids.

Antipsychotic drugs block dopamine and 5-hydroxytryptamine and have serious extrapyramidal side effects (EPSs). Acute dystonia, which presents as either a cramped and spastic neck (torticollis) or as the more dramatic opisthotonos, is fortunately rare in older adults. More common is akathisia, a sensation of motor restlessness. An older adult who is cognitively intact will say they must fidget all the time and that they can't seem to sit down. If the patient has dementia, this side effect is easy to miss because the patient may just become more physical and walk all the time.

Like Parkinson's Disease, drug-induced parkinsonism, another EPS, presents with stiffness, bradykinesia, and tremor, and like PD it is easy to misdiagnose. All patients taking antipsychotics should be assessed for parkinsonism, which often presents several months after treatment is started. Clinicians typically make formal assessments at 3 and 6 months after starting the atypical antipsychotics to test for any sign of parkinsonism.

Tardive dyskinesia, which usually presents as abnormal involuntary movements of the face such as lip smacking or other tics, is markedly more common in older adults than in the young. Unfortunately, this often does not remit if the antipsychotic is stopped; it can progress and become socially disabling.

Finally, monitor for the development of the rare but significant neuroleptic malignant syndrome (NMS), which occurs when an antipsychotic drug is started at too high a dose or is increased very fast. NMS presents as fever, stiffness, and confusion, eventually progressing to rhabdomyolysis, acute renal failure, disseminated intravascular coagulation, and death. If a patient taking an antipsychotic develops a fever, always think of NMS as a possibility and consider getting a creatine phosphokinase level and holding the drug.

Because of this panoply of side effects, and because the drugs have limited effectiveness in treating behavioral complications of dementia, consider consulting with a psychiatrist, geropsychiatrist, or geriatrician before initiating or maintaining these drugs.

Anxiolytics

Drugs in this class include benzodiazepines and a host of other medications. In older adults, try to avoid long-acting benzodiazepines, such as diazepam (Valium), chlordiazepoxide (Librium), and clorazepate (Tranxene). These drugs are strongly associated with confusion, weakness, slurred speech, ataxia, and falls due to the delirium, euphoria, and other mood change they can bring. If they must be used, monitor closely and use the lowest possible dose. Particularly avoid flurazepam (Dalmane).

Shorter-acting benzodiazepines are safer, especially those with a moderate half-life and no active metabolites, such as lorazepam (Ativan), temazepam (Restoril), or oxazepam (Serax), but even these have the same toxicities, just at a lower rate.

Other pharmacological choices with less toxicity than benzodiazepines include buspirone (BuSpar) and SSRIs. However, because buspirone does not produce the euphoria of benzodiazepines, it is often hard for the clinician to wean people off them. It is also not recommended that drugs with high-risk for abuse, such as meprobamate or barbiturates, be used to treat anxiety in older adults. Consider nonpharmacological therapy for anxiety, such as psychotherapy, relaxation, tai chi, and regular office visits.

Corticosteroids

Corticosteroids may be life-saving in older adults, but making sure the benefits justify their use is a fine balancing act because of their many side effects. Clinicians today routinely do not give corticosteroid dose-packs for nonspecific syndromes such as back pain because even a single course of steroids in older adults can cause aseptic necrosis of the joints.

All older adults receiving steroids for a chronic condition will develop serious side effects, especially Addison's disease and cataract formation. A partial list of long-term steroid side effects includes sodium retention (this may worsen hypertension or congestive heart failure), agitation and psychosis, diabetes, skin ecchymosis, and osteoporosis. All older adults on chronic steroids should have an assessment of their bone density and receive adequate amounts of calcium and vitamin D.

Digoxin

Digoxin has multiple toxicities, including GI, ocular, and cardiac side effects. But the two major side effects in older adults are anorexia and confusion. These are easy to miss and can occur in patients who have normal serum digoxin levels.

Digoxin is only useful for two conditions: systolic heart failure (HF) and rate control of atrial fibrillation. If the patient has neither of these, discontinue the drug.

In older adults with HF, question the accuracy of the diagnosis. Rales at the lung base and peripheral edema do not equal HF. Most HF in older adults is diastolic (normal ejection fraction), and in these patients, digoxin is ineffective. In patients who do have systolic HF, digoxin should be considered only after using a vasodilator, diuretic, and beta blocker. If digoxin is used, monitor the patient closely for side effects, and keep the serum digoxin level less than 1 ng/mL.

In many older adults with atrial fibrillation, rate control is not necessary because the heart rate is already at the target of 60 to 90 bpm. Beta blockers and the calcium channel blocker diltiazem are better choices than digoxin, which should be reserved for use when other agents have failed. Its dosage should rarely exceed 0.125 mg/day. The dosage in a manufacturer's daily tablet (Lanoxin) is either 0.125 mg/day or 0.25 mg/day. In most frail older adults, there is almost always a better choice than digoxin.

NSAIDs

NSAIDs have serious toxicity in older adults, particularly their GI system, such as gastric bleeding, perforation, and obstruction. Acute renal failure, interstitial nephritis, and nephritic syndrome are also common. NSAIDs frequently raise the blood pressure and may worsen volume overload in diseases such as heart failure.

A conscientious clinician will use these drugs sparingly in older adults, tearing up more prescriptions than writing new ones. Before using NSAIDs for conditions such as degenerative joint disease (DJD), make sure the diagnosis is correct. X-ray the most affected joint(s), and check a complete blood count (CBC), sedimentation rate, chemistry panel, and 25(OH)-vitamin D level: You don't want to miss malignancy, an osteoporotic compression fracture, hyperparathyroidism, Paget's disease of bone, osteomalacia, or non-bone causes of pain such as an aortic aneurysm or retroperitoneal lymphadenopathy.

Most older adults diagnosed with DJD are able to tolerate some degree of joint pain. Patients should only be treated if the pain interferes with motor function. For these patients relief may come from warm baths, use of methyl salicylate rubs, and resting the affected joint. Clinicians may also consider referral to a physical therapist for lower extremity DJD or to an occupational therapist for upper extremity pain. Joint injections and joint replacement, which are safer than several years of treatment with NSAIDs, may also be considered.

If pharmacological treatment is necessary, consider using acetaminophen first, at 650 mg per dose, up to 3,000 mg per day in healthy older adults, and up to 2,000 mg per day in the frail. A next choice might be glucosamine/chondroitin; its efficacy is uncertain, but it is very safe. Over-the-counter lineaments and creams are also safe. Tramadol (Ultram) may also be tried before resorting to NSAIDs. To learn more about treatment guidelines for rheumatoid arthritis and osteoarthritis refer to Chapter 4, Drugs Used in the Treatment of Bone and Joint Disorders.

NSAIDs may be used for chronic pain, but their efficacy is limited. If clinicians prescribe these drugs, they should use the lowest possible dose. For some patients, using naproxen 250 mg once or twice daily, only when it rains or when the patient mows the lawn, may be appropriate. It is reasonable to use generic, inexpensive short-acting NSAIDs first, such as ibuprofen.

Ask patients if the NSAID is clearly making them feel better. NSAIDs treat pain, not arthritis. If the patient is unsure if the pain is better, recommend a trial off the drug. For patients who clearly receive analgesia from these drugs, many clinicians add a proton pump inhibitor to reduce GI side effects rather than use a COX-2 inhibitor such as celecoxib (Celebrex) in older adults. However, other COX-2 inhibitors were withdrawn from the market when FDA acted on these drugs' ability to increase cardiac mortality.

Opioid Analgesics

When used appropriately in the older adult, opioid analgesics may be markedly safer and effective than the alternatives. For example, treating pain in an 85-year-old woman with moderate dementia and severe spinal stenosis with MS Contin 15 mg twice a day is likely to be safer and more effective than large doses of acetaminophen, NSAIDs, or tramadol given long term. However, dosing with acetaminophen should always be a first-line consideration for simple pain in the elderly. The World Health Organization (WHO) Pain Ladder provides guidelines for managing pain (WHO, 1986).

The major toxicities of opioids in older adults are CNS and respiratory side effects. CNS effects include sedation and confusion, which can usually be mitigated by altering the dose or timing of the drug. Respiratory depression is a possibility, but it is very rare when drugs are slowly and carefully titrated. Constipation is universal in older adults taking opioids, and it can be recalcitrant. This side effect needs to be routinely prevented, looked for, and managed. Stool softeners alone are generally not effective in managing opioid-induced constipation, but they are useful adjuncts when combined with stimulant laxatives (Goodheart & Leavitt, 2006). Some clinicians first treat the constipation with diet changes that include more fiber and hydration, next with stimulant products such as senna, and then use osmotic laxatives such as sorbitol or polyethylene glycol (PEG), emollient, and bulk laxatives. However, osmotic and saline laxatives will worsen a patient's constipation if it has been induced by dehydration. Prostaglandin agents have also been used because they change the way the intestines absorb water and electrolytes, changing transit time and adding bulk to stools. The drug methylnaltrexone (Relistor) is particularly effective in opiate-induced constipation that is resistant to standard measures. This drug is available as a subcutaneous injection (8 mg and 12 mg). It reverses the peripheral opioid side effect of constipation, but because it does not cross the blood-brain barrier, it does not interfere with opioid-induced pain relief (Van Meerveld, 2008).

Do not use meperidine (Demerol) or pentazocine (Talwin) in older adults. These drugs are relatively ineffective and have serious side effects. Oral meperidine is a particularly poor choice because it is unreliably absorbed and has been associated with seizures and many other side effects such as confusion, sedation, hypotension, constipation, nausea, and vomiting.

Tricyclic Antidepressants

Tricyclic antidepressants, which include amitriptyline (Elavil) and others, are very rarely indicated in older adults because there are safer and more effective alternatives. These drugs commonly cause dry mouth, blurred vision, constipation, and urinary retention through their anticholinergic effects. They are also associated with orthostatic hypotension and quinidine-like effects, including serious ventricular arrhythmias. In all cases, try to find an effective alternative such as Abilify (dapiprazole) to Zyban (bupropion) (see Chapter 15, Practical Pharmacotherapy of Drugs Used to Treat Psychiatric Disorders, for more information on tricyclic antidepressants).

PREVENTING POLYPHARMACY AND MANAGING DRUG-RELATED PROBLEMS

A U.S. Government Accountability Office study estimated that 1 in 6 Medicare recipients receives inappropriate drugs resulting in adverse drug event–related hospital admissions being 6 times greater in the older adult as compared to the younger adult. This practice of inappropriate prescribing accounts for as many as a quarter of hospital admissions for older adults resulting in a tremendous cost burned to patients and to society (Berenbeim, 2002). Yet in the intervening years, little has been done to implement an effective means of curbing this high use of pharmaceuticals.

Because the most important pharmacokinetic change in older adults is a decrease in the capability of the kidney to excrete drugs, more so than the declining rate of hepatic drug metabolism, it is important for clinicians to always be wary of drug-drug interactions when several drugs are "on board" a patient with declining kidney function. At the same time, pharmacodynamic changes in the older adult are common and seen as shifts in an older adult's sensitivity to a drug; this happens irrespective of changes in drug excretion. An example of this would be the shift in sensitivity of the cardiovascular system to beta-adrenergic agonists and antagonists, a shift in sensitivity that decreases over time and manifests as the increases seen in orthostatic episodes when an elderly person responds differently to the prescribed antihypertensive medication. Thus, these hypotensive episodes can become the source for many of the falls that plague the older adult. Additionally, the CNS in older adults becomes more sensitive to agents that affect brain function (e.g., opioids, benzodiazepines, and psychotropic drugs), required the clinician to be ever more conscientious when using these agents in the elderly. All of this can be complicated even more by the plague of polypharmacy and drug-drug interactions. The complexity of the interactions between polypharmacy, comorbidity, altered pharmacodynamic sensitivity, and even modest changes in pharmacokinetics in elderly necessitate the clinician heed the admonishment to "start low and go slow" for aged subjects, especially if drug therapy is considered beneficial or absolutely necessary for them.

Polypharmacy is the act of prescribing more medications than are clinically necessary. Although many have tried to define it more succinctly, it is still considered to be either "use of at least one potentially inappropriate drug" or "the presence of six or more concurrent medications" (Bushart, Massey, Simpson, Ariail, & Simpson, 2008). Disabled older adults living in the community are likely the greatest population at risk for adverse drug events (ADE) initiated by polypharmacy. In fact, a study of older women who fit this category revealed not only did they take five or more prescription medications putting them at high risk for ADEs, but they were also frail, had congestive heart failure, diabetes mellitus, angina, COPD, cancer, and needed help with activities of daily living; thus they were at the greatest risk for the ravages of polypharmacy (Crentsil, Ricks, Xue, & Fried, 2010). Thus, it is a general maxim that drug therapy for older adults should be tailored to the individual patient. However, in many cases, clear, evidence-based guidelines for medication use in older adults are lacking. Thus, the wise clinician should consider obtaining answers to these questions before prescribing any new medication for their older adult patients:

1. Do I have a comprehensive list of all medications (including OTC, vitamins, and herbal preparations) this patient is taking? Ask your older patients to bring along all of their

medications to each visit, including drugs prescribed by other clinicians.

2. Is he/she taking the currently prescribed medications as instructed? Some patients reduce the dose or otherwise modify their medications due to side effects, costs, or other reasons. Ask your patients if they are taking the drugs as prescribed. Older adults may be reluctant to tell you that they cut the pill in half because they are afraid the dose is too high. Patients are often fearful of drugs and may take them as needed rather than on a regular basis. Review how patients are taking their drugs. For example, bisphosphonates must be taken first thing in the morning, with a large glass of water, while upright, with no more medications or food or drink for the next 30 minutes; if not, the drug is not well absorbed. Ask your patients if they can open a child-resistant cap. Use calendars, medication boxes, and family or caregivers as reminders for proper medication use. Use generic drugs whenever possible, and know the costs of the drugs you prescribe.

3. Does this patient need a new drug? In this particular patient, do the benefits of the proposed drug outweigh its risks? Is an older, generic drug that is just as effective available, or is there a newer drug that is safer? Avoid treating every minor symptom with another drug, and set priorities in drug therapy. For example, for a very old, frail, diabetic patient, adding a drug to lower the hemoglobin A1c below 8 is more likely to lead to hypoglycemia and a fall than to reduce future vascular events. Conscientious clinicians set reasonable treatment goals tailored to the individual patient.

4. Could the patient's new symptom be the side effect of a medication? When an older adult presents with any new symptom or laboratory test result abnormality, the first consideration should be whether or not this anomaly could be the side effect of a drug. For example, if a patient on a calcium blocker develops edema, stop the calcium blocker. If a patient with hypertension taking a diuretic develops hypokalemia, rather than automatically prescribing a potassium supplement, consider whether substituting an ACE inhibitor or ARB for the diuretic makes more sense. Constantly review each patient's medication list for contraindications and possible drug interactions; for example, patients with chronic kidney disease should not take metformin. Be wary of using new medications in frail older adults.

5. Could this patient be a victim of polypharmacy? Taking multiple medications is not by itself a problem because older adults often have multiple medical problems, and evidence-based treatment of diseases such as systolic heart failure requires using several medications. Rather, as the medication list grows, keep asking if each medication is still indicated. Could you treat more than one disease with a single drug? For example, if the patient has hypertension and heart failure, could the patient use an ACE inhibitor? If you are unsure of cause and effect, advise a "therapeutic untrial" of a drug. Stop or taper the drug and reassess if the medication is still needed. Drugs do not need to be continued forever: Ask if this drug is still helpful in your patient, especially as the patient ages and accumulates comorbidities and functional limitations. Try to reduce the number of medications and simplify dosing.

6. Is the patient being undermedicated? For example, older adults with established vascular disease should generally be on aspirin. Selected patients with chronic atrial fibrillation should be on warfarin. Aggressively detect and treat depression in older adults. Be careful in dosing older adults, but also titrate doses upward to gain maximal effect. Other conditions for which older adults frequently are not treated with appropriate polypharmacy include systolic heart failure, osteoporosis, and chronic pain. Both quantity and quality of life can be enhanced by appropriate medication prescription.

Clinicians should be cautious and "light-handed" in prescribing for patients older than 75 to 80 years. In most cases, there is a lack of appropriate evidence-based guidelines for this age group. Assume that there is progressive decline in renal and hepatic clearance, and look at the overall goals of care for the patient. Take the time to continually re-assess the medication list for older patients.

7. Clinicians should ask themselves if the prescription that they are prescribing, and any other medications the older adult is taking, is on the list of medications now considered inappropriate according to the National Guideline for Determining Potentially Inappropriate Medication Use By the Elderly, or the "Beers List" (Beers, 1997). These practice-based guidelines list medication therapy inappropriate for all elderly over the age of 65 and are divided into two categories: (1) medications to avoid or to use within specific dosages and durations in the elderly and (2) medications to avoid in the elderly with concomitant diseases. Now in use for nearly two decades, the Beers List is considered a world standard to help guild the clinician to help older adults get the best use of their medications.

LEARNING EXERCISES

Case 1

An 86-year-old man on Medicaid is admitted to the nursing home with advanced Parkinson's Disease for terminal care. He also has hypertension, DJD, and had severe delirium during recent hospitalizations for aspiration pneumonia and a hip fracture. He is able to speak very softly, and although he is hard to understand, he is "cognitively intact." He has lost 25 pounds, has dysphagia, and also has severe stiffness, cogwheel rigidity, and bradykinesia. His current medications include lisinopril 20 mg/day, hydrochlorothiazide 25 mg/day, naproxen 250 mg twice daily, risperidone 1.5 mg once a day, Sinemet 25/250 three times a day, and pramipexole 0.5 mg in the morning.

1. Stopping which medication(s) is likely to cause the most functional improvement?

2. At nursing home admission, DIP was suspected. Write an order for gradually discontinuing the risperidone.

3. What clinical signs would you follow to see if the withdrawal of the antipsychotic is safe and effective?

Case 2

You see a vigorous 76-year-old woman in the clinic for follow-up of hypertension, coronary artery disease, and osteoporosis. She is asymptomatic, with no signs of cognitive or functional impairment. She has had no falls in the last year. On your examination, you palpate and auscultate an irregularly irregular rhythm, and ECG confirms new-onset of atrial fibrillation. Her chronic medications include amlodipine, aspirin, simvastatin, vitamin D, calcium, and once-a-week alendronate. She had bleeding from a peptic ulcer 20 years ago, without recurrence. Her heart rate is 80 bpm, and when you walk her around the clinic for a few minutes, it increases to about 105 bpm, and she remains asymptomatic.

You consult with your physician supervisor about the new diagnosis and decide to check an echocardiogram, thyroid-stimulating hormone, CBC, chemistry panel, and a baseline INR. Rate control doesn't seem to be necessary. All the tests come back normal, except for left ventricular hypertrophy documented by echo.

1. Is this patient a good candidate for anticoagulation with warfarin?

2. Write a prescription for starting her warfarin anticoagulation.

3. Over the next several years, the patient develops Alzheimer's dementia, becomes functionally impaired, loses weight, and has frequent falls. Is she now a suitable candidate for warfarin anticoagulation?

References

ALLHAT or Coordinating Center for Clinical Trials. (2006). The Antihypertensive and Lipid Lowering Treatment to Prevent Heart Attack Trial, The University of Texas. Retrieved March 1, 2013, from http://allhat.sph.uth.tmc.edu/

Atri, A., Shaughnessy, L. W., Locasio, J. J., Growden, J. H. (2009). Memantine in combination with AChEI: Long-term course and effectiveness. *Alzheimer Disease and Associated Disorders.* 22(3), 209-221. Accessed March 4, 2013, from www.ncbi.nlm.nih.gov/pubmed/18580597

Aymanns, C., Keller, F., Maus, S., Hartmann, B., & Czock, D. (2010). Review of pharmacokinetics and pharmacodynamics and the aging kidney. *Clinical Journal of the American Society of Nephrology,* 5(2), 314-327.

Beers, M. H. (1997). Explicit criteria for determining potentially inappropriate medication use in the elderly. *Archives of Internal Medicine,* 157, 1531-1536.

Berenbeim, D. (2002). Polypharmacy: Overdosing on good intentions. *Managed Care Quarterly,* 10(3), 1-5.

Briesacher, S. A., Limcangco, M. E., Simoni-Wastila, L., Doshi, J. A., Levens, S. R., Shea, D. G., et al. (2005). The quality of antipsychotic drug prescribing in nursing homes. *Archives of Internal Medicine,* 165(11), 1280-1285.

Burgio, K. L., Goode, P. S., Richter, H. E., Markland, A. D., Johnson, T. M., 2nd, Redden, D. T. (2010). Combined behavioral and individualized drug therapy versus individualized drug therapy alone for urge urinary incontinence in women. *Journal of Urology,* 184(2), 598-603.

Bushart, R. L., Massey, E. B., Simpson, T. W., Ariail, J. C., & Simpson, K. N. (2008). Polypharmacy: Misleading but manageable. *Journal of Clinical Interventions in Aging,* 3(2), 383-389.

Carr, W., Weir, P. L. & Azar, D. (2013). Universal Design: A Step towards Successful Aging, *Journal of Aging Research.* Retrieved March 5, 2013, from www.ncbi.nlm.nih.gov/pubmed/23431446

Centers for Disease Control and Prevention (CDC). (2011). National Health and Nutrition Examination Survey (NHANES). Retrieved March 3, 2013, from http://www.cdc.gov/nchs/nhanes.htm

Crentsil, V., Ricks, M. O., Quan Li Xue, & Fried, L. P. (2010). A pharmacoepidemiological study of community dwelling older women: Factors associated with medication use. *American Journal of Geriatric Pharmacotherapy,* 8(3), 215-224.

Dahlof, B., Lindholm, L. H., Hasson, L., Scherstein, B. (1991, November, 23). Morbidity and Mortality in the Swedish Trial in Old Patients with Hypertension. Lancet, 338(8778), 1281-5. Retrieved March 4, 2013, from www.ncbi.nlm.nih.gov/pubmed/1682683

Furberg, C. D., Cutler, J. A., Probstfield, J. L., et al. (1987). *The systolic hypertension in the elderly program. Mild hypertension: From drug trials to practice* (pp. 59-63). New York: Raven Press.

Glynn, L. G., Murphy, A. W., Smith, A. M., Schroeder, K., & Fahey, T. (2010). Interventions used to control blood pressure in patients with hypertension. *Cochrane Database Systematic Review,* 17(3), CD005182. Retrieved March 3, 2013, from http://www.ncbi.nlm.nih.gov/pubmed/20238338

Goodheart, C. R., & Leavitt, S. B. (2006). *Managing opioid-induced constipation in ambulatory-care patients.* Glenview, IL: Paint Treatment Topics. Retrieved March 3, 2013, from http://pain-topics.org/pdf/Managing_Opioid-Induced_Constipation.pdf

Howland, R. H. (2009). Effects of aging on pharmacokinetic and pharmacodynamic drug processes. *Journal of Psychosocial Nursing and Mental Health Services,* 47(10), 15-16.

Lazarou, J., Pomeranz, B. H., & Corey, P. N. (1998). Incidence of adverse drug reactions in hospitalized patients: A meta-analysis of prospective studies. *Journal of the American Medical Association,* 279, 1200-1205.

Lotrich, F. E., & Pollock, B. G. (2005). Aging and clinical pharmacology: Implications for antidepressants. *Journal of Clinical Pharmacology,* 45, 1106-1122.

Messerli, F. H., Beevers, D. G., Franklin, S. S., & Pickering, T. G. (2003). Beta blockers in hypertension—The emperor has no clothes: An open letter to present and prospective drafters of new guidelines for the treatment of hypertension. *American Journal of Hypertension,* 16(10), 870-873.

Quato, D. M., Alexander, G. B., Conti, R. M., Johnson, B. A., Schumm, P., & Lindau, S. T. (2008). Use of prescription drugs and over the counter drugs among older adults. *Journal of the American Medical Association,* 300(24), 2867:28.

Ripley, T. L., Chonlahan, J. S., & Germany, R. E. (2006). Candesartan in heart failure. *Journal of Clinical Interventions in Aging,* 1(4), 357-366.

Robinson-Cohen, C., Katz, R., Mozaffarian, D., Dalrymple, L. S., de Boer, I., Sarnak, M., et al. (2009). Physical activity and rapid decline in kidney function in older adults. *Archives of Internal Medicine,* 169(22), 2113-2116.

Sacco, R. L., Diener, H. C., Yusuf, S., Cotton, D., Ôunpuu, S., Lawtonet, W. A., et al. (2008). Aspirin and extended release dipyridamole vs. clopidogrel for prevention of recurrent stroke. *New England Journal of Medicine,* 359(12), 1238-1251.

Sawyer, P., Bodner, E. V., Richie, S. C., & Allman, R. M. (2006). Pain and pain medication use in community dwelling older adults. *American Journal of Geriatric Pharmacotherapy, 4*(4), 316-324.

Slone Epidemiology Center. (2006). *Patterns of medication use in the United States 2006: A report from the Slone Survey.* Retrieved March 3, 2013, from www.bu.edu/slone/SloneSurvey/AnnualRpt/Slone SurveyWebReport2006.pdf

Stokes, G. S. (2009). Management of hypertension in the elderly patient. *Journal of Clinical Interventions in Aging,* (4), 379-389.

U. S. Census Bureau. (2009). Projections of the population by selected age groups and sex for the United States 2010-2050, Table 2. Population Division, U.S. Census Bureau. Accessed March 4, 2013, from www.census.gov/population/projections/data/national/2009/2009cnmsSumTabs.html

Van Meerveld, B., & Standifer, K. M. (2008). Methylnaltrexone in the treatment of opioid-induced constipation. *Journal of Clinical and Experimental Gastroenterolgy, 1*, 48-49. Retrieved March 3, 2013, from www.ncbi.nlm.nih.gov/pmc/articles/PMC3108626/

Vilarino-Guell, C., Ross, O. A., Wider, C., Jasinska-Myga, B., Cobb, S. A., Soto-Ortolaza, A. I., et al. (2010). *LINGO1* rs9652490 is associated with essential tremor and Parkinson's disease. *Parkinsonism and Related Disorders, 16*(2), 109-111. Retrieved March 13, 2013, from www.ncbi.nlm.nih.gov/pmc/articles/PMC2844122/

World Health Organization (WHO). Cancer: *WHO's Analgesic ladder.* (2013). Accessed March 4, 2013, from www.who.int/cancer/palliative/painladder/en/

World Health Organization (WHO). (Medicines: Rational use of medicines. Fact Sheet No. 338. Retrieved March 13, 2013, from www.who.int/mediacentre/factsheets/fs338/en/index.html

Prescribing for the Pediatric Patient

chapter 23

Justin Beverly, Edward Clark

CHAPTER FOCUS

The focus of this chapter is twofold: first, it addresses six unique challenges clinicians must face in the selection of a drug for a pediatric patient, and second, it describes how various agents are applied to treat common pediatric disorders. An underlying premise of this chapter is that differences in decision-making do exist when making choices for medications for children, adolescents, and adults. Attention is also given to special caretaker and family situations, drug contraindications, dosage forms, and black box warnings, using examples to illustrate the drug selection challenges of dealing with pediatric patients.

OBJECTIVES

After reading and studying this chapter, the student should be able to:

1. Recall the challenges in administering various pharmaceuticals to a pediatric population.
2. Describe how to calculate the correct dosages for various common medications for different pediatric age groups.
3. Describe how taste, texture, drug delivery, and other factors greatly influence pediatric compliance with medications.
4. Describe and discuss some common drugs that are contraindicated or have black box warnings in the pediatric population.
5. Describe and discuss the drugs used in the treatment of some of the most common outpatient pediatric disorders by body system, with emphasis on pediatric otolaryngology, pulmonology, gastroenterology, genitourinary, behavior (attention deficit-hyperactivity disorder), and neurology.

Key Terms

Atopy
Black box warning
Epistaxis
Gasping syndrome
Gray-baby syndrome
Inspiratory stridor
Kernicterus
Laryngotracheitis
Metered dose inhaler (MDI)
Milligrams per kilogram (mg/kg) dosing
Nonallergic rash
Pseudomembranous colitis
Reye's syndrome
Steroid rage
Stratum corneum

KEY DRUGS IN THIS CHAPTER

For Infectious Conjunctivitis

Topical Antibiotics: Miscellaneous
neomycin + polymyxin + bacitracin (Neosporin): drops and ointment
polymyxin B + bacitracin (Polymyxin) ointment
polymyxin B + trimethoprim (Polytrim) drops

Topical Antibiotics: Aminoglycosides
gentamicin (Garamycin, Genoptic): drops and ointment
tobramycin (Tobrex): drops and ointment

Topical Antibiotics: Fluoroquinolones
ciprofloxacin (Ciloxan): drops and ointment
moxifloxacin (Vigamox): drops
ofloxacin (Ocuflox): drops

For Allergic Conjunctivitis

Topical Antihistamines
naphazoline (Vasocon, Naphcon, Clear Eyes)
oxymetazoline (Visine LR, Afrin)
azelastine (Optivar)
olopatadine (Patanol)

Topical Corticosteroids
fluticasone (Veramyst and Flonase)
mometasone (Nasonex)

Oral Antihistamines
diphenhydramine (Benadryl)
loratadine (Claritin)
desloratadine (Clarinex)
fexofenadine (Allegra)

For Bacterial Infections

Oral Antibiotics
amoxicillin (Amoxil)
amoxicillin + clavulanic acid (Augmentin and Augmentin ES-600)
azithromycin (Zithromax)
cefuroxime (Ceftin)
ceftriaxone (Rocephin)
cephalexin (Keflex)
clarithromycin (Biaxin)
clindamycin (Cleocin)
sulfamethoxazole + trimethoprim (Septra, Bactrim)

Topical Antibiotics
hydrocortisone + polymyxin + neomycin (Cortisporin Otic Suspension)

continued

KEY DRUGS IN THIS CHAPTER—cont'd

ofloxacin (Floxin Otic soln.)
ciprofloxacin + dexamethasone (Ciprodex
Otic Suspension)
ciprofloxacin + hydrocortisone (Cipro HC
Otic Suspension)

For Viral Infections
oseltamivir (Tamiflu)
zanamivir (Relenza)
acyclovir (Zovirax)

For Yeast Infections (Thrush)
fluconazole (Diflucan)
nystatin

For Rhinitis and Common Cold
Antihistamines
azelastine (Astelin)
brompheniramine (Dimetane, Dimetapp),
cetirizine (Zyrtec)
clemastine (Tavist OTC)
chlorpheniramine (Chlor-Trimeton, Chlor-
Phen)
desloratadine (Clarinex)
diphenhydramine (Benadryl)
fexofenadine (Allegra)
loratadine (Claritin)
Decongestants
pseudoephedrine (Sudafed)
Antitussives
dextromethorphan (DM, Delsym)

Expectorants
guaifenesin (Mucinex, Robitussin)

For Asthma and other Pulmonary Disorders
Inhaled Bronchodilators
Short-Acting Beta Agonists (SABA)
albuterol (Ventolin, Proventil)
racemic epinephrine (racepinephrine)
Long-Acting Beta Agonists (LABA)
salmeterol (Serevent)
Anticholinergics
ipratropium (Atrovent)
**Inhaled Corticosteroids (Long-Term
Anti-Inflammatory Agents)**
beclomethasone (QVAR)
budesonide (Pulmicort)
fluticasone (Flovent)
triamcinolone (Azmacort)
**Systemic/Oral Steroids (Short-Term
"Burst" Therapy)**
methylprednisolone (Medrol)
prednisolone
prednisone
dexamethasone (Decadron)
Anti-Inflammatory Agents
**Leukotriene Receptor Antagonists
(Inhibitors)/Mast Cell Inhibitors**
montelukast (Singulair)

Combination Products
salmeterol/fluticasone (Advair)

For Gastrointestinal Disorders
Oral Antiemetics
promethazine (Phenergan)
ondansetron (Zofran)
prochlorperazine (Compazine)
Flatulence
simethicone (Mylicon)

For Pinworms
mebendazole (Vermox)

For Control of Pain/Analgesics
acetaminophen
codeine (Paveral)
hydrocodone/acetaminophen (Lortab)

For Headache
sumatriptan (Imitrex)
rizatriptan (Maxalt)

For Behavioral and Psychiatric Disorders (ADHD)
methylphenidate (Ritalin)
dexmethylphenidate (Focalin)
dextroamphetamine with amphetamine
(Adderall)
atomoxetine (Strattera)
lisdexamfetamine (Vyvanse)

For Iron Deficiency Anemia
ferrous sulfate (Fer-in-Sol)

The pharmacology relative to pediatric patients presents a constantly changing set of challenges to clinicians in the specialty of pediatrics and primary care. Knowledge of pediatric pharmacology has been undergoing sweeping growth in the last 10 years because of an expansion of public and private funded research. Much of this research has been pharmacokinetic studies and multisite controlled efficacy trials so that treatment of children and adolescents can be done using better information and be based on "best evidence." Additionally, federal regulatory agencies have offered incentives to the pharmaceutical industry to conduct pediatric trials on the use of pharmaceuticals. At the same time, public funding has been supporting research into off-patent medications. With the growth in pediatric drug research, the role of government as a clearing agency to help avoid duplication and to ensure better integration of efforts and utilization of resources has also grown. Thus, today's clinicians have greater insight into the complexities of drug use in children and know that when it comes to medications, children are *not* to be treated as little adults.

Prescribing for children is a complex process. Drug therapy in pediatric patients must be individualized, taking into consideration the patient and his or her medical history, the patient's caregiving network and support structure, and the pharmacology of the drug(s) under consideration. This is important because adults typically receive the same dosage of a medicine as other adults, regardless of their age or weight, but this is not the case

in children. Children constantly undergo rapid changes in their body mass, metabolism, excretion, and ability to absorb medicines. Thus, dosing of medicines in children is a specialty wherein the following seven questions must be well thought through and answered by the clinician before prescribing any drug:

1. How does the age of the child affect the drug's pharmacokinetics and pharmacodynamics?
2. Has the drug dosage using "milligrams per kilogram" been carefully calculated?
3. Has the taste, texture, and ease of administration of the drug been considered?
4. Have the drug's contraindications in a pediatrics population been considered?
5. Have any black box warnings for use of the drug in pediatric populations been considered?
6. Have the risks and benefits been carefully considered?
7. Has the ability of the caretaker to administer the medication and to adhere to the medication schedule been considered?

These seven questions constitute the limbs of a good decision tree for pediatric prescribing. Each of these questions addresses a topic that must be answered on a case-by-case basis to ensure the safety and effectiveness of medication use in a population where much clinical decision-making has been based on extrapolation of adult data and personal experience.

Pharmacodynamic and Pharmacokinetic Considerations

From a pharmacological perspective, the process of growth and development represents an unstable and dynamic condition leading to many challenges for the prescribing clinician. The continuous development of body and organ functions in pediatric patients influences drug effects and drug disposition. Age-related differences in drug pharmacokinetics and drug pharmacodynamics occur throughout childhood and influence drug dosing across the life span. Differences in drug dosing are not purely dependent upon body mass; they also have to do with the processes controlling the absorption, distribution, metabolism, excretion, and pharmacological effects of drugs.

Pharmacodynamics

At one time, drug testing in infants, children, and adolescents was considered morally wrong, and until recently testing was not required of a manufacturer before bringing a drug into the market. Clinicians prescribed to children smaller doses of drugs that were safe for adults and observed them for unexpected reactions. Much information about drug use in children and infants was discovered when that drug use resulted in poor outcomes. For example, infants are deficient in the glucuronide enzymes necessary to detoxify chloramphenicol. Children who took chloramphenicol developed high levels of the drug, which produced **gray-baby syndrome**. They became cyanotic, and eventually died as a result of chloramphenicol buildup.

Another example occurred when sulfonamide drugs were found to displace bilirubin from plasma proteins, which caused infants to develop **kernicterus**, neurological damage to the brain and spinal cord as a result of too much bilirubin in the bloodstream. Finally, when antihistamines and barbiturates are given to children, rather than producing sedation, the combination produces hyperactivity.

Pharmacokinetics

Drug absorption, metabolism, and excretion vary widely throughout infancy, childhood, and even well into puberty. Thus, neonates, infants, toddlers, children, and adolescents all process drugs differently.

Drug Absorption

Among children, drug absorption is affected by blood flow at the site of administration, gastrointestinal (GI) function, and a thinner **stratum corneum** or (outer layer of the epidermis) than adults. Neonates exhibit blood flow variability among their muscles, which affects drug absorption from intramuscular or subcutaneous injection sites. If drug absorption is rapid, it may lead to toxic doses of the drug in the bloodstream.

GI functioning among children is also variable. For example, gastric pH does not reach adult levels until a child is between 18 and 36 months of age. Additionally, the gastric emptying time of a child is longer than that of an adult and does not reach adult levels until a child is least 9 months old. These developmental differences in a child's gastric functioning alter drug absorption in predictable ways. For example, the oral bioavailability of compounds such as the acid-labile beta-lactam antibiotics (cephalosporins and penicillins) is increased, whereas the oral bioavailability of weak organic acids such as phenytoin is decreased.

Finally, because infants and children have a thinner stratum corneum than do adults, as well as a larger body surface area in relation to their size, they tend to absorb medicines placed onto their skin more readily than adults. This characteristic has led to toxicity in children due to increased absorption of drugs such as topical anesthetics (lidocaine), antihistamines, diphenhydramine (Benadryl), and topical corticosteroids. In some cases, the topical steroids have been absorbed to levels high enough to induce cushingoid symptoms. As a result, several cortisone creams have been relabeled "to be used in adults only."

Drug Distribution

Drug distribution among children is different than it is in adults. This is because changes in body composition occur as children grow through infancy and adolescence and their levels of total body water and lean muscle-to-fat ratio shifts. Total body fat typically decreases in adult males between the ages of 10 and 20 by about 50%, and lean body mass increases. Thus, it becomes hard to predict a drug's pharmacokinetic outcomes during puberty. This becomes critical for a clinician monitoring an adolescent taking an anti-seizure medication such as phenytoin, where dosing is paramount to preventing seizures. The clinician has an ongoing task of assuring continuous monitoring of the adolescent with epilepsy throughout his or her pubertal development.

Drug Metabolism

A child's metabolic pathways to detoxify drugs develop sporadically during the first year of life. Additionally, a large number of variations in drug metabolism occur because of the ability of the small bowel to metabolize drugs. Among adults much is known about the cytochrome P450 enzyme system and its several isomers, but among neonates, children, and adolescents much is still to be learned. What is known is that for some drugs, such as caffeine, limited enzyme metabolism occurs until a newborn is about 4 months of age. Then drug metabolism increases until it reaches normal adult levels between 1 to 2 years and continues to rise beyond adult levels until puberty is reached. After puberty, metabolic clearance of drugs by cytochrome P450 enzymes (CYP450) begins to decline to adult levels. In females this decline occurs faster than in males.

Diseases such as cystic fibrosis can affect CYP450 isomers and require larger than normal dosing. In addition, grapefruit juice, charbroiled foods, cruciferous vegetables, and cigarette smoking all affect therapeutic levels of medications requiring cytochrome isoenzymes to metabolize them. It is important to note that NSAIDs, macrolides, antihistamines, oral contraceptives, antiepileptics, and many other common pediatric medications are metabolized by CYP450 enzymes and its isomers, causing pediatric care professionals to be vigilant about prescribing when more than one drug competes with these enzymes for metabolism.

Drug Excretion

The glomerular filtration rate of newborns is about 30% to 40% that of adults and does not reach adult values until the newborn is about 1 year old. For newborns, dosage adjustments of drugs (strength and intervals) that depend on renal excretion (aminoglycosides, ampicillin) must be carefully made because these drugs are more slowly cleared than in infants than they are in an older person.

Drug Dosing Considerations in Pediatric Patients

The vast majority of pediatric medicines are typically dosed on a milligram per kilogram basis. Many drugs are available in a variety of formulations. A classic example is amoxicillin, which is available in several different formulations (Table 23-1).

With over a dozen commercial formulations of amoxicillin to choose from, the clinician has many options when choosing one for a child. Yet, it is typical for pediatricians to prescribe only a few formulations to help avoid dosing errors.

Dosing charts are available for many commonly prescribed drugs. One such resource is the Pedibiotic Card, a laminated reference card for clinicians that provides essential data for dosing antibiotics and pain medications for children. It is available at Amazon.com, www.amazon.com/Pedibiotic-Card-Intellicard/dp/1888411066, or at www.intelli-card.com/pedifan.html. These types of charts greatly simplify and streamline pediatric dosing for a variety of weights and ages. However, these charts, and others like them, are simply guidelines, and clinicians should always individualize doses for pediatric patients.

Exact dosages of pediatric medications are rarely achieved, but some minimal rounding of numbers should not affect clinical results. In some situations the calculated dose of a pediatric medicine may be greater than the recommended adult dose. For example, for an 80-kg adolescent with otitis media, the recommended dose of amoxicillin is 90 mg/kg of amoxicillin. Thus, the 80-kg adolescent theoretically would need 80 × 90 or 7,200 mg or 7.2 gm. This far exceeds the maximum daily dose of amoxicillin, which is (2,000 to 3,000 mg). In such situations, the clinician should prescribe the recommended adult dose. Three more examples of common dosing scenarios when treating otitis media follow:

CASE 1 15-month-old male, weight of 13.4 kg, using amoxicillin. Amoxicillin is usually dosed at 80 to 90 mg/kg/day divided into two doses to be administered twice daily for otitis media (OM). You decide to dose at 90 mg/kg/day divided to dose two

times a day. Total dose required is 1,206 mg. You select amoxicillin at a dose form of 400 mg/5 mL. Performing some quick math, you see that 1,206 mg/400 mg/5 mL = 15.075 mL. Round this number down to 15 mL for ease of delivery. Finally, divide this amount (15 mL) into a twice-daily schedule, and you arrive at 7.5 mL (1.5 teaspoons) of amoxicillin, 400 mg/5 mL strength, two times a day.

CASE 2 4-year-old male, weight of 18 kg, using amoxicillin. Amoxicillin is usually dosed at 80 to 90 mg/kg/day divided into two doses to be administered two times a day for OM. You decide to dose at 90 mg/kg/day divided to dose two times a day. Total dose required is 1,620 mg. You select amoxicillin at a dose form of 400 mg/5 mL. Performing some quick math, you see that 1,620 mg/400 mg/5 mL = 20.25 mL. Round this number down to 20 mL for ease of delivery. Finally, divide this amount (20 mL) into a twice-daily schedule and you arrive at 10 mL (2 teaspoons) of amoxicillin, 400 mg/5 mL strength, two times a day.

CASE 3 16-year-old male, weight of 70 kg, using amoxicillin. Amoxicillin is usually dosed at 80 to 90 mg/kg/day divided into two doses to be administered two times a day for OM. However, a quick calculation reveals that this would give 6,300 mg of amoxicillin per day, whereas the maximum usual adult dose is 2 to 3 gm per day. Accordingly, you select the adult dose and give a 500-mg to 875-mg tablet two times a day.

For liquid products, caretakers should always use the measuring device (dropper, dosing cup, or dosing spoon) that is packaged with each formulation because they are marked to deliver the recommended dose. Kitchen teaspoons or tablespoons are not appropriate measuring devices for giving medicines to children because they vary considerably (2.5 mL to -6 mL) in how much liquid they hold. Using a household teaspoon or tablespoon can result in underdosing or overdosing a child.

Drug Formulations: Being Creative and Flexible

The clinician must also be aware of the various formulations and strengths of a particular agent before prescribing it. This allows for flexibility, but it can also be a source of confusion and subsequent dosing errors. It takes the average practitioner years to remember which drugs are well tolerated, which ones children simply won't take, and which ones burn or feel cold when administered topically. Creativity and flexibility on the part of the clinician is important when dealing with young children because their determination to spit out a medicine is often greater than the patience of the caretaker or clinician.

Some medications have a well-accepted, pleasing taste (Amoxil), whereas others have an unpleasant taste (Prelone). Another example is polyethylene glycol 3350 (MiraLax), which is used to treat constipation. This is a relatively tasteless medication, but children often don't like the gritty texture of it after it is mixed in juice. Whether or not children would prefer "gritty MiraLax" to a glycerin rectal suppository is something that varies from child to child. Pediatric patients are individuals, and what they prefer or will tolerate varies from one to another. The following case illustrates how drug taste, delivery, adherence,

TABLE 23-1	Available Commercial Formulations and Dosing Strengths of Amoxicillin
FORM	DOSAGES
Capsules	250 mg, 500 mg
Scored tablets	500 mg, 875 mg
Chewable tablets (banana, cherry, peppermint)	125 mg, 200 mg, 250 mg, 400 mg
Bubble gum-flavored drops (pediatric)	50 mg/mL
Bubble gum-flavored powder (oral suspension)	125 mg/5 mL, 200 mg/5 mL, 250 mg/5 mL, 400 mg/5 mL

and a host of other factors must be considered during a typical pediatric encounter.

CASE 4 Asthma exacerbation in a 5-year-old boy. A 5-year-old boy comes to the office with a moderately severe asthma exacerbation, his second this year. After improvement with several in-office nebulizer albuterol treatments, which he tolerates quite well, the clinician prescribes albuterol aerosols via a nebulizer machine and a 5-day course of methylprednisolone (10 mg/day) to be taken at home.

Unfortunately, the generic methylprednisolone tastes so awful (the mother describes it as something close to nail polish remover) that the child refuses to take it and vomits it up after each dose despite multiple efforts to administer it. As a remedy, the clinician can prescribe an alternative and much better-tasting steroid (Orapred, for example); or advise the pharmacy to add cherry flavor to the syrup; or even consider other options, such as crushing a single 10-mg prednisone tablet and sprinkling it in applesauce to hide the flavor.

When the mother attempts to administer the albuterol nebulizer treatment at home, the child kicks and screams throughout the 20-minute treatment (despite tolerating it well in the office), but seems to tolerate his brother's spacer/mask/**metered dose inhaler (MDI)** combination just fine. Accordingly, the clinician changes the prescription to an MDI for better compliance.

It is also important to remember that as children grow, their tolerance to medications and preferences may change. For instance, because a patient may have tolerated Amoxil syrup for treatment of otitis media when he or she was 8 years old, that does not mean that he or she will do the same age 12. At age 12 many children prefer the chewable tablet or a pill version, because it is viewed as being more grown-up. The clinician must take the time to communicate with the child as well as the caretaker to get a full understanding of what will and will not work when prescribing for children at any age.

Drug Contraindications in Pediatric Patients

Many drugs are safe for adult and pediatric use, but they have age restrictions or other caveats. Many drugs that were initially developed for adults were later approved by the U.S. Food and Drug Administration (FDA) for use in pediatrics. Other drugs have not been approved by the FDA for children and likely never will. This is due to a variety of reasons, but it is mostly because clinical trials on children do not exist. However, drugs may be widely used in children as experience and clinical judgment reveal things about their safety. In addition, some medicines once routinely used in pediatric populations are no longer used due to contraindications that have recently come to light. These include aspirin, over-the-counter cold medications, fluoroquinolones, tetracyclines, metoclopramide, and antimigraine serotonin 5-HT receptor agonists.

Aspirin, once used universally for a variety of ailments, has disappeared from pediatric use because of its association with Reye's syndrome and GI side effects. Notable exceptions include children who have Kawasaki syndrome, rheumatic fever, or have had surgical correction of complex congenital heart disease.

Over-the-counter cough/cold preparations have recently lost favor in the pediatric community. For children under the age of 2, there are some cough/cold medications still available with a prescription, but they are generally discouraged because they are not efficient and have the potential for adverse reactions. The FDA has warned caretakers not to give children younger than 2 years of age over-the-counter cough or cold medicines unless given specific directions to do so by a clinician.

Fluoroquinolones, such as Cipro and Levaquin, are effective antimicrobials against a wide range of pathogens. However, they have been shown to have potentially adverse effects on the growth of immature cartilage, joints, and surrounding tissues. As such, they are not routinely used in patients under 18 years of age and are generally reserved for those patients with severe infections with resistant organisms.

Tetracyclines, such as doxycycline, should not be used in children less than 8 years old due to dental discoloration, enamel hypoplasia, and skeletal development problems.

Metoclopramide (Reglan) was commonly used as an antiemetic just a few short years ago, but it now is contraindicated in pediatrics because it can cause extrapyramidal symptoms (EPS) and tardive dyskinesia; these serious movement disorders are often irreversible.

The antimigraine serotonin 5-HT receptor agonists such as sumatriptan (Imitrex), rizatriptan (Maxalt), and zolmitriptan (Zomig) are not officially indicated for use in the pediatric population owing to serious adverse effects such as myocardial infarction, stroke, death, and vision loss. Although widely used without FDA approval, studies are lacking in demonstrating their efficacy and advantages, and thus careful use of these agents by pediatric neurologists is highly recommended.

Pediatric Drugs with Black Box Warnings

A **black box warning** is the most severe warning the FDA can require of a prescription drug and is often the first step the FDA takes when it is considering pulling a drug off the market. If untoward usage continues or if prescribing habits show the black box warnings are going unheeded, the FDA calls on its special Pediatric Advisory Committee to help decide the necessary next steps to either continue a black box warning or recommend pulling the drug off the market. In recent years the FDA has issued black box warnings for the following:

■ Drugs used for the treatment of depression
■ Drugs used for the treatment of eczema
■ Drugs used for the treatment of asthma
■ Drugs used for the treatment of attention deficit-hyperactivity disorder (ADHD)

Some examples of drugs that have black box warnings indicating they may cause adverse events in children follow. Clinicians should be cautious when using these medications.

■ Promethazine (Phenergan): Routinely used as an antiemetic in children for decades, in children younger than 2 years old it has the potential for severe or fatal respiratory depression, even with recommended doses. In children older than

2 years, caution should still be used, and the lowest effective dose should be given.

- Pimecrolimus (Elidel) and tacrolimus (Protopic, Prograf): Used in the treatment of severe eczema, these drugs may increase susceptibility to infection and development of lymphoma owing to immunosuppression. In addition, use in children younger than 2 years of age is not recommended.
- Metformin (Glucophage): This biguanide antidiabetic agent may cause lactic acidosis, a rare but potentially severe consequence of therapy.
- Lisinopril (Zestril) and other ACE inhibitors (Captopril, Enalapril, etc.): These drugs can cause injury to and death of a developing fetus.
- Salmeterol (Advair, Serevent): Increased risk of asthma-related deaths occurs. Accordingly, Advair and Serevent should only be used when other asthma drugs, such as low- to medium-dose inhaled corticosteroids, do not work or if the patient's asthma symptoms are severe enough to merit the use of two medications.
- Methylphenidate (Concerta, Metadate, Methylin, Ritalin) and other behavioral medicines: Drug dependency may develop with use of these drugs.
- Amphetamines (Adderall and Adderall XR, Vyvanse): Misuse may cause sudden death and serious cardiovascular adverse events.

The list of drugs with black box warnings regarding their use in pediatric populations continues to grow. Clinicians who treat children must be knowledgeable and vigilant regarding adverse effects caused by any drug.

Patient-Family Issues Affecting Adherence in Pediatrics

Poor adherence to a prescription medicine's regimen is a factor in treatment failure. More often than not it is due to the caretakers' failure to understand some important aspect of the drug regimen. For example, antibiotics should be dosed at regular intervals, such as every 6 hours around the clock. For some caretakers this regimen is difficult to remember and to follow. Thus, at times the child may not receive all doses necessary in a 24-hour period. Furthermore, caretakers may experience difficulty actually administering a medication to a child due to the amount (1 to 2 teaspoons), taste, or texture. However, because medications come in differing strengths, clinicians can prescribe a stronger strength and a smaller amount can be administered. If a child has trouble swallowing a whole teaspoonful of medicine, then a more concentrated drug strength could be chosen so that only 0.5 teaspoonful needs to be administered. In addition, some drugs are available in a crushable tablet form, allowing the drug to be sprinkled on the child's favorite food, such as applesauce, a commonsense approach to improving medication adherence. Caretakers do not always know about these options and solutions. It is up to the clinician to make wise choices for both caretaker and child and to educate the caretaker.

Motivational and reminder aids for caretakers can help improve adherence. For example, many pediatric offices prepare printed handouts for common and frequent conditions that they see in the practice. They know that the child's caretaker may forget instructions given in the office due to the anxiety, fear, and/or worry of the moment. Reinforcing what has been said with a printed handout increases the probability of a positive outcome. Typical handouts have a few brief statements in lay language about any disease, process, and therapy and a blank space to put additional notes about any drug. It is not uncommon for these notes to show the dosage, calculated using **milligrams per kilogram (mg/kg) dosing**, showing caretakers how the dose is set in relation to the child's weight. It is also the custom of many pediatricians to use telephone reminders to check up on treatment progress. Such calls are an opportunity to reinforce any teaching that took place in the office.

Drugs That Increase the Risk of Suicidal Thinking in Children and Adolescents

Some antidepressants and antipsychotics increase the risk of suicidal thinking and behavior (suicidality) in children and adolescents with major depressive disorder (MDD) and other psychiatric disorders. This was discovered when analysis of esearch done on children and adolescents using antidepressant drugs for periods totaling 4 to 16 weeks demonstrated that children and adolescents with MDD, obsessive compulsive disorder, or other psychiatric disorders are at a greater risk for suicidal thinking or behavior (suicidality), and that risk is twice what it would be if the child or adolescent were given a placebo. The average risk of such events on a depressant drug is 4%, twice that of a placebo (Bridge, Barbe, Birmaher, Kolko, & Brent, 2005; Bridge et al., 2007; Jick, Kaye, & Jick, 2004; Olfson, Marcus, & Shaffer, 2006; Simon, Savarino, J., Operskalski, B., & Wang, 2006; Zito et al., 2003). As a result of this research, done for the American Academy of Child and Adolescent Psychiatry, the FDA now requires makers of antidepressants to place a black box warning in their promotional material and requires that a medication guide be distributed with each supply of antidepressant medication. This guide lays out specific warning signs of antidepressants in lay language for caretakers.

Examples of drugs that are commonly used in adolescent psychiatry are the selective serotonin reuptake inhibitors (SSRIs) escitalopram (Lexapro), citalopram (Celexa), paroxetine (Paxil), fluoxetine (Prozac), and sertraline (Zoloft). Because of their black box warnings, it is strongly recommended that a pediatric psychiatrist and/or a behavioral specialist manage these drugs when children and adolescents are involved. Antipsychotics such as aripiprazole (Abilify) and quetiapine (Seroquel) also carry black box warnings similar to those for the SSRIs.

DRUG TREATMENT OF COMMON PEDIATRIC OUTPATIENT DISORDERS

Because the majority of drugs used in pediatric patients are also used in adults, one approach to understanding their use is to study the drugs is by using a systems-based approach, which is commonly used with drugs for adults, that is, studying drug therapies by reviewing how commonly seen diseases and disorders in the pediatric population are treated, system by system. The following discussion provides a broad overview and important caveats in the use of medications to treat common pediatric diseases and disorders, but it is not meant to be all inclusive. Clinicians vary in their choices of treatment options for these disorders. Even though there may be some agreement with treatment protocols offered here, there may also be some disagreements, depending on the experience of the provider. Also, drugs being mentioned in this section are discussed more fully in Chapter 5, Drugs Used in the Treatment or Eye and Ear Disorders.

Treatment of Common Pediatric Eye Disorders

Conjunctivitis, also known as pink eye, is the most common eye disorder seen in primary care. The majority of conjunctivitis occurs among school-age children, beginning in one eye and then typically spreading to the other. Most school-age children who present with this complaint have a simple infection rather than an allergy, and it is easily treated with topical antibiotic drops. These types of infections are highly contagious and must be treated in a timely manner.

Infectious Conjunctivitis

Typically symptoms of infectious conjunctivitis include infected sclera and conjunctiva; varying (but mild) lid edema; a yellow, usually copious discharge, especially upon waking; and often a minor upper respiratory infection (URI). Many children are overtreated with topical antibiotics because it is difficult to determine whether a child has bacterial or viral conjunctivitis. The vast majority of children with bacterial conjunctivitis respond adequately regardless of the type of antibiotic drops used. Sample treatment choices and dosing for infectious conjunctivitis follow.

Dosage and Administration

Generic Name	Trade Name	Dosage
polymyxin B + trimethoprim	Polytrim drops	1–2 drops every 4–6 hr for 7 days
polymyxin B + bacitracin	Polysporin ointment	Apply ointment every 3–4 hr for 7–10 days
bacitracin+ neomycin + polymyxin B	Neosporin drops and ointment	Apply up to 3 times a day
ciprofloxacin, garamycin, moxifloxacin, tobramycin, ofloxacin drops	Ciloxan, Gentamicin, Vigamox, Ocuflox, Tobrex	1–2 drops 3 times/day, then every 6 hours for a total of 7 days

Allergic Conjunctivitis

During allergy season, children (especially those with a history of **atopy** or a genetic predisposition towards immediate hypersensitivity reactions, especially common inhaled allergens which result in conditions such as asthma, hives, and hay fever) may present with allergic conjunctivitis. Here, the conjunctiva appears to be mildly infected, has a cobblestone appearance, a discharge that is somewhat clear and watery, and the patient has a history of sneezing, itching, and a seasonal recurrence. Several

treatments for allergic conjunctivitis, their dosing, and special considerations follow.

Dosage and Administration

Generic Name	Trade Name	Dosage	Special Considerations
naphazoline + pheniramine)	Naphcon-A (OTC)	1 drop 4 times/day for 3–5 days.	Longer use may cause rebound congestion to occur. Its use is limited to children older than 6 years of age, because marked sedation can occur in infants with large doses
azelastine	Optivar	1 drop in each eye 2 times/day	Emergency medical help is needed if any signs of allergic reactions occur (hives, difficult breathing, swelling of lips)
olopatadine	Patanol 0.1% solution	1–2 drops 2 times/day	Safety and effectiveness has not been established in children <3 years

Installation of eyedrops can be quite challenging in the pediatric patient. It occasionally requires two people, one to hold the patient and another to instill the drops. Many eyedrops sting or burn on contact, and children will often squeeze their eyes shut while thrashing about. One technique to help with administering eyedrops is to place the drops in the medial corner of the closed eyes so that when the patient opens his or her eyelids, the drops roll into the eye. Another technique to avoid use of drops in children is to use ointments, but caretakers can have as much or more difficulty instilling ointments as they do drops.

The real challenge for any clinician is to determine if the child with conjunctivitis, or pink eye, actually has a more serious condition for which topical antibiotics or antihistamines are not appropriate and if consultation with an ophthalmologist is necessary.

Treatment of Common Pediatric Ear Disorders

Obtaining an accurate ear assessment of a child can be among the most challenging but important aspects of a pediatric ear examination because not all cases of ear pain (otalgia) are caused by an infection, nor is a "red ear drum" sufficient to make a diagnosis of an infection. As always, signs and symptoms must be taken in context. Two common pediatric conditions affecting the ear are otitis media (OM) and otitis externa (OE).

Otitis Media

Otitis media is an acute inflammation and infection of the middle ear that frequently accompanies an upper respiratory infection. It typically presents when an otherwise minimally ill child has a sudden onset of pain, irritability, and fever. With today's concerns about bacterial resistance to drugs caused by overuse of antibiotics, proper selection of those children that should be treated is essential. Most children with otitis media do *not* require antibiotic therapy, and a policy of watchful waiting, with adequate pain control measures, is appropriate. But once the diagnosis of otitis media is established and a decision to treat is made, a variety of antibiotics can be given. The American Academy of Pediatrics (AAP) recommends a step-wise approach to antibiotic selection for children between 2 months and 12 years old who have uncomplicated otitis media, with careful attention to whether or not the patient is allergic to penicillin (PCN) (AAP, 2004). Should a treatment failure occur after using the first choice, a selection of an antibiotic having a different mechanism of action should be made. Treatment failure generally means no improvement within 48 to 72 hours. The AAP guidelines for otitis media are summarized in Table 23-2.

In most cases, amoxicillin remains the first choice for otitis media, and it is important to understand its dosing options and strengths. In general, children like the taste of amoxicillin syrup (bubble gum flavor), and any side effects are usually mild, generally a rash or diarrhea. However, a nonallergic amoxicillin rash, which is a nonpruritic, maculopapular rash that begins on the trunk and spreads to the rest of the body, can occur in up to 10% of all patients. It often appears 3 to 14 days after beginning treatment. In these patients, there is no need to discontinue treatment with the drug as the rash will clear without any further intervention. This distinction between allergic and **nonallergic rash** is important because a typical allergic reaction is usually intensely pruritic and requires discontinuation of the drug. When choosing an amoxicillin suspension, the clinician should remind the caretakers that it is only stable for about 2 weeks, and it must be refrigerated.

Probably outnumbered only by amoxicillin in the sheer numbers of prescriptions written each year for pediatric patients is Augmentin, a combination of amoxicillin and clavulanate potassium. The clavulanic acid binds and inhibits beta-lactamases so that amoxicillin is not rendered inactive by beta-lactamase-producing organisms such as *Moraxella catarrhalis, Haemophilus influenzae*, methicillin-sensitive *Staphylococcus aureus* (MSSA), and *Neisseria gonorrhoeae*. Augmentin is dosed based on its amoxicillin component and Augmentin

tablets all contain the same amount of clavulanic acid (125 mg). Various formulations and pediatric recommended dosages of Augmentin follow.

Dosage and Administration

Drug Name	Formulations	Dosage for Infants and Children
Augmentin (amoxicillin/ clavulanate potassium)	Powder for oral suspension: 125 mg/5 mL, 200 mg/5 mL; 250 mg/mL; 400 mg/5 mL; 600 mg/5 mL plus 125 mg of clavulanic acid in each Tablets: 125 mg, 250 mg, 500 mg, 875 mg amoxicillin plus 125 mg of clavulanic acid in each Chewable tablets: 125 mg (lemon-lime), 200 mg (cherry-banana), 250 mg (lemon-lime), 400 mg (cherry-banana), amoxicillin plus 31.5 mg of clavulanic acid	Infants <3 months: Use 30 mg/kg/day divided, 2 times/day of the 125 mg/ 5 mL suspension. For children weighing <40 kg: Use 45 mg/kg/day divided, 2 times/day of the 200 mg/5 mL or 400 mg/5 mL suspension.

Side effects with Augmentin are more common than with plain amoxicillin because both amoxicillin and clavulanic acid are involved. Of course, patients can have the same nonallergic and allergic rashes as they do with amoxicillin. Augmentin is not tolerated as well by children because it doesn't taste as good as amoxicillin and it tends to cause a much higher incidence of GI side effects (nausea/vomiting, abdominal pain/diarrhea), as well as vaginal candidiasis. GI side effects can be lessened if it is administered prior to a meal. Like amoxicillin, the suspension of Augmentin must be refrigerated.

Otitis Externa (Swimmer's Ear)

Otitis externa usually results from excessive moisture in the ear canal leading to an overgrowth of bacteria (*Pseudomonas* spp., *S. aureus*) or occasionally a fungus. Abrasions or trauma to the ear canal can further predispose a child to OE. Otitis externa causes intense pain, especially with physical manipulation of the

TABLE 23-2	American Academy of Pediatrics (AAP) Clinical Practice Guidelines for the Diagnosis and Management of Acute Otitis Media (AOM)					
TEMP >39°C OR SEVERE OTALGIA	RECOMMENDED INITIAL THERAPY	IF PCN ALLERGIC (NOT TYPE 1)	IF PCN ALLERGIC (TYPE 1)	RECOMMENDED THERAPY AFTER TREATMENT FAILURE	IF PCN ALLERGIC (NOT TYPE 1)	IF PCN ALLERGIC (TYPE 1)
No	amoxicillin at 80–90 mg/kg/ day	cefdinir, cefuroxime, cefpodoxime	azithromycin, clarithromycin	Augmentin ES 600 at 90 mg/ kg/day	ceftriaxone for 3 days	clindamycin
Yes	Augmentin ES 600 at 90 mg/ kg/day	ceftriaxone for 1 or 3 days	ceftriaxone for 1 or 3 days or clindamycin	ceftriaxone for 3 days	ceftriaxone for 3 days	clindamycin

American Academy of Pediatrics (2004). American Academy of Pediatrics and American Academy of Family Physicians clinical practice guidelines: diagnosis and management of acute otitis media. Pediatrics, 113(5), 1459. Reproduced with permission from American Academy of Pediatrics.

ear. A thick, white discharge is also usually seen, the canal being erythematous and edematous, whereas the tympanic membrane, if able to be seen, is normal. Topical therapy is often difficult to achieve without the use of a cotton wick, which may be saturated with the topical agent and inserted in the ear canal. The wick should be replaced every 24 hours along with any antibiotic. However, it is important to treat the intense pain that accompanies OE. Very mild cases of OE can be treated with a simple mixture of one-third white vinegar and two-thirds rubbing alcohol (30% to 10% water plus 70% to 90% ethyl or isopropyly alcohol created unfit to drink), and applying 5 to 10 drops 3 times a day. However, it is more than likely that by the time a patient has presented to a clinician, a prescription antibiotic and analgesic are necessary.

Treatment of Common Nose and Throat Disorders

Disorders of the nasal and sinus passages make up a large and disproportionate share of all sick visits for pediatric patients. These disorders include upper respiratory infections, allergic rhinitis, and sinusitis. Differentiating the nasal discharge of a URI from that of allergic rhinitis or even sinusitis can be difficult because they look very much the same.

Rhinitis/The Common Cold

The common cold with its associated rhinitis is responsible for nearly 40% of all sick visits to clinicians in the United States. Although the common cold is usually mild, with symptoms lasting 1 to 2 weeks, it is a leading cause of doctor visits and missed days from school and work. According to the Centers for Disease Control and Prevention, 22 million school days are lost annually in the United States owing to the common cold. In the course of a year, people in the United States suffer 1 billion colds, and children have about 6 to 10 colds a year (CDC, 2010b).

Despite many years of educating the general public about the benign course of a common cold, patients continue to seek treatment and often request either an antibiotic or a cold medicine for a cure. The common cold and various treatment regimens probably constitute some of the most exhaustively studied medical conditions in all of pediatrics. Whether OTC or in prescription form, antihistamines, decongestants, cough suppressants, mucolytics, and the vast array of combination drugs have consistently failed to show improvement in symptoms or overall cure of disease. In addition, they can be dangerous in younger children, especially children under 2 years of age. To that end, the AAP and the FDA have recommended that these products not be given to children under 2 years of age, and that caution be exercised when used in older children (AAP, 2008)

Dextromethorphan (DM) is an antitussive agent found in a wide array of OTC and prescription cough/cold preparations. A nonnarcotic, nonaddicting chemical relative of morphine, it suppresses cough by depressing the medullary cough center. It is usually used for the symptomatic relief of cough caused by minor URI, but should not be used when the patient has a productive cough or one that is accompanied by significant mucus production. A 2:1 rule of thumb is that 15 to 30 mg of DM is equivalent to 8 to15 mg of codeine for its cough suppression efficacy. Although its efficacy has been demonstrated in adults, caution should be used when giving this medication to children between the ages of 2 to 12 years because quality studies regarding their efficacy and safety in children are lacking. Dosage forms are numerous, and the clinician is strongly advised to use caution when prescribing DM. Adverse reactions to DM include drowsiness, dizziness, nausea, and rarely a rash/edema.

Guaifenesin (Mucinex, Robitussin) is an expectorant used in a wide variety of both OTC and prescription cold formulations. As with other cold preparations, rare but serious adverse events (including deaths) have been reported with its use, and the FDA does not approve its use in children younger than 2 years of age. Its mechanism of action is uncertain, but it is thought to act by stimulating respiratory tract secretions and thus decreasing the viscosity of the mucus/phlegm production. Usual dosage in children old than 2 years is 2 mg/kg dose every 4 to 6 hours as needed. Side effects include drowsiness, dizziness, headache, rash, nausea, vomiting, and abdominal pain.

Codeine is a narcotic antitussive available by itself or in combination with a wide variety of medicines. The Institute for Safe Medication Practices (ISMP) has included this medicine in its list of high-alert medications because it has a high risk of causing harm when used improperly. As an antitussive, it should be used only in cases of nonproductive cough.

Codeine's mechanism of action is typical of narcotics in that it binds to opiate receptors in the central nervous system (CNS), causing inhibition of pain pathways and cough suppression by direct action on the medulla cough center. Onset of action is rapid, usually within 30 minutes, and its half-life is approximately 3 hours.

Side effects are extensive and typical for a narcotic, including bradycardia and hypotension, pruritis from histamine release, CNS sedation and depression, respiratory depression, nausea, vomiting, constipation, urinary tract spasms, elevated liver enzymes, as well as physical and psychological addiction and extensive interactions with other medications. Codeine is transmitted in a very small amount in breast milk, but it is generally considered to be compatible with breastfeeding.

Allergic Rhinitis (AR)

Differentiating between allergic rhinitis, hay fever, and other similar conditions is often difficult in children. A remarkable 10% to 20% of the entire pediatric population has allergic rhinitis (AR). Common symptoms of AR include frequent nose blowing, **epistaxis** (i.e., nosebleed), nasal pruritus, throat clearing, and a chronic cough that is generally worse at night. This constellation of symptoms often leads to disturbed sleep and daytime fatigue.

A variety of oral and topical agents, both OTC and prescription, can be used for symptom control. Intranasal application of medicines for the control of allergic rhinitis in pediatrics can be challenging. The metered actuators are designed to be used with active patient inhalation, which is often difficult in the small child. Thus, administration usually requires a caretaker learning to time a nasal spray application with the child's inhalation to achieve good drug delivery into the nasal passages.

As is often the case with AR, if a single agent doesn't adequately control symptoms, then a combination of agents can be used. A three-step approach, such as beginning with an oral antihistamine diphenhydramine (Benadryl) or loratadine (Claritin), then adding nasal steroids (Flonase), and finally adding an oral leukotriene inhibitor (Singulair), is considered best.

Pediatricians often begin treatment with diphenhydramine (Benadryl), which is well tolerated and inexpensive. Liquid Benadryl is available as 12.5 mg/5 mL, and 0.5 teaspoon is administered every 4 to 6 hours for children 2 to 6 years of age and 1 to 2 tsp every 4 to 6 hours for ages 6 to 12. Because of its common side effect of sedation, Benadryl is often helpful for children with primarily nighttime symptoms. However, OTC use is not approved by the FDA for children under the age of 2. Larger doses (1 mg/kg/dose every 6 to 8 hours) can be used for moderate to severe exacerbations of allergies. Adverse reactions, in addition to typical anticholinergic effects of sedation and dry mouth, include paradoxical excitation and rare photosensitivity reactions. If oversedation with antihistamines is a problem, the nonsedating H1 blockers can be used. The anticholinergic side effect profiles are otherwise quite similar for all of the nonsedating H1 blockers.

Montelukast (Singulair) is a leukotriene receptor antagonist that helps diminish vascular permeability, mucus production, and mucosal edema. Montelukast is especially helpful to add to the treatment of those patients with refractory AR and who have failed other therapies. Many of these patients also have other atopic conditions (asthma and eczema) and montelukast helps to attenuate these other conditions, as well. Side effects are rare, and it is well tolerated. Dosing for children between 6 months and 5 years is 4 mg/day, 6 to 14 years is 5 mg/day, and 14 years and older is 10 mg/day. Dosage forms include 4-mg chewable tablets, 5-mg chewable tablets, 10-mg tablets, and 4-mg granule packets. The granule packets are especially helpful in young children, but it is important to remember that the granules should *not* be dissolved in liquids; rather, they must be sprinkled on applesauce or ice cream and must be used within 15 minutes of opening the packet.

Over-the-counter agents for allergic rhinitis may include vasoconstrictors and antihistamines, which often provide dramatic improvement of symptoms in adults; however, their use is discouraged in pediatrics because of their side effect profiles. Exceptions may be naphazoline (Naphcon), a common OTC topical vasoconstrictor for adults but not one recommended for children younger than 6 years. Children older than 6 years may receive one spray every 6 hours or as needed, but it should never be used for more than 3 to 4 days to avoid rebound congestion. CNS side effects are common, and

marked sedation can also occur. Local mucosa irritation and stinging are usually mild.

Azelastine (Astelin) is another OTC nasal antihistamine spray used in children aged 5 to 12 years who receive one spray two times a day. Children over the age of 12 receive two sprays two times a day. Along with typical side effects of antihistamines, azelastine can actually induce bronchospasm (especially in asthmatics) and can produce local burning of the nasal mucosa, epistaxis, rhinitis, and laryngitis.

Intranasal topical corticosteroids often provide excellent relief for both seasonal and perennial allergic (and nonallergic) rhinitis by controlling cellular protein synthesis, decreasing inflammation, and decreasing capillary permeability. Topical nasal steroids generally are most effective when used on a regular basis (daily, two times a day), but some older children and adolescents find that taking it as needed may be effective. The lowest effective dose should be used to minimize side effects. Various formulations of intranasal spray steroids exist, each with similar efficacy and side effect profiles. Several are listed below.

Dosage and Administration

Generic Name	Trade Name	Dosage
fluticasone furoate	Veramyst	Children 2 years and over: 1–2 sprays to each nostril daily, then reduce to 1 spray once symptoms are controlled.
fluticasone propionate	Flonase	Children 4 years and older: 1–2 sprays to each nostril daily, then reduce to 1 spray once symptoms are controlled
mometasone	Nasonex	Children 2–11 years: 1 spray in each nostril daily; children 12 years and older: 2 sprays in each nostril daily

Adrenal suppression due to the use of these drugs, although possible, is generally not a problem for otherwise healthy patients; the risk increases with high doses over longer periods of time and with younger children. Reduction in growth and bone density has been studied in children and have been found to be not statistically significant. CNS side effects such as hyperactivity, anxiety, restlessness, and behavioral changes, and a type of **steroid rage/"roid rage"** (i.e., a sudden, uncontrollable, aggressive and often violent outburst induced by excessive use of anabolic steroids) that is commonly associated with oral steroids can also be seen with topical applications, especially in children.

Sinusitis

The significance of sinusitis in young children is not well grasped by clinicians asked to treat it. Sinus development continues throughout early and middle childhood, causing the definition of sinusitis to be restrictive and not practical for young children because the clinical overlap between sinusitis, allergic rhinitis, and recurrent URIs is very hard to distinguish, even for seasoned and experienced clinicians. For example, 3 to 5 days of copious nasal congestion and cough in a toddler may simply be a cold, but 10 days of worsening congestion and daytime cough is more likely sinusitis. In clinical practice, any child with more than

7 days of copious nasal congestion accompanied by chronic cough (especially during the day) often is diagnosed with sinusitis and should be treated with antibiotics, usually amoxicillin at 50 to 90 mg/kg/day, two times a day, for 10 to 14 days (or more). Another excellent option is Augmentin at 45 mg/kg/day or Augmentin ES-600 at 90 mg/kg/day for severe infections. Cephalosporins are a fine alternative, and the macrolides or clindamycin can be used for true type 1 penicillin allergies.

Streptococcal Pharyngitis (Strep Throat)

Despite protests to the contrary, no amount of clinical experience can consistently and accurately distinguish between strep throat (group A beta-hemolytic streptococcus, or GABHS) and other causes of pharyngitis. Classic symptoms of strep throat include the relatively sudden onset of fever, pharyngitis, exudative/erythematous tonsils, cervical adenopathy, headache, and stomach ache (may include vomiting), with little or no cough or congestion symptoms. To make a definitive diagnosis of strep pharyngitis, a rapid strep test and/or a culture is essential because between 10% to 20% of all children are *asymptomatic carriers* of GABHS, and as such, they will have recurrent positive rapid screens and cultures, despite no true infection (Martin, 2010). These children should not be treated repeatedly without clinical evidence their illness is a true strep infection.

Although for many years oral penicillin (penicillin V potassium [Pen-Vee K]) was recommended for treatment of strep throat, recent studies show that 10 days of amoxicillin results in better efficacy than Pen-Vee K, and does so likely because of better compliance (Colletti & Robinson, 2005; Martin, 2010). The medical literature is now advocating that 5 days of cephalosporins, regardless of specific agent, demonstrate better efficacy than 10 days of amoxicillin in overall clinical cure (Zepf, 2005). Regardless of the agent chosen, it is important to administer the medication for the entire course of therapy and not just until the child's symptoms resolve. For those in whom compliance will be a problem, a single dose of Bicillin LA given intramuscularly is helpful.

Although expensive, third-generation cephalosporins and Augmentin are often prescribed for strep pharyngitis. However, there is no demonstrated advantage to using these agents over less-expensive agents. Also, their use contributes to increased resistance of other bacterial species. Because GABHS has near universal sensitivity to all forms of penicillin and cephalosporins, clinical failures are more often due to failure of the clinician to provide a formulation that a child will tolerate for the prescribed course of therapy.

Clindamycin or azithromycin may be prescribed for children with a true type 1 allergy to penicillin. However, resistance to azithromycin is rising in some areas, which makes clindamycin the more acceptable choice. Side effects to clindamycin are uncommon, but they can include rash, urticaria, Stevens Johnson syndrome, prolonged QT times, thrombocytopenia, and neutropenia. GI side effects, such as nausea, vomiting, and diarrhea can also occur. Development of significant diarrhea with blood or mucus in the stool and severe abdominal pain could herald the onset of **pseudomembranous colitis** (or as it is also known "*c.difficile colitis*," i.e., foul smelling diarrhea, abdominal pain, fever caused by broad spectrum antibiotics which kill off competing bacteria in the intestine and allow the bacterium *clostridium difficile* to flourish and to colonize the GUT with toxins), a complication of this and other antibiotics that can be severe or fatal. A black box warning has been added to clindamycin because of its ability to cause this condition. Treatments for strep pharyngitis follow.

Dosage and Administration

Generic Name	Trade name	Form	Dosage	Special Considerations
amoxicillin	Amoxil	Tabs, caps, IM	50 mg/kg/day divided 2 times/day for 10 days	Do not exceed recommended dose
cephalexin	Keflex	Tabs, caps IM	2,550 mg/kg/day divided 2 times/day	Not recommended for use in those <6 months of age
cefuroxime	Ceftin	250- and 500-mg tabs	20 mg/kg/day divided doses 2 times/day for 10 days	Not recommended for use in those <3 months of age; give with food.
clindamycin	Cleocin	Granules: 75 mg/5 mL Capsules: 75 mg, 150 mg, and 300 mg	20 mg/kg/day 3 times/a day for 10 days	Good to use for patients with PCN allergies **Black Box Warning**
azithromycin	Zithromax (Z-Max)	Oral suspension as 100 mg/5 mL or 200 mg/5 mL in cherry flavor	60 mg/kg either as 12 mg/kg daily for 5 days or 20 mg/kg daily for 3 days	These schedules, rather than the usual 5-day course provide the best rate of GABHS eradication.
penicillin G benzathine	Bicillin LA	IM	25,000–50,000 units/kg as single dose IM Alternative regimen: children <27 kg: 300,000–600,000 units IM; children >27 kg: 900,000 units IM Adults/late adolescents: 1.2 million units IM.	Monitor for serum sickness and anaphylaxis

Infectious Mononucleosis

Infectious mononucleosis (mono), caused by the Epstein-Barr (EB) virus, is one of the more frustrating conditions in pediatrics owing to its dramatic presentation and lack of effective treatment.

Mono is often overlooked as a diagnosis in younger children because of its milder symptoms compared to symptoms of older children and teenagers. The illness usually begins with several days of general malaise, followed by fever, cervical adenitis, and an intensely painful pharyngitis, often with marked tonsilar hypertrophy. Posterior cervical adenopathy is common, and splenomegaly occurs in up to 50% of patients.

With few exceptions, children with mono require a multipronged approach to treatment, which includes use of steroids. Markedly edematous tonsils with no obvious abscess can be treated with dexamethasone (Decadron), but it has a side effect profile similar to other corticosteroids. However, if a clinician prescribes an antibiotic in an otherwise clear-cut case of mono, amoxicillin (Amoxil) will cause a rash 95% to 99% of the time.

Herpetic Gingivostomatitis

Primary herpetic gingivostomatitis (HSV) in children and young adults presents as extremely painful and extensive ulcers affecting the entire oral cavity, including the palate, tongue, and lips, with fever and irritability often preceding the actual ulcers. Oral lesions tend to last anywhere from 10 to 14 days, and a clinician should prepare the family in advance for the extended duration of this illness. Many clinicians prescribe narcotics for the intense pain because a complete refusal to take anything by mouth is common and prevention of dehydration is paramount.

Thrush

Oral thrush is a common infection (mycosis) caused by the fungus *Candida albicans*. It presents as white plaque-like lesions within the mouth, usually on the tongue and inner buccal mucosa. The lesions can be painful and may occasionally bleed. It usually infects infants, owing to the relative immaturity of the infant's immune system. Treatment for thrush is to give caretakers clear directions on how to administer an antifungal drug, such as nystatin, as follows:

1. Feed the baby its normal bottle, or if breastfeeding, avoid feeding 5 to 10 minutes prior to administration.
2. Wipe the plaques out of the baby's mouth with a moist rag.
3. Administer the nystatin. For infants: Administer 2 mL of suspension by placing half of the dose in each side of the mouth and avoid any feedings for another 10 minutes. For children: Administer 4 to 6 mL four times a day by placing half the dose into each side of the mouth and instruct the child to hold the dose in the mouth for as long as possible.

This three-step process ensures the longest contact time between the medicine and the plaques before being diluted with saliva.

Failure of nystatin to cure thrush occasionally occurs. In these cases, a reasonable second choice is fluconazole (Diflucan). Fluconazole works by interfering with the fungal cell membranes by decreasing their ergosterol synthesis. Unlike nystatin, fluconazole is well absorbed from the GI tract, and adverse reactions, although rare, are important. Rare cases of side effects, including fatalities due to hepatotoxicity, have occurred with Diflucan. It is of note that the oral Diflucan suspension contains sodium benzoate, an additive found in many drugs but of particular importance in this scenario. When benzoate is given to neonates it may precipitate **gasping syndrome**. This describes a potentially fatal toxicity of sodium benzoate involving metabolic acidosis, respiratory distress, gasping respirations, CNS convulsions, CNS hemorrhage, hypotension, and cardiovascular collapse. Treatment options for oral thrush follow.

Dosage and Administration

Generic Name	Trade name	Form	Dosage	Special Considerations
nystatin,	Mycostatin Nilstat	60 mL of the oral suspension containing 100,000 units/mL Oral lozenges (pastilles) containing 200,00–400,00 units per lozenge	Swish and swallow 1 mL PO 4 times/day Suck 4 or 5 lozenges per day for up to 30 minutes each per lozenge	Nystatin is poorly absorbed from the mucous membranes of the GI tract so adverse reactions are uncommon, but they may include mild GI symptoms.
fluconazole	Diflucan	10 mg/mL or 40 mg/mL suspension; Tablets (orange flavor) are available in 50-, 100-, 150-, and 200-mg strengths	6 mg/kg on day 1, then 3 mg/kg days 2–14	If symptoms do not start to clear in 3 days, dosage and drug adjustments may be needed. Use cautiously in neonates because safety has not been established.

Treatment of Common Pulmonary Disorders

Pediatric pulmonary disorders are a large segment of the typical clinician's daily workload, and understanding them and their therapies is essential for optimal outcomes. It is tempting to apply routine adult diagnoses (asthma, bronchitis, etc.) to children, but it is important to remember that children are not small adults. For example, the common diagnosis of bronchitis is seldom used by the pediatric community, because bronchiolitis, sinusitis, allergic rhinitis (with prominent cough), asthma, and reactive airway disease are more accurate definitions of most pediatric cases. Additionally, it is tempting to diagnose an infant who presents with wheezing in winter months as having asthma and then to prescribe albuterol and steroids, when in actuality the child most likely has bronchiolitis, for which neither albuterol nor steroids are indicated. Thus, when faced with a child in respiratory distress, it is critical that the clinician first determine whether it is a process affecting the upper or lower airways. Once the level of involvement has been determined, other signs and symptoms can be helpful in determining the exact cause. For example, a child with severe distress involving stridor caused by upper airway obstruction will not respond to the same pharmacological agents used to treat a child in severe distress with wheezing, which is likely caused by lower airway obstruction.

Asthma

According to the Asthma and Allergy Foundation, every day in the United States 40,000 people miss school or work, 30,000 people have an attack, 5,000 people visit an emergency room, 1,000 people are admitted into a hospital, and 11 people die because of asthma (AAFA, n.d.). In cases of asthma, over 80% will be diagnosed before the age of 5 years, so an understanding of how to treat it at a young age is imperative to the quality of life of its young victims (AAFA, n.d.). Asthma and its related pharmacology is discussed extensively in Chapter 10, Drugs Used in the Treatment of Pulmonary Diseases and Disorders, and will not be repeated here; however, a few pediatric-centered points are in order.

The goals of asthma therapy among a pediatric population are to prevent symptoms, minimize morbidity when an attack occurs, and allow a child to live as close to a "normal" lifestyle as possible. To accomplish these goals a stepwise approach is taken, and the severity of symptoms determines the intensity of the treatment. Charts that help clinicians and patients categorize the chronicity and severity of asthma are widely available and help guide therapy. For example, when asthma attacks are only occasional, short-acting beta agonists (SABAs) such as albuterol can be used. If it becomes necessary to use SABA agents more than 2 days a week, therapy should be stepped up to include inhaled corticosteroids. After several months of stepped-up treatment with no attacks, therapy can be stepped down as appropriate.

Inhaled corticosteroids are considered the cornerstone of long-term management and are delivered by the following devices:

1. A nebulizer machine
2. A dry powder inhaler (DPI)
3. A pressurized metered dose inhaler (pMDI)
4. A breath-actuated metered dose inhaler (pMDI) (an alternative technology for a pressurized MDI that delivers a mist of medicine automatically to a patient as they breath in thus it is helpful for those who can not master the technique of a regular MDI which requires breathing in while at the same time pressing a button on the canister to release the medicine)

For children below the age of 4 years, an MDI with a mask/spacer is the most appropriate combination. Children aged 4 to 6 years should use an MDI and a valved holding chamber. Children over 6 years can use a pMDI, a breath-actuated pMDI, or a DPI. A nebulizer machine with a mask is an acceptable alternative for children under 4 years. As always, consideration should be given to the cost and convenience of any chosen therapy. Studies have clearly shown that using MDIs are just as effective, and perhaps more so, than nebulizer machines for all but the most severe of hospitalized asthma attacks (Broeders, Molema, Hop, & Folgering, 2003). However, only 5% to 20% of children will properly use the inhaler without a detailed

and supervised teaching session (Broeders, Molema, Hop, & Folgering, 2003). It is important for clinicians to be actively involved in ensuring that a patient can demonstrate proper care and use of an MDI prior to obtaining one. Finally, as with any inhaler, children must be reminded to rinse their mouths after use to avoid tooth erosion.

Bronchiolitis

Bronchiolitis is an infectious condition that primarily affects infants during the winter. It causes intense inflammation of the bronchioles, resulting in varying degrees of wheezing, tachypnea, hypoxia, fever, copious nasal discharge, and cough. It is often misdiagnosed as asthma or bronchitis, and children are inappropriately treated like asthmatics, in that they are given bronchodilators and steroids that are inhaled or taken by mouth. Respiratory syncytial virus is the most common pathogen, but others can cause the clinical picture of bronchiolitis, including metapneumovirus, influenza, parainfluenza, rhinovirus, and others.

Unfortunately, there are very few medications to treat bronchiolitis with the exception of administering oxygen if the patient is hypoxic or in respiratory distress. Despite millions of sick visits each year and near universal treatment by clinicians, studies over the last few decades have shown that SABA bronchodilators and steroids are of no use in treating bronchiolitis, except in a very small subset of patients (approximately 10% to 15%) who clearly have underlying asthma tendencies (children of atopic families, etc.) (AAP, 2006). According to the latest AAP guidelines, while steroids are almost never indicated in bronchiolitis, a trial of a SABA is reasonable. The SABA should only be continued if objective evidence of clinical improvement is noted, such as improvement in oxygenation or a decrease in respiratory rate or the overall work of breathing (AAP, 2006).

Frequent nasal suctioning, whether by bulb syringe or suction device, can have a dramatic effect on patient comfort and hospitalization rates. For children who may require hospitalization, an in-office trial of racemic epinephrine (discussed in the following section on croup) may provide some benefit. Otherwise, treatment of the vast majority of children with bronchiolitis is supportive.

Croup

Croup, also known as **laryngotracheitis** or laryngotracheobronchitis, is an infection causing inflammation and edema in the larynx, trachea, and bronchi. Parainfluenza virus type 1 is the most common pathogen, but a variety of other infectious agents can be responsible. The illness is most often seen in children aged 6 months to 3 years and usually begins with mild rhinorrhea, cough, sore throat, and fever. Inflammation and edema reduces the diameter within the upper airways, resulting in limited airflow with subsequent hoarseness, a "seal-like" barking cough, stridor, chest retractions, and varying degrees of respiratory distress. Treatments vary depending on the phase of illness the patient is in and the accompanying symptoms.

Dosage and Administration

Phase of Illness	Symptoms	Treatment	Drug Treatments
Mild croup	A Barky cough (lung sounds known as mild **inspiratory stridor**) with crying	Most cases improve within 24 hr with no therapy	None
Mild to moderate croup	Inspiratory stridor at rest, but no respiratory distress	Decadron (0.6 mg/kg for 1 dose, max of 10 mg) by mouth is recommended, along with close follow-up	Decadron: Either IM or PO at 0.15–0.6 mg/kg as a single dose (max of 10 mg). Due to occasional "rebound" after 24 hr, clinicians sometimes give a single dose in the office, followed by another dose 24 hr later.
Moderate to severe croup	Biphasic stridor, retractions	Decadron and nebulized racemic epinephrine, followed by at least 2–3 hr of observation to watch for the so-called rebound phenomenon (worsening of stridor after effects of epinephrine wear off).	Racemic epinephrine: The usual dose is 0.25 mL of a 2.25% solution in 3 ml NS (normal saline) for patients <6 months; 0.5 mL of a 2.25% solution in 3 ml NS in older patients. Racemic epinephrine can be repeated every 2–3 hr as needed for respiratory distress.

   Racemic epinephrine stimulates both alpha- and beta-adrenergic receptors resulting in both relaxation of smooth muscles in the bronchial tree as well as a decrease in local airway edema with resultant decrease in the work of breathing. Results are often dramatic after treatment. Adverse reactions to nebulized racemic epinephrine are potentially dangerous, and there is a heightened risk of causing significant patient harm if it is used inappropriately. It is therefore essential to consider these risks and weigh the benefits prior to administration, especially in any patient with preexisting cardiac or lung disease. Because potential complications include cardiac irritability, tachycardia, hypertension, and dysrhythmias, most clinicians suggest continuous cardiovascular monitoring during treatment. Other, more common side effects include palpitations, tremor, agitation, nausea, vomiting, and headache.

Influenza

Classic influenza, or flu, usually begins with abrupt onset of high fever, headache, malaise and myalgia, and respiratory symptoms such as cough, sore throat, conjunctival injection, and rhinitis. Younger children tend to have higher fevers (which can lead to febrile seizures) and GI symptoms of nausea, vomiting, and anorexia. Although the most common complication of influenza is otitis media, bacterial pneumonia complicates the course of influenza in approximately 15% of cases and is a major cause of morbidity and mortality.

   Antiviral agents such as zanamivir (Relenza) and oseltamivir (Tamiflu) are neuraminidase inhibitors and are structurally related compounds used for both prophylaxis and treatment of influenza. They help prevent infection by competitively inhibiting the neuraminidase on the surface of both influenza A and B viruses, minimizing the release of the virus from infected cells

and diminishing the spread of infection. Although these medications can prevent anywhere from 70% to 90% of influenza infections if given very early after symptoms start, when given for the treatment of influenza these agents decrease the illness only by about 1 day. Popular anti-flu medications and dosing in children follow.

Dosage and Administration

Generic Name	Trade Name	Form	Dosage
oseltamivir	Tamiflu	75 mg capsules and a 12 mg/mL oral suspension	**TREATMENT** For children 1–12 years old: Children <15 kg: 2 mg/kg/dose (max 30 mg) 2 times a day for 5 days 15–23 kg: 45 mg/dose 2 times a day for 5 days <15 kg: 2 mg/kg/dose (max 30 mg) 2 times a day for 5 days; 23–40 kg: 60 mg/dose 2 times a day for 5 days >40 kg: 75 mg/dose 2 times a day for 5 days Adolescents older than 12 years: 75 mg 2 times a day for 5 days Must begin within 48 hr of exposure **PROPHYLAXIS** Children 13 years and older: 75 mg daily for 10 days Must begin within 48 hr of exposure
zanamivir	Relenza	Powder inhalation: Package contains a Diskhaler delivery device, 5 Rotadisks, each with 4 blisters (5 mg/blister).	**TREATMENT** Children 7 years and older: 2 inhalations (10 mg) 2 times/day for 5 days **PROPHYLAXIS** Children 5 years and older: 2 inhalations (10 mg) daily for 10 days

   Neuropsychiatric adverse events, including hallucinations, confusion, delirium, and self-injury with fatalities, have been seen in children who have taken Tamiflu. Thus, clinicians and caretakers must monitor patients closely for signs of any unusual behavior. Although rare, other adverse reactions, including arrhythmia, dizziness, headache, fatigue, insomnia, vertigo, seizure, confusion, delirium, self-injury, rash, toxic epidermal necrolysis, nausea, vomiting, diarrhea, anemia, hepatitis, and facial and oral swelling, have been reported.

   In patients taking Relenza, anaphylaxis, allergic reactions, edema, rashes, and neuropsychiatric events including hallucinations, confusion, delirium, and self-injury have been reported. Relenza is not to be used in patients with underlying respiratory disorders such as asthma.

Pneumonia

True bacterial pneumonia is a serious cause of morbidity and mortality in the pediatric population. Because many conditions can mimic pneumonia, especially in children with underlying asthma or other pulmonary comorbidities, it is important to differentiate upper from lower respiratory tract infections. Typically, pneumonia is defined as an infectious condition associated with fever, respiratory symptoms, and evidence of direct parenchymal involvement, supported by both physical examination and the presence of infiltrates on chest radiography. Pneumonia often follows an otherwise routine upper respiratory tract illness, which allows invasion of the lower respiratory tract by viruses, bacteria, or other organisms. These pathogens then trigger an intense immune response and produce inflammation; the air spaces fill with inflammatory cells, fluid, and other cellular debris. This entire process may obstruct smaller airways, and lead to air trapping and ventilation/perfusion mismatches with resultant hypoxemia. Usual pathogens that cause pneumonia in children and the recommended antibiotics to treat it are described in Table 23-3.

Treatment of Common GI Disorders

Regardless if rare or common, any functional GI disorder that affects GI motility and structure can be very painful to a child and very distressing to both child and family. Additionally, functional disorders cannot be diagnosed in traditional ways. For example, inflammation of the GI tract is usually diagnosed by its symptoms. Childhood functional disorders causing abdominal pain, nausea, vomiting, diarrhea, and constipation are usually age dependent, chronic, and recurring.

Nausea and Vomiting

Nausea and vomiting are common among the pediatric population and should never be taken lightly or treated readily with antiemetics without a thorough evaluation and consideration of their etiology. More caution should be taken with younger patients, and there should be more concern for organic causes other than gastroenteritis. Vomiting may be caused by a wide range of etiologies and can originate from several systems, including gastrointestinal, neurological, renal, metabolic, endocrine, and respiratory. Treatment of vomiting with antiemetics should be reserved for the child older than 2 years of age, the child with gastroenteritis, or the child with dehydration. When a clinician is uncertain of the etiology of vomiting, it is best to observe the child rather than to mask the natural course of the process by use of medications.

Promethazine (Phenergan) and ondansetron (Zofran) may help alleviate symptoms of nausea and vomiting. When using promethazine, it is important not to overdose the child. Clinicians should start with one-half the recommended adult dose to decrease the possibility of side effects such as sedation, respiratory depression, dystonic reactions, or ataxia. It is also recommended that the medication be given every 8 to 12 hours and that the clinician monitor the efficacy of the drug before giving at any shorter intervals. Drugs for nausea and vomiting and their pediatric dosing schedules follow.

Dosage and Administration

Generic Name	Trade Name	Form	Pediatric Dose
ondansetron	Zofran	Liquid: 4 mg/5 mL	8kg-5 kg: 2 mg one time
		Tabs: 4 mg, 8 mg, 16 mg, 24 mg	15kg-30 kg: 4 mg one time
		Tabs, orally disintegrating: 4 mg, 8 mg	>30 kg: 8 mg one time
		Injection: 2 mg/mL	IV: 0.1–0.5 mg/kg/dose for one time ; max dose 4 mg/dose
prochlorperazine	Compazine	Syrup: 5 mg/5 mL	PO or PR: 0.4 mg/kg/day divided 3–4 times a day; max dose: 15 mg/day
		Suppository: 2.5 mg, 5 mg, 25 mg	
		Tabs: 5 mg, 10 mg	IM: 0.1–0.15 mg/kg/dose 3–4 times a day; max. dose: 40 mg/day
		Slow-release caps: 10 mg, 15 mg	
		Injection: 5 mg/mL	
promethazine	Phenergan	Syrup: 6.25 mg/5 mL	Child > 2 years: 0.25–1 mg/kg/dose every 4–6 hours as needed; max. dose 25 mg
		Suppository: 12.5 mg, 25 mg, 50 gm	
		Tabs: 12.5 mg, 25 mg, 50 mg	
		Injection: 25 mg/mL or 50 mg/mL	

Diarrhea

Diarrhea is a common childhood problem. Most cases are of viral etiology and of short duration, thus most clinicians provide reassurance and recommend over-the- counter (OTC) medications. However, neonates and young infants with diarrhea should have a thorough workup if the following occurs:

- It is accompanied by high fever and or blood in the stools.
- It causes dehydration and/or weight loss.
- The patient presents with altered mental status.
- It lasts more than 2 weeks.

These are likely signs of infections in the gastrointestinal tract caused by a wide variety of entero-pathogens, including bacteria, viruses, and parasites. Clinical manifestations depend on the organism and the host response. Thus, patients with diarrhea

TABLE 23-3 Recommended Therapies for Bacterial Pneumonia Diagnosed in Children	
DIAGNOSES	USUAL OUTPATIENT TREATMENT
Uncomplicated Community Acquired Pneumonia: providing coverage for S. Pneumonia	First-line: High dosages of amoxicillin (100 mg/kg/day) Second line: Macrolides or third-generation cephalosporins
School-aged children	Macrolides (azithromycin) (because they cover most common pathogens)
Hospitalized patients	IV administration of third-generation cephalosporin in combination with macrolide) plus clarithromycin or azithromycin
Patients who are toxic	Vancomycin plus second-or third-generation cephalosporin if MRSA suspected.

need fluid and electrolyte therapy as well as other nonspecific support, and some may need antimicrobial therapy.

One form of chronic diarrhea affecting children between 1 and 3 years of age is toddler's diarrhea. This chronic diarrhea often follows a distinct enteritis and treatment with an antibiotic. Its loose, nonbloody stools of two or more per day without fever or pain may also be caused by consumption of fruit juices. The diagnosis is made by exclusion, and treatment consists of removing any offending agents, decreasing or changing fruit juice consumption, reassurance, and using psyllium bulking agents.

When the cause of the diarrhea is found to be bacterial or parasitic in nature, restraint should be used in use of antimicrobials and their use justified and susceptibility testing performed unless it is deemed "medically necessary."

Gastroesophageal Reflux Disease (GERD)

Gastroesophageal reflux (GERD) is the most common esophageal disorder in children of all ages. GERD is the return of stomach contents into the esophagus as a result of increased relaxation of the lower esophageal sphincter. Infant reflux peaks at about 4 months of age; 75% resolve by 1 year of age, and 95% resolve by 18 months of age. A small degree of reflux is physiological and considered normal, but it becomes pathological in children who have episodes that are more frequent or persistent, produce esophagitis, esophageal symptoms, or go on to produce respiratory sequelae.

When diagnosing GERD, history taking is very important. GERD may be accompanied by effortless vomiting, aspiration pneumonia, and apnea in infants, and by belching and mid-epigastric pain in older children. In infants, GERD is usually associated with spitting up and not projectile vomiting; it often occurs after feedings and results from positioning during feeding. Reflux is more likely to occur in the infant that is supine or sitting up, not burped frequently, and overfed.

If the evaluation points toward a diagnosis of GERD, then a trial period of empiric therapy, lifestyle modification, and pharmacotherapy may be used as a confirmation of diagnosis. However, failure to respond to such empirical treatment, or a prolonged requirement for the treatment should mandate a formal diagnostic evaluation.

A stepwise approach in which different categories of therapy are added to each other is the preferred treatment of GERD. In the patient with mild to moderate reflux, dietary and feeding techniques are usually adequate to help the child. If the reflux persists, then a histamine-2 receptor antagonist, which selectively inhibits histamine receptors on gastric parietal cells, may be indicated. These are recommended as first-line therapy because of their excellent overall safety profile. Ranitidine (Zantac) and famotidine (Pepcid) have been widely used in the pediatric populations. Proton pump inhibitors are used in severe esophagitis and GERD. They are superior to the histamine-2 receptor antagonists. Once a proton pump inhibitor has been started, then the patient should be weaned off the histamine-2 receptor antagonist over approximately a 2-week period. In severe cases, the patient may benefit from using both at the same time. As a general rule, the proton pump inhibitors should not be used

longer than 4 to 12 weeks at a time, depending on which is used. Proton pump inhibitors have a potent effect by blocking the hydrogen-potassium ATPase channels of the final common pathway in gastric acid secretion. Examples of histamine-2 receptor antagonists, proton pump inhibitors, and their pediatric dosages are listed below.

Dosage and Administration

	Generic Name	Trade Name	Liquid Strength	Pediatric Dose
HISTAMINE-2 RECEPTOR ANTAGONISTS	ranitidine	Zantac	15 mg/1 mL	5–10 mg/kg/day 2–3 times/day
	famotidine	Pepcid	40 mg/5 mL (8 mg/1 mL)	<3 months, 0.5 mg/kg/dose daily
				≥3 months to 1 year, 0.5 mg/kg/dose every 12 hr
				≥1 year, 1–2 mg/kg/day 2 times/day
	cimetidine	Tagamet	300 mg/5 mL (60 mg/1 ml)	<3 months, 5–20 mg/kg/day: every 6–12 hr
				≥3 months to 1 year, 10–20 mg/kg/day every 6–12 hr
				≥1 year 20–40 mg/kg/day every 6 hr
	nizatidine	Axid	15 mg/1 mL	<12 years, 10 mg/kg/day every 12 hr
PROTON PUMP INHIBITORS	lansoprazole	Prevacid	3 mg/1 mL 15 mg SoluTab	<10 kg, 7.5 mg PO daily
				11—30 kg, 15 mg 1–2 times a day
				>30 kg, 30 mg 1–2 times a day
	esomeprazole	Nexium	20-mg, 40-mg packets	10–12 years, 20 mg 2 times/day
				1–10 years, 10 mg 2 times/day
	omeprazole	Prilosec	2 mg/mL	0.2 mg–0.5 mg/kg/day 1—2 times a day
				5–10 kg, 5 mg daily
				10–20 kg, 10 mg daily
				>20 kg, 20 mg daily
	rabeprazole	AcipHex		>12 years, 20 mg daily
	pantoprazole	Protonix	2 mg/1 mL	0.5–1 mg/kg/day daily

Pinworms

Enterobiasis, or pinworms, is caused by the helminth *Enterobius vermicularis*. Once a host's GI tract is infected, the gravid females migrate at night to the perianal and perineal regions where they deposit their eggs. Symptoms are caused by allergic reactions to the eggs and by irritation as the worms migrate. Usually a child presents with a pruritic complaint in their perianal area that worsens in the evening and at night. Worms may be seen in the rectal area or stool and eggs may be found in skinfolds and the perianal and vaginal regions. Pinworms can be treated with one mebendazole (Vermox) 100-mg tablet by mouth, then repeated in 2 weeks. The incidence of reinfection is high. In a child that will not take a pill, the tablet can be crushed and put it in apple-sauce or peanut butter. It is important to treat the other children at home. Good hygiene is critical in eradication of this organism.

Flatulence

Whether the child is a newborn or infant, clinicians will be asked what to do with the child that has a lot of gas. Other than explaining that this is a normal body function, if it is a breastfed baby, clinicians may recommend diet changes for the mother and trying such remedies as the following:

- Making sure that the infant is not swallowing too much air when feeding.
- Burping frequently and positioning the infant in the prone position while awake.

Simethicone (Mylicon) drops may help or at least may make the caretakers feel like they are able to do something. Simethicone drops are generally safe to use and have few side effects. However, it must be noted that Mylicon infant drops contain sodium benzoate, which may precipitate gasping syndrome, described earlier in this chapter. Details about simethicone dosing follow.

Dosage and Administration

Trade Name	Generic Name	Liquid Supply	Dose
simethicone drops	Mylicon Infant, Gas-X drops	20 mg/0.3 mL	<2 years, 20 mg PO 4 times/day
		40 mg/0.6 mL	2–12 years, 40 mg PO 4 times/day; maximum dose is 240 mg/day

Management of Pediatric Pain

Pain control in children needs to be taken seriously because it may be due to a variety of reasons, ranging from teething pain to the pain of otitis media. Managing pediatric pain should be based on the following two tenets:

- Children experience real pain and they should not have to suffer unnecessarily.
- Medicating a child for pain needs to be done cautiously so that the patient isn't overdosed. It is best to underdose and work up than to start at too high a dose and cause side effects.

The majority of pain management in pediatric patients can be treated with either acetaminophen (Tylenol) or ibuprofen (Advil, Motrin). However, it is essential for the safety of the child and the efficacy of these medicines that caretakers know how these medications should be properly administered by following these instructions:

- Aspirin should *never* be given to children under the age of 19 years for pain management because it may induce **Reye's syndrome** (the potentially fatal disease that attacks body mitochondria, especially in the liver and brain following a viral illness and the simultaneous ingestion of aspirin and aspirin-containing products. Its seriousness is underscored

by the U.S. government recommending no person under 19 years of age be given aspirin products if they also have a fever producing illness). The U.S. Surgeon General, the FDA, the CDC, and the American Academy of Pediatrics all recommend that aspirin and combination products containing aspirin not be given to children under 19 years of age while they have any fever-causing illnesses. Aspirin may be listed in combination products as acetylsalicylate, acetylsalicylic acid, salicylic acid, or salicylate. Clinicians must carefully educate caretakers about the contents of medications.

- Acetaminophen and ibuprofen come in oral drops, oral liquids of different flavors, and chewable tablets for infants, toddlers, and children who can't swallow a tablet or capsule. Acetaminophen also comes in suppository form as well as combination forms with different opioids.
- Acetaminophen given in suppository form will relieve pain in 30 to 60 minutes.
- Acetaminophen is to be used with caution with patients with G6PD deficiency (an inherited deficiency of the enzyme glucose-6 phosphate dehydrogenase, which is found in red blood cells and results in neonatal jaundice and acute hemolytic anemia). Acetaminophen overdose can complicate this type of anemia.
- Ibuprofen may be the drug of choice for night pain because of its longer duration.
- Ibuprofen is contraindicated in any patient, whether pediatric or not, if there is history of GI distress, dehydration, and hepatic or renal insufficiency.
- Opioid-containing medications should be reserved for intense pain caused by such disorders as ulcers from herpetic gingival stomatitis, postfracture management, after removal of a toe nail, and significant coughs. They can also be used for chronic conditions such as sickle cell disease.

Treatment of Pediatric Psychiatric/Behavioral Disorders

Attention Deficit-Hyperactivity Disorder (ADHD)

Attention-deficit/hyperactivity disorder (ADHD) is a chronic childhood disorder that, according to the CDC, afflicts 5.5% to 9.3% of all children between 5 and 17 years of age (CDC, 2010a). ADHD usually causes difficulty in controlling behavior and results in children failing to achieve their academic potential. The child may present with symptoms of hyperactivity, impulsivity, and/or inattention, is easily distracted, is unable to pay attention and follow directions, and/or has poor self-control. The *Diagnostic and Statistical Manual of Mental Disorders*, 4th edition (*DSM-IV*) (2000) describes three subtypes of ADHD:

- Inattentive only: Children with this form of ADHD are not overly active. This form is most common in girls and accounts for 30% to 40% of children diagnosed with ADHD.
- Hyperactive/impulsive ADHD: These children can pay attention but show hyperactive and impulsive behavior.

This subgroup accounts for about 10% of the children diagnosed with ADHD.

- Combined inattentive/hyperactive/impulsive: Children diagnosed with this type of ADHD show all three symptoms. This is the most common type of ADHD and accounts for 50% to 60% of children with ADHD.

Once the diagnosis has been made, a multitherapeutic approach is recommended, which includes psychotropic medication, behavior modification, family education and counseling, and educational intervention. Drug treatment for ADHD is typically focused on the use of the psychostimulant medications, including methylphenidate (Ritalin, Methylin, Metadate, Daytrana, Concerta); dexmethylphenidate HCL (Focalin); amphetamine and/or dextroamphetamine (Dextrostat, Dexedrine, Adderall); atomoxetine (Strattera); and lisdexamfetamine dimesylate (Vyvanse). Short-duration and long-duration formulations of these medications exist, but the long-duration, or once-daily, dosage formulations facilitate compliance. These drugs significantly decrease the core ADHD symptoms of inattentiveness, hyperactivity, and impulsivity in 75% to 95% of treated individuals. If a child doesn't respond to one medication, about half of children will respond to another stimulant.

Methylphenidate is a mild CNS stimulant that blocks the reuptake of norepinephrine and dopamine into presynaptic neurons and appears to stimulate the cerebral cortex and subcortical structures in a manner similar to amphetamines. Its side effects are minor and typically do not result in stopping the medication. The most common side effects are decreased appetite, insomnia, increased anxiety and/or irritability, and mild stomachaches or headaches. Rebound agitation or exaggeration of premedication symptoms may be seen as the medication is wearing off. Infrequent side effects are weight loss, increased heart rate and blood pressure, dizziness, growth suppression, hallucinations/mania, exacerbation of tics and Tourette syndrome. Decreased appetite may be worse in the middle of the day and more normal in the evening. Insomnia can be helped by taking the medication earlier in the day or by adding an antidepressant.

The overall approach when starting a child on treatment for ADHD is to start with methylphenidate (Ritalin, Concerta, Daytrana), an amphetamine, and/or a dextroamphetamine combination, and preferably one of a long-acting duration. The long-acting preparations of methylphenidate have either 20 mg, 30 mg, or 40 mg (Ritalin); 18 mg, 27 mg, 36 mg, 54 mg (Concerta); or 15 mg, 20 mg, 30 mg (Daytrana) of active methylphenadate allowing for individualization and titration of dosage regimens. Amphetamines (generic) also are produced in several immediate release and delayed release dosage forms (e.g.: 5 mg, 7.5 mg, 10 mg, 12.5 mg, 15 mg, 20 mg, and 30 mg). The immediate release has an onset of effects within about 30 to 60 minutes and the delayed release, depending on the preparation, has a duration of 8 to 14 hours.

A wide variety of psychostimulant formulations is available, but as a general rule clinicians should begin by prescribing a low dose and every 1 to 2 weeks, over a 4-week period, gradually increase the dose if tolerated and if side effects are minimal. One caveat for those treating children with ADHD is to increase the dose to achieve maximum benefit as long as few or no side effects are seen. If the patient has reached the maximum dose or has encountered side effects, preventing further dose adjustment in the presence of persistent symptoms, then an alternate class of stimulant should be chosen. If use of a second stimulant does not bring satisfactory results, then the clinician may consider prescribing an alternative medication, such as guanfacine or tricyclic antidepressants, bupropion, and atomoxetine. It should be noted that medication alone is not always sufficient treatment for ADHD in children, especially when children have comorbidities. When children do not respond appropriately to medication, the next step may be referral to a mental health specialist, psychiatrist, or psychologist.

The majority of the time clinicians spend with an ADHD patient is spent adjusting the ADHD medication, switching from methylphenidate to amphetamine and vice versa, and changing from short-acting to long-acting preparations to improve compliance and decrease rebound. As the patient gets older and needs better control of their symptoms in the afternoon in order to do homework, the clinician will need to extend the duration of the medication. Additionally, once a patient's regimen is stable, ongoing follow-up and monitoring of therapy for side effects and efficacy of treatment should be carried out every 3 to 6 months.

Treatment of Common Neurological Disorders

Headaches

Headache is a common presenting complaint, especially in the older pediatric age group and in febrile children. Headache can be caused by tension and migraine or secondary causes such as sinus disease, tumors, and febrile illnesses (meningitis, viral infections)

A majority of pediatric patients that present with headaches are diagnosed with migraine headaches. The clinician's goal, then, should be to eliminate the headache within 1 to 2 hours of its presenting. If the initial medication does not eliminate the headache, then the clinician should consider repeating the initial medication or start a possible rescue drug with the goal to eliminate all pain by 4 hours. However, for children under 12 years of age, the headache may only last for a few hours. If the frequency of migraine headaches continues, a preventative medication plan may need to be started. The goal is to decrease both frequency and severity of the migraine by at least 50%. Once a child is on a preventative plan, the clinician needs to reevaluate the patient every 6 months to consider weaning or tapering the drug owing to the high rate of remission of migraines in children. It is also important to counsel patients and caretakers about eliminating triggers of headaches as part the management plan.

As a general rule, headaches in children tend not to last as long as headaches in adults. Triptans are useful in treating young adolescents and to abort headaches in the majority of patients. Triptans may be taken via subcutaneous, oral, oral disintegrating, and nasal spray formulation. One general algorithm for dosing triptans follows:

- Start with a dose where the intent is to abort the headache within 2 hours.

■ If the headache has not aborted after 2 hours, then repeat, but use double the same dose as the first in the hope that the patient may be symptom free in 4 hours.

■ Most symptoms of migraine such as nausea and photophobia are relieved with the use of triptans, but in some instances treatment with a rescue medication such as acetaminophen, ibuprofen, or an opioid will be necessary. Opioids (over the age of 6 years) may be used as an escape or rescue medication when triptan drugs are not tolerated, contraindicated, or ineffective. However, these drugs may be associated with tolerance, rebound, or dependence.

■ Promethazine (Phenergan) and ondansetron (Zofran) may help alleviate migraine headaches and/or symptoms of nausea and vomiting. When using promethazine, start with half the recommended dose to decrease the possibility of side effects.

Although the triptans have revolutionized the treatment of migraine among adults, and several of them are available in several dosage formulations, the FDA has not approved their use in children. These agents are available in a variety of forms.

Dosage and Administration

Generic Name	Trade Name	Dosage and Form
sumatriptan	Imitrex	Injection: 4 mg/0.5 mL, 6 mg/0.5 mL
		Tab: 25 mg, 50 mg, 100 mg
		Nasal spray: 5 mg, 20 mg
zolmitriptan	Zomig	Nasal spray: 5 mg (0.1 mL)
		Tab: 2.5 mg, 5 mg; Tab, disintegrating: 2.5 mg, 5 mg
rizatriptan	Maxalt	Maxalt Tabs: 5 mg, 10 mg;
		Maxalt -MLT (oral disintegrating wafer/tablet): 5mg, 10mg
almotriptan	Axert	Tab: 6.25 mg, 12.5 mg
eletriptan	Relpax	Tab: 20 mg, 40 mg
frovatriptan	Frova	Tab: 2.5 mg

Over time, only a few formulations have been evaluated for use in children. One promising study is the use of sumatriptan (Imitrex) as a subcutaneous injection; however, children are quite loath to use a needle or give an injection during a headache attack. In fact, 27% of pediatric patients are affected by needle anxiety (trypanophobia) so they, like adults, prefer oral administration of medications (Simmons et al., 2007). Over 15 years ago, an effective oral dose for sumatriptan (Imitrex) was found to be 0.06 mg/kg, the dose at which 72% of headaches were relieved (Linder, 1995). Similar research using the nasal spray formulation of sumatriptan found the 20-mg dose to be effective (Winner et al., 2000). Rizatriptan (Maxalt) has been evaluated in 12 to 17 year olds, and it was found that the drug was very effective when using both 2.5-mg and 5-mg doses (Winner et al., 2002).

When children and adolescents do not respond to acute management of migraine headaches and/or are having frequent headaches, or are missing excessive amounts of school, or have debilitating headaches, they should be considered candidates for a prophylactic medication. There are many options to choose from, ranging from anticonvulsants, antidepressants, antihistamines, beta blockers, calcium channel blockers, and NSAIDs. Once a preventative medication has been started, the typical treatment period is from 3 to 18 months, with an average length of 6 months.

Treatment of Common Hematological Disorders: Iron Deficiency Anemia

Although many hematological disorders occur in the pediatric population, one of the most common is iron deficiency anemia. Many medical practices routinely screen for this type of anemia among toddlers and adolescent females with heavy menstruation.

Once iron deficiency anemia is diagnosed, iron replacement is the therapy of choice. This can be challenging due to the undesirable taste of the medicine and frustrating to the clinician due to the multiple preparations to choose from and the confusion of making dosage calculations based on milligrams of elemental iron and not the overall milligrams of the iron preparation. Iron overdose is also an issue; family teaching with regards to its safety should be thoroughly explained.

Iron replacement therapy is based on the dose of elemental iron (Fe). The dose for children is 3 to 6 mg of elemental Fe/kg/day and divided into three or four doses per day. There are many iron preparations in the marketplace, and each preparation has a different percentage of elemental Fe. The preparation most commonly used in the pediatric population is ferrous sulfate, which contains 20% elemental Fe and is formulated as drops, elixir, oral liquid, and tablets. One liquid drops preparation is Fer-in-Sol drops, which contains 75 mg of ferrous sulfate per 0.6-mL dropper or 15 mg elemental Fe per 0.6 mL. Liquid iron preparations may stain teeth, so they should be given with a dropper or drunk through a straw. Iron therapy may cause constipation, dark stools, nausea, and epigastric pain. Due to the bioavailability of iron being increased by ascorbic acid, replacement iron may be administered with a vitamin C–fortified fruit juice 30 minutes before a meal.

LEARNING EXERCISES

Case 1

You have recommended an unpleasant-tasting medication for a child. The medication is going to be administered by the child's caretaker, and the child is 2 years of age. The child's mother asks the question, "Is it OK to mix this medicine in with the child's favorite food?" How would you respond?

Case 2

You would like a child to receive acetaminophen (Tylenol) drops. A recommended dose is 15 mg/kg as needed every 6 hours. The child weighs 33 lbs. How many milligrams (mg) of Tylenol would the child receive in 24 hours, and is this safe?

References

American Academy of Pediatrics (AAP). (2004). American Academy of Pediatrics and American Academy of Family Physicians Clinical Practice Guidelines: Diagnosis and management of acute otitis media. *Pediatrics*, *113*(5), 1459.

American Academy of Pediatrics. (October, 2006). Diagnosis and Management of Bronchiolitis. *Pediatrics, 118*(4). Retrieved March 5, 2013, from http://pediatrics.aappublications.org/content/118/4/1774.full?sid=64208328-70d3-43a5-9c90-d5d1963c89f0

American Academy of Pediatrics (AAP). (January, 2008). Treating Coughs and Colds. Retrieved March 5, 2013, from www.aap.org/new/kidcolds.htm

American Psychiatric Association. (2000). *Diagnostic and statistical manual of mental disorders* (4th ed., rev.). Arlington, VA, American Psychiatric Publishing, Inc.

The Asthma and Allergy Foundation of America (AAFA). (n.d.). Asthma Facts and Figures. Retrieved February 28, 2011, from www.aafa.org/display.cfm?id=8&sub=42

Bridge, J. A., Barbe, R. P., Birmaher, B., Kolko, D. J., & Brent, D. A. (2005). Emergent suicidality in a clinical psychotherapy trial for adolescent depression. *The American Journal of Psychiatry, 162*, 2173-2175.

Bridge, J. A., Iyengar, S., Salary, C. B., Barbe, R. P., Birmaher, B., Pincus, H.A., et al. (2007). Clinical response and risk for reported suicidal ideation and suicide attempts in pediatric antidepressant treatment. A meta-analysis of randomized controlled trials. *Journal of the American Medical Association, 297*, 1683-1696.

Broeders, M. E., Molema, J., Hop, W. C., & Folgering, H. T. (2003). Inhalation profiles in asthmatics and COPD patients: reproducibility and effect of instruction. *Allergy, 58*, 602-607.

Centers for Disease Control and Prevention (CDC). (2010a). Attention deficit/hyperactivity disorder. Retrieved March 5, 2013, from www.cdc.gov/ncbddd/adhd

Centers for Disease Control and Prevention (CDC). (2010b). The common cold: rhinitis vs. sinusitis: Physician information sheet (pediatrics). Retrieved March 5, 2013, from www.cdc.gov/getsmart/campaign-materials/info-sheets/child-rhin-vs-sinus.html

Colletti, T., & Robinson, P. (2005). Strep throat: guidelines for diagnosis and treatment. *Journal of the American Academy of Physician Assistants, 18*(9), 38-44.

Gilbert, D. N., Moellering, R. C. Jr., Eliopoulos, G. M., Chambers, H. F., Saag, M. S. (eds.) (2010). *The Sanford guide to antimicrobial therapy 2010* (40th ed.). Sperryville, VA: Antimicrobial Therapy Inc.

Jick, H., Kaye, J. A., & Jick, S. S. (2004). Antidepressants and the risk of suicidal behaviors. *Journal of the American Medical Association, 292*, 338-343.

Linder, S. L. (1995). Subcutaneous sumatriptan in the clinical setting: the first fifty consecutive patients with acute migraine in a pediatric neurology office practice. *Headache, 35*, 291-292.

Martin, J. M. (2010). Pharyngitis and streptococcal throat infections. *Pediatric Annals, 39*(1), 22-27.

Olfson, M., Marcus, S. C., & Shaffer, D. (2006). Antidepressant drug therapy and suicide in severely depressed children and adults. *Archives of General Psychiatry, 63*, 865-872.

Simmons J. H., McFann, K. K., Brown, A. C., Rewers, A., Follansbee, D., Temple-Trujillo, R. E. et al. (April, 2007). Reliability of the diabetes fear of injection and self-testing questionnaire in pediatrics. *Diabetes Care, 30*(4), 987-988.

Simon, G. E., Savarino, J., Operskalski, B., & Wang, P.S. (2006). Suicide risk during anti-depressant treatment. *American Journal of Psychiatry, 163*, 41-47.

Winner, P., Rothner, D., Saper, J., Nett, R., Asgharnejad, M., Laurenza A, et al. (2000). A randomized, double-blind, placebo-controlled study of sumatriptan nasal spray in the treatment of acute migraine in adolescents. *Pediatrics, 106*, 989-997.

Winner, P., Lewis, D., Visser, W. H., Jiang, K., Ahrens, S., & Evans, J. K. (2002). Rizatriptan 5 mg for the acute treatment of migraine in adolescents: A randomized, double-blind, placebo-controlled study. *Headache, 42*, 49-55.

Zepf, B. (2005). Cephalosporins vs. penicillin for treatment of strep throat. *American Family Physician, 71*(6), 1208-1210.

Zito, J. M., Safer, D. J., Dos Reis, S., Gardner, J. F., Magder, L., Soeken, K., et al. (2003). Psychotropic practice patterns for youth: A 10-year perspective. *Archives of Pediatric & Adolescent Medicine, 157*(1), 17-25.

Drugs Used to Manage Pain

chapter 24

Steven A. House

CHAPTER FOCUS

Medications to alleviate pain, acute or chronic, nociceptive or neuropathic, malignant or nonmalignant, are presented in this chapter. The pathophysiology of the pain response and the various receptors involved in pain sensation and transmission are discussed as well as the pharmacology of pain relief using opioid and nonopioid analgesics and adjuvant medications. The need for clinicians to be aware of potential adverse effects of opioid medications, especially respiratory depression and death, is emphasized. Clinicians also need to be aware of the patient's concomitant medical conditions and that use of other medications may affect treatment benefits or result in a potential life-threatening drug interaction.

OBJECTIVES

After reading and studying this chapter, the student should be able to:

1. Describe the signs, symptoms, and management of pain as well as the effects of poorly managed pain.
2. Describe the role of the five receptors involved in the sensation of pain and which receptors respond to opioids.
3. Recall the consequences of poorly controlled pain.
4. Compare and contrast the different classes of analgesics, their mechanism of action, relative potency, clinical use, side effect profile, drug interactions, conscientious prescribing rules, and patient advisories.
5. Differentiate between nociceptive and neuropathic pain, chronic pain and acute pain, and malignant and nonmalignant pain.
6. Perform equal analgesic dosing calculations.
7. Recall how the use of adjuvant medications can maximize relief and minimize side effects.
8. Define salicylism and how it occurs and how it can be reversed.

Key Terms

Adjuvant medications
Bone pain
Breakthrough pain
Controlled substances
Incident pain
Neuropathic pain
NMDA (*N*-methyl D-aspartate) receptors
Nociceptive pain
Nonopiate
Opiate
Opioid receptors (mu, delta, kappa, sigma
Visceral pain

KEY DRUGS AND CLASSES IN THIS CHAPTER

Opioids (Narcotics)
hydromorphone (Dilaudid)
meperidine (Demerol)
codeine (Tylenol with Codeine)
oxycodone (OxyContin, Percocet)
hydrocodone (Vicodin, Lortab)
fentanyl (Duragesic, Sublamaze)
methadone (Dolophine)

Opioid Antagonists
naloxone (Narcan)
methylnaltrexone (Relistor)
naltrexone (ReVia)
nalmefene (Revex)

Non-Opiate Analgesics
tramadol (Ultram)
tapentadol (Nucynta)
ziconotide (Prialt)

NSAIDS
celecoxib (Celebrex)
etodolac (Lodine)
diclofenac (Voltaren)
ibuprofen (Advil, Motrin)
indomethacin (Indocin)
ketoprofen (Orudis)
ketorolac (Toradol)
meclofenamate (Meclomen)

mefenamic acid (Ponstel)
nabumetone (Relafen)
naproxen (Aleve)
oxaprozin (Daypro)
piroxicam (Feldene)
sulindac (Clinoril)
aspirin
acetaminophen

According to the American Pain Foundation, more than 80 million people (68% of all full-time employees) suffer from pain-related conditions, and more than 17 million people took sick days in 1995 due to pain conditions, resulting in 50 million lost workdays (American Pain Foundation, 2008). The Centers for Disease Control and Prevention (CDC, 2006) provides the following statistics:

- One-fifth of adults 65 years and older experienced low back pain within the past 3 months.
- Three-fifths of adults 65 years and older said their pain had lasted for 1 year or more.
- Fifteen percent of adults experienced migraine or severe headache in the past 3 months.
- Reports of severe joint pain increased with age, and women reported severely painful joints more often than men (10% versus 7%) (CDC, 2006).

Arthritis, back pain, cancer, and headache are major contributors to the onset of pain (Pas, 2006). Twenty-six million women suffer from arthritis, and an equal number of Americans between the ages of 20 and 64 experience frequent back pain. A majority (68%) of adults in the United States experience back pain during their lifetime. About 25 million Americans suffer from migraines, whereas 90% of Americans have non-migraine headaches every year. Although 70% of cancer patients suffer from significant pain, only half receive adequate treatment for their pain, and some of them avoid taking pain medication out of fear they may become addicted to pain-killing drugs. Yet, when pain is intolerable, 67% of Americans use high doses of pain medications such as morphine, despite being warned of the high risk of addiction. NSAIDs are the most common prescription medications used for pain relief, and 70% of pain sufferers self-medicate with NSAIDS or illegal substances.

Understanding and Defining Pain

Random House Dictionary defines pain as "bodily, mental or emotional suffering due to injury or illness." However, Margo McCaffrey, an internationally known nurse who is responsible for pioneering work in pain management, defines pain as follows: "Pain is whatever the experiencing person says it is, existing whenever he says it does" (McCaffrey & Beebe, 1989). The International Association for the Study of Pain (IASP) states that "pain is an unpleasant sensory and emotional experience arising from actual or perceived tissue damage or described in terms of such damage" (Gallager, 2005; American Pain Society, 2003). In a medical context, the word *pain* comes from the Latin word *poena* meaning "a fine or a penalty," but most clinicians accept that the experience of pain includes the interaction of physical, mental, emotional, and spiritual/existential pain in the context of the patient's life and family relationships. As such, clinicians accept that pain is not a simple thing, and they accept a patient's report of having pain as being valid.

Chronic pain is pain that lasts longer than 3 months and for which it may be difficult to identify an exact cause. This is different from acute pain, which has an identifiable cause and cure or end point: for example, after an injury has healed, the pain disappears. With chronic pain, however, those pain messages can replay over and over again, even if the acute pain has been properly treated. Many patients find chronic pain debilitating.

Both adults and children experience pain; however, children are often less able to describe their pain. Children may cling to or desire to be held by a caregiver because they do not understand why they are uncomfortable and can't express their feelings of pain. Illustrations can be used to determine the severity of a child's pain (e.g., a series of circle faces, usually 10, that show eyes and mouth in various stages from happy to a serious grimace). Children experiencing pain may find relief in distraction, such as playing a video game. In infants it has been found that feeding the infant a 25% sucrose solution produces an analgesic response as the sucrose stimulates release of endogenous endorphins. Although numerous studies demonstrate the presence of acute pain in a pediatric population, chronic pain is also significant because it is conservatively estimated to affect 15% to 20% of all children (The American Pain Society, 2011a).

Acute Pain

Acute pain is generally considered **nociceptive** pain. This means it is pain that follows the usual pain sensory pathways and will often manifest with characteristic hypersympathetic findings such as elevations of blood pressure and pulse, diaphoresis, and mydriasis. Acute pain is the result of actual or pending tissue damage, and its duration is short. A person's perception of acute pain is a function of its inciting event and the reality that it will resolve as healing progresses.

Chronic Pain

It is estimated that about 35% of the American population has some degree of chronic pain, and up to 50 million Americans are partially or totally disabled due to chronic pain. According to the International Association for the Study of Pain (IASP), chronic pain involves suffering from pain in a particular area of the body (e.g., in the back or the neck) for at least 3 to 6 months (AMA, 2003).

Because pain is considered a symptom rather than a diagnosis, there are no valid incidence figures available for chronic pain itself. Chronic pain can be associated with a known cause or an unknown cause (e.g., fibromyalgia). A considerable amount of controversy surrounds chronic pain, especially its definitions, causes, diagnoses, and cures. A person's perception of chronic pain is a function of his or her personality and character traits, cultural and ethnic background, presence of support systems, satisfaction with work and home, level of formal education, and motivation or desire for feeling pain or not feeling pain.

Seven Tenets for Conscientious Prescribing of Drugs for Pain

Medical care clinicians of all kinds have always had trouble accurately assessing the severity of a patient's pain. Most clinicians ask patients to rate their pain on a scale of 1 to 10 and then try to assess their flexibility, strength, and reflexes. This often results in an exasperating experience for both the patient and the clinician. There are seven tenets that have proven to be helpful in making an assessment of pain before committing to prescribed therapy.

1. *Remove the barriers that render pain management ineffective.* There are barriers to the effective treatment of pain on the parts of both patient and clinician. Morphine and other opiates may have a stigma connected with being too strong, too addictive, or too harmful. Furthermore, the patient may associate the death of a loved one with the use of morphine rather than with the underlying disease. Some patients may want to save the "strong" medications for when their condition gets "really bad." Clinicians and patients share concerns about addiction and dependence, and many clinicians are concerned about regulatory reprisals from the DEA if they prescribe opioid analgesics regularly. Clinicians as well as law enforcement officials are concerned about the possibility of drug diversion. The laws in many states are being changed in an attempt to strike more of a balance between regulation and appropriate pain management.

2. *Never forget the consequences resulting from pain being poorly managed.* These include the following:
   - Impaired function and poor quality of life.
   - Depression.
   - Polypharmacy through treatment of other manifestations of pain, for example, agitation, confusion, sleep disturbances, impaired ambulation, falls, cognitive dysfunction, depression and decreased socialization, and anorexia.
   - Uncontrolled acute pain can lead to the development of chronic pain that often takes on a neuropathic component through neurochemical and neurophysiological changes that can make the pain much more difficult to tolerate and manage.

3. *Properly assess pain before prescribing any drug.* Before pain medications, especially **controlled substances**, are prescribed, a detailed history and physical is imperative. Controlled substances are drugs that are controlled under the Controlled Substance Act under federal law into "schedules" depending on its medical use, its potential for abuse, and its safety. The pain has to be assessed before it can be managed appropriately. Identification of the source (nerve damage, neuropathic; kidney stones, visceral; bone metastases, somatic) of the pain may save the patient's life. Clinicians should institute diagnosis-specific therapy and treat the pain while completing the diagnostic evaluation. Furthermore, clinicians should discuss realistic goals with the patient and identify the limitations of pain therapy related to specific pain diagnoses. Lastly, clinicians should reassess, re-examine, and adjust therapy as needed.

   Multiple scales for the assessment of pain have been designed and validated. There are visual analogue scales for which patients mark their pain on a line ranging from no pain to extremely severe pain. Pain can be rated on a scale of 0 to 10 (1 to 3, mild; 4 to 6, moderate; 7 to 10, severe). Faces rating scales determine the pain score by identifying the facial expressions of children (used because of developmental stage) and is useful as well for adults (e.g., those with dementia) who may not be able to verbalize the severity of the pain.

4. *Remember the goal of using medications for acute pain.* One of the primary goals of acute pain management is to restore function as soon as possible and to prevent the development of a chronic pain syndrome. With increasing pain, medications can be added to drugs used for lower levels of pain or substituted for less potent medications. For example, morphine can be added to acetaminophen (APAP) and gabapentin (Neurontin) if pain is escalating, or it can be substituted for a hydrocodone/acetaminophen (Lorcet, Lortab) preparation if a sustained release or more potent medication is required for adequate analgesia or if the intravenous route becomes a necessity. This principle applies to the treatment of chronic pain as well.

5. *Remember to use different prescribing algorithms for mild, moderate, and severe acute pain.* For mild pain, treatment may consist of an NSAID or acetaminophen plus or minus an adjuvant medication. This type of pain may respond to measures as simple as repositioning the patient (elevating a swollen limb or turning the patient in bed) and may not require medications at all.

   Other options for mild pain may include topical salicylates (Ben-Gay, sport creams) or capsaicin cream. Capsaicin cream is made from hot peppers and works by depleting substance P. Prescribers should not be fooled into thinking that these topical medications are benign. They are generally very safe, but if overused, the topical salicylates can cause systemic salicylate toxicity, and the capsaicin creams *escalate* the pain before they help. The lower concentration of capsaicin should be used first, and over time the higher concentration may be initiated to maintain and improve pain control. If the patient cannot understand (pediatrics, dementia patients) that there will be benefit gained through the initial pain with repeated applications, capsaicin should not be used.

   For moderate pain, the provider may prescribe tramadol (Ultram), hydrocodone/APAP (Norco, Lortab, Lorcet, Vicodin); hydrocodone/ibuprofen (Vicoprofen); oxycodone/APAP (Percocet, Tylox); or codeine (Tylenol #3, Tylenol #4). These medications may be used in combination with NSAIDs and/or adjuvant medications.

   For severe pain the pure opiates may be used. Due to the increase in all-cause mortality associated with higher dose opioids, dosages should be limited to less than 200 mg morphine equivalent per day, especially in the elderly (Solomon et al, 2010a & 2010b).

6. *Use a different algorithm when prescribing for chronic pain.* Chronic pain is defined as lasting longer than 3 months, and it often includes a significant neuropathic component that usually requires the use of adjuvant medications to manage the pain. This comes about through the hyperstimulation of **NMDA receptors** (*N*-methyl D-aspartate receptors) that ultimately decrease the effectiveness of the opiates upon mu receptors, possibly through down-regulation of the mu receptors or excessive pre- and postsynaptic

substance P. This ultimately leads to central sensitization or "wind up pain" that is characterized by hyperalgesia (pain out of proportion to the injury), allodynia (non-noxious stimuli produce a pain response), and/or prolonged pain response (pain lasts longer than expected). In this situation, the clinician may choose to start with an adjuvant medication, add an adjuvant to an opiate, or choose opiate that has activity at receptors other than or in addition to the mu receptor (methadone has effects upon the NMDA receptor as well as the reuptake of norepinephrine and serotonin, whereas tramadol has two enantiomers that impact the reuptake of norepinephrine and serotonin).

Chronic pain may not manifest in the usual hypersympathetic responses exhibited during acute pain. Rather, the vegetative signs of depression, fatigue, or anorexia are more common. Chronic pain may be multifactorial, with an unidentifiable cause or indeterminate duration.

7. *Remember there is a role for adjuvant medications.* **Adjuvant medications** are those that may be used in the management of pain but whose primary indication is not for analgesia; that is, the use of the medications for pain is often off-label. These may include tricyclic antidepressants, anticonvulsants, corticosteroids, anesthetics (e.g., ketamine), bisphosphonates, radiopharmaceuticals, muscle relaxants, antiarrhythmics (lidocaine, mexiletine), and others. These medications will not be discussed in detail in this chapter, but they will be mentioned in relation to the types of pain for which they may be used as well as the rationale for their use in those conditions.

The same stepwise escalation of medications is useful in chronic pain; however, the use of adjuvant medications is much more likely to be necessary for adequate analgesia in chronic pain. Adjuvant medications have demonstrated benefit in chronic neuropathic pain, visceral pain, and bone pain. Chronic **neuropathic pain** is described as burning, lancinating (stabbing pain, pain as if a cut from a sharp instrument), stinging, or tingling. It can be treated with opiates such as methadone or tramadol (Ultram). Tricyclic antidepressants are also useful in the treatment of neuropathic pain. Amitriptyline is the most studied drug, but nortriptyline (Pamelor, Elavil), imipramine (Tofranil), and desipramine (Norpramin) are as effective and often better tolerated. The higher doses used to treat depression are not necessary and only add to toxicity. Amitriptyline given at 10 to 25 mg at bedtime is usually adequate. It likely works by increasing central inhibition by increasing synaptic serotonin.

The antidepressant duloxetine (Cymbalta) is indicated for the treatment of diabetic neuropathic pain, and venlafaxine (Effexor) seems to work as well. These medications can be thought of as tricyclics without as many side effects. The mechanism of action is again related to increasing central inhibition of pain signal transmission.

The anticonvulsants gabapentin, pregabalin, and carbamazepine have the most supporting data for their use in neuropathic pain, but valproic acid and lamotrigine have also demonstrated some benefit. Gabapentin and pregabalin are usually first-line choices because of their tolerability, safety, and efficacy. Monitoring of blood levels or signs of toxicity (bone marrow, liver) is not necessary with these two drugs. The likely mechanism for benefit is the decrease in neuronal excitability. Ketamine may be used for refractory cases. Full anesthetic doses of 0.4 to 0.5 mg/kg/hr are not necessary. These doses may be associated with significant side effects such as dysphoria or hallucinations. Usually 0.1 to 0.2 mg/kg/hr is adequate to shut down the NMDA receptors and augment the efficacy of the opiates.

Antiarrhythmics such as lidocaine and mexiletine are the most studied for the treatment of neuropathic pain, but cardiac monitoring is necessary if these drugs are to be used, and the clinician needs to insure that the risk does not outweigh the potential benefits. Finally, corticosteroids have also been used in the treatment of neuropathic pain. There is significant risk to using corticosteroids long term, but in the acute setting they may be helpful in the case of nerve/spinal cord compression by decreasing perineural edema.

Visceral pain is described as colicky, cramping, or sharp, for example, the pain of pancreatitis or kidney stones. Opiates can be used in the treatment of this type of pain. Furthermore, smooth muscle relaxants such as hyoscyamine and scopolamine are also useful. Finally, octreotide is used only for malignant bowel obstruction.

Bone pain is described as aching, dull, and/or throbbing. Often it is mediated by prostaglandins. Similar to visceral and neuropathic pain, opiates can be used. Also useful are NSAIDs, corticosteroids, and bisphosphonates such as zoledronic acid, pamidronate, and ibandronate. Radiopharmaceuticals such as strontium-89, samarium, and others are used in the treatment of malignant bone pain. Finally, calcitonin is effective for pain caused by osteoporotic fractures but not for pathological fractures.

Pharmacology of Drugs Used to Alleviate Pain

Medications used to alleviate pain are usually grouped into two classes: the opiates and the nonopiates. **Opiates** are the natural drugs derived from alkaloids of opium or are synthetic derivatives of these alkaloids. **Nonopiates** are the synthetic drugs that alleviate pain and also alleviate inflammation, such as the NSAIDs.

The Roles of Opioid Receptors in Responding to Pain

As long as pain continues to plague people, opioids will continue to be one of the best means to relieving it. However, their side effects, especially in tolerant patients who increase their dosages, and the concerns over their addictive qualities interfere with their use. Until recently, all opioids were considered to be equivalent to morphine, but research has shown that is not the case. No longer can they be said to differ only in duration of action, dosage form, side effects, and oral availability because there are seven distinct subtypes of opioid receptors found in the human body, of which six are capable of modulating some type of pain. Compounds that act through these subtypes are being made available as the science of opioid receptors advances and allows the development of new, highly selective analgesics with fewer side effects.

Since World War II, scientists have worked to better understand why the perception of pain is highly dependent upon the situation in which it occurs. It is now believed the brain and central nervous system (CNS) have the ability to filter pain through the use of pain-filtering systems throughout the CNS. Evidence now concludes that upon pain stimulation there is the release of morphine-like, or endogenous opioid, peptide compounds composed of the enkephalins, dynorphins, and beta-endorphin, which, together with their highly selective receptors, constitute a complex system capable of influencing the subjective sensation of pain. The criteria for activating these systems physiologically remains unclear, but pharmacologically these systems are activated by the opioid analgesics.

The discovery that multiple subclasses of **opiate receptors** exist was soon followed by the demonstration that a number of discrete analgesic systems exist, each capable of independently relieving pain. These are the Mu_1, Mu_2, $kappa_1$, $kappa_2$, $kappa_3$, $delta_1$, and $delta_2$ receptors with the Mu_1 and Mu_2 receptors being the most sensitive (Table 24-1) and most important for managing general analgesia. As endogenous opioid receptor research continues, the existence of other opioid receptors will likely be discovered or suspected, but today those listed in Table 24-1 are the most important.

All of the receptor types listed in Table 24-1 (i.e., μ_1, μ_2, δ_1, δ_2, κ_1, κ_2, κ_3) are members of the G protein–coupled group of receptors and are found on free nerve endings on most tissues throughout the body. This includes skin, muscle, joints, connective tissue, and organs. Once activated, these pain receptors release neurotransmitters that send information about the sensation of pain through the spinal cord and into the brain. This process of pain perception and transmission is called *nociception*, and receptors that send the pain sensation along nerves are called *nociceptors*. Pain-relieving drugs (analgesics) such as the opiates function as either agonists, partial agonists, or antagonists at one or more types of receptor to stunt or dull the transmission of the pain sensation to the brain (Table 24-2). Thus, analgesic drugs are capable of diverse pharmacological effects in both their efficacy and tolerability.

TABLE 24-1 Classification of the Opioid Receptors

RECEPTOR	ANALGESIA	LOCATION	OTHER ACTIONS
Mu_1 (μ_1)	Supraspinal	Brain	
Mu_2 (μ_2)	Spinal	CNS	Respiratory depression, decreased heart rate, euphoria, physical dependence
$Delta_1$ (δ_1)	Spinal	CNS	Modulate mu receptor
$Delta_2$ (δ_2)	Supraspinal	Brain	Modulate mu receptors
$Kappa_1$ (κ_1)	Spinal	Brain, spinal cord	Diuresis (due to negative deregulation of antidiuretic hormone (ADH)
$Kappa_2$ (κ_2)	Unknown	Brain, spinal cord, pain neurons	Produce dysphoria and psychotomimetic effects
$Kappa_3$ (k_3)	Supraspinal	Brain, spinal cord, pain neurons	Produce dysphoria and psychotomimetic effects

TABLE 24-2 Selectivity of Opioid Medications on mu Receptors

TYPE OF OPIOID MEDICATION	GENERIC NAME	TRADE NAME
NATURALLY OCCURRING OPIUM ALKALOIDS	morphine	MS Contin, Avinza, Kadian, Duramorph
	codeine	Tylenol #3 or #4
	oxycodone	OxyContin, OxyIR, OxyFast, Roxicodone
SEMISYNTHETIC DERIVATIVES OF OPIUM	hydromorphone	Dilaudid
	hydrocodone	Norco, Lortab, Lorcet
SYNTHETIC AGENTS	meperidine	Demerol
	fentanyl	Duragesic patches or Actiq lozenges
	propoxyphene	Darvon
	methadone	Methadose, Dolophine
MU AGONIST-ANTAGONIST	pentazocine	Talwin
	butorphanol	Stadol
	nalbuphine	Nubain
MU PARTIAL AGONISTS	buprenorphine	Buprenex
MU ANTAGONIST	naloxone	Narcan
	methylnaltrexone	Relistor
	naltrexone	ReVia
	nalmefene	Revex

Conscientious Prescribing of Opiates for Pain Management

■ Equivalencies of opiates for pain management are approximate, particularly if switching from an oral drug to its subcutaneous or intravenous equivalent. Thus, clinicians routinely use 70% to 75% of the equal-analgesic dose unless the pain is poorly controlled. The dose may also be decreased because of limited cross-tolerance.

■ Hydromorphone is more potent than morphine and is available in a more concentrated solution. It may be beneficial to administer it as a substitute for morphine if the patient requires more than 20 mg/hr of morphine by the subcutaneous route because the volume of fluid administered will be smaller.

■ Use oral dosage forms when possible. Avoid intramuscular administration because it is more painful and offers no benefit over subcutaneous forms.

■ The appropriate dose of an opioid is the dose that relieves the pain with minimal side effects. Use enough drug and do so often enough.

■ Because there is no ceiling dose when it comes to the use of opioids, this can become a major safety hazard. Thus, limits are imposed by the combination of acetaminophen or ibuprofen with an opioid, not by the opioid. An exception is Avinza, where the dose is limited to 1,600 mg/day because of the fumaric acid contained in the formulation. Higher doses of the fumaric acid may be nephrotoxic.

■ Schedule medications around the clock, not just as needed, especially for chronic pain.

■ **Breakthrough pain** is pain that comes on suddenly, lasts for 3 to 30 minutes, and can occur at any time. These are flares that typically occur in people taking pain medications for cancer or in persons experiencing chronic pain. Supplemental opioid medication (10% to 15% of the daily dose) is warranted, and it may be added to the original regimen and given every 2 hours as needed.

■ For **incident pain** (an episodic increase in pain intensity), an opioid dose calculation is the same as for breakthrough pain (10% to 15% of daily dosage), but incident pain can be pretreated by administering the drug 1 hour before the regular dose is scheduled if it is by mouth or 10 to 15 minutes before the regular intravenous dose. Examples of events that can induce a specific incident of pain are changing a wound or surgical dressing, eating, defecating, socializing, walking, or repositioning a patient with bone metastasis.

■ Constipation is the main side effect of opiates that will not resolve on its own. It has to be treated and prevented as long as the patient is on opiates. Prevention of constipation is much better than treating impactions. Generally, treatment of constipation requires daily stimulants such as sennosides (Senakot) because they are safe to use long term. Avoid chronic bisacodyl because it can damage myenteric plexus. Polyethylene glycol, sorbitol, or milk of magnesia may be added if necessary. Prunes can be helpful because they are converted to sorbitol. Avoid the bulking agents or fiber laxatives because these will worsen the constipation if the motility issue is not addressed with sennosides.

■ Myoclonus (a sudden spasm or twitching of a muscle or parts of a muscle) is rare, but if it occurs, the patient can change opioids. Also, treat the patient with lorazepam, or use enough subcutaneous or intravenous fluids (approximately 40 mcg/hr) to maintain creatinine clearance and remove metabolites (morphine-3-glucuronide or hydromorphone-3-glucuronide).

■ Pruritus can be encountered with all of the opiates, but especially morphine and codeine. This *is not* an allergic response. It is due to direct histamine release (much like red man syndrome that occurs with vancomycin) and can be treated and prevented with diphenhydramine, cetirizine, loratadine, or fexofenadine.

■ Nausea from opiates is common and is mediated through the chemoreceptor trigger zone, a primarily dopaminergic pathway. Therefore, medications such as promethazine, prochlorperazine, metoclopramide, or even low-dose haloperidol are the drugs of choice. The nausea should subside after 3 to 4 days of opiate treatment, at which time the need for antiemetics will be limited.

■ AVOID MEPERIDINE. Because meperidine (Demerol) has a high incidence of neurotoxicity/seizures, premature death, especially in the frail or elderly, worse bioavailability, and lower efficacy than other opiates, it should be avoided in these populations. It should never be used in patients who are being treated with monoamine oxidase inhibitors.

■ Opioid overdose is treated with the opioid antagonist naloxone (Narcan). The typical dose is 0.2 to 0.8 mg intravenously, but as much as 2 mg is often given. Smaller doses are usually sufficient and help temper withdrawal symptoms.

Patient/Family Education for Patients Taking Opiates

■ Instruct the patient on how and when to ask for pain medication.

■ Instruct the patient to take these medications *exactly* as directed. If the dosage seems less effective after a few weeks of use, the dose should not be increased unless the patient talks with the clinician who prescribed it.

■ Instruct patients that these drugs are known to cause drowsiness or dizziness, thus they should ask for help when walking until they adjust. Patients should avoid driving a car or operating machinery that requires being alert.

■ As orthostatic hypotension is a probable, patients should be advised to change positions slowly, especially getting up from a sitting position.

■ Instruct patients to avoid use of alcohol or any other CNS depressant while on these pain relievers.

■ Advise patients that any nausea and vomiting are side effects that may be minimized by lying down.

■ Instruct patients on opiates that every 2 hours they should turn over, cough, and breathe deeply to help avoid/allay any respiratory depression caused as an adverse effect of the opiate's central analgesia.

The Antagonist Agonist Opiate Analgesics: Morphine and Its Derivatives

Morphine is still the prototype agent in this class of analgesics. Due to the difficulty in synthesizing it in the laboratory, it is still obtained from the alkaloids found in the poppy plant *Papaver somniferum* (*Papaver* means "poppy," *somniferum* means "to induce sleep" in Latin). Today there are synthetic and semisynthetic analogues, but unfortunately none have been found to be superior to morphine itself. For this reason, dosing of the semisynthetics and synthetics is based on an equivalency scale using morphine as the standard. For 6,000 years humans have cultivated opium poppies and all morphine, and codeine legally used today begins with its extraction from the poppy plant to make pain-killing, cough suppressing, and antidiarrheal medicine. Illegally grown plants are used to produce highly addictive mind-altering and abused substances such as heroin.

Mechanism of Action

Morphine and other opioids have activity at pre- and postsynaptic mu receptors as well as at presynaptic kappa and delta receptors where they reduce neurotransmitter release from nociceptive primary afferent terminals. The postsynaptic mu activity evokes an inhibitory postsynaptic potential by hyperpolarizing the membrane of pain transmission neurons.

Pharmacokinetics

■ Absorption: Generally well absorbed by oral, subcutaneous, and intramuscular routes, except fentanyl is not usually given orally because it is broken down by mucosal as well as hepatic P450 3A4.
■ Distribution: Medications distribute widely into CNS and other tissues. The lipophilic opioids have excellent CNS penetration.
■ Metabolism: Morphine and hydromorphone undergo glucuronidation, fentanyl is metabolized by P450 3A4, and most of the others are metabolized primarily by the P450 2D6 isozyme.
■ Excretion: Opioids are primarily eliminated in the urine.
■ Half-life: 2 to 3 hours, prolonged in patients with hepatic impairment.

When dosing these agents, two helpful online resources are the End of Life/Palliative Education Resource Center (www.eperc.mcw.edu) and the Narcotic Equivalence Converter (www.medcalc.com/narcotics.html). The Narcotic Equivalence Converter site has a calculator that enables a clinician to enter the name of a currently used narcotic, its dose, and its route of administration and the calculator will automatically provide the equivalent dose and route for administering a different narcotic (see Special Case: Opiate Equianalgesic Tables).

SPECIAL CASE: Opiate Equianalgesic Tables

Many narcotic equivalence converters are available, mostly on the Internet, and many institutions develop their own conversion chart to convert the dosage of one opiate to another. Although equianalgesic tables provide clinically sound estimates, the conscientious clinician will also consider other information, such as the patient's metabolism and clinical condition. Some patients cannot convert codeine to morphine, and some metabolize drugs faster than others. If pain is poorly controlled, patients may require a larger dose when changing drugs. If the pain is well controlled, the patient may need a lower dose of the new agent, perhaps 25% lower. The patient's history of exposure to narcotics is important because some patients are more sensitive than others.

To use a conversion table:

1. *Create a conversion factor for switching one drug to another:* Take the drug you are using and use the table below to select the denominator (IV hydromorphone = 1.5). Take the drug you want to use and set its conversion factor as the numerator (morphine tablets = 30). Then divide the two numbers (30/1.5 = 20). This gives the conversion factor 20.

2. *Calculate the daily dose of the agent currently being used:* IV hydromorphone given as 1 mg/hour or 24 mg/day. If the patient has also had 6 doses of 0.5 mg as added boluses, they have been given 27 mg/day.

3. *Multiply the daily dose of the current drug by the conversion number to get the dose of the new drug:* 27 mg/day of IV morphine × 20 (the conversion factor) = 540 mg/day of PO morphine.

4. *Divide the 24 hour total dose by the usual dosing schedule of the formulation you wish to give. Rounding up or down is acceptable per patient situation.* This is not an exact science, but rounding down is done more often: 540 mg PO morphine per day/200 mg sustained release (SR) caps = 3 caps per day, perhaps 1 SR cap A.M., then 1 SR cap P.M. or at bedtime, with one 100 SR cap at noon as needed.

Drug	Trade Name	Dosage Form Available	Parenteral	Oral
morphine	MS Contin	PO, SC, IV, PR	10	30
oxycodone	OxyContin	PO, PR	N/A	20
hydrocodone	Lortab Vicodin	PO	N/A	60
hydromorphone	Dilaudid	PO, SC, IV, PR	1.5	7.5
codeine	codeine generic	PO, IV, SC	120	200
fentanyl	Duragesic	Transdermal patch		Multiply patch strength by 2 for daily oral morphine equivalent.

Dosage and Administration

Opioid	Parenteral	Oral	Properties
hydromorphone (Dilaudid) 1, 2, 3, 4, 8 mg tabs; 5 mg/mL liquid; 3 mg suppositories Exalgo SR 8, 12, 16 mg	1.5 mg	7.5 mg	Good alternative to morphine, especially if using SC by continuous infusion (>20 mg/hr) due to higher potency (lower volume). Active glucuronide metabolites.
morphine 10, 15, 30 60, 100, 200 mg tabs; 15, 30, 60, 100, 200 mg capsules; 10, 20, 100 mg/mL liquid (Roxanol); SR tabs 15, 30, 60, 100, 200 mg SR caps (Kadian) 20, 50, 100 mg SR caps (Avinza) 30, 60, 90, 120 mg SR caps w/naltrexone (Embeda) 20, 30, 50, 60, 80, 100 mg Suppositories 5, 10, 20, 30 mg	10 mg	30 mg	Versatile: PO, SL, PR, IV, SC, intrathecal, epidural. Very cheap, readily available, available in IR and SR versions. Active metabolites, morphine-6-glucuronide 10 times more potent than morphine.
meperidine (Demerol) 50, 100 mg tabs 50 mg/5 mL syrup	100 mg	300 mg	Indicated for ACUTE use ONLY (i.e., <48 hours). Very weak, but heavy on side effects and adverse effects. Contraindicated with renal disease: a neurotoxic metabolite normeperidine can cause seizures and death.
methadone (Dolophine) 5, 10 mg tabs 1, 2, 10 mg/mL liquid		Variable conversion ratios; converted by oral morphine equivalent dose. See below.	At least three mechanisms: mu agonist, NMDA receptor antagonist, norepinephrine-serotonin reuptake inhibition. The only "long-acting" opiate and no active metabolites. Metabolized by P450 3A4. CHEAP at 1 cent/mg. Can cause QT prolongation; caution with other medications that can affect the QT interval. Torsades de pointes more likely with IV dosing.
levorphanol (Levo-Dromoran) 2-mg tabs, generic only		Variable conversion ratios; converted by oral morphine equivalent dose. See below.	Much like methadone, it works on mu and NMDA receptors and inhibits uptake of neurotransmitters. L-enantiomer of dextromethorphan with 50% first-pass metabolism via conjugation.
codeine 15, 30, 60 mg tabs 15 mg/5 mL solution	130 mg	180 mg	Prodrug converted by liver to morphine. About 10% of people lack the P450 2D6 enzyme for conversion. Ceiling dose of 60 mg/dose is due to the need to convert to morphine; enzymes saturate.
hydrocodone 2.5, 5, 7.5, 10 mg with 325, 500, or 650 mg APAP or 200 mg ibuprofen 7.5/500 per 15 mL	N/A	20 mg	Can refill, but only available in combination with acetaminophen or ibuprofen. Metabolized to hydromorphone and others.
oxycodone 5, 10, 20, or 30 mg tabs 5 mg/5 mL or 20 mg/mL liquid SR tabs 10, 15, 20, 30, 40, 60, 80 mg Multiple combinations with APAP	N/A	20 mg	Equal potency but a little more bioavailable than morphine. Bioavailability increased with ethyl alcohol consumption. Caution in liver disease: $T_{1/2}$ extends to 4 times normal. Metabolized to oxymorphone, which is 40 times more potent than oxycodone.
fentanyl (Duragesic) Patch, Actiq or Oralet lozenges Patch 12.5, 25, 50, 75, 100 mcg/hr 100, 200, 300, 400, 800, 1,200, 1,600 mcg lozenges Buccal patch (Onsolis) 200, 400, 600, 800, and 1,200 mcg (dose every 2 hr as needed, max 4 doses/day); requires FOCUS program enrollment.	~100 mcg/hr No conversion for lozenges or buccal patches. MUST start at lowest dose and titrate.	~ 1 to 2 times daily morphine dose; e.g.,200 mg morphine PO/day = 100 mcg/hr patch.	Patch for those who cannot swallow. MUST have subcutaneous fat due to drug's lipophilicity. Lozenge or buccal patch for transmucosal use. No cheap forms available. Very short $T_{1/2}$, can reverse without naloxone. Buccal ONLY indicated for breakthrough cancer pain in the opioid tolerant.
oxymorphone (Numorphan, Opana) 5, 10 mg in naive starting dose; >20 mg/day not recommended. SR tabs (Opana ER) 5, 7.5, 10, 15, 20, 30, 40 mg tabs dosed every 12 hr	1 mg	10 mg	Potentiated by cimetidine, MAOIs, and other CNS depressants. 10% bioavailability increased by 57%–65% in moderate to severe renal impairment. Caution with CrCl <50 or with liver impairment. Take 1 hr before or 2 hr after food (food increases AUC, area under the plasma concentration time curve, by 38%).
buprenorphine (Butrans patch) 5, 10, 20 mcg/hr weekly transdermal patches SL tabs & film 2, 8 mg Subutex, Temgesic IV Buprenex	0.3 mg (IV) Patch minimal effective dose <30 mg/day = 5 30–80 mg/day = 10 >80 mg/day (don't use)	Oral buprenorphine, with or without naloxone is usually limited to treatment of opiate addiction; requires training, approval, and new DEA number.	Partial agonist. Can cause QT prolongation; caution with other medications that can affect the QT interval. Has abuse potential. C-III

Adverse Reactions to Opiates

CV: Orthostatic hypotension, decreased blood pressure (BP).

DERM: Occasional allergic rash/pruritus.

EENT: Visual changes.

GI: Constipation, nausea, vomiting, abdominal cramps, dry mouth.

GU: Urine retention.

META: Decrease in appetite, urine glucose increases.

NEURO: Sedation, diaphoresis, facial flushing, somnolence, dizziness.

PUL: Overdose results in RESPIRATORY DEPRESSION, accompanied by skeletal muscle flaccidity, cold and clammy skin, cyanosis, extreme somnolence progressing to seizures, stupor, coma, and DEATH.

Interactions

■ Any medication that can be sedating or cause respiratory depression (benzodiazepines, phenobarbital, etc.).

■ Medications that cause QT prolongation only if using methadone (agonist) or buprenorphine (partial agonist).

Patient/Family Education

■ Patients should be taught to change positions slowly to avoid orthostatic hypotension.

■ Patients should be advised to avoid alcohol and any other CNS depressants.

■ Patients should be advised of the potential for physical dependency.

The Mixed/Partial Agonist-Antagonist Analgesics

The mixed or partial agonist-antagonist medications derive their name from being agonist agents at kappa and delta receptors and agonist antagonists at the mu receptor. Thus their use will precipitate withdrawal symptoms in patients who are dependent upon mu antagonism for pain relief, just as if they were taking morphine. Four mixed agonist-antagonist analgesics are available today: buprenorphine (Buprenex, Subutex) is a partial agonist. Others such as pentazocine (Talwin), nalbuphine (Nubain) and butorphanol (Stadol) are agonist-antagonists. Buprenorphine (Buprenex) is a partial agonist and has a high affinity for the mu receptor but low analgesic activity because of its partial antagonism at delta and kappa receptors. Thus, it binds with mu-opioid receptors in the CNS and alters the perception of and emotional response to pain. Because of its slow dissociation from the mu receptor, buprenorphine is used as an alternative to methadone in the management of opioid detoxification.

Pentazocine (Talwin) and nalbuphine (Nubain) are two other examples of this class of agents. They find use in treating moderate to severe pain, but they have a higher rate of hallucinations, nightmares, and anxiety than do other opioids. Talwin is used as a supplement to surgical anesthesia or as a sedative prior to surgery as either an intramuscular or intravenous administered agent.

Butorphanol (Stadol) is the fourth mixed antagonist-agonist opioid analgesic that is available as a nasal spray as well as intravenous injection. Typical uses of Stadol are to manage moderate to severe pain, such as migraine headache pain; as a supplement to balanced anesthesia; and to manage pain during labor. These medications can precipitate withdrawal symptoms in patients taking chronic opiates.

THE SYNTHETIC OPIATE ANTAGONISTS

The basic structure of morphine can be altered in minor ways, which can produce significant changes to the effects of the drug. A good example of this is the acetylation of its hydroxyl groups, which changes morphine into heroin. Another example is oxycodone. This agent was created because morphine is glucuronidated in the liver. If the morphine's phenolic hydroxyl group is protected with a methyl group, it will dull the first-pass effect in the liver and make this new product less susceptible to glucuronidation. Thus, oxycodone and codeine and its derivatives can retain analgesic activity following oral administration. Similarly, the opiate antagonists naloxone (Narcan), methylnaltrexone (Relistor), nalmefene (Revex), and naltrexone (ReVia) are created by relatively minor changes in the morphine structure. These agents are created by substituting one of the piperidine nitrogen methyl group for a longer chain, which changes the drug from an agonist to an antagonist. The opioid antagonists bind to the same opioid receptors as morphine but with high affinity, thus blocking the effects of the opioid. All opioid antagonists precipitate withdrawal symptoms in opioid-dependent patients. Interestingly, when given alone to those who are not addicts, no pharmacological effects are seen.

Conscientious Prescribing of Opiate Antagonists

■ A clinician may overestimate a patient's degree of pain and give an amount of opiate drug that exceeds the amount necessary to dull the pain, which may produce euphoria or respiratory depression. Patients on chronic opioids may experience withdrawal symptoms if treated with an opiate antagonist.

■ Patients must have respiratory rate, rhythm, and depth; pulse and ECG blood pressure; and level of consciousness monitored for 3 to 4 hours AFTER the expected peak of the antagonist concentrations in the blood.

■ Assess patients for signs of opioid withdrawal (vomiting, restlessness, abdominal cramps, increased blood pressure, increased temperature). These symptoms may begin in a few minutes to 2 hours. The severity of withdrawal symptoms is a function of the dose given, the opioid involved, and the degree of addiction.

■ Lack of significant improvement is a sign that symptoms are caused by another disease process or another nonopioid depressant.

Patient/Family Education for Patients Taking Opiate Antagonists

■ Patients who are taking the opioid for pain relief should be told that respiratory depression will be reversed but the drug also reverses analgesia.

Naloxone (Narcan)

Because of its fast onset (a few minutes), this agent is administered intravenously and is done so more frequently than any other for the reversal of opioid overdose. However, it fails to block some of the side effects of the opioids, such as hallucinations. The rapid onset of naloxone (Narcan) requires the drug to be repeatedly administered until the opioid agonist has cleared the system, otherwise a relapse into the overdose mode can occur.

Mechanism of Action

This medication has a high affinity for the mu receptor but has antagonistic effects at delta and kappa sites as well.

Pharmacokinetics

- Absorption: Very poor absorption from the GI tract. When given SC or IM, it is well absorbed
- Distribution: Rapidly distributed to all tissues, crosses the placenta
- Metabolism: Glucuronide conjugation in the liver
- Excretion: Urine
- Half-life: 1 to 2 hours

Dosage and Administration

Generic	Trade Name	Formulation	Administration
naloxone	Narcan	SC or IM	0.4 mg SC or IM and can increase to 0.8 mg if necessary. It can also be given down an endotracheal tube.

Clinical Uses

- To rapidly reverse effects of opiates, especially respiratory depression

Adverse Reactions

CV: Hypertension, hypotension, ventricular fibrillation, and tachycardia
GI: Nausea, vomiting
MISC: Severe opiate withdrawal

Interactions

- Opiates and naloxone have minimal interaction with tramadol.

  Will antagonize postoperative opioid analgesics

Conscientious Considerations

- Use cautiously in female patients who are pregnant because it may cause withdrawal symptoms in both mother and fetus.

Methylnaltrexone (Relistor)

This newer agent is approved for treating opioid-induced constipation caused by narcotic medications that have been used over time in chronically ill patients, such as those with cancer, when the drug is a part of the palliative care regimen. It is a drug with no risk of abuse or dependency.

Mechanism of Action

Methylnaltrexone is a peripherally acting mu-opioid receptor antagonist with a permanently charged tetravalent nitrogen atom that does not allow it to cross the blood-brain barrier. This property allows the drug to have opioid antagonistic effects throughout the body, counteracting opioid effects such as itching and constipation, but without affecting opioid effects and analgesia in the brain.

Pharmacokinetics

- Absorption: Medication is administered SC with peak concentrations occurring in 30 minutes.
- Distribution: Methylnaltrexone undergoes moderate tissue distribution.
- Metabolism: Only slightly via methylation in the liver.
- Excretion: 85% is excreted unchanged, almost half in the urine, the rest in the feces.
- Half-life: 8 hours

Dosage and Administration

Drug	Trade	Dosage Form	Administration*
methylnaltrexone	Relistor	SC	8 mg for patients weighing 38 to <62 kg (84 to <136 lb) or 12 mg for patients weighing 62–114 kg (136–251 lb). Patients whose weights fall outside of these ranges should be dosed at 0.15 mg/kg. Give 1 dose every other day.

*Methylnaltrexone has not been studied in pediatric patients, and no age-adjusted dosages are necessary for geriatric patient.

Clinical Uses

- Methylnaltrexone is indicated for the treatment of opioid-induced constipation in patients with advanced illness and in whom any response to laxative therapy has not been sufficient.

Adverse Reactions

DERM: Hyperhidrosis
GI: Abdominal pain, flatulence, nausea, severe and/or persistent diarrhea
NEURO: Dizziness

Interactions

- Although methylnaltrexone is a weak inhibitor of cytochrome P450 (CYP) isozymes, it does not significantly affect the metabolism of other drugs that use the CYP isozymes.

Contraindications

- Methylnaltrexone is contraindicated in patients with known or suspected mechanical gastrointestinal obstruction.
- It is rated a category B because it is safe in pregnancy, but it should be used with caution in nursing mothers because this population has not been adequately studied.

Conscientious Considerations

- Methylnaltrexone is expensive and only indicated for opiate-induced constipation and should only be used when cheaper and safer laxatives such as sennosides, polyethylene glycol, bisacodyl, etc. have failed.

■ Safety and efficacy of methylnaltrexone have not been established in pediatric patients.

Patient/Family Education

■ Contact a clinician if severe or persistent diarrhea develops.
■ Methylnaltrexone is a peripherally acting mu-opioid receptor antagonist with no known risk of abuse or dependence and will not precipitate opiate withdrawal.

Nalmefene (Revex) and naltrexone (ReVia, Trexan)

Nalmefene and naltrexone are opioid antagonists with similar chemical structures, but since their use is not related to pain management or side effects of pain management, they will only be mentioned briefly. Naltrexone has been most recently used in the procedure known as "rapid detox" for opiate addicts, but is also used in alcoholics. It is three to five times as potent as naloxone (Narcan) with excellent oral bioavailability, and a duration of action up to 48 hours. As a long-acting injectable pure opioid antagonist, it can be used to decrease the craving for opioids in highly motivated recovering addicts. Nalmefene is also a long-acting injectable opioid antagonist effective in preventing alcoholics from relapsing. It may be used in much the same way as naloxone (Narcan), but its longer half-life, of around 8 to 10 hours, makes it preferred for treatment of opioid overdose, especially with opioids with longer half-lives. Nalmefene (Revex) does not produce morphine-like effects and has low potential for abuse.

Pharmacology of Nonopiate Analgesics

Several novel nonopiate analgesics are available for treatment of pain; however, these agents are not chemically related to the opioids. Thought of as medications for the treatment of pain, such medications are often used as adjuvant treatments for neuropathic, visceral, or bone pain. Three such agents are tramadol (Ultram), ziconotide (Prialt), and tapentadol (Nucynta).

Tramadol (Ultram)

Tramadol (Ultram) is a centrally acting synthetic agent that has analgesic properties, but it is not chemically related to any agent in the opioid family. Like the opioids, however, it can be a drug subject to abuse; thus it is not recommended for persons with any history of drug addition, opioid allergy, or drug dependence.

Mechanism of Action

Tramadol binds to mu-opioid receptors in the CNS causing inhibition of ascending pain pathways, thus altering the perceptions and response to pain. It also inhibits the reuptake of serotonin and norepinephrine, which modifies the ascending pathways of pain. Its onset of action is 1 hour and its pain relief lasts up to 9 hours.

Pharmacokinetics

■ Absorption: Tramadol has good absorption from the GI tract.
■ Distribution: Distributes widely.
■ Metabolism: It is metabolized in the liver.

■ Excretion: Excreted in the urine.
■ Half-life: 6 to 8 hours

Dosage and Administration

■ Dosage is 50 to 100 mg by mouth, four times a day. No IV form.

Clinical Uses

■ Analgesia of moderate to moderately severe pain.
■ It may have a particular niche in treating neuropathic pain.

Adverse Reactions

CV: Flushing
DERM: Rash
EENT: Blurry vision, miosis
GI: Nausea, constipation
MISC: Flu-like symptoms
NEURO: Dizziness (usually transient), headache, insomnia, somnolence, weakness, and seizures are a possibility.

Interactions

■ Selective serotonin reuptake inhibitors and cyclobenzaprine can lead to serotonin syndrome, and tramadol may lower the seizure threshold; thus, it should be used with caution in combination with other medications that lower seizure threshold.
■ Antagonized by ondansetron (5-HT3 antagonist).

Contraindications

■ Seizures or concomitant use of tramadol with other medications that lower the seizure threshold

Conscientious Considerations

■ Tramadol has relatively low addictive potential, which makes it an attractive alternative to the pure opioids for first-line or even second-line treatment.

Patient Family Education

■ Instruct patient on how and when to ask for pain medication.
■ Instruct patient not to drive or operate machinery until response to this medication is known.
■ Advise patients to change sitting to standing positions slowly because this drug may induce orthostatic hypotension.
■ Encourage patients to avoid alcohol while on this medication.
■ In order to avoid atelectasis, advise patients to move about, cough, and breathe deeply every 2 hours.

Ziconotide (Prialt)

Ziconotide is a synthetic form of a natural toxin found in the cone snail's (*Conus magus*) whiplike appendage (flagella). The snail inserts the toxin into passing prey so it can stun and capture them.

Mechanism of Action

Ziconotide is a selective N-type voltage-gated calcium channel blocker used to inhibit the release of pro-nociceptive neurochemicals such as glutamate, calcitonin gene-related peptide, and substance P in the brain and spinal cord. By binding to these sensitive calcium channels located on the afferent nerves of the dorsal horn of the spinal cord, it blocks excitatory neurotransmitter release and reduces their sensitivity to painful stimuli.

Pharmacokinetics

- Absorption: The drug is administered intrathecally (IT) directly into cerebral spinal fluid.
- Distribution: About 50% is distributed bound to protein.
- Metabolism: Metabolized by several enzymes present in multiple organs (kidney, liver, lung), which degrade it to peptide fragments and free amino acids.
- Excretion: In the urine.
- Half-life: When given IT, half-life is 2.9 to 6.5 hours.

Dosage and Administration

- Because of the profound side effects or lack of efficacy when delivered through more common routes, such as orally or intravenously, ziconotide must be administered intrathecally (directly into the spine).
- Dose for adults is 2.4 mcg/day given intrathecally using an ambulatory infusion pump (Medtronic SynchroMed, Medtronic, Minneapolis, Minnesota) attached to the patient.

Clinical Uses

- Appropriate only for management of severe chronic pain in patients for whom IT therapy is warranted and who are intolerant of or refractory to other treatment, such as systemic analgesics, adjunctive therapies, or IT morphine.

Adverse Reactions

EENT: Abnormal vision.
GI: Nausea, anorexia.
NEURO: Dizziness, confusion, headache, hypertonia, ataxia, somnolence, unsteadiness on feet, and memory problems. The most severe but rare side effects are hallucinations, thoughts of suicide, new or worsening depression, and seizures.

Drug Interactions

- None are known, but ziconotide may increase the effects of other CNS depressants.

Contraindications

- Ziconotide is contraindicated in people with a history of psychosis, schizophrenia, clinical depression, bipolar disorder, and seizures.
- It may enhance the adverse effects of other CNS depressants.

Conscientious Considerations

- Monitor for signs of psychological or neurological impairment.

Patient/Family Education

- This agent is administered by an intrathecal pump (Medtronic SynchroMed) requiring naïve pump priming, initial pump fill, and pump refills. The patient must be fully aware of the ambulatory infusion pump system and its care.

- Teach patients to watch for signs of meningitis or other infection in the spinal cord area.

Tapentadol (Nucynta)

Tapentadol is similar to, though more expensive than, tramadol. This medication is similar to oxycodone in its ability to relieve severe pain, but it is more expensive than oxycodone. It is metabolized by glucuronidation and sulfate conjugation with extensive first-pass metabolism and renal elimination. Half-life is approximately 24 hours.

Pharmacology of NSAIDs

There are several dozen NSAIDs available for human consumption, and many of the same chemical entities are sold under differing trade names. However, these drugs all exert a similar mechanism of action, similar pain-alleviating effects, and have similar adverse reaction profiles. Even though there are certain differences that distinguish one form from the others, no one NSAID is superior to another. However, patients will relate that one drug works better for them than does another.

Most of the NSAIDS are extensively metabolized, even though that varies greatly by chemical structure. This characteristic makes it hard for the clinician to determine effective dosing and to extrapolate effective outcomes when switching patients from one NSAID to another.

Conscientious Prescribing of NSAIDs

- Hypersensitivity reactions can occur with NSAIDs, thus the prescriber must be vigilant for a history of asthma, urticaria, aspirin-induced allergies, and nasal polyps.
- NSAIDs cause renal damage, thus the clinician must watch for renal impairment.
- NSAIDs should not be used during late pregnancy because they may cause closure of ductus arteriosus.
- Safety of NSAID usage has not been established in people under age 18.
- Because of NSAIDs' ability to prolong bleeding times, the conscientious clinician checks for bleeding and bruising; additionally NSAID usage should be stopped 1 week before surgery.
- Administration in higher than normal doses does *not* provide increased effectiveness as an analgesic, but it may increase the side effects.

Patient/Family Education for Patients Taking NSAIDs

- Take medicines with food or antacids if GI symptoms appear.
- Take these medications with a full glass of water and remain upright for 15 to 30 minutes after dosing.
- Take as directed; increasing the dose does not increase effectiveness, thus a missed dose should be taken when remembered, but *not* if it is almost time for the next dose.
- Notify clinician if there is any sign of GI toxicity, such as abdominal pain, black stool, skin rash, weight gain, and edema.

- Notify clinician if there are any signs of hepatotoxicity, such as nausea, fatigue, lethargy, pruritus, jaundice, upper right quadrant pain, and flu-like signs.
- Patients should be asked about pregnancy and told to notify their clinician if pregnancy is suspected.
- Warn patient that NSAIDs taken with three glasses of any alcohol may increase the risk of GI bleeding.
- Caution patients to wear sunscreen and protective clothing to prevent photosensitivity reactions.
- Caution patients that these are not long-term drugs and use should be for no more than 10 days if taking for pain or 3 days if for fever.
- Advise patients that side effects such as rash, itching, visual disturbances, tinnitus, weight gain, black stools, headache that is persistent, or anything like a flu symptom are indications they should contact their clinician.

Mechanism of Action

All of the NSAIDs share a common mechanism of action; that is, they inhibit the cyclooxygenase enzyme (COX) (Fig. 24-1). Decreasing this enzyme results in a decreased formation of prostaglandin precursors (PGE_2, prostacyclin, and thromboxane) and an inhibition of phospholipids. Inhibition of lipoxygenase may also occur. The major effect is the inhibition of cyclooxygenase-1 and -2. COX-1 is found in the GI mucosa, and COX-2 is a function of inflammation. The extent of this inhibition varies with each chemical category. For example, NSAIDs also produce vasodilation by acting on the heat-regulation center of the hypothalamus. Thus, they are used to reduce fever.

The impact of NSAIDs on prostaglandin precursors results in a number of bodily effects because as normal agents in the body, the prostaglandins have a number of functions, such as the following:

- Causing pain when they come in contact with certain nerve fibers

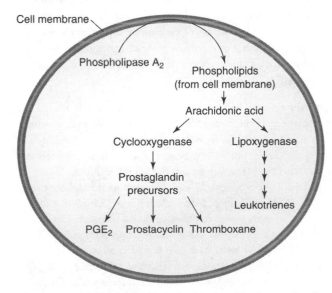

- Helping to protect the stomach lining against acid and digestive enzymes
- Participating in both blood flow and blood-clotting regulation

By inhibiting the COX enzyme, which produces prostaglandins, NSAIDs help to prevent and reduce pain and inflammation. The inhibition of the COX enzyme is also responsible for many of the side effects of NSAIDs, especially their notoriety for inducing GI distress.

Clinicians like to view NSAIDS as two main types: nonselective and selective. Nonselective NSAIDs inhibit stomach enzymes, blood platelets, and blood vessels (COX-1) as well as the enzymes found at sites of inflammation (COX-2) to a similar degree. Nonselective NSAIDs include agents such as aspirin, ibuprofen, naproxen, and diclofenac. Selective NSAIDs, also called COX-2 inhibitors, inhibit the COX enzyme found at sites of inflammation (COX-2) more so than the type of enzyme found in the stomach, blood platelets, and blood vessels (COX-1). Celecoxib is an example of a selective NSAID.

Pharmacokinetics

- Absorption: Rapidly absorbed for the GI tract.
- Distribution: Protein binding is greater than 90%, and the NSAID is carried to the site of inflammation on albumin.
- Metabolism: Metabolized in the liver by oxidation to water-soluble conjugates so that they can be cleared.
- Excretion: 99% in the urine.
- Half-life: Mostly 2 to 4 hours, but differences in clearance rates account for the variability in half-life among these agents (see Dosage and Administration).

Clinical Uses

- Relief of pain (analgesic effect)
- Reduction of inflammation
- Reduction of fever

Adverse Reactions

CV: Edema
DERM: Itching, rash
EENT: Tinnitus
ENDO: Fluid retention
GI: Dyspepsia, vomiting, abdominal pain/cramps, heartburn, nausea, diarrhea, constipation, flatulence, epigastric pain, appetite suppression
NEURO: Dizziness, headache, nervousness

Interactions

- Antihypertensives (alpha blockers, angiotensin-converting enzyme inhibitors [ACEIs], angiotensin II-receptor blockers, beta blockers, diuretics) are inhibited by the presence of NSAIDs, leading to unfavorable hemodynamic events.
- Decreased platelet aggregation occurs in the presence of anticoagulants, leading to increased risk of GI bleeding.
- Decreased renal clearance with aminoglycosides, leading to potential toxicity.
- Corticosteroid use concurrent with NSAIDs increases risk of GI bleeding.

FIGURE 24-1 NSAID Mechanism of Action: The Prostaglandin Cascade Inside a Cell.

Dosage and Administration

Chemical Class	Generic Name	Trade Name	Usual Adult Dosage	Half-Life
PROPIONIC ACIDS	naproxen	Naprosyn, Anaprox	500 mg initially followed by 250 mg every 6–8 hours	Short (2–3 hr)
	ketorolac	Toradol	Adults younger than 65, 20 mg STAT, then 10 mg every 4–6 hr	4.5 hr
	ibuprofen	Motrin	400–800 mg 3–4 times/day	2–4 hr
	oxaprozin	Daypro	1,200 mg 1 time/day	42–50 hr
	flurbiprofen	Ansaid	200–300 mg/day in 2–3 divided doses	5.7 hr
IN-DOLEACETIC ACIDS	sulindac	Clinoril	200 mg every 12 hr	Short (2 hr)
	indomethacin	Indocin	25–50 mg every 8 hr	2.6–11 hr; prolonged in neonates up to 60 hr.
	etodolac	Lodine	200–40 mg, every 6–8 hr	6–7 hr
PHENYLACETIC ACID	diclofenac	Cataflam, Voltaren	50 mg, every 8 hr	Short (2–3 hr)
NAPHTHYLALKANONE	nabumetone	Relafen	1,000–2,000 mg/day	Long (24 hr)
OXICAM	piroxicam	Feldene	10–20 mg/day, 1 time/day	Long (45–50 hr)
FENAMATES	mefenamic acid, meclofenamic acid	Ponstel	500 mg to start, then 250 mg every 4 hr	Short (3.5 hr)

Contraindications

■ People with active peptic ulcers, chronic inflammation of the GI tract, GI bleeding, history of ulceration, and a history of sensitivity to aspirin or other NSAIDs should not use these medicines.

Aspirin and Acetaminophen: The Non-Narcotic Analgesics

Aspirin and acetaminophen are over-the-counter drugs that are sold as single agents or in combination with many other agents.

Aspirin

Acetylsalicylic acid (aspirin) serves as the prototype drug for the non-narcotic analgesics. It possesses analgesic, antipyretic, anti-inflammatory, and antiplatelet properties. It is also considered an NSAID. Aspirin (acetylsalicylic acid) is a weak organic acid with a pK_a of 3.5. The breakdown of acetylsalicylic acid into

acetic acid and salicylate often leads to the vinegar-like odor of old aspirin tablets.

Mechanism of Action and Clinical Use

■ Aspirin has an analgesic action. It relieves low-to-moderate intensity pain such as headache, myalgia, arthralgia, and other pains arising from integumentary structures. Aspirin may also be effective against chronic postoperative pain or pain associated with inflammation. Aspirin also has an antipyretic action. Aspirin lowers elevated body temperature. Body temperature is maintained at a "set point" regulated by the hypothalamus; during fever, the set point is at a higher level. The salicylates reset the "thermostat" for normal temperature, and heat loss is enhanced as a result of cutaneous vasodilation and sweating. However, salicylates do not reduce exercise-induced hyperthermia.

■ Aspirin also has anti-inflammatory effects. The salicylates are used in the treatment of rheumatic diseases. Again, inhibition of prostaglandin and thromboxane synthesis is the mechanism of anti-inflammatory action. Generally, higher doses are required for effective anti-inflammatory action, as compared to analgesic and antipyretic doses. This may be related to the concept that COX-2 plays a more prominent role than COX-1 in the inflammatory process and that aspirin is a much more effective inhibitor of COX-1 than COX-2. Evidence suggests that COX-2 is induced by cytokines and other mediators of inflammation. Aspirin does not inhibit the formation of leukotrienes via the lipoxygenase pathway.

■ Aspirin further has an antiplatelet effect. Aspirin significantly reduces the incidence of stroke and myocardial infarction in patients at risk. In even the lowest therapeutic doses, aspirin produces a measurable prolongation of bleeding time. This effect is due to alteration of platelet aggregation. Aspirin covalently acetylates a serine at the active site of platelet cyclooxygenase, thereby reducing the formation of thromboxane A_2, which promotes platelet aggregation. Because the acetylation of the enzyme is irreversible, the inhibitory effect of aspirin on platelet aggregation lasts for up to 8 days, until new platelets are formed.

Pharmacokinetics

■ Absorption: Orally ingested salicylates are rapidly absorbed, partly from the stomach and mostly from the small intestine. Significant plasma concentrations are found at 30 minutes; peak concentrations may be seen at 1 to 2 hours. Absorption occurs by passive diffusion of the nonionized form.

■ Distribution: Salicylates rapidly distribute throughout the body, primarily by pH-dependent passive diffusion. Salicylate is highly bound to plasma proteins (primarily albumin but also ß-globulins). At a concentration of 20 mg/mL, 85% is bound, whereas 50% is bound at 50 mg/mL.

■ Metabolism: Metabolism of salicylates takes place primarily in the liver microsomal system and mitochondria. The primary metabolites are conjugates with glycine (salicylic acid) and glucuronic acid (an ether glucuronide and an ester glucuronide). Salicylic metabolism demonstrates biphasic kinetics; at high and toxic doses, metabolism is limited and occurs according to zero-order kinetics, whereas at lower doses metabolism proceeds according to first-order kinetics. This difference in rate of metabolism is very important from the standpoint drug accumulation with repeated administration of high doses.

■ Excretion: Salicylate is excreted in the urine as the free compound and as conjugated metabolites. The amount of unchanged salicylate excreted may vary between 10% (acid urine) and 85% (alkaline urine). Excretion of the metabolites is not pH dependent. Alkalinization of the urine by various procedures can markedly enhance salicylate clearance.

■ Half-life: The half-life for salicylate is 3 to 6 hours in low doses and 15 to 30 hours at high doses.

Dosage and Administration of Aspirin

Drug	Use	Dose
aspirin	analgesic/antipyretic	Adults: 325–650 mg every 4–6 hr up to 4 gm per day Children: 10–15 mg/kg dosed every 4–6 hr up to 4 gm per day
	anti-inflammatory	Adults: 2.4–3.6 gm/ day in divided doses Children: 60–90 mg/kg/day in divided doses

Adverse Reactions

GI: Gastric intolerance is the main adverse effect associated with normal aspirin usage. Salicylates may induce nausea and vomiting owing to stimulation of gastric mucosal receptors and the medullary chemoreceptor trigger zone. The mechanism of salicylate-induced gastric bleeding and damage also involves inhibition of prostaglandin synthesis. PGI_2 and PGE_2 serve as cytoprotective agents in the gastric mucosa. They inhibit acid secretion, increase mucosal blood flow, and enhance secretion of protective gastric mucus.

HEM: The primary effect of the salicylates on this system is the antiplatelet effect.

META: The salicylates may cause several changes in acid-base balance and electrolyte patterns. In situations of poisoning by as few as 10 aspirin tablets, respiratory acidosis and metabolic acidosis can exist simultaneously. Among infants and children, toxicity often develops beyond respiratory alkalosis before they are seen by a physician because dehydration also occurs because of water loss through the lungs during hyperventilation and salicylate-induced sweating.

PUL: Salicylates stimulate respiration directly and indirectly. High toxic doses depress respiration. The direct stimulation is due primarily to an action on medullary respiratory neurons that control rate. Respiratory alkalosis nearly always occurs at some stage of salicylate poisoning. The indirect effect is due to salicylate-induced uncoupling of oxidative phosphorylation. If the toxic dose is high enough, the salicylates depress the medulla and cause central respiratory paralysis and circulatory collapse (vasomotor depression).

NEURO: In toxic doses, salicylates produce CNS stimulation (including convulsions) followed by depression. Confusion, dizziness, tinnitus, high tone deafness, delirium, psychosis, stupor, and coma may occur. The hearing loss is completely reversible.

RENAL: Uric acid excretion is altered by salicylates. Low doses (2 gm or less) decrease urate excretion by competing with urate for the organic acid secretory mechanism. The possibility of reduced urate excretion is of significance in patients with gout. Prostaglandins are involved in maintenance of renal blood flow under certain conditions. Inhibition of prostaglandin synthesis by salicylates can lead to decreased renal blood flow with salt and water retention, especially in the elderly. Box 24-1 discusses salicylism and its treatment.

Interactions

■ The effects of ACEIs may be blunted with aspirin, as well as the effects of beta blockers and loop and thiazide diuretics.

■ Alcohol and ethanol may induce gastric mucosal damage.

■ Aspirin and NSAIDs together increase GI adverse effects.

■ Aspirin and antiplatelet agents increase bleeding times.

BOX 24-1 Salicylism: Salicylate Poisoning

Mild chronic salicylate intoxication occurring after repeated administration of high doses of salicylate is termed *salicylism*. Symptoms consist of headache, dizziness, tinnitus, hearing loss, mental disturbances, sweating, thirst, hyperventilation, nausea, vomiting, and sometimes diarrhea.

With more severe intoxication, more marked CNS effects develop, as well as skin eruptions and marked changes in acid-base balance. The CNS effects may include excess stimulation, incoherent speech, vertigo, tremor, delirium, hallucinations, convulsions, and coma. The skin eruptions may be of various types. Hyperthermia is usually present, and dehydration often occurs. Nausea, vomiting, and abdominal pain are commonly present. A key point to remember is that in acute toxicity, the initial hyperventilation is due to the drug and not the patient's acid-base status, so early in the course the patient may have a respiratory alkalosis before developing the typical anion gap acidosis that would be expected. Hyperventilation may persist but will not compensate adequately for the metabolic acidosis.

Treatment of severe salicylate poisoning must be immediate. Gastric lavage or induction of emesis will prevent further absorption if performed within a few hours after ingestion. Activated charcoal may be given to adsorb drug left in the stomach.

Source: Kreplick, L. W., & Tarabar, A. (2010, December 7). Salicylate Toxicity in Emergency Medicine. Medscape Reference. Retrieved March 9, 2013, from http://emedicine.medscape.com/article/818242-overview.

Contraindications

■ Hypersensitivities to salicylates, other NSAIDS.

Conscientious Considerations

■ The U.S. Food and Drug Administration (FDA) recommends Aspirin or aspirin-containing products NOT be given to any child under the age of 12 who has a fever. The British Medicine and Healthcare Products Regulatory Agency makes the same recommendation but raises the age to children under the age of 16. Interestingly many American special interest groups are advocating no aspirin products should be given to anyone under the age of 19. FDA data shows the 93% of Reye's Syndrome cases occurred 3 weeks after a child with a fever also had a respiratory infection, chicken pox, or diarrhea. Thus there is a great opportunity for clinicians to be conscientious about treating the young an young adults (Box 24-2).

■ Clinicians should have a complete drug history of their patients so that they can check for the many drug interactions that exist with aspirin

---

BOX 24-2 Aspirin And Reye's Syndrome

An association exists between the administration of aspirin to children with acute febrile illness (influenza and chickenpox) and concomitant development of Reye's syndrome with its severe hepatic injury and encephalopathy (swelling in brain). Reye's syndrome is quite rare and mostly affects children and adolescents recovering from a febrile influenza who also may have a metabolic disorder. Its onset of symptoms (confusion, seizures, and loss of consciousness) require immediate medical care. Although aspirin is approved for children over the age of 2, clinicians must warn caregivers that if their child or teenager is suffering from chickenpox or recovering from influenza, it is wise not to administer aspirin.

From a physiological basis, the child's blood sugar levels drop, he or she experiences a swelling in the liver in which fatty deposits develop and a swelling of the brain, which results in seizures and loss of consciousness. The first signs may be rapid breathing and diarrhea in younger children and persistent vomiting and lethargy in older children. As the syndrome progresses, the child experiences irritable behavior, confusion, paralysis in arms and legs, seizures, and loss of consciousness.

The exact cause of Reye's syndrome remains unknown, although its trigger is the use of aspirin to treat a viral infection. Its incidence is higher in children with a fatty acid oxidation disorder, although exposure to insecticides, herbicides, and paint thinners may also be triggers. Treatment will take place in an intensive care unit (ICU) in a hospital, with supportive therapy to maintain blood pressure (glucose and electrolytes IV); drugs to decrease intracranial pressure (diuretics); antiseizure medications; medications to prevent bleeding (vitamin K, plasma, platelets) if liver damage is suspected, and perhaps a ventilator if breathing is impaired.

Patient/Family Education

■ Adults should not take 325-mg doses of aspirin for any longer than 10 days unless recommended by their clinician. Adolescents should take it no longer than 5 days, and even then do so cautiously, because of the risk of Reye's syndrome. Adolescents should not take aspirin if they are febrile or have viral symptoms. Since there is no cure, no test, and no way to predict Reye's Syndrome, the clinician has a great responsibility to inform all patients with young children about Reye's Syndrome, as too many parent's know little of it or about it. FDA states that children under the age of 12 who have a fever should not take aspirin or aspirin-containing products. The British Healthcare Regulatory Agency recommends that children under the age of 16 should not take aspirin unless they are under the care of a clinician.

■ Adults should be warned against concurrent use with alcohol because they may have GI distress.

■ Aspirin should be explained as a drug that also "thins the blood" and should not be taken concurrently with antiplatelet therapy such as Coumadin.

Acetaminophen: The Aspirin Alternative

Acetaminophen (Tylenol) is an alternative to aspirin for analgesic and antipyretic properties. Its pain-relieving effects are equivalent to aspirin, but it does not have any antiplatelet effects. This agent is ineffective as anti-inflammatory agent. It is recommended by the Rheumatological Association for non-inflammatory osteoarthritis. Acetaminophen lacks several of the undesirable effects of aspirin (gastritis, ulceration, inhibition of platelet function). However, in *acute overdose, acetaminophen can cause fatal hepatic necrosis.*

Mechanism of Action

The analgesic and antipyretic actions of acetaminophen are similar to those of aspirin, but the inhibition of arachidonic acid metabolism is not necessary to produce the effect as it is with aspirin or other NSAIDs. It produces little or no effect on respiration, cardiovascular function, acid-base balance, platelet aggregation, or uric acid excretion. It does not produce the gastric irritation, erosion, and bleeding characteristic of aspirin, nor does it show cross-hypersensitivity.

The exact site and mechanism for analgesic action is uncertain, but it appears to raise the pain threshold, possibly by inhibiting the nitric oxide pathway mediated by multiple neurotransmitter receptors, most notably substance P and NMDA receptors. Essentially, acetaminophen blocks the production and release of prostaglandins (notably PGE) into the central nervous system and thereby blocks their effects in the heat-regulating areas of the anterior hypothalamus that would otherwise lead to increased heat production and decreased heat loss.

Pharmacokinetics

■ Absorption: Acetaminophen is almost completely absorbed (85% to 98% bioavailability) from the gastrointestinal tract, and the rate of absorption is dependent upon the rate of gastric emptying. Peak plasma concentrations are reached within 1 hour after oral administration of immediate-release preparations and within 2 hours for extended-release preparations. Disease states or medications that delay gastric emptying can slow the rate of absorption.

■ Distribution: Acetaminophen distributes widely into all fluids throughout the body, but it does not distribute into fat. It crosses the placenta and is excreted in very small amounts into breast milk, but acetaminophen is safe in pregnancy and breastfeeding.

■ Metabolism: Metabolism occurs by way of liver microsomal enzymes primarily to conjugates of glucuronic acid and sulfuric acid, but a small amount is converted via the cytochrome P450 system (CYR2E1, CYP1A2, and CYP3A4) to a hepatotoxic metabolite, N-acetyl-p-benzoquinone imine), which is in turn conjugated by glutathione to a nontoxic metabolite when therapeutic doses of acetaminophen are given.

■ Excretion: Inactive glucuronate and sulfate conjugates are excreted into the urine.

■ Half-life: Acetaminophen's plasma half-life is 1 to 4 hours.

Dosage and Administration

Drug	Trade Name	Adult Dosing to Remove Mild to Moderate Pain and Reduce Fever*	Child Dosing
acetaminophen	Tylenol	650–1,000 mg by mouth, every 4–6 hr as needed or 1,300 mg every 8 hr as needed (extended release formulas), not to exceed 3 gm/day.	Children 10 mg/kg, every 4–6 hr as needed. Available in 80- and 160-mg tablets (children's dissolving tabs), 160 mg/5 mL suspension, and infant drops 80 mg/0.8 mL. No more than 5 doses/day. Suppositories are also available.

*Acetaminophen dosage forms are many and varied, including 500-mg caplets and extended release caplets, 650 mg; elixirs 160 mg/5 mL; liquid, 500 mg/5 mL; solutions oral drops 100 mg/0.9 mL, and 80 mg/0.8 mL; suppositories 120 mg, 325 mg, 500 mg; tablets of 325 mg, 500 mg, and chewable tabs 80 mg. The most recent dosage form is a 10-mg/mcg IV injection (Ofirmev), the first and only of its kind.

Clinical Uses

■ Analgesic
■ Antipyretic in adults and children
■ Mild forms of arthritis (osteoarthritis); aspirin or NSAIDs are preferred for rheumatoid arthritis
■ Analgesic in patients taking anticoagulant medications or in those allergic to aspirin or in children with fever and flu because it is not associated with Reye's syndrome

Adverse Reactions

DERM: Rash and urticaria
GI: Hepatic failure (overdose)
GU: Renal failure (high dosages and chronic use)

Interactions

■ Warfarin effects may be enhanced in the presence of acetaminophen, especially when acetaminophen is given at doses in excess of 2 gm/day.

■ Alcohol intake may increase the risk of acetaminophen-induced hepatotoxicity.

■ Drugs that increase the action of liver enzymes that metabolize acetaminophen. For example, carbamazepine (Tegretol), isoniazid (INH, Nydrazid, Laniazid), and rifampin (Rifamate, Rifadin, Rimactane) reduce the levels of acetaminophen and may decrease the action of acetaminophen.

■ Cholestyramine decreases absorption from the gut.

Contraindications

■ Liver disease, especially in high doses
■ Allergy to medication or use of other acetaminophen-containing compounds that may exceed the toxic acetaminophen dosage

Conscientious Considerations

■ Assess the patient's health and use of alcohol because patients who are malnourished and abuse alcohol have the highest risk for hepatotoxicity.

■ Assess amounts and types of prescription and over-the-counter drugs being taken.

■ Whenever possible assess the location and intensity of pain 30 to 60 minutes following administration of acetaminophen.

■ Acetaminophen is considered safe in pregnant and breastfeeding patients.

Patient/Family Education

■ Use only when necessary for pain or fever.
■ Keep a diary of how many doses per day are used to monitor the total daily dose so as not to exceed the maximum recommended daily dose.
■ Keep this medication out of the reach of children.
■ Patients should be advised to use the drug only as indicated on the label or as instructed by their clinician.

Medical Emergencies Involving Acetaminophen Overdosing

In acute overdose, acetaminophen produces a dose-dependent, potentially fatal hepatic necrosis. Renal tubular necrosis may also occur. Nephrotoxicity was more common with acetaminophen's predecessor, phenacetin, which was taken off the market by the FDA in 1983 because of nephrotoxic and carcinogenic tendencies (most notably urothelial tumors such as transitional cell carcinoma). Normally, acetaminophen is conjugated either as a sulfate or a glucuronide. With toxic doses, this system is saturated and microsomal enzymes produce other metabolites that can bind sulfhydryl groups on cell constituents. These metabolites are normally inactivated by glutathione. If glutathione stores are depleted by large amounts of metabolites resulting from toxic doses, then hepatic damage ensues.

Treatment of acute overdose of acetaminophen must begin immediately and includes removal of the remaining drug from the stomach, supportive therapy, and initiation of therapy to protect against hepatic damage. The hepatotoxicity caused by acetaminophen is delayed, and the patient may appear to improve after initial GI symptoms subside (24 to 48 hours after ingestion). However, after 36 to 72 hours, hepatic enzymes, bilirubin, and prothrombin time become abnormal as hepatic injury occurs. Protection against hepatic damage may be obtained by early administration of sulfhydryl compounds to inactivate the toxic metabolites. N-acetylcysteine (Mucomyst, Mucosol; 10% or 20% solution) is effective if given less than 24 hours after ingestion of acetaminophen, and it is even more effective when administered within 10 hours.

SPOTLIGHT ON ALTERNATIVE PAIN MANAGEMENT

Because the majority of clinicians have little training in pain management, it should not be surprising that many patients seek alternative ways to manage their pain, especially because it gives them a sense of being in control of what is happening with their bodies. Thus, the relief of pain by aromatherapy (basil clove, camphor, menthol eucalyptus, black pepper, peppermint oil, rosemary oil, wintergreen oil); acupuncture; traditional Chinese medicine; ayurvedic medicine; homeopathy (arnica); hydrotherapy; diet, exercise, and lifestyle changes; plus a host of other alternatives that may or may not include use of herbals, have come to earn the testimony of millions who have used them over the centuries and found relief. Chapter 25 discusses many of the remedies that have been recorded for centuries and, according to the ancient writings of the Greeks, Phoenicians, Egyptians, Native Americans, Persians, Hebrews, and others, bring relief from pain. Still today, herbs like boswellia, bromelain, cayenne pepper, devil's claw, ginger and ginger tea, glucosamine, licorice root, tumeric, and white willow bark remain as popular remedies for relief of chronic pain, even though they may take days to weeks to bring that relief.

Implications for Special Populations

Pregnancy Implications

When prescribing any drugs, clinicians should carefully consider their choices as they relate to their assigned FDA Safety Category.

FDA SAFETY CATEGORY	DRUGS
B	acetaminophen, naloxone (Narcan), nalmefene (Revex), NSAIDs (e.g., ibuprofen) in first trimester
C	aspirin, nalbuphine (Nubain), morphine, fentanyl morphine (Dilaudid), meperidine (Demerol), codeine (Tylenol with codeine), oxycodone (OxyContin, Percocet), hydrocodone (Vicodin, Lortab), fentanyl (Duragesic), methadone (Dolophine), methylnaltrexone (Relistor), naltrexone (ReVia), tramadol (Ultram), tapentadol (Nucynta), ziconotide (Prialt)

Pediatric Implications

Children and teenagers under the age of 16 (FDA recommendation) should avoid aspirin when used to relieve fever or symptoms of a virus. Additionally, NSAIDS use should also be avoided in children and young people under 16 but liquid ibuprofen (bubble-gum flavor 100mg/5ml suspension; $7.50 for 8 oz) has found common use among pediatrician's recommendations and in institutionalized children where expert medical supervision is available.

Geriatric Implications

Older adults should not take large doses of NSAIDs for long periods of time nor should they take them more frequently than prescribed because there is a danger of nephrotoxicity if they have any decline in liver function. Older adults also may have slowed liver metabolism of many drugs resulting in higher blood plasma levels of drug than anticipated or healthy. By 2014 FDA regulations will cause changes in prescription combinations of acetaminophen and opiates such that these products will contain no more than 325 mg acetaminophen per dose unit.

LEARNING EXERCISES

Case 1

IP, a 50-year-old white female, has worsening pain associated with her ovarian cancer. She rates the pain 8/10, aching in her lower abdomen despite hydrocodone/APAP 10/325, every 4 hours. Her last bowel movement was 2 days ago and was difficult to pass. You want to convert her to a sustained-release preparation of morphine and continue her other medication for breakthrough pain.

1. **Write a prescription for the morphine SR that takes into account her current use of hydrocodone.**

    Rx: _____

    #: _____

    Sig: _____

2. **How did you decide on your dosing of morphine SR?**

3. **Based upon the history given, what side effect of the morphine will you be most concerned about?**

4. **When would you like to see her again?**

Case 2

SM, a 32-year-old male, is seen in follow-up for his chronic low back pain, which until recently had been controlled with hydrocodone. The pain began to worsen after he worked in his yard, and he now has lancinating, tingling, burning pain down the left leg, rated 7/10. He has tried some naproxen in addition to his hydrocodone with mild benefit. The pain is keeping him awake at night.

1. **What are some other nonopioid options that may help with this patient's pain?**

2. **Why did you select this medication?**

3. **What precautions would you give him regarding the medication you selected?**

References

American Medical Association. (2003). Pathophysiology of pain and pain assessment. www.amacmeonline.com/pain_mgmt/printversion/ama_painmgmt_m1.pdf

American Pain Foundation. (October, 2008). A reporter's guide: Covering pain and its management. www.painfoundation.org/learn/publications/files/reporters-guide.pdf

American Pain Society. (2008). *Principles of analgesic use in the treatment of acute and cancer pain* (6th ed.) Skokie, IL: American Pain Society.

American Pain Society. (April, 2011a). Pediatric Chronic Pain: A Position Statement. www.ampainsoc.org/advocacy/pediatric.htm

American Pain Society. (2011b). Pediatric Chronic Pain. www.ampainsoc.org/advocacy/pediatric.htm

Centers for Disease Control and Prevention (CDC). (2006). New Report Finds Pain Affects Millions of Americans. Retrieved March 9, 2013, from www.cdc.gov/nchs/pressroom/06facts/hus06.htm

Gallagher, R. M. (2005). Rational integration of pharmacologic, behavioral, and rehabilitation strategies in the treatment of chronic pain. *American Journal of Physical Medicine and Rehabilitation, 84*(Suppl. 3), S64-76.

Kreplick, L. W., & Tarabar, A. (December, 2010). Salicylate Toxicity in Emergency Medicine. Medscape Reference. Retrieved March 10, 2013, from http://emedicine.medscape.com/article/818242-overview

McCaffrey, M., & Beebe, A. (1989). *Pain: Clinical manual for nursing practice* (p. 4). Toronto: The C.V. Mosby Company.

Pas, S. (2006). Prevalence of Americans suffering from pain. *US Pharmacist* (5), 211.

Solomon, D. H., Rassen, J. A., Glynn, R. T., Lee, J., Levin, R., Schneeweiss, S. (2010a). The Comparative Safety of Analgesics in Older Adults with Arthritis. *Arch. Int. Med. 170*(22):1968-1978.

Solomon, D. H., Rassen, J. A., Glynn, R. T., Garneau, K., Levin, R., Lee, J., et al. (2010b). The Comparative Safety of Opioids for Non-malignant Pain in Older Adults. *Arch. Int. Med. 170*(22) 1979-1986.

The Integrative Medicine Pharmacopeia: Herbals, Vitamins, and Dietary Supplements

Roberta Weintraut, Monique Davis-Smith

CHAPTER FOCUS

This chapter introduces common, naturally sourced dietary supplements, including botanicals (herbals) and vitamins, and reviews their risks and benefits. With the growth of evidence-based integrative medicine, many health professionals are now trained to use herbals and other dietary supplements and include these in treatment plans along with more conventional medications. These products are also frequently used without medical advice by patients because dietary supplements are now widely available over the counter. Although an increasing body of evidence is available to the clinician to guide safe use of natural products, patients often rely on testimonials and unfiltered Internet resources to initiate supplement use. Even though natural products in many cases offer patients significant benefits, like conventional pharmaceuticals, they may also carry the risk of potential drug interactions or side effects. Thus, the conscientious clinician must have a working knowledge of commonly used herbals, vitamins, and supplements, and their interactions and side effect profiles.

This chapter also reviews the role of the FDA in dietary supplement regulation, including the Dietary Supplement and Health Education Act (DSHEA) of 1994, which broadened widespread availability of over-the-counter supplements.

OBJECTIVES

After reading and studying this chapter, the student should be able to:

1. Recall the usage, risks, and benefits associated with commonly used dietary supplements, including botanicals and vitamins.
2. Distinguish among alternative medicines, complementary medicines, integrative medicines, and phytomedicines.
3. State three general tactics that will help patients use alternative supplements correctly.
4. Recall the current federal safety and regulatory standards associated with supplements.
5. Describe the differences between the fat-soluble and water-soluble vitamins.
6. Describe the significant drug interactions that can occur between prescription medication and herbals.
7. Recall the uses and typical doses of common natural remedies in use today.
8. Name three commercial resources a clinician can use to research information about dietary supplements.

KEY HERBALS, VITAMINS, AND DIETARY SUPPLEMENTS USED IN THIS CHAPTER

Natural Product Adjuncts to Fight Infections
- echinacea
- cranberry juice
- elderberry
- vitamin C

Probiotics to Prevent Infections
- yogurt

Herbals for Menopause and Menstrual Disorders
- black cohosh
- dong quai
- red clover
- chaste tree berry
- evening primrose oil
- soy
- calcium and vitamin B_6

Herbals for Benign Prostate Hyperplasia (BPH)
- stinging nettle
- pumpkin seed
- saw palmetto
- pygeum

Supplements Used to Promote Well-Being
- panax ginseng
- American ginseng
- dehydroepiandrosterone (DHEA)
- ashwagandha

Supplements for Memory Enhancement/Cognitive Function
- ginkgo biloba
- docosahexaenoic acid (DHA)

Herbals for Reflux Esophagitis
- slippery elm
- deglycyrrhizinated licorice (DGL)

Herbals for Nausea
- ginger
- caffeine

Herbals for Bloating and Flatulence
- fennel
- caraway seed

Herbs for Intestinal Cramping
- chamomile
- peppermint oil

Herbals for Constipation
- aloe vera latex
- triphylla
- senna
- cascara
- konjac glucomannan
- phosphorus/phosphate

Herbals for Diarrhea
- black and green tea
- cinnamon
- rhubarb
- probiotics for acute diarrhea (*Lactobacillus, Saccharomyces boulardii*)
- zinc

Supplements for Sleep and Sedation
- melatonin
- valerian
- chamomile
- hops

Herbals for Anxiety
- passion flower
- kava kava

Supplements for Depression
- St. John's wort
- SAM-e
- saffron

Herbals for Arthritis
- chondroitin/glucosamine
- methylsulfonylmethane (MSM)
- turmeric
- ginger
- omega 3-fatty acids (fish oil, alpha linoleic acid)
- borage seed

Herbals for Erectile Dysfunction
- yohimbe
- American ginseng

Supplements to Prevent or Mitigate Headache
- feverfew
- riboflavin
- magnesium
- butterbur
- caffeine
- topical peppermint oil

Herbals to Improve Glycemic Control
- cinnamon
- alpha-lipoic acid
- konjac glucomannan
- Beta-glucanase

Supplements to Improve Lipids
- omega-3 fish oils
- olive oil
- red rice yeast
- phytosterols
- guar gum
- garlic
- niacin

Herbs for Wounds and Burns
- aloe vera
- tea tree oil

Natural Supplement Adjuncts to Prevent Cancer
- melatonin
- omega-3 oils
- ashwagandha
- cruciferous vegetables

Food Supplements and Vitamins

Fat-Soluble Vitamins
- vitamin A
- vitamin D
- vitamin E
- vitamin K

Water-Soluble Vitamins
- vitamin B_1
- vitamin B_2
- vitamin B_3
- vitamin B_6
- vitamin B_9
- vitamin B_{12}

Natural products are used for a wide variety of indications in current practice, and especially in the growing field of integrative medicine. For many patients, they are a reasonable alternative to conventional pharmaceuticals. For example, a patient may choose to use cranberry juice as a preventative for recurring *Escherichia coli* urinary tract infections (UTI) instead of using low-dose sulfa drugs. For some patients, integrative treatment plans include using natural products to amplify the benefits of conventional therapy, such as adding cinnamon to a regimen including glyburide for a diabetic patient. For others, integrative practice uses dietary supplements to decrease the toxicity of necessary conventional drugs, such as adding coenzyme Q10 (CoQ10) to a regimen that includes a statin for a patient with hyperlipidemia.

When use them conscientiously and cautiously, natural product offer low-risk enhancement to conventional prescription therapy. However, two challenges to the conscientious clinician may occur with natural product use by patients. First, many patients erroneously believe that natural substances are inherently safer than a synthetic drug and thus may risk delaying definitive conventional therapy. This results in an opportunity cost—a loss of health resulting from delay in care—for example, by delaying conventional surgery or chemotherapy for cancer. Although supplements may be used to relieve a patient's symptoms during cancer therapy, thereby keeping the treatment course on track, there is no herbal cure for cancer! The second challenge is that out of fear or embarrassment, nearly half of patients using dietary supplements do not tell their clinician that they are using both conventional medicines and dietary supplements. Testimonials from family, friends, the media, and on the Internet influence patient choice of supplement use. The wide availability of these products in grocery stores, large retail chains, and even gyms fosters patient empowerment to select supplements to promote health and manage symptoms. With this empowerment, however, not all patients have acquired sufficient health literacy to recognize the risks as well as the benefits of these supplements. The conscientious clinician who is supportive of recommending integrative treatment plans will recognize these potential challenges and also keep patient-centered communication with his/her patients open and nonjudgmental. This is because patients turning to alternative therapies often do so because they have found conventional treatments ineffective or have experienced adverse effects.

Defining Alternative, Complementary, and Integrative Medicine

In this chapter the term **integrative medicine** is used to refer to the combination of conventional pharmaceutical therapy with evidence-based use of natural products in designing treatment plans for patients. This term is reflective of a progression from the traditional terms *alternative* and *complementary* medicine used over the last two decades and often referred to as CAM.

Complementary and Alternative Medicine (CAM)

Alternative medicine is defined as medicine that is not conventionally taught in medical schools. It customarily includes a wide range of therapies, including herbal therapy, megavitamins, acupuncture, alternative systems of medicine such as Ayurveda, and many mind-body therapies.

As more research and information have been accumulated regarding their use, some alternative therapies are now mainstreamed into conventional therapeutics (e.g., Lamaze techniques, use of fish oil, etc.) and are no longer considered to be alternative. Therapies that continue to be used only as alternatives may include those that may have no evidence in science, or even those that have been disproved or are regarded as unsafe. Alternative practitioners may include nonphysicians whose standards of training and licensure requirements vary from state to state.

The terms *complementary medicine* and *alternative medicine* are often used together and are known as complementary and alternative medicine, or CAM. However, **complementary medicine** is generally considered the use of alternative medications *within* or alongside conventional medical practice. Using complementary medicine, a clinician may prescribe a regimen that includes fish oil supplements, a conventional statin by prescription, and COQ10 for hypertriglyceridemia. In some cases, a clinician may work in partnership with a provider of alternative therapy, such as an orthopedist working with a licensed acupuncturist to manage fibromyalgia.

Integrative Medicine

Integrative medicine seeks to combine the best of conventional therapy with evidence-based alternative therapeutics. It is patient-centered and incorporates recognition of the role of the "body, mind and spirit" in wellness and disease. An integrative clinician may include a low-glycemic diet, cinnamon, metformin, aerobic exercise, and mindfulness meditation in caring for a patient with type 2 diabetes.

Clinicians who also complete postgraduate work in the integrative medicine use of natural herbs and supplements develop a broad pharmacopeia that includes natural products and conventional pharmaceuticals. Typically, clinicians trained in integrative medicine use natural products that have evidence of efficacy based on extensive usage and peer-reviewed studies. Because of their competency with dietary supplements and natural products, integrative medicine clinicians often serve as consultants for both specialists and primary care clinicians. For those interested in CAM and integrative medicine, the National Center for Complementary and Alternative Medicine (NCCAM) conducts and supports research, trains CAM researchers, and provides information about CAM. Additionally, the NCCAM offers 10 video lectures with CME credits free to nurses and physicians as part of its CAM online lecture series.

Defining Dietary Supplements

Several types of **dietary supplements** are commonly used. These include herbal (botanical) medicines, vitamin therapy, biologically based supplements, and homeopathic remedies.

Botanical Medicines

Botanical medicines (or **phytomedicines**) include preparations of whole herbs, herb parts (root, rhizome, flower, leaf, seed or stem), or extracts of herbs. In traditional Western and Ayurvedic herbal supplement use, plants are used in dosages of milligrams to grams, sometime singly or in combination with a few other herbs. In traditional Chinese medicine, these same herbs are used in much smaller doses, and in combination with a multitude of other herbs. When reviewing a patient's botanical or herbal usage, the conscientious prescriber should carefully note the type of product used. When properly labeled, the herbal supplement should include the common and botanical names of the herbs; the part used (root, leaf, etc.); the extraction ratio and solvent (if an extract); the amount in each capsule or tablet; usual dosage; and contact information for the manufacturer. These botanicals should be routinely evaluated as part of the medication review on each patient visit.

Vitamin Therapy

Vitamin therapy is widely used in both conventional and integrative treatment plans. Multivitamin supplements are routinely used to minimize the risk of vitamin deficiency in at-risk populations such as pregnant patients or dieters. Single vitamin supplements may be necessary when specific deficiencies are noted. Integrative medicine providers often prescribe specific vitamin therapy to correct deficiencies resulting from malabsorption, intestinal dysbiosis, and pharmaceutical depletion. For example, metformin causes vitamin B_{12} deficiency and can produce neuropathy in diabetic patients. Clinicians prescribing metformin, then, will recommend prophylactic vitamin B_{12} therapy. The conscientious clinician will also review the patient's use of vitamins for excess use of potentially toxic vitamins, particularly vitamin A.

Biologically Based Therapies

Biologically based therapies include nonbotanical, nonvitamin supplements such as fish oil, glucosamine, and melatonin. These products are generally available in single or combination forms. Dose ranges for specific supplements may vary widely, as does risk of drug-supplement interaction.

Homeopathic Remedies

Homeopathic remedies are prepared according to the homeopathic *law of minimum*, or principle of *least dosing*. The selection of the remedy is not based solely on its accurate homeopathic use but also on its dosing. The homeopathic remedy is designed for a gentle effect, using drugs in a process called potentiation or dilution. Homeopathic remedies are prepared by making a series of 1:10 dilutions of an active ingredient, which may be a plant, mineral, or animal part. A 1:10 dilution is labeled 1X. A *potentiated dilution* of this 1X dilution is made by taking an aliquot of the 1X and further diluting it 1:10, thus making a 2X dilution. In homeopathic therapy, the most potent remedy is the most dilute, and beyond the 24X dilution, it will not even contain Avogadro's number of the remedy's named active substance.

The use of homeopathic remedies is generally safe. Because active ingredients in these remedies are extensively diluted, no risk of allergic reaction or drug interaction is found unless the homeopathic remedy is combined with measurable amounts of other supplements. Pure homeopathic remedies have been regulated as OTC drugs since the 1920s and therefore meet federal quality, purity, and safety standards.

When reviewing a patient's dietary supplement usage, whether botanical, vitamin, biologic, or homeopathic, a standardized reference such as Natural Medicines Comprehensive Database, a pharmaceutical collaborative on dietary supplements offering the latest updates on natural medicine, is useful (Jellin et al., 2000). It is available as a book or as an online subscription, and many hospitals and medical schools offer group access.

Regulation of Dietary Supplements

The manufacture of nonhomeopathic dietary supplements, including botanicals and biologically based supplements is regulated in the United States by the FDA. In general, this regulation includes the Dietary Supplement and Health Education Act (1994), the Medwatch surveillance system, and generally recognized as safe (GRAS) status determination.

The **Dietary Supplement and Health Education Act (DSHEA)** was passed in 1994 as a first step in the federal regulation of dietary supplement manufacturing. At the time, it guaranteed availability to the consumer of all dietary supplements on the market as of October 1994. Although it required label accuracy, it did not guarantee safety, efficacy, or purity of products sold. It permitted a claim on bodily structure and function, but disallowed claims of treatment or cure for disease. Specifically, each supplement is also required to carry the following wording on its label: "This product has not been evaluated by the FDA. This product is not intended to diagnose, treat, cure or prevent any disease." Supplements brought to the market after October 1994 were subject to the more rigorous safety and efficacy standards of OTC medications. The Final Rule of DSHEA (2007) requires that dietary supplement manufacturers follow good manufacturing practices. This now provides a modicum of consumer protection because it encourages better product quality in dietary supplement manufacture. It is important to remember that the FDA is a regulatory agency and has no enforcement capabilities. When violations of DSHEA are noted, it is generally the Federal Trade Commission (FTC) that enforces these regulations. The FTC also regulates dietary supplement advertising and enforces fraudulent advertising regulations.

The FDA *Medwatch Reporting System* is used by clinicians to report suspected adverse events caused by dietary supplements, just as it is used to report adverse events caused by conventional pharmaceuticals. Although the DSHEA does not include FDA evaluation of individual supplement premarket safety, upon receipt of MedWatch reports from clinicians in postmarket experience the FDA may convene an investigatory panel to evaluate risks of a suspect supplement. If evidence of clear patient risk is noted, the FDA may ban the supplement from the market or further regulate available dosage forms.

When a substance has been found through a long history of common usage to be safely consumed as a food substance, it may be granted **generally recognized as safe (GRAS)** status by the FDA. Many herbals and spices meet these criteria. It is important to distinguish that use as a food flavoring, for instance, may differ substantially in amount and route from use of the same substance as an alternative medication. Cinnamon, for instance, has GRAS status as a spice used in food flavoring, but it is generally used in much higher doses for medicinal purposes. GRAS therefore confers a degree of comfort with a given substance, but does not preclude possible significant side effects or drug interactions at these medicinal doses.

Dietary supplements, when used medicinally, pose several unique safety concerns, including inherent toxicity, contamination, and drug interactions. Inherent toxicities may include hepatotoxic chemicals, such as pyrrolizidine alkaloids, safrole, etc., that are components of the plant itself. Careful review of the safety profile of the supplement should be included in the evaluation for use by a patient, regardless of the assumption of safety. Contamination is a potential risk for all supplements because regulation of quality and purity is less rigorous for supplements than for prescription medications. Contamination with heavy metals, toxins, bacteria, fungi, other botanicals, and even prescription medications has been found in supplements sold in the United States. Although such contamination is unusual, patients should be cautioned to choose products that are produced in the United States by well-known supplement manufacturers. Products that meet United States Pharmacopeia or Consumer Lab independent testing laboratory standards are preferred when possible.

Drug interactions with dietary supplements are common. These may be trivial or life threatening, as in the case of transplant failure when St. John's wort is used with posttransplant immune suppressants. Some supplement-drug interactions vary depending on the mode of preparation of a supplement. Licorice, for instance, may be prepared in a deglycyrrhizinated form, which contains little glycyrrhizinic acid and few drug interactions. When this chemical is not removed, licorice use produces hypokalemia, which can have serious interactions with digoxin. Drug interactions should be routinely reviewed when evaluating a patient's medical regimen, and patients should be cautioned not to add or change supplements without reviewing possible interactions with their clinician. Adverse events from dietary supplement use should be reported to the FDA using the FDAs MedWatch Safety and Adverse Event Reporting System and FDA form 3500.

Conscientious Use of Natural and Alternative Medicines

Patients are often hesitant to discuss their use of dietary supplements and alternative therapies with their clinician. Some fear that the provider will be angry with them or lecture them on the evils of such therapies. Owing to this fear, many times a patient's medical chart and drug history is incomplete because the patient withholds vital information from the clinician. This can lead to serious drug-to-drug interactions or even devastating illnesses such as liver or kidney failure.

It is important that clinicians establish a rapport with their patients that allows the patient to share this information freely and to ask questions. First, always ask nonjudgmentally about any vitamins, tonics, or other supplements a patient may be using to keep healthy. Framing their use in acceptable terms allows patients a comfort level in revealing use. Do not assume the supplement is good or bad, right or wrong for the patient until the exact supplement and patient scenario are fully evaluated. Let the patient know there are potential benefits and risks with each supplement and that these can be evaluated. Congratulate the patient on making choices for better health, even if it is necessary to encourage the patient to change the use of supplements.

Review each supplement and the conventional medicine list of the patient. Review goals of care, cultural and social preferences, and patient literacy. Assess the safety and appropriateness of each supplement individually, keeping in mind drug interaction, cost, and evidence. If there is minimal risk and likelihood of benefit, encourage use. If risk is minimal and benefit is potential, patients may be able to decide themselves. Often, patients will bring in several supplements, of which one or two

are inappropriate. Commend the patient on those that are good choices, and explain the reasoning behind discontinuing the inappropriate ones. Often the phrase "each patient is unique, and in your individual case I would not recommend this supplement" allows the patient to understand that the choice is in his or her best interest.

Clinicians should educate themselves and their patients about the dietary supplements patients are taking. Private and public Web-based resources are updated frequently and are more helpful than outdated print-only resources. Private resources charge user fees but many larger hospitals and clinics maintain site licenses. Public resources are less encyclopedic, but are also available for patient use, so may be used for patient education. It is best practice to become familiar with the public resources and establish familiarity with any private resources that may be available at the local medical facilities.

Three widely used commercial resources are available to the clinicians seeking to research a question asked by a patient about alternative medicines. These include the following:

1. *Natural Medicines Comprehensive Database:* The Natural Medicines Comprehensive Database is an encyclopedic source of information on natural medicines, brand name products, and ingredients. It is created by teams of pharmaceutical experts at The Therapeutic Center and is available in print, electronic, and Web-based formats (www.naturaldatabase.com/nd/products.aspx).

2. *Natural Standard:* This site was founded by clinicians and researchers to provide high-quality, evidence-based information about complementary and alternative therapies. This international multidisciplinary collaboration now includes contributors from more than 100 eminent academic institutions (www.naturalstandard.com).

3. *Consumer Laboratory:* ConsumerLab provides independent testing results online about vitamins, supplements, and nutrition products to consumers and clinicians (www.consumerlab.com).

Three highly respected public databases and resources also exist for the health professional to use to gain a better understanding of complementary and alternative medicines.

1. *National Center for Complementary and Alternative Medicine* (NCCAM): This is a U.S. government agency specifically dedicated to exploring complementary and alternative healing practices and provides an authoritative resource and knowledge base for professionals and patients (http://nccam.nih.gov).

2. *Office of Dietary Supplements* (ODS): Located within the National Institutes of Health (NIH), the ODS supports research and disseminates research results in the area of dietary supplements. It also provides advice to other federal agencies regarding the use and manufacture of vitamins. Clinicians have access to its online searchable database of scientific literature (http://dietary-supplements.info.nih.gov).

3. *MD Anderson Cancer Center.* MD Anderson Cancer Center sponsors CIMER, the Complementary/Integrative

Medicine Education Resource, free for physician and patient use. This site includes an extensive database of dietary supplements as well as other alternative practices. Web access is available at the CIMER link at www.mdanderson.org.

A GUIDE TO COMMONLY USED HERBALS AND SUPPLEMENTS

Today, the use of dietary supplements in the United States is thriving and growing. In 2007 a government survey found that 38% of adults had used natural products during the past year, but that number climbs to over 70% if multivitamins are included (NCCAM, 2011). It is important that all clinicians have a working knowledge of the practice of using botanicals and other dietary supplements in therapeutic treatment plans. This is because they are likely to encounter patients who use them and colleagues who prescribe or promote them.

Herbals Used for Infections: Echinacea, Cranberry Juice, Elderberry

Conscientious prescribing for infections mandates that the following be considered as adjuncts to conventional medications. Because there is no current conventional drug therapy for the common cold, Echinacea offers treatment not otherwise available. Cranberry may be used to help prevent infection, especially *Helicobacter pylori*, and should be considered for use in combination with conventional drugs for prophylaxis treatment of urinary tract infections. Elderberry can reduce the severity of influenza, but is best considered as an adjunct for influenza therapy. Use of reliable antivirals and antibiotics should not be deferred or delayed when employing these supplements.

Echinacea (Echinacea purpurea, Echinacea angustifolia, Echinacea pallida)

Echinacea is the common term used to represent the botanical supplements derived from three different species: *E. purpurea*, *E. angustifolia*, and *E. pallida*. These also are known popularly by the term *purple coneflower* and are native American wildflowers. All three species contain moieties that produce a stimulation of immune system response, although varying degrees of this stimulation are found in the roots and aerial parts of the three species. Most common supplements contain *E. purpurea* or *E. angustifolia* root extract or whole herb.

Echinacea is generally used as a stimulant to enhance the immune response to a viral illness and thus is used both as a preventative of upper respiratory infections and as a treatment. Use of 1 to 3 grams a day for 3 days taken at onset of illness stimulates an increase in production of interferons and interleukins, which in turn limits spread of viral infection and shortens the duration of illness modestly. This herb may be reasonably used to shorten the duration of a mild viral illness such as a cold, but should be avoided during a severe viral illness that has already produced high interleukin and interferon levels, such as influenza. Side effects may include low-grade malaise as interferon levels rise.

Drug interactions are rare because of limited induction of cytochrome P450 3A4 in rare patients. This herb should also be avoided during pregnancy (safety data is absent), by patients with autoimmune disease, and by HIV patients or others with high risk for lymphoproliferative disorders (safety data are absent for these subgroups), as well as by patients with ragweed allergy.

Cranberry (Vaccinium macrocarpon)

Cranberry fruit juice and cranberry extract are used to prevent infection in the oral cavity, urinary tract, and skin surrounding stoma sites. Vaccinia species contain proanthocyanidins and flavonols, which neutralize the ability of *E. coli* pili to attach to urothelium and skin, thereby actively limiting the ability of *E. coli* to invade the urinary tract and skin surrounding stoma sites. These moieties also have bacteriostatic effects on oral *diphtheroid* populations and *Klebsiella* and *Pseudomonas* species. Regular intake of cranberry low-sugar juices reduces the incidence of both oral caries and urinary tract infections in nursing home populations. Cranberry is generally very well tolerated, and some people like its tart taste. Drug interactions with warfarin are theoretical, but have not been noted even with very large doses of the juice. Adverse side effects of nausea and diarrhea have been noted at doses of 3 L daily. Effective doses of juice in studies range from 15 mL twice daily to 300 mL daily of cranberry juice cocktail with 26% cranberry, or 400 mg twice daily of encapsulated dried cranberry fruit. For oral health, sugar-free juice is more effective than encapsulated or sugar-containing formulas.

Elderberry (Sambucus nigra)

Elderberry fruit is used in a syrup-based extract as an adjunct to treat influenza. The active ingredients include flavonoid anthocyanidins as well as the lectin *Sambucus nigra* agglutinin IVf and salicylic acid. These anthocyanidins produce a mild anti-inflammatory effect and a mild immunomodulating effect, increasing production of cytokines and interleukins as well as tumor necrosis factor. In addition, agglutinin IVf and the anthocyanidins bind hemagglutinins associated with influenza A and B, and limit viral replication. When used for 3 to 5 days, elderberry extract syrup in a dose of 15 mL four times daily in adults, twice daily in children, significantly reduces the duration of influenza symptoms. Elderberry is well tolerated and is also used in jellies and wines. Unripe and raw fruit is toxic, however, and produces diarrhea, nausea, and dizziness, so patients should not use fresh elderberry juice.

Dosing of Herbals Used to Fight Infections

Common Name	Active Agent	Indication	Common Dose for Adults
Echinacea (Purple coneflower)	E. purpurea, E. angustifolia, E. pallida	Enhance immune system	1–3 gm/day
Cranberry juice	V. macrocarpon	Bacteriostatic for UTA	15 mL, 2 times/day
Elderberry	S. nigra	Adjunct treatment for influenza	15 mL, 4 times/day of extract syrup for 3–5 days

Probiotics Used to Fight Infections

Probiotics are live microorganisms that help maintain the natural balance of the microflora in the gastrointestinal tract. Probiotics such as *Streptococcus thermophilus* and *Lactobacillus bulgaricus* in fermented milk have been used for millennia. Research has shown that probiotics are beneficial in some diseases, with viable bacteria having favor over nonviable bacteria. Most commercially available probiotics are made from human strains of *Bifidobacterium or Lactobacillus* species. Nonbacterial microorganisms such as yeasts from the genus saccharomyces are also used in commercial products.

Probiotics are used for ailments ranging from simple upset stomach, to gastritis, to antibiotic-induced diarrhea, and inflammatory bowel disease. They are sold as food supplements rather than herbals, medicines, or pharmaceuticals, often in yogurt-type products, although they can be acquired in capsule form. Sepsis is the greatest concern with probiotic use, but research indicates that probiotic-induced sepsis occurs only in patients who have a compromised immune system, especially premature infants, or a preexisting condition such as a short intestine. Probiotics are generally safe in healthy people, but the results will vary from patient to patient and from disease to disease.

Herbals Used for Menopause and Menstrual Disorders

Dietary supplements used for menopause and premenstrual syndrome (PMS) may include phytoestrogens, although black cohosh is now thought to activate serotonin receptors. Patients often choose these supplements instead of conventional hormonal medications. Particular care should be taken to review the safety of these commonly used herbals for patients with breast cancer.

Black Cohosh

Black cohosh, also known as bugbane, is *Cimicifuga (Actaea) racemosa*. This herb has been used for centuries for mood disorder and hot flushes, and is now thought to have activity at the $5\text{-}HT_7$ serotonin receptor. (Note that the $5\text{-}HT_7$ receptor is a member of the superfamily cell receptors known as G-Protein-Coupled Receptors (GPCRs) which are activated by serotonin, the neurotransmitter. Once activated a cascade of events is induced by the $5\text{-}HT_7$ receptor which result in thermoregulation, circadian rhythm, learning, memory, sleep, and mood regulation.)

Ongoing NIH studies indicate little if any effect by black cohosh at estrogen receptors, so this herb should not generally be considered a phytoestrogen. The use of 40 to 160 mg per day results in reduction of hot flushes in many women, although German Commission E safety data includes safe usage of up to 200 mg per day for up to 6 months. This herb will not reverse vaginal atrophy and does not improve bone density, but it does offer improvement in mood, night sweats, and sleep disturbance in addition to hot flush relief. In doses used for hot flushes, black cohosh does not cause the anorgasmia seen with other serotonin activity modulators. Few side effects are reported, and drug interactions are generally unseen. There is a putative inhibition of cytochrome P450 2D6, although human case reports are lacking. However, the NIH has reported several cases of liver toxicity involving black cohosh, which have now led to warning labels regarding possible hepatotoxicity in several countries (NIH, 2011). These reports have been difficult to substantiate, and in many cases, actual identification of the herb itself is lacking. Best practice is to consider black cohosh for the patient with menopausal dysphoria and hot flushes, establish normal baseline liver function, and monitor liver function periodically while the patient is using the herb. In terms of alternate supplements or pharmaceuticals used to relieve these symptoms, black cohosh has a superior safety and side effect profile.

Dong Quai *(Angelica sinensis)*

Dong quai is found in many products used for PMS, dysmenorrhea, and menopause. Its constituents include ferulic acid and ligusticide, as well as many coumarins and safrole, which confer anti-inflammatory and antiplatelet effects. Few large studies support effectiveness for PMS or menopausal complaints; however, a few animal studies show anti-inflammatory and antispasmodic activity that may reduce dysmenorrhea. Doses of 3 to 6 gm daily have been used. Adverse effects of dong quai include an increase in menstrual blood loss and photosensitivity. Phytoestrogenic activity has also been noted. The safety of dong quai in patients at high risk of breast cancer is unknown; however, the herb has been noted to increase breast cancer cell line growth in vitro and should be avoided by patients with breast cancer. Drug interaction with warfarin and toxic international normalized ratio (INR) elevations has been reported with customarily used doses.

Red Clover *(Trifolium pratense)*

Red clover is a phytoestrogen marketed primarily for hot flushes. Red clover's effect on breast tissue does not seem to increase tissue density, but it should be used cautiously by patients with breast cancer and those at high risk for breast cancer because few studies demonstrate safety in this group (Geller et al., 2009). As a treatment for menopause, red clover should be considered second line after failure of black cohosh. If a patient is not a good candidate for HT owing to an estrogen-sensitive tumor, an alternative for red clover use should be considered. Usual doses range from 40 to 160 mg daily. Although many theoretical effects on levels of drugs metabolized through the cytochrome P450 system have been suggested, none have been reported in humans at this time. Both procoagulant and anticoagulant activity have been attributed to red clover in case reports. Patients should discontinue use of red clover 10 to 14 days prior to elective surgery.

Chaste Tree Berry *(Vitex agnus castus)*

Chaste tree berry is commonly found in PMS and menopause remedies. The active ingredients are unclear, with multiple ingredients possibly contributing to its actions. Chaste tree berry has been noted to bind to dopaminergic receptors as well as to estrogen receptors, making it a phytoestrogen. Theoretically, dopaminergic suppression of prolactin contributes to improved leutenizing hormone (LH) production, which in turn modulates PMS and perimenopausal symptoms connected with luteal phase function. For PMS and mild premenstrual dysphoric disorder, chaste tree berry provides relief of mood symptoms as well as relief of breast tenderness and bloating. The usual dose is 500 mg per day of the berry, with extracts containing standardized extracts of agnuside and casticin dosed at 40 to 80 mg per day. Because the exact nature of the phytoestrogen effect on breast tissue is unclear, chaste tree berry should generally not be used by patients with breast cancer. The dopaminergic agonist/antagonist effect of the herb may also interact with pharmaceuticals modulating the dopaminergic system, and patients taking them should avoid it.

Evening Primrose Oil (Oenothera biennis)

Evening primrose oil (EPO) is commonly found in PMS and menopausal remedies. Its active constituent is thought to be gamma-linolenic acid, which reduces interleukin production, and produces anti-inflammatory effects. EPO is effective in reducing mastalgia associated with PMS, but has limited data for efficacy in menopause. Dosage range is 2 to 4 gm daily, with lower doses effective in reducing arthritis pain, and higher doses used for mastalgia or PMS. EPO is usually well tolerated with occasional side effects of nausea. Due to the effect on the arachidonic acid cascade, EPO may interfere with platelet aggregation at high doses and should not be used with anticoagulant therapy. Evidence for estrogenic action is mixed, with both inhibition and stimulation of breast cancer cell lines noted and potentiation of some forms of chemotherapy also noted. EPO should be used by patients with breast cancer only under supervision of a physician familiar with the specific effect of the supplement on the chemotherapy regimen used by the patient.

Soy (Glycine max)

Soybeans have been a dietary mainstay for centuries, and soy is generally well tolerated as a protein source. Lifelong soy food intake historically correlates well with lower risk of breast cancer, menopausal symptoms, and osteoporosis. Soy isolates have been used in PMS and menopausal formulas because of their phytoestrogen content as well, and they may provide relief of hot flushes in the menopause. Two isoflavones, genistein and daidzein, are widely included in soy isolate products. These are converted in up to 50% of women to more potent estrogen compounds (including equol). Variable results of soy trials are thought to be due to variations in equol conversion among different women. Side effects include occasional nausea and bloating. In patients with iodine deficiency, excessive use of soy may cause hypothyroidism. Usual dose of soy dietary protein to control hot flushes is 20 to 40 gm daily. Drug interactions are rare, although when used with tamoxifen, theoretical concern exist that the soy may preferentially bind to estrogen receptors, thus blocking the full effect of tamoxifen from occurring. Therefore, soy use should be limited to occasional dietary protein sources (1 to 2 weekly) for patients with breast cancer using estrogen receptor antagonists.

Dosing of Common Herbals for Menopause and Menstrual Disorders

Common Name	Active Ingredient	Indication	Adult Dose
Black cohosh (bugbane)	C. (Actaea) racemosa	Reduce hot flushes*	40–60 mg/day
Dong quai	A. sinensi	Dysmenorrhea	3–6 gm/day
Red clover	T. pratense	Hot flush	40–60 mg/day
Chaste tree berry	V. agnus castus	PMS	500 mg/day
Evening primrose oil	O. biennius	PMS	3–4 gm/day
Soy	Glycine max	Hot flushes	20–40 gm/day

*Hot flushes/flashes are the most frequent symptom of menopause. They manifest as a sudden mild wave of heat on the upper part of the body that lasts from 30 seconds to a few minutes.

Herbals Used for Benign Prostate Hyperplasia (BPH)

Herbals for BPH have mixed efficacy, with saw palmetto the best studied and with the most benefit noted. Many formulations of mixed herbals are available. Patients should be cautioned to avoid use if they have a history of undiagnosed prostate symptoms or prostate cancer.

Stinging Nettle (Uritica dioica)

Stinging nettle is in some compound products used for BPH, usually in compounds that include saw palmetto. The mechanism of action appears to be anti-inflammatory, with multiple ingredients including vitamin C and beta sitosterol conferring possible ability to decrease prostate hyperplasia. Diuretic effects are also noted, and some patients experience lowered blood pressure with prolonged use of the product. Adverse effects include nausea, diarrhea, and skin irritation. There are potential drug interactions with warfarin, hypoglycemic agents, antihypertensives, and sedatives. Compounds with saw palmetto generally contain 120 mg per dose of stinging nettle.

Pumpkin Seed Extract (Cucurbita pepo) or Pumpin Seed Oil (curcurbotacin)

Pumpkin seed oil is occasionally used for BPH, either as a single agent or in combination with stinging nettle and saw palmetto. The oil contains omega-3 fatty acids, phytosterols, as well as carotenoid moieties and the enzyme acyl-CoA oxidase. The primary action appears to be diuretic, with usual doses of 480 mg per day used in combination formulas. Pumpkin seed as a food source is generally well tolerated.

Saw Palmetto (Serenoa repens)

Serenoa repens is primarily used for benign prostatic hypertrophy. This herb contains beta-sitosterol as well as other components with weak estrogen agonist/antagonist activity. Most importantly it is used as a 5-alpha reductase inhibitor, preventing the conversion of free testosterone to dihydrotestosterone (DHT) at the target tissue. In most instances this effect is used to shrink prostatic tissues, as is the case with BPH. A secondary usage is in the treatment of benign postmenopausal hirsutism. This herb should not be used by women of childbearing age due to the risk of damage during male fetal development. This botanical is generally well tolerated, with few side effects, primarily occasional nausea. There are no significant drug interactions reported; however, little data are available to predict the effect of long-term saw palmetto use on hormone-sensitive tissues beyond the simple effect of inhibition of DHT production. Saw palmetto may lower the baseline PSA. Men should have routine PSA screening before starting the herb, and routine follow-up to detect elevations during usage. Men with known prostate cancer should be cautioned not to use this herb because there is a theoretical risk that its use would mask PSA evidence of recurrence or spread of disease. Effective dose is generally considered to be 320 mg daily.

Pygeum (African Plum Tree)

Pygeum africanum is a 30- to 75-foot tree that grows in high altitudes in Africa and Central Asia. The bark of the tree has shown properties to reduce an enlarged prostate, which is speculated to be the result of its natural ingredient interfering with the binding sites for dihydrotestosterone. Although not studied as much as saw palmetto and nettle root, this agent increases urine flow by reducing the size of the prostate, and some believe that it improves sexual functioning. In areas were the tree grows, it is known by many names, including stinkwood or African plum, cherry, almond or plum, because its fruit is favored by gorillas.

Dosing of Herbals for Benign Prostate Hyperplasia

Common Name	Active Ingredient	Indication	Dosage
Stinging nettle	U. dioica	BPH	120 mg/day
Pumpkin seed	C. reponens semen	BPH	480 mg/day
Saw palmetto	S. repens	BPH	320 mg/day
Pygeum	Several phytosterols including beta-sitosterol and pentacyclic terpenes	BPH	100 mg/day in 6- to 8-week cycles

Herbals Used for Energy and Well-Being (Adaptogens)

Many patients choose the following herbals for energy and wellness. They are termed *adaptogens* because they may help patients adapt to their environmental stressors. Each should be used cautiously, and the conscientious clinician will determine if, in fact, they are being used inappropriately to cope with underlying illnesses such as depression, vitamin deficiency, or sleep disturbance, which may require additional therapy.

Ginseng (Panax)

Panax ginseng, and its botanical cousin, *Panax quinquefolius* (American ginseng), are two widely used adaptogenic herbals. They contain beta-sitosterol as well as multiple ginsenosides, which can produce measurable increases in adrenocorticotropic hormone, endothelial nitric oxide production, and decreases in blood glucose. These herbals are generally used as tonics for energy and have been recognized as having mild stimulant effects. They are used for the patient with easy fatigability after steroid taper, and are successfully used over 2 to 4 weeks to encourage adrenal recovery. However, they are often found in combination products with other stimulant botanicals, such as caffeine, bitter orange, and guarana, and are widely included in energy drinks and "pep pills" sold at truck stops.

Drug interactions with the panax botanicals include counteraction of antihypertensives and potentiation of hypoglycemic agents. Side effects are primarily nausea and insomnia, although anxiety and frank psychosis may also occur with prolonged usage or at higher doses. In general, side effects are more severe in younger patients, a phenomenon that has resulted in the recommendation by the German Commission E to limit its use to patients over 50 and for a maximum of 6 months. Some alteration of bleeding time is also noted as measured in platelet function assays. The usual dose of *Panax ginseng* is 200 mg daily.

Dehydroepiandrostenedione (DHEA)

Dehydroepiandrostenedione (DHEA) is used as an adrenal tonic by patients who complain of fatigue and generalized malaise. DHEA levels in humans decline gradually after mid-adulthood adrenopause, and DHEA has been used in an effort to promote patient stamina and energy levels. If dehydroepiandrosterone sulfate (DHEA-S) is measured to be low, replacement with DHEA often produces good clinical results, including resolution of poor libido and overall energy levels. Although generally well tolerated, at high doses mild hirsutism and dyslipidemia may occur with chronic use, and estrogenic potential precludes its use in those with breast cancer. Dose ranges from 10 to 25 mg daily in women to 50 to 100 mg per day in men. Conscientious clinicians monitor lipid levels, DHEA-S, and blood pressure periodically in all patients using DHEA.

Ashwagandha

Ashwagandha is an Indian botanical supplement commonly used as a general tonic and for well-being and energy. It contains several alkaloids and lactones, some of which are similar to those found in ginseng. In general, the root and berries are used medicinally, and have broad-ranging effects from sedation, to immunomodulation, to smooth muscle relaxation and thyroid stimulation. Ashwagandha is also used to assist recovery of bone marrow after chemotherapy regimens. Side effects are uncommon and consist mainly of gastrointestinal upset with high doses. Drug interactions with other sedating agents may result in enhanced sedative effects. Caution should also be used with immunomodulating drugs, because Ashwagandha may decrease desired immunosuppression. Thyroid-stimulating hormone should be monitored in patients taking thyroxine supplements when adding Ashwagandha. Patients should stop this medication 2-3 weeks prior to surgery to minimize central nervous system (CNS) depressant effects with anesthesia. Usual doses range from 1 to 3 gm daily taken in capsule form.

Dosing of Herbals Used to Promote Well-Being

Common Name	Active Ingredient	Indication	Dosage
Panax ginseng	Ginsenosides	Fatigue	200 mg/day y
American ginseng	*Panax quinquefolius*	Fatigue	1–2 gm/day (whole herb)
DHEA	Dehydroepiandrostenedione	Fatigue	10–25 mg daily in women
			50–100 mg daily in men
Ashwagandha	ashwagandha	Fatigue	1–3 gm/day

Herbals Used for Memory Enhancement and Cognitive Function

Although no drug, conventional or alternative, can reverse dementia, Ginkgo biloba may be used to minimize progression. Docosahexaenoic acid (DHA) may be best used as preventive agent. Patients taking these should be monitored for concurrent use of blood thinners and should be advised to optimize other strategies to maintain neural health, normalizing blood pressure, reducing lipids, and considering anti-inflammatory agents.

Ginkgo biloba

Ginkgo is one of the oldest plants on earth, and it has been used for its antioxidant properties for centuries. More recently, Ginkgo has been widely used both for memory impairment in elders and by students preparing for major exams. Efficacy data for memory improvement is minimal, and professional literature states it is not effective nor does it delay or worsen Alzheimer's dementia in patients using the recommended dose of 240 mg/day (DeKosky et al., 2008). Efficacy in dementia of other etiologies has not been definitively evaluated. The primary pharmacological effects include vasodilation, decrease in platelet aggregation, and antioxidant effects, thought to be mediated by a combination of bilobalides. Although the herb is generally well tolerated, with minimal side effects (primarily nausea), it does significantly inhibit platelet aggregation and can potentiate bleeding complications after falls, especially when used with aspirin or clopidogrel. In premenopausal women it is a common cause of menorrhagia.

Docosahexaenoic acid (DHA)

DHA is an omega-3 fatty acid, which has been used for mood, memory, and for neural recovery after trauma. DHA's first metabolite is a peroxisome proliferator-activated receptor gamma agonist, which stimulates the effect of brain-derived neurotrophic growth factor. At doses of 200 mg/day, few side effects are noted, and improvement in mood and attention have been noted. DHA dietary intake averaging 200 mg daily is correlated with a 17-fold reduction in all causes of dementia. Side effects include fishy taste if taken as fish oil. At doses of 200 mg daily, no change in coagulation status is noted; however, if the dose is obtained by taking high-dose multi-omega-3 supplements, anticoagulant effects may be noted. For vegan patients, an algae-derived DHA is available. Children and pregnant women may prefer to use algae or fish oil sources of DHA rather than eating fish to minimize mercury load.

Dosing of Herbals for Memory Enhancement

Common Name	Active Ingredient	Indication	Dosage
Ginkgo biloba	*Ginkgo biloba*	Memory enhancement	240 mg/day
DHA	Docosahexaenoic acid	Memory enhancement	200 mg/day

Herbals Used for Reflux Esophagitis

Patients often reach for OTC antacids as well as histamine blockers for reflux disease. The following alternatives are often used in reflux remedies as well and are generally well tolerated.

Slippery Elm

Slippery elm bark is a demulcent, which is soothing to irritated oral and esophageal tissue. Acting topically, slippery elm contains mucilage, which coats irritated mucous membranes and stimulates secretion of additional mucus to soothe irritated tissues. Two forms are widely available, lozenges and powdered inner bark, which is prepared in a slurry and taken orally (1 to 2 teaspoons three times daily).

Deglycyrrhizinated Licorice (DGL)

Deglycyrrhizinated licorice is available in chewable tablets, which are used before meals to minimize reflux symptoms. DGL reduces gastric inflammation (reducing PGE and PGF$_2$) and decreases gastric and esophageal spasms. DGL has more than 90% of the glycyrrhizinic acid removed, greatly reducing mineralocorticoid activity normally found with pure licorice. When used three times a day in 300 to 400 mg doses, no significant drug interactions or adverse effects are noted. Adverse effects may be noted at higher doses, and hypertension or hypokalemia may be noted in products with higher glycyrrhizic acid content. DGL licorice products are standardized to contain less than 3% of glycyrrhizin, although standard licorice contains 7% to 10%. Drug interactions are based on mineralocorticoid content, and possible induction of cytochrome P450 2A6, with warfarin interaction the most problematic in non-DGL licorice.

Dosing of Herbals for Acid Reflux

Common Name	Active Ingredient	Indication	Dosage
Slippery elm	Polysaccharide mucilage	Acid reflux	1–2 teaspoons 3 times/day
DGL	Deglycyrrhizinated licorice	Acid reflux	300–400 mg 3 times/day

Herbals Used for Nausea

Although many antiemetics are available over the counter, most also have antihistaminic effects and can cause significant sedation. Ginger combines good antiemetic effect without debilitating side effects.

Ginger *(Zanzibar officinalis)*

Ginger is most widely used to treat nausea and has good evidence for the reduction of emesis in naval cadets, for chemotherapy, for gastroparesis, and for mild morning sickness. Recent studies have identified ginger's activity at the odansetron receptor. Ginger is also a potent anti-inflammatory at higher doses and has been shown to reduce the pain of osteoarthritis when used consistently. Ginger's effect on the gut is to increase the pyloric opening and reduce gastric irritability, effectively resulting in caudal movement of stomach contents. When used in low doses (250 mg to 1 gm daily), such as in tea or candy form, ginger has an antiemetic effect without sedation. At higher doses (2 to 3 gm/day), ginger exerts an anti-inflammatory effect on joints and soft tissues. Generally, raw ginger is less effective than dried ginger. Low dose ginger can be taken as a food source, by dosing as a tea, or including it in curried foods, candies, etc. Higher doses, however, can irritate the esophageal mucosa, so it is recommended that for anti-inflammatory purposes ginger be used in capsule form. Side effects of ginger at low doses are minimal, and no drug interactions with ginger in usual food amounts are reported. However, when used in amounts greater than 4 gm daily, ginger may alter bleeding times and blood pressure. Mild hypertensive and hypotensive effects have been reported.

Dosing of Herbals for Nausea

Common Name	Active Ingredient	Indication	Dosage
Ginger	Z. officinalis	Nausea/antiemetic	250 mg–1 gm as tea, candy

Herbals Used for Bloating and Flatulence

Many patients seek an alternative to over-the-counter simethicone for flatulence. Both fennel and caraway seed may be chewed or prepared as teas and are common Indian and European culinary remedies.

Fennel (Foeniculum vulgare)

Fennel seeds are used for postprandial bloating and flatulence. Fennel has a GRAS status in the United States and can be found in Indian restaurants and food stores. Patients use fennel to aid digestion, either chewing the seed or preparing a tea from the crushed seed. Fennel contains anethole, as well as beta-carotene and vitamin C. Fennel is a weak phytoestrogen and should not be used in large amounts by those with estrogen-sensitive disease unless under a clinician's supervision. The usual dose is 1 to 2 gm crushed or ground and steeped in 5 to 6 ounces of hot water as a tea.

Caraway Seed

Caraway seed is used for bloating and flatulence. Seeds may be chewed or crushed and prepared as a tea. Caraway contains limonene and carvone, and the isolated oil is sold in capsules as well for the purpose of reducing gastrointestinal motility. Side effects are unusual but include nausea and heartburn when combined with peppermint. Adverse effects may include hypoglycemia at high doses, and possible drug interaction with hypoglycemic agents may occur. Usual doses range from 50 to 100 mg daily, crushed or ground and prepared as tea.

Dosing of Herbals for Bloating and Flatulence

Common Name	Active Ingredient	Indication	Dosage
Fennel	F. vulgare	Bloating/flatulence	1–2 gm prepared as tea
Caraway seed	Carvone in its volatile oil	Bloating/flatulence	50–100 mg/day prepared as tea

Herbals Used for Intestinal Cramping

Chamomile and peppermint are found in numerous enteric calmative formulas. Although chamomile may be used with good results as a tea, peppermint may induce reflux if used as a tea and should be used only in enteric-coated format for enteric cramping.

Chamomile (Matricaria recutita)

Chamomile (German) is used in tea form to reduce gastrointestinal cramping, as well as colic and other gastric and oral irritation. Containing quercetin, apigenin, bisabolol and essential oils, chamomile exerts an anti-inflammatory effect on enteric mucosa by inhibiting both cyclooxygenase (COX) and lipoxygenase (LOX). Many patients note some sedation, thought to be due to apigenin. Adverse effects include sedation at higher doses and possible allergy (related to ragweed allergy). At high doses (several cups of tea daily) interaction with warfarin is possible. Patients on warfarin therapy should be cautioned to limit chamomile products to once daily. Oral dosing is often accomplished as tea (one teabag steeped in hot water after meals) and is also available in combination products including fennel.

Peppermint Oil (Mentha piperita)

Peppermint oil acts as an enteric calmative once past the pylorus and relaxes bowel motility and spasticity. It is widely used by patients with irritable bowel syndrome to relieve painful cramping and flatulence. For this purpose it is taken in enteric capsules 90 mg or 0.2 to 0.4 mL in capsule form three times a day. It is also effective for barium-induced colon spasm. Adverse effects include heartburn, nausea, and anal burning. Peppermint oil should never be given orally to infants because it may induce laryngospasm. Drug interactions are generally limited to antacid effects on the enteric capsules, resulting in peppermint oil being released too early in the GI tract. Patients using peppermint for irritable bowel syndrome should not use antacids or H_2 blockers to avoid prepyloric dissolution of enteric dose forms.

Dosing of Herbals for Intestinal Cramping

Common Name	Active Ingredient	Indication	Dosage
Chamomile	bisabolol, apigenin	Cramps	One tea bag steeped for 5 minutes, used as needed
Peppermint oil	M. piperita	Cramps	90-mg capsules taken 3 times/day

Herbals Used for Constipation

Some of the most common uses of alternative therapies are as laxatives. The most common are aloe, senna, and cascara. Of these, consider aloe (with aloin, or whole-leaf latex) the least likely to induce dependence or electrolyte imbalance. Be sure to note that aloin-free aloe has few, if any, laxative effects.

Aloe (Aloe vera latex)

Aloe vera latex contains anthraquinone laxative aloin. This substance is quite cathartic and is sold by the gallon in health food stores. In general, patients should not use aloe for long-term laxative effect because hypokalemia and dehydration can result. For laxative effect, 100 to 200 mg is generally used at night. This product should be distinguished from aloe gel and aloin-free aloe juice, which do not contain anthraquinone laxative effects but contain antibradykinin and antibacterial properties. Adverse effects of Aloe vera latex with aloin include abdominal pain, cramps, diarrhea, and hypokalemia. Drug interactions include potentiation of both diuretic potassium depletion and other stimulant laxatives.

Triphala (Emblica officionalis, Termialia chebula, Terminalia belerica)

Triphala is an Ayurvedic botanical blend containing pectins and other soluble fibers from three fruits. Triphala provides a combination of a very gentle stimulant laxative and bulk laxative effect. Doses range from 250 to 500 mg, usually in capsule form; however, the powder may also be mixed in juice or water. Triphala is not habit-forming and is available widely at Indian food stores as well as at health food stores. No drug interactions are reported.

Senna

Senna contains anthraquinone and is a powerful stimulant laxative. Senna has FDA safe and effective status as an over-the-counter drug. Senna should not be used long term owing to the risk of laxative dependence. Both the leaf and fruit are used, with the leaf having more potent effect. Sennosides increase colonic motility and fluid secretion about 8 hours after the dose is taken. The usual dose is 15 to 17 mg per day. Side effects include cramping, nausea, and excessive potassium depletion. Drug interactions may increase bleeding risk with warfarin use. Senna should be used with a regular bowel regimen that includes adequate stool softeners, liquid, and bulk laxatives.

Cascara (Frangula purshiana)

Cascara bark contains anthraglycosides, which cause stimulation of the large intestine. Cascara lost FDA approval in 2002. Long-term use is associated with diarrhea, cramping, hypokalemia, and dependence. Drug interactions with agents that cause hypokalemia or increase bleeding time are possible. Patients should be cautioned not to use cascara for more than a few days, and the smallest amount needed to maintain soft stools should be used, generally 20 to 30 mg daily. Like senna, cascara should only be used in combination with a regular bowel regimen that includes stool softeners and adequate fluid and bulk as needed.

Konjac Glucomannan

Konjac glucomannan is the most viscous water-soluble fiber in nature. It is a polysaccharide that is the main ingredient in several Japanese foods when it is extracted from the roots of corn or the konjac plant. Its main use in food is as an emulsifier and thickener. In Japan it is known as the "broom of the intestine" for its centuries of use as a preventative or curative for constipation. It can block the throat and cause choking if not consumed with a full glass of water. It also may have some effect in improving a person's cholesterol profile.

Phosphate Salts

Phosphates are normally absorbed from food and are important elements in the body. As laxatives, they cause water to be drawn into the gut. Hence, they stimulate the gut to increase its peristaltic action and push out feces much quicker. Phosphate salts are used as fecal stimulants to cleanse the bowel before surgery or endoscopies. They can irritate the GI tract and cause more upset and/or diarrhea.

Dosing of Herbals for Constipation

Common Name	Active Agent	Indication	Common Dose for Adults
Aloe vera latex	Anthraquinone laxative aloin	Cathartic	100–200 mg as a laxative
Triphala	Ayurvedic botanical blend containing pectins	Constipation	250–500 mg daily
Senna	Anthraquinone sennosides	Constipation	15–17 mg/day
Cascara	Anthraquinone cascarosides	Constipation	20–30 mg daily
Konjac glucomannan	Water-soluble polysaccharide	Constipation	4 gm in a cup of water 3 times/day
Phosphate salts	Sodium bisphosphate/ sodium phosphate	Constipation	Oral solutions taken with water or enemas

Herbals Used for Diarrhea

Antidiarrheal supplements contain tannins, which slow bowel contractility and increase fluid reabsorption in the large bowel. They are generally well tolerated and disturb normal bowel function recovery less than do kaolin or opium-based antidiarrheals.

Black and Green Tea

Tea contains tannins and polyphenols, which can be used to treat mild diarrhea. Tea for diarrhea should be made with decaffeinated teabags, if possible, to reduce the stimulant effect of caffeine. Both black and green teas are effective. If decaffeinated teabags are unavailable, tea may be made by using regular teabags, discarding the hot liquid from the first cup made, then reusing the same teabags and allowing the hot water to steep for 5 to 10 minutes. Caffeine elutes almost immediately and so can be easily separated from the tea to be used. Patients may drink 1 cup of decaffeinated tea for each diarrheal stool and may include a small amount of sugar to facilitate water absorption in the large intestine.

Cinnamon (Cinnamonum verum, Cassia cinnamonum)

Cinnamon is used orally for diarrhea. Tannins in the cinnamon reduce fluid excretion in the large intestine. Cinnamon has a

GRAS status and may be added as a food spice to applesauce or toast to achieve the desired effect as tolerated. Use as food spice is generally free of adverse effects, but use of cinnamon oil concentrate may produce skin irritation, dizziness, and sedation, and should not be used for diarrhea. The usual effective dose of cinnamon as a food spice is 1 to 2 gm daily, equivalent to 0.25 to 0.5 teaspoon. This is particularly effective when mixed with applesauce or bananas because the pectin and soluble fiber help reduce diarrhea loss. Either cinnamon spice may be used with efficacy for bowel regulation.

Rhubarb (Rheum officinale)

Rhubarb root and rhizome have GRAS status and are commonly found in pies and preserves. Rhubarb contains anthraquinones, pectin, and tannins, and the effect of the herb depends on the concentration used. At high doses, anthraquinone effects produce diarrhea. Tannin effects are noted at doses as low as 100 to 300 mg daily and are effective at relieving diarrhea. Baked rhubarb may be flavored with cinnamon to increase antidiarrheal effect.

Dosing of Herbals for Diarrhea

Common Name	Active Agent	Indication	Common Dose for Adults
Black and green tea	Tannins and polyphenols	Mild diarrhea	One cup steeped 5-10 minutes/loose stool
Cinnamon	C. cinnamonum	Mild diarrhea	0.25–0.5 tsp as food spice/day
Rhubarb	Tannins	Mild diarrhea	100–300 mg/day

Supplements Used for Sleeping and Sedation

All sedatives should be treated with respect. Patients who choose to take supplements for sleep or sedation should be cautioned that although they are natural supplements, significant sedation may result from their use. They should not be used except in the setting of anticipated sleep induction.

Melatonin

Melatonin is normally produced in the pineal gland, and is formed in response to daytime light exposure and secreted in response to dark. Melatonin helps regulate circadian rhythm and sleep cycles and is generally used to facilitate sleep in cases of insomnia or jet lag. Melatonin is most effective when taken within 30 minutes of bedtime in a low dose (0.5 to 1 mg). As most tablets are 3 to 5 mg, patients should be instructed to cut the tablets in half, then half again, or to use liquid products that allow low-dose titration. Patients should also be instructed to get 15 to 20 minutes of sun exposure daily (which facilitates melatonin receptor production) and to reduce indoor light sources late in the evening, as well as to reduce sources of electromagnetic radiation near the bed at night, to reduce interference of native melatonin function. This may involve moving phones, alarm clocks, weather alarms, and TVs away from the head of the bed. Few side effects are noted in melatonin use at this low dose, and drug interaction effects are not seen. At higher

doses it is used for solid tumor therapy, nausea may be noticed and potential for drug interactions with nifedipine, immunosuppressants, and antidepressants may be noted at very high doses (over 15 mg daily). Melatonin is not habit-forming, and when used in low dose, it does not disturb the sleep cycle.

Valerian (Valeriana officinalis)

Valerian is a sedative used largely in tincture or capsule form. Valerian has a GRAS status in the United States and acts at gamma-aminobutyric acid (GABA) receptors, although its effect is not as rapid in onset on or as potent as benzodiazepine effects. Adverse effects include sedation and CNS depression. Valerian in rare cases may be habit-forming, and drug interactions with other CNS depressant drugs are noted. When used at usual doses of 400 to 800 mg 2 hours before bedtime, valerian does not inhibit cytochrome P450, but at higher doses it may cause 3A4 inhibition. Its primary use is to help initiate the sleep cycle. Because it has a pungent, unpleasant odor, it is normally taken in capsule or tincture form, not as a tea.

Chamomile

Chamomile tea is often used as a mild sedative (see section on GI cramping) and may be used in combination with valerian, with additive effects. The dose is generally 1 cup of tea steeped 5 to 10 minutes, with mild muscle relaxation and sedation noted within 30 minutes of ingestion.

Hops (Humulus lupulus)

Hops, a flavoring traditionally used to brew beer, has intrinsic sedative properties. Hops has GRAS status and contains many anti-inflammatory flavonoids. It does not appear to affect GABA or melatonin. Side effects include sedation and drug interactions, including CNS depressant potentiation. The usual dose is 40 to 80 mg at bedtime.

Dosing of Herbals to Help with Sleep

Common Name	Active Agent	Indication	Common Dose for Adults
Melatonin	Melatonin	Sleep aid	0.5–1 mg within 30 min before sleep
Valerian	V. officinalis	Sedative	400–800 mg at least 2 hr before sleep
Chamomile tea	Chamomile apigenin	Mild sleep aid, mild stress reliever	1 cup of tea, steeped 5–10 min 30 min before sleep
Hops	H. lupulus	Mild sedative	40–80 mg at night

Herbals Used for Anxiety

Patients often seek nerve tonics. Chamomile and passionflower are often found in teas formulated to relieve stress. Kava kava is often found in tablet form, but it has potential for liver toxicity if aerial parts are used. Patients should be encouraged to avoid it unless they are certain they are using a root source.

Passionflower (Passiflora incarnata)

Passionflower contains many flavonoids, including apigenin, also found in chamomile, that cause sedation. They can also be used in low doses for anxiety and in higher doses for sedation and opiate withdrawal. The primary side effect of the herb is CNS depression, and drug interactions include primarily potentiation of CNS depression. Passionflower is generally found in combination products containing melatonin or hops and may also be found as a combination in tea. Patients should be cautioned regarding sedation and should be advised to avoid driving or cooking when using these combined agents. Generally 1 gm is used in tincture, tea, or extract form.

Kava Kava

Kava kava is a South Sea island herb that relieves anxiety and in high doses has anticonvulsant properties. Prolonged use at high doses results in kani, a kava-induced dermopathy. Kava kava is effective in producing sedation, but liver failure is a known complication of use of the aerial portions of the herb. Patients should be advised not to use this herb unless they are certain of using a root-sourced product.

Dosing of Herbals for Anxiety

Common Name	Active Agent	Indication	Common Dose for Adults
Passionflower	apigenin flavonoids	Mild anxiolytic	For mild anxiety 1 gm daily
Kava kava	Kavalactone from kava root	Mild anxiolytic	For mild anxiety: 250 mg at night
			For anxiety: 250 mg of plant root 3–4 times/day

Supplements Used for Depression

Patients desiring to use supplements for depression should be fully evaluated for severity of depression as well as risk of suicidal ideation and homicidal ideation. Although many patients will experience good results with these supplements, they should be used under medical supervision, with frequent reassessment of suicide risk and efficacy.

St. John's Wort *(Hypericum perforatum)*

St. John's wort contains several ingredients, which act on the monoamine oxidase (MAO) and GABA systems. Although it is an effective antidepressant for mild to moderate depression, this herb also is known to induce multiple enzymes in the cytochrome P450 system, as well as the glycoprotein P transport system. This effectively means that patients taking St. John's wort will not be absorbing and benefiting from a wide variety of other therapeutic drugs, including many common anticonvulsants, antineoplastics, antiretrovirals, oral contraceptives, statins, cyclosporine, and antibiotics. St. John's wort also causes photosensitivity. For these reasons, patients should be cautioned not to use the herb if they are on any regular drug regimen known to interact with these systems. Other options for patients considering this herb include SAM-e and DHEA.

S-adenosylmethionine (SAM-e)

SAM-e is a molecule found in many synthesis pathways of neurochemicals and hormones in the body. It is well tolerated in intravenous formulations in Europe, where it is used to initiate rapid response to antidepressant oral agents. In the United States, it is widely available in oral form, and doses from 400 to 1,600 mg/day are well tolerated, with efficacy for mild to moderate depression. A starting dose of 200 mg twice daily is recommended, but an antiarthritic effect is also noted at low doses (200 mg, three times/day). Drug interactions with selective serotonin reuptake inhibitors (SSRIs) and monoamine oxidase inhibitors (MAOIs) are possible, and SAM-e should not be used in combination with these agents because of the risk of serotonin syndrome.

Dosing of Herbals for Depression

Common Name	Active Agent	Indication	Common Dose for Adults
St. Johns wort	H. perforatum	Depression	300 mg, 3 times/day to start; may increase up to 500 mg 3 times/day
SAM-e	S-adenosyl-methionine	Depression	400–1,600 mg/day

Oral Herbals Used for Arthritis

Patients with chronic joint pain often choose these supplements to manage pain. Although slower in onset of analgesic effect, they offer fewer side effects than do NSAIDs.

Chondroitin Sulfate/Glucosamine Sulfate

Glucosamine and chondroitin are glycosaminoglycans, which produce a chondrocyte-stimulating effect. These supplements are effective in reducing the pain associated with moderate to severe arthritis when used consistently for 3 to 4 weeks. Dosages of 1,500 mg of glucosamine sulfate and 1,200 mg of chondroitin sulfate per day are used. Patients should be told to use the product consistently for at least 2 weeks before anticipating pain relief and may use a gradual taper of NSAID or acetaminophen therapy to provide pain management during this run-in period. Benefits of glucosamine and chondroitin include pain management without NSAID side effects such as renal impairment, hypertension, and gastric ulceration. They are generally well tolerated. Patients should read labels to avoid possible shellfish sources if allergy is an issue. No significant drug interactions are reported.

Methylsulfonylmethane (MSM)

Methylsulfonylmethane (MSM) is an anti-inflammatory often included in combination with glucosamine and chondroitin. It provides more rapid onset of pain relief and allows earlier taper of NSAIDs. It is generally well tolerated, and there are no known drug interactions. Long-term safety of chondroitin and glucosamine is established; MSM safety data is limited to 12 weeks. Therefore, consider recommending that patients limit their use of MSM for the first 2 to 3 months of conversion to chondroitin and glucosamine from NSAIDs.

S-adenosylmethionine (SAM-e)

SAM-e is an excellent choice for the patient with both body aches and depression, often resulting in improvement in both symptoms simultaneously. (Also see antidepressant section.)

The effective dose for arthritis is much lower than that used for depression, so care should be taken to optimize the dose for both symptoms. Side effects, including nausea, sleep disturbance, and anorgasmia are uncommon, and drug interactions are limited to concomitant use of SSRI and MAOI drugs.

Turmeric/Curcumin

Turmeric has a GRAS status. It contains curcuminoids, which act as COX-2 inhibitors, inhibiting prostaglandins, leukotrienes, and thromboxanes. It also causes apoptosis in some cancer cell lines and inhibits angiogenesis as well as platelet aggregation. When taken orally, turmeric remains in the enteric tract acting as a local anti-inflammatory. When taken with fat sources or black pepper, turmeric is easily absorbed and reaches significant serum concentrations. Side effects are limited to occasional nausea. Drug interactions are limited to antiplatelet effects. Patients should be advised to use 2,000 mg daily in divided doses, with 94% curcuminoid extract. Absorption and systemic levels are maximized by taking curcumin with fat-containing food or black pepper.

Ginger

Ginger can be used in doses of 1 gm three times a day to reduce inflammation in arthritis, and it is effective at reducing CRP at these doses. Capsule form should be used to prevent heartburn at these higher doses, and patients should understand that high doses may prolong the bleeding time. (Also see the GI section.)

Dosing of Oral Herbals Used for Arthritis

Common Name	Active Agent	Indication	Common Dose for Adults
Chondroitin Glucosamine	Chondroitin sulfate	Anti-arthritic	1,500/1,200 mg of each taken daily
	Glucosamine sulfate		
MSM	Methylsulfonyl-methane	Anti-arthritic	Limit use to 12 weeks
Tumeric	Curcuminoids	Anti-arthritic	200 mg/day in divided doses
Ginger	Terpenes and oleoresins (ginger oil)	Anti-inflammatory	1 gm PO, 3 times/day

Topical Herbals Used for Arthritis

Several botanicals, including wintergreen, capsaicin (hot pepper), ginger, and turmeric can be used in lotion, paste, ointment, or liniment form for pain relief. These are traditionally used for arthritis, but may also be used on areas of postherpetic neuralgia, hypesthesia, and chronic neuropathy. Care should be taken not to use these treatments on broken skin, not to heat the skin or dressing after application, and not to use them near the eyes or mucous membranes. Many topical botanicals may irritate the skin, so the area in use should be closely monitored for signs of inflammation and allergic reaction. Wintergreen and capsaicin are widely available in commercial forms; ginger and turmeric are easily prepared at the bedside by the patient or family. Although all are effective for mild arthritic pain and neuropathic pain, there are differences in action and side effects with each.

Capsaicin

Capsaicin causes substance P release and thereby depletion with recurrent use, resulting in a diminished pain signal over time. Capsaicin produces an intense burning sensation when first applied to the affected area, which is not well tolerated by many patients. The burn diminishes with recurrent use as the pain control increases. Severe burning when touching mucous membranes may occur even with careful hand washing after use.

Ginger and Tumeric

Ginger and turmeric may also be used topically. Their mode of action is thought to be anti-inflammatory because both are COX inhibitors. Simple water- or olive oil-based pastes may be prepared from food-grade ginger and turmeric for home use. The area to be treated is coated in a thin layer of paste, and the area is covered with a light dressing. Although these will stain clothing and skin, they offer pain relief without the risk of the burning sensation caused by capsaicin.

Wintergreen Oil

Wintergreen oil contains methyl salicylate, and this is used as an ointment to achieve anti-inflammatory effect, again without the burning that capsaicin causes. Methyl salicylate will be absorbed transdermally, and with extensive use serum salicylate levels can rise measurably. Drug interactions, especially with warfarin, are possible with use over large surface areas. The table below provides a summary of topical herbals used for arthritis.

Borage

Known as starflower or bee bread, borage is an herb from the Middle East that was originally cultivated as a food (tastes like a cucumber), but is used today as an anti-arthritic for the oil (starflower oil) expressed from its seeds. The seeds contain gamma-linoleic acid and several other fatty acids. Naturopathic practitioners use it for PMS and menopausal symptoms, bronchitis, colds, and its anti-inflammatory properties.

Dosing of Topical Herbals Used in Arthritis

Common Name	Active Agent	Indication	Common Dose for Adults
Chili peppers	Capsaicin	Anti-inflammatory	0.025% cream applied 4 times a day
Ginger/tumeric	Terpenes and oleoresins (ginger oil)	Anti-inflammatory	25–100 mg of tincture per day (2–3 droppers)
Wintergreen oil	Methyl salicylate	Anti-inflammatory	5% cream/ointment applied 3 times/day
Borage	Oleic and palmitic fatty acids	Anti-inflammatory	500 mg of seed oil capsules taken 3 times/day

Herbal Used for Impotence

Yohimbe is the herbal most commonly used for impotence. It contains the alkaloid yohimbine, which is used for erectile dysfunction. It acts as an alpha-2 adrenergic receptor blocker and also blocks peripheral serotonin receptors and has MAOI activity. The bark of the plant also has hallucinogenic properties.

While effective for erectile dysfunction, yohimbe's side effects are significant and include hypertension, excitability, dizziness, and fluid retention at low doses, with hypotension, cardiac failure, and death at high doses. Multiple drug interactions and food interactions with tyramine-containing compounds are noted. This herb should be used only with extreme caution, and physician supervision should be strongly considered. Dose range is generally 15 to 30 mg daily. Drug interactions with antidepressants, antihypertensives, and naloxone have been reported.

Dosing of Herbal Used for Erectile Dysfunction

Common Name	Active Agent	Indication	Common Dose for Adults
Yohimbe	Yohimbine	Erectile dysfunction	15–30 mg daily

Herbals Used for Headaches

Chapter 24, Drugs used to Manage Pain, deals with medications such as the analgesic NSAIDS and triptans for migraine headache. However, increasingly patients seek "natural means" of finding relief. Diet and lifestyle changes are included in these integrative approaches to headache; for example, dehydration can trigger a headache, and food sensitivities are also a common cause (alcohol, artificial sweeteners, chocolate, pickled foods, shellfish, monosodium glutamate, nitrites, excess tyramine). Common natural remedies used today include magnesium, riboflavin, feverfew, coenzyme Q10, and melatonin.

Feverfew (Tanacetum parthenium)

Feverfew leaf contains parthenolide, which inhibits COX-2 as well as tumor necrosis factor-alpha and interleukin-1 production. It is used by patients to reduce the frequency of migraine headaches, but not to stop an acute attack. Although feverfew inhibits cytochrome P450 enzymes at high doses, drug interactions with feverfew have not been reported in humans at the doses used for headache. Usual doses are 50 to 100 mg daily or a product containing 250 to 500 mcg of active parthenolides. Adverse effects include heartburn and oral ulceration if leaves are chewed; however, the drug does appear to be quite safe. Patients should be encouraged to use capsule forms and to avoid opening capsules.

Riboflavin

Vitamin B_2 is a water-soluble vitamin used in a dose of 200 mg per day to prevent headache. Although its mechanism in preventing migraines is unknown, it is well tolerated, inexpensive, and effectively reduces headache attacks in most patients. It has no drug interactions, and side effects are limited to a deep yellow coloration to sweat and urine. For patients with chronic migraines, riboflavin supplementation is a good first choice to use as a prophylactic agent.

Magnesium

Magnesium is often used as a migraine prophylactic. Magnesium supplementation helps relax smooth muscle and effectively reduces frequency and severity of attacks. Patients who have triptan-resistant migraine often recover triptan sensitivity when magnesium is added to the regimen, and magnesium levels should be checked in all refractory migraine patients. The oral dose should be titrated to at least keep the patient at normal range and may be increased slowly until unacceptable softening of stool occurs. Starting doses of 200 to 400 mg a day of magnesium citrate are well tolerated, with efficacy noted between 600 and 1,500 mg daily in most cases. Magnesium may interfere with the absorption of other medications, so it should not be taken along with many other medications. Its most common side effect is diarrhea, which can be improved when the dosage is lowered.

Dosing of Herbals Used to Prevent or Relieve Headache

Common Name	Active Agent	Indication	Common Dose for Adults
Feverfew	Parthenolide	Headache	50–100 mg/day
Riboflavin	Vitamin B_2	Headache preventative	200 mg/day
Magnesium	Magnesium citrate	Migraine preventative	200–1,500 mg/day titrated slowly

Herbals Used for Glycemic Control

Cinnamon bark (from *Cinnamomum verum*) and *Cassia cinnamomum* are most commonly used for glycemic control. They contain methylhydroxychalcone polymer that improves insulin function. Taken in doses of 1 gm two to three times daily, improvement in glycemic control is noted. Drug interaction is noted in potentiation of hypoglycemic medications, so patients taking prescription medications for diabetes should closely monitor their glucose levels and anticipate possible hypoglycemia when adding cinnamon to their regimen.

Dosing of Herbals for Glycemic Control

Common Name	Active Agent	Indication	Common Dose for Adults
Cinnamon	*C. cinnamomum*	Glycemic control	1–3 gm/day

Herbals Used for Lipid Control

Although cholesterol is an essential component of every cell in the body and is part of the manufacturing process of hormones, excessive cholesterol in the blood accumulates in artery walls leading to plaque buildup and strokes. Thus, cholesterol-lowering drugs are frequently prescribed to prevent or halt the buildup of plaque. Dietary supplements to lower cholesterol include red yeast rice extract, plant sterols, garlic, niacin, omega-3 fish oils, and green tea.

Omega-3 Fish Oils

Omega-3 fatty acids include alpha linolenic acid (ALA), eicosapentaenoic acid (EPA), and docosahexaenoic acid (DHA). EPA and DHA are derived from deepwater fish, such as wild salmon, tuna, and mackerel, and from algae. ALA is found in plant sources such as flaxseed oil. EPA/DHA containing fish oil reduces triglycerides in patients with dyslipidemia, decreases cardiac arrhythmias, and promotes neural regeneration in both the central and peripheral nervous systems. A small amount of

ALA is converted to EPA and DHA (5% to 15%) depending on dietary omega-6 fat intake and patient genetics, and although not an efficient method of obtaining EPA or DHA, is used by some vegans. Effective doses of EPA, DHA, and ALA range from 1 to 3 gm daily. Side effects include fishy odor to the breath and increased bruising. Drug interactions include potentiation of anticoagulants and antihypertensives. Excessive doses (more than 4 to 6 gm daily) of fish oils can increase bleeding times and should be avoided unless taken under clinician supervision. Omega-3 fish oil is not equivalent to fish liver oil, and patients should be cautioned to avoid large doses of the latter to avoid the risk of vitamin A overdose.

Olive Oil

Olive oil contains monounsaturated fatty acids and reduces cholesterol levels when used in place of saturated fats in the diet. Olive oil also is an anti-inflammatory, with both COX-1 and -2 inhibition noted. When used in a diet that replaces saturated fat with olive oil, significant reduction in pain and inflammation is also noted by arthritis patients. Olive oil is well tolerated as a food source. Excessive use may result in mild diarrhea. Because it may reduce blood pressure and glucose, patients using high doses should carefully monitor these. Drug interactions primarily involve antihypertensives and hypoglycemics, which may need to be reduced.

Red Yeast Rice

Red yeast rice is the fermented product of rice on which red yeast has been grown. It is a dietary staple in Japan and China. Red yeast rice contains several monacolin, which inhibit HMG CoA reductase in the liver. Although the statin compound lovastatin (monacolin K) occurs as the active ingredient in red yeast rice, it is only one of several monacolin moieties found in the supplement. Red yeast rice lowers total cholesterol (11% to 32%) and LDL cholesterol and triglycerides (12% to 19%) using the same mechanism as do statin drugs. Potential liver toxicity and drug interactions are similar to those of the statin class. Liver enzymes should be monitored periodically while patients use red yeast rice consistently for lipid management. Doses range from 600 to 1,200 mg, two to three times a day for a total daily monacolin dose of 5 to 15 mg. Generally, less myalgia is reported with red yeast rice than with conventional statins, and myopathy is rare but possible. Drug interactions similar to those seen with statins are possible, but they are generally minimal. As with statins, patients should consider taking 200 mg CoQ10 daily while using red yeast rice to minimize myalgia and prevent CoQ10 deficiency. Red yeast rice side effects are mild and may include heartburn, dizziness, and flatulence.

Phytosterols (Plant Sterols)

Phytosterols (plant sterols) include plant stanol esters. These act as adsorbents in the gut lumen to prohibit enterohepatic recirculation of conjugated cholesterol. They decrease serum cholesterol levels by trapping and eliminating them. Plant sterol and stanol esters are generally found in food sources, including margarines and liquid fiber sources, nuts, seeds, cereals, legumes,

and vegetable oils. Two servings daily helps reduce cholesterol in the setting of a low-fat diet. These are generally well tolerated, with few side effects (bloating at high doses), and they have few drug interactions. With excessive use, some blockage of drug absorption may be noted, so patients should be cautioned not to use more than 2 to 3 servings daily. Today, some foods such as margarines, salad dressings, and snack bars qualify for claims of *cholesterol lowering* based on their having plant sterols. Most phytosterol supplements are currently derived from soy and should be used only with caution by patients with soy allergies.

Gum (Guar)

Guar gum is a resin that provides a soluble fiber source to allow enteric trapping of cholesterol and fats, thus preventing enterohepatic recirculation of lipids. It is effective in lowering LDL and improving postprandial glucose. It is an ingredient in many dietary supplements and may also be used as a powder. The usual starting dose is 4 gm daily, and the dose may be titrated to 12 gm daily. Side effects include nausea and bloating. Drug interactions include reduced absorption of drugs, including antibiotics, hypoglycemics, digoxin, and oral contraceptives.

Dosing of Herbals Used for Lipid Control

Common Name	Active Agent	Indication	Common Dose for Adults
Red yeast rice	Multiple monacolins	Lowering cholesterol	5–15 mg of monacolins daily in 2–3 divided doses
Phytosterols	Soy cell membrane sterol esters	Lowering cholesterol	2–3 servings/day
Guar gum	Fatty alcohol sulfates from the legume, *Cyamopsis*	Lowering LDL	4 grams daily state, may move up to 12 gm/day
Omega-3 fish oils	eicosapentaenoic acid (EPA), and docosahexaenoic acid (DHA)		1–3 gm/day

Herbals Used for Topical Wound Treatment

Healing of the skin after an injury is a process that is as old as humankind. The capacity of a wound to heal is not only a function of the type and extent of the wound, but also of the person's overall health and nutritional status. Over the millennia, wound healing has been aided by herbals such as flowering plants, shrubs, moss, fruits, leaves, twigs, barks, and seeds. Following injury, an inflammatory process occurs, and the cells below the dermis begin to increase collagen production. Later, the epithelial tissue is regenerated. Herbal supplements may improve the quality of wound healing by influencing the reparative process or by limiting the effects of inflammation. Two agents that do this are tea tree oil and aloe vera.

Tea Tree Oil

Tea tree oil is used topically for skin infections including acne, minor cuts and scrapes, and tinea infections. The active ingredients include terpinen-4-ol and alpha-terpineol, which disrupt microbial walls but in general have no effect on intact skin tissue. In vitro activity has been noted against a wide variety of bacteria and fungi, including *Candida, Malassezia, Trichophyton, Staphylococcus, Enterococcus,* and *Pseudomonas* and *Propionibacterium* species. Adverse effects include mild estrogenic activity with extensive topical use. Chronic use can cause drying of skin. Full-strength oil may be ototoxic and should not be used in the ear canal for otitis externa (2% concentrations are well tolerated). Allergic reactions include eczema-like skin lesions.

Tea tree oil is used full strength twice daily on nails for onychomycosis, but diluted to 5% to 10% strength for topical use on skin, and generally used once daily. It is not used on mucous membranes unless very dilute and should not be used internally due to toxicity. Dizziness, nausea, and coma have resulted from ingestion of full-strength tea tree oil.

Aloe Vera

Aloe vera gel contains antibradykinins, antimicrobials, and antifungal ingredients. It is widely used in sunburn preparations and provides infection control and pain management. Topical use of the gel may cause irritation, however this is rare. No known drug interactions exist for topical use. Aloe should not be used on severe burns (large second-degree or any third-degree burns). For small second-degree burns, aloe gel may be used alternating with Silvadene to provide antibacterial coverage and limit skin contracture caused by Silvadene.

Dosing of Topical Herbals Used for Wounds and Burns

Common Name	Active Agent	Indication	Common Dose for Adults
Tea tree oil*	98 kinds of cyclic terpenes, collectively known as Melaleuca oil	Skin infections as an antiseptic, antibiotic, antifungal, antiviral	5% solutions and shampoos
Aloe vera	Aloe vera gel	Antiseptic, pain relief	Use purified gel on skin as many times as patient thinks is necessary

Do not confuse with the tea seed oil, obtained from the tea plant, and used for cooking.

Antioxidant and Anticancer Supplements

When patients with cancer desire to use botanicals and dietary supplements, the fundamental idea is to determine whether the aim of treatment is curative or palliative. If the goal is cure, patients should refrain from using supplements until the chemotherapy round is completed. Supplements, even vitamins, may interfere with desired effects of chemotherapy, so the rule of thumb is to avoid interference. In some instances, if symptoms caused by chemotherapy or radiation are intolerable and threaten completion of oncology treatment protocols, the integrative clinician will use specific herbals known to be free of significant drug interactions (such as ginger or aloe) to provide relief of symptoms, thus allowing completion of the protocol. This must be done cautiously and in partnership with the oncologist to maximize patient benefit while minimizing risk. After chemotherapy is completed, the patient may consider some of the agents in the following dosing table for specific indications.

Dosing of Common Herbal Antioxidants Used for Cancer Prevention

Common Name	Active Agent	Indication	Common Dose for Adults
Melatonin	N-methyl-5 methoxytryptamine	Impede tumor growth	20 mg/day
Omega-3 oils	Eicosapentaenoic acid (EPA), and docosahexaenoic acid (DHA)	Polyp growth inhibitor	1–4,000 mg/day
Ashwagandha	Alkaloids, steroidal lactones, saponins, and with anolides	Reduces doxorubicin toxicity	1-2 gm/day after treatment course completed
Cruciferous vegetables	Indole-3-carbinoles	Reduces estrogen metabolite toxicity	400 mg/day tablet 0.5 cup broccoli

Melatonin

In addition to its sedating properties, a high dose of melatonin (20 mg/day) has also been noted to slow solid tumor growth. This dose far exceeds the recommended sleep-inducing dose and should be used with caution by patients under clinician direction. (Also see sleep and sedation section.)

Ashwagandha

Ashwagandha has been noted to decrease chemotherapy-induced cardiomyopathy in patients receiving doxorubicin. It is generally used after completion of chemotherapy and should be used with physician guidance. Dose ranges from 1 to 6 gm per day of whole herb. Drug interactions are minor and include CNS depressants and sedatives.

Omega-3 Fatty Acids

Omega-3 oils are also noted to reduce the progression of adenomatous polyps in the colon. A diet rich in healthy omega-3 sources and low in omega-6 and saturated fats is prudent for colon cancer patients. If dietary omega-3 sources are not tolerated, the dose range for fish oil supplements is 1 to 4 gm daily, containing both EPA and DHA. This dose may increase bleeding time, so caution should be used by patients using aspirin, warfarin, or other anticoagulant drugs. (Also see the lipid control section.)

Indole-3-Carbinole (I3C)

Indole-3-carbinole, or I3C, is a compound found in broccoli and other cruciferous vegetables. I3C induces cytochrome P450 1A1 and 1A2, which acts to increase estrogen metabolism into the lower potency 2-alpha hydroxyestrone instead of 16-alpha hydroxyestrone, thereby reducing stimulation of hormone-sensitive tissue. I3C is therefore used as a chemopreventive agent by patients at risk of breast cancer, but clinical trials have yet to be published that establish efficacy. It is generally well tolerated in food sources, although the recommended dose (400 mg/daily) requires an average of 0.5 cup daily intake of cruciferous vegetables, raw or lightly cooked. It is also available in tablet form. Drug interactions include lowered serum concentrations of drugs metabolized by 1A2. Efficacy is thought to be reduced if stomach acid is not adequate because an acidic gastric milieu is required to convert I3C to its active metabolite.

THE VITAMINS: AN OVERVIEW

Vitamins were discovered by Dutch physician Christiaan Eijkman who won the 1929 Nobel Prize in Physiology and Medicine. The term *vitamin* may refer to any of the organic compounds required by the body in small amounts (micronutrients) to protect health and for proper growth in living creatures. In general, although the vitamins are not biochemically related, they are divided into two groups: fat-soluble vitamins and water-soluble vitamins (Table 25-1). Each group shares some basic physiological characteristics.

The U.S. Food and Nutrition Board of the National Research Council has published recommended dietary allowances (RDAs) for vitamins, minerals, and other nutrients. RDAs are normally expressed in international units (IU) or milligrams. For adults and children of normal health, these recommendations are useful guidelines not only for professionals in nutrition but also for the growing number of families and individuals who eat irregular meals and rely on prepared foods (many of which are now required to carry nutritional labeling). Unfortunately, these RDAs give only the bare minimum required to ward off deficiency diseases such as rickets, beriberi, scurvy, and night blindness. What they do not account for are the amounts needed to maintain maximum health.

All vitamin supplements work best when taken along with food. Typically, fat-soluble vitamins should be taken before

TABLE 25-1	Vitamins Used as Dietary Supplements: Classification, Active Compound Use, Recommended Daily Allowance (RDA)		
NAME	**ACTIVE COMPOUND**	**USE**	**RECOMMENDED DIETARY ALLOWANCE (RDA)***
Fat-Soluble Vitamins			
Vitamin A	Retinoic acid	Promotes growth, promotes healthy skin, and prevents night blindness	Men: 5,000 IU Women: 4,000 IU
Vitamin D	1,25 dihydroxychole-calciferol, calcitriol	Regulates Ca, Mg, and P metabolism Use to treat rickets and osteomalacia. Postmenopause supplementation for osteoporosis and fall prevention in elderly Treatment of muscle pain and weakness Replacement therapy for high level of deficiency seen in northern United States in winter months	AI for adults: 400–1,000 IU, 10–25 mcg/day; lower range based on historical dose necessary to prevent rickets, higher based on recent Institute of Medicine recommendations
Vitamin E	Four forms of toco-pherols and four forms of tocotrienols	Antioxidant properties, improves endothelial function, and fibrocystic breast symptoms	60–75 IU daily
Vitamin K	Phytonadione	Deficiency leads to bleeding	2.5–25 mg/day
Water-soluble vitamins			
Vitamin C	Ascorbic acid	Necessary to form collagen in bone, cartilage, muscle, blood vessels, heart. Symptoms of mild deficiency may include faulty bone and tooth development, gingivitis, bleeding gums, and loosened teeth.	Prevention of scurvy 70–150 mg/day, if scurvy appears, 300-100 mg per day
		Wound healing	300–500 mg daily for 10 days
Vitamin B$_1$	Thiamine	Carbohydrate metabolism, nerve cell function Deficiencies found in alcoholism, cirrhosis, overactive thyroid tobacco use decreases thiamine	Men: 1.5 mg Women: 1.1 mg (Note: Average person gets 9 mg/day in diet; multivitamins have 20–25 mg/day)
Vitamin B$_2$	Riboflavin	Use to reduce symptoms of fatigue, eye fatigue, headache, cataracts, as antioxidant that scavenges free radicals	Men: 1.7 mg Women: 1.3 mg

Continued

TABLE 25-1	Vitamins Used as Dietary Supplements: Classification, Active Compound Use, Recommended Daily Allowance (RDA)—cont'd		
NAME	ACTIVE COMPOUND	USE	RECOMMENDED DIETARY ALLOWANCE (RDA)*
Vitamin B_6	Pyridoxine	Use to treat PMS and neonatal jaundice	Men: 2 mg Women: 1.6 mg
Vitamin B_9	B_9 (folate)	Deficiency increases risk of neural tube defects. Mild deficiencies occur in celiac disease, alcohol consumption, irritable bowel syndrome.	Women of childbearing age: 400 mcg daily Pregnant women with history of children with neural tube defects: 4,000 mcg daily Men: 160 mg Women: 200 mg
Vitamin B_{12}	Methylcobalamin and 5-deoxyadeno-sylcobalamin	Required for proper red blood cell formation, neurological function, and DNA synthesis	Men: 2.4 mcg Women: 2.4 mcg
Vitamin B_3	Niacin	Required for energy production processes. Deficiency leads to pellagra.	Men: 19 mg Women: 15 mg

*See http://dietary-supplements.info.nih.gov/factsheets/vitamind.asp for more detailed information.

meals, and water-soluble vitamins should be taken after meals. Vitamins are compounds that act as cofactors in essential biochemical reactions. Although they are needed in microgram or milligram amounts, deficiencies can produce severe, even lethal disease. Oversupplementation, however, also carries the risk of disease. To provide some estimate of safe supplementation, the U.S. Food and Nutrition Board of the National Research Council, the National Academy of Sciences, and the Institute of Medicine periodically review recommendations for the daily amount of each vitamin that will prevent overt deficiency states and provide wellness.

In general, the AI (adequate intake) recommendation provides an age-based guideline for safe but adequate intake of each vitamin to prevent deficiency. However, these guidelines often change as more evidence is found to help our understanding of the consequences of low-normal vitamin levels. In addition, these recommendations are based on the assumption that the recommended intake will be universally absorbed with equal efficiency by the population, an assumption we now know to be wrong. In many instances, such as with malabsorption syndromes, serum vitamin levels rather than RDA guidelines must be used to properly maintain normal vitamin levels.

The Fat-Soluble Vitamins as Food Supplements

Fat-soluble vitamins A, D, E, and K are best absorbed with food and may be difficult to absorb by patients with gallbladder disease or on severe fat-restricted diets. Excess intake by patients with no fat malabsorption or deficiency may result in toxicity syndromes. Because they can be stored in the body's adipose tissue, deficiency syndromes may be slow in onset.

Vitamin A (Retinoic Acid)

Retinoic acid is the primary form of vitamin A found in most supplements. Retinoic acid belongs to a family of chemicals derived from carotene—the carotenoids. Vitamin A is essential for the normal development of the retina as well as the cornea, skin, bones, and teeth, and for normal function of the immune system. Vitamin A deficiency is the most common cause of childhood blindness in the world and contributes to the lethality of childhood measles in undeveloped countries. In addition, retinoic acid mobilizes iron from its storage sites in the liver, so a deficiency in vitamin A can lead to a limitation of the body's ability to use stored iron, resulting in iron deficiency anemia. In both children and adults, deficiency results in night-blindness and Bitot spots, superficial, irregularly-shaped, foamy gray or white patches that appear on the conjunctiva and are composed of keratinized epithelial cells. Progression of untreated vitamin A deficiency will result in keratosis of the cornea, called xerophthalmia, and blindness.

Because vitamin A and carotenoids are readily found in red, yellow, orange, and dark green vegetables, as well as in milk, butter, cheese, and eggs, a well-rounded diet is generally adequate to prevent deficiency. Patients with severe fat malabsorption, however, may develop deficiency states and require high-dose oral replacement. This should be managed by following serum levels and should not be undertaken by patients without expert guidance to prevent the risk of toxicity. Acute vitamin A toxicity can result in liver failure, hemolysis, and headaches. Chronic vitamin A toxicity induces osteolysis and increases the risk of some malignancies.

Dietary carotenoids other than retinoic acid have generally not been associated with these toxicity syndromes. Conversely, consistent dietary intake, not supplementation by ingestion of pills, has been linked to reduction in the risk of prostate cancer, macular degeneration, and cataracts. These carotenoids include alpha and beta carotene, zeaxanthin, lutein, and lycopene, among others. Although widely sold as supplements, dietary intake of these in the form of tomatoes, pumpkin, broccoli, sweet potatoes, etc., is inexpensive and readily obtainable. Keeping in mind that fat enhances their absorption, spaghetti sauce prepared with a small amount of olive oil is a very affordable, tasty way to recommend adequate intake to patients!

Vitamin D (Calcitriol)

Calcitriol is the active metabolite of vitamin D. Vitamin D, unlike most other vitamins, can be made in the body under optimal circumstances. Sterol precursors in the skin, upon exposure to sunlight (UVB), form cholecalciferol, which then undergoes two hydroxylation reactions: first in the liver, resulting in 25-hydroxyvitamin D, or 25(OH) D, and the second in the kidney, resulting in 1,25-dihydroxy vitamin D. Thus, native production of adequate vitamin D requires a combination of healthy skin, adequate sunlight exposure, normal liver and kidney function, normal skin/body mass ratio, and adequate nutritional reserves for sterol production. Any impairment of any of these prerequisites may cause inadequate production. Patients with severe eczema, hepatitis, renal insufficiency, obesity, or who avoid sun exposure will be predictably deficient, and this risk may include the inadvertent lack of sunlight among people who live in northern areas during winter. Vitamin D may also be absorbed from foods rich in the vitamin, such as cod liver oil or fortified cow's milk, and from oral supplements. Excess calcium intake limits the intestinal absorption of vitamin D, so combined calcium/vitamin D supplements are not generally used to correct a vitamin D deficiency state. Disruptions of small intestinal absorptive function, such as Crohn's disease or celiac sprue, also result in vitamin D deficiency.

Vitamin D deficiency syndrome includes myalgias, hypertension, depression, hyperkeratotic skin lesions (psoriasis), insulin resistance, and osteopenia. Patients with these syndromes are followed by 25(OH) D levels (the most accurate storage form of the vitamin), and oral replacement is generally used to obtain normalization of levels over a 4- to 6-week period. Below a 25(OH) D level of 30 mg/dL, parathyroid hormone activation occurs, which triggers osteopenia. Below 20 mg/dL, clinical deficiency states are noted. Therefore, most treatment regimens target levels between 40 and 80 mg/dL. Replacement is most efficiently and economically obtained by using vitamin D_3 (cholecalciferol), which may be used in oral doses of 1,000 IU two to three times daily to remedy a deficiency state. Ergocalciferol (vitamin D_2), which has approximately 70% of the biological activity of cholecalciferol, tends to cause more nausea, and must be used in higher doses to achieve the same effect. Both of these supplements require further hydroxylation to the 1,25(OH) form; therefore they will not be effective in the setting of hepatic or renal failure.

Calcitriol (Rocaltrol) is a pharmaceutical prescription that can be used for patients unable to use the over-the-counter vitamin D forms. These high doses should be used under clinician supervision for correction of deficiency and are not for general public use. Excessive intake of vitamin D in the absence of deficiency can result in hypercalcemia and arrhythmia and should be discouraged.

Vitamin E (Tocopherols/Tocotrienols)

Vitamin E actually includes eight forms: alpha, beta, gamma, and delta tocopherol and alpha, beta, gamma, and delta tocotrienol. Alpha-tocopherol is the most commonly found form in dietary supplements, but food sources generally are rich in delta and gamma forms, as well as in tocotrienols. Dosing and daily allowance recommendations for vitamin E are often provided in alpha-tocopherol equivalents to account for the different biological activities of the various forms of vitamin E, or in international units, which food and supplement labels tend to use.

Vitamin E has been proposed for the prevention or treatment of numerous health conditions, often based on its antioxidant properties. However, aside from the treatment of vitamin E deficiency, which is rare, there are no clearly proven medicinal uses of vitamin E supplementation beyond the recommended daily allowance. There is ongoing research in numerous diseases, particularly in cancer and heart disease.

Vitamin E naturally occurs in whole grains, nuts, fruits, eggs, poultry, vegetables, and grain and vegetable oils, particularly wheat germ oil. Vitamin E deficiency produces muscle weakness and decreased red blood cell survival; it occurs primarily in patients with severe dysregulation of fat absorption. More commonly, vitamin E is used in an effort to prevent atherogenesis and inflammatory disease states. This use is based on food diary studies, including large reviews of the Nurse's Health Study, correlating decreased risk of heart disease with dietary, not supplemental, intake of vitamin E sources. Subsequent trials using alpha-tocopherol, the most widely used and easily synthesized vitamin E form, have failed to demonstrate the benefits seen in food use studies. Although vitamin E deficiency is uncommon, excessive use can produce nausea, diarrhea, and fatigue. High doses of alpha-tocopherol can also increase bleeding time and have been associated with increased risk of all-cause mortality in recent studies of patients with cardiovascular disease. Therefore, patients should be advised to obtain their vitamin E in food sources. If deficiency is suspected, supplements containing mixed tocopherols and tocotrienols should be used rather than isolated alpha-tocopherol.

Vitamin K (Phytonadione)

Vitamin K is the term used for a group of five compounds produced by intestinal bacteria in the ileum or absorbed from dark green leafy vegetables, which have a central ring structure in common and which function as coenzymes for gamma-carboxylation of multiple clotting factors as well as osteocalcin. Vitamin K is essential for normal blood clotting and bone growth and maintenance because it is used by the liver for the formation of prothrombin. Deficiency of vitamin K owing to impaired or delayed absorption is caused by long-term use of antibiotics or the presence of drugs such as warfarin or dicoumarol, or aspirin, and leads to bleeding.

Deficiency of vitamin K is seen occasionally in newborns, with lethal hemorrhagic disease resulting. Therefore, most newborns receive one dose of phytonadione shortly after delivery. Deficiency can also occur with chronic bowel inflammation (Crohn's disease) and chronic antibiotic use.

Vitamin K toxicity may include hypercoagulability, soft tissue calcification in dialysis patients, and hemolysis in patients with glucose-6-phosphate dehydrogenase deficiency. Intravenous use in infusion therapy may result in anaphylaxis if not adequately diluted. Use will also counteract anticoagulant use and result in potential failure of warfarin and aspirin therapy. Replacement of vitamin K should include monitoring of coagulability, bone density, and review of dietary choices to optimize availability when possible. Because this is best absorbed with food containing fat, patients using dark leafy greens as their source should be counseled to include a healthy oil or fat source such as olive oil, avocado, or tree nuts in their meals containing greens. In the United States, only K_1 (phytonadione) is currently available and can be used to correct overdose of warfarin. Several combination vitamin products contain vitamin K and should not be used by patients on anticoagulant therapy.

The Water-Soluable Vitamins

With the exception of vitamin B_{12}, water-soluble vitamins are generally more easily absorbed than fat-soluble vitamins. They are more readily excreted if taken in excess, with lower risk of toxicity. The water-soluble vitamins include the eight B vitamins and vitamin C. The water-soluble vitamins are not stored in the body, and thus short periods of inadequate dietary consumption of their sources can lead to deficiency-induced disease.

Vitamin B1 (Thiamine)

Thiamine, or vitamin B_1, acts as a catalyst in carbohydrate metabolism, enabling pyruvic acid to be absorbed and carbohydrates to release their energy. Thiamine also plays a role in the synthesis of nerve-regulating substances. Deficiency in thiamine causes beriberi, which is characterized by muscular weakness, swelling of the heart, and leg cramps and may, in severe cases, lead to heart failure and death. Many foods contain thiamine, but few supply it in concentrated amounts. Foods richest in thiamine are pork, organ meats (liver, heart, and kidney), brewer's yeast, lean meats, eggs, leafy green vegetables, whole or enriched cereals, wheat germ, berries, nuts, and legumes. Milling of cereal removes those portions of the grain richest in thiamine; consequently, white flour and polished white rice may be lacking in the vitamin. Widespread enrichment of flour and cereal products has largely eliminated the risk of thiamine deficiency, although it still occurs today in nutritionally deficient alcoholics. Wernicke's encephalopathy, Korsakoff's psychoses, and Wernicke-Korsakoff syndrome develop in the alcoholic patient.

Vitamin B2 (Riboflavin)

Riboflavin, or vitamin B_2, like thiamine, serves as a coenzyme in the metabolism of carbohydrates, fats, and respiratory proteins.

It also serves in the maintenance of mucous membranes. Riboflavin deficiency may be complicated by a deficiency of other B vitamins; its symptoms include perioral dermatitis and photosensitivity. The best sources of riboflavin are liver, milk, meat, dark green vegetables, whole grain and enriched cereals, pasta, bread, and mushrooms.

Vitamin B₃ (Niacin)

Niacin, known as nicotinic acid and vitamin B_3, also works as a coenzyme in the release of energy from nutrients. A deficiency of niacin causes pellagra, which is manifested as a photosensitive rash, glossitis, diarrhea, mental confusion, and irritability. Depression and dementia may occur in late cases. The best sources of niacin are liver, poultry, meat, canned tuna and salmon, whole grain and enriched cereals, dried beans and peas, and nuts. The body also makes niacin in a limited amount from the amino acid tryptophan. In large amounts (500 to 1,500 mg daily), it reduces levels of cholesterol in the blood, and it is used routinely as part of an antihyperlipidemic regimen. Niacin preferentially lowers triglycerides, and at higher doses it lowers LDL. Rash, flushing, and gastric upset are common with niacin use at these doses and may be minimized by using slow-acting agents. Hepatic irritation is noted more often with the long-acting agents.

Vitamin B₆ (Pyridoxine)

Pyridoxine, or vitamin B_6, is necessary for the absorption and metabolism of amino acids, including methionine and homocysteine. It is essential for the production of vitamin B_{12} and folate. Pyridoxine deficiency is characterized by skin disorders, cracks at the mouth corners, smooth tongue, seizures, dizziness, nausea, anemia, and kidney stones. The best sources of pyridoxine are whole, but not enriched, grains, cereals, bread, liver, avocados, spinach, green beans, and bananas. Pyridoxine is unique among the water-soluble vitamins in that it causes irreversible peripheral neurotoxicity when taken in high doses, over 300 mg daily. Patients should be cautioned not to use doses in excess of 50 mg daily unless under clinician supervision.

Vitamin B₉ (Folate)

Folic acid serves as a methyl donor, and is critical in methionine and homocysteine metabolism. Folic acid deficiency results in a high incidence of neural tube defect and impaired hematopoiesis, resulting in anemia. Folic acid deficiency can cause poor growth, tongue inflammation, gingivitis, loss of appetite, shortness of breath, diarrhea, irritability, forgetfulness, and mental sluggishness. The U.S. Public Health Service recommends that women of childbearing age take 0.4 mg of folic acid daily. Women should continue to take that dose through the first 3 months of pregnancy. The RDA for men is 200 mcg and for postmenopausal women is 180 mcg. Dietary sources are organ meats, leafy green vegetables, legumes, nuts, whole grains, and brewer's yeast. In the United States, a folate fortification program fortifies many cereal and grain-based foods with extra folate to be sure Americans get adequate intake in their diets. Folic acid is lost in foods stored at room temperature and during cooking.

Malabsorption syndromes such as celiac disease and Crohn's disease may result in folate deficiency. Drugs such as methotrexate also interfere with folate metabolism, which is an issue for patients who take methotrexate for long periods to allay rheumatoid arthritis (RA). Disorders that cause high marrow turnover, such as sickle cell disease or spherocytosis, may consume folate, raising the daily requirement more than 1 mg daily. Women who have had infants with neural tube defects should consume 4 mg of folate daily during their childbearing years. Patients with hyperhomocysteinemia owing to impaired folate metabolism may require 1 to 4 mg of folate daily. Cancer chemotherapy may deliberately deplete folate reserves; these are replaced by oncologists with leucovorin, and patients undergoing chemotherapy should not be given replacement folate until cleared by their oncologist.

Vitamin B₁₂ (Cyanocobalamin)

Cyanocobalamin, or vitamin B_{12}, is necessary in minute amounts for the formation of nucleoproteins, proteins, and red blood cells, and for the functioning of the nervous system. Cobalamin deficiency is often due to the inability of the stomach to produce intrinsic factor or acid, which aids in the absorption of this vitamin. This may be caused by antibodies to parietal cells (pernicious anemia), prolonged use of proton pump inhibitors and H_2 blockers, or the normal aging process. When a deficiency results, it produces ineffective production of red blood cells, faulty myelin (nerve sheath) synthesis, and loss of epithelium (membrane lining) of the intestinal tract. Cobalamin is obtained only from animal sources—liver, kidneys, meat, fish, eggs, and milk. Vegetarians are advised to take vitamin B_{12} supplements because they are at a higher risk of developing vitamin B_{12} deficiency.

Vitamin C (Ascorbic Acid)

Vitamin C is an antioxidant vitamin essential for collagen synthesis. As such, normal levels are critical for maintenance of soft tissue structures, hemostasis, as well as wound healing. Vitamin C also enhances iron absorption. Deficiency of vitamin C produces scurvy, characterized by bleeding gums, loosened teeth, and hemorrhagic lesions. Although Linus Pauling and others have suggested vitamin C prevents viral infections when used in high doses, this has not been clearly demonstrated in humans. Maintenance of normal vitamin C levels is impaired by poor diet, stress, trauma, and infection, and requirements during acute illness increase. Trauma, intensive care unit, and burn patients require supplemental vitamin C in excess of the usual RDA for optimal support of tissue regeneration. Customarily, this is given in oral or enteric doses ranging from 500 mg to 1,000 mg. As ascorbic acid in excess of 500 mg in one dose is quickly excreted in the urine; large and prolonged doses can result in the formation of bladder and kidney stones, and should be avoided. If doses higher than 500 mg are required, as for severe trauma patients, multiple doses may be timed through the day. Sources of vitamin C include citrus fruits, fresh strawberries, cantaloupe, pineapple, and guava. Good vegetable sources are broccoli, Brussels sprouts, tomatoes, spinach, kale, green peppers, cabbage, and turnips. Most patients can easily meet daily requirements with moderate fruit and vegetable intake, and excess vitamin C use on a routine basis should be discouraged.

Vitamin Coenzyme Q10 (CoQ10)

Although not a true vitamin, CoQ10 is a fat-soluble compound present in every cell in the body. It is also known as ubiquinone. It is an essential component of mitochondrial ATP electron transport as a coenzyme for several of the key enzymatic steps in the production of energy within the cell. Because it is manufactured by the human body in large amounts, it is normally not considered an essential nutrient. Under certain circumstances, however, CoQ10 production is markedly impaired by a deficiency in diet, an impairment in biosynthesis, or excessive utilization, or a combination of the three impairments. Decreased dietary intake is presumed in chronic malnutrition and cachexia, extreme bodily decline, and weakness.

HMG-CoA reductase inhibitors used to treat elevated blood cholesterol levels by blocking cholesterol biosynthesis also block CoQ10 biosynthesis; thus, all patients on statin drugs will have predictably decreased CoQ10 levels. In addition, diabetes and metabolic syndrome also reduce the production of the CoQ10 enzyme. Symptoms of deficiency include fatigue, myalgia, and exercise intolerance, which may be mistaken for statin-induced rhabdomyolysis. If a patient on a statin develops this combination of symptoms, and the serum CPK is within normal range, empiric supplementation of CoQ10 (200 mg daily) is indicated. Serum levels are available from referral laboratories and may be considered if improvement in symptoms on 200 mg/day is not adequate. Doses of CoQ10 up to 400 mg daily have been well tolerated, with no drug interactions noted. It is naturally present in small amounts in a wide variety of foods, but it is particularly high in organ meats such as heart, liver, and kidney, as well as beef, soy oil, sardines, mackerel, and peanuts. To put dietary CoQ10 intake into perspective, 1 pound of sardines, 2 pounds of beef, or 2.5 pounds of peanuts provide 30 mg of CoQ10.

The Role of the Clinician in Integrative Prescribing

Dietary supplements and herbal medicine have become widely available and are widely used by the general public. The role of the integrative clinician is one of a supportive guide helping patients make safe, informed decisions regarding their dietary supplement choices. The conscientious clinician can help patients review these choices during each patient encounter if they remember to do so as a routine part of history taking and/or patient counseling. It is important to help patients evaluate potential clinically significant interactions between dietary supplements and prescription drugs. This would also include their interference with dosing, laboratory tests, and nutritional status. Clinicians should encourage patients in choosing appropriate supplements when the evidence exists that indicates these supplements provide appropriate benefits that far outweigh any risk.

Implications for Special Populations
Pregnancy Implications

When prescribing for the pregnant or lactating female, clinicians should carefully consider their choice of all natural and prescribed and OTC drugs, especially considering the increased nutritional demands of pregnancy and the probability of developing nutritional deficiencies. Following is a selected list of vitamins with their assigned FDA Safety Category. Herbals and other dietary supplements generally have not been assigned an FDA Pregnancy category, although those with GRAS status are generally considered safe to use as foods during pregnancy.

FDA CATEGORY (FOR DOSES EXCEEDING THE RDA)	VITAMIN
A	Thiamine, pyridoxine, folic acid
B	
C	Vitamin D, cyanocobalamin (B_{12}), ascorbic acid
X	Vitamin A
Unclassified	Niacin, riboflavin, vitamin K, vitamin E

Pediatrics

Children who eat a balanced diet should be getting all the vitamins they need for healthy growth. However, some children are "picky" about what they eat and also may not be obtaining adequate vitamin D, especially during the winter months. Children's multivitamins are usually dosed for children under 12, and thus parents should avoid use of adult vitamins or megadose vitamins, vitamin A, those with iron, and those with vitamin D in children because they can cause a toxic effect. Many of the foods a child will eat are fortified with vitamins, especially bread (B vitamins and extra iron), milk (vitamin D), breakfast cereals (most vitamins and minerals), and orange juice (vitamin C), but fortified foods often contain only about 20% of the RDA, counting on diet to supply the rest. Children and menstruating adolescents may need iron supplements to prevent anemia.

Geriatrics

Because aging adults typically take multiple prescription medications, they are likely to have drug-associated nutrient deficiencies. They may also be taking herbals and supplements, not realizing many of these agents are interacting with their prescription medications. The seven most common products taken by older adults are a multivitamin; vitamins B, C, D, and E; calcium; and glucosamine/chondroitin. Women are more than twice as likely to take calcium and vitamin D and more likely to take magnesium. As age and function decline, elderly patients may use these products to restore their health and function. The conscientious integrative clinician prescribing for the elderly takes a thorough drug history, including OTC and dietary supplements (which may not be considered medicine in the eye of the elderly). The conscientious clinician should also be aware of the increased incidence of nutritional deficiencies that exist in the elderly population owing to the aging process, the presence of chronic disease, and the associated increased nutritional demands and nutrient depletion associated with some prescription medications. The decreased ability to prepare healthy meals owing to budget limitations or decreased mobility may also limit the ability of the elderly patient to have a well-rounded diet. A combination of any of these factors may contribute to the increased incidence of nutritional deficiencies.

LEARNING EXERCISES

Case 1

Mrs. M is a 55-year-old female with a history of inflammatory bowel disease and osteoporosis, and who has been faithfully coming into your clinic for 10 years for her annual check-up. She always has presented as being healthy and says she eats well, exercises regularly, and takes her vitamins to ward off disease. This year, however, she presents with symptoms that include nausea, anorexia, hair loss, unusual fatigue, joint pain, and frequent headaches. She states that initially she felt her symptoms were because of aging or even a thyroid problem, but over the last 2 months she hasn't felt like herself. Also, she states that although she has been taking her vitamins and herbs to improve her health and specifically her vision, she now has started to experience blurry vision. Further history reveals that she began to double some of her vitamin doses over the last 3 months because she read in a magazine article that people with chronic diarrhea do not always absorb vitamins well.

1. What is causing Mrs. M's symptoms?

2. What patient education should Mrs. M. be given?

Case 2

Mrs. J. is a 75-year-old female. She presents for a routine follow-up for her hypertension and you note elevated blood pressure, some ankle swelling, and some face redness. She also states she is having a few headaches. Her past medical history (PMH) includes hypertension, atrial fibrillation, CAD, and a stroke 4 years ago. Her daily medications include warfarin 2 mg daily, HCTZ 25 mg daily, lisinopril 5 mg twice daily, paroxetine 5 mg daily, and digoxin 0.025mg daily.

Laboratory results reveal the patient's INR to be 1.5. However, because of her elevated blood pressure and her nontherapeutic INR, some changes to her medications are made. Specifically, warfarin is increased to 4 mg daily; hydrochlorothiazide is increased to 50 mg daily; and lisinopril is increased to 10 mg twice daily.

Five days after taking the increased dosages, the patient's son notices that she is wandering around the house in a state of confusion. Because she had a stroke several years ago, the son calls the Rescue Squad and the patient is taken to the local emergency department for evaluation. Mrs. J. is diagnosed with altered mental status and a probable transient ischemic attack (TIA) and admitted for observation. Following admission, a pharmacist attempts to gather details of her medications. Deep questioning reveals Mrs. J. has been taking some herbs after reading about them in a magazine. These herbals include ginkgo biloba and St. John's wort. When asked how much she has been taking, she admits to taking 240 mg of ginkgo biloba, and 1,000 mg of St. Johns wort every day.

1. What should the clinician do in this case?

References

DeKosky, S. T., Williamson, J. D., Fitzpatrick, A. L., Kronmal, R. A., Ives, D. G., Saxton, J. A., et al. (2008). Ginkgo biloba for dementia: a randomized controlled trial. *JAMA, 300*(19), 2253-2262.

Geller, S. E., Shulman, L. P., van Breeman, R. B., Banuvar, S., Zhour, Y., Epstein, G., et al. (2009). Safety and efficacy of black cohosh and red clover for management of vasomotor symptoms. *Menopause, 16*(6), 1156-1166. Retrieved March 13, 2013, from www.ncbi.nlm.nih.gov/pubmed/19609225

Jellin, J., Gregory, P., Batz, F., Hitchen, K., Burson, S., Shaver, K., et al. (eds.) (2000). *Natural medicines comprehensive database* (3rd ed.). Stockton, CA: Therapeutic Research.

National Center for Complementary and Alternative Medicine (NCCAM) of the National Institutes of Health (NIH). (2011). Using Dietary Supplements Wisely. Retrieved March 13, 2013, from http://nccam.nih.gov/health/supplements/wiseuse.htm

National Institutes of Health, Office of Dietary Supplements. (2011). Dietary Supplement Fact Sheet: Black Cohosh. Retrieved March 13, 2013, from ods.od.nih.gov/factsheets/blackcohosh

Agents Used to Manipulate the Immune Response

Fred S. Girton

chapter 26

CHAPTER FOCUS

This chapter describes the manipulation of host defenses by pharmaceutical agents to better control immune reactions and/or to enhance them. The chapter presents the use of antihistamines, corticosteroids, mast cell stabilizers, and leukotriene modifiers in the treatment of allergies and hypersensitivities such as allergic conjunctivitis and atopic dermatitis. While these agents are discussed in Chapter 10, Drugs Used in the Treatment of Pulmonary Diseases and Disorders, and in Chapter 16, Drugs Used in the Treatment of Skin Disorders, here we more fully focus on their use in the treatment of common allergic conditions. Treatment of less common allergic reactions and hypersensitivities such as insect venom allergy, drug allergies, food allergies, urticaria, angioedema, contact dermatitis, and anaphylaxis are also discussed. Finally, the vaccinations are introduced as to help clinicians gain insight into the immunization for disease prevention and immunotherapy for desensitization.

Key Terms

Allergens
Allergic reactions
Allergy
Anaphylaxis
Antigens
Antibodies
Atopy
Hypersensitivity
Immunization
Immunoglobulins (Ig)
Immunotherapy
Inflammation
Vaccine

OBJECTIVES

After carefully reading and studying this chapter, the student should be able to:

1. Explain how antigens can become allergens.
2. Describe the role that pharmaceuticals play in manipulating the immune system and its primary reaction, inflammation.
3. Distinguish between the four types of hypersensitivity reactions and provide examples of each.
4. Describe how clinicians know which drug treatment to use in various hypersensitivities and allergies.
5. Provide examples of allergen avoidance.
6. Describe the benefit of topical corticosteroids in inflammation.
7. Discuss the complications of corticosteroid medication.
8. Explain how to treat an anaphylactic reaction.
9. Distinguish between live attenuated vaccines, inactivated vaccines, and immunotherapy.

KEY DRUGS IN THIS CHAPTER

Topical Corticosteroids
Class 1: Super Potent
  betamethasone 0.5%
  clobetasol propionate 0.05% (Temovate)
  halobetasol propionate 0.05% (Ultravate)
Class 2: Potent
  amcinonide 0.1% (Cyclocort)
  betamethasone dipropionate 0.05% (Diprosone)
  desoximetasone 0.25% (Topicort)

  fluocinonide 0.05% (Lidex, Fluonex)
  halcinonide 0.1% (Halog)
Class 3: Moderate or Upper Mid-Strength
  betamethasone dipropionate 0.05% (Diprosone)
  betamethasone valerate 0.1%
  diflorasone diacetate 0.05% (Florone, Maxiflor)
  fluticasone propionate 0.005% (Cutivate)

Class 4: Mid-Strength
  amcinonide 0.1% (Cyclocort)
  desoximetasone 0.05% (Topicort LP)
  flucinolone acetonide 0.2% (Synalar HP)
  hydrocortisone valerate 0.2% (Westcort)
  triamcinolone acetonide 0.1% (Kenalog, Aristocort)
Class 5: Lower Mid-Strength
  betamethasone dipropionate 0.05% (Diprosone)

continued

Proper prescribing for immunological disorders begins with a firm understanding of how the body deals with immunity, the system of protecting the body from assault by foreign invaders (microbes). The human body is surrounded by pathogens of many kinds, in the air, in water, on the skin, in mucous linings, and along the gastrointestinal (GI) and respiratory tract. Although some are harmless and some beneficial, some are pathogenic. The body needs protection from extracellular organisms seeking to reproduce at the expense of their host. Innate/passive immunity and acquired/adaptive immunity provide protection through the immune response.

Innate immunity is the body's natural immunity system. It is nonspecific, always present, and does not change in action or strength. The innate immune system comprises skin, gastric acid, bronchial mucus, and certain nonspecific white blood cells such as phagocytes and leukocytes. It is capable of recognizing only a limited number of molecular patterns common to a wide variety of pathogens, called pathogen-associated molecular patterns (PAMPs). Because pathogens and other invading organisms are constantly evolving to protect themselves by blocking the innate immune system, the acquired immune system adapts to foreign bodies to maintain the effectiveness of the immune response and protect the human body. The acquired, or adaptive, immune system recognizes unique molecular structures that are present in foreign substances or pathogens and those not shared with any other pathogen. Originally, the cells of the body's immune system with this ability were called *antigens*. However, the meaning of the term *antigen* has evolved, and it is now defined as molecular structures that are targeted by either a cell-mediated or a humoral adaptive response. Thus, a foreign microbe is likely to be recognized as such by leukocytes that recognize either its PAMPs or its antigens. Innate responses occur throughout the body, but mostly below the skin and on mucous membranes where microbes attempt to gain access. If a microbe invades the body and overwhelms the innate immune response, the adaptable immune response takes over, usually starting in the lymphoid tissues.

Humans develop their adaptive immune response by exposure to various foreign substances (antigens). Once exposed, the body develops immunity specific to that antigen. The adaptive immune response to an antigen is beneficial when the antigen represents a threat and the immune response destroys the antigen, but if the antigen is benign or nonharmful, as is the case of pollen or dander, the resulting immune response is unwanted and results in inflammation such as in allergic rhinitis. When the resulting immune response is too strong, even if it is an appropriate response, it is considered **hypersensitivity**, as is often the case in poison ivy or an asthma attack. The tendency to develop an **allergy**, or hypersensitivity, is greatly determined by inheritance and is referred to as **atopy**. This genetic tendency to develop an allergy is why certain people are more prone to develop allergies such as atopic dermatitis, allergic rhinitis, and hay fever.

No one is born with an allergy, nor does one inherit an allergy, but the tendency to develop allergies is inherited. The immune system, like all bodily functions, begins to wane as it becomes older; for this and several other reasons, allergies are more prevalent in young children and adolescents and tend to decrease as people reach their 60s. This decreasing immunity with aging also puts geriatric populations at greater risk for infections and malignancies than their younger counterparts.

Understanding Immunity

A key to a healthy immune response is the body's ability to recognize its own cells and the cells of a foreign microbe. Thus, the body's immune system coexists peacefully with its own cells, but when it encounters cells that are foreign, because of their PAMPs, it attacks and attempts to eliminate them. Anything that triggers this response is called an antigen. Any invading agent, toxin, chemical, or virus may have only one or a few recognizable antigens whereas bacteria and parasites may have hundreds or even thousands, making the role of the adaptive immune response easier when it comes to recognizing them. This is because in humans, the adaptive immunity is triggered when a pathogen evades the innate immune system but generates a threshold level of antigen which in turn is uniquely expressed on each individual lymphocyte. Because the gene rearrangement leads to an irreversible change in the DNA of the lymphocyte, all of the progeny of that cell inherits gene encoding having the same receptor specificity, which in turn is the reason why adaptive immunity is specific and long lived. Antigens, once recognized as foreign, initiate an immune response within the body first by releasing cytokines and chemokines, which induce inflammation. **Inflammation** is a process with five distinguishing signs and symptoms:

- *rubor* (redness)
- *tumor* (swelling)
- *dolor* (pain)
- *calor* (warmth)
- *functio laes* (loss of function)

When the invasion is large or widespread, inflammation can become systemic, resulting in large quantities of cytokines, which in turn can cause fever, tachycardia, and organ failure, possibly leading to shock or death. Thus, inflammation can be destructive, not only to the invading agent but also to the body as well.

After initiation of the inflammatory response, the adaptive immune system splits into humoral immunity and cellular immunity. Humoral immunity involves special lymphocytes, white blood cells called B cells that produce specific antibodies. **Antibodies** are large protein molecules released from the lymphocytes that bind with and help destroy an offending antigen by marking it for destruction. An antibody binds with an antigen much in the same way as a key fits into a lock. The shape of its chemical structures allows interlocking, making antibodies specific for a particular antigen. An antibody that is a protein is called an **immunoglobulin (Ig)**, and there are distinct subclasses of them: four kinds of IgG, and two kinds of IgA, IgM, IgD, and IgE. Each class has different properties, but they all bind to the specific antigen for which they were made. IgG is the most abundant immunoglobulin among internal body fluids, and it is mostly found in the blood where it combats microorganisms and their toxins.

IgA is found in the seromucous secretions (tears, saliva, respiratory tract, and GI tract) where it defends the gut and mucous surfaces of the body. IgM is the most common immunoglobulin and is capable of binding five antigens at once. IgM is found mostly in the blood where it is most effective against bacteria. IgD is mostly present on lymphocyte surfaces where it regulates the cell's activation. IgE is found primarily on the skin and external surfaces of the body in trace amounts. Although it is the smallest percentage of total body immunoglobulin (0.002%), IgE is the predominant immunoglobulin responsible for allergy and allergic diseases.

Cellular immunity is performed mainly by white blood cells. These cells either destroy the invading agent or direct and assist other cells in performing that function. Both humoral and cellular immunity are managed by lymphocytic T cells, which regulate the intensity, type, and duration of the immune response. When an individual has been immunologically primed by exposure to an antigen, repeat exposures result in a much more rapid and effective response. Repeat exposures, particularly by patients who are atopic, can result in excessive immune reactions with possible tissue damage. These hypersensitivities are called type I allergies when they are IgE mediated. Most hypersensitivity reactions involve IgE, but there are other hypersensitivities that are not IgE mediated; these hypersensitivities are mediated by other immunoglobulins or by specific immunologic cells. For example, type II hypersensitivities of allergies are IgM and IgG mediated. This differentiation is important to know because selecting the proper drug treatment depends on knowing what type of hypersensitivity is present. Coombs and Gell defined four types of hypersensitivity (Rabson, Arthur, Roitt, & Delves, 2005) (Table 26-1):

- Type I (immediate or anaphylactic) or Ig E mediated: Treatment requires antihistamines, epinephrine, or corticosteroids (penicillin allergy). Type I is called *immediate* because its reaction can occur immediately upon exposure (15 to 30 minutes) and involves release of vasoactive amines and lipid mediators. It can also be a *late-phase* reaction and occur 2 to 4 hours or more after exposure, but now includes the release of cytokines. The reaction may involve the skin (urticaria, eczema); eyes (conjunctivitis); nasopharynx (rhinorrhea); bronchopulmonary tissue (asthma); or GI tissue (gastroenteritis). The reaction is further complicated by release of histamine, heparin, and vasoactive amines.
- Type II (cytotoxic hypersensitivity): This is type IgM and IgG mediated, with reactions occurring minutes to hours after exposure to an exogenous antigen. Drug-induced conditions such as agranulocytopenia, thrombocytopenia, and pernicious anemia are examples.
- Type III (immune complex hypersensitivity): This is mediated by the IgG class and somewhat by IgM. It takes 3 to 10 hours after exposure to see a reaction in individual organs or general reactions such as skin (systemic lupus, allergic contact dermatitis); lung (aspergilloses); blood vessels (polyarteritis); or joints (rheumatoid arthritis).
- Type IV (delayed-type hypersensitivity [DTH]): This type involves cell-mediated T cells. Type IV delayed-hypersensitivity reactions are inflammatory reactions initiated by mononuclear leukocyte T cells and macrophages rather than antibodies. The term *delayed* differentiates them from *immediate* hypersensitivities in that a secondary cellular response appears 48 to 72 hours after an antigen challenge. Delayed hypersensitivity is a major mechanism of defense against various intracellular pathogens, including mycobacteria,

TABLE 26-1	Gell and Coombs Classification of Hypersensitivity
HYPERSENSITIVITY	**DEFINITION**
TYPE I: IMMEDIATE ANAPHYLACTIC	• Often referred to as atopic disease, hypersensitivity, or allergy. It is the result of overproduction of IgE antibodies, which are attached to mast cells. When the specific antigen is present, it reacts with the IgE antibodies to degranulate the mast cells, resulting in release of histamine, heparin, tryptase, and various chemotactic factors. These inflammatory agents result in the classic symptoms of common allergies, depending on where they occur. • When localized to the skin or mucosa this hypersensitivity results in local inflammation of the mucosa or skin (irritating but seldom life threatening). • When IgE is widely attached to mast cells throughout the body, this hypersensitivity can be severe and systemic, resulting in bronchospasm, vascular collapse, organ failure and death. **Examples: Allergic rhinitis, asthma, atopic dermatitis, urticaria, food allergies, and insect venom sensitivity.**
TYPE II: CYTOTOXIC	• Occurs because of the development of abnormal antibody, usually IgG or IgM, directed against a particular cell or tissue. • May be an autoimmune sensitivity, with antibodies being directed against a cell or tissue in the body, or it can be a drug that is attached to a cell stimulating antibodies that attack both the cell and the drug (e.g., chlorpromazine seen in hemolytic anemia and quinidine associated with agranulocytosis; when the drug is removed, these sensitivities are no longer evident). **Other examples: Autoimmune hemolytic anemias, myasthenia gravis with antibodies directed at acetylcholine receptors, Graves' disease, and probably some cases of diabetes.**
TYPE III: IMMUNE COMPLEX	• Occurs when there is an excess of antigen, which may result in antibodies and antigens forming insoluble complexes. These complexes can become fixed at various sites in the body, in particular the kidneys and liver. When antigens combine with antigens, inflammatory cytokines are released and inflammation can occur. • Because the complex is fixed, it can cause damage to the tissue to which it is affixed. **Examples: Serum sickness, glomerulonephritis, vasculitis of the skin and joints.**
TYPE IV: DELAYED HYPERSENSITIVITY	• Does not involve immunoglobulins but is a result of an exaggerated interaction between antigen and the normal cell-mediated immune response. • Often called delayed-type hypersensitivity because it often takes several days to manifest itself. • The most well-known cell-mediated hypersensitivity is the Mantoux TB skin test. If the person has been previously infected with tuberculosis, he or she will manifest a cell-mediated immunity to the tuberculin and within 24–48 hours the classic red (erythematous, rubor), raised (indurated, tubor) skin lesion will be seen. **Examples: Contact dermatitis (poison ivy, nickel allergy), certain insect bites, certain organ-specific autoimmune diseases (diabetes type 1), and the skin lesions of measles and herpes simplex.**

From Gell, P. G. H., & Coombs, R. R. A. (Eds.). (1963). Clinical aspects of immunology, (1st ed.). Oxford, England: Blackwell.

fungi, and certain parasites, and it occurs in transplant rejection and tumor immunity. The central role of T cells in delayed hypersensitivity is seen in AIDS where, because of the loss of CD4+ T cells, the host response against intracellular pathogens such as *Mycobacterium tuberculosis* is impaired. Type IV delayed hypersensitivity reactions are normal physiological events, but if anything alters these events, such as T-cell dysfunction, opportunistic infections can arise. The traditional and most accepted classification of hypersensitivity reactions is attributed to Gell and Coombs (see Table 26-1). Despite its widespread decades of use, it may be too general for some clinicians who prefer a more recent classification proposed by Sell et al. (1996), which classifies hypersensitivities (immunopathological responses) as being in one of the following seven categories:

■ Inactivation/activation antibody reactions
■ Cytotoxic or cytolytic antibody reactions
■ Immune complex reactions
■ **Allergic reactions**
■ T-cell cytotoxic reactions
■ Delayed hypersensitivity reactions
■ Granulomatous reactions.

The Sell Classification has its proponents because it allows for multiple components of the immune system being involved in a hypersensitivity response.

Making a diagnosis of hypersensitivity reaction requires a complete history, with an emphasis on the type and triggers surrounding the hypersensitivity response, and a series of physical examinations to document the patient's state of health before, during, and after a hypersensitivity reaction. Diagnostic tests are not always necessary if an antigen is strongly suspected and treatment is effective. Two main types of diagnostic tests are available for diagnosing hypersensitivities: skin testing (prick, patch, and intradermal) and in vitro blood analysis for antibodies (usually IgE). Skin testing can be expensive, may require stopping certain medications to prevent false negatives, can be somewhat uncomfortable, is time-consuming, and occasionally, in the case of intradermal skin testing, can carry a risk of anaphylaxis.

Performing skin tests requires specialized knowledge on the part of the clinician, whereas in vitro testing of serum for antibodies (radioallergosorbent test, also known as a RAST) is easily performed with a simple blood draw and no special preparations or risks are involved. Although the in vitro blood test is much simpler than skin testing, many allergists consider in vitro testing less sensitive. Both types of diagnostic testing require correlation with the patient's clinical symptoms. Many patients will have positive diagnostic tests demonstrating IgE antibodies to specific antigens but will have no clinical allergic symptoms, and the reverse is also common. Nonetheless, diagnostic testing can be helpful in difficult cases and in preparation for immunotherapy.

Management of the Immune Response

The goal of the immune system is to destroy an invading agent (antigen) and repair any damage that it may have caused. The primary means of destroying an invading agent is through inflammation; however, it is often necessary for inflammation to destroy normal, healthy tissue in its attempt to destroy the invader. The clinician's challenge is management of this normal immune response (inflammation) when it becomes inappropriately excessive or persistent. The clinician can assist the body in minimizing the effects of dealing with its immune response by prescribing medications or can enhance the normal immune system through effective immunization or vaccination (i.e., the stimulation of the immune system in order to fortify the body against foreign molecules. This is typically done with vaccines.).

TREATMENT OF ALLERGIC RHINITIS

Allergic rhinitis is one of the most common chronic conditions affecting humans and is the most common immunologic disease. It may occur at almost any age, but the majority of patients develop the disorder before they are 30, with the highest incidence between the ages of 15 and 25. Symptoms are variable and can be extremely irritating and difficult to control to mildly bothersome and easily subdued. Depending on the type of allergy and the exposure to the specific allergens, the symptoms may be continual as in perennial allergic rhinitis (such as mold and dust mites) or periodic, as in seasonal (owing to pollens such as ragweed). The symptoms of allergic rhinitis, although seldom life threatening, can affect school, work, and leisure activities.

The classic symptoms of allergic rhinitis are sneezing, itching, nasal discharge, and congestion. Swelling from inflammation can result in nasal, sinus, and eustachian tube blockage, which can then lead to sinusitis, otitis media, rhino sinusitis, conjunctivitis, and other ear, eye, nose, and throat disorders.

The pathophysiology of allergic rhinitis is based on the IgE type 1 hypersensitivity; that is, a genetically predisposed individual is exposed to an allergen, which in normal individuals may cause little, if any, immunoglobulin E (IgE) antibody response. However, the atopic person generates a great amount of IgE specific to this allergen. The IgE antibody then binds and sensitizes mast cells throughout the body, but in this case predominately in the mucous membranes of the nose and sinuses. Upon subsequent exposure to the allergen, the IgE antibodies attached to the mast cells are cross-linked and they stimulate mast cell degranulation. This degranulation results in the allergic symptoms. Histamine, leukotrienes, proinflammatory cytokines, and other immediate hypersensitivity agents are released, resulting in sneezing, itching, production of excess mucus, and swelling of the nose and sinuses. In other words, excess and undesirable inflammation, usually annoying, but in some cases so severe that systemic symptoms such as aches, low-grade fever, and fatigue can occur. Because this is a condition that individuals may be genetically predisposed to developing, it is not surprising that 38% of patients with allergic rhinitis also have asthma and 78% of asthmatics have allergic rhinitis. Not all rhinitis is allergic, however, and other causes of the symptoms must be ruled out. For example, rhinitis can be the result of infection (usually viral), pregnancy, nonallergic rhinitis with eosinophilia syndrome, changes in temperature, hormonal changes, anatomical abnormalities, foreign bodies, exercise, and medication. The conscientious clinician will consider these causatives and rule them out before making the diagnosis of allergic rhinitis.

Nonpharmacological treatment of allergic rhinitis is best obtained by minimizing exposure to the offending allergens. Once the likely allergens have been determined, patients should be educated to avoid them whenever possible. Seasonal allergens can, in some cases, be controlled by limiting outdoor exposure to certain activities such as cutting grass and yard work, or by staying indoors and using an air conditioner. Perennial allergies are more difficult to control and, of course, require year-round avoidance. Box 26-1 summarizes suggestions for avoiding allergen exposure.

Pharmacological treatment of allergic rhinitis is primarily based on treating the inflammatory response that occurs with the release of histamine, leukotrienes, and other inflammatory reactive substances. Oral antihistamines, the primary class of medications used for allergic rhinitis, are commonly used because of their relative inexpensiveness, availability without a prescription, and reasonable efficacy in controlling symptoms. To bypass the side effects of oral systemic antihistamines, several nasal spray antihistamines that are fairly effective are available: azelastine nasal (Astelin, Astepro) and olopatadine nasal (Patanase). All presently require prescriptions and are expensive. After antihistamines, the intranasal corticosteroids are the preferred prescription treatment of allergic rhinitis. Intranasal steroids are now used extensively by young and old, with few side effects or problems.

Often combined with decongestants and analgesics, antihistamines come in a multitude of forms and dosages. See Chapter 10,

Drugs Used in the Treatment of Pulmonary Diseases and Disorders, for more information on antihistamines. Besides antihistamines and intranasal corticosteroids, nasal mast cell stabilizers, decongestants, anticholinergics, and leukotriene receptor antagonists all have a place in therapy of allergic rhinitis.

Intranasal Corticosteroids

Intranasal corticosteroids for allergic rhinitis are usually applied directly to the nasal passages via nasal spray and are absorbed within 10 minutes. The corticosteroid is a human glucocorticoid receptor agonist. These agents inhibit mast cells, eosinophils, basophils, lymphocytes, macrophages, and eicosanoids, all of which contribute to inflammation. In the case of allergic rhinitis, these agents reduce nasal congestion, sneezing, nasal itching, and rhinorrhea.

The side effects of intranasal corticosteroids are usually minimal and may be preferred to the side effects of oral systemic drugs, such as the sedation of antihistamines. Intranasal corticosteroids do not work immediately and require at least 1 to 2 weeks of continuous usage to obtain adequate response. Systemic corticosteroids (oral or injectable) are seldom used in allergic rhinitis, and because of their systemic adverse effects, are only recommended in intractable allergic rhinitis not responding to other therapy.

Corticosteroids are slower to act than antihistamines, and it may be 3 to 5 days before response is noted.

Dosage and Administration

Generic Name	Trade Name	Route	Usual Adult Daily Dose
beclomethasone dipropionate*	Beconase Vancenase	Intranasal	1–2 inhalations each nostril 2–4 times/day
budesonide	Rhinocort	Intranasal	2 sprays each nostril 2 times/day or 4 sprays in a.m.
flunisolide	Nasarel, Nasalide	Intranasal	2 sprays each nostril 2–3 times/day
fluticasone furoate	Veramyst	Intranasal	2 sprays each nostril daily
fluticasone propionate	Flonase	Intranasal	2 sprays each nostril 1 time/day or 1 spray each nostril 2 times/day
mometasone furoate	Nasonex	Intranasal	2 sprays each nostril once daily
triamcinolone acetonide	Nasacort	Intranasal	2–4 sprays each nostril once daily

Beclomethasone dipropionate is sold as an inhalant with a special adapter for intranasal delivery, hence the use of the term inhalation rather than spray.

Adverse Reactions

In general, there are almost no serious side effects occurring with the use of nasal corticosteroids. Some patients experience headaches, pharyngeal candidiasis, pharyngitis, nasopharyngeal irritation, epistaxis, and septal perforation.

Interactions

- There are very few proven interactions of inhaled corticosteroids. When taken systemically, adverse reactions are more likely.

Contraindications

- Hypersensitive to medication

Nasal Mast Cell Stabilizer

The *mast cell stabilizers* prevent the release of histamine from mast cells by stabilizing their membranes. This decreases the tendency to release inflammatory mediators from mast cells when allergenic stimulation occurs. Considered moderately effective, cromolyn is safe and some intranasal preparations are available over the counter (OTC), but it must be used three to six times a day for effectiveness. Cromolyn is prophylactic and must be used prior to allergic antigen exposure, because once the mast cell releases its inflammatory mediators, cromolyn is of little use.

Dosage and Administration

Generic Name	Trade Name	Route	Usual Adult Daily Dose
cromolyn sodium	Nasalcrom	Intranasal	1 spray each nostril 3–6 times/day

Adverse Reactions and Contraindications

In general, there are almost no serious or common adverse reactions or drug interactions occurring with the use of nasal inhaled mast cell stabilizers other than their bad taste. Like all medications, the risk of allergic reaction and anaphylaxis is possible, and no one allergic to cromolyn-like medications should take them.

Decongestants

Decongestant agents are sympathomimetics (alpha-adrenergic agonists) that cause vasoconstriction in the superficial mucosal blood vessels and as a result decrease swelling of the nasal mucosa and rhinorrhea. Available orally and intranasally, several decongestant agents are available in a myriad of OTC formulations. The use of topical decongestants avoids the side effects of systemic decongestants, tachycardia, sweating, nausea, dizziness, headache, unusual sweating, or tremors. However, local side effects such as temporary burning, stinging, tearing, dry nose, and runny nose can be a concern. Use of topical decongestants for greater than 3 to 4 days can result in *rhinitis medicamentosa*, which is a rebound effect resulting in return and worsening of original symptoms. To prevent this rebound congestion, intranasal decongestants are labeled for use for no more than 3 days out of every 7.

Anticholinergic Agents

Although not a first-line treatment like decongestants, anticholinergic medications are considered an adjunctive medication for allergic rhinitis. Topical nasal anticholinergic agents such as ipratropium bromide (Atrovent) are quite effective in reducing nasal hypersecretion and congestion in allergic rhinitis. The other symptoms of allergic rhinitis such as itching and sneezing are less affected by anticholinergic medication. Atrovent nasal spray is currently the only available agent for this use. The Atrovent nasal spray comes in two concentrations, 0.03% and 0.06%. The dosage is two sprays in each nostril two to four times a day.

Leukotriene Receptor Antagonists

Leukotriene receptor antagonists such as montelukast (Singulair) in a dose identical to that for treating allergic asthma has been approved for treatment of allergic rhinitis. Not considered a mainline treatment, it may provide relief for some patients. The leukotriene modifiers are discussed in greater detail in the allergic asthma section.

TREATMENT OF ALLERGIC CONJUNCTIVITIS

Although allergens are a common cause of conjunctivitis, viral or bacterial infections can also cause it. Conjunctivitis can be seasonal, perennial, acute contact type, or nonallergic, thus requiring an in-depth history identifying triggering events and timelines of symptoms. Ocular itching is a key distinguishing feature of allergy and should be differentiated from burning, scratchy, or sandy sensation in the eyes. A history of other allergic diseases is also common and helpful.

Care must be taken in making the diagnosis of acute allergic conjunctivitis because serious conditions such as viral infections, acute glaucoma, vernal conjunctivitis, giant papillary

conjunctivitis (associated with contact lenses), and other conditions must be ruled out. Failure to make the correct diagnosis in an acute case of a bacterial or viral infection can result in significant loss of vision and other serious complications. The use of topical steroids can be dangerous when dealing with viral or bacterial infections of the eye, and they should be prescribed with caution. The close association with other allergic diseases is so great that all individuals diagnosed with allergic conjunctivitis should be evaluated for other atopic conditions such as asthma, food allergies, atopic dermatitis, and so on. The most effective management of allergic conjunctivitis is avoiding exposure to the offending allergens. If the allergen is a cosmetic or foreign body, irrigation with saline solution or artificial tears may help. Cold compresses may provide symptomatic relief.

Pharmacological treatment of allergic conjunctivitis is primarily the treatment of the symptoms, not the underlying antigen-antibody IgE reaction. Almost all pharmacological treatments are in the form of eyedrops. Because topical medications for the conjunctivae are limited to the eye, little or no systemic effect or absorption is noted in the use of these preparations. Systemic drugs are seldom used for treatment of the conjunctivae except in the case of oral antihistamines, which are used in standard doses and provide only partial relief. Several classes of drugs are used to treat allergic conjunctivitis.

Artificial tears/lubricants are used to treat dryness and irritation associated with allergies. *Topical vasoconstrictors* constrict arterioles when applied topically by stimulating alpha-adrenergic receptors in the sympathetic nervous system. Topical vasoconstrictor agents have been found to be helpful in treating conjunctivitis. They do little to treat the underlying pathophysiology but can reduce eye redness and ocular itching. Topical vasoconstrictors are often combined with other medications such as topical antihistamines. Vasoconstrictor topical medications can have a rebound vasodilatation after prolonged use.

Antihistamines compete with histamine on H1 effector cells inhibiting the release of histamine and its resultant local irritation caused by the hyperactivity of histamine release during the allergic response. The class of drugs called NSAIDs, used widely in treating inflammatory diseases of the musculoskeletal system and rheumatological diseases, are also found to be helpful in treating conjunctivitis. Topical eyedrops of various NSAIDs have been very beneficial in controlling allergic conjunctivitis.

Mast stabilizers prevent the release of histamine from cells to decrease the frequency and intensity of allergic reactions. Finally, *topically applied steroids* are a potentially effective treatment for allergic conjunctivitis because, through multiple mechanisms, they mediate the inflammation resulting from the allergic response. Although effective, the use of topical steroids for allergic conjunctivitis should be avoided if at all possible. If used, close ophthalmological monitoring must be done because adverse reactions such as glaucoma, cataracts, and viral infections can be aggravated by steroid use.

Dosage and Administration

Drug Class	Generic Name	Trade Name	Dose
ARTIFICIAL LUBRICANTS	hydroxypropyl cellulose	Comfort Tears	1–2 drops 4–8 times/day
		Lubrifilm	
		Lacril	
VASOCONSTRIC-TORS	tetrahydrozoline hydrochloride	Visine	1–2 drops affected eye 4 times/day
VASOCON-STRICTOR/ ANTIHISTAMINE	antazoline phosphate	Vasocon-A	Instill 1 or 2 drops in conjunctival sac 3–4 times/day
	naphazoline hydrochloride	Naphcon	Instill 1 drop 3–4 times/day
ANTIHISTAMINES	emedastine difumarate 0.05%	Emadine	1 drop in affected eye 4 times/day
	levocabastine hydrochloride 0.05%	Livostin	1 drop in affected eye, 4 times/day
	azelastine hydrochloride 0.05%	Optivar	1 drop in affected eye, 2 times/day
NSAIDS	ketorolac tromethamine 0.5%	Acular	1 drop in affected eye, 4 times/day
	diclofenac sodium 0.1%	Voltaren	1 drop in affected eye, 4 times/day
MAST CELL STABILIZERS	ketotifen fumarate 0.025%	Zaditor	1 drop in affected eye, 2–3 times/day
	cromolyn sodium 4%	Crolom	1–2 drops in affected eye, 4–6 times/day
	olopatadine hydrochloride 0.1%	Patanol	1 drop in affected eye, 2 times/day
	olopatadine hydrochloride 0.2%	Pataday	1 drop in affected eye daily
	lodoxamide tromethamine 0.1%	Alomide	1–2 drops in affected eye 4 times/day
CORTICOS-TEROIDS	dexamethasone 0.1%	Maxidex	1–2 drops in affected eye, 4 times/day
	prednisolone acetate 0.12%	Pred Mild	1–2 drops in affected eye 4 times/day
	prednisolone acetate 1%	Omnipred	1–2 drops in affected eye, 4 times/day

Adverse Reactions

The side effects and adverse reactions of ocular medications are seldom systemic and seldom involve reactions with other medications. Any preparation applied topically, however, especially to the cornea or conjunctiva, is likely to produce some stinging and/or blurring of vision. The potential for an allergy to the drug itself or some of its constituents is possible, and use of such medication in someone with an allergy to the drug is contraindicated.

Conscientious Considerations

■ In general, topical ocular medications prescribed in appropriate doses are safe, with the possible exception of topical steroids, which require close monitoring of intraocular pressure because prolonged use has been associated with glaucoma.

■ Lifestyle modifications to avoid allergens can be traumatic and in some cases difficult for some patients to do, such as putting a pet outdoors. Compassion and understanding are necessary.

■ Prior to referral for immunotherapy for either conjunctivitis or rhinitis, be certain the patient is unable to respond adequately to nonpharmacological and pharmacological treatment. Immunotherapy has risks, complications, failures, and expenses that may not be in the patient's best interest.

■ Patient and family should be made aware of the importance of avoiding nonallergenic environmental irritants such as smoke, fumes, strong cleaners, and so on.

■ Proper use of eyedrops may require explanation and even demonstration to patients who have never used them. Family members should be educated if the patient is too young or unable to understand.

TREATMENT OF ATOPIC DERMATITIS

Atopic dermatitis is a chronic and/or recurrent allergic inflammation of the skin. It also is described briefly in Chapter 16, Drugs Used in the Treatment of Skin Disorders. Generally beginning in the first few years of life, atopic dermatitis is the most common childhood skin disorder. Most children outgrow the condition by early adolescence, but when associated with early onset, severe widespread disease, asthma or hay fever, and/or a strong family history, the disease can persist into adulthood. The etiology of atopic dermatitis is quite complex, but we know it is related to early IgE production and later allergen/IgE reactivity.

The symptoms of atopic dermatitis, while not life threatening, are extremely irritating and consist of intense itching (pruritus), eczema and skin inflammation, and reactivity. These symptoms can have a serious impact on a patient's life, affecting his/her ability to sleep, perform normal life functions owing to the irritation and need for constant application of medication, as well as the embarrassment of visible skin inflammation. Pruritus often is intermittent during the day, but in the evenings and at night it can be extremely bothersome, resulting in significant loss of sleep with complications of drowsiness, irritability, and mood changes. The usual areas of skin involvement are the face, buttocks, and extensor areas in children whereas neck, hands, and flexor surfaces are common in any age group. The groin and axilla are usually spared. Lesions and symptoms can be chronic or relapsing, but they are almost always associated with dry skin (xerosis). Skin irritation and breakdown can allow microorganism invasion, resulting in recurrent bacterial, fungal and viral skin infections.

Accurate diagnosis is important because treatment for atopic dermatitis might exacerbate such conditions as scabies or fungal infections. Unlike allergic rhinitis and asthma, food allergies, especially in children, are common in atopic dermatitis, and a basic elimination diet with an attempt to identify offending allergens should be made, although success is limited.

Atopic dermatitis is one of the allergic triad (allergic asthma, rhinitis, dermatitis) diseases, and other atopic conditions should be considered and treated if present. The mainstay of pharmacological treatment for flare-ups of atopic dermatitis is the topical corticosteroids, for which professional guidelines recommend application two times a day (Buys, 2007). There is no compelling evidence that increasing applications beyond twice a day will enhance effectiveness. Using the lowest potency topical steroid for the shortest duration is always best. Options for topical steroid treatment are many because over 30 topical corticosteroids compounds are available. No studies have shown any superiority of one corticosteroid over another; however, strength, dose, and vehicle of application all affect results.

After flare-ups have been controlled, treatment should revert back to preventative strategies, because topical steroids do not cure atopic dermatitis. Significant local side effects have limited the use of the more potent topical corticosteroids and thus they are only used for serious flare-ups, and then for a limited amount of time.

Calcineurin inhibitors, tacrolimus (Protopic ointment), and pimecrolimus (Elidel cream) are topical immunosuppressive agents considered to be second-line agents for atopic dermatitis. Introduced in 1983, their limitation is the high degree of severe burning and itching at the application site. Because of their potent immunosuppressant effect, these topical agents have been suspected of causing local or distant malignancies. Although this relationship is unclear, the U.S. Food and Drug Administration limited their use and issued an enhanced warning statement in 2006 and again in 2010 that these agents in their topical format might cause cancer (FDA, 2006, 2010).

Rarely is the use of oral corticosteroid therapy indicated for severe disease. The use of systemic corticosteroids has been demonstrated to be effective, but long-term, high-dose use should be restricted because of the significant side effects and adverse reactions that can occur. If used, oral corticosteroids should be restricted to a short period of time of no more than 2 weeks. Certain chemotherapeutic drugs such as cyclosporine (Sandimmune) and interferon gamma-1b (Actimmune) may be considered in severe atopic dermatitis, but prescription should be by someone trained and familiar with their use. Other chemotherapeutic agents, immunoglobulins, immunotherapy, antihistamines, and leukotriene inhibitors have shown either conflicting or poor evidence of efficacy in treating atopic dermatitis.

The comorbidities of atopic dermatitis include skin infection, lack of sleep, depression, and intense pruritus; therefore, use of antibiotics, antifungals, antivirals, antidepressants, and antihistamines may be beneficial in treating the comorbidities of atopic dermatitis. Because of their sedative and antihistamine effects, first-generation antihistamines are particularly helpful in patients with pruritus that prevents sleep.

Conscientious Prescribing of Drugs for Atopic Dermatitis

■ Allergens may not always be easily determined, but once determined they should be avoided.

■ Oral antihistamines are of little value in the reversal of atopic dermatitis, but they will assist in symptom reduction by easing itching. The older antihistamine agents are sedating, and for this reason may assist the patient in sleeping.

■ Atopic dermatitis often is cosmetically embarrassing, and patients should be evaluated concerning how they feel about their appearance.

■ Often stress and emotional problems will aggravate the symptoms of atopic dermatitis and can occasionally become more problematic than the atopic condition. Psychological treatment and counseling should be considered in these patients.

■ Be aware of potential infections within the atopic dermatitis area and treat accordingly with appropriate antifungal, antiviral, and antibiotics.

■ Food allergies should be considered, and this may require a referral for testing, even though skin testing and immunotherapy have been of questionable value.

■ In atopic dermatitis, skin testing and immunotherapy are indicated only if there is accompanying allergic rhinitis or allergic asthma.

Patient and Family Education Regarding Use of Drugs to Treat Atopic Dermatitis

■ Patient education is crucial in treating all allergic diseases, but especially so in atopic dermatitis. Ideally, a handout of recommendations should be available to the patient and family so that they can discuss with you or one of your staff.

■ Advise patients to avoid scratching where it itches by trimming their nails and wearing gloves at night. Making patients aware they must resist the urge to scratch because doing so may worsen the irritation and open the skin to infections.

■ Proper skin care is imperative in patients with atopic dermatitis, and time should be spent in giving skin care guidelines to the patient and family.

■ Patients should be told that atopic dermatitis is not curable and should be informed of the limitations of therapy.

■ Avoid frequent, prolonged (3 to 5 minutes), and hot water bathing; hydrating emollients should be applied as soon as possible after bathing.

■ Avoid drying, strong, heavily perfumed soaps, chemicals, and detergents on skin.

■ Wash all new clothing prior to wearing.

■ Use minimal fabric softener and avoid harsh detergents (liquid is best).

■ Wear loose fitting cotton or cotton-blend clothing; avoid wool and abrasive or heavy clothing.

■ Avoid sunburns, especially if on calcineurin inhibitors.

- Avoid sunscreen with irritating components.
- Use air conditioning in hot weather.
- Use adequate amounts of topical medications, but apply only as frequently as prescribed.

Topical Corticosteroids

In the United States there are seven categories of topical corticosteroids with class 1 being the most potent and class 7 the least (Table 26-2). To minimize local adverse side effects, only low-potency (class 6 and 7) agents should be used on the face, groin, and axillae. Methods of application as well as the vehicle in which the corticosteroid is presented can also affect potency. In general, ointments are more potent than creams, but they are greasy. Creams may have preservatives that can precipitate contact dermatitis but are more acceptable to patients. Lotions lack the hydrating properties helpful in treating atopic dermatitis. Occlusion of topical steroids will also enhance potency, as will warmth and application on areas of thin skin.

Mechanism of Action

The methods by which topical steroids exert their anti-inflammatory effect is quite complex. They have specific and nonspecific effects that result in them being anti-inflammatory, immunosuppressive, antiproliferative, and vasoconstrictive. Most effects are caused by the corticosteroid acting at the molecular level by crossing the cell membrane and binding to a cell's nuclear DNA and cytoplasmic receptors. Inflammation is reduced when it inhibits adjacent genes to regulate the inflammatory process through release of a phospholipase A, an enzyme responsible for formation of leukotrienes, prostaglandins, and other elements in the arachidonic pathway. Topical steroids also prevent macrophage accumulation at inflamed sites.

Pharmacokinetics

- Absorption: Absorption into the skin is variable depending on the drug used, the formulation (lotion, cream, ointment, gel), the extent of the area being treated, and the condition

TABLE 26-2 Topical Corticosteroids

CLASS	DRUGS
1 SUPER POTENT	betamethasone 0.5%
	clobetasol propionate 0.05% (Temovate)
	halobetasol propionate 0.05% (Ultravate)
2 POTENT	amcinonide 0.1% (Cyclocort)
	betamethasone dipropionate 0.05% (Diprosone)
	desoximetasone 0.25% (Topicort)
	fluocinonide 0.05% (Lidex, Fluonex)
	halcinonide 0.1% (Halog)
3 MODERATE OR UPPER MID-STRENGTH	betamethasone dipropionate 0.05% (Diprosone)
	betamethasone valerate 0.1%
	diflorasone diacetate 0.05% (Florone, Maxiflor)
	fluticasone propionate 0.005% (Cutivate)
4 MID-STRENGTH	amcinonide 0.1% (Cyclocort)
	desoximetasone 0.05% (Topicort LP)
	flucinolone acetonide 0.2% (Synalar HP) hydrocortisone valerate 0.2% (Westcort)
	triamcinolone acetonide 0.1% (Kenalog, Aristocort)
5 LOWER MID-STRENGTH	betamethasone dipropionate 0.05% (Diprosone)
	betamethasone valerate 0.1% (Beta-Val)
	fluocinolone acetonide 0.025% (Synalar)
	flurandrenolide 0.05% (Cordran SP)
	fluticasone propionate 0.05%
	hydrocortisone butyrate 0.1% (Locoid)
	hydrocortisone valerate 0.2% (Westcort)
	triamcinolone acetonide 0.025%–0.1% (Kenalog)
6 MILD	alclometasone dipropionate 0.05% (Aclovate)
	desonide 0.05% (Tridesilon, DesOwen)
	fluocinolone acetonide 0.01% (Synalar)
7 LEAST POTENT	hydrocortisone 0.5%, 1%, 2.5% (many OTC brands at 1%, Hytone Cream 2.5%)

of the skin. There is little or no systemic effect or absorption noted.

■ Distribution: They remain primarily at their site of application.
■ Metabolism and excretion: Topical corticosteroids are metabolized in the skin. Some have been altered chemically to prolong local metabolism and so have a prolonged half-life.
■ Half-life: If applied topically, their half-life can be as little as 8 hours or as much as 2 to 4 days.

Dosage and Administration

All topical steroids are applied two to four times a day in a thin film or layer. Children should be given the lower potency classes, and treatment with the higher potency classes should not exceed 2 weeks of use or a dosage of more than 50 gm/week. High potency agents should be used on areas like palms and soles where there is a smaller surface area and treatment resistance is more likely.

Adverse Reactions

Short-term topical corticosteroid use is usually safe, but long-term use can be associated with local and in some cases systemic adverse effects.

DERM: Striae, petechia, telangiectasia, skin thinning, atrophy, worsening acne, burning, contact dermatitis, hyperpigmentation, folliculitis, irritation, and itching
EENT: Cataracts, glaucoma
ENDO: Primary hypothalamic-pituitary-adrenal axis suppression
MS: Bone density changes in adults, reduced linear growth in children
NEURO: Headaches

Interactions

■ The topical nature of application and poor systemic absorption make drug interactions unlikely.

Contraindications

■ Hypersensitivity to the drug or any of its components in vehicles (cream base, ointment base, preservatives, alcohol)
■ Lesions of skin caused by tuberculosis, fungal, or viral agents
■ Untreated bacterial infections
■ Concomitant skin infections of any type
■ Rosacea or perioral dermatitis

Conscientious Considerations

■ Patients tend to underestimate the amount of corticosteroid and emollients needed for adequate treatment. Adequate quantity of medication is essential for proper response.
■ Always start with the lowest potency that gives control. This may take a bit of trial and error, but usually topical steroids in the medium-potency range are best for adults, quickly switching to less-potent agents or nonsteroidal medications when control is achieved.

Patient/Family Education

■ Demonstration of the application procedure is usually very helpful, that is, application of a pea-sized amount in the affected area and applied thinly over the affected area.
■ Patients should also be taught some of the serious side effects that can occur with overuse and prolonged use.

■ Patients also need teaching on use of the higher potency corticosteroids and what makes them different from the common 1% or 0.5% over-the-counter creams.
■ If occlusion is to be used, the patient needs instruction in exactly how to do it and when to change the dressing.

Topical Calcineurin Inhibitors

The adoption of calcineurin inhibitors (CNI) as the mainstay of immunosuppression has resulted in a significant decrease of the acute rejection associated with allografts, a tissue transplant between two humans who are genetically distinct. The use of calcineurin inhibitors has led to an improvement in short-term graft survival; however, because of the irreversible nephrotoxicity associated with the chronic use of these drugs, improvement of long-term graft survival has been more modest.

Cyclosporine and tacrolimus are two potent immunosuppressives that inhibit calcineurin, a phosphatase, resulting in inhibition of pro-inflammatory cytokines and interruption of the downstream sequence of events leading to allograft rejection. However, despite their limitations of severe burning and itching at the application site, two of these CNI agents, tacrolimus (Elidel) and pimecrolimus, are useful as topical agents to effectively reduce inflammation.

Mechanism of Action

These agents inhibit calcineurin in the skin and thus are able to block T-cell activation and the subsequent release of inflammatory causing cytokines.

Pharmacokinetics

■ When absorbed into skin, there is little or no systemic absorption.

Dosage and Administration

Generic Name	Trade Name	Route	Usual Daily Adult Dose
pimecrolimus 1%	Elidel	Topical	Apply to affected areas 2 times/day.
tacrolimus 0.03%, 0.1%	Protopic	Topical	Apply to affected areas 2 times/ day.

Adverse Reactions

DERM: Redness and burning sensations of the skin

Interactions

■ Topical nature of their application makes drug interactions unlikely.

Contraindications

■ Hypersensitivity to drug or its components
■ Infected or abraded skin
■ Premalignant skin lesions

Conscientious Considerations

■ Rare cases of malignancy (skin and lymphoma) have been reported in patients treated with topical calcineurin inhibitors. Although no proof of causality has yet been determined, it is recommended that treatment with topical calcineurin inhibitors should be avoided long term and use should be limited to areas of involvement with atopic dermatitis.

▪ These topical agents are not indicated for children less than 2 years of age.

Introduction to Allergen Immunotherapy

Allergen **immunotherapy**, also called allergy **vaccine** therapy, consists of injecting ever-increasing amounts of the offending antigen/allergen subcutaneously into a patient over several months to years, attempting to reach a dose that will reduce the patient's allergic reaction when exposed naturally. With infectious disease vaccination, the goal is to induce a reaction against the antigen; with immunotherapy, the goal is to induce a tolerance for the allergen.

Allergen immunotherapy therefore would seem counterintuitive because you are giving increasingly greater doses of the very antigen that causes the IgE allergic reaction. Although the exact mechanism of restoring the immune system's adaption to foreign or external antigens is not fully understood (Huggins & Looney, 2004; Akdis & Akdis, 2009), allergen immunotherapy is efficacious, especially in allergies, asthma, and autoimmune diseases. Also, unlike use of antiallergic medication, immunotherapy can actually alter the course of the allergic response/disease. Possible mechanisms suggest that injection of the antigen/allergen as opposed to inhalation, may provoke production of antibodies of other classes that are not involved in hypersensitivity or allergies, blocking the allergen from combining with IgE and thereby preventing an allergic reaction.

Candidates for Immunotherapy

Allergy immunotherapy is most beneficial for those who have IgE-mediated allergic rhinitis, asthma, or insect hypersensitivity. It is not helpful in atopic dermatitis, urticaria, or in food or antibiotic allergies. Allergy immunotherapy is not without difficulties; it is potentially dangerous, not guaranteed to work, can be uncomfortable for the patient, may not be permanent, and can be expensive. For those reasons, allergen avoidance, pharmacotherapy, and time are often desired over immunotherapy. However, for the individual who is not responding to allergen avoidance, is unresponsive or unable to take conventional medications, is having significant quality-of-life issues, or developing serious medical problems, allergy immunotherapy is worth considering. Prior to any immunotherapy, an experienced clinician should be enlisted to diagnose the offending allergen(s) and prescribe a proper allergen immunotherapy protocol. Diagnosis of the offending allergens is crucial and requires an in-depth allergic history with proper testing (skin, in-vitro, challenge, etc.).

Immunotherapy Regimen

Once a protocol has been developed, the patient is required to come in at regular time intervals (usually weekly) to receive increasing doses or concentrations of the allergen vaccine. If the patient experiences a significant reaction to the dose or misses a dose, the next dose may not be increased or it may be lowered based on the protocol. Although it is not necessary to be seen by an allergist to receive allergy shots, it should be done in a medical facility where trained personnel familiar with the protocol and capable of managing a severe anaphylactic reaction are readily available. For this reason, patients should wait 20 to 30 minutes after an injection before leaving the clinic. Life-threatening reactions are rare, but they can occur, and one must be prepared to manage them. Maximum or maintenance dose is usually reached in about 6 months, at which time the patient will begin receiving maintenance doses at 4- to 6-week intervals. The effect of allergen immunotherapy is variable, but significant improvement should be observed before maintenance has been reached. Once maintenance dose has been reached, treatments are usually continued for several years.

Prognosis With Immunotherapy Treatment

Upon cessation of treatments, symptoms usually do not return for at least 3 years if at all. If symptoms return, one must again determine the offending allergen(s) as often new allergens have come in to replace the allergies of the past. As allergy immunotherapy has the potential to alter the course of allergic disease, and since allergies are more common in children it is thought that early treatment of children over 3 with allergy vaccine therapy may benefit their atopic diseases (Huggins & Looney, 2004).

ANAPHYLAXIS AND ANAPHYLACTOID REACTIONS

Anaphylaxis is the most severe form of allergic reaction. **Anaphylaxis** is an explosive and massive activation of mast cells through a systemic IgE-mediated type I immune response to **antigens** and **allergens** to which the patient has previously been exposed. The mast cells are primed with IgE antibodies that degranulate the mast cell when it comes into contact with the antigen again. Anaphylaxis must be differentiated from anaphylactoid reactions. An anaphylactoid reaction is an immediate systemic reaction that mimics anaphylaxis but is not IgE mediated. Because anaphylactoid reactions are not dependent on previous exposure, they can occur at first exposure to an antigen. Most anaphylactoid reactions require systemic exposure and more antigen than that needed for anaphylaxis, but the antigens are often similar. Fortunately, clinical symptoms and treatment are the same for both.

Any allergen capable of stimulating antibody (IgE) formation can cause anaphylaxis. This includes antibiotics, insulin, vaccines, latex, blood components, food allergies, insect stings, allergen extracts, exercise, and those without definable cause (idiopathic). Patients with an atopic history or a family history of atopy or anaphylaxis are at greater risk of developing anaphylaxis.

Anaphylaxis is IgE mediated. It can occur rapidly and is identified by systemic signs and symptoms. Because of the systemic effects of histamine release, anaphylaxis can present with many different symptoms, but it usually begins within minutes of exposure to the allergen with the following symptoms:

▪ Difficulty breathing, wheezing
▪ Changes in consciousness, including confusion, lightheadedness, or stupor

- Rapid swelling throughout the body
- Hives
- Cyanosis
- Severe abdominal pain, nausea, or diarrhea

Signs and symptoms may begin within seconds to minutes after exposure, but usually within 1 to 2 hours. Signs and symptoms may persist and progress for several hours despite treatment.

Management of Anaphylaxis

Treatment of anaphylactic and anaphylactoid reactions is a medical emergency. As in all medical emergencies, maintaining an adequate airway and blood pressure are crucial. The following should be done:

- Monitor vital signs frequently and treat as needed to ensure adequate blood pressure and oxygenation.
- Administer adrenalin (epinephrine) 0.2 mL to 0.5 mL of a 1:1000 (wt/vol) dilution (0.2 to 0.5 mg) intramuscularly or subcutaneously.
- Repeat adrenalin dose every 10 to 15 minutes as needed for first hour.

Adrenalin (epinephrine) is a sympathomimetic catecholamine that acts on both alpha- and beta-adrenergic receptors. Epinephrine is a potent alpha receptor and, as a result, causes rapid vasoconstriction and bronchodilation. Side effects include palpitations, ventricular fibrillation, and dysrhythmias, but the beneficial effects in this emergency situation far outweigh the risks. Additional steps in the medical management of anaphylaxis include:

- If the patient remains hypotensive, he or she may require intravenous fluids.
- Patients on beta blockers may have epinephrine resistance and require glucagon injection to counter resistance. Administer 1 mg of glucagon, followed by consideration for a 1 to 5 mg per hour continuous infusion.
- Administer diphenhydramine parenterally 25 to 50 mg, or consider starting oral diphenhydramine 25 mg every 4 to 6 hours.
- Consider starting ranitidine (Zantac) 50 mg intramuscularly or intravenously or 150 mg orally 2 times a day.
- Consider starting corticosteroids if initial response is inadequate or severe; 0.5 to 1 mg/kg/day of prednisone or equivalent.
- Treat bronchospasm with inhaled beta-2 agonists (as described in Chapter 10, Drugs Used in the Treatment of Pulmonary Diseases and Disorders).
- Monitor for at least 4 to 6 hours and consider hospitalization if not responding adequately.

Patients at risk for anaphylaxis from certain foods, exercise (rare), hymenoptera (bees, wasps, yellow jackets, hornets) stings, and ants should be provided with an epinephrine kit and instruction in its use. Several kits (Epi E-Zpen auto-injector and EpiPen) have preloaded syringes that can be self-injected by patients immediately upon an allergen exposure. Patients should be instructed to self-inject 0.3 to 0.5 mg intramuscularly of a 1:1,000 solution of aqueous epinephrine and may repeat the dose in 15 to 20 minutes if needed. Immediately thereafter, they should call 911 and seek medical attention. Anaphylaxis can have a late phase several hours after the initial reaction; thus, medical care and observation are required. Medical alert identification is also essential, and all such patients should have medical alert tags or some form of identification to alert emergency personnel if unconscious. Patient education, awareness, and compliance are crucial to a satisfactory outcome in those who suffer from anaphylactic reactions.

Management of Drug Hypersensitivity

Adverse drug reactions (ADR) are predictable (related to the action of the drug), unpredictable (related to the patient's immunological system and its response), or genetic (differences in susceptibility among patients). True drug hypersensitivity, reproducible outcomes in individuals exposed to a dose that is normally tolerated by nonhypersensitive people, accounts for only 5% to 10% of all drug reactions. This includes IgE-mediated (immediate) and non-IgE-mediated (delayed) drug allergies (deShazo & Kemp, 1997). However, the number of drug hypersensitivities is increasing and now accounts for 3% to 6% of all hospital admissions and affects 10% to 15% of hospitalized patients (Gomes & Demoly, 2005).

Most drug reactions are not immunologically mediated. To properly treat adverse allergic drug reactions, the clinician must obtain a complete history and time sequence of drug usage and resulting symptoms. Although an immunologic reaction to drugs can occur at any time, it is much more likely to occur early in the drug exposure (days) rather than years after a patient has been using a medication.

Adverse drug reactions that are immunologic in etiology fall into the four classifications of hypersensitivities outlined by Gells and Coombs (see Table 26-1). Knowing which type of reaction is common for certain drug hypersensitivities can assist in determining cause and effect and, therefore, treatment.

Penicillin allergy is an example of a type I (IgE mediated) drug hypersensitivity; heparin-induced thrombocytopenia is an example of type II (cytotoxic) drug hypersensitivity. Serum sickness and drug-induced lupus syndromes with procainamide or phenytoin are examples of type III (immune complex) drug hypersensitivity. The contact dermatitis caused by treatment with topical lidocaine is an example of a type IV (delayed, cell-mediated) drug hypersensitivity.

The first line of treatment is to determine the offending drug and discontinue it. Depending upon the severity of the reaction, removing the drug may be all that is required. For mild to moderate drug hypersensitivities, types I, II, and III, treatment will depend on symptoms and severity. Antihistamines, bronchodilators, and corticosteroids are all potential and effective treatments. In type III reactions, which often involve muscle-skeletal and joint pain, the use of NSAIDs may be of value. For more serious reactions, hospitalization should be considered for monitoring, diagnosis, and in some cases transfusions, systemic corticosteroids, and even plasmapheresis. Plasmapheresis is a process whereby blood is taken from a person and separated in a device to remove the plasma. The remaining cell components of the blood are then returned to the body as a purification process, enabling the body to treat its own autoimmune diseases using its own red and white blood cells because circulating antibodies have been removed. Type IV hypersensitivity, because it is cell mediated, will not respond to all the treatments for types I, II, and III. Corticosteroids, either topical or systemic, are the best treatment. Antihistamines are of limited value but may help in controlling some of the symptoms such as itching.

Immunotherapy and desensitization are treatment modalities that should be considered if a person requires the medication that they have become hypersensitive to, such as insulin or an antibiotic. Penicillin and insulin desensitization have been found to be quite effective but must be performed by someone familiar with the technique. Premedication to prevent an immunologic reaction has also been found to be effective, such as diphenhydramine and steroids prior to an injection of radio contrast media. Caution should be used as premedication does not guarantee against an allergic reaction. Most patients who are hypersensitive to a drug should simply avoid using it if possible and be sure the hypersensitivity is well known by family and clinician. Wearing a medical alert bracelet or necklace is also prudent.

Management of Insect Stings (Hypersensitivity)

Biting insects can occasionally cause local allergic swelling and pruritus, but systemic or anaphylactic reactions are extremely rare. Stinging insects on the other hand can cause severe allergic reactions and even anaphylaxis. Stinging insects belong mainly to the Hymenoptera family, and in the United States the yellow jacket is most commonly associated with sting reactions. The family includes honeybees, bumblebees, yellow-faced hornets, paper wasp, fire ants, and harvester ants. Prior exposure is necessary to develop an allergy.

If the stinging apparatus is detected in the skin, attempt to remove it by flicking or scraping it off; do not squeeze it. Squeezing may actually inject more of the venom.

Large local reactions can be treated with ice or cold compresses. Antihistamines and analgesics in the usual dosage may be helpful to control symptoms. A burst of oral corticosteroids (prednisone, methylprednisone) can be helpful if started within 2 hours of the sting. An initial dose of 40 to 60 mg of prednisone is commonly given daily for 3 to 5 days with some clinicians tapering the dose starting on the third day. Anaphylactic reactions are medical emergencies requiring immediate medical treatment.

Venom immunotherapy is highly effective. Patients who have experienced a systemic reaction after an insect sting should be tested for IgE sensitivity and referred for immunotherapy if positive. Like all allergies, the best treatment is avoidance of the antigen.

Management of Food Hypersensitivity

The terms food *intolerance* and food *hypersensitivity* are often applied inappropriately. Food intolerance is a nonimmunologic abnormal physiological response to ingested food. Toxins, poisons, caffeine, and lactic acid in lactase-deficient individuals are examples of food intolerance. Food allergy is an immunologic reaction, which is much less common than food intolerance, and usually an IgE-mediated type I hypersensitivity; however, other sensitivity types can be involved as well. Food allergies affect about 8% of children and less than 5% of adults (Wilson & Bahna, 2005; Chafen et al., 2010). Any food can be an antigen and thus potentially an allergen, but by far the majority (over 90%) of food allergies in adults come from crustaceans (shellfish), tree nuts, peanuts, and fish.

Patients with food allergies are often not atopic, and they do not have a strong family history of food allergies or other atopic diseases. Symptoms in IgE-mediated food allergies usually occur within a few minutes to hours after food ingestion, whereas non-IgE mediated immunologic reactions may take several hours or days to become evident. Food allergies can result in anaphylactic reactions requiring immediate medical treatment. Peanut and shellfish allergies are well-known causes of food antigen anaphylaxis.

A specific syndrome called the *oral allergy syndrome* is the most common food allergy and can be seen in up to 10% of patients with atopic disease. The syndrome is brief in duration, involves only the mouth and throat, and usually involves fruits and vegetables that cross react with aero-antigens (dust, pollen, airborne antigens) to which the patient has already developed allergies. Fortunately, the condition is usually mild and usually resolves by swallowing or removing the food from the mouth.

Strict avoidance of offending food allergens is the only proven therapy that works. Fortunately, reactivity to food allergens often is lost over time, but avoidance must be complete. Monitoring processed foods is of particular importance because these foods often may change over time, and patients are advised to be meticulous in observing labels on food packages. Similar care must be taken when eating out.

Symptomatic treatment for food allergy symptoms is helpful but does not affect the immunologic response. Examples of these treatments include antiemetics for vomiting, antidiarrheals, and antihistamines for pruritus and skin inflammation. Fortunately, food allergies usually do not persist once the offending food has been withdrawn.

Immunotherapy has been shown to be of limited effect in the treatment of food allergies. Novel new treatments are being investigated, including oral tolerance induction, injection of monoclonal IgG to bind the offending IgE, and a specific Chinese herbal tea formula (Kurowski & Boxer, 2008).

Management of Contact Dermatitis (Hypersensitivity)

Contact dermatitis (also discussed briefly in Chapter 16) is a common condition in which an immunologic hypersensitivity reaction occurs on the skin. Most contact dermatitis reactions are mediated by sensitized T cells and are of the type IV delayed cell-mediated hypersensitivity reaction. Other types of hypersensitivity reactions can also cause contact dermatitis, such as the latex IgE-mediated reaction above, but most are of the type IV hypersensitivity. Because of the use of latex in medical equipment (gloves, stoppers, tubes, etc.), latex hypersensitivity has become an important health concern for healthcare professionals, rubber industry workers, and patients. It also occurs with condom use. Contact dermatitis in susceptible individuals can occur with almost any substance applied to the skin, although common causes include poison ivy, household cleaners, and topical antimicrobials, anesthetics, and antihistamines. Most cases are localized, but in very sensitized individuals, reactions can be widespread. Most reactions will occur within 24 to 48 hours after exposure. In contact dermatitis, the epidermal route of exposure to the allergens favors the development of a T-cell-mediated response, thus effective therapy for these reactions is suppression of the T-cell function. Corticosteroids are presently the best treatment for this type of therapy. Treatment of contact dermatitis is done in stages based on its severity; in many cases removal of the allergen and local skin care is all that is needed. Following are some recommended steps in treatment:

■ Remove offending allergen.
■ Apply wet compress of water, saline, or Domeboro solution if acute eruption is present.
■ Topical application of a class 2 or class 3 corticosteroid cream is advised for a brief period of time not to exceed 2 weeks. Class 1 (most potent) is seldom needed. Discontinue if dermatitis resolves; if resolving but persisting, you may need to continue topical corticosteroid but taper with a class 4 or 5 corticosteroid and monitor for adverse reactions.
■ Avoid class 1, 2, 3 topical steroids on face, axillae, breast, and genitals. Some topical corticosteroids contain preservatives that can be sensitizing as well; triamcinolone 0.1%, fluocinolone acetonide 0.025%, and betamethasone valerate 0.1% are several that do not.
■ If the reaction is severe, widespread, or the individual is known to have serious reactions, consider oral corticosteroids. The usual dose is prednisone or equivalent 0.5 to 1 mg/kg/day tapering over 6 to 14 days. Shorter courses of oral or topical corticosteroids often result in recurrence of symptoms.
■ For very severe contact dermatitis or patients extremely sensitive to the allergen, it may be necessary to use injectable steroids for the first 1 to 3 days followed by oral steroids. Usually 30 to 60 mg prednisone equivalent one to two times a day will be adequate.
■ Treat any skin infection that may develop as a result of inflamed and abraded skin. Avoid topical antibiotics because they can act as contact sensitizers on the inflamed skin.
■ Oral antihistamines can help relieve associated pruritus. Nonsedating antihistamines are preferred during the day, but the older sedating antihistamines can assist in sleeping as well as pruritus at night. Avoid topical antihistamines because they can be contact sensitizers, such as topical calamine preparations containing diphenhydramine.

■ Recalcitrant cases may require adjuvant therapy with psoralen and ultraviolet light, coal tar in petrolatum, or tar bath soaks.
■ Referral or consultation may be necessary if patient fails to respond, has significant complications, needs hospital admission, or requires consideration for desensitization.

Patients need to be educated in avoiding offending allergens. Patients should wear appropriate clothes to avoid contact, avoid burning of such plants because the agents can become aerosolized, and wash skin immediately with soap and water after exposure. Patients also need to remove and wash all exposed clothes before wearing then again. Patients often suspect the fluid in bullae and vesicles to contain antigen, but this is not true; contact dermatitis is not spread by exposure to bullae, vesicles, or their contents. The late appearance of dermatitis, up to 2 weeks after the first exposure, is the result of lesser exposure to an antigen or in skin areas of decreased reactivity; once the antigen has been washed from the skin, it is no longer of concern. It does not spread after initial exposure.

URTICARIA AND ANGIOEDEMA

Urticaria (hives) and angioedema are manifestations of mast cell activation and, although not specific to any allergen, they are immunologically mediated and involved in common pathways of potent inflammatory mediators released from mast cells. Urticaria and angioedema have 20% prevalence in the United States (Schaefer, 2011).

Urticaria is a cutaneous eruption consisting of polymorphic, round or irregularly shaped, erythematous, pruritic, raised wheals. Though usually transient, such reactions can persist for weeks to months. Angioedema, which can occur with or without urticaria, is an episodic, asymmetric, nonpitting swelling of loose tissue, involving subcutaneous tissues, abdominal organs, and the upper airway. Angioedema tends to occur on the face and can become a medical emergency if airway obstruction occurs. Both urticaria and angioedema are usually a result of IgE antibody-mediated reactions and usually occur within an hour of exposure to the offending antigen. Offending antigens are the commonly expected type I hypersensitivity agents: drugs, foods, insect venom, aeroallergens. Urticaria and angioedema may also have nonimmunologic causes, but treatment should focus on suppression of inflammatory mediators, with histamine being the most prominent. Emergency measures are obvious if the patient presents with airway obstruction or potential obstruction by an enlarged tongue, uvula, or epiglottis. Treatment much like that for anaphylaxis with epinephrine may be of benefit, and in severe cases, intubation may be required. Assuming mild to moderate symptoms, treatment of urticaria and angioedema should progress in a step-wise manner.

■ Begin with nonsedating second-generation antihistamines such as fexofenadine (Allegra), desloratadine (Clarinex), loratadine (Claritin), or cetirizine (Zyrtec) in doses as described earlier in the chapter. See Chapter 10 for more information on these medications.

■ Consider adding older, sedating first-generation antihistamines such as diphenhydramine (Benadryl), brompheniramine (Dimetapp), or chlorpheniramine (Chlortrimeton) if symptoms persist or nighttime pruritus and lack of sleep are a problem.

■ Consider hydroxyzine (Atarax, Vistaril), an antihistamine/antianxiety/sedative agent, which works centrally, 25 mg by mouth four times a day.

If symptoms persist, consideration for H_1 and H_2 (blocker) receptor antagonists is indicated.

■ Add anti-depressant doxepin (Sinequan), which has H_1 and H_2 receptor agonist effects, 10 to 50 mg at night or serotonin and histamine antagonist cyproheptadine (Periactin), 4 mg by mouth three times a day.

■ Consider H_2-receptor antagonists such as cimetadine (Tagamet), 400 mg by mouth, three times a day or ranitidine (Zantac), 150 mg by mouth, two times a day. These medications are discussed in detail in Chapter 10.

If symptoms are still not adequately controlled, consider the following:

■ Add leukotriene modifiers, montelukast (Singulair), 10 mg daily, or zafirlukast (Accolate), 20 mg daily.

■ Oral corticosteroids such as prednisone burst of 10 to 20 mg followed by a short-term 1 to 10 mg daily may help to control symptoms, but should not be used for more than 2 weeks.

■ Failure to respond to the above therapy requires referral or consultation for possible other therapy such as immunoglobulin therapy, immunotherapy, plasmapheresis, or cyclosporine.

The multiple medications used to treat urticaria and angioedema speak for the difficulty in its control. Patients with a history of isolated angioedema that may compromise the airway should be prescribed an epinephrine kit and instructed in its proper use.

IMMUNIZATION: DEVELOPING AND MANIPULATING IMMUNE REACTIONS

Antigens, such as pollens, foods, drugs, and venom, are not usually life threatening unless they stimulate a vigorous immune reaction, and they are treated by diminishing or controlling the allergic or immunologic response. The other means of immune manipulation is to enhance weak immune responses or develop immune reactions that did not exist previously. This is usually done by supplying immunoglobulins (antibodies) to the body by injection (passive immunity) or exposing the body to weakened or dead antigens called vaccines (active immunity) to create immunity.

Providing immunoglobulins (passive immunity) is quick, effective, and lifesaving when immunity is needed immediately, such as on exposure to dangerous antigens (rabies or hepatitis) when there is no time for the body to develop its own natural immunity. Unfortunately, immunity obtained by injecting immunoglobulins is temporary, has no memory, and does not involve the cell-mediated immunologic defense mechanisms. Within a few months, at most the immunoglobulins of passive immunity are gone and the antigen forgotten. This is the type of immunity conferred by vaccines for hepatitis B, varicella, pertussis, polio, tuberculosis, and herpes zoster.

Active immunization usually requires up to 2 weeks for immunity to become adequate, results in the body making its own antibodies, and develops cell-mediated responses, which allow for memory cells. These memory cells allow the body to mount a rapid and strong defense at the next exposure to the antigen. Historically, vaccines have been made to immunize the body from viruses and bacteria, but modern immunology has and is developing vaccines for all kinds of undesired invaders of the body, including parasites, cancers, toxins, and poisons.

Saving Lives: The Success Story of Vaccines

All current routine vaccines have been created to fight infectious disease. The dramatic drop in infectious disease mortality is a tribute to the success and safety of these vaccines.

Vaccines can be inhaled, taken orally, provided in a patch, and administered intradermally, as well as by standard injection. The antigens in these vaccines range from the actual weakened organism itself to biochemical compounds that mimic antigens of the offending agent. Along with these antigens, vaccines contain various compounds, adjuvants, and stimulants to enhance their immunogenic response. Although vaccines are varied and complicated, understanding the two main classifications (live attenuated and inactivated) are important in vaccine use.

Live Attenuated Vaccines (Active Immunity)

Live attenuated vaccines, such as in yearly influenza vaccines, are considered more potent than inactivated or dead vaccines because the organism in the vaccine actually reproduces and creates a small infection in the host. The immune response to a live attenuated vaccine is virtually identical to the natural infection. Although the live vaccine is attenuated (weakened), it can potentially cause a serious and very rarely fatal reaction in patients who are immunocompromised. The other problem with live attenuated vaccines is that certain blood products such as immunoglobulins can restrict the reproduction of the attenuated organism and decrease the development of immunity. Although live attenuated vaccines are considered more effective than inactivated vaccines and usually require only one or two doses, there are complications that make them more problematic as to who receives them and under what circumstances. For example a live vaccine could become underattenuated and thus render the vaccination ineffective. The organism could have undergone a mutation that leads to reversal of virulence. Also, the preparation could be unstable or could be rendered useless because of heat lability resulting from not being refrigerated. Finally, these vaccines should not be given to pregnant women or anyone who is immune compromised.

Dosage and Administration

Vaccine	Brand Name	Dosage
Measles	Usually in combination with mumps, and rubella	Measles usually should be given in combination vaccine of MMR (measles, mumps, rubella) subcutaneously. Children should be given the first dose of mumps vaccine soon after their first birthday (12–15 months of age). The second dose is recommended before they start kindergarten. Worldwide over 500,000 children still die of measles.
Mumps	Mumpsvax (single antigen) Usually in combination with measles and rubella (MMR)	Mumps should be given usually in a combination vaccine of MMR (measles, mumps, rubella) subcutaneously. Children should be given the first dose of mumps vaccine soon after their first birthday (12–15 months of age). The second dose is recommended before they start kindergarten.
Varicella	Varivax (single antigen) Also several combination vaccines	Children 12 months through 12 years of age should receive two 0.5 mL doses of varicella-containing vaccine administered subcutaneously, separated by at least 3 months. First dose is recommended soon after first birthday, second dose before kindergarten. Persons 13 years of age and older should receive two 0.5 mL doses of the single-antigen varicella vaccine subcutaneously 4–8 weeks apart.
Rubella	Usually given as part of the MMR vaccine (protecting against measles, mumps, and rubella)	Rubella is recommended usually in combined MMR (measles, mumps, rubella) vaccine given subcutaneously at 12–15 months (not earlier) and a second dose when the child is 4–6 years old (before kindergarten or first grade). Rubella vaccination is particularly important for nonimmune women who may become pregnant because of the risk for serious birth defects if they acquire the disease during pregnancy.
Combination vaccine of measles, mumps, rubella, and varicella	ProQuad, MMRV	MMRV is approved for use only among healthy children 12 months through 12 years of age. Dose as for Varivax and MMR. MMRV is not approved for use in persons 13 years of age and older.
Herpes zoster	Zostavax	Herpes zoster (shingles) vaccine was recently recommended by the Advisory Committee on Immunization Practices (ACIP) to reduce the risk of shingles and its associated pain in people 50 years old or older. This is a one-time vaccination given subcutaneously. Zostavax does not treat shingles or postherpetic neuralgia (pain after the rash is gone) once it develops. Zostavax is the same antigen as in Varivax, but contains 14 times more antigen.
Rotavirus	RotaRix RotaTeq	Rotavirus can cause severe acute gastroenteritis with diarrhea and vomiting in infants and young children. Rotavirus vaccine can protect children from this disease in about 75% of cases. About 600,000 children die from rotavirus infections each year worldwide. The usual schedule is to administer the vaccine orally at 2, 4, and 6 months of age.
Nasal influenza	FluMist	FluMist is an intra-nasal spray flu vaccine for healthy people between 2 and 49 years of age and contains the same live, attenuated strains of three viruses believed to be most virulent in the upcoming season as used in the inactivated vaccine. Nasal flu vaccine can be given starting in late August and as far along as late March.

Adverse Reactions

When given by injection, it is fairly common for these agents to cause pain, soreness, and swelling at the injection sites. In addition they can induce systemic effects such as fever, general malaise, and headache. Serious or long-term adverse reactions are extremely rare, and despite recent studies attempting to link immunizations with autism, diabetes, etc., vaccines have been repeatedly vindicated as truly lifesaving interventions.

Interactions

- Live attenuated vaccines do not interact with drugs, but certain blood products such as immunoglobulins may restrict the attenuated vaccine's ability to reproduce and should not be given less than 2 weeks prior to immunoglobulin therapy or at least 3 months after immunoglobulin therapy.
- Depending on blood product and amount given, the period to wait will vary, and in most cases it is recommended to seek guidance from some authority, such as the Centers for Disease Control and Prevention (CDC).
- Because reproduction of the attenuated virus is required in live attenuated viral vaccines, concern has arisen over the use of antivirals when giving live attenuated viral vaccines such as varicella, MMR, Zostavax, and nasal flu. For that reason it is recommended that the patient wait 24 to 48 hours after cessation of antiviral treatment before receiving a live attenuated viral vaccine. Patients may be given attenuated vaccines even if they are on antibiotics.
- Live attenuated vaccines may be given simultaneously, but once given, another live attenuated vaccine should not be given for at least 4 weeks.

Contraindications

- Allergy to the vaccine or its components
- Pregnancy
- Immunosuppression by disease
- Immunosuppression by medication (20 mg or more/day of prednisone, 2 mg/kg/day of prednisone or chemotherapeutic drugs)

Conscientious Considerations

Warnings for live attenuated vaccine administration include the following:

- Moderate to severe illness
- Recent blood products
- Recent live attenuated vaccine (within 4 weeks)
- Antiviral medication

Patient/Family Education

- All patients, their parents, and/or guardians should be given standard CDC-VIS (Vaccine Information Statements), which are available in many languages. This is a requirement by law.
- Should any patient suffer an adverse event or reaction, he or she should be told to report this incident to the clinician, who must, by law, fill out a government form called a Vaccine Adverse Event Reporting System form (VAERS, n.d.).
- If pain or discomfort at the injection site occurs, acetaminophen may be taken for relief.

Inactivated Vaccines (Active Immunity)

Inactivated vaccines come in numerous types: polysaccharides, toxoids, conjugated, and recombinant, among others. Their main commonality is that they are all dead, do not reproduce, and cannot cause disease.

Toxoid vaccines (tetanus, diphtheria, and pertussis) have antigens that induce creation of antibodies against the toxin of the organism, not the organism itself. Other inactivated vaccines are made of organism parts or replicas made from other organisms such as yeast cells in the case of the human papilloma virus vaccine.

Polysaccharide vaccines are created from pure cell wall polysaccharides, the coating that surrounds bacteria. They are unable to stimulate T cells and thus make poor vaccines for children, but conjugating them with protein antigens helps to make them more immunogenic. A good example is the pneumococcal polysaccharide vaccine known as Pneumovas-23 or PPV-23. These inactivated vaccines are not as effective at stimulating an immune response as live attenuated vaccines; therefore, three to five doses may be required to boost the immune response to an adequate protective level.

Conjugated Vaccines/Recombinant Vaccines/DNA Vaccines

These are experimental vaccines. They use an attenuated virus or bacterium to introduce microbial DNA cells to the body by determining the microbe's genetic material that codes for important antigens. Once the genes/DNA from a microbe are introduced into the body, certain cells take up those genes/DNA and begin to develop the antigens molecule. The cell excretes the antigen and attaches it to its surface. Then when the body is introduced to the offending agent, the body has its own factory for making antigens and stimulating the body's immune response. These vaccines will likely be the future of bacterial and viral vector vaccines because they are currently being researched for HIV, rabies, and measles. The Centers for Disease Control lists its recommendations for inactivated vaccines (CDC, 2010).

CDC Recommended Administration of Inactivated Vaccines

Vaccine	Trade Name	Route
Hepatitis A	Havrix Vaqta Twinrix (combo A&B)	Two-dose schedule of 1 mL (adults), and 0.5 mL (children under 19) given IM.
Hepatitis B	Engerix-B Recombivax HB	Three-dose schedule for all children and for adults whose travel, occupation, or lifestyle put them at risk; dose at 0, 1, and 6 months using IM route
Hepatitis A & B	Twinrix Comvax Pediarix	Combination with other antigens; dose as per vaccine insert.
Human papilloma virus (HPV)	Gardasil Cervarix	Three-dose IM series for both vaccines recommended for women 11–12 years of age; Gardasil recommended for men also.

Vaccine	Trade Name	Route
Diphtheria, tetanus, pertussis (3) for adults	Adacel Boostrix	No recommendations for booster dose yet approved; may give to all 10 years old and older; 1 dose IM.
Diphtheria, Tetanus, pertussis (DTaP) for children	Daptacel Infanrix TriHIBit Many combo vaccines	Usual 3-dose initial series followed by 2 boosters. Given IM, 90% of all patients develop protective immunity that persists for 10 years, but immunity wanes after 4–6 years, leading to the need for a booster.
Inactivated poliovirus vaccine (IPV)	Most are combo vaccines, Pedirix, Pentacel	IM dose depending on vaccine. Polio is on the verge of extinction, but it still exists in parts of the world today.
Haemophilus influenzae type B (HiB)	ActHIB Hiberix PedvaxHIB Combo vaccines, Pentacel, TriHIBit, ComVax	Three-dose series with booster, given IM. Haemophilus influenzae used to be a serious infection of infants resulting in meningitis and other deep infections. Although still present, it is not nearly as devastating as it once was. Combination vaccines may have different doses and schedules.
Influenza (injectable)	Afluria Agriflu Fluarix FluLaval Fluvirin Fluzone	Each year the FDA decides which three flu virus strains to use. Given IM, the vaccine produces antibodies to the selected strains within 10–14 days. Immunity lasts probably several years. Flu vaccine can be started in late August and given throughout the end of March. Immunity lasts throughout the season, and it is always best to get the shot when it is available.
Pneumococcal PCV13 PPSV	Prevnar 13 Pneumovax 23	Prevnar13 (PCV13), 3-dose series followed by booster, all IM, targets 13 common strains of pneumococcus, which account for 80% of invasive pneumococcal disease in children. Pneumovax 23 (PPSV) given SC once to all 65 or older; may give earlier and booster dose in certain cases; targets 23 strains of pneumococcal commonly found in adults.
Meningococcal (MCV4)	Menactra Menveo	One-dose IM vaccination recommended for adolescents 11–12 years old, and then a booster dose prior to college.

Adverse Reactions

Adverse reactions to these vaccines are usually mild and consist of pain and tenderness at the injection site, which may persist for 1–2 days.

Interactions

- Inactivated vaccines do not interact with drugs and are not affected by blood products such as immunoglobulins because they do not reproduce.
- Any vaccine, including live attenuated vaccines, may be given in any time relation to inactivated vaccines.

Contraindications

- Allergy to the vaccine or its components
- Encephalopathy within 7 days of a previous pertussis vaccine

■ Although not contraindicated, the new inactivated vaccine Tdap has yet to be approved for routine use in pregnant women.

Conscientious Considerations

■ Warnings for inactivated vaccine administration include patients with moderate to severe illness.

Patient/Family Education

■ Same as those recommended for live attenuated vaccines.

Recommended Schedules for Immunizations

The Advisory Committee for Immunization Practices (ACIP), a function of the federal government's Centers for Disease Control and Prevention (CDC), each year publishes its annual recommended immunization schedule for healthy children, adolescents, and adults (CDC, 2011). For those who miss their recommended scheduled immunizations, a catch-up schedule is also available, and for patients who have certain medical problems or conditions, a fifth schedule is available. It should be noted that several vaccines, mainly inactivated ones, require a series of vaccinations for someone to become fully immunized. It is important to monitor the time between immunizations in a series because any vaccine given too soon or at too early an age will be considered invalid and must be repeated at the proper time or age. Vaccines given late are considered valid regardless of length of time since the last dose. The next appropriate dose in a series is determined by the time of the last dose; there is no need to repeat the series even if a dose is very late.

Other vaccines that are available for individuals with special needs, such as travelers to exotic places or people working in such areas as veterinary science and research biology, include the following:

■ Anthrax (inactivated)
■ Oral typhoid (live attenuated)
■ Injectable typhoid (inactivated)
■ Japanese encephalitis (inactivated)
■ Rabies (inactivated)
■ Yellow fever (live attenuated)

Vaccine Safety

Vaccination is among the most significant public health success stories of all time. Like any pharmaceutical product, no vaccine is completely safe or always totally effective; however, vaccine-adverse events reported today are for the most part minor and self-limiting, with only rare exceptions. The CDC, through its Vaccine Adverse Event Reporting System (VAERS), maintains close monitoring of untoward reactions to vaccines. With vaccine-preventable diseases at or near record lows, it is the occasional adverse vaccine event or coincidental adverse event that is reported, not the dramatic eradication of disease (VAERS, n.d.). Still, patients are correct to question the safety and efficacy of anything prescribed, and it remains the clinician's job to reassure them of the great benefits vaccines have brought.

Monoclonal Antibodies

The science of immunology has brought new ways to control and manipulate the immune system, making it possible to lead healthier and longer lives. Although it is beyond the scope of this chapter, monoclonal antibodies warrant mention because new techniques in producing antibodies have allowed production of specific antibodies to specific antigens in large quantities. This allows greater specificity of these antibodies to bind to specific antigens, making them excellent vehicles for pinpointing the destruction of certain cells (tumors) or the delivery of certain medications (attached to the antibodies).

These new antibodies are referred to as monoclonal antibodies, and their names end in the letters "mab." Two examples are infliximab and adalimumab, which are used in inflammatory arthritis, Crohn's disease, and ulcerative colitis because of their ability to bind with and inhibit alpha-TNF (tumor necrosis factor). Basiliximab and daclizumab are two others used to inhibit acute rejection of kidney transplants by inhibiting interleukin-2 on activated T cells. Omalizumab is yet another monoclonal antibody, which is used to inhibit human immunoglobulin and has application in treating moderate to severe allergic asthma. Gemtuzumab is another monoclonal antibody that targets myeloid cell surface antigens, making it helpful in treating acute myeloid leukemia that has relapsed. The potential to use these monoclonal antibodies in virtually all areas of medicine and biology is growing and limited only by our imagination to use them.

Implications for Special Populations

Pregnancy Implications

Pregnancy is unique in that a genetically and immunologically foreign fetus survives to full term without rejection by the mother's immune system. It is now known that recognition of the foreign fetus does occur, and several mechanisms have been discovered that explain why the mother does not reject her "foreign" fetus. These mechanisms include fetal factors such as trophoblastic cell properties and maternal factors such as specialized uterine cells and a shifting of the helper T-cell cytokine profile from a type 1 to a type II array. While immunomodulators are expressed in the uterus to aid in fetal survival, fetal cells also persist in the mother's circulation long after pregnancy is over, and this may have implications for the etiology and treatment of some autoimmune diseases. For the preceding reasons the use of immunologic medications should be done thoughtfully in pregnancy, weighing the risks (often not known) versus benefits very carefully.

Pregnant women should not receive most vaccines, mainly due to theoretical concerns for the fetus. Women of childbearing age should be up to date on their immunizations before becoming pregnant so they may pass on antibodies to their child. If a woman contracts rubella (German measles) or varicella (chickenpox) while pregnant, the risk of birth defects rises dramatically for the child and the risk for pneumonia increases for the mother. When pregnant women do need vaccines, it is thought that inactivated vaccines are safer than live attenuated ones; in fact, injectable influenza is recommended (not live attenuated nasal flu) for women during pregnancy (Table 26-3).

TABLE 26-3	Vaccines Recommended in Pregnancy
IMMUNIZATIONS BEFORE PREGNANCY	Varicella (chickenpox) Human papilloma virus
IMMUNIZATIONS DURING PREGNANCY	Influenza Tetanus, diphtheria, pertussis
IMMUNIZATIONS FOR HIGH-RISK PREGNANCIES	Hepatitis A Hepatitis B Poliomyelitis Pneumococcus Other local infections *(yellow fever, smallpox, meningococcus, Japanese encephalitis, typhoid, cholera)

*Depending upon the mother's travel schedule and risk of exposure.

Source: National Library of Medicine. Infections and Pregnancy. (2013). Available at www.nlm.nih.gov/medlineplus/infectionsandpregnancy.html

As with all medications, clinicians must weigh the risk versus the benefits of vaccines. The new Tdap vaccine, although inactivated, has yet to be approved for pregnant women; however, it is recommended that women considering pregnancy obtain the vaccine before pregnancy or as soon after as possible. Two Tdap vaccines (toxoid diphtheria and acellular pertussis) are available in the United States. Their brand names are Adacel, licensed for people age 16 to 64, and Boostrix, licensed for those 10 to 18 years. No harm is known to come to the baby of a breastfeeding mother who receives these vaccinations. The Advisory Committee on Immunization Practices (ACIP) of the CDC (2011) recommends that Tdap be given to women during the late second trimester or third trimester rather than waiting until immediately after delivery as a means of better protecting the newborn against pertussis. This practice provides protection for the mother and indirectly to the child through transplacental antibodies. Children are at higher risk until about 2 months, when they start their series of vaccines. This practice offers the advantage of protecting children at birth.

The use of monoclonal antibodies, steroids, NSAIDs, antihistamines, and other immunologically active medications requires careful consideration in pregnancy at all times.

Pediatric, Geriatric, and Immunocompromised Implications

Prescribing of immunologically active medications is no different from prescribing other medications. The clinician must perform a careful and complete history and physical examination and understand the benefits, potential risks, and contraindications to the medications used. The very young, the very old, those on other medications, those who are immunologically compromised, and those who are incapacitated for one reason or another provide unique issues and concerns that the clinician must consider when prescribing. It is not the purpose nor the capability of this chapter to discuss all the implications of immunologic medications; however, in view of the rapidly changing field of immunologic

biologicals, it is crucial that anyone prescribing immunizations, monoclonal antibodies, and immunologic-altering medications should be familiar with the most recent updates of their uses.

LEARNING EXERCISES

Case 1

PW is an 18-year-old female who is starting college. Recently she bought some new clothes and is certain some of the fabrics are causing her to break out in a red, itchy, dry rash around her neck where everyone can see it. She is quite anxious about starting college and is now distraught that she has this to contend with as well. You have cared for PW for many years and know that she has atopic dermatitis, but it has eased over the years. Her mother has been very careful to remind PW to keep her skin moist and avoid allergens or rough, irritating materials. You realize that, with PW now going to school, she will have to take over the care of her skin herself. Examination reveals the typical, red, dry, pruritic rash of atopic dermatitis in the neck, waist, and elbows. She is on no medications and except for a history of irritable bowel syndrome a few years ago, her record is clear.

1. Write a prescription for the medication you would recommend.

   Rx: _____

   #: _____

   Sig: _____

2. Why did you choose this medication?

3. What patient advisories would you give?

4. What recommendations would you make for follow-up?

Case 2

GW is a 46-year-old scout master who recently took his troop camping in the woods. GW is extremely hypersensitive to poison ivy, and although he and his scouts are very careful about avoiding the noxious plant, the troop mascot, a long-haired retriever, is not. That evening after many loving licks and hugs from the dog, GW realized that he was beginning to break out in his typical contact dermatitis rash. When he came to see you the next day, you observed several areas on his chest, legs, and especially the inside of his arms, where the classic red inflamed skin with bullae formation of dermatitis was seen. Mr. GW was concerned as it was spreading. From past experience both you and he realized that he was very sensitive to poison ivy and this was going to be a serious dermatitis. He has no other medical problems and takes no medications.

1. Write a prescription for the medication you would recommend.

   Rx: _____

   #: _____

   Sig: _____

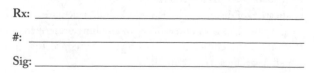

2. Why did you choose this medication?

3. What patient advisories would you give?

4. What recommendations would you make for follow-up?

References

Akdis, M., & Akdis, C. A., (August, 2009). Therapeutic manipulation of immune tolerance in allergic disease. *Nature Reviews Drug Discovery, 8*(8) 645-660. Available at www.ncbi.nlm.nih.gov/pubmed/19644474

Buys, L. M. (2007). Treatment options for atopic dermatitis, *American Family Physician, 75*(4), 523-528.

Centers for Disease Control and Prevention (CDC). (March, 2010). U.S. vaccines. Table. Retrieved March 14, from www.cdc.gov/vaccines/pubs/pinkbook/downloads/appendices/B/us-vaccines.pdf

Centers for Disease Control and Prevention (CDC). (2011). Appendix D, diphtheria. In *Epidemiology and prevention of vaccine-preventable diseases. The pink book: Course textbook* (12th ed., pp. 59-70). Available at www.cdc.gov/vaccines/pubs/pinkbook/downloads/dip.pdf

Centers for Disease Control and Prevention (CDC). (2013). Vaccines & immunizations. Immunization schedules. Retrieved March 19, 2012, at www.cdc.gov/vaccines/recs/default.htm

Chafen, J. J. S., Newberry, S. J., Riedl, M. A., Bravata, D. M., Maglione, M., Suttorp, M. J., et al. (2010). Diagnosing and managing food allergies: A systematic review. *JAMA, 303*(18), 1848 1856.

deShazo, R. D., & Kemp, S. F. (1997). Allergic reactions to drugs and biologic agents. *JAMA, 278*, 1895-1906.

Gell, P. G. H., & Coombs, R. R. A. (eds.). (1963). *Clinical aspects of immunology* (1st ed.). Oxford, England: Blackwell.

Gomes, E. R., & Demoly, P. (2005). Epidemiology of hypersensitivity drug reactions. *Current Opinion in Allergy and Clinical Immunology, 5*, 309–316.

Huggins, J. L., & Looney, R. J. (2004). Allergen immunotherapy. *American Family Physician, 70*(4), 689-696.

Kurowski, K., & Boxer, B. W. (2008). Food allergies: Detection and management. *American Family Physician, 77*(12), 1678-1686.

Sur, K., & Sandale, S. (June, 2012). Treatment of Allergic Rhinitis, *Am. Family Phys. 81*(12):1440-1446. Available at www.aafp.org/afp/2010/0615/p1440.html

Resources

Muller, B. A. (2004). Urticaria and angioedema: A practical approach. *American Family Physician, 69*(5), 1123-1128.

Nebeker, J. R. (2004). Clarifying adverse drug events: A clinician's guide to terminology, documentation, and reporting. *Annals of Internal Medicine, 140*, 795-801.

Rabson, A. R., Roitt I., Delves P., (2005). *Really essential medical immunology* (2nd ed., pp. 148-163). Oxford, England: Wiley-Blackwell.

Rich, R. R., Fleisher, T. A., Schearer, W. T., Schroeder, H., Frew, A. J., Weyand, C. M., (Eds.). (2013). *Clinical Immunology: Principles and Practice 4th ed* (pp. 449-477). Elsevier-Saungers, Philadelphia.

Schaefer, P. (2011). Urticaria and treatment. *American Family Physician, 83*(9).

U. S. Food and Drug Administration (FDA). (January, 2006). FDA approves updated labeling with boxed warning and medication guide for two eczema drugs, Elidel and Protopic. *FDA News.* Available at www.fda.gov/NewsEvents/Newsroom/PressAnnouncements/2006/ucm108580.htm

U. S. Food and Drug Administration (FDA). (2010). Tacrolimus (marketed as Protopic ointment) information. *Drugs.* Available at www.fda.gov/Drugs/DrugSafety/PostmarketDrugSafetyInformationforPatientsandProviders/ucm107845.htm

Wilson, B. G., & Bahna, S. L. (2005). Adverse reactions to food additives. *Annals of Allergy, Asthma, & Immunology, 95*(6), 499-507.

The Vaccine Adverse Event Reporting System (VAERS). (n.d.). Available at http://vaers.hhs.gov/index

Answers and Rationales for Learning Exercises

Chapter 1

1. The legal distinction between a prescription drug and an over-the-counter (OTC) drug is not founded on relative safety of the agent but rather involves a government decision on whether or not the OTC package will contain "adequate directions for a layperson to safely use it." Similarly, the prescription packaging will contain a summary of the chemical and physical nature of the product's ingredients, its pharmacological indications, its administration, its dosing ranges, and other information pertinent to how a clinician could safely choose it for a particular patient that results in it being safe and effective. Thus the FDA has had the legend or prescription only medication undergo tests that assure the public it is what its labels says it is, it does not have labeling that has not been approved by FDA officially, and the drug is effective for the use and dosages so stated. The FDA does not dictate how, what, when, and where a clinician should practice; that is a prerogative left to state licensing boards. However, the FDA does recognize that clinicians make decisions "one patient at a time" and are well equipped to recommend usage of both OTC and Rx (legend) products. Thus, Mrs. Jones needs to be made assured and comfortable that her prescription medication is right for her and that her clinician has not abridged that responsibility.

2. The FDA has regulatory jurisdiction over all drugs, including how they are to be named, how they are approved for sale to the public, their official labeling, and how they are to undergo surveillance for adverse drug reactions, as well as their methods and means of manufacture and distribution. The matter of whether or not a drug is sold over the counter or prescription only is also a matter of federal law. If the FDA determines it is to be prescription only, it will contain the legend, "Caution: Federal Law prohibits dispensing without a prescription" and will require that statement on all its packaging and labeling (and this includes advertising). Hence, the term *legend drug*.

Chapter 2

1. Assuming the drug elimination is linear, then after 1 hour the 100-mg tablet will be reduced to 50 mg, after 2 hours there will be 25 mg left, and after 3 hours there will be 12.5 mg left.

2. The small intestine may be the primary site of drug absorption from tablet dosage forms, but this is not always the case. The small intestine offers a large surface area and a high level of blood perfusion; however, not all drugs are absorbed from the small intestine. Much drug absorption occurs in the stomach and large intestine as well. But because of their relatively smaller surface area, more acidic environment, and gastric emptying times, these factors will increase or decrease absorption of a drug from the stomach. In addition, alterations in gastric motility affect the amount of time a drug spends in any area of the GI tract. The presence of food can also cause decreased absorption from the stomach. Certainly presence of some ions (Ca, Fe Mg) can bind a drug, and pH is always a factor in tablet dissolution. Additionally, changes in drug formulations can alter absorption by how they affect dissolution rates of the tablet.

3. There is a general rule of thumb that approximately five half-lives are to be reached before a drug reaches a level where it is no longer active or causing adverse effects. Because this new drug has a half-life of 20 hours, it will require almost 100 hours (5×20), or nearly 4 days, before the patient is probably clear of adverse effects. In practice, however, a patient's personal characteristics, such as body mass index, may alter this general rule. For example, many drugs cause nausea, vomiting, diarrhea, and a skin rash. The selective serotonin reuptake inhibitors can induce nausea and vomiting, which is typically transitory and disappears as the person adjusts to the medicine. There is no rule regarding how long this adjustment period may last; if the nausea and vomiting do not cease, the drug is discontinued.

   Patients given Vicodin (acetaminophen and hydrocodone) to relieve moderate pain may become nauseated within the first hour of taking the first tablet and be fine thereafter, or they may experience nausea and vomiting for a day or two longer. In this instance the nausea has nothing to do with the half-life; it is a patient-specific event.

   Some of its less serious side effects of hydroxychloroquine (Plaquenil), which is used to treat or prevent malaria, are nausea, vomiting, ringing in the ears, and headache. Its more serious side effects may include visual disturbance (blurry vision, light sensitivity, seeing halos around lights) and muscle weakness (with uncontrolled twitching or movement), which may persist for weeks, months, or years before they resolve, or they may become irreversible despite stopping the medicine and despite knowing its half-life falls in the range of 41 days plus or minus 14 days.

Chapter 3
Case 1

1. First, establish a good communication pattern with the patient. If you know the patient well, ask about his family, job, hobbies, etc. Make an effort to show you are truly interested in his life and well being. Use open-ended

questions to ask him the reason for his visit, as well as general questions regarding his overall health.

2. Every practitioner handles this type of situation differently. If you have established a good relationship with the patient, you will feel more at ease, as will your patient, when you discuss his general health, medications, diet, and exercise at every visit. It is wise to assess the patient's state of mind and his willingness to have an open discussion with you. It may be overwhelming to discuss all his health issues at every visit, thus choosing your topics for discussion is a wise approach. For instance, at this first visit you could discuss weight and exercise; at the next, diet; and during a future visit bring up the topic of smoking.

   Although you do not want to be afraid to discuss important issues with your patient, you must understand that each patient is unique in their ability and willingness to address all their health issues at one visit. Begin the conversation and ask the patient what his preferences are and what, if anything, he is concerned about. Tell him your concerns and give him options on how you should address them together.

3. To gain a patient's trust, the clinician must show that he or she is truly interested in the patient as a whole individual and not as a cancer, hypertension, or diabetes. In other words, you must first establish a relationship and earn trust over time. Being honest with patients is critical, as is being nonjudgmental. Taking the time to educate and involve patients in their own care as well as giving them a say in their own care is vital. Using patient-centered communication techniques is a great way to begin.

Case 2

1. It is important to recognize your patient's understanding of the English language. This patient's frustration may be due to either his difficulty understanding the English language or it may be due to your use of medical jargon. As the patient's clinician, you must slow down and assess where the communication breakdown is happening and then correct the issue.

2. Begin by speaking slower, using less medical jargon, and checking frequently with the patient to ensure that he understands. If the problem appears to be due to language, ask if there is someone with him in the waiting room who could translate or someone he could call that could translate. Use diagrams if necessary. You could also give him written instructions that he could take to a friend or relative who could explain. Or you could purchase translation software that is now available for mobile electronic devices and use this in your clinic.

Case 3

1. To achieve high-quality interpersonal communication with all patients, clinicians need to develop an accurate understanding of each patient's lifestyle, health beliefs, home setting, and support systems.

2. When communication is impaired owing to diminished intellect or senses and/or psychosocial factors, the clinician can still offer patient-centered care by asking questions of a family member, making a visit to the home, or talking with other clinicians, such as a family pharmacist. The clinician can also order appropriate tests to evaluate the patient's hearing, sight, gait, and so on. Social service providers, a church pastor, or other support group can also be of help in evaluating the home situation and providing assistance.

   Mechanical and digital aids are available to assist older adults in understanding and retaining medication information. Clinicians can individualize a care plan and put it into motion with follow-up that provides feedback on a timely basis so that the plan can be modified as needed.

Chapter 4
Case 1

It has been well documented in the medical literature that ibuprofen interacts with different groups of antihypertensive drugs (beta-adrenergic blockers, alpha-adrenergic blockers, diuretics, and angiotensin-converting enzyme inhibitors), reducing their antihypertensive activity. The mechanism of action of ibuprofen involves inhibition of the enzyme cyclooxygenase, thereby inhibiting the synthesis of inflammatory prostaglandins and vasodilatory prostaglandins that increase renal blood flow and thus favor the excretion of water and sodium. More than 5 days of treatment with both drugs are normally required for the interaction to manifest. Although the changes in blood pressure resulting from this interaction are typically small, some patients can experience substantial elevations in both systolic and diastolic blood pressure.

Case 2

1. AB is at a relatively high risk of renal impairment because of changes in blood flow through the kidney mediated by prostaglandins, which in turn are affected by NSAIDS and angiotensin-converting enzyme inhibitors (ACEIs). Prostaglandins cause vasodilation of afferent arterioles, and by blocking this effect with NSAIDS (Tylenol) and ACEIs, the patient is at risk of renal failure.

2. The Mylanta may be hiding GI irritation. The COX-2 selective NSAIDS have a better safety profile in short-term treatments, but for long-term use there are concerns. They are as effective as any nonselective NSAID or acetaminophen for reducing joint pain and inflammation, but there are concerns when they are used in patients with cardiovascular issues. Thus, the clinician has to weigh carefully the benefits to risks by considering the patient's intolerance to other NSAIDS, history of GI bleed, cardiovascular risk, renal disease, preferences, and cost. A.B. should be cautioned about his use of Mylanta and be given a nonselective NSAID with misoprostol or a proton pump inhibitor as an alternative.

Chapter 5
Case 1

Any commercial strength of pilocarpine that works (0.04% up to 8%) is likely to continue working. Common side effects of pilocarpine are blurry vision upon application and other effects that are transitory, but after 2 years with no complaint of any discomfort from the drug, a lack of patient compliance to the drug regimen is likely in this case, despite what the patient states.

Noncompliance or nonadherence must be evaluated because it has caused many patients to undergo unnecessary eye surgeries and switching medications. Additionally, patients will typically tolerate some side effects rather than report these effects to the clinician, which in turn can lead to inadequate care.

Case 2

1. Because ocular allergies are common, this is the likely cause.
2. Ocular allergies do have a large number of treatment options. Many patients will be well managed if placed on either antihistamines or mast cell stabilizers. Oral antihistamines reduce the response to allergens, whereas many topical ocular antihistamines have more than one active ingredient, usually an antihistamine and a decongestant.
3. The side effects of the ocular use of topical antihistamines reflect their anticholinergic activity, and include mydriasis, decreased accommodation, increased intraocular pressure, and dry eyes. The mast cell stabilizers prevent the release of histamine from its storage sites, the mast cells. If the disease is chronic and threatens sight, prolonged treatment with mast stabilizers, short courses of topical steroids, and oral NSAIDs may be needed. As the underlying pathophysiology of allergies is not fully understood, work is still being done to understand its processes and develop medications having different mechanisms of action to combat a condition that affects millions of people.

Chapter 6
Case 1

This is a common scenario when a patient comes to the urgent care center without his or her medications and can't remember the specific diagnoses or pills he or she is taking. A simple call to the patient's pharmacy can often determine the prescriptions that were filled the last time the patient picked up prescriptions.

Based on the history of having a fast heart rate, this patient probably has atrial fibrillation. Because she has not been able to get around, she has probably not been eating well and has lost some weight. Therefore, the medications she is taking may be too strong. A call to her pharmacy reveals that she is taking metoprolol XL 50 daily, amlodipine 10 mg daily, and digoxin 0.25 mg daily.

Her ECG reveals a junctional escape rhythm most likely secondary to excessive digoxin. This patient should be transferred to the hospital for further evaluation and treatment. Laboratory tests should be obtained to rule out myocardial infarction, as well as to assess other causes of her problem, including her nutritional status, electrolytes, and thyroid status. Digibind can be used to treat digoxin overdose, but it is usually not necessary. Careful observation and electrocardiographic monitoring of this patient for 2 to 3 days should be sufficient to allow the digoxin to clear from the body. During that time, her medications can be adjusted safely and nutritional status can be addressed.

Case 2

Furosemide helps heart failure patients feel better, but lisinopril is more likely to decrease mortality. In this case, a reasonable approach should be to increase lisinopril to at least 20 mg and possibly 40 mg daily. While increasing the lisinopril, careful attention must be paid to the blood pressure, and the furosemide should be decreased accordingly. Additionally, the use of beta blockers has been shown to reduce mortality associated with congestive heart failure. Once the patient is stabilized on the lisinopril and furosemide, a beta blocker such as carvedilol should be started at a very low dose and gradually increased over 3 to 6 weeks. The gradual increase is necessary because increasing beta blockers too quickly can cause an exacerbation of congestive heart failure.

Chapter 7
Case 1

1. Sample RX
   RX: hydrochlorthiazide 12.5 mg
   M: 24
   Sig: take one tablet every day

   RX: Atenolol 25 mg
   M: 24
   Sig: Table one table every day for 2 weeks
   Note: doses of more than 25 mg of hydrochlorthiazide are associated with greater risk of electrolyte abnormalaties. Studies indicate 12.5 mg is just as effective as higher doses. Patient should return after 2 weeks of therapy on atenolol to have BP checked and dosage strength adjusted if necessary. Once everything is checked out, patient may have a 90 day supply which meets most insurance payment standards.
2. Choice of medication and advise the patient: as per JNC 7, first line medications are diuretics or beta blockers such as hydrochlorthiazide and any beta blocker whose generic name ends with -olol such as propranolol. Advise the patient to eat a low-salt diet and avoid canned and frozen foods, diet, and exercise. Advise the patient to lose weight. Advise the patient to take this medication in the morning to prevent nocturnal diuresis. Advice the patient that for first few days he needs to be careful standing up or sitting up suddenly (postural hypotension).
3. Side effects: Common side effects that need to be discussed are postural hypotension and hypokalemia. Potassium levels need to be monitored periodically.

Case 2

1. The answer is **D**. JC is on Norvasc and lisinopril. JC's blood pressure is well controlled on the current regimen, and her echocardiogram report is normal except for left ventricular hypertrophy, which appears from the hypertension. But JC is having swelling in legs and constipation, which are common side effects of the Norvasc (CCB). JC is tolerating the lisinopril. Stop the Norvasc and increase the dose of the lisinopril. Having one blood pressure agent will also increase compliance. Adding either hydrochlorothiazide or Lasix will increase the probability of side effects such as postural hypotension and hypokalemia and may not cure the swelling in legs. Both can also increase constipation.

Chapter 8
Case 1

1. It would seem that the dosage of simvastatin is not working at 40 mg. Increasing the simvastatin to a dosage of 80 mg by mouth daily would seem in order, but the patient does not meet the FDA guideline of having been on the drug for 12 months or more and not reporting any muscle toxicity. Thus, switching to another class of drug or using combination therapy is recommended.
2. Council patient on the need for compliance to the drug regimen, diet, and exercise program.
3. 6 weeks

Case 2

1. Change to atorvastatin.
2. Intensify diet, adding fiber, soy, omega-3 fatty acids (fish oil).
3. Intensify regular exercise routine.

Chapter 9
Case 1

1. This patient is an excellent candidate for outpatient treatment of thromboembolism. Randomized controlled trials show that outpatient low molecular weight heparin (LMWH), followed by warfarin, is as effective and as safe as inpatient management, with substantial cost savings.

   In your office, give him LMWH (for example, enoxaparin 80 mg (1 mg/kg) subcutaneously twice daily) and send him for the outpatient ultrasound study. If the study is normal, then you have wasted one or perhaps two doses of LMWH, and you can pursue alternative diagnoses. If the study is diagnostic for deep venous thrombosis (DVT), then start warfarin at 5 mg daily, and check the international normalized ratio (INR) daily. Titrate the warfarin as needed, and discontinue the LMWH when the INR is greater than 2 on two consecutive days.
2. Probably 3 to 6 months. He has a clear reason for the DVT—the immobility associated with his prolonged hospitalization, which is now resolved. If there was no reversible cause of his DVT, for example in a frail patient with severe congestive heart failure, you should treat for a longer period, probably at least 6 to 12 months. If this DVT was a second episode, then the warfarin should probably be continued indefinitely.

Case 2

1. Yes. Although this man is not at high risk, all hospitalized patients should be considered for venous thromboembolism (VTE) prophylaxis. Unless there is a contraindication, prescribe either unfractionated heparin, 5,000 units SC, every 8 to 12 hours; enoxaparin, 40 mg SC, once daily; dalteparin 5,000 units SC, once daily; or fondaparinux, 2.5 mg SC, once daily. All of these agents reduce the risk of VTE by at least 50%.
2. In this case anticoagulation would be contraindicated, but he would still be a good candidate for physical means to prevent VTE, such as graduated compression stockings or intermittent pneumatic compression, or both. In any case, you should also promote early ambulation and encourage him to flex his ankles and knees while lying in bed. Remove oxygen, IV lines, cardiac monitors, and other devices as soon as possible to enhance mobility and reduce the risk of DVT.

Chapter 10
Case 1

The triggering event in this patient's history is the addition of oral theophylline to his asthma medications. Theophylline has a long-standing reputation for producing wildly swinging plasma concentrations. Theophylline interferes with the metabolism of warfarin, and as warfarin levels get elevated, bleeding becomes an issue. However, withdrawing any asthma medication is likely to spin the asthma out of control. Warfarin levels should already be monitored more frequently in this patient and adjusted to maintain levels within the therapeutic range.

Case 2

Student D is correct. In all asthma treatment regimens, the inhaled beta-agonists are used as bronchodilators to relieve acute symptoms as needed. But because asthma is an inflammatory disease, inhaled corticosteroids are also used to control symptoms in all but the mildest cases. The drug theophylline, because of its potential for side effects and drug interactions, is used only rarely today, and if used at all, it is in cases in which it is difficult to control asthma symptoms. The beta receptor agonists can be used alone as monotherapy, but in very mild cases.

Chapter 11
Case 1

1. Patient education is the key to successfully managing constipation. First review what are "normal" bowel habits as to frequency and the effect of diet. Modest exercise also affects the regularity of bowel movements, and this factor should be discussed with the patient. Finally, it may be helpful to have the patient keep a diary of his movements, their size, shape, and consistency, and any experience of discomfort.
2. In addition to bulk laxatives, treatment options include lubricating laxatives (mineral oil), stimulating laxatives (surface acting agents such as docusate or bisacodyl), and anthraquinones (senna, cascara, and rhubarb). Fiber agents are typically effective when transit time is normal, but it may not be normal for this patient; thus, another agent may be tried. Stimulant laxatives irritate colonic mucosa and promote peristalsis. They may also affect fluid and electrolyte absorption resulting in colonic fluid accumulation. Bisacodyl is a useful rescue agent when managing chronic constipation. Stool softeners such as docusate soften stools by reducing the surface tension at the oil-water interface of fecal matter allowing water to penetrate. They are of marginal value in treating constipation.

Case 2

1. Diarrhea is usually a symptom caused by another health issue, such as an infection by bacteria or a parasite, or a virus picked up in food or water. It may also be caused by reactions to medications or in people who are lactose intolerant. Diarrhea that persists for a month is usually a serious health

issue such as inflammatory bowel disease (IBS) or Crohn's disease, especially if there is any blood seen in the stool. Thus, BJ needs a thorough workup to rule out anything serious.

2. In most cases diarrhea will go away on its own. However, in this case if we assume BJ has a normal case of diarrhea, a drug such as diphenoxylate/atropine (Lomotil) is likely in order. If the diarrhea is caused by a bacterial infection, an antibiotic may be prescribed, but the danger here is bacterial overgrowth, which may be *Clostridium difficile*. Because diarrhea is the body's way of getting rid of toxins, it is best to let it run its course. However, in this case it is important that a more thorough history regarding frequency and aggravating factors as well as a travel history be taken before prescribing. BJ may have IBS or even IBD, thus a thorough history, physical, and diagnostic testing may be called for.

Chapter 12

Case 1

1. When this patient first presented, a total team approach to the initial differential diagnosis included severe anxiety disorder, sepsis, neuroleptic malignant syndrome, thyroid storm, recreational drug overdose, and meningitis. Because laboratory data came in demonstrating an extremely elevated free T4 and T3 in the setting of a decreased TSH, a diagnosis of thyroid storm was confirmed. The elevated thyroid-stimulating immunoglobulin indicated that there was new hormone synthesis likely from Graves' disease. Graves' disease can also cause a transient leukopenia and thrombocytopenia. Thyroid storm can cause nonspecific abnormalities in the liver enzymes, which usually resolve after the acute crisis. On further probing it was concluded that the patient had been suffering from hyperthyroidism for years because he indicated he had seen his appetite increase and was eating a lot of junk food, but without any significant weight gain. He also reported increased frequency of his bowel movements and had noticed his palpitations.

2. Once a diagnosis of thyroid storm was established, the patient's tachycardia was treated with propranolol, a beta blocker. Propanolol is frequently used because it can be given intravenously initially and then switched to oral tablets upon discharge. His fever was managed with acetaminophen and a cooling blanket. It is important to remember to avoid salicylates because they compete with T3 and T4 for binding of thyroid-binding globulin and can therefore increase the free hormone levels in the body. The patient was also started on high-dose intravenous steroids. Glucocorticoids work by blocking peripheral conversion of T4 to T3 (T3 being the active form of thyroid hormone). In addition, the patient received methimazole, preventing new thyroid hormone synthesis. Once the patient's condition was more stable, he was evaluated for total thyroid removal. With all factors considered, it was decided that a total thyroidectomy would serve as the best treatment option. The patient underwent surgery without any complications and was started on thyroid hormone replacement after surgery.

Case 2

1. and 2. This is an ethical issue as well as a medical issue because in the United States, entitlement to a medical treatment is generally understood to mean inclusion of the treatment in a basic health care plan, whether specified by the government, insurance companies, or managed care program. It has long been assumed that there is an entitlement to growth hormone (GH) therapy for children with documented growth hormone deficiency (GHD), but not necessarily for others who may be equally short. Some have argued, however, that fairness requires clinicians to offer GH treatment to all children whose predicted adult height is below a certain level. Thus, this would extend the entitlement to all children whose predicted height is viewed as some sort of handicap or whose shortness may result in psychological impairment or social functioning.

Chapter 13

Case 1

1. This patient is presenting with the classic signs of hyperglycemia associated with type 2 diabetes. With a BMI of 31 (obesity) and glucose over 400, pharmacological and nonpharmacological interventions are indicated because of the risk factors and the need to obtain specific glycemic goals that will substantially reduce the patient's morbidity. Choice of an antihyperglycemic agent is going to be based on: (a) its effectiveness in lowering glucose, (b) extra glycemic effects that will reduce the risk of long-term complications of the diabetes (especially eye and foot issues), (c) safety profile, (d) tolerability, (d) ease of administration and adherence to the regimen, and (f) expense to patient as self-pay or insurance copay and plan limitations/regulations (i.e., generic only).

2. As of today there is enough information that is supportive of certain "guidelines" that are aimed at improving the probability that a patient will have better long-term control of his or her diabetes. There is also good evidence that metformin should be the first-line therapy in most cases of type 2 diabetes. The greatest contributor to improving that probability is not any drug or intervention per se, but the impact of an early diagnoses when the metabolic abnormalities of diabetes are less severe.

The major modifiable factors that increase type 2 diabetes risk factors are obesity and sedentary lifestyle. Thus, in this overweight patient, a lifestyle intervention program to promote weight loss and increase activity should be included as part of the patient's diabetes management program. The patient should be encouraged to set goals as a weight loss of 5% to 10% will improve glycemia. In most cases, metformin, a biguanide drug, will lower HbA1c by 1.5%, especially when it is administered concurrently with lifestyle modifications. Sulfonylureas are as effective as metformin, but unlike metformin, they cause hypoglycemia and may increase cardiovascular disease mortality. Thus, they are not recommended as first-line therapy. Alpha-glucosidase inhibitors reduce the rate of digestion of polysaccharides in the proximal small intestine, thus they lower postprandial glucose levels without causing hypoglycemia. They are less effective than the biguanides or sulfonylureas, and because they are absorbed distally, they may produce gas and GI symptoms but do not impact weight loss. TZD or glitazones increase the sensitivity of muscle, fat, and liver to endogenous and exogenous insulin but come with an increased risk of cardiovascular issues, thus they are often used as add-on medications in combination with metformin, sulfonylureas, glinides (TZD), and insulin.

3. This patient has a prime need for an intervention with a caring and conscientious health professional who will explain all the risk factors and what glycemic goals are and why it's important to meet them, not just with a drug, but with a commitment to lifestyle changes that will guarantee him living longer than both parents. In this case, he needs to get his glucose under control with a goal of HbA1C under 7. However, lowing HbA1c too quickly can be dangerous. Initial treatment with insulin is often used in cases of high glucose associated with symptoms with subsequent addition of metformin followed by a tapering of insulin based on frequent self-assessment of finger-stick glucose. This patient should also undergo intense education regarding diabetes treatment, including lifestyle modifications, medication use and side effects, glucose monitoring, recognizing hypoglycemia and how to treat it, exercise planning, including risks of exercise during hypoglycemia and hyperglycemia, and interventions that can improve health and longevity in diabetes.

Case 2

1. Glyburide (DiaBeta) is somewhat effective in this age group, yet the dizziness, sweating, and afternoon agitation could be signs of an adverse drug reaction between the Lipitor and the DiaBeta. His family history of type 2 diabetes and his BMI of 28 put him at risk for type 2 diabetes, but it also may be an indication that he is not adhering to his drug regimen or making lifestyle modifications to get his glucose under control.

   COMMON side effects when using DiaBeta include a feeling of stomach fullness, heartburn, and nausea. However, SEVERE side effects when using DiaBeta include severe allergic reactions (rash; hives; itching; difficulty breathing; joint or muscle pain; tightness in the chest; swelling of the mouth, face, lips, or tongue; unusual hoarseness); blisters on the skin; confusion; fainting; fever, chills, or persistent sore throat; irregular heartbeat; low blood sugar symptoms (e.g., anxiety, dizziness, drowsiness, fast heartbeat, headache, lightheadedness, tremors, unusual sweating, weakness); severe or persistent blurred vision or other vision problems; symptoms of liver problems (e.g., dark urine, loss of appetite, pale stools, stomach pain, yellowing of the eyes or skin); unusual bruising or bleeding; unusual tiredness or weakness. These do not seem to be evident in this case.

2. The following recommendations should be discussed with this patient.
   - Change to metformin which is recommended as first-line therapy

- Addition of an antihypertensive medication starting at a low dose with gradual increase to help achieve blood pressure less than 130/80
- Increase of Lipitor to 20 mg/day
- Improvement in lifestyle, with specific goals for weight loss and exercise
- As in Case 1, intensive counseling on diabetes outcomes, treatments, and so on

Chapter 14
Case 1

1. This patient may be beginning to show signs of mild dementia but is it truly Alzheimer's Disease (AD).
2. Mrs. P.T. needs a thorough behavioral assessment plan and an examination of any environmental factors that could be causing her issues *before* any pharmacotherapy is recommended, especially because she is taking six drugs now and may be a victim of polypharmacy.
3. Remember drug therapy is only to allay symptoms and is not a cure, so non-drug therapy and social support systems should be in place as the primary intervention for both family and patient. Patient education is also part of the intervention, but referral to social services and legal support services may also be needed. Remember reversing cognitive decline is the goal of any pharmacotherapy, but all choices have limitations. Medication dosing should be done slowly and with careful titration to avoid adverse effects. Finally, pharmacotherapy for behavioral symptoms should also be self-limiting and be discontinued in patients with stable symptoms.

Case 2

1. The woman is likely a migraine patient and as migraine is one of the top 10 presenting complaints in primary care and it presents with or without aura, women are two to three times more likely to present with it than are men.
2. Migraine-specific medications are now available to provide relief from moderate to severe attacks; however, a thorough evaluation of the headache history is necessary to determine if a patient will benefit from these agents. Although migraines appear to be a result of neuronal dysfunction, the precise etiology is unknown; however, serotonergic neurotransmission plays an important role. A careful patient workup is a must, and a wellness program aimed at avoiding triggers should be included in the management plan. Patients should be taught to use abortive therapy early in the attack, and once an effective agent and dosage have been identified, patients should adhere to that medication and dosage. Attack severity varies, and patients may be advised to use nonspecific agents in mild attacks (NSAIDs) and hold off using serotonin agonists (triptans) for the more moderate to severe attacks.
3. "Preventive therapy", as opposed to "abortive therapy", should be considered if the patient experiences migraines more than twice a week. The goals of preventive therapy are to reduce the incidence of migraines, their pain, and their duration as neither therapy is a cure. If preventive therapy is

to be considered effective, a trial of 2 to 3 months duration will be needed. The beta-blocker drugs have been used as prophylaxis therapy especially if there is comorbid anxiety, angina, or hypertension. Other medications, such as the tricyclic antidepressants, NSAIDs, vitamin B_2, valproic acid, and topiramate have also been used prophylactically. In addition, preventive management may include nonpharmacological interventions such as use of biofeedback, relaxation, and cognitive therapy. Any of the ergotamine preparations, triptans, and valproate should be avoided in pregnant women.

Chapter 15
Case 1

1. Sample RX: Fluoxetine 10 mg
   M: 50
   Sig: 1 tab every day for 1 week; increase to 2 tabs per day after the first week
2. Although you may have chosen either a benzodiazepine or a tricyclic agent for this patient, you first must consider the patient that is going to be using this drug because side effects can affect not only outcomes, but also adherence to any agent or regimen. A once a day tablet is preferred over multi-tab dosing. Remember also that benzodiazepines are Schedule drugs (controlled substances) and are subject to abuse. Additionally, they depress all levels of the central nervous system. Thus, it is important to know when their use is appropriate and when it is not.
3. The advisories for patients who are taking tricyclic antidepressants, benzodiazepines, or selective serotonin reuptake inhibitors (SSRIs) are the same as for patients taking any other antianxiety disorder medication. The SSRIs are a more popular choice today because of the better risk-benefit profile and lower incidence of adverse events.

Case 2

1. and 2. The medication history of HG's brother, sister, and mother are clues regarding where to start. If all three responded to one of the SSRIs or tricyclic antidepressants, begin with that drug. A newer SSRI may work best because of their favorable side effect profiles. Therefore, you might try prescribing sertraline (Zoloft) as follows:
   RX: Zoloft 50 mg tabs
   M: 50 tabs
   Sig: 1 tab by mouth a.m. for 6 weeks, DO NOT REFILL
3. Advise HG that it may take several weeks before he is feeling "up" again but that he should return in 6 weeks for an assessment and perhaps a dosage adjustment (should he need a new prescription). Explain that he might feel nausea, have loose stools, and experience some insomnia, dizziness, fatigue, dry mouth, and even sexual dysfunction, assuming he is active. (Explaining too many side effects, though, may create anxiety about them and cause HG to be noncompliant.) Reinforce the importance of adhering to the prescription regimen and explain that since this is the first time he has been depressed, he may need to take the medication for longer than this initial period to prevent

recurring episodes but that you are there to help him. **Note:** Although this patient is slightly over the age recommended for young people to be counseled about the risk of suicide ideation, it is advisable to discuss it with him, give him an FDA-approved pamphlet about it, and instruct him to call if necessary.

Chapter 16
Case 1

1. Any elderly patient who complains of pruritus (intense itching) should be assessed for scabies. The main symptoms are intense itching, especially at night. The itching may take between 4 to 6 weeks to develop because this is the amount of time it takes for a mite to burrow under skin folds. Elderly people, young children, and anyone who is immunocompromised are the most vulnerable. The elderly also may develop a rash on the back and neck. The two most widely used treatments are permethrin cream and malathion lotion, which should be applied to cool, dry skin (if the skin is too hot the drug may be absorbed and lose its local potency by not staying on the skin). Adults should not apply lotion above the neck, but the very elderly or immunocompromised should apply the treatment to the whole body including the face, neck, and scalp. Permethrin needs to be kept on the skin for 8 to 12 hours, malathion for 24 hours. A follow up treatment after 7 days is always a good recommendation to prevent reinfection because it assures that any eggs left over from the first treatment are killed.
2. It is important that not only the patient be treated, but also anyone who has had close contact with the patient, especially sexual contact, even if he or she shows no signs and symptoms.

Case 2

1. The patient, a child, may need a topical corticosteroid, but there are a number of reasons that patients with suspected eczema, especially children, do not respond appropriately to topical corticosteroids. These reasons include (a) inadequate potency of the preparation, (b) an insufficient amount being applied to the affected area, (c) possibility of an infection, especially *S. aureus,* (d) a contact allergy to the steroid, and (e) nonadherence to the treatment regimen. As with any chronic disease, caregivers or patients often expect a quick and permanent resolution of their illness, but this is not one of those times. Prescribers may mistakenly assume that the potency of a topical corticosteroid is defined by the percentage stated after the compound's name, rather than by the specific compound. Prescribing "the least potent corticosteroid that is effective" is the best axiom to follow. Thus for a moderate to severe atopic dermatitis or eczema that is not on the hands, face, groin, or axillae, a stepped care approach could be followed. For example, start with a moderately potent corticosteroid such as betamethasone valerate cream and lotion 0.1% (Valisone), fluocinolone acetonide cream 0.025% (Synalar), flurandrenolide cream 0.05% (Cordran), hydrocortisone butyrate cream 0.1% (Locoid), hydrocortisone valerate cream 0.2% (Westcort), or triamcinolone

acetonide cream and lotion 0.1% (Kenalog), then taper this off to a lower potency preparation upon seeing clinical improvement. High-potency topical corticosteroids should be used cautiously by a specialist, and used only for severe eczema of the hands or feet, which is not the case here.

2. In children the fingertip unit (FTU) or the amount of a topical medication that extends from the tip to the first joint on the index finger, is a good measure for applying topical corticosteroids. It takes approximately one FTU to cover the hand or groin, 2 FTUs for the face or foot, 3 FTUs for an arm, 6 FTUs for the leg, and 14 FTUs for the trunk. Caregivers who have to refill prescriptions frequently may undertreat a patient's eczema. Topical corticosteroids are typically applied twice daily; using them more frequently may increase side effects and cost without significant clinical benefit. On the other hand, once daily treatment has been shown to be effective for certain corticosteroid preparations, including fluticasone propionate and mometasone furoate, adherence to the treatment regimen could improve. Children with chronic and severe eczema should have their growth monitored because in such cases sufficient steroid may be absorbed and begin to affect the child's normal growth. Occlusive dressings are not suitable for covering corticosteroids to a child's skin because the dressing will increase absorption of the steroid into the body, and by doing so increase the risk of steroid side effects.

Chapter 17
Case 1

1. MG should be educated about the urinary tract infection (UTI) disease process and the need to report to the office with any worsening of signs and/or symptoms such as fever, chills, and/or flank pain that may be indicative of pyelonephritis. She should also avoid sexual intercourse until symptoms have resolved and return to the clinic if she has noticed no improvement within 48 hours. She should void immediately after sexual intercourse if she does have intercourse.

2. A prescription for Bactrim DS (trimethoprim/ sulfamethoxazole) with instruction to take one tablet twice per day with food for 7 days would be good. A longer period of treatment is warranted here because of the recurrence. She should also be made aware of the potential side effects of Bactrim DS and any adverse effects that would require her to stop it or return to the clinic. Measures to prevent future UTIs, such as the need to maintain adequate hydration by increasing fluid intake (particularly with acidic fruit juices, like cranberry juice), should be explained. A follow-up appointment in 2 weeks and a repeat urinalysis (multistix) at that time is recommended. If there are any further signs or symptoms, a urology consultation should be requested.

Case 2

1. This situation requires trust and open communication between patient and prescriber. This is especially important when there is evidence that antibiotics are not always

indicated in treating otitis media. Typically, a clinic has a written policy on how it will handle routine requests for antibiotics, and because the mother wants to do what is best for her children, it becomes an opportunity to explain in simple terms why it is better to treat the discomfort and pain of the ear rather than the infection itself.

Chapter 18
Case 1

1. His tapeworm is likely caused by ingestion of raw fish; other sources of tapeworm are beef, pork, rodents, dogs, and other humans. It could be treated with Ivermectin. In addition you may want to treat for vitamin B_{12} deficiency because the tapeworm can absorb vitamin B_{12} from the diet and cause pernicious anemia in the patient. Eating undercooked pork and salmon is still a problem in the United States. The pork tapeworm often grows to 20 or more feet after several months. The methods of prevention are washing hands before preparing food and not eating raw or undercooked food. A round of antihelminth medication is usually sufficient, along with a laxative to help expel the tapeworm. If no tapeworm segments are found in the stool after 4 months, a cure has been accomplished.

Case 2

1. For any clinician to provide effective care for their HIV-infected patients, they must have a detailed knowledge of the pharmacology of antiretroviral drugs. Because the effectiveness of these agents can be greatly affected by HIV drug resistance, it is vital that clinicians understand the mechanisms of HIV drug resistance, as well as factors that contribute to the emergence of resistance and ways to overcome it. HIV drug resistance is a complicated and dynamic topic, and new information regarding mechanisms and prevalence of HIV drug resistance is appearing almost daily in the literature. The ever-changing nature of this subject requires keeping abreast of the latest clinical and scientific developments in this area because emerging HIV drug resistance has driven the search for new classes of drugs that target different components of HIV and its life cycle.

2. Clinicians can play an important role in preventing the emergence of HIV drug resistance and its symptoms by stressing to their patients the need for strict adherence to their drug regimen. Many antiretroviral agents have relatively short half-lives, and missed doses can reduce blood levels of drugs and allow for viral proliferation and the development of resistance. This is important to remember because studies correlate good adherence to drug regimens with an improvement in virological response. The patient could be noncompliant or nonadherent for many reasons.

Chapter 19
Case 1

1. The adverse events that Mrs. H will experience could be any and all effects from a list of events that result from having her drug therapy affect normal rapidly dividing cells in the

body as well as the cancer cells. These adverse events may affect the blood system (e.g., thrombocytopenia); GI system, especially by nausea, vomiting, and diarrhea; skin and hair; the respiratory system; genitourinary system (because most chemotherapy is excreted renally); cardiotoxicities; and the reproductive system (because they induce teratogenicity). They can also induce hypersensitivities and a serious set of symptoms associated with delayed recall dermatitis.

2. Mrs. H. should be carefully instructed in the events that are likely to affect her and especially to avoid becoming pregnant, should she be sexually active. She also should be instructed as to general health issues, such as diet and exercise, and that she will need to get plenty of rest and uninterrupted sleep to fight fatigue. She especially will need help in understanding how best to take care of her skin and nails and to avoid the risk of any infections. Instructions regarding hair loss and help with wigs and resources are always very supportive, as well as helping her directly or indirectly deal with the psychology of the cancer experience so that a positive attitude will help with the healing.

Case 2

1. Tell Mr. G. that the risk factors for prostate cancer include the following:
   - Increasing age.
   - Race: This is likely not a risk factor for him because prostate cancer tends to occur more often in African-American men.
   - Lifestyle factors such as smoking and a high-fat diet increase his risk of prostate cancer as well as other diseases such as diabetes, hypertension, and stroke.
   - Genetics may be an important factor given his father's history.
     Recommend that Mr. G. have a PSA test done at today's visit as a baseline along with a digital rectal exam.
2. Informative websites for obtaining more information on the latest advances in chemotherapy:
   - World Health Organization, www.who.int/cancer/en
   - National Cancer Institute, www.cancer.gov/cancertopics/types/prostate
   - Prostate Cancer Foundation, www.pcf.org/site/c.leJRIROrEpH/b.5699537/k.BEF4/Home.htm

Chapter 20
Case 1

1. Recommend Fosamax 70 mg weekly by mouth for at least 5 years.
2. Patient advisories would include the following: Take medication with a full glass of water while staying upright for 30 minutes after taking the medication. If esophagitis develops, stop the medication. In addition, the patient should increase her weight-bearing exercise, calcium, and vitamin D intake, and decrease her alcohol consumption and quit smoking. Fall prevention will also be important.

Case 2

1. Rifampin is a CYP34A inducer, which results in significant drug interactions, especially when coadministered with combination oral contraceptives that contain norethindrone and ethinyl estradiol. In effect, it reduces circulating levels of steroid drugs and thus compromises their efficacy as oral contraceptives. Given the serious nature of having an unplanned pregnancy Mary Jane should have been offered the opportunity to use alternative forms of contraception during her term on antibiotic therapy because her abstinence from sex was not likely.

Chapter 21
Case 1

1. RX: Viagra 50 mg
   #: 6 (six)
   Sig: 1 tab by mouth 30 to 60 minutes prior to sexual activity; no more than 1 tab daily
2. You might consider Cialis or Levitra, but the patient specifically asked for Viagra. It may be that he saw it on TV. Viagra is also the oldest of the three and has proven to be safe and effective. Certainly, the patient should be informed of the other two and advised that if Viagra does not work, he might try the others. The patient should also be told that his insurance may not pay for this medication. Although he is not taking nitrates, the patient should be made aware of potential interactions with nitrates and advised that if he is ever being treated for chest pain he needs to let the attending physicians know of his Viagra use, especially within the previous 48 hours. He should also be made aware of several of the common side effects of PDE5 inhibitors, in particular change in color vision, headache, and flushing.
3. The patient should be advised to follow up if after several attempts the medication does not work or if he feels he is having side effects from the medication. It may be possible to adjust the medication, including lowering the dose if the 50 mg is effective or increasing it if it is not.

Case 2

1. RX: Propecia (Finasteride) 1 mg
   #: 30 (thirty)
   Sig: 1 tab by mouth daily
2. You really have little else to offer of a pharmacological treatment for male pattern (androgenic alopecia) baldness. Topical minoxidil (Rogaine) and finasteride (Propecia) are the only two recognized effective pharmacological treatments for male pattern baldness. The patient should also be told insurance seldom pays for either of these medications when prescribed for this purpose.
   Finasteride is a 5-alpha-reductase inhibitor, which decreases the amount of dihydrotestosterone in the scalp skin. The small dose of only 1 mg daily makes side effects unlikely, but patients should be advised that in a few cases decreased libido and erectile dysfunction have been seen. Finasteride (Propecia) is usually most effective in younger

men under 40, and the major effect is prevention of hair loss rather than regrowth. Although some regrowth is probable, the growth of a full head of hair should not be expected. This patient should also be told that, because it is a 5-alpha-reductase inhibitor, finasteride might lower the diagnostic value of the prostate-specific antigen (PSA) level in screening for prostate cancer. He should also be informed that pregnant women should not handle the drug because it may cause harm to the fetus.

3. It may take 3 to 6 months for the medication to reach its full effect, and unless the patient is having concerns or side effects, he need not follow up until then. He should be advised that upon stopping the medication, hair loss usually returns within 4 to 6 months. Finally, as his clinician you should be sensitive to the underlying emotional issues associated with his male pattern baldness.

Chapter 22
Case 1

1. This patient is taking two drugs to treat Parkinson's disease: Sinemet, which is a combination of levodopa and carbidopa, and pramipexole (Mirapex), a dopamine agonist. But he is also taking a drug that directly blocks the dopamine receptor, risperidone (Risperdal), an atypical neuroleptic used to treat psychoses. It is possible that he does not have Parkinson's disease, but rather drug-induced parkinsonism (DIP), which is potentially reversible. As an alternative, perhaps he has idiopathic Parkinson's disease, which has been shown to become worse by the dopamine-blocking drug, risperidone.

2. Change risperidone to 2 mg in the a.m. and 1 mg in the p.m. for 1 week, then prescribe the following:
1 mg twice daily for 1 week, then
1 mg in the a.m. and 0.5 mg in the p.m. for 1 week, then
0.5 mg twice daily for 1 week, then
0.5 mg in the a.m. and 0.25 mg in the p.m. for 1 week, then
0.25 mg twice daily for 1 week, then
0.25 mg in the a.m. only for 1 week, then
discontinue

3. There are two major areas to monitor: First is whether the parkinsonian side effects of the antipsychotic drug will abate as the dose or risperidone is reduced, and second is whether stopping the antipsychotic drug will lead to exacerbation of any behavioral complications.

For the Parkinson's side effects, monitor for bradykinesia, cogwheel rigidity, and tremor. See if the patient's function will improve, such as his ability to swallow, gain weight, and walk.

For the behavioral issues, ask the nurses to monitor for signs of agitation, such as confusion, physical behavior such as hitting, and psychological signs such as crying, yelling, delusions, or hallucinations.

As the neuroleptic was reduced, the patient's bradykinesia, rigidity, and dysphagia, all improved and eventually completely resolved. Sequentially the pramipexole and then the Sinemet were reduced. After several months, the patient was found to have underlying Parkinson's disease, moderate in severity, well managed by Sinemet 25/100 three times daily. He regained his lost weight, was able to walk again, with a dramatic improvement in quality of life. He improved enough for hospice to be discontinued.

His final diagnosis was moderate Parkinson's disease, dramatically exacerbated by risperidone (drug-induced parkinsonism).

Case 2

1. She is an excellent candidate for warfarin anticoagulation. She has structural heart disease and hypertension without cognitive or functional impairment and a reasonable medication list. Her remote history of bleeding from peptic ulcer disease is of concern, but overall her risk of bleeding from warfarin is small.

2. There is no rush to treat her with an anticoagulant, no indication to hospitalize her, or to start heparin or a low-molecular-weight heparin. The average warfarin dose in a 76-year-old woman to achieve the goal INR of 2 to 3 is about 4 mg/day. A loading dose is not used when starting warfarin anticoagulation.
Write: D/C the aspirin.
Start warfarin 5 mg; take 0.5 tablet (2.5 mg) daily.
Check INR weekly until stable.
(Titrate warfarin until a stable therapeutic range of 2 to 3 is achieved.)

Discontinuing the aspirin is a little controversial; –it is mainly to protect the patient from recurrent myocardial infarction (MI) due to her coronary disease, and the warfarin is meant to prevent stroke and peripheral embolism from the atrial fibrillation. However, combining aspirin and warfarin substantially increases the risk of bleeding. Individualize this decision, depending on the risk factors of the patient.

Warfarin has a small therapeutic-toxic ratio. If the dose is too low, the patient is not protected against stroke and peripheral embolism, and if the dose is too high, bleeding risk rises. Consider always using the 5-mg warfarin tablet in older adults. Titrate the patient's warfarin by using part or all of these 5-mg tablets. For example, some patients may need 0.5 tablet (2.5 mg) every day, whereas some patients may need 1 tablet (5 mg) alternating with 1.5 tablets (7.5 mg) every day. All patients prescribed warfarin should be instructed to take it exactly as prescribed, particularly to take the medication at the same time every day. They should also review their diets to be sure they have limited or no intake of foods with vitamin K because these foods would act as an antidote to the warfarin and cause fluctuations in the blood test results. Other instructions to patients would include use of a soft toothbrush to prevent bleeding gums and to shave with an electric razor to avoid bleeding nicks and cuts. They should also be made aware that any signs of bleeding (excessive bruising, black tarry stools) will require immediate medical attention.

3. This is a difficult question, but probably not. Discuss the role of the warfarin with the patient (if she is still able to comprehend) or with her family. Is prevention of stroke and

prolongation of life still a reasonable goal of care? Her risk of serious bleeding is now much higher. Weigh the pros and cons of anticoagulation and be willing to start and stop warfarin, depending on the circumstances of the individual patient.

Chapter 23

Case 1

Several choices are available to the clinician in responding to this question. However, not telling the caretaker and the child that the medicine may taste bad will likely result in both of them losing trust in their clinician. Mixing the medicine in the child's favorite food will likely cause the child to begin disliking the favorite food, and if the child does not understand why the food tastes bad, he or she will likely gag or spit it out. A better approach would be to tell the caretaker that you have recommended a stronger dose of the medicine so that if a medicine dropper is used and drawn up about 0.5 mL (marked on the side of the dropper), that would enable placing a small volume of the medicine between the cheek and the gum. Placement there will promote swallowing and prevent the child from spitting out or aspirating the medicine.

Case 2

First: Determine the child's weight in kilograms. For example: A 33-lb child weighs 33/2.2 or 15 kg

Second: Determine the milligrams per dose. For example: 15 kg × 15 mg/kg = 225 mg per dose

Third: Determine the daily amount of Tylenol. For example: 24 hr/6 = 4 doses per day × 225 mg per dose = 900 mg/day

The recommended dosage of acetaminophen is 10 to 15mg/kg, thus this dosage is near the upper limits, but is safe. The caretaker should be cautioned about long-term use of this medication.

Chapter 24

Case 1

1. RX: Morphine SR 30 mg
   #: 60 NR
   Sig: 1 by mouth twice daily

2. In the Special Case box, hydrocodone and morphine are interchanged on a 1:1 ratio. Therefore, she is taking 60 mg hydrocodone per day, and her morphine equivalent, especially since her pain is unrelieved, is 60 mg. Morphine SR 30 mg, two times a day provides the right amount of medication. An alternative would be Avinza 60 mg by mouth daily. Another prescription could be written for hydrocodone to continue for breakthrough pain.

3. Constipation. She has already been 2 days without a bowel movement and her last one was difficult to pass. She should be treated with a stimulant laxative such as senna on a scheduled basis. Bisacodyl should only be used on an as-needed basis because it can damage the myenteric plexus of the gut. Opioids increase bowel wall tension (decreased compliance) and decrease the propulsive contractions.

4. She could be seen in 1 to 2 weeks to follow up on her pain control and adjust her medications as necessary. Checking up on bowel function and other side effects is a must as well.

If she is still requiring three hydrocodone tablets per day on a fairly regular basis, the morphine SR could be increased to three times a day.

Case 2

1. Other options are a low-dose tricyclic antidepressant; gabapentin or pregabalin; or possibly a short course of steroids.

2. Tricyclics are effective and very cheap, and they have sedation as a side effect that will help him sleep. Gabapentin is cheaper than pregabalin and seems to work as well. These can cause some initial sedation, which can help with sleep. For an acute exacerbation of the pain, steroids may be beneficial to decrease swelling around discs and/or nerves. Steroids should not be used for chronic pain because of side effects and long-term risks.

3. For tricyclics, advise him of the possible side effects: somnolence, dry mouth, urinary retention, constipation. For anticonvulsants, possible side effects are somnolence and ataxia (if he escalates dose too quickly). Steroids can stimulate appetite and aggravate insomnia and may cause psychosis if the dose is high.

Chapter 25

Case 1

1. Vitamin A toxicity. Because vitamin A is fat soluble, disposing of any excesses taken in through diet is much harder than with water-soluble vitamins B and C. Vitamin A toxicity causes the symptoms Mrs. M. is experiencing—nausea, jaundice, irritability, anorexia (not to be confused with anorexia nervosa, the eating disorder), vomiting, blurry vision, headaches, hair loss, muscle and abdominal pain and weakness, drowsiness, and altered mental status.

   Despite Mrs. M.'s chronic malabsorption, she may be experiencing vitamin A toxicity. A serum retinol level should be drawn to firmly establish her diagnosis, and to guide future safe supplementation. Best practice would also include determining serum thiamine, niacin, vitamin B_{12} and 25-H vitamin D levels, because deficiency of these can produce similar symptoms. The integrative clinician will review her supplement labels to determine actual dosages taken.

2. Acute toxicity generally occurs at doses of 25,000 IU/kg of body weight, with chronic toxicity occurring at 4,000 IU/kg of body weight daily for 6 to 15 months. However, liver toxicity can occur at levels as low as 15,000 IU per day to 1.4 million IU per day, with an average daily toxic dose of 120,000 IU per day.

   It has been estimated that 75% of people may be ingesting more than the RDA for vitamin A on a regular basis in developed nations. Intake of twice the RDA recommendations chronically may be associated with osteoporosis and hip fractures. High vitamin A intake has been associated with spontaneous bone fractures in animals.

   Vitamin A is readily found in red, yellow, orange, and dark green vegetables, as well as in milk, butter, cheese, and eggs; a well-rounded diet is generally adequate to prevent deficiency. Patients with severe fat malabsorption, however, may develop deficiency states and require high-dose oral replacement. This should be managed by following serum levels and should not be undertaken by patients without expert guidance to prevent the risk of toxicity.

Case 2

1. During a careful review of this case, the integrative clinician will note several sources of concern in the treatment plan. Pharmaceutical usage of potential concern includes (1) use of digoxin, a drug with a very narrow therapeutic window, which is often responsible for confusion in the elderly and in this case may cloud the patient's judgment; (2) an excessively high dose of hydrochlorothiazide (50 mg), which may cause dehydration and increase her risk of uremia and hypercoagulability, another potential cause of altered mental status; (3) a doubled dose of lisinopril (20 mg daily) in a frail elder who is also on a diuretic may cause hypotension and impaired cerebral circulation; (4) warfarin use in a patient with potential uremia or altered mental status is difficult to safely dose. Dietary supplement usage also is a source of concern for this patient: 1) Ginkgo biloba used in combination with warfarin may predispose to bleeding diatheses, a particular risk in a frail elder; (2) St. John's wort can affect the absorption, metabolism, and disposition of other drugs by inducing the cytochrome P450, glycoprotein P transport system, and multidrug-resistant cassette systems.

St. John's wort therefore lowers blood concentrations of many drugs, including cyclosporine, amitriptyline, digoxin, indinavir, warfarin, theophylline, and some statins. It may also cause delirium and serotonin syndrome when used concomitantly with selective serotonin-reuptake inhibitors.

In light of the multiple sources of risk for this patient, the conscientious integrative clinician will recommend consideration of the following: discontinuation of both the herbals and digoxin (now rarely used for atrial fibrillation in the absence of congestive heart failure), decrease of the hydrochlorothiazide (which has increased toxicity but no more effectiveness at the 50 mg dose), monitoring of the blood pressure, potassium, and creatinine on the increased lisinopril dose, monitoring of the warfarin, and consideration of an alternative such as dabigatran. A dietary supplement such as omega-3 fish oil should be considered to facilitate neural recovery after the transient ischemic attack and to protect the cardiac function.

Chapter 26

Case 1

1. RX: Fluocinolone acetonide, 0.2% (Synalar HP Cream)
   #: 30 grams
   Sig: Apply topically to affected area twice daily for 2 weeks
2. The treatment for a mild atopic dermatitis flare-up is topical steroids. Numerous topical steroids are available, but the lowest potency prescription that works should be used. Other popular choices for topical corticosteroids are betamethasone or dexamethasone, however clinicians must be prepared to watch for hypersensitivities or intolerance to any corticosteroid or the components that make up its vehicle (e.g., ointment, cream, preservatives, alcohols, etc.). If the patient is a child, the unfluorinated corticosteroids are recommended (e.g., fluticasone, hydrocortisone, methylprednisone, and triamcinolone). Synalar HP 0.2% cream is level 4 potency and is a good starting point for mild dermatitis. Although ointments are more lubricating and perhaps more effective, they are greasy and less cosmetically pleasing, which may be of concern in a young woman going to college.

3. This patient must be educated about her condition. A hand out is helpful in explaining allergen and skin irritation avoidance, as well as ways to avoid skin dryness and irritation, but a face-to-face discussion may be the best means to get the message across. The patient's new clothes need to be evaluated as well as her new living area at college. Although this potency of steroid is low, one should always instruct the patient to avoid using the steroid on the face or eyes.

4. The patient's understandable anxiety over entering college may also be an area of concern and need for treatment. You may wish to ask her how she feels about going away to college and set up some counseling to assist her in her transition.

   The dermatitis should resolve relatively quickly, but if it does not, stronger steroids may be needed, as might further evaluation of triggers such as different allergens encountered at college as well as the ongoing stress that accompanies going to college. PW should follow up in 2 weeks if she is no better, but if the rash resolves, she can decrease use of Synalar and return at fall break. One might consider a lesser potency topical steroid if she is better but still having problems.

Case 2

1. RX: Prednisone 20 mg.
   #: 20 tablets
   Sig: 4 tabs by mouth daily for 2 days, then
   3 tabs by mouth daily for 2 days, then
   2 tabs by mouth daily for 2 days, then
   1 tab by mouth daily for 2 days.
2. The treatment of contact dermatitis is different from other allergies in that it is cell mediated, requiring the action of specific cells, not immunoglobulins, to provide the allergic response. For that reason contact dermatitis usually takes longer to manifest itself than other allergies or anaphylaxis, and its treatment is different from those allergies caused by immunoglobulins. Although the treatment in this example is an 8-day regimen, there is some research to show that 2 weeks of steroid use may be more effective. However, clinicians will continue to use what works best in their clinical judgment until research proves otherwise.

   Antihistamines, although they may be minimally helpful for sedation and itching, are of little or no help in the treatment of the allergic reaction. Steroids are best for cell-mediated contact dermatitis, and strong (class 1, 2, 3) potency topical steroids can be used for short periods of time if the rash is localized and the patient is not highly sensitized. Mr. GW, however, needs more than just topical treatment because of the severity of his condition, and either oral or injectable steroids should be used. Topical antihistamines and antibiotics should be avoided because they are of little help and can become contact skin sensitizers themselves. Injectable steroids or oral steroids given for short periods of time (less than 2 weeks) are considered safe and unlikely to affect the adrenal-pituitary axis.

3. Mr. G.W. can be reassured that once he has taken a bath and washed off the poison ivy oil (urushiol), washed his clothes, and given the troop mascot a bath, his dermatitis will not spread. It is not spread by the fluid in the bullae, but certain areas of skin may have gotten lesser allergen or are slower to react, and this is why he may continue to be having a break out of vesicles. Topical application with compresses of tap water, saline, or Domeboro solution is often soothing. The patient should be warned not to scratch excessively because he can aggravate the dermatitis and possibly cause a skin infection.

4. The condition should resolve in 3 to 6 days, but he should complete the course of medication because stopping too soon or giving too short a course can result in the allergic reaction recurring. He should return if the rash is getting worse or if he develops what appears to be a skin infection or if the rash persists beyond the medication treatment period of 8 days.

Index

Please note: page numbers followed by b indicate box; f, figure; and t, table.